# Hurst's The Heart
## Manual of Cardiology

# Notice

Medicine is an ever-changing science. As new research and clinical experience broaden our knowledge, changes in treatment and drug therapy are required. The editors and the publisher of this work have checked with sources believed to be reliable in their efforts to provide information that is complete and generally in accord with the standards accepted at the time of publication. However, in view of the possibility of human error or changes in medical sciences, neither the editors nor the publisher nor any other party who has been involved in the preparation or publication of this work warrants that the information contained herein is in every respect accurate or complete, and they disclaim all responsibility for any errors or omissions or for the results obtained from use of the information contained in this work. Readers are encouraged to confirm the information contained herein with other sources. For example and in particular, readers are advised to check the product information sheet included in the package of each drug they plan to administer to be certain that the information contained in this work is accurate and that changes have not been made in the recommended dose or in the contraindications for administration. This recommendation is of particular importance in connection with new or infrequently used drugs.

# Hurst's The Heart
## Manual of Cardiology

Thirteenth Edition

### EDITORS

**Richard A. Walsh, MD, FACC, FAHA**

John H. Hord Professor
Chair, Department of Medicine
Case Western Reserve University
Physician-in-Chief
University Hospitals Health System
Cleveland, Ohio

**James C. Fang, MD**

Professor of Medicine
Division of Cardiovascular Medicine
Case Western Reserve University
Irving B. and Virginia Spitz Master Clinician Chair in Cardiology
University Hospitals Case Medical Center
Cleveland, Ohio

**Valentin Fuster, MD, PhD, MACC, FAHA**

Physician-in-Chief, The Mount Sinai Medical Center
Director, Mount Sinai Heart Center
Professor of Cardiology
The Mount Sinai Medical Center
New York, New York

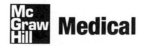

New York   Chicago   San Francisco   Lisbon   London   Madrid
Mexico City   Milan   New Delhi   San Juan   Seoul   Singapore   Sydney   Toronto

The **McGraw·Hill** Companies

**Hurst's The Heart, Thirteenth Edition**
**Manual of Cardiology**

Copyright © 2013, 2009, 2005, 2001, by The McGraw-Hill Companies, Inc. All rights reserved. Printed in the United States of America. Except as permitted under the United States Copyright Act of 1976, no part of this publication may be reproduced or distributed in any form or by any means, or stored in a data base or retrieval system, without the prior written permission of the publisher.

1 2 3 4 5 6 7 8 9   DOC/DOC   18 17 16 15 14 13 12

ISBN 978-0-07-177315-7
MHID 0-07-177315-0

This book was set in Minion Pro by Cenveo Publisher Services.
The editors were Christine Diedrich and Christie Naglieri.
The production supervisor was Catherine Saggese.
Project management was provided by Ridhi Mathur, Cenveo Publisher Services.
RR Donnelley was printer and binder.

This book is printed on acid-free paper.

**Library of Congress Cataloging-in-Publication Data**

Hurst's the heart manual of cardiology / editors, Richard A. Walsh,
Valentin Fuster, James Fang.—13th ed.
      p. ; cm.
  Heart manual of cardiology
  Companion handbook to: Hurst's the heart. 13th ed. c2011.
  Includes bibliographical references and index.
  ISBN 978-0-07-177315-7 (pbk. : alk. paper)—ISBN 0-07-177315-0
(pbk. : alk. paper)
  I. Hurst, J. Willis (John Willis), 1920-  II. Walsh, Richard A., 1946-
III. Fuster, Valentin.  IV. Fang, James C.  V. Hurst's the heart.  VI. Title: Heart
manual of cardiology.
  [DNLM: 1. Cardiovascular Diseases—Handbooks.   WG 39]
  616.1'2—dc23
                                  2012006519

McGraw-Hill books are available at special quantity discounts to use as premiums and sales promotions, or for use in corporate training programs. To contact a representative please e-mail us at bulksales@mcgraw-hill.com.

# CONTENTS

---

[†]Deceased.

[†]Deceased.

[†]Deceased.

# CONTRIBUTORS

**Jamil A. Aboulhosn, MD**
Assistant Professor of Medicine, Co-director, Ahmanson/UCLA Adult
Congenital Heart Disease Center, David Geffen School of Medicine at
UCLA, Los Angeles, California
Chapter 45


**William T. Abraham, MD, FACP, FACC, FAHA**
Professor of Medicine, Physiology, and Cell Biology, Chair of Excellence in
Cardiovascular Medicine, Director, Division of Cardiovascular Medicine,
Deputy Director, Davis Heart and Lung Research Institute, The Ohio State
University, Columbus, Ohio
Chapter 19


**David H. Adams, MD**
Professor and Chairman, Department of Cardiothoracic Surgery,
Marie-Josée and Henry R. Kravis Center, The Mount Sinai School of
Medicine, New York, New York
Chapter 33


**Samuel J. Asirvatham, MD**
Professor, Division of Cardiovascular Diseases and Internal Medicine,
Division of Pediatric Cardiology, Mayo Clinic College of Medicine,
Rochester, Minnesota
Chapter 14


**G. Brandon Atkins, MD, PhD, FACC**
Assistant Professor, Department of Medicine, Case Western Reserve
University School of Medicine, Case Cardiovascular Research Institute,
University Hospitals Case Medical Center, Harrington-McLaughlin Heart &
Vascular Institute, Cleveland, Ohio
Chapter 28


**Usman Baber, MD, MS**
Assistant Professor of Medicine, Mount Sinai Heart, The Mount Sinai
Medical Center, New York, New York
Chapters 36, 55

**Sameer Bansilal, MD, MS**
Cardiovascular Medicine, Boston VA Healthcare System & Brigham and
Women's Hospital, Harvard Medical School, Boston, Massachusetts
Chapters 48, 57

**Robyn J. Barst, MD**
Professor Emerita, Columbia University College of Physicians and
Surgeons, New York, New York
Chapter 29

**Antoni Bayés de Luna, MD, FESC, FACC**
Director of Cardiac Service, Hospital Quiron, Emeritus Professor,
Universitat Autónoma de Barcelona, Barcelona, Spain
Chapter 2

**Antoni Bayés-Genis, MD, PhD, FESC**
Chair, Cardiology Department, Hospital Germans Trias i Pujol,
Professor, Department of Medicine, Universitat Autònoma de Barcelona,
Barcelona, Spain
Chapter 2

**Michael J. Blaha, MD, MPH**
The John Hopkins Ciccone Center for the Prevention of Heart Disease,
Baltimore, Maryland
Chapter 20

**Roger S. Blumenthal, MD**
Director, Johns Hopkins Ciccarone Center for the Prevention of Heart
Disease, Baltimore, Maryland
Chapter 20

**Wendy M. Book, MD**
Emory Healthcare, Emory University, Atlanta, Georgia
Chapter 42

**Michael R. Bristow, MD, PhD**
Professor of Medicine (Cardiology), Co-director CU Cardiovascular
Institute,University of Colorado, Aurora, Colorado
Chapter 38

**Craig S. Broberg, MD, FACC**
Assistant Professor of Cardiovascular Medicine, Director, Adult
Congenital Heart Disease Program, Oregon Health and Science University,
Portland, Oregon
Chapter 51

**Ramon Brugada, MD, PhD, FACC**
Director, Medical School, University of Girona, Director, Cardiovascular
Genetics Center, Girona, Spain
Chapter 44

**Louis R. Caplan, MD**
Senior Neurologist, Beth Israel Deaconess Medical Center, Boston,
Professor of Neurology, Harvard Medical School, Boston, Massachusetts
Chapter 53

**Blasé A. Carabello, MD**
Professor, Department of Medicine, Baylor College of Medicine,
Houston, Texas
Chapters 32, 33

**Mark D. Carlson, MD, MA**
Chief Medical Officer, Cardiac Rhythm Management Division, St. Jude
Medical, Sylmar, California
Chapter 16

**Alain Carpentier, MD, PhD**
Professor of Cardiothoracic and Vascular Surgery, University of Paris
Descartes, Assistance Publique-Hôpitaux de Paris, Hôspital Européen,
Paris, France
Chapter 35

**Javier G. Castillo**
Cardiothoracic Surgery Resident, Department of Cardiothoracic Surgery,
The Mount Sinai School of Medicine, New York, New York
Chapter 33

**Pamela Charney, MD**
Weill Medical College of Cornell University, Professor of Clinical Internal
Medicine, Associate Professor of Clinical Obstetrics and Gynecology,
New York, New York
Chapter 50

**Joanna Chikwe, MD, FRCS**
Assistant Professor, Department of Cardiothoracic Surgery, The Mount
Sinai Medical Center, New York, New York
Chapter 35

**John S. Child, MD**
Streisand Professor of Medicine/Cardiology, Director, Ahmanson UCLA
Adult Congenital Heart Disease Center, David Geffen School of Medicine at
UCLA, Los Angeles, California
Chapter 45

**Jason S. Chinitz, MD**
Fellow, Cardiovascular Disease, Mount Sinai Heart, The Mount Sinai
Medical Center, New York, New York
Chapter 54

**Jayer Chung, MD**
Vascular Surgery Fellow, Division of Vascular Surgery and Endovascular
Therapy, Emory University Hospital, Atlanta, Georgia
Chapter 56

**Jennifer Conroy, MD, MBE**
Fellow, Cardiovascular Disease, Mount Sinai Heart, The Mount Sinai
Medical Center, New York, New York
Chapter 51

**Rebecca B. Costello, PhD**
National Institute of Health, Office of Dietary Supplements, Bethesda,
Maryland
Chapter 60

**James A. de Lemos, MD**
J. Fred Schoelkopf Jr, Chair in Cardiology, Coronary Care Unit and
Fellowship Director, University of Texas Southwestern Medical Center,
Dallas, Texas
Chapter 24

**Thomas F. Dodson, MD**
Professsor of Surgery, Associate Chairman, Program Director, Department
of Surgery, Emory University, Atlanta, Georgia
Chapter 56

**John S. Douglas, Jr, MD**
Professor of Medicine, Director of International Cardiology and Cardiac Cathetertization Laboratory, Emory University School of Medicine, Atlanta, Georgia
Chapter 25

**Kim A. Eagle, MD**
Albion Walter Hewlett Professor of Internal Medicine, Chief of Clinical Cardiology, Director, Cardiovascular Center, Ann Arbor, Michigan
Chapter 46

**Kenneth A. Ellenbogen, MD**
Vice Chair, Division of Cardiology, Virginia Commonwealth University School of Medicine, Richmond, Virginia
Chapter 11

**Sammy Elmariah, MD, MPH**
Interventional Cardiology and Structural Heart Disease, Massachusetts General Hospital Harvard Medical School, Boston, Massachusetts
Chapter 52

**Alan D. Enriquez, MD**
Fellow, Cardiovascular Disease, Mount Sinai Heart, The Mount Sinai Medical Center, New York, New York
Chapter 58

**Gordon A. Ewy, MD**
Professor and Chief Cardiology Director, Sarver Heart Center, University of Arizona College of Medicine, Tucson, Arizona
Chapter 18

**Michael E. Farkouh, MD, MSc, FACC**
Director, Cardiovascular Clinical Trials, University of Toronto, Toronto, Canada, Director, FREEDOM Trial Office, Mount Sinai School of Medicine, New York, New York
Chapters 48, 57

**Peter F. Fedullo, MD**
Professor of Medicine, University of California San Diego Medical Center, San Diego, California
Chapter 30

**Farzan Filsoufi, MD**
Billy S. Guyton Distinguished Professor, Professor of Physiology and
Medicine, Dean, School of Graduate Studies in the Health Sciences,
University of Mississippi Medical Center, Jackson, Mississippi
Chapter 35

**Miquel Fiol, MD**
Chief, Coronary Care Unit, Son Dureta University Hospital, Palma de
Mallorca, Spain
Chapter 2

**Richard I. Fogel, MD**
Clinical Electrophysiologist, St. Vincent Medical Group, Indianapolis,
Indiana
Chapters 8, 9, 12, 13

**Rosario V. Freeman, MD**
Associate Professor of Medicine, Division of Cardiology, Director,
Echocardiography Laboratory, University of Washington School of
Medicine, Seattle, Washington
Chapters 31, 52

**Valentin Fuster, MD, PhD, MACC, FAHA**
Richard Gorlin, MD/Heart Research Foundation, Professor of
Cardiology, Director, Mount Sinai Heart, Director, The Zena and
Michael A. Wiener Cardiovascular Institute and Marie-Josée and Henry
R. Kravis Center for Cardiovascular Health, The Mount Sinai Medical
Center, New York, New York
Chapters 22, 36, 48, 57

**Bernard J. Gersh, MD, ChB, DPhil**
Professor of Medicine, Mayo Medical School, Consultant, Cardiovascular
Diseases and Internal Medicine, Mayo Clinic, Rochester, Minnesota
Chapter 23

**Gary Gerstenblith, MD**
Professor, Department of Medicine, Johns Hopkins University School of
Medicine, Johns Hopkins Hospital, Baltimore, Maryland
Chapter 59

**Edward M. Gilbert, MD**
Professor of Medicine, University of Utah School of Medicine, Salt Lake City, Utah
Chapter 38

**Robert C. Gilkeson, MD**
Director of Cardiothoracic Imaging, University Hospitals Case Medical Center, Professor, Case Western Reserve University School of Medicine, Cleveland, Ohio
Chapter 3

**Ty J. Gluckman, MD, FACC**
Director, Coronary Care Unit, Providence St. Vincent Heart and Vascular Institute, Portland, Oregon
Chapter 20

**Judith Z. Goldfinger, MD**
Fellow, Cardiovascular Disease, Mount Sinai Heart, The Mount Sinai Medical Center, New York, New York
Chapter 50

**Diego Goldwasser, MD**
Institut Català de Ciències Cardiovasculars, Hospital Sant Pau, Barcelona, Spain
Chapter 2

**Blair P. Grubb, MD**
Professor of Medicine and Pediatrics, Health Science Campus, The University of Toledo, Toledo, Ohio
Chapter 16

**Scott M. Grundy, MD, PhD**
Director, Center for Human Nutrition, UT Southwestern Medical Center at Dallas, Dallas, Texas
Chapter 47

**Saptarsi M. Haldar, MD**
Assistant Professor of Medicine, Department of Medicine, Harrington-McLaughlin Heart & Vascular Institute, Case Western Reserve University School of Medicine, University Hospitals Case Medical Center, Cleveland, Ohio
Chapter 37

**Robert A. Harrington, MD, FACC, FAHA**
Arthur Bloomfield Professor of Medicine and Chairman of the Department
of Medicine at Stanford University, Stanford, California
Chapters 1, 24

**Ayesha Hasan, MD**
Ohio State University Medical Center, Ross Heart Hospital Ohio State
University, Columbus, Ohio
Chapter 19

**Emily E. Hass, MD**
Fellow, Division of Cardiology, University of North Carolina at Chapel Hill,
Chapel Hill, North Carolina
Chapter 23

**Brian D. Hoit, MD**
Professor of Medicine and Physiology and Biophysics, Case Western
Reserve Univeristy, Director of Echocardiographic Services, University
Hospitals Health Systems, Cleveland, Ohio
Chapters 40, 43

**Jooby John, MD, MPH**
Chief Fellow, Cardiology, Department of Medicine, The University of
Arizona, Tucson, Arizona
Chapter 18

**Mark E. Josephson, MD**
Professor of Medicine, Harvard Medical School, Director,
Harvard-Thorndike Electrophysiology Institute and Arrhythmia Service,
Beth Israel Deaconess Medical Center, Boston, Massachusetts
Chapter 17

**Samir R. Kapadia, MD**
Director Sones Cardiac Catheterization Laboratory, Director Interventional
Cardiology Fellowship, Professor of Medicine, Cardiovascular Medicine,
Cleveland Clinic, Cleveland, Ohio
Chapter 54

**Mala S. Kaul, MD**
Fellow, Division of Rheumatolotgy, Department of Medicine, Duke
University Medical Center, Durham, North Carolina
Chapter 49

**Richard E. Kerber, MD**
Professor of Medicine, Interim Director of Cardiovascular Medicine, University of Iowa Hospitals, Iowa City, Iowa
Chapter 15

**Morton J. Kern, MD, FSCAI, FAHA, FACC**
Professor of Medicine, Chief Cardiology Long Beach Veterans Administration Hospital, Associate Chief of Cardiology University of California, Irvine, University of California, Irvine Medical Center, Orange, California
Chapter 7

**Michael C. Kim, MD, FACC**
Professor of Medicine, Coronary Care Unit, Mount Sinai Heart, The Mount Sinai Medical Center, New York, New York
Chapter 22

**Spencer B. King III, MD, MACC**
President, Saint Joseph's Heart and Vascular Institute, Professor of Medicine Emeritus, Emory University School of Medicine, Atlanta, Georgia
Chapters 7, 25

**Annapoorna S. Kini, MD**
The Mount Sinai Medical Center, Mount Sinai Hosptial, New York, New York
Chapter 22

**Kerunne S. Ketlogetswe, MD**
The John Hopkins Ciccone Center for the Prevention of Heart Disease, John Hopkins Hospital, Baltimore, Maryland
Chapter 20

**Amar Krishnaswamy, MD**
Fellow, Division of Cardiology, Cleveland Clinic, Cleveland, Ohio
Chapter 54

**Mitchell W. Krucoff, MD**
Professor of Medicine, Division of Cardiology, Department of Medicine, Duke University Medical Center, Durham, North Carolina
Chapter 60

**Megan C. Leary, MD**
Harvard Clinical Research Institute, Boston, Massachusetts
Chapter 53


**Brian D. Lowes, MD**
Associate Professor, Division of Cardiology, University of Colorado Health
Sciences Center, Denver, Colorado
Chapter 38


**Donna M. Mancini, MD**
Professor of Medicine, Columbia University, New York, New York
Chapter 41


**Ali J. Marian, MD**
Professor of Molecular Medicine and Internal Medicine (Cardiology),
Director, Center for Cardiovascular Genetics, Institute of Molecular
Medicine, Professional Staff, Texas Heart Institute at St. Luke's Episcopal
Hospital, The University of Texas Health Science Center, Houston, Texas
Chapter 44


**Daniel B. Mark, MD, MPH**
Duke University Medical Center, Professor of Medicine, Duke Clinical
Research Institute, Director, Outcomes Research, Durham, North Carolina
Chapter 60


**Pedro Martinez-Clark, MD**
Assistant Professor of Medicine, Cardiovascular Division, Miller School
of Medicine, University of Miami, Miami, Florida
Chapter 26


**John H. McAnulty, MD, FACC, FAHA**
Professor Emeritus of Medicine, Division of Cardiology, Oregon Health and
Sciences University, Good Samaritan Hospital, Portland, Oregon
Chapter 51


**Luisa Mestroni, MD, FACC, FESC, FACP**
Professor of Medicine, Director, Molecular Genetics, Cardiovascular
Institute, University of Colorado, Aurora, Colorado
Chapter 38

**James Metcalfe, MD**
Professor of Medicine (Retired), Oregon Health and Science University, Portland, Oregon
Chapter 51

**Marc A. Miller, MD**
Assistant Professor of Medicine, Mount Sinai Heart, The Mount Sinai Medical Center, New York, New York
Chapters 47, 50, 52, 58

**Debabrata Mukherjee, MD, MS**
Professor, Division of Cardiology, Department of Medicine, University of Kentucky, Lexington, Kentucky
Chapter 46

**Samer S. Najjar, MD**
Medical Director, Heart Failure and Heart Transplantation, Washington Hospital Center and MedStar Health Research Institute, Washington, DC
Chapter 59

**Ira S. Nash, MD, FACC, FAHA, FACP**
Chief Medical Officer, Senior Vice President for Medical Affairs, The Mount Sinai Medical Center, Associate Professor of Medicine, Associate Professor of Health Policy and Evidence, Mount Sinai School of Medicine, New York, New York
Chapter 57

**Chiadi E. Ndumele, MD**
Post Doctoral Fellow, Division of Cardiology and Johns Hopkins Ciccarone Center for the Prevention of Heart Disease, Johns Hopkins University School of Medicine, Baltimore, Maryland
Chapter 20

**Rick A. Nishimura, MD, FACC**
Mayo Clinic College of Medicine, Consultant, Division of Cardiovascular Diseases, Rochester, Minnesota
Chapter 39

**Patrick T. O'Gara, MD**
Associate Professor of Medicine, Harvard Medical School, Director, Clinical
Cardiology, Brigham and Women's Hospital, Boston, Massachusetts
Chapter 37

**Gbenga Ogedegbe, MD, MPH, MS, FAHA**
Associate Professor of Medicine, Director of the Center for Healthful
Behavior Change, Division of General Internal Medicine, Department of
Medicine, New York University School of Medicine, New York,
New York
Chapter 27

**Gerard O. Oghlakian, MD**
Cardiovascular Fellow, Case Western Reserve University, Department of
Medicine/Cardiology, Cleveland, Ohio
Chapter 58

**Steve R. Ommen, MD**
Professor of Medicine, Mayo Clinic, Rochester, Minnesota
Chapter 39

**William W. O'Neill, MD**
Executive Dean for Clinical Affairs, Chief Medical Officer, University of
Miami Health System, Professor of Medicine and Cardiology, University of
Miami Miller School of Medicine, Miami, Florida
Chapter 26

**Robert O'Rourke, MD, MACP, MACC, FAHA†**
Professor of Medicine Emeritus, University of Texas Health Science Center
at San Antonio, San Antonio, Texas
Chapters 3, 21, 23, 24

**Catherine M. Otto, MD**
J. Ward Kennedy-Hamilton Professor of Cardiology, Director, Fellowship
Programs in Cardiovascular Disease, University of Washington School of
Medicine, Seattle, Washington
Chapters 31, 52

---

†Deceased.

**Richard L. Page, MD**
George R. and Elaine Love Professor, Chair, Department of Medicine, University of Wisconsin School of Medicine and Public Health, Madison, Wisconson
Chapter 10

**Thomas G. Pickering, MD, DPhil†**
Assistant Professor of Medicine, Center for Behavioral Cardiovascular Health, Columbia Presbyterian Medical Center, New York, New York
Chapter 27

**Ileana L. Piña, MD, MPH**
Associate Vice Chief for Academic Affairs, Albert Einstein College of Medicine, Division of Cardiology, Montefiore Medical Center, Bronx, New York
Chapter 58

**Sean P. Pinney, MD**
Director, Advanced Heart Failure & Cardiac Transplant Program, Associate Professor of Medicine, Mount Sinai School of Medicine,
New York, New York
Chapter 41

**Duane S. Pinto, MD, MPH**
Associate Director, Interventional Cardiology Section, Director, Cardiology Fellowship Training Program, Beth Israel Deaconess Medical Center, Assistant Professor, Harvard Medical School, Boston, Massachusetts
Chapter 17

**Ian Del Conde Pozzi, MD**
Fellow, Cardiovascular Disease, Mount Sinai Heart, The Mount Sinai Medical Center, New York, New York
Chapter 47

**Eric N. Prystowsky, MD, FACC, FAHA, FHRS**
Consulting Professor of Medicine, Duke University Medical Center, Director, Clinical Electrophysiology Laboratory, St. Vincent Hospital, Indianapolis, Indiana
Chapters 8, 9, 12, 13

---

†Deceased.

**Mahboob Rahman, MD, MS**
Associate Professor Medicine, Case Western Reserve University, University Hospitals Case Medical Center, Louis Stokes Cleveland VA Medical Center, Cleveland, Ohio
Chapter 28

**Elliot J. Rayfield, MD**
Clinical Professor of Medicine (Endocrinology, Diabetes and Bone Disease), Mount Sinai School of Medicine, New York, New York
Chapter 48

**Matthew R. Reynolds, MD, SM**
Division of Cardiology, Beth Israel Deaconess Medical Center, Assistant Professor of Medicine, Harvard Medical School, Boston, Massachusetts
Chapter 17

**Robert W. Rho, MD**
Associate Professsor, University of Washington School of Medicine, Director, Cardiac Electrophysiology Ablation Program, University of Washington Medical Center, Seattle, Washington
Chapter 10

**Robert Roberts, MD, FRCP(C), MACC, FAHA**
President and CEO, University of Ottawa Heart Institute, Professor of Medicine and Director, The Ruddy Canadian Cardiovascular Genetics Centre, Ottawa, Ontario, Canada
Chapter 44

**Thom W. Rooke, MD**
Krehbiel Professor of Vascular Medicine, Mayo Clinic, Rochester, Minnesota
Chapter 55

**Lewis J. Rubin, MD**
Professor of Medicine, University of California, San Diego School of Medicine, La Jolla, California
Chapter 29

**Steven P. Schulman, MD**
Professor of Medicine, Department of Medicine, Johns Hopkins University
School of Medicine, Director, Coronary Care Unit, Johns Hopkins
University, Baltimore, Maryland
Chapter 59

**Pravin M. Shah, MD, MACC**
Chair, Medical Director, Hoag Hospital's Heart and Vascular Institute,
Newport Beach, California
Chapter 34

**Mark E. Silverman, MD, MACP, FRCP, FACC[†]**
Emeritus Professor of Medicine, Emory University, Chief of Cardiology,
Fuqua Heart Center of Atanta, Piedmont Hospital, Atlanta, Georgia
Chapter 1

**Sidney C. Smith, Jr, MD**
Professor of Medicine, Center for Cardiovascular Science and Medicine,
University of North Carolina School of Medicine, Chapel Hill, North
Carolina
Chapter 47

**Andrew L. Smith, MD**
Associate Professor of Medicine, Division of Cardiology Harbor UCLA
Medical Center, David Geffen UCLA School of Medicine, Los Angeles,
California
Chapter 42

**E. William St. Clair, MD**
Professor of Medicine and Immunology, Department of Medicine, Division
of Rheumatology and Immunology, Duke University Medical Center,
Durham, North Carolina
Chapter 49

**William G. Stevenson, MD**
Cardiovascular Division, Brigham and Women's Hospital, Harvard Medical
School, Boston, Massachusetts
Chapter 14

---

[†]Deceased.

**Joseph M. Sweeny, MD**
Assistant Professor of Medicine, Cardiac Catheterization Laboratory,
Mount Sinai Heart, The Mount Sinai Medical Center, New York, New York
Chapter 56

**A. Jamil Tajik, MD**
Thomas J. Watson Jr Professor, Professor of Medicine and Pediatrics,
Chairman Emeritus, Sheikh Zayed Cardiovascular Center, Mayo Clinic,
Rochester, Minnesota, Consultant, Cardiovascular Division, Mayo Clinic,
Scottsdale, Arizona
Chapter 39

**Victor F. Tapson, MD**
Duke University Medical Center, Durham, North Carolina
Chapter 49

**Usha B. Tedrow, MD, MSc**
Director, Clinical Electrophysiology Program, Brigham and Women's
Hospital, Boston, Massachusetts
Chapter 14

**Amit J. Thosani, MD**
Clinical Fellow in Cardiac Electrophysiology, Beth Israel Deaconess Medical
Center, Boston, Massachusetts
Chapter 17

**Torsten Vahl, MD**
Interventional Cardiology Fellow, Columbia University Medical Center,
New York, New York
Chapter 53

**Prashant Vaishnava, MD**
Department of Internal Medicine, Division of Cardiovascular Medicine,
The University of Michigan Health System, Ann Arbor, Michigan
Chapter 49

**Rajesh Vedanthan, MD, MPH**
Assistant Professor of Cardiology, Mount Sinai Heart,
The Mount Sinai Medical Center, New York, New York
Chapter 60

**Pugazhendhi Vijayaraman, MD**
Program Director, Cardiac Electrophysiology Fellowship, Geisinger Medical
Center, Danville, Pennsylvania
Chapter 11

**John H. K. Vogel, MD, MACC, SCAI, ESC**
Honorary Faculty, Santa Barbara Cottage Hospital, Staff, North Hawaii
Community Hospital, Santa Barbara, California
Chapter 60

**Richard A. Walsh, MD, FACC, FAHA**
John H. Hord Professor & Chairman, Department of Medicine, Case
Western Reserve University, Physician-in-Chief, University Hospitals of
Cleveland, Cleveland, Ohio
Chapter 21

**Paul W. Wennberg, MD**
Gonda Vascular Center, Department of Cardiovascular Diseases, Mayo
Clinic, Rochester, Minnesota
Chapter 55

**Charles F. Wooley, MD†**
Professor of Medicine Emeritus, Division of Cardiology, Department of
Internal Medicine, The Ohio State University, Heart Lung Research
Institute, Columbus, Ohio
Chapter 1

**Jackson T. Wright, Jr, MD, PhD**
Professor of Medicine, Director, Clinical Hypertension Program, Division
of Nephrology and Hypertension, Program Director, William T. Dahms
Clinical Research Center, Case Western Reserve University, Cleveland, Ohio
Chapter 28

**Jay Yadav, MD**
Staff Interventional Cardiologist, Piedmont Heart Institute, Atlanta, Georgia
Chapter 54

†Deceased.

**Eric H. Yang, MD, FACC**
Assistant Professor of Medicine, Director of the Coronary Care Unit,
University of North Carolina at Chapel Hill, Chapel Hill, North Carolina
Chapter 23

**Wilson Young, MD, PhD**
Fellow, Cardiovascular Disease, Mount Sinai Heart, The Mount Sinai
Medical Center, New York, New York
Chapter 59

# PREFACE

The 13th edition of *the Manual of Cardiology* provides an up-to-date practical summary of the diagnosis and management of the wide spectrum of patients with cardiovascular disease. It contains useful clinical information relating to heart disease patients for all health care providers, and meets the needs of physicians and students for a concise, portable handbook that can be used any time, day or night, when there is no access to larger reference material (such as the recently published 13th edition of *Hurst's The Heart*).

Written by many of the same experts who contributed to the larger textbook, the manual has been extensively revised to include additional material such as myocardial imaging and genetic causes of cardiovascular disease. The manual can also be used as a stand-alone source for quick information concerning the presentation, natural history, and treatment of various cardiovascular disorders. Important information from the ACC/AHA *Clinical Practice Guidelines* is included in many chapters, and this book contains tables and algorithms not available in the larger text, in order to provide the reader with appropriate, easily accessible indications for specific therapy.

We express our gratitude to the authors of the individual chapters of this practical concise resource for cardiovascular diagnostics and therapeutics.

Finally we wish to thank our families for their support and the many sacrifices they made to make this manual possible. We sadly mourn the recent loss of the former editor, friend, and colleague Robert A. O'Rourke.

The Editors:
*Richard A. Walsh, MD, FACC, FAHA*
*James C. Fang, MD*
*Valentin Fuster, MD, PhD, MACC, FAHA*

# CHAPTER 1
# HISTORY, PHYSICAL EXAMINATION, AND CARDIAC AUSCULTATION

## Robert A. Harrington, Mark E. Silverman[†], and Charles F. Wooley[†]

The history and physical examination should be the foundation for evaluating any patient with known or suspected heart disease. Integration of these data often results in accurate diagnoses and appropriate decisions regarding further diagnostic studies, therapeutic options, or both.

## HISTORY

The history is the first step in the assessment of the patient. A common complaint among patients with heart disease is chest pain; however, other symptoms are also prevalent and may include exercise intolerance, shortness of breath (particularly with exertion), orthopnea, and paroxysmal nocturnal dyspnea. Symptoms of edema, ascites, cough, hemoptysis, palpitation, fatigue, and peripheral embolization can be consistent with heart disease.

Distinguishing cardiac from noncardiac chest discomfort is the primary challenge in clinical practice. Cardiovascular chest discomfort may originate from the myocardium, pericardium, or vascular (eg, aorta) structures. The differential diagnosis of chest pain is extensive and is listed in **Table 1-1**.

Angina pectoris is defined as chest pain or discomfort of cardiac origin that usually results from a temporary imbalance between myocardial oxygen supply and demand. The important characteristics of angina include the quality of the pain, precipitating factors, mode of onset, duration, location, and pattern of disappearance.

The quality of the pain is typically described as "tightness," "pressure," "burning," "heaviness," "aching," "strangling," or "compression." The description of the quality may be influenced by the patient's intelligence, social background, and education.

The most common precipitating factor is physical exertion or emotional stress. Angina can also be provoked by emotional distress, cold weather, or eating. It typically has a crescendo pattern, but can also occur acutely, as with the acute coronary syndromes. An episode may last up to several minutes; discomfort that is fleeting or lasting seconds is rarely angina. Most patients have relief of symptoms within 5 minutes after cessation of physical activity, or by the use of nitroglycerin lingual spray or sublingual tablets. Localizing the site of chest discomfort is helpful in determining the cause. Angina pectoris is usually retrosternal or slightly to the left of midline, but rarely localized to a discrete (eg pinpoint) precordial area. Pain tends to radiate into the arms (both or left), neck, and jaw. Severity of angina is traditionally defined by the vigor of the activities that produce the symptoms (**Table 1-2**).

---

[†]Deceased.

**TABLE 1-1.** Differential Diagnosis of Chest Pain

1. Angina pectoris/myocardial infarction
2. Other cardiovascular causes
   a. Ischemic in origin
      (1) Aortic stenosis
      (2) Hypertrophic cardiomyopathy
      (3) Severe systemic hypertension
      (4) Severe right ventricular hypertension
      (5) Aortic regurgitation
      (6) Severe anemia/hypoxia
   b. Non-ischemic in origin
      (1) Aortic dissection
      (2) Pericarditis
      (3) Mitral valve prolapse
3. Gastrointestinal
   a. Esophageal spasm
   b. Esophageal reflux
   c. Esophageal rupture
   d. Peptic ulcer disease
4. Psychogenic
   a. Anxiety
   b. Depression
   c. Cardiac psychosis
   d. Self-gain
5. Neuromusculoskeletal
   a. Thoracic outlet syndrome
   b. Degenerative joint disease of cervical/thoracic spine
   c. Costochondritis (Tietze's syndrome)
   d. Herpes zoster
   e. Chest wall pain and tenderness
6. Pulmonary
   a. Pulmonary embolus with or without pulmonary infarction
   b. Pneumothorax
   c. Pneumonia with pleural involvement
7. Pleurisy

**TABLE 1-2.** The Old New York Heart Association Functional Classification

Class 1. No symptoms with ordinary physical activity.
Class 2. Symptoms with ordinary activity. Slight limitation of activity.
Class 3. Symptoms with less than ordinary activity. Marked limitation of activity.
Class 4. Symptoms with any physical activity or even at rest.

Data compiled from the Criteria Committee of the New York Heart Association. *Diseases of the Heart and Blood Vessels: Nomenclature and Criteria for Diagnosis of the Heart and Great Vessels.* 6th ed. New York, NY: New York Heart Association/Little Brown; 1964.

Other cardiovascular diseases can also precipitate chest pain in the absence of coronary atherosclerosis. Increased oxygen demand resulting in myocardial ischemia can occur with aortic stenosis and regurgitation, hypertrophic cardiomyopathy, and systemic arterial hypertension. Significant chest pain that is not related to myocardial ischemia can be caused by pericarditis, aortic dissection, and mitral valve prolapse.

# PHYSICAL EXAMINATION

The physical examination of a patient with definite or suspected heart disease includes a general inspection, an indirect measurement of the arterial blood pressure in both arms and one or both lower extremities, an examination of the central and peripheral arterial pulses, an evaluation of the jugular venous pressure and pulsations, palpation of the precordium, and cardiac auscultation. This brief and efficient evaluation may suggest the diagnosis and is useful for guiding further diagnostic testing and therapeutic interventions.

## ■ ARTERIAL PRESSURE PULSE

The arterial pulse wave begins with the aortic valve opening and the onset of left ventricular ejection. The rapid-rising portion of the arterial pressure curve is often termed the *anacrotic limb* (from the Greek, meaning "upbeat"). During isovolumic relaxation, reflection of propagated waves from the central arteries toward the ventricle just prior to aortic valve closure is associated with an incisura on the descending limb of the aortic pressure pulse.

A small weak pulse, *pulsus parvus*, is common in conditions with a diminished left ventricular stroke volume and is characterized by a narrow pulse pressure, and increased peripheral vascular resistance. Such a pulse may be due to hypovolemia, left ventricular failure, restrictive pericardial disease, or mitral stenosis. In aortic stenosis, the delayed systolic peak, *pulsus tardus*, results from obstruction to left ventricular ejection. In contrast, a large, bounding pulse is usually associated with an increased left ventricular stroke volume, producing a wide pulse pressure and a decrease in peripheral vascular resistance. This pattern occurs characteristically in patients with hyperdynamic circulation or with a rapid runoff of blood from the arterial system—such as with an arteriovenous (AV) fistula. Patients with mitral regurgitation or a ventricular septal defect may also have a bounding pulse. In aortic regurgitation, the rapidly rising, bounding arterial pulse results from an increased left ventricular stroke volume and an increased rate of ventricular ejection. The *bisferiens* pulse, which has 2 systolic peaks, is characteristic of aortic regurgitation and hypertrophic cardiomyopathy.

*Pulsus alternans* is a pattern in which there is regular alteration of the pressure pulse amplitude, despite a regular rhythm. It denotes severe impairment of the left ventricular function and commonly occurs in patients who also have a loud third heart sound. In *pulsus paradoxus*, the decrease in systolic arterial pressure that normally accompanies inspiration is accentuated. In patients with pericardial tamponade, airway obstruction (asthma), or superior vena cava obstruction, the inspiratory decrease in systolic arterial pressure may exceed the normal decrease of 10 mm Hg—the palpable peripheral pulse may disappear completely during inspiration.

## ■ JUGULAR VENOUS PULSE

The 2 main objectives of the examination of the neck veins are inspection of their waveforms and estimation of the central venous pressure (CVP). In most patients, the right internal jugular vein is best for both purposes. Usually, the pulsation of the

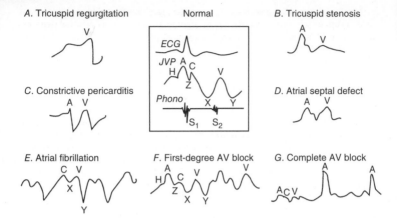

**FIGURE 1-1.** Schematic representation of the normal jugular venous pulse (JVP), 4 types of abnormal JVPs, and the JVPs in 3 arrhythmias. See text under "Jugular Venous Pulse" for definitions of h, a, z, c, x, v, and y.

internal jugular vein is optimal when the trunk is inclined less than 30 degree. In patients with elevated venous pressure, it may be necessary to elevate the trunk further, sometimes to as much as 90 degree. Simultaneous palpation of the left carotid artery aids the examiner in determining which pulsations are venous and in relating the venous pulsations to their timing in the cardiac cycle.

The normal jugular venous pulse (JVP) consists of 2 to 3 positive waves, and 2 negative troughs (**Fig. 1-1**). The positive, presystolic *a wave* is produced by venous distention due to right atrial contraction and is the dominant wave in the JVP. Large *a* waves indicate that the right atrium is contracting against increased resistance, as it occurs with tricuspid stenosis or more commonly with increased resistance to right ventricular filling. Large *a* waves ("cannon" *a* waves) also occur during arrhythmias whenever the right atrium contracts while the tricuspid valve is still closed. The *a* wave is absent in patients with atrial fibrillation, and there is an increased delay between the *a* wave and the carotid arterial pulse in patients with first-degree atrioventricular block.

The *c* wave is a positive wave produced by the bulging of the tricuspid valve into the right atrium during right ventricular isovolumetric systole and by the distention of the carotid artery located adjacent to the jugular vein. The *x* descent is due to both atrial relaxation and the downward displacement of the tricuspid valve during ventricular systole. It is lost in tricuspid regurgitation. The positive late systolic *v* wave results from right atrial filling during ventricular systole and reflects atrial compliance. Tricuspid regurgitation causes the *v* wave to become more prominent; when tricuspid regurgitation becomes severe, the combination of a prominent *v* wave and the obliteration of the *x* descent results in a single large, positive systolic wave. The negative descending limb, the *y* descent of the JVP, is produced by the opening of the tricuspid valve and the rapid inflow of blood into the right ventricle. A venous pulse characterized by a sharp *y* descent, a deep *y* trough, and a rapid ascent to the baseline is seen in patients with constrictive pericarditis or with severe right heart failure and a high venous pressure.

As mentioned before, the right internal jugular vein is the best vein to use for accurate estimation of the CVP. The sternal angle (where the manubrium meets the sternum) may be used as a reference point, because the center of the right atrium lies approximately 5 cm below the sternal angle. The clavicle may also be used as a reference, and may be preferable due to its ease of identification; it lies 10 cm from the right atrium. The patient is best examined at the optimal degree of trunk elevation for visualization of the jugular venous pulsations. The vertical distance between the top of the oscillating venous column and the level of the sternal angle is determined; generally it is less than 3 cm (3 cm + 5 cm = 8 cm blood or water; multiply by 0.8 to convert to mm Hg). In case the clavicle is used as a reference, venous pulsations should not be visible in the seated position, eg, less than 10 cm blood or water. In patients suspected of having right ventricular failure who have a normal CVP at rest, the abdominojugular reflux test may be helpful. The palm of the examiner's hand is placed over the abdomen, and firm pressure is applied for 10 seconds or more. When the right heart function is impaired, the upper level of venous pulsations usually increases. A positive abdominojugular reflux test is best defined as an increase in the JVP during 10 seconds of firm midabdominal compression followed by a rapid drop in pressure by 4 cm blood on release of the compression.

*Kussmaul sign*—an increase rather than the normal decrease in the CVP during inspiration—is most often caused by severe right-sided heart failure; it is also a frequent finding in patients with constrictive pericarditis or right ventricular infarction.

## ■ PRECORDIAL PALPATION

The location, amplitude, duration, and direction of the cardiac impulse can usually be best appreciated with the fingertips. Left ventricular hypertrophy (LVH) results in exaggeration of the amplitude, duration, and often size (normal diameter is < 3 cm) of the left ventricular thrust. The impulse may be displaced laterally and downward into the sixth or seventh interspace, particularly in patients with an LV volume load, as in the case of aortic regurgitation or dilated cardiomyopathy (**Fig. 1-2**).

Additional abnormal features detectable at the left ventricular apex include (1) a marked presystolic distention of the LV, which is often accompanied by a fourth heart sound ($S_4$) in patients with an excessive LV pressure load (eg, during myocardial ischemia or infarction) and (2) a prominent early diastolic rapid-filling wave, which is often accompanied by a third heart sound ($S_3$) in patients with LV volume overload.

Right ventricular hypertrophy often results in a sustained systolic lift at the lower left parasternal area that starts in early systole and is synchronous with the LV apical impulse.

A left parasternal lift is frequently present in patients with severe mitral regurgitation. This pulsation occurs distinctly later than the LV apical impulse, is synchronous with the *v* wave in the left atrial pressure curve, and is due to the anterior displacement of the right ventricle by an enlarged, expanding left atrium. Pulmonary artery pulsation is often visible and palpable in the second left intercostal space. Although this pulsation may be normal in children or in thin young adults, in others, it usually denotes pulmonary hypertension, increased pulmonary blood flow, or pulmonary artery dilation.

## CARDIAC AUSCULTATION

To optimize cardiac auscultation, the observer should keep several principles in mind:

1. Auscultation should be performed in a quiet room.

2. Attention must be focused on the phase of the cardiac cycle during which the auscultory event is expected to occur.

3. The timing of a heart sound or murmur can be determined accurately from its relation to other observable events in the cardiac cycle.

4. It is often necessary to observe alterations in the timing or intensity of a heart sound during various physiologic and/or pharmacologic interventions (dynamic auscultation).

**Graphic Representation**
(Palpable features in heavy line)

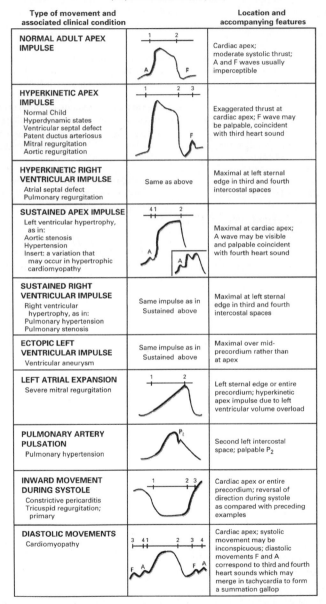

| Type of movement and associated clinical condition | | Location and accompanying features |
|---|---|---|
| **NORMAL ADULT APEX IMPULSE** | | Cardiac apex; moderate systolic thrust; A and F waves usually imperceptible |
| **HYPERKINETIC APEX IMPULSE**<br>Normal Child<br>Hyperdynamic states<br>Ventricular septal defect<br>Patent ductus arteriosus<br>Mitral regurgitation<br>Aortic regurgitation | | Exaggerated thrust at cardiac apex; F wave may be palpable, coincident with third heart sound |
| **HYPERKINETIC RIGHT VENTRICULAR IMPULSE**<br>Atrial septal defect<br>Pulmonary regurgitation | Same as above | Maximal at left sternal edge in third and fourth intercostal spaces |
| **SUSTAINED APEX IMPULSE**<br>Left ventricular hypertrophy, as in:<br>Aortic stenosis<br>Hypertension<br>Insert: a variation that may occur in hypertrophic cardiomyopathy | | Maximal at cardiac apex; A wave may be visible and palpable coincident with fourth heart sound |
| **SUSTAINED RIGHT VENTRICULAR IMPULSE**<br>Right ventricular hypertrophy, as in:<br>Pulmonary hypertension<br>Pulmonary stenosis | Same impulse as in Sustained above | Maximal at left sternal edge in third and fourth intercostal spaces |
| **ECTOPIC LEFT VENTRICULAR IMPULSE**<br>Ventricular aneurysm | Same impulse as in Sustained above | Maximal over mid-precordium rather than at apex |
| **LEFT ATRIAL EXPANSION**<br>Severe mitral regurgitation | | Left sternal edge or entire precordium; hyperkinetic apex impulse due to left ventricular volume overload |
| **PULMONARY ARTERY PULSATION**<br>Pulmonary hypertension | | Second left intercostal space; palpable $P_2$ |
| **INWARD MOVEMENT DURING SYSTOLE**<br>Constrictive pericarditis<br>Tricuspid regurgitation; primary | | Cardiac apex or entire precordium; reversal of direction during systole as compared with preceding examples |
| **DIASTOLIC MOVEMENTS**<br>Cardiomyopathy | | Cardiac apex; systolic movement may be inconspicuous; diastolic movements F and A correspond to third and fourth heart sounds which may merge in tachycardia to form a summation gallop |

**FIGURE 1-2.** Graphic representation of apical movements in health and disease. Heavy line indicates palpable features. ($P_2$) pulmonary component of second heart sound; A: atrial wave, corresponding to a fourth heart sound ($S_4$) or atrial gallop; F: filling wave, corresponding to a third heart sound ($S_3$) or ventricular gallop. (From O'Rourke RA, Shaver JA, Silverman ME. The history, physical examination, and cardiac auscultation. In: Fuster V, Alexander W, O'Rourke RA, eds. *The Heart.* 10th ed. New York, NY: McGraw-Hill; 2001.)

# ■ HEART SOUNDS

The intensity of the first heart sound ($S_1$) is influenced by (1) the position of the mitral valve leaflets at the onset of ventricular systole, (2) the rate of rise of the LV pressure pulse, (3) the presence or absence of structural disease of the mitral valve, and (4) the amount of tissue, air, or fluid between the heart and the stethoscope. The $S_1$ sound is louder if the diastole is shortened (tachycardia) or if atrial contraction precedes ventricular contraction by an unusually short interval, reflected in a short PR interval. The loud $S_1$ in mitral stenosis usually signifies that the valve is pliable (**Fig. 1-3**).

A reduction in the intensity of $S_1$ may be due to poor conduction of sound through the chest wall, a long PR interval, or imperfect closure, as in mitral regurgitation.

Splitting of the 2 high-pitched components of $S_1$ is a normal phenomenon. The first component of $S_1$ is attributed to mitral valve closure, and the second to tricuspid valve closure. Widening of $S_1$ is most often due to complete right bundle branch block.

Splitting of the second heart sound ($S_2$) into aortic ($A_2$) and pulmonic ($P_2$) components normally occurs during inspiration. Physiologic splitting of $S_2$ is accentuated in conditions associated with right ventricular volume overload and a distensible pulmonary vascular bed. However, in patients with an increase in pulmonary vascular resistance, narrow splitting of $S_2$ is present. Splitting that persists with expiration (heard best at the pulmonic or left sternal border) when the patient is in the upright position is usually abnormal. Such splitting may be due to delayed activation of the right ventricle (right bundle branch block), pulmonary embolism or pulmonic stenosis, or atrial septal defect.

In pulmonary hypertension, $P_2$ is increased in intensity, and the splitting of $S_2$ may be diminished, normal, or accentuated. Early aortic valve closure, which occurs with mitral regurgitation or a ventricular septal defect, may also produce splitting

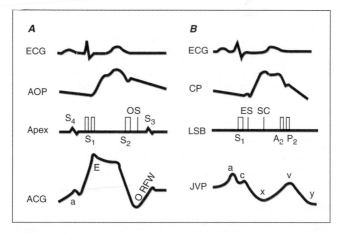

**FIGURE 1-3.** (A) Schematic representation of ECG, aortic pressure pulse (AOP), phonocardiogram recorded at the apex, and apex cardiogram (ACG). On the phonocardiogram, $S_1$, $S_2$, $S_3$, and $S_4$ represent the first through fourth heart sounds; OS represents the opening snap of the mitral valve, which occurs coincidently with the O point of the apex cardiogram. $S_3$ occurs coincidently with the termination of the rapid-filling wave (RFW) of the ACG, while $S_4$ occurs coincidently with the $a$ wave of the ACG. (B) Simultaneous recording of ECG, indirect carotid pulse (CP), phonocardiogram along the left sternal border (LSB), and indirect jugular venous pulse (JVP). ES, ejection sound; SC, systolic click.

that persists during expiration. In patients with an atrial septal defect, the volume and duration of right ventricular ejection are not significantly increased by inspiration, and there is little inspiratory exaggeration of the splitting of $S_2$. This phenomenon, termed as *fixed splitting* of the second heart sound, is of considerable diagnostic value.

A delay in aortic valve closure, causing $P_2$ to precede $A_2$, results in reversed (*paradoxic*) splitting of $S_2$. Splitting is then maximal during expiration and decreases during inspiration. The most common causes of reversed splitting of $S_2$ are left bundle branch block and delayed excitation of the LV from a right ventricular ectopic beat. Mechanical prolongation of LV systole, resulting in reversed splitting of $S_2$, may also be caused by severe aortic outflow obstruction, a large aorta-to-pulmonary artery shunt, systolic hypertension, and ischemic heart disease or cardiomyopathy with left ventricular failure. A $P_2$ that is greater than $A_2$ suggests pulmonary hypertension, except in patients with an atrial septal defect.

The third heart sound ($S_3$) is a low-pitched sound produced in the ventricle after $A_2$. In patients over 40 years of age, an $S_3$ usually indicates impairment of the ventricular function, AV valve regurgitation, or some other condition that increases the rate or volume of ventricular filling. The left-sided $S_3$ is best heard with the bell of the stethoscope at the left ventricular apex during expiration and with the patient in the left lateral position. The right-sided $S_3$ is best heard at the left sternal border or just beneath the xiphoid. It is usually louder with inspiration. Third heart sounds often disappear with the treatment of heart failure and improvement in volume status.

The *opening snap* (OS) is a brief, high-pitched, early diastolic sound that is usually due to stenosis of an AV valve, most often the mitral valve. It is generally best heard at the lower left sternal border and radiates well to the base of the heart. The $A_2$–OS interval is inversely related to the mean left atrial pressure.

The fourth heart sound ($S_4$) is a low-pitched, presystolic sound produced in the ventricle during ventricular filling; it is associated with an effective atrial contraction (and thus absent in atrial fibrillation), and is best heard with the bell of the stethoscope. The $S_4$ is frequently present in patients with systemic hypertension, aortic stenosis, hypertrophic cardiomyopathy, and ischemic heart disease. Most patients with an acute myocardial infarction and sinus rhythm have an audible $S_4$. It is best heard at the LV apex when the patient is in the left lateral position, and is accentuated by mild isotonic or isometric exercise in the supine position. In patients with chronic obstructive pulmonary disease (COPD) and increased anteroposterior (AP) diameter of the chest, $S_4$ (and often $S_3$) may be best heard at the base of the neck or in the epigastrium.

The *ejection sound* is a sharp, high-pitched sound occurring in early systole and which closely follows the first heart sound. They occur in the presence of semilunar valve stenosis and in conditions associated with dilatation of the aorta or pulmonary artery. The aortic ejection sound is usually best heard at the LV apex and the second right intercostal space; the pulmonary ejection sound is strongest at the upper left sternal border. The latter, unlike most other right-sided acoustical events, is heard better during expiration. *Nonejection* or *midsystolic clicks*, occurring with or without a late systolic murmur, often denote prolapse of 1 or both leaflets of the mitral valve.

## ■ HEART MURMURS

The evaluation of a patient with a heart murmur may vary greatly and depends on the intensity of the murmur; its timing, location, and radiation; and its response to changing loading conditions. The context of the murmur is also critical, eg, the presence or absence of concomitant symptoms and other physical findings, to its clinical significance.

Although 2-dimensional echocardiography and color Doppler flow imaging can provide additional information about the origin of a cardiac murmur, they are not necessary tests for all patients with cardiac murmurs. Many murmurs are functional. For example, in a recent study of 200 healthy Japanese subjects, some degree of mitral regurgitation could be detected by the Doppler in up to 45% of individuals, tricuspid regurgitation in up to 70%, and pulmonic regurgitation in up to 88%, even though these subjects were healthy, had no auscultatory evidence of heart disease, and had normal ECGs. "Normal" aortic regurgitation is encountered much less frequently, and its incidence increases with increasing age.

In general, echocardiography is not necessary for the evaluation of asymptomatic patients with short grade I to grade II midsystolic murmurs, and with otherwise normal physical findings, and no history suggestive of cardiac disease.

The intensity of murmurs may be graded from I to VI. A grade I murmur is so faint that it can be heard only with special effort and takes several beats of ausculation to appreciate; a grade VI murmur is audible with the stethoscope removed from contact with the chest. The configuration of a murmur may be a crescendo, decrescendo, or a plateau. The precise time of onset and cessation of a murmur depend on the instant in the cardiac cycle at which an adequate pressure difference between 2 chambers arises and disappears (**Fig. 1-4**).

The location on the chest wall where the murmur is best heard and the areas to which it radiates can be helpful in identifying the cardiac structure from where the murmur originates. In addition, by noting changes in the characteristics of the murmur during maneuvers that alter cardiac hemodynamics (dynamic auscultation), the auscultator can often identify its correct origin and significance.

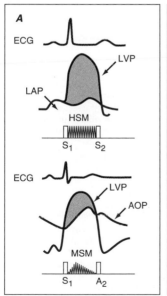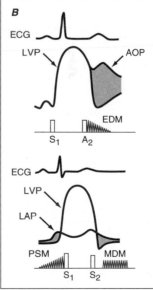

**FIGURE 1-4.** (**A**) Schematic representation of ECG, aortic pressure (AOP), left ventricular pressure (LVP), and left atrial pressure (LAP). The shaded areas indicate a transvalvular pressure difference during systole. HSM, holosystolic murmur; MSM, midsystolic murmur. (**B**) Schematic representation of ECG, aortic pressure (AOP), left ventricular pressure (LVP), and left atrial pressure (LAP), with shaded areas indicating transvalvular diastolic pressure difference. EDM, early diastolic murmur; MDM, mid-diastolic murmur; PSM, presystolic murmur.

Accentuation of a murmur during inspiration implies that the murmur originates on the right side of the circulation due to the inspiratory increase in venous return. The Valsalva maneuver reduces the intensity of most murmurs by diminishing both right and left ventricular filling. The systolic murmur associated with hypertrophic cardiomyopathy and the late systolic murmur due to mitral valve prolapse are exceptions and may be paradoxically accentuated during the Valsalva maneuver. Murmurs due to flow across a normal or obstructed semilunar valve increase in intensity in the cycle following a premature ventricular beat or a long RR interval in atrial fibrillation. In contrast, murmurs due to AV valve regurgitation or a ventricular septal defect do not change appreciably during the beat following a prolonged diastole. Standing accentuates the murmur of hypertrophic cardiomyopathy and, occasionally, the murmur due to mitral valve prolapse. Squatting increases most murmurs, except those caused by hypertrophic cardiomyopathy and mitral regurgitation due to a prolapsed mitral valve. Sustained hand-grip exercise often accentuates the murmurs of mitral regurgitation, aortic regurgitation, and mitral stenosis, but usually diminishes those due to aortic stenosis or hypertrophic cardiomyopathy.

## ■ SYSTOLIC MURMURS

*Holosystolic* (pansystolic) murmurs are generated when there is flow between 2 chambers that have high-pressure gradients throughout systole. Therefore, holosystolic murmurs accompany mitral or tricuspid regurgitation, and ventricular septal defect. Although the typical high-pitched murmur of mitral regurgitation usually continues throughout systole, the shape of the murmur may vary considerably. The holosystolic murmurs of mitral regurgitation and ventricular septal defect are augmented by transient exercise and diminished by inhalation of amyl nitrate. The murmur of tricuspid regurgitation associated with pulmonary hypertension is holosystolic and frequently increases during inspiration.

Midsystolic murmurs, also called *systolic ejection murmurs*, which are often crescendo-decrescendo in shape, occur when blood is ejected across the aortic or pulmonic outflow tracts. When the semilunar valves are normal, an increased flow rate, ejection into a dilated vessel beyond the valve, or increased transmission of sound through a thin chest wall may be responsible for this murmur. Most benign functional murmurs are midsystolic, originate from the pulmonary outflow tract, and are typically grade 1–2.

Aortic (AS) and pulmonic (PS) stenosis produce prototype crescendo systolic murmurs. In valvular AS, the murmur is usually maximal in the second right intercostal space, with radiation into the neck, clavicles, and apex. When the aortic valve is immobile (calcified), the aortic closure sound ($A_2$) may be soft and inaudible, so that the length and configuration of the murmur are difficult to determine. In supravalvular AS, the murmur is occasionally loudest above the second intercostal space, with disproportionate radiation into the right carotid artery. In hypertrophic cardiomyopathy, the midsystolic murmur originates in the LV cavity and is usually maximal at the lower left sternal edge and apex, with relatively little radiation to the carotids.

Midsystolic aortic and pulmonic murmurs are intensified after amyl nitrate inhalation and during the cardiac cycle following a premature ventricular beat, while those due to mitral regurgitation are unchanged or softer.

Early systolic murmurs begin with the first heart sound and end in midsystole. Patients with acute mitral regurgitation into a noncompliant left atrium and a large *v* wave often have a loud early systolic murmur that diminishes as the pressure gradient between the left ventricle and the left atrium decreases in late systole.

Late systolic murmurs are faint or moderately loud, high-pitched apical murmurs that start well after ejection and do not mask either heart sound. Late systolic murmurs following midsystolic clicks are often due to late systolic mitral regurgitation caused by prolapse of the mitral valve into the left atrium. The timing of the murmur does not necessarily correlate with its severity.

## ◼ DIASTOLIC MURMURS

Early diastolic murmurs begin with or shortly after $S_2$. The high-pitched murmurs of aortic regurgitation or of pulmonic regurgitation are generally decrescendo. They are difficult to hear unless they are specifically sought by applying firm pressure on the diaphragm over the left midsternal border while the patient sits leaning forward and holds a breath in full expiration. The diastolic murmur of aortic regurgitation may be best heard over the sternal borders and apex.

Mid-diastolic murmurs, usually arising from the AV valves, occur during early ventricular filling. Such murmurs are usually subtle; the murmurs may be soft or even absent despite severe obstruction if the cardiac output is markedly reduced. When the stenosis is marked, the diastolic murmur is prolonged. So as an index of the severity of valve obstruction, the duration of the murmur is more reliable than its intensity.

The low-pitched, mid-diastolic murmur of mitral stenosis characteristically follows the OS. It should be specifically sought by placing the bell of the stethoscope at the site of the left ventricular impulse, which is best localized with the patient in the left lateral position. Frequently, the murmur of mitral stenosis is present only at the left ventricular apex. It may be increased in intensity by mild supine exercise or by inhalation of amyl nitrate.

A soft, mid-diastolic murmur may sometimes be heard in patients with acute rheumatic fever (Carey–Coombs murmur). In acute, severe aortic regurgitation, the left ventricular diastolic pressure may quickly exceed the left atrial pressure, resulting in rapid truncation of the diastolic murmur. In chronic, severe aortic regurgitation, a second diastolic apical murmur may be present (Austin Flint murmur) and is related to the premature closure of the mitral valve.

Presystolic murmurs begin during the period of ventricular filling that follows atrial contraction, and therefore occur in sinus rhythm. They are usually due to stenosis of the AV valve and have the same quality as the mid-diastolic filling rumble, but they are usually crescendo, reaching peak intensity at the time of a loud $S_1$. It is the presystolic murmur that is most characteristic of tricuspid stenosis and sinus rhythm.

## ◼ CONTINUOUS MURMURS

Continuous murmurs are louder in systole, wane in diastole, and do not discretely cease with either systole or diastole. They generally reflect the continuous flow of blood from the arterial into the venous circulation. Continuous murmurs may result from congenital or acquired systemic arteriovenous fistulas, coronary arteriovenous fistula, pulmonary arteriovenous malformations, and communications between the sinus of Valsalva and the right side of the heart.

A patent ductus arteriosus causes a continuous murmur as long as the pressure in the pulmonary artery is much lower than that in the aorta. The murmur is intensified by elevation of the systemic arterial pressure and reduced by amyl nitrate inhalation.

## ◼ PERICARDIAL RUBS

These adventitious sounds may have presystolic, systolic, and early diastolic scratchy components; they may be confused with a murmur or extracardiac sound when they are heard only in systole. A pericardial friction rub is best appreciated with the patient upright and leaning forward, and may be accentuated during inspiration.

# SUGGESTED READINGS

Harrington RA, Silverman ME, Wooley CF. A History of the heart, cardiac diseases, and the development of cardiovascular medicine as a specialty. In: Fuster V, Walsh R, Harrington RA, et al, eds. *Hurst's The Heart*. 13th ed. New York, NY: McGraw-Hill; 2011; 1:1-16.

Ewy GA. Venous and arterial pulsations: bedside insights into hemodynamics. In: Chizner M, ed. *Classic Teachings in Clinical Cardiology: A Tribute to W. Proctor Harvey*. Cedar Grove, NJ: Laennec; 1996.

O'Rourke RA. Approach to the patient with a murmur. In: Goldman L, Braunwald E, eds. *Primary Cardiology*. 2nd ed. Philadelphia, PA: Saunders; 2003.

O'Rourke RA, Braunwald E. Physical examination of the cardiovascular system. In: Fauci AS, Braunwald E, Isselbacher KJ, et al, eds. *Harrison's Principles of Internal Medicine*. 15th ed. New York, NY: McGraw-Hill; 2007.

# CHAPTER 2
# THE RESTING ELECTROCARDIOGRAM

Antoni Bayés de Luna, Diego Goldwasser,
Miquel Fiol, and Antoni Bayés-Genis

The electrocardiogram (ECG) has many uses. It may function as an independent marker of myocardial disease; it may reflect anatomic, hemodynamic, molecular, ionic, and drug-induced cardiac abnormalities; and it may provide essential information for the proper diagnosis and therapy of many cardiac problems. In fact, it is the most commonly used laboratory procedure for the diagnosis of heart disease.

## VENTRICULAR DEPOLARIZATION AND REPOLARIZATION

Depolarization occurs with an endocardium-to-epicardium *sequence*. It has been described as a moving wave *with the positive charges in front* of the negative charges. The unipolar lead records a positivity because it consistently faces positive charges throughout the entire depolarization sequence. On the other hand, the *sequence* of ventricular repolarization is from the epicardium to the endocardium, but with the negative charges in front. M cells play a determining role in the inscription of the T wave, since currents flowing down voltage gradients on either side of the usual (but not necessarily) midmyocardial cells determine both the height and the width of the T wave, as well as the degree to which the ascending or descending limbs of the T wave are interrupted. A transmural dispersion of repolarization is created by differences in the repolarization time among the 3 myocardial layers, with the M cells having the longest repolarization time. The greater the transmural dispersion of repolarization (the difference between repolarization times between midmyocardium and endo/epicardium), the greater the risk for arrhythmic events.

### ■ NORMAL ACTIVATION OF THE HEART: VENTRICULAR DEPOLARIZATION

After emerging from the sinus node, the cardiac impulse propagates throughout the atria toward the atrioventricular (AV) node. The sequence of atrial depolarization occurs in an inferior, leftward, and somewhat posterior direction. The PR interval (used to estimate AV conduction time) includes conduction through the "true" AV structures (AV node, His bundle, bundle branches, and main divisions of the left bundle branch) as well as through those parts of the atria located between the sinus and AV nodes. The onset of ventricular depolarization (defined as the beginning of the normal Q wave) reflects activation of the left side of the interventricular septum.

Hence, the normal initial depolarization is oriented from left to right, explaining the small Q wave in lead $V_6$ and the small R wave in $V_1$. Thereafter, the interventricular septum is activated in both directions. Septal activation is encompassed within or neutralized by subsequent free-wall activation. The greater mass of the left ventricular (LV) free wall explains why LV free-wall events overpower those of the interventricular septum and the right ventricular free wall.

## ■ CARDIAC MEMORY

The term *memory* has been applied to gradual adjustments of action potential duration (roughly corresponding to QT intervals) after abrupt changes in cycle lengths (events influenced by past history), without necessarily requiring previous abnormal ventricular repolarization. Cardiac memory can be seen in the surface electrocardiogram as persistent abnormal repolarization (T waves), for example, after disappearance of preexcitation, resolution of bundle branch block, RV pacing, and wide QRS complex tachycardias.

## ELECTRICAL AXIS

The electrical axis (EA) may be defined as a vector originating in the center of Einthoven's equilateral triangle. When applied to the EA of the QRS complexes, the vector that represents it also gives the direction of the activation process as projected in the plane of the limb leads. The classic approach recommends calculating the net *areas* enclosed by the QRS complex in leads I to III. A simpler, though less precise, method of calculating the quadrant (or part of the quadrant) in which the EA is located consists of using the maximal QRS deflection in leads I and aVF and, when necessary, lead II. A normal QRS axis orientation in the frontal plane lies between +90 and –30 degrees.

## ST-SEGMENT CHANGES

In orthodox ECG language, *injury* implies *abnormal ST-segment changes*; *necrosis* or *fibrosis* implies *abnormal Q waves*; *and ischemia* implies *symmetrical T-wave inversion* (or elevation). Various hypotheses have been postulated to explain how injury-related diastolic hypopolarization is manifested as abnormal ST-segment shifts. One hypothesis is based on the existence of a *diastolic* current of "injury," and the other presupposes a true, active, *systolic* displacement. Most likely, injury reflects both the disappearance of diastolic baseline shifts and active ST-segment elevation. In addition, loss or depression of the action potential dome in the epicardium, but not in the endocardium, underlies the development of a prominent ST-segment elevation. Some authors consider ST-segment changes in ventricular aneurysms to be a result of the earlier repolarization of a ring of persistently viable tissue surrounding the aneurysm; however, others believe that they reflect functional (echocardiographic) dyskinesia. ST-segment elevation from epicardial injury due to pericarditis should be differentiated from the benign "early repolarization" pattern (**Fig. 2-1**), a normal variant characterized by J-point elevation with an upwardly concave ST-segment and tall R waves with a distinct notch on the downstroke commonly seen in the precordial leads and affected by exercise and hyperventilation. Although the mechanism of early repolarization has not been fully elucidated, it has been related to enhanced activity of the right sympathetic nerves.

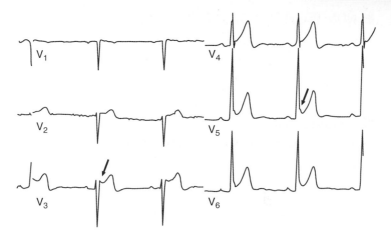

**FIGURE 2-1.** Early repolarization. This normal variant is characterized by narrow QRS complexes with J-point and ST-segment elevation in the chest leads. Left chest leads often show tall R waves with a distinct notch or slur in their downstroke (arrow in $V_5$), while the right chest leads may display ST-segments having a "saddleback" or "humpback" shape (arrow in $V_3$).

High-takeoff ST segments of either the caved or saddleback type localized to the right chest leads, associated with different degrees of right bundle-branch block (RBBB) with or without T-wave inversion, are seen in the Brugada syndrome (see Chapters 8, 11, and 16). Strong sodium channel-blocking drugs can produce ST-segment elevations even in patients without any evidence of syncope or ventricular fibrillation. Slight ST-segment elevation with an incomplete RBBB pattern showing an epsilon wave has been described in some patients with arrhythmogenic right ventricular dysplasia. Hyperkalemic "injury" can produce an anteroseptal myocardial infarction (MI) pattern (dialyzable current of injury).

## ◼ ISCHEMIC T-WAVE CHANGES

Symmetrical T waves, inverted or upright (as in "hyperacute" T waves), characteristic of ECG "ischemia" have been considered to reflect a type or degree of cellular affection resulting in action potentials of increased and different duration with regional alterations of the duration of the depolarized state. T-wave inversions do not always reflect "physiologic" ischemia (due to decreased blood supply), since they can also be seen in evolving pericarditis, myocardial contusion, and increased intracranial pressure, and in the right chest leads of young patients (persistent juvenile pattern).

## ◼ SECONDARY ST–T-WAVE CHANGES

Alterations in the sequence of (and sometimes delay in) ventricular depolarization (as produced by BBBs, ventricular pacing, ectopic ventricular impulse formation, pre-excitation syndromes, and ventricular hypertrophy) result in an obligatory change in the sequence of ventricular repolarization. This causes non-ischemic T-wave inversions (secondary T-wave changes) in leads showing predominantly positive QRS deflections. Disappearance of these alterations in ventricular depolarization may be followed by narrow QRS complexes with negative T waves due to cardiac memory, as previously stated.

## ■ NONSPECIFIC ST–T-WAVE CHANGES

Nonspecific (or rather, nondiagnostic) ST–T-wave changes are the most commonly diagnosed ECG abnormalities. When ECGs were analyzed without clinical information, this diagnosis was made in 40% of 410 abnormal ECGs, with the number reduced to 10% when clinical data became available. In the absence of structural heart disease, these changes can be due to a variety of physiological, pharmacological, and extracardiac factors.

# ACUTE MYOCARDIAL INFARCTION

Myocardial infarctions are classified as non–ST-segment elevation (NSTEMI) or ST-segment elevation (STEMI). In the thrombolytic era, the prevalence of non–ST-segment elevation MI seems to be greater. The prethrombolytic "classic" evolution of acute ST-segment elevation MI has been transformed by pharmacological therapy and interventional techniques. The succession of events in the course of a classic ST-segment elevation MI is from hyperacute positive T waves (on occasion) to ST-segment elevation to abnormal Q waves to T-wave inversion. Acceleration of these phases can occur with effective reperfusion. The time course of ST-segment elevation is a good predictor of reperfusion. Sensitivity increases as frequency of monitoring increases. Resolution of ST-segment elevation has been defined as a progressive decrease, within 40 to 60 minutes, to less than 50% of its maximally elevated value. The subsequent development of pathologic Q waves is dependent on the site of coronary occlusion, reperfusion, and ultimate extent of infarction.

The electrocardiographic criteria for STEMI include new ST-segment elevation in 2 or more contiguous leads of:

1. $\geq 0.2$ mV in leads $V_1$, $V_2$, or $V_3$
2. $\geq 0.1$ mV in other leads (eg, I and aVL or II, aVF, and III)

The site of coronary occlusion can be reliably predicted from the pattern of ST-segment elevation in the surface electrocardiogram , which reflects the location of the myocardial injury (**Table 2-1, Figs. 2-2** and **2-3**).

The location of the ultimate myocardial infarction can be gleaned from the pattern of abnormal Q waves. However, Q waves may reflect other processes as well (**Table 2-2**).

# ABNORMAL Q WAVES

Abnormal Q waves appearing several hours after total occlusion of a coronary artery result from necrosis secondary to decreased blood supply. The number of affected cells has to be large enough to produce changes that are reflected at the body surface, and abnormal Q waves can occur in MIs that are not completely transmural. The following changes have been said to be equivalent to Q waves in non–Q-wave MIs: R/S ratio changes, acute frontal-plane right-axis deviation, new left-axis deviation or left bundle branch block (LBBB), initial and terminal QRS notching, and some types of "poor R-wave progression" not related to precordial lead misplacement.

# PERICARDITIS

In acute pericarditis, ST-segments can be elevated in all leads except aVR (**Fig. 2-4**) and, rarely, $V_1$. Symmetrical T-wave inversion (due to epicardial "ischemia") usually develops after the ST-segments have returned to the baseline (but it can appear during

**TABLE 2-1.** Site of Coronary Artery Occlusion in ST-segment Elevation Myocardial Infarction

1. Right coronary artery occlusion
   - ST depression in lead I
   - ST elevation in lead III greater than in lead II
   a. Proximal occlusion
      - ST elevation more than 1 mm with positive T wave in lead $V_4R$
   b. Distal occlusion
      - ST isolectric with a positive T wave in lead $V_4R$
2. Left circumflex artery occlusion
   - ST elevation in lead II greater than lead III
   - ST isoelectric or elevated in lead I
   - ST isoelectric or depressed with negative T wave in $V_4R$
   a. Extension to posterior wall
      - ST depression in precordial leads
   b. Extension to lateral wall
      - ST elevation in leads I, aVL, $V_5$, and $V_6$
3. Left anterior descending artery occlusion
   a. Proximal to first septal branch and first diagonal branch
      - ST elevation in leads aVR and aVL
      - ST depression in leads II, III, and aVF
      - ST elevation in lead $V_1$ (> 2 mm) and leads $V_2$ to $V_4$
      - ST isolectric or depressed in leads $V_5$ and $V_6$
      - Acquired intra-Hissian or RBBB may occur
   b. Distal to first septal branch, proximal to first diagonal branch
      - ST elevation in lead I and aVL
      - ST depression in lead III (lead II is isoelectric)
      - ST elevation in leads $V_2$ to $V_6$ but not in lead $V_1$
   c. Distal to first diagonal branch, proximal to first septal branch
      - ST depression in lead aVL
      - ST elevation in inferior leads, highest in lead III
      - ST elevation in leads $V_1$ to $V_4$
   d. Distal LAD
      - ST depression in aVR
      - ST elevation in inferior leads, highest in lead II
      - ST elevation in leads $V_3$ to $V_6$
4. Left main coronary artery occlusion
   - ST elevation in lead aVR
   - ST elevation in lead $V_1$ (lower than that of lead aVR)
   - ST depression in leads II and aVF
   - ST depression in the precordial leads to the left of $V_2$

the injury stage). Neither reciprocal ST-segment changes nor abnormal Q waves are seen. In most cases of acute pericarditis, the PR segment is depressed (or elevated in aVR). ST-segment resolution generally occurs within 2 weeks (see also Chapter 44).

# QRS COMPLEX WIDENING

The most common causes of QRS complex widening are conduction delays due to fibrosis or infarction of the conduction system (**Table 2-3**).

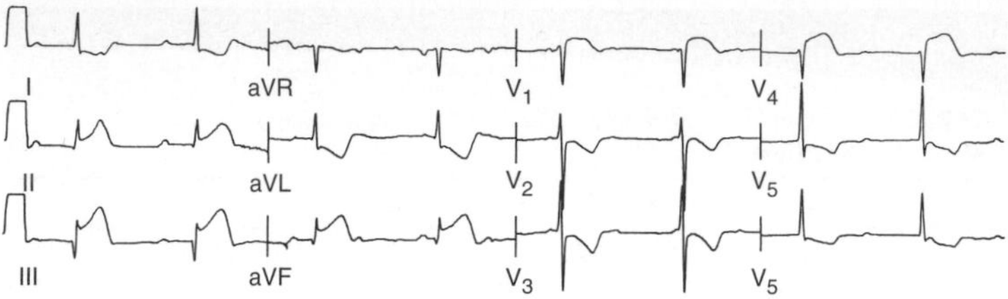

I　　aVR　　$V_1$　　$V_4$

II　　aVL　　$V_2$　　$V_5$

III　　aVF　　$V_3$　　$V_5$

**FIGURE 2-2. Acute inferior myocardial infarction.** Acute inferior (diaphragmatic) injury showing ST-segment elevation in the inferior leads as well as in $V_1$ (due to right ventricular infarction). There are reciprocal changes from $V_2$ to $V_6$ as well as an AV junctional rhythm due to complete AV block. These changes were caused by proximal right coronary artery occlusion.

## Wolff–Parkinson–White Syndrome

In this syndrome where the ventricular myocardium is activated by both the normal conduction system and through an accessory pathway (eg "preexcited"), the ventricular complex is a fusion beat resulting from ventricular activation of these 2 wavefronts. The degree of preexcitation (amount of muscle activated through the accessory pathway) is variable and depends on many factors, including the distance between the sinus node and the atrial insertion of the accessory pathway, and more importantly the differences in the refractory periods and conduction times through the normal and accessory pathways. If there is total block at the AV node or His–Purkinje system, the impulse will be conducted using the accessory pathway exclusively. Consequently, the QRS complexes are different from fusion beats, although the direction of the delta wave remains the same. Moreover, the QRS complexes are as wide as those produced by artificial or spontaneous beats arising in the vicinity of the ventricular end of the accessory pathway. Initial noninvasive determination of the anatomic position of the accessory pathway is of great clinical importance because surgical and catheter ablative techniques are used for symptomatic cases of preexcitation. Many ECG algorithms have been proposed to determine the location of accessory pathways (see Chapter on WPW).

## Ventricular Pacing

In determining the location of the stimulating electrodes, what is relevant is the polarity of the *properly positioned* $V_1$ and $V_2$ electrodes and the direction of the EA.

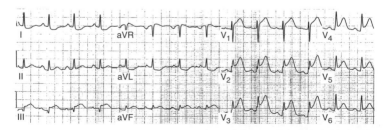

I　　aVR　　$V_1$　　$V_4$

II　　aVL　　$V_2$　　$V_5$

III　　aVF　　$V_3$　　$V_6$

**FIGURE 2-3. Acute anterior myocardial infarction.** Changes produced by a "wrapped up" distal left anterior descending coronary artery showing ST-segment elevation in all precordial leads as well as inferior leads.

**TABLE 2-2.** Electrocardiographic Location of Infarction Sites Based on the Presence of Abnormal Q Waves

| Site | Leads | False Patterns |
|---|---|---|
| Inferior (diaphragmatic) | II, III, aVF | WPW (PSAP), HCM |
| Inferolateral | II, III, aVF, VL, $V_4$–$V_6$ | |
| "True" posterior (posterobasal) | $V_1$ | RVH, "atypical" incomplete RBBB, WPW (LFWAP) |
| Inferoposterior | II, III, aVF, $V_1{}^a$ | WPW (left PSAP), HCM |
| Inferior–right ventricular | II, III, aVF plus $V_4R$–$V_6R$ or $V_1$–$V_3$ | ASMI |
| Anteroseptal | $V_1$, $V_2$, $V_3$ | LVH, chronic lung disease, LBBB, chest electrode misplacement, right ventricular MI |
| Extensive anterior | I, aVL, $V_1$–$V_6$ | |
| High lateral | I, aVL | Extremely vertical hearts with aVL resembling aVR |
| Anterior (apical) | $V_3$–$V_4$ | WPW (LFWAP) |
| Posterolateral | $V_4$–$V_6$, $V_1$ | |
| Right ventricular | $V_4R$ with $V_4R$–$V_6R$ or $V_1$–$V_3$ | ASMI |

ASMI, anteroseptal myocardial infarction; HCM, hypertrophic cardiomyopathy; LBBB, left bundle-branch block; LFWAP, left free-wall accessory pathway; PSAP, posteroseptal accessory pathway; WPW, Wolff–Parkinson–White syndrome; RVH, right ventricular hypertrophy.

$^a$Tall R wave, "reciprocal" to changes in "indicative" back leads.

For example, endocardial or epicardial stimulation of the *anteriorly* located right ventricle at any site—apical (inferior) or mid/outflow tract (superior)—yields predominantly negative deflections in the right chest leads because of the *posterior* spread of activation. The reverse (positive deflections in $V_1$ and $V_2$) occurs when the epicardial stimulation of the superior and lateral portions of the posterior left ventricle by catheter electrodes in the distal coronary sinus, or great and middle cardiac veins (or by implanted electrodes in the nearby muscle) results in *anteriorly* oriented forces. Right ventricular apical pacing may rarely produce positive deflections in

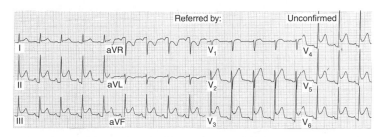

**FIGURE 2-4. Pericarditis.** Acute nonspecific pericarditis showing ST-segment elevation in all leads except aVR and $V_1$.

**TABLE 2-3.** Intraventricular Conduction Delays

1. Left anterior fascicular block
   a. Abnormal left superior (rarely right superior) axis with RS complexes in II, III, and aVF. Peak of R in aVL occurs before that in aVR. S wave deeper in III than in II.
   b. Left precordial leads may show RS complexes when the electrical axis is markedly superior.
   c. Other causes of left axis deviation—such as extensive inferior wall MI, Wolff–Parkinson–White syndrome (posteroseptal accessory pathway), hyperkalemia, ventricular pacing, and pulmonary emphysema—should be excluded.
   d. QRS widening (over normal values) does not exceed 0.025 seconds.
   e. Usually there are no interferences with the diagnosis of MI or RBBB.
2. Left posterior fascicular block
   a. Usually diagnosed only when coexisting with complete RBBB.
   b. Right (and inferior) axis deviation should not be due to right ventricular hypertrophy or lateral MI.
   c. The QRST pattern resembles that of inferior ischemia or infarction.
3. Complete right bundle-branch block
   a. Does not deviate the electrical axis (determined by maximal deflections) abnormally to the left or to the right.
   b. Although true posterior MI cannot be diagnosed in its presence, it does not interfere with the diagnosis of MI of other locations.
   c. It may masquerade as LBBB when the expected wide S wave is not present in lead I, presumably because the terminal vectors are perpendicular to this lead.
   d. An upright T wave in the right chest leads may be reciprocal to posterior ischemia or may reflect a primary change in repolarization in anteroseptal leads.
4. Incomplete right bundle branch block
   a. An r' or R' in $V_1$ with QRS duration of less than 0.10 second may be referred to as a normal incomplete RBBB (IRBBB) "pattern."
   b. It need not always reflect a conduction delay in the trunk of a normal right branch, since it has been attributed to an increased conduction time due to a right ventricular enlargement or to stretch-related delay in an elongated right branch, or in the Purkinje–myocardial junction; an interruption of a subdivision of the right bundle branch; or a physiological later-than-usual arrival of excitation at the crista supraventricularis.
5. Complete left bundle branch block
   a. May simulate anteroseptal MI.
   b. Interferes with the diagnosis of lateral and inferior MI but not anteroseptal MI.
   c. A normal Q wave before an otherwise typical wide R wave indicates anteroseptal, not lateral, MI.
   d. MI of any location may be present without any change in its basic features.
   e. Acute inferior and anterolateral MIs can be diagnosed by characteristic ST-segment changes.
   f. A positive T wave always reflects a primary change in repolarization.
6. Nonspecific intraventricular conduction delay
   This condition is associated with a wide QRS complex (with repolarization abnormalities) that does not have a characteristic left or right BBB pattern. The EA may be normal, left, or right.

$V_1$, specifically if this lead is (mis)placed above its usual level. On the other hand, *superior* deviation of the electrical axis only indicates that a spatially *inferior* ventricular site has been stimulated, regardless of whether this site is the apical portion of the right ventricle or the inferior part of the left ventricle, the latter being paced through the middle cardiac vein. Conversely, an *inferior* vertical axis is simply a

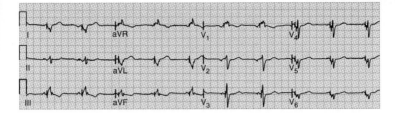

**FIGURE 2-5.** Effects of biventricular pacing on the QRS. Note the rightward axis and prominence of the R waves in $V_1$ and $V_2$ reflecting early activation of the left ventricular posterolateral wall as a consequence of stimulation from a lead placed in a posterolateral coronary vein.

consequence of pacing from a *superior* site, which can be the endocardium of the right ventricular outflow tract or the epicardium of the posterosuperior and lateral portions of the left ventricle. Ventricular capture of the left ventricular lead in subjects with biventricular pacing is suggested by an R/S ratio $\geq 1$ in $V_1$ and a rightward axis (**Fig. 2-5**). Lead location can also be determined from the anteroposterior and lateral chest x-ray.

# LEFT VENTRICULAR HYPERTROPHY

Multiple ECG criteria have been proposed to diagnose left ventricular hypertrophy (LVH) using necropsy or echocardiographic information (**Table 2-4**). Of these, the Sokolow–Lyon criterion ($SV_1 + RV_{5-6} \geq 35$ mm) is the most specific (> 95%), although it is not very sensitive (around 45%). The Romhilt–Estes score has a specificity of 90% and a sensitivity of 60% in studies correlated with echocardiography. The Casale (modified Cornell) criterion (RaVL + $SV_3$ > 28 mm in men and > 20 in women) is somewhat more sensitive, but less specific than the Sokolow–Lyon criterion. The Talbot criterion (R $\geq 16$ mm in $aV_L$) is very specific ( > 90%), even in the presence of MI and ventricular block, but not very sensitive. The Koito and

**TABLE 2-4.** Electrocardiographic Criteria for Left Ventricular Enlargement

| Voltage Criteria | Sensitivity (%) | Specificity (%) |
|---|---|---|
| 1. $R_I + S_{II}$ > 25 mm | 10.6 | 100 |
| 2. RVL > 11 mm | 11 | 100 |
| 3. RVL > 7.5 mm | 22 | 96 |
| 4. $SV_1 + RV_5 - V_6 \geq 35$ mm (Sokolow–Lyon) | 22 | 100 |
| 5. $RV_6 - V_6$ > 26 mm | 25 | 98 |
| 6. RVL + $SV_3$ > 28 mm (men) or > 20 mm (women) (Cornell voltage criterion) | 42 | 96 |
| 7. Cornell voltage duration measurement QRS duration × Cornell voltage > 2436 mm/seg | 51 | 95 |
| 8. In $V_1$–$V_6$, the deepest S + the tallest R > 45 mm | 45 | 93 |
| 9. Romhilt–Estes score > 4 points | 55 | 85 |
| 10. Romhilt–Estes score > 5 points | 35 | 95 |

Spodick criterion ($RV_6 > RV_5$) claims a specificity of 100% and a sensitivity of more than 50%. According to Hernandez Padial, a total 12-lead QRS voltage > 120 mm is a good ECG criterion for LVH in systemic hypertension and is better than those most frequently used. The electrocardiographic diagnosis of LVH in the presence of complete LBBB or left anterior fascicular block (LAFB) is difficult, but most patients with these patterns will have echocardiographic LVH.

# RIGHT VENTRICULAR HYPERTROPHY

The ECG manifestations of right ventricular hypertrophy (RVH) include (1) the posterior and rightward displacement of the QRS forces associated with low voltage, as seen in patients with pulmonary emphysema; (2) the incomplete RBBB pattern *with right axis deviation* occurring in patients with chronic lung disease and congenital heart defects, particularly when there is right ventricular volume overload; (3) true posterior wall MI pattern with prominent R wave in $V_1$ (seen in mitral stenosis with abnormal P waves); and (4) the classic RVH and strain pattern seen in young patients with congenital heart disease (in the presence of pressure overload) or in adult patients with high right ventricular pressures, such as "primary" pulmonary hypertension. (See also Chapter 30.)

# QT INTERVAL

The QT interval (considered by some to be a surrogate for action potential duration) is manually measured from the beginning of the Q wave to the point at which the T-wave downslope crosses the baseline. However, there has been considerable debate and speculation regarding the accurate measurement of the QT interval. For example, according to Coumel and associates, the human interobserver variability is 30.6 milliseconds. Similarly, the machine interautomatic comparison of 19 systems yielded standard deviations as great as 30 milliseconds. At present there seems to be a trend toward acceptance of the (automatic) values obtained with the QT Guard package (Marquette). With this system, the end of the T wave is determined using the intersection of the isoelectric line with the tangent to the *inflection point* of the descending part of the T wave. The QT interval is affected by autonomic tone and catecholamines, and has day–night differences. It varies with heart rate and sex. Several formulas (most commonly Bazett) have been proposed to take these variables into account and provide a corrected measurement (eg $QT_c$ interval). In general, the unadjusted resting QT interval decreases linearly from ± 0.42 second at rates of 50/minutes to ±0.32 second at 100/minutes to ±0.26 second at 150/minutes. However, during exercise when the rate becomes faster, the $QT_c$ first increases until it reaches a maximum at approximately a rate of 120/minutes and thereafter decreases again.

Regardless of the method of correction of QT, its measurement should be done accurately. Recommendations from an expert panel established that the QT interval should be measured manually, preferably by using one of the limb leads that best shows the end of the T wave on a 12-lead ECG. The QT interval should be measured from the beginning of the QRS complex to the end of the T wave and averaged over 3 to 5 beats. *U waves* possibly corresponding to the late repolarization of cells in the midmyocardium should be included in the measurement *only if they are large enough to seem to merge with the T wave.*

As the 12-lead ECG shows a normal degree of QT and $QT_c$ variability, indexes have been used to quantify the extent of what has been called "the heterogeneity in ventricular repolarization." The difference between the longest and shortest QT interval is referred to as *QT dispersion*. Since 1990, it has been used as a prognostic marker not only in patients with congenitally prolonged QT intervals, but also in

**TABLE 2-5.** Causes of QT Prolongation

Acquired
1. Cardiomyopathies (dilated, hypertrophic, takotsubo)
2. Myocardial infarction
3. Electrolyte disturbances (hypokalemia, hypomagnesium, hypocalcemia)
4. Drugs (Type I antiarrhythmics, antipsychotics, antibiotics, tricyclic antidepressants)
5. Toxins (organophosphates)
6. Metabolic (hypothyroidism, hypothermia, starvation)
7. Stroke and brain death

Congenital
1. Long QT syndromes 1–12
   a. Jervell and Lange–Nielson syndrome (autosomal recessive, congenital deafness)
   b. Romano–Ward syndrome (autosomal dominant)
   c. $LQT_1$, $LQT_2$, $LQT_3$ most common

those with acute MI and those taking drugs with proarrhythmic properties; it has also been used to predict mortality in general epidemiological studies. However, recent reports have challenged the values of QT dispersion. The upper limits of the normal vary with different investigators, but a value of 60 to 65 milliseconds may be an acceptable compromise.

QT prolongation is common and has both acquired and congenital causes (**Table 2-5**). Drugs are one of the most common causes of QT prolongation and should always be reviewed when QT prolongation, especially if complicated by torsades de pointes, is present (see www.qtdrugs.org).

# ELECTROLYTE IMBALANCES

## ◼ HYPERKALEMIA

Peaked T waves are the initial effect of acute hyperkalemia. The diagnosis is almost certain when the duration of the base is less than 0.20 second at normal heart rates. As hyperkalemia increases, the QRS complex widens and the electrical axis deviates abnormally to the left and rarely to the right. Additionally the PR interval prolongs and the P wave flattens until it disappears. Rarely, hyperkalemia can simulate acute MI with anteroseptal ST elevation in the absence of coronary artery disease or a Brugada pattern.

## ◼ HYPOKALEMIA

Hypokalemia manifests as QU rather than QT prolongation. With major degrees of hypokalemia, the ST-segment becomes progressively more depressed, and there is a gradual blending of the T wave into what appears to be a tall U wave.

## ◼ HYPOMAGNESEMIA AND HYPERMAGNESEMIA

Isolated hypomagnesemia does not produce QU prolongation unless severe hypokalemia is also present. Long-standing and severe magnesium deficiency lowers the amplitude of the T wave and depresses the ST segment. The ECG findings of hypomagnesemia are difficult to differentiate from those of hypokalemia, which is commonly concomitant. Similarly, the effects of hypermagnesemia on the ECG are difficult to identify because the changes are dominated by calcium. Intravenous magnesium given to patients with torsades de pointes can control the arrhythmia without changing the prolonged QT interval significantly.

## ■ HYPERCALCEMIA AND OTHER CAUSES OF SHORT QT INTERVALS

Hypercalcemia produces a short QT interval during normal sinus rhythm, characterized by a short Q-to-apex-of-T interval (so-called "QaT" interval). Occasionally the ST segment disappears and the T waves become inverted. Digitalis also shortens the QT interval with the characteristic effects in leads where the R waves predominate. In addition, short QT intervals have been reported in hyperthermia, hyperkalemia, and altered autonomic tone. A congenital short QT syndrome has also been described, characterized by a $QT_c$ shorter than 300 milliseconds and associated with malignant ventricular arrhythmia and sudden death.

## SUGGESTED READINGS

Bayés de Luna A, Goldwasser D, Fiol M, Bayés-Genis A. Surface electrocardiography. In: Fuster V, Walsh R, Harrington RA, et al, eds. *Hurst's The Heart*. 13th ed. New York, NY: McGraw-Hill; 2011; 15:307-370.

Ammann P, Sticherling C, Kalusche D, et al. An electrocardiogram-based algorithm to detect loss of left ventricular capture during cardiac resynchronization therapy. *Ann Intern Med*. 2005;142:968-973.

Wagner GS. *Marriott's Practical Electrocardiography*. 10th ed. New York, NY: Lippincott Williams & Wilkins; 2000.

Wellens HJJ, Conover M. *The ECG in Emergency Decision Making*. 2nd ed. St. Louis, MO: Saunders, Elsevier; 2006.

# CHAPTER 3
# CARDIAC ROENTGENOGRAPHY

Robert A. O'Rourke[†] and Robert C. Gilkeson

In addition to the electrocardiogram, the chest roentgenogram is one of the primary and most widely available cardiovascular diagnostic studies to all clinicians. Unfortunately, it is less commonly used than in the past as a primary diagnostic technique for determining the presence and severity of cardiac disease, despite its simple diagnostic utility. The approach to the chest roentgenogram should be thorough and objective so that no clue is overlooked and no bias is incorporated in the process of radiographic analysis.

Familiarity with the altered anatomy and pathophysiology of a diseased heart are the cornerstones to appropriate interpretation of its radiographic manifestations.. For example, a secundum atrial septal defect can be incorrectly diagnosed as mitral stenosis (MS) because of their similar physical signs. The split second sound can be misinterpreted as the opening snap. The diastolic rumble caused by the increased flow through a normal tricuspid valve can mimic the murmur of MS. The radiographic signs of the 2 entities, however, are quite different (**Fig. 3-1** vs **Fig. 3-2**).

The radiological examination for heart disease consists of 5 major steps (**Table 3-1**).

## ROENTGENOGRAPHIC EXAMINATION FOR ANATOMY

The first step in a radiological examination is to survey the roentgenogram and assess all the structures, searching particularly for noncardiac conditions that can reflect heart disease (Table 3-1). For instance, a right-sided stomach with an absent image of the inferior vena cava suggests the possibility of congenital interruption of the inferior vena cava with azygos continuation. A narrowed anteroposterior (AP) diameter of the thorax can be the cause of an innocent murmur.

### ■ PULMONARY VASCULATURE

The lung can often reflect the underlying pathophysiology of the heart. For example, if uniform dilation of all pulmonary vessels is present, the diagnosis of a left-to-right shunt is more likely than a left-sided obstructive lesion. The latter typically shows a cephalic pulmonary blood flow pattern.

### ■ LUNG PARENCHYMA

With right-heart failure, the lungs become unusually radiolucent because of decreased pulmonary blood flow (PBF). Conversely, significant left-heart failure is characterized by the presence of pulmonary edema and/or a cephalic blood

[†]Deceased.

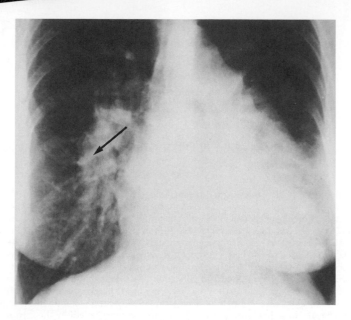

**FIGURE 3-1.** Roentgenographic assessment of the volume of pulmonary blood flow. A patient with a secundum atrial septal defect showing uniform increase in pulmonary vascularity bilaterally. The right descending pulmonary artery is markedly enlarged, measuring 27 mm.

flow pattern. Long-standing, severe pulmonary venous hypertension can lead to hemosiderosis and/or ossification of the lung. When right-heart failure results from severe left-heart failure, the preexisting pulmonary congestion can improve because of the decreased PBF. However, it should be recognized that the chest x-ray is not sensitive, though specific for left-sided heart failure.

## ■ CARDIAC SIZE

An enlarged heart is always abnormal; however, mild cardiomegaly can reflect a higher-than-average cardiac output from a normal heart, as seen in athletes with slow heart rates. The cardiothoracic ratio remains the simplest yardstick for assessment of cardiac size; the mean ratio in the upright posteroanterior (PA) view is 44%.

The nature of cardiomegaly can often be determined by the specific roentgen appearance. As a rule, when the PBF pattern remains normal, volume overload tends to present a greater degree of cardiomegaly than lesions with pressure overload alone. For example, patients with aortic stenosis (AS) typically show features of left ventricular hypertrophy (LVH) without dilation. Conversely, the left ventricle both dilates and hypertrophies in the case of aortic regurgitation (AR), producing a much larger heart (eg, cor bovinum) even before the development of heart failure.

## ■ CARDIAC CONTOUR

Any significant deviation from the normal cardiovascular contour can be a clue to the correct diagnosis. For instance, *coeur en sabot*, a "boot-shaped heart," is characteristic

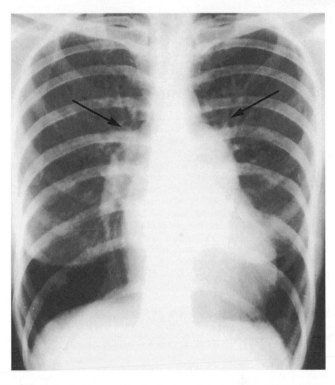

**FIGURE 3-2.** Abnormal pulmonary blood flow patterns. *Cephalization*. A patient with severe mitral stenosis (MS) showing dilation of the upper vessels with constriction of the lower vessels.

**TABLE 3-1.** Major Steps of Roentgenologic Examination

Roentgenographic examination for anatomy
    Overview (eg, rib notching)
    Pulmonary vascularity (eg, shunt vascularity in ASD)
    Lung parenchyma (eg, ossification in critical MS)
    Cardiac size (eg, huge right heart in Ebstein anomaly)
    Cardiac contour (eg, boot-shaped heart in TOF)
    Abnormal densities (eg, calcification of LV aneurysm)
    Abnormal lucency (eg, conspicuous fat stripes in PE)
    Cardiac malpositions (eg, dextrocardia with SS)
    Other abnormalities (eg, Holt–Oram syndrome)
Fluoroscopic observation for dynamics
Comparison of serial studies
Statistical guidance
Clinical correlation
Conclusion

ASD, atrial septal defect LV, left ventricle; MS, mitral stenosis; PE, pericardial effusion; SS, situs solitus; TOF, tetralogy of Fallot.

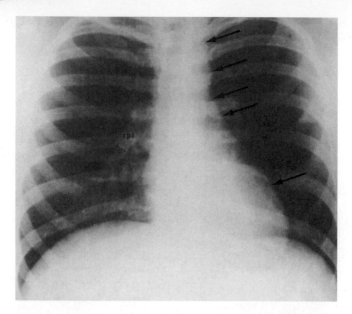

**FIGURE 3-3.** Normal chest x-ray. The components of the mediastinal left-heart border include (1) the vertical left subclavian artery, (2) the concave aortic knob, (3) the convex pulmonary artery window, (4) the convex left atrial appendage, and (5) the concave left ventricle.

of tetralogy of Fallot. A bulge along the left cardiac border with a retrosternal double density is virtually diagnostic of left ventricular (LV) aneurysm. A markedly widened right cardiac contour with a straightened left cardiac border is seen frequently in patients with severe MS leading to tricuspid regurgitation (TR). The classic components of the left border of the mediastinum, cranial to caudad, include (**Fig. 3-3**) (1) the vertical left subclavian artery, (2) the concave aortic knob, (3) the convex pulmonary artery window, (4) the convex left atrial appendage, and (5) the concave left ventricle.

## ■ ABNORMAL DENSITIES

Besides the familiar double density cast by an enlarged left atrium (LA), other increased densities can be found within the cardiac shadow, indicating a variety of dilated vascular structures (eg, tortuous descending aorta, aortic aneurysm, coronary artery [CA] aneurysm, pulmonary varix). Furthermore, large cardiac calcifications are readily seen in lateral and oblique views. If smaller calcific deposits are suspected, they should be verified promptly, or ruled out by cardiac fluoroscopy or CT. Any radiologically detectable calcification in the heart is clinically important. In general, the denser the calcification, the more significant it becomes.

## ■ ABNORMAL LUCENCY

The abnormal lucent areas in and about the heart include (1) displaced subepicardial fat stripes caused by effusion or thickening of the pericardium, (2) pneumopericardium, and (3) pneumomediastinum. Pneumomediastinum is differentiated from pneumopericardium by the fact that the former shows a superior extension of the air strip beyond the confines of the pericardium.

# ■ PULMONARY VASCULARITY

## Normal

The normal roentgen appearance of the pulmonary vasculature of an upright human being is typified by a caudal flow pattern because of gravity. The pressure differential between the apex and the base of the lung is approximately 22 mm Hg in adults in the upright position. Therefore, under higher distending pressure, more flow is expected in the lower-lobe vessels than in the upper. Normally, one sees very little vascularity above the hilum, whereas more and larger vessels are found below the hilum. Because the pulmonary resistance is normal, all vessels taper gradually in a tree-like manner from the hilum toward the periphery of the lung. The right descending pulmonary artery measures 10 to 15 mm in diameter in males and 9 to 14 mm in females.

## Abnormal

Abnormal pulmonary vascularity can be classified into 2 categories, either in terms of volume or in terms of distribution.

**Abnormalities in Volume**   In the evaluation of pulmonary vasculature, the caliber of the vessels is more important than the length or the number. As long as the PBF pattern remains normal, with a greater amount of flow to the bases than to the apices, the volume of the flow is proportional to the caliber of the pulmonary arteries. Besides measuring the right descending pulmonary artery, pulmonary blood volume can be assessed by comparing the size of the pulmonary artery with that of the accompanying bronchus, where they are viewed on end. Normally, the 2 structures have approximately equal diameters. When the artery–bronchus ratio is greater than unity, increased blood flow is suggested. Conversely, when the ratio is smaller than unity, decreased flow is likely.

**Increased Pulmonary Blood Flow**   In the case of mild to moderate left-to-right shunts, for example, the vessels dilate in proportion to the increased flow with no significant change in pressure, resistance, or flow pattern. This phenomenon is also called *shunt vascularity* or *equalization*. Equalization of the PBF between the upper and lower lung zones is more apparent than real; however, the lower lobes still receive a great deal more blood than the upper lobes, although the ratio of PBF between the 2 zones has changed—for example, from 5:1 to 4:1 or 3:1. A mild increase in pulmonary vascularity with slight cardiomegaly is commonly found in pregnant women and trained athletes with increased cardiac output.

**Decreased Pulmonary Blood Flow**   Patients with tetralogy of Fallot frequently show decreased pulmonary vascularity with smaller and shorter pulmonary arteries and veins, and more radiolucent lungs. Marked reduction in PBF is also encountered in patients with isolated right-sided heart failure without a right-to-left shunt. This is attributed to the significant decrease in cardiac output from both ventricles.

**Abnormalities in Distribution**   An abnormal distribution of PBF (or an abnormal PBF pattern) always reflects a changed pulmonary vascular resistance, either locally or diffusely.

**Cephalization**   In the presence of postcapillary pulmonary hypertension (PH), physiological disturbances begin when the total intravascular pressure exceeds the oncotic pressure of the blood. As a result, fluid leaks out of the vessels and collects in the interstitium before filling the alveoli.

Pulmonary edema interferes with gas exchange, resulting in a state of hypoxemia. Alveolar hypoxia has a profound influence on the pulmonary vessels, causing them to constrict. Because there is greater alveolar hypoxia in the lung bases than in the apices, the basilar vessels constrict significantly, forcing the blood to flow upward. This phenomenon actually represents a reversal of the normal PBF pattern—redistribution or cephalization of the pulmonary vascularity.

Cephalization occurs in any of 3 conditions: (1) left-sided obstructive lesions—for example, MS or AS, (2) LV failure—for example, coronary heart disease or cardiomyopathies, and (3) severe mitral regurgitation (MR) even before pump failure of the left ventricle occurs. It should be emphasized that unless there is obvious *constriction* of the lower-lobe vessels, a diagnosis of cephalization should not be made. Dilation of the upper-lobe vessels is of secondary importance and can be found without narrowing of the basilar vessels in a number of entities, most noticeably left-to-right shunts.

**Centralization** In the presence of precapillary PH, the pulmonary trunk and central pulmonary arteries dilate, whereas the distal pulmonary arteries constrict in a concentric fashion from the periphery of the lung toward the hilum. This phenomenon is called *centralization of the pulmonary vascularity*. It occurs in patients with primary PH, Eisenmenger syndrome, recurrent pulmonary thromboembolic disease, or severe obstructive emphysema.

**Lateralization** Massive unilateral pulmonary embolism can cause a lateralized PBF pattern. Because one major pulmonary artery is obstructed, the blood is forced to flow only through the healthy lung. The paucity of pulmonary vascularity in the diseased lung with the obstructed pulmonary artery is termed the *Westermark sign*. In the case of congenital valvular pulmonary stenosis, a jet effect from the stenotic valve can cause a lateralized PBF pattern in favor of the left side.

**Localization** A localized abnormal flow pattern is exemplified by a congenital pulmonary arteriovenous fistula in a cyanotic child.

**Collateralization** Patients with markedly decreased PBF (eg, severe tetralogy) tend to show numerous small, tortuous bronchial arterial collaterals in the upper medial lung zones near their origin from the descending aorta. The native pulmonary arteries are extremely small, although smooth and gracefully branching.

# ■ HEART FAILURE

In addition to specific chamber enlargement, the pulmonary vasculature uniquely portrays the underlying pathophysiology of heart failure. In the chronic setting, decreased flow with increased pulmonary lucency is the hallmark of right-heart failure; striking cephalization of the pulmonary vasculature is typical for left-sided decompensation.

## *Left-Sided*

**Acute** Acute left-sided heart failure is characterized by alveolar edema in a "bat-wing" appearance without cardiomegaly (**Fig. 3-4**). Generally, the pulmonary vasculature has not had time to accommodate an increase in flow to produce a radiographic change. Such findings can be seen in large acute myocardial infarction or acute mitral regurgitation due to chordal rupture.

**Chronic** Chronic left-sided heart failure is characterized by gross cardiomegaly, striking cephalization of the pulmonary vasculature, and interstitial pulmonary edema or fibrosis with multiple distinct Kerley B lines. Pulmonary hemosiderosis, ossification, or both can result from long-standing severe postcapillary PH.

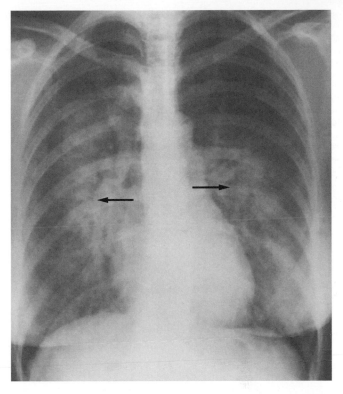

**FIGURE 3-4.** Acute left-heart failure (eg, acute pulmonary edema). Note the alveolar infiltrates in a bat-wing appearance in this patient with acute mitral regurgitation from chordal rupture. The heart is of normal size.

## *Right-Sided*

**Acute**  Acute right-sided heart failure most commonly results from massive pulmonary embolism. The typical radiographic signs are rapidly developing centralization of the pulmonary vasculature and dilation of the right-sided cardiac chambers and venae cavae. In addition, the lungs can show localized or lateralized oligemia. Eventually, opacities in either or both lungs can develop as a result of pulmonary infarction.

**Chronic**  Chronic right-heart failure has many causes. The common ones include congenital pulmonary stenosis, Ebstein anomaly, severe chronic obstructive pulmonary disease, and recurrent pulmonary thromboembolic disease. Diffusely decreased pulmonary vascularity with unusually lucent lungs is seen in patients with right-heart failure without PH. Centralized PBF pattern is encountered when the right-sided heart failure is secondary to precapillary PH. A cephalized flow pattern with unusually lucent lungs is found in patients with right-sided heart failure secondary to long-standing severe left-heart failure. The degree of right-sided chamber enlargement is proportional to the severity of TR.

## Combined

Right-heart failure is caused most often by severe left-heart failure. This is exemplified by patients with severe MS leading to severe TR. Other examples of bilateral heart failure are cardiac tamponade and constrictive pericarditis.

# SUGGESTED READINGS

O'Rourke RA, Gilkeson RC. Cardiac radiography. In: Fuster V, Walsh R, Harrington RA, et al, eds. *Hurst's The Heart*. 13th ed. New York, NY: McGraw-Hill; 2011; 17:388-410.

Chen JTT. *Essentials of Cardiac Imaging*. 2nd ed. Philadelphia, PA: Lippincott-Raven; 1997.

Woodley K, Stark P. Pulmonary parenchymal manifestations of mitral valve disease. *Radiographics*. 1999;19:965-972.

# CHAPTER 4
# NONINVASIVE TESTING FOR MYOCARDIAL ISCHEMIA

Michael J. Lipinski, Victor F. Froelicher,
Daniel S. Berman, Sean W. Hayes, Rory Hachamovitch,
Leslee J. Shaw, and Guido Germano

Myocardial ischemia is commonly detected using diverse electrocardiographic and imaging modalities. Dramatic developments in the field of cardiac imaging have paralleled improvements in microprocessor speed as well as progress in new contrast and radio-pharmaceutical agents, resulting in improved resolution, image quality, processing time, and quantitative interpretation programs.

## PATHOGENESIS OF STRESS-INDUCED MYOCARDIAL ISCHEMIA

*Myocardial ischemia* is defined as a discord between oxygen supply and demand within the cardiac myocyte. Most commonly, the mechanism for demand ischemia is reduced coronary blood flow from a fixed stenosis, although impaired coronary flow reserve in nonobstructive coronary disease as a result of endothelial dysfunction may also elicit ischemic responses to stress. Resting blood flow is generally maintained up till 90% stenosis. When oxygen delivery fails to meet regional demand, myocardial ischemia ensues, characterized by a shift from aerobic metabolism as a dominant energy source toward anaerobic substrates and the accumulation of metabolic end products (eg, lactate). The shift toward anaerobic metabolism quickly results in a depletion of high-energy phosphate stores followed by impaired mechanical function.

The aim of stress testing is to provoke myocardial ischemia within a controlled environment with incremental increases in the metabolic requirements for graded physical work or as a response to a drug stressor. The manifestations of myocardial ischemia may be commonly documented through examination of regional myocardial perfusion or left ventricular wall motion, the surface electrocardiogram (ECG), and clinical observations, including angina-like symptoms, exertional hypotension, or chronotropic incompetence. The sequence of occurrences, and the ensuing consequences and timing of reductions in blood flow, is defined as the ischemic cascade. This model for elucidating myocardial ischemia will allow us to understand the expected utility of various imaging risk markers, such as reductions in myocardial perfusion or regional wall-motion abnormalities. **Figure 4-1** depicts the cascade of events that occur during myocardial ischemia and the type of test that is currently applied to document each facet of the ischemic cascade. An understanding of the ischemic cascade and how it interfaces with present-day imaging allows for a more precise understanding of ischemia risk markers, their predictive accuracy, and patient populations that benefit from each type of imaging modality. The initial manifestation of myocardial ischemia is decreased perfusion followed by documented shifts toward glucose as a more prominent substrate for metabolic activity, and then by diastolic and systolic dysfunction, electrocardiographic ST–T-wave

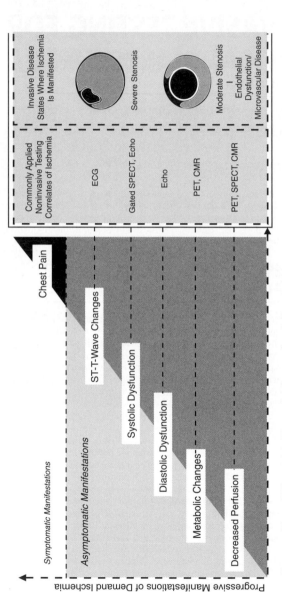

**FIGURE 4-1.** Progressive manifestations of myocardial ischemia as illustrated by the ischemic cascade.

ECG = Electrocardiogram, SPECT = Single Photon Emission Computed Tomography, PET = Positron Emission Tomography, Echo = Echocardiogram, CMR = Cardiovascular Magnetic Resonance Imaging changes, and finally the provocation of angina-like symptoms. Intermediate stenoses may provoke perfusion abnormalities. With more prolonged ischemia, regional wall-motion abnormalities and systolic dysfunction occur. ECG and symptomatic manifestations of myocardial ischemia occur later on in this cascade.

# BASICS OF PROBABILISTIC AND RISK-BASED DECISION MAKING

## ■ OPTIMAL CANDIDATE SELECTION FOR STRESS TESTING— UNDERSTANDING PRINCIPLES OF BAYESIAN THEORY

Effective referral to noninvasive stress testing requires integrating numerous parameters from a careful patient history. Upon presentation, the type, quality, and characteristics of a patient's symptoms are an important risk stratification tool. Angina with typical exertional components generally has a higher likelihood of obstructive coronary artery disease (CAD). A thorough integration of risk markers into a global risk score comprises risk factors, symptoms, past medical history, laboratory and physical examination parameters, as well as electrocardiographic results, and is a central component in decision making for noninvasive stress testing choice. **Table 4-1** provides a simple approach to risk estimation based on the patient's symptom presentation. Determining risk or a patient's pretest likelihood of CAD provides the basis for referral for a noninvasive stress test or for invasive coronary angiography. As illustrated in **Fig. 4-2**, only patients with an intermediate to high likelihood of CAD are candidates for stress testing. This is based on Bayesian theory by which CAD posttest likelihood is a function of the initial pretest risk assessment. Using this reasoning, the predictive accuracy of a test is related to disease prevalence. In low-risk populations, high rates of false positives can be expected, and the shift from pretest to posttest risk is minimal. Specifically, the overall likelihood of CAD remains relatively low in the setting of an abnormal exercise ECG, for example, for a low-risk patient. Thus, the ability to shift posttest likelihood is directly related to pretest likelihood of disease. In a low-risk population where the pretest probability of CAD is ≤ 20%, there is exceptional near-term event-free survival exceeding 99%. Thus, testing and the initiation of any intervention would yield trivial improvements in the outcome. The greatest shift in posttest likelihood of disease occurs in those patients with an intermediate pretest likelihood of CAD. Using our risk-based thresholds, this population has an annual cardiac death or myocardial infarction rate ranging from 1% to 3% and expected pretest probability ranging from about 20% to 80%. Theoretically, the major benefit of stress testing in this population is that a negative test will result in a reclassification to a low-risk subset and an abnormal test will result in a reclassification to a higher-risk cohort. High-risk patients, on the other hand, are often referred to stress testing for evaluation of ischemic burden as an aid to medical management decisions.

Additional key decision points in the workup of patients with stable chest pain symptoms are illustrated in **Fig. 4-2**; these include knowledge of the patient's functional capabilities, coronary anatomy, and resting ECG abnormalities. In addition to selecting symptomatic women and men with an intermediate to high likelihood of CAD, the second tier of decisions is an estimation of the patient's ability to perform activities of daily living. Patients who are capable of performing maximal exercise or ≥ 4 to 5 metabolic equivalents (METs; A MET is a metabolic equivalent and is equal to an oxygen consumption of 3.5 cc/kg/min.) should generally be referred to treadmill or bicycle exercise testing (**Table 4-2**). A patient incapable of performing ≥ 4 to 5 METs of work can undergo pharmacological stress imaging. In addition to the functionally impaired, patients with a prior CAD history or those with resting ST–T wave are often referred directly for an imaging stress test (most commonly stress echocardiography or single-photon emission computed tomography [SPECT]).

**TABLE 4-1.** Comparing Pretest Likelihood of CAD in Low- to High-Risk Symptomatic Patients—Results From the ACC Guidelines for Exercise Testing

| | Nonanginal Chest Pain | | Atypical/Probable Angina | | Typical/Definite Angina | |
|---|---|---|---|---|---|---|
| | Men | Women | Men | Women | Men | Women |
| < 40 y old | Low | Very low | Intermediate | Very low | Intermediate | Intermediate |
| 40-49 y old | Low | Very low | Intermediate | Low | High | Intermediate |
| 50-59 y old | Intermediate | Low | Intermediate | Intermediate | High | Intermediate |
| 60-69 y old[a] | Intermediate | Intermediate | Intermediate | Intermediate | High | High |

[a]Candidates who are ≤ 70 years of age are at intermediate to high likelihood of CAD.

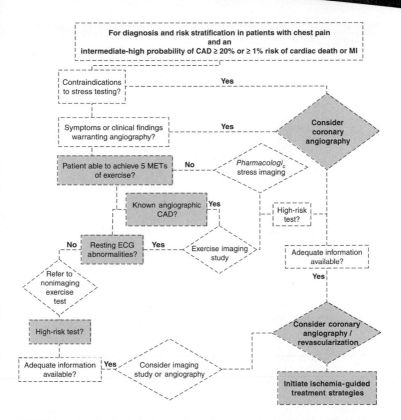

**FIGURE 4-2.** Choosing the appropriate candidates for stress testing—modification of the ACC/AHA Guidelines for the Evaluation of Stable Angina.

# ■ DIAGNOSTIC ACCURACY AND ISSUES OF VERIFICATION BIAS

Test accuracy has historically been defined by calculating diagnostic sensitivity and specificity. *Sensitivity* is the proportion of patients with an abnormal test that have obstructive CAD (or true positives/[true positives + false negatives]), while *specificity* is the proportion of patients who have a negative test and no obstructive CAD (or true negatives/[true negatives + false positives]). Tests where the sensitivity and specificity values exceed 80% are considered highly accurate. The diagnostic accuracy (uncorrected for workup bias) of exercise ECG, echocardiography, single-photon emission computed tomography (SPECT), and cardiac magnetic resonance (CMR) is detailed in **Table 4-3**. During our routine workup of patients, those with abnormal studies comprise the vast majority of referrals to coronary angiography, with few patients with negative stress test results proceeding to catheterization. The differential referral to coronary angiography for patients with negative and positive stress testing results in a workup or verification bias. Thus, measures such as diagnostic sensitivity and specificity in current clinical practice more often reflect how we are applying the test as a gatekeeper to angiography (where perfect gatekeeping would

**TABLE 4-2.** Estimated Energy Requirements for Various Activities Derived From the AHA Exercise Testing Guidelines and Duke Activity Status Index (DASI)

| | | | |
|---|---|---|---|
| 1 MET | Can you take care of yourself—for example, eat, dress, or use the toilet? | 4 METs | Climb a flight of stairs or walk up a hill? |
| | Walk indoors around the house? | | Walk on level ground at 4 mph? Run a short distance? |
| | Walk a block or two on level ground at 2-3 mph? | | Do heavy work around the house, such as scrubbing floors or lifting or moving heavy furniture? |
| | | | Participate in moderate recreational activities such as golf, bowling, dancing, doubles tennis, or throwing a baseball or football? |
| 4 METs | Do light work around the house like dusting or washing dishes? | 10 METs | Participate in strenuous sports such as swimming, singles tennis, football, basketball, or skiing? |

**TABLE 4-3.** Compilation of Meta-analyses and Reviews on the Diagnostic Accuracy of Contemporary Noninvasive Stress Testing Including Exercise ECG, SPECT, and Echocardiography as well as Pharmacological Stress SPECT, Echocardiography, and MRI[a]

| Modality | No. Studies | No. Patients | Sensitivity (%) | Specificity (%) |
|---|---|---|---|---|
| Exercise ECG | 58 | 11 691 | 67 | 72 |
| Exercise SPECT | | | | |
| Tc-99m agents only | 22 | 2360 | 87 | 73 |
| | | | 88 | 72 |
| Adenosine SPECT | | | | |
| Tc-99m agents only | 11 | 3539 | 89 | 77 |
| | | | 87 | 86 |
| Dobutamine SPECT | | | | |
| Tc-99m agents only | 20 | 1419 | 85 | 79 |
| | | | 83 | 76 |
| Exercise echocardiography | 13 | 741 | 83 | 84 |
| Dobutamine stress echocardiography | 13 | 436 | 75 | 83 |
| Stress magnetic resonance | | | | |
| Dobutamine stress wall motion | 10 | 644 | 84 | 89 |
| Adenosine/ dipyridamole perfusion | 3 | 108 | 84 | 85 |

[a]The diagnostic sensitivity and specificity values presented here are uncorrected for verification bias. (Note that these are average values and wide ranges exist for most modalities.)

result in an observed sensitivity of 100% and specificity of 0%). Methods are available for correcting verification bias.

## ■ WHY DO STRESS TESTING RESULTS WORK SO WELL TO ESTIMATE PROGNOSIS?

The rationale for using prognosis as a measure of test performance is that an accurate assessment of patient risk is a strong determinant of the intensity of patient management. Thus, estimating prognosis has become a new standard for evaluating test performance—an evidence-based approach that requires a *larger body of evidence* on the role of testing in patient management and therapeutic decision making. This latter notion expands beyond the idea of correlating stress testing results to a "gold standard" such as angiographic CAD extent and severity to include assessing coronary physiology, metabolism, and function that may provide added information for estimating clinical outcomes. That is, angiographic CAD extent is a major driver of prognosis, but additional measures such as regional and global ventricular function, and myocardial perfusion are supplemental components to a risk assessment, as well as major drivers in ischemia-guided medical management.

Simplistically stated, the estimation of prognosis is commonly defined as risk stratification, where the overall event rate is calculated for patients with normal (ie, low risk) to severely abnormal (ie, high risk) stress testing results. These event rates may be compared to the larger body of evidence from population studies or observational registries on CAD. Low-risk and high-risk event rate thresholds have been defined using these larger datasets; for example, an annual risk of cardiac death or nonfatal myocardial infarction of ≥ 2% is equivalent to the annual risk of those with established cardiovascular disease or diabetes. These thresholds may then be applied to the review of outcome results for stress testing data (**Fig. 4-3**). Those with suspected CAD have an annual rate of death or myocardial infarction < 2% per year; with established CAD, of about 2% per year; and with severe or high-risk CAD, in the range of 3% to 5% or more.

# SYNOPSIS OF AVAILABLE EVIDENCE ON STRESS TESTING FOR MYOCARDIAL ISCHEMIA

## ■ PREDICTIVE ACCURACY OF EXERCISE ECG—OPTIMIZING EXERCISE TREADMILL DATA

Candidates for a routine exercise treadmill test include patients with suspected CAD, an interpretable 12-lead ECG, and normal physical work capacity. According to the recent stable angina guidelines, those patients with established CAD, functional disability, or resting ST–T-wave changes (that preclude interpretation of peak exertional changes) are appropriate candidates for cardiac imaging testing, including stress echocardiography, SPECT, and increasingly, magnetic resonance (MR) imaging. Of the current indications for a nonimaging stress test, the most challenging decision is discerning whether a patient is capable of maximal exercise. A guide to this decision-making process is whether or not a patient is capable of performing ≥ 4 to 5 METs, equivalent to routine activities of daily living (**Table 4-2**). A test should be considered adequate if ≥ 85% predicted maximal heart rate and ≥ 5 METs of exercise have been achieved. An accelerated heart rate response at low levels of exercise can lead to premature fatigue; consideration should then be given to repeat testing using pharmacological stress imaging.

An impaired heart rate or blunted blood pressure response to exercise is associated with an increased risk of events. An impaired chronotropic response to exercise

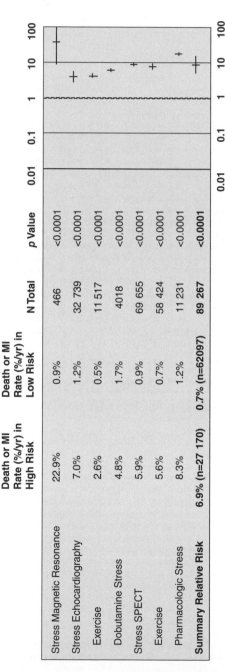

|  | Death or MI Rate (%/yr) in High Risk | Death or MI Rate (%/yr) in Low Risk | N Total | p Value |
|---|---|---|---|---|
| Stress Magnetic Resonance | 22.9% | 0.9% | 466 | <0.0001 |
| Stress Echocardiography | 7.0% | 1.2% | 32 739 | <0.0001 |
| Exercise | 2.6% | 0.5% | 11 517 | <0.0001 |
| Dobutamine Stress | 4.8% | 1.7% | 4018 | <0.0001 |
| Stress SPECT | 5.9% | 0.9% | 69 655 | <0.0001 |
| Exercise | 5.6% | 0.7% | 58 424 | <0.0001 |
| Pharmacologic Stress | 8.3% | 1.2% | 11 231 | <0.0001 |
| **Summary Relative Risk** | **6.9% (n=27 170)** | **0.7% (n=62097)** | **89 267** | **<0.0001** |

**Source:** CMR data is for dobutamine stress wall motion derived from SCMR and ESC Consensus Panel report (9) and related publications. Echocardiographic data is ACC/AHA guidlines for Stable angina (5) and related publications (88-97), SPECT data is ACC/AHA guidlines for SPECT imaging (5) and a recent metanalysis (30).

**FIGURE 4-3.** Forest plot illustrating results of a meta-analysis on the prognostic value of stress echocardiography, SPECT, and CMR. This figure examines the annual cardiac death or myocardial infarction rate in patients with low- and high-risk studies and a calculation of the relative risk (95% confidence interval) of high-risk ischemia by CMR or echocardiographic wall motion and SPECT perfusion imaging. The largest body of evidence is for stress SPECT imaging, where overall event rates are higher for patients with known CVD or diabetes and for those referred to pharmacological stress imaging. The results for stress echocardiography have been published in several smaller series, but recently the Echo Persantine International Cooperative (EPIC) study and the American Society of Echocardiography (ASE) outcome registries have been published on its prognostic value in 7333 and 11 132 patients. Overall event rates in these larger series vary by type of stress, where annual event rates are 0.3% to 1% for low- to high-risk exercising patients and about 3% to 12% for low- to high-risk patients undergoing pharmacological stress echocardiography. The preliminary evidence from 3 reports on dobutamine stress MR wall motion is promising but will require additional validation in larger series for a more definitive comparative analysis.

should be considered when peak heart rates are < 110 to 120 bpm (beats per minute), and is often related to impaired myocardial contractility and left ventricular dysfunction. Similarly, hemodynamic impairment, defined as a blunted rise or drop in systolic blood pressure (eg, ≤ 5 mm Hg), is also associated with a greater frequency of multivessel CAD and a depressed ejection fraction.

During stress, ECG changes with exercise should be documented, including the time of onset and offset, as well as the extent and severity of ST-segment depression. A test is considered positive when there is ≥ 1 mm of horizontal or downsloping ST-segment depression at 60 milliseconds post-J point, but a threshold of ≥1.5 mm is applied for upsloping ST-segment depression. Anti-ischemic drugs (eg, β-blockers or nitrates) should be discontinued prior to testing if the purpose of the test is to establish the diagnosis of ischemic heart disease, as they interfere with the provocation of ischemia. High-risk patients are those who present with ST-segment changes at a low workload (ie, < 5 METs), exhibit ≥ 2 mm ST-segment depression, and for whom the time to resolution of ≥ 1 mm ST-segment depression is ≥ 5 minutes into recovery. A change of ≥ 1 mm of ST-segment deviation may be applied to patients with resting ST–T-wave abnormalities. ST-segment elevation is a rare (occurring in about 1 in 10 000 patients tested), but serious occurrence during exercise testing, reflecting transmural ischemia, and consideration should be given to immediate angiography. ST-segment elevation in a Q-wave lead, however, is a marker for a preexisting wall-motion abnormality.

Care should be taken when interpreting the exercise ECG, as there are many factors that confound its interpretation, including medications (ie, anti-ischemics and other vasoactive drugs), hormonal status, resting ST–T-wave changes, prior myocardial infarction, and, importantly, functional capacity. Evidence supports the fact that there are certain patient subsets where the exercise ECG is of diminished value. False-positive results can be due to lower QRS voltage, ECG abnormalities (such as left ventricular hypertrophy, left bundle-branch block, or Wolff–Parkinson–White syndrome), and drug effects (eg, digoxin); these patients should be referred to cardiac imaging. The highest relative proportion of false-positive test results is in premenopausal female patients; however, marked ST abnormalities are associated with an improved predictive accuracy. False-negative results are commonly the result of a submaximal stress test and occur commonly in patients with limited functional capacity.

Use of ΔST/Δ heart rate indices (abnormality is defined as ≥ 1.6 mV/bpm), available on most commercial equipment, improves the sensitivity and specificity of imaging, in particular for women. Additionally, the Duke Treadmill Score (exercise time – [5 × ST deviation] – [4 × chest pain index (0 = none, 1 = nonlimiting, 2 = limiting)]) is readily calculable, and has been shown to estimate a 5-year survival and the presence and extent of significant CAD in men and women alike. Using this score, low-risk (> +5), intermediate-risk (–10 to +5), and high-risk (< –11) patients have 5-year mortality ranges from 3% to 10% for women and 9% to 30% for men.

Electrical instability, defined as a ≥ 3-beat run of ventricular tachycardia or ventricular fibrillation, is also a high-risk marker. The occurrence of premature ventricular contractions with exercise or in recovery has been studied frequently and is associated with an increased risk of coronary disease or cardiac events. Other ischemic markers, such as exertional chest pain symptoms, especially when they mimic the patient's historical symptoms, increase diagnostic certainty, particularly when concurrent with ECG changes, but are of limited value in women.

Of all the risk markers available to the physician, 2 factors are of high priority: heart rate profile during exercise and recovery, and maximal exercise capacity. A patient's physical work capability, commonly measured in METs, is a potent predictor of survival. For example, patients with impaired physical work capacity who cannot achieve > 5 METs of exercise, are at increased risk of death. Additionally, a large body of evidence is available supporting the substantial prognostic value of baseline heart rate, heart rate response during exercise, and the fall in heart rate following peak exercise (ie, heart rate recovery). Because heart rate responses to

**TABLE 4-4.** Low- to High-Risk Noninvasive Stress Testing Markers From the ACC/AHA Stable Angina Guidelines

High risk ( > 3% annual mortality rate or > 5% annual cardiac death, or nonfatal myocardial infarction rate)
1. Severe resting left ventricular dysfunction (LVEF < 35%).
2. High-risk Duke Treadmill Score (score ≤ –11).
3. Severe exercise left ventricular dysfunction (exercise LVEF < 35%).
4. Stress-induced large perfusion defect (particularly, if anterior).
5. Stress-induced multiple perfusion defects of moderate size.
6. Large, fixed perfusion defect with LV dilation or increased lung uptake (thallium-201 only).
7. Stress-induced moderate perfusion defect with LV dilation or increased lung uptake (thallium-201 only).
8. Echocardiographic wall-motion abnormality (involving > 2 segments) developing at low dose of dobutamine (≤ 10 mg/kg/min) or low heart rate (< 120 bpm).
9. Stress echocardiographic evidence of extensive ischemia.

Intermediate risk (1%-3% annual mortality rate or 3%-5% annual death, or myocardial infarction rate)
1. Mild/moderate resting left ventricular dysfunction (LVEF = 35%-49%).
2. Intermediate risk Duke Treadmill Score (–11 < score < 5).
3. Stress-induced moderate perfusion defect without LV dilation or increased lung uptake (thallium-201).
4. Limited stress echocardiographic ischemia with a wall-motion abnormality involving ≤ 2 segments, only at higher doses of dobutamine.

Low risk ( < 1% annual mortality rate or < 1% annual death, or myocardial infarction rate)
1. Low-risk Duke Treadmill Score (score ≥ 5).
2. Normal or small myocardial perfusion defect at rest or with stress.[a]
3. Normal stress echocardiographic wall motion or no change of limited resting wall-motion abnormalities during stress.[a]

[a]Although the published data are limited, patients with these findings should be considered at higher risk in the presence of a high-risk Duke Treadmill Score, left ventricular dysfunction, known coronary artery disease (or its risk equivalent, such as diabetes or peripheral arterial disease), or severe resting LVEF < 35%.

exercise are controlled by the autonomic nervous system, abnormalities in these parameters reflect abnormal autonomic balance and portend decreased survival due to cardiovascular disease. The risk of sudden death from myocardial infarction is increased in subjects with a resting heart rate above 75 beats per minute; in subjects with an increase in heart rate of less than 89 beats per minute during exercise; and in subjects with a decrease in heart rate of less than 25 beats per minute after the termination of exercise.

A thorough interpretation of the exercise stress test (with or without imaging) should include an evaluation of functional capacity, ECG responses to stress, ventricular ectopy, and heart rate recovery, as well as hemodynamic and chronotropic responses to stress. A synopsis of high-risk exercise test parameters is given in **Table 4-4**.

# ■ DECISIONS REGARDING USE OF EXERCISE VERSUS PHARMACOLOGICAL STRESS IMAGING

An important decision for the referring clinician and supervising physician in the exercise testing laboratory is whether the patient is capable of performing maximal stress. A careful history and inquiry into the performance of activities of daily living (eg, using the Duke Activity Status Index) can provide insight into a patient's MET capacity. Patients capable of most common household activities, generally, meet this criterion and may be able to perform a graded treadmill or bicycle exercise test. However, those with activity limitations and who are incapable of 5 METs of exercise should be referred to a pharmacological stress test.

A major reason for preferring exercise is to gain insight into the actual capabilities of the patient as well as the co-occurrence and timing of inducible ischemia. For a growing segment of the population, including obese or diabetic patients, choosing the correct exercise protocol is paramount to elicit a maximal myocardial stress. Although the standard Bruce protocol is commonly employed, the first stage in the protocol begins at 4.7 METs (ie, 1.7 mph/10% grade) and is challenging for numerous subsets of the population. A modified Bruce protocol begins at about 3 METs (1.7 mph/0% or 5% grade) and may be helpful when employed in modestly impaired patients. Not only is the Bruce protocol initially demanding, but each successive 3-minute stage increases metabolic demands by about 2 to 3 METs. Other protocols with less aggressive physical work demands include the Naughton and Balke protocol. Linear protocols, which increase exercise demands by about 1 MET/stage with shorter exercise stages (about a minute), are commonly employed in heart failure populations, but may also be of value to other patients. Many laboratories favor the use of the Bruce protocol for purposes of standardization.

For functionally impaired patients, vasodilator or inotropic pharmacological stress testing with imaging is recommended. For SPECT imaging, vasodilator stress testing includes a short infusion of intravenous adenosine, dipyridamole, and regadenoson (an $A_{2a}$-specific adenosine receptor agonist). Because of the vasodilatory actions of these drugs, heart rate increases by around 10 to 25 beats per minute and systolic blood pressure measurements drop modestly. Side effects are common but mostly mild and transient due to the short half-life of the agents. With dipyridamole, in the event of any severe side effects, aminophylline is given to reverse the effects. Because of the short half-life of adenosine, aminophylline is seldom employed. Although side effects are more common with adenosine and regadenoson, they rapidly diminish following drug infusion (generally 30-45 seconds). Chest discomfort during dipyridamole or adenosine infusion is considered nondiagnostic, as it can be a side effect of the drug unrelated to ischemia.

In patients able to walk, low-level exercise can be combined with pharmacological stress, and has become the preferred approach to vasodilator stress because it reduces drug side effects and improves image quality due to decreased hepatic uptake of radioactivity following stress injection.

All the agents act by inducing arteriolar dilation. They also induce hyperemia or an increase in blood flow within the normal vasculature. In the presence of a hemodynamically significant stenosis, coronary steal—a shifting of blood toward areas of normal arterial dilation from arteries with impaired flow reserve—will result in inducible ischemia and a heterogeneity of coronary blood flow. Additionally, there is a modest increase in myocardial oxygen demand from reflex tachycardia. Both adenosine and dipyridamole precipitate bronchoconstriction, and should be avoided in patients with severe lung disease. Patients with severe obstructive lung disease should be referred for dobutamine SPECT or echocardiographic imaging. There is a growing body of evidence as to the accuracy of using this pharmacological stress agent in varying patient populations. However, regadenoson is specific for the adenosine $A_{2a}$ receptor and consequently associated with lower rates of side effects, including bronchoconstriction, and may be helpful in lung disease patients.

Dobutamine is employed as an inotropic stress agent for echocardiographic imaging. Graded infusions of dobutamine elicit incremental increases in heart rate and myocardial contractility. The goal of dobutamine stress is to achieve a maximal heart rate response (ie, ≥ 85% predicted maximal heart rate [220 – patient age]). Atropine may be given in order to augment heart rate and contractility responses during the latter stages of an infusion protocol. Ventricular arrhythmias (ie, frequent premature ventricular contractions) are common during dobutamine infusion but rarely require treatment. The frequency of serious side effects (3/1000) is somewhat greater than in other groups that undergo coronary vasodilator stress.

# STATE-OF-THE-ART CARDIAC IMAGING

## ■ STRESS ECHOCARDIOGRAPHY

### Basics of Interpretation

Stress echocardiography is based on the premise that the contractile response of ischemic segments is less than normal segments. This has important implications that limit sensitivity (the myocardium must be sufficiently underperfused to be dysfunctional), but optimize specificity (few conditions other than ischemia cause stress-induced wall-motion abnormalities). Echocardiographic imaging is performed in conjunction with exercise or pharmacological stress, most commonly in the United States, with incremental dosing of dobutamine. Multiple views are obtained at rest and immediately poststress. Traditional views include the long axis, short axis, and 2- and 4-chamber views (**Fig. 4-4**). For ease of comparing and evaluating changes in regional wall motion, rest and stress images are viewed in a side-by-side continuous loop format. A normal stress echocardiogram results in a decrease in left ventricular cavity size, and in regional myocardial segments becoming hyperdynamic as a response to stress. Thus, a normal stress echocardiogram would include normal resting ventricular function without wall-motion abnormalities associated with a hyperkinetic peak/poststress regional contractile response.

Reduction in either the amplitude or speed of thickening denotes an abnormal echocardiographic contractile response. That is, for patients without a prior CAD diagnosis, an ischemic test is defined as a new or worsening wall-motion abnormality or delayed contraction. Contractile responses are characterized by regional wall motion. This function is generally classified as normal, hypokinetic, akinetic, or dyskinetic. Most laboratories also employ some qualitative or semi-quantitative estimate of global left ventricular function (ie, normal, mildly depressed, moderately depressed, or severely depressed). Although abnormal regional function is often described as "wall-motion abnormality," wall thickening is a more reliable parameter, because wall motion is subject to translational movement. A segment is considered abnormal if a wall-motion abnormality is viewed in more than 1 echocardiogram view, apart from the basal inferior and septal segments, which are frequent sites of false-positive interpretations, and should therefore be identified as abnormal only in the presence of an abnormality in an adjacent segment.

Resting regional wall-motion abnormalities indicate a prior myocardial infarction—these findings are relatively specific if the segment is thinned and akinetic; hypokinesis is less specific. For example, cardiomyopathies commonly demonstrate regional hypokinesis in the absence of infarcted myocardial segments. In the setting of resting wall-motion abnormalities, discerning stress-induced changes becomes more difficult. In segments with resting wall-motion abnormalities, ischemia is defined as (1) a deterioration from hypokinesis to akinesis or dyskinesis, or (2) a biphasic response (ie, increased contractility at low dobutamine doses followed by a worsening of the contractile function). The biphasic response is suggestive of viability of a myocardial territory that is hypokinetic at baseline. When there is concomitant left ventricular dilation during stress, multivessel or left main coronary disease is probable.

Based on the extent and severity of inducible wall-motion abnormalities, the clinician can estimate the site and extent of obstructive CAD. A 17-segment myocardial

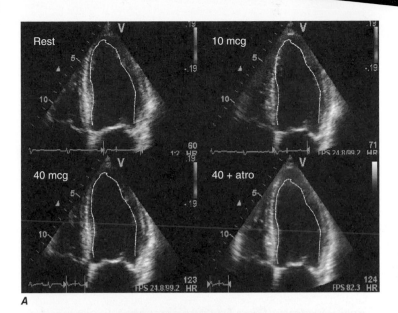

*A*

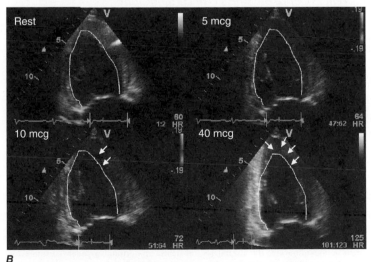

*B*

**FIGURE 4-4.** Appearance of a normal (**A**) and abnormal (**B**) response to dobutamine echocardiography. The display demonstrates end-systolic freeze frames at rest (*upper left*), low dose (*upper right*), prepeak (*lower left*), and peak stress (*lower right*). The resting end-systolic contour has been superimposed on subsequent images, showing no change in systolic cavity size in the normal study, but showing reduction in apical and anterior wall thickening (and hence shape change) in the abnormal study.

model has been used to quantify the extent (number of vascular territories or segments with abnormalities) and severity (ranking of wall-motion abnormalities from normal, hypokinetic, akinetic, to dyskinetic) of ischemia, similar to nuclear imaging. These scores may be integrated with clinical and stress data to produce a composite score analogous to the Duke Treadmill Score.

## Intravenous Contrast Enhancement

A number of intravenous contrast agents are commercially available and approved for left ventricular opacification and endocardial border delineation in patients with initial suboptimal acoustic window, for example, those with lung disease or obesity. These contrast agents are encapsulated gas-filled microbubbles that are generally administered as a constant infusion. For the less experienced echocardiographers and sonographers, contrast enhancement may allow for a more prompt visualization of regional function in poststress evaluation. In patients with limited image quality, contrast enhancement has been shown to improve differentiation of low-risk and high-risk patient subsets.

Another application for contrast agents, currently under development, is the evaluation of myocardial perfusion. To evaluate myocardial perfusion, microbubbles are applied as intravascular tracers for imaging microcirculation. Myocardial contrast perfusion may provide new information such as the detection of subendocardial ischemia.

## Current Evidence on Stress Echocardiography

**Diagnostic Accuracy** Echocardiographic visualization of left ventricular performance during stress results in dramatic improvements in diagnostic accuracy when compared with the evaluation of ST-segment changes alone. The diagnostic sensitivity and specificity for exercise echocardiography are 83% and 84%, respectively, a rate that is approximately 10% to 20% greater than that for the ECG alone (see **Table 4-3**). In a recent head-to-head comparison, the improved diagnostic characteristics of stress echocardiography resulted in incremental cost-effectiveness when compared with exercise treadmill testing alone.

**Risk Stratification** The "general tenet" of risk stratification derived from patients with stable chest pain is that low risk is defined by an annual risk of myocardial infarction or cardiac death of < 1%, intermediate risk is 1% to 5%, and high risk is > 5%. Similar to risk stratification with SPECT imaging, stress echocardiography has there is prognostic value. Using large prognostic series, a summary of relative risk ratios for stress echocardiography has been plotted in **Fig. 4-3**. This summary includes data obtained from 32 739 patients who underwent stress echocardiography—figures taken from several large outcome data registries, including the Echo Persantine International Cooperative (EPIC) and the American Society of Echocardiography (ASE). The annual risk of death or myocardial infarction was 0.5% for patients with a negative exercise echocardiogram. In women with a normal stress echocardiogram, the annual risk of death or nonfatal myocardial infarction was 0.5% ($n = 5971$), and increased to 5.8% ($n = 1425$) for those with a moderate to severely abnormal study.

Similar to SPECT imaging, patients undergoing pharmacological stress echocardiography have a greater comorbidity and cardiovascular disease burden, which is associated with a higher rate of events, even in the setting of a normal dobutamine stress study. However, effective risk stratification is still possible in these generally higher-risk patients. That is, the event rate of a low-risk study is approximately 1.5%, which is decidedly lower than average risk in this population (~2%-3%), and dramatically lower than the 5% annual risk of events in those with high-risk echocardiography results.

## Candidates for Cardiac Catheterization

For diagnostic patient subsets, in the setting of an inducible wall-motion abnormality, anti-ischemic therapies and risk-factor modification would be initiated. Consideration would also be given to coronary angiography. Of course, referral to coronary angiography is dependent on the symptom status, treatment response, comorbidities, and risk—the latter being determined in part by the extent and severity of the inducible wall-motion abnormalities. Clinicians may prefer to treat patients with discrete small areas of ischemia medically. They may not refer patients who are not good revascularization candidates (eg, very elderly patients with serious comorbidity). Angiography is advised in patients with evidence of high risk (see **Table 4-4**), including those with global left ventricular dysfunction with stress or multiple vascular territories (ie, evidence of multivessel disease), or extensive wall-motion abnormalities across the anterior myocardium (reflecting proximal left anterior descending [LAD] disease). Abnormalities in the left anterior descending coronary artery distribution had a higher event rate than abnormalities elsewhere (3.2% vs 2.1% at 3 years and 10.8% vs 2.1% at 5 years; $p = 0.009$); this risk is independent of the resting ejection fraction and the extent of wall-motion abnormalities during exercise.

Stress echocardiography, when compared to exercise ECG testing, can result in cost-effective testing as a result of improved detection of CAD. In a study of exercise echocardiography cost-effectiveness involving 7656 patients, echocardiographic imaging identified more patients as low (51% vs 24%; $p < 0.0001$) and high (22% vs 4%; $p < 0.0001$) risk when compared to exercise ECG. Although initial procedural cost was higher, echocardiography was associated with a greater incremental life expectancy (0.2 years) and a lower use of additional diagnostic procedures when compared with exercise ECG. Echocardiography was more cost-effective than exercise ECG testing at $2615 per life-year saved (eg, dialysis is associated with $50 000 per life-year saved).

## ■ STRESS-GATED NUCLEAR (SPECT/PET) IMAGING

Today, state-of-the-art multidetector single-photon emission computed tomography (SPECT) systems can acquire rest and stress ejection fractions, and regional wall motion, as well as assess regional myocardial perfusion. In contrast to 2-dimensional echocardiography, SPECT and positron emission tomography (PET) provide true tomographic imaging, where all segments of the myocardium are visualized. More than 7 million patients undergo nuclear stress testing per year in the United States, with annual growth rates exceeding 20%.

### Basics of Interpretation

Generally, a 17- or 20-segment myocardial model is used to describe regional perfusion. It utilizes visual estimates of segmental perfusion defect severity (normal to absent perfusion on a 5-point scale; **Fig. 4-5**). For rest and stress images, individual myocardial segment severity scores are summed to give a global perfusion score. This semiquantitative method has been extensively evaluated and correlates well with prognosis. A percentage of fixed or reversible myocardium can also be reported by normalizing the score to the highest possible value, which is clinically intuitive. Gated SPECT imaging also provides quantitative rest and postexercise left ventricular ejection fractions, segmental wall-motion assessment, and left-ventricular volumes, which all add further prognostic information. Transient ischemic dilation (TID) of the left ventricle and increased lung uptake of the tracer can also be reported. They are markers of significant ischemic heart disease and increased pulmonary capillary wedge pressure, respectively.

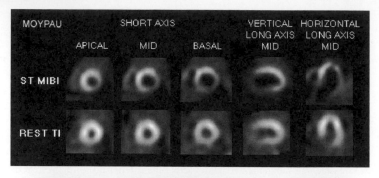

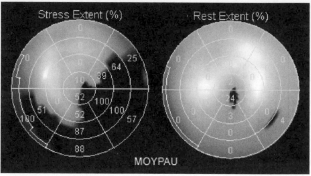

**FIGURE 4-5.** An example of myocardial perfusion SPECT (54-year-old man, asymptomatic, 9 minutes of exercise, ischemic ECG, reversible defect, TID 1.52, cath: LM 70%, LAD 80% prox, LCX 100% prox, RCA 100% mid).

## Current Evidence on Gated SPECT Imaging

**Diagnostic Accuracy** Table 4-3 summarizes the superiority of SPECT imaging to exercise ECG alone. For exercise SPECT, the sensitivity and specificity were 87% and 73%, respectively and similar for both Tl-201 and Tc-99m. For adenosine SPECT, the diagnostic sensitivity was 89% and the specificity was 77%.

The principal factor affecting the specificity of myocardial perfusion SPECT is soft-tissue attenuation (ie, breast tissue artifacts in women and diaphragmatic attenuation in men) but occurs less commonly with Tc-99m agents. It is also important to note that physiologically and prognostically important decreases in perfusion may occur with less severe stenoses than 50% to 75%, which are the traditional values used for hemodynamic significance. Therefore, "false positives" may in fact be clinically relevant. Specificity per se, as a measure of diagnostic test performance, fails to incorporate the prognostic value of a perfusion defect. For this and other reasons noted previously (eg, workup bias), accuracy in estimating risk is as important in guiding management as diagnostic accuracy.

**Risk Stratification** Similar to stress echocardiography, SPECT imaging is an excellent prognostic tool. In a meta-analysis of 19 reports in 39 173 patients, those with a normal or low-risk (eg, summed stress score < 4) myocardial perfusion study had an annual cardiac event rate of 0.6%. In a multicenter registry of 10 408 patients, cardiac death rates were similar for a normal Tl-201 and Tc-99 sestamibi or tetrofosmin SPECT. In patients with normal perfusion findings, measures of left ventricular size, function, and dilation following stress can provide additional prognostic information. For example, TID with exercise or pharmacological stress is associated with an increased risk of cardiac events, even in the setting of a normal perfusion scan.

The excellent survival rates in patients with normal stress SPECT findings reveals the value of evaluating the physiology of the patient's disease as supplemental information. However, there are higher-risk subsets such as the elderly, diabetics, and those with vascular disease, who would be expected to have major adverse cardiac event rates (eg, 1.5%-2% per year) with normal scans. Because of this higher risk, patients with CAD or its risk equivalent (eg, diabetics or those referred for pharmacological stress imaging) may be considered for closer surveillance with reimaging sooner (about 1.5 years) than in lower-risk patients with normal stress scans. With any of the stress modalities, a normal stress study implies a low risk over a relatively short term (1-2 years) but does not imply the absence of risk for CAD progression over a longer time.

An abnormal study is determined by the presence of perfusion defects, either fixed or reversible. Using summed stress scores (from the 17-segment models), higher-risk subsets may be defined as mildly abnormal (4-8), moderately abnormal (9-13), or severely abnormal (> 13). When considered as a percentage of the myocardium, patients with minimal perfusion defects but < 5% of the myocardium involved are generally considered normal and those with 5% to 9% as having a mild perfusion abnormality. A cutoff of ≥ 10% of the myocardium ischemic improves the likelihood of benefit from revascularization since there is a greater prevalence of more extensive CAD or proximal LAD disease. In addition to the application of semiquantitative scores, a high-risk study may be defined as patients with (1) severe exercise left ventricular dysfunction (exercise LVEF < 35%), (2) stress-induced large perfusion defect (particularly if anterior), (3) stress-induced multiple perfusion defects of moderate size, (4) large, fixed perfusion defect with LV dilation or increased lung uptake, or (5) stress-induced moderate perfusion defect with LV dilation or increased lung uptake (see **Table 4-4**).

The annual rate of cardiac death or nonfatal myocardial infarction for those with high-risk perfusion findings is 5.9% and consistent with studies of angiographically severe CAD whose annualized event rates are approximately 5% per year. Those with high-risk SPECT results, diabetic patients, and those referred to pharmacological stress will have higher event rates than other cohorts.

Serial changes in stress SPECT also has prognostic value in patients with known CAD and may reflect disease progression. In the Clinical Outcomes Using Revascularization and Aggressive Drug Evaluation (COURAGE) trial, a failure to reduce ischemia by at least 5% of the myocardium or residual ischemia following 1 year of treatment is associated with a high rate of death or nonfatal myocardial infarction.

There is an inverse relationship between left ventricular ejection fraction and cardiac event rates. There is a "threshold" of risk for any given degree of perfusion defect abnormality when there is a concomitant decrease in ejection fraction ≤ 45%. Increases in ventricular volumes indicate remodeling and are also associated with increased cardiovascular risk. For example, end-systolic volume measurements > 70 mL have been associated with worsening event-free survival.

## Candidates for Cardiac Catheterization

Coronary angiography should be considered in the setting of high risk SPECT findings which include

1. Moderate to severely abnormal perfusion abnormalities
2. Multivessel perfusion abnormalities

3. ≥ 10% myocardial perfusion defect

4. Summed stress score >8 [for the 20-segment model

5. Poststress left ventricular ejection fraction < 45%

6. Transient ischemic dilation

7. Larger ventricular volumes

8. Increased lung uptake

For patients with known angiographic CAD, referral to coronary angiography should also be considered when there is persistent or worsening myocardial perfusion SPECT ischemia despite intensive medical management or prior coronary intervention. Patients with mild defects have good outcomes and may be effectively managed medically.

With either stress myocardial perfusion SPECT or echocardiography, the decision to proceed with coronary angiography is complex and should integrate clinical observations with imaging data. Factors associated with increased risk for any degree of scan abnormality include a brief duration of exercise, a high Duke Treadmill Score, an abnormal heart rate recovery, an abnormal peak/rest heart rate with adenosine stress, comorbidity (eg, diabetes), symptoms such as chest pain or shortness of breath, and exertional hypotension. Prognostic score systems that integrate the clinical stress test findings and imaging information are available. Selective use of coronary angiography based on the extent and severity of SPECT abnormalities is cost-effective and may lower costs as much as 35%.

# ■ PET STRESS MYOCARDIAL PERFUSION

Cardiac PET imaging is a growing and well-validated technique to assess myocardial perfusion, LV function, and viability. In addition to fluorine-18 fluorodeoxyglucose (FDG) viability studies, PET stress myocardial perfusion imaging with rubidium-82 can now be performed with a commercially available Rb-82 generator, obviating the need for a cyclotron. PET stress myocardial perfusion imaging utilizes radionuclide tracers (Rb-82 and a to lesser extent, N-13 ammonia) which decay with the emission of a positron. The positron interacts with an electron to combine mass that is converted into the energy of photons and detectable by a PET camera. The new generation of high-performance dedicated PET cameras features high instrument sensitivity (10-20 times greater than SPECT), high resolution (4-5 vs 20-25 mm for SPECT), high speed, and larger fields of view. These technical advantages give PET stress imaging better diagnostic accuracy than traditional SPECT imaging. PET stress myocardial perfusion can also assess regional myocardial blood flow, thus extending the scope of conventional scintigraphic imaging by providing subtler details of transmural myocardial perfusion.

# ■ CURRENT EVIDENCE ON CARDIOVASCULAR MAGNETIC RESONANCE IMAGING

The improvement in CMR technology has led to dramatic high spatial and temporal resolution of both static and dynamic imaging. Currently, 1.5 Tesla CMR scanners applying rapid-gradient systems enable acquisition of cine imaging of the heart at rest and under stress, allowing comparison of global as well as segmental heart function. Furthermore, assessment of a contrast agent (usually gadolinium) injected at rest and stress can provide high-quality information about the pattern of myocardial perfusion.

Because exercise is not a practical option in the scanner bore, and patient movement may severely affect image quality, pharmacological stress agents (such as adenosine) have been used mainly to elicit stress. Dobutamine is rarely used due to its unfavorable side effects profile, especially in the limited monitoring surrounding of the MR scanner.

Stress perfusion CMR studies have the capability to provide comprehensive and complementary information, that is, rest and stress cardiac function, and wall motion as well as myocardial perfusion using nonionizing radiation technology that has better resolution and is attenuation freeing in comparison to SPECT. Delayed enhancement images may give additional information about the presence, extent, and pattern of myocardial fibrosis The diagnostic performance for stress perfusion CMR in comparison with coronary angiography and SPECT is excellent and equivalent if not better than SPECT.

However, stress perfusion CMR is costly, a time-consuming study, highly dependent on operator and patient cooperation, and requires an experienced technical team with cutting-edge hardware. Also, because exercise stress is not an option, information about functional capacity and electrocardiographic and physiological response to exercise is virtually always unavailable.

## SUGGESTED READINGS

Lipinski MJ, Froelicher VF. ECG exercise teating. In: Fuster V, Walsh RA, Harrington RA, et al, eds. *Hurst's The Heart.* 13th ed. New York, NY: McGraw-Hill. 2011;16:371-387.

Berman DS, Hayes SW, Hachamovitch R, Shaw LJ, Germano G. Nuclear cardiology. In: Fuster V, Walsh RA, Harrington RA, et al, eds. *Hurst's The Heart.* 13th ed. New York, NY: McGraw-Hill. 2011;21:562-598.

ACCF/ASNC/ACR/AHA/ASE/SCCT/SCMR/SNM 2009 appropriate use criteria for cardiac radionuclide imaging. *Circulation.* 2009;119;e561-e587.

Gibbons RJ, Balady, GJ, Bricker JT, et al. ACC/AHA 2002 guideline update for exercise testing—summary article. *J Am Coll Cardiol.* 2002;106:1883-1892.

Jouven. Heart-rate profile during exercise as a predictor of sudden death. *N Engl J Med.* 2005;352:1951-1958.

Mieres JH, Shaw LJ, Arai A, et al. Diagnostic performance of stress cardiac magnetic resonance imaging in the detection of coronary artery disease: a meta-analysis. *J Am Coll Cardiol.* 2007;50:1343-1353.

Noninvasive coronary artery imaging: a scientific statement from the AHA. *Circulation.* 2008;118:586-606.

Pennell DJ, Sechtem UP, Higgins CB, et al. Clinical indications for cardiovascular magnetic resonance: consensus panel report. *J Cardiovasc Mag Res.* 2004;6:727-765.

Redberg RF, Taubert K, Thomas G, et al. American Heart Association, Cardiac Imaging Committee consensus statement: the role of cardiac imaging in the clinical evaluation of women with known or suspected coronary artery disease. *Circulation.* 2005;111:682-696.

Shaw LJ, Berman DS, Maron DJ, et al. Prognostic value of gated myocardial perfusion SPECT. *J Nucl Cardiol.* 2004;11:171-185.

# CHAPTER 5
# NONINVASIVE TESTING FOR CARDIAC DYSFUNCTION

Anthony N. DeMaria, Daniel G. Blanchard, Daniel S. Berman, Sean W. Hayes, Rory Hachamovitch, Leslee J. Shaw, and Guido Germano

Accurate, noninvasive assessment of global and regional left ventricular (LV) function is critical in managing most types of heart disease. The most common clinically useful parameter is the left ventricular ejection fraction (LVEF), which is the LV stroke volume normalized by LV end-diastolic volume. EF is most often *estimated* echocardiographically, but radionuclide angiography (RNA), computed tomography (CT), single-photon emission computed tomography (SPECT), positron emission tomography (PET), and cardiac magnetic resonance imaging (CMR) may be employed. Whereas EF measures ventricular chamber properties, tissue velocity and strain—characterized most notably by echocardiography and CMR—measure myocardial contractility. LV diastolic function is also a clinically relevant parameter of function, which encompasses various measures of diastolic filling, myocardial relaxation, and ventricular stiffness, which are assessed by echocardiography, RNA, and CMR. In addition, various CT techniques (electron beam CT, multidetector CT) allow noninvasive coronary atherosclerosis risk stratification, complementary to the traditional methods of echocardiographic and nuclear stress testing. This chapter discusses the various imaging modalities available for noninvasive assessment of cardiac function.

## ECHOCARDIOGRAPHY

Echocardiography remains the most popular cardiac imaging modality because of its efficacy, relatively low cost, portability, versatility, and widespread availability without compromising spatial and temporal resolution. However, limitations include the need for adequate acoustic windows, operator dependence, use of geometric assumptions in computing volumes, and inter-reader variability.

Myocardial function may be quantified using a variety of echocardiographic techniques. The M-mode (**Fig. 5-1A**) can be used to measure myocardial shortening and radial thickening with excellent temporal resolution, but can be used in only a limited number of myocardial segments, since the ultrasound beam has to be perpendicular to the segments being assessed. Although M-mode echocardiography can be used to assess LV morphology, the technique is optimally suited only for ventricles with uniform geometry and wall motion. Two-dimensional echocardiography (2DE) overcomes these limitations and quantifies accurately global and regional ventricular functions (**Fig. 5-1B**). However, errors due to off-axis imaging, reduced interobserver variability and reproducibility, and the subjectivity inherent in mental reconstruction of tomographic 2DE images are problematic.

*A*

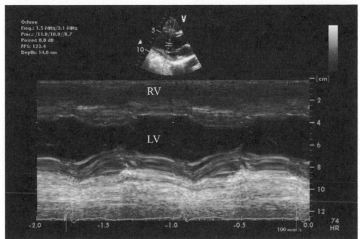

*B*

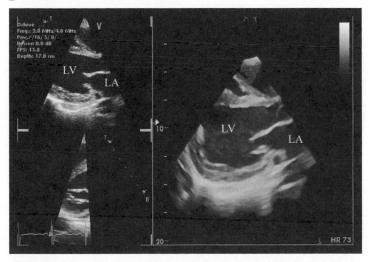

**FIGURE 5-1.** Left ventricular imaging by M-mode (**A**), 2D-echocardiography (**B**, *left*), and 3D-echocardiography (**B**, *right*). Annotations represent left ventricle (LV), left atrium (LA), and right ventricle (RV).

## ■ THREE-DIMENSIONAL ECHOCARDIOGRAPHY

Three-dimensional echocardiography (3DE) has added literally a new dimension to the evaluation of LV function and addresses these limitations. Although early 3DE approaches were cumbersome—involving prolonged and tedious data acquisition, time-consuming digitization, spatiotemporal registration of images, and volume rendering—advances in transducer technology, software, and computing power have made possible rapid acquisition of data from multiple, simultaneous lines of sight (matrix imaging). In this fashion, a volume of ultrasound data is reconstructed in near real time from a pyramidal ultrasound beam providing a more accurate quantification of global and regional cardiac functions (see **Fig. 5-1B**). To display the entire LV, a series of component volumes of the heart are acquired over 4 to 7 consecutive cardiac cycles and combined (or "stitched" together), making respiration and movement artifact a limitation in such full-volume acquisitions.

Noninvasive assessment of regional myocardial function plays a critical role in the management of ischemic heart disease. Although the echocardiographic evaluation of regional myocardial function relies largely on the visual detection of endocardial wall-motion abnormalities, this technique is subjective and demands complete visualization of the endocardium. Tissue (myocardial) velocities during systole and diastole are used to quantify ventricular function, but *measurement of strain and strain rate* (using Doppler-derived strain imaging or speckle-tracking echocardiography) *offers 2 important advantages*. First, within a myocardial segment, strain and strain rate (the magnitude and rate of tissue deformation, respectively), unlike tissue velocity, are less affected by translational (whole heart) movement and unaffected by "tethering" of adjacent segments; thus strain, unlike tissue Doppler, discriminates akinetic segments that are pulled (or tethered) from actively contracting segments. Second, strain and strain rate tend to be uniformly distributed across the myocardium, whereas tissue velocities tend to decrease from base to apex, making the establishment of reference values more difficult. These observations make strain and strain rate particularly well suited for the assessment of regional myocardial performance. These measures may also be useful for the determination of myocardial viability.

Diastolic function can be evaluated using M-mode and 2DE by measurement of the timing and extent of LV wall motion, wall thinning rate, and the duration of early relaxation and atrial contraction. LV filling dynamics can also be assessed by 2DE using frame-by-frame measurements of LV volume in either short-axis or apical 4-chamber views; however, 2DE is limited by a low sampling rate and suboptimal lateral resolution. More commonly, Doppler echocardiographic measurements are employed. Assessment of transmitral flow (LV filling), pulmonary vein flow (LA filling), and longitudinal motion of the mitral annulus during early diastole (myocardial relaxation) are used to evaluate LV diastolic function and pressure. The normal pattern of transmitral flow is biphasic consisting of early (peak E) and late (peak A) atrial filling velocities, which is expressed as the E/A ratio and is >1 in a normal individual. The variations in this pattern along with deceleration time of E velocity (DT) and isovolumic relaxation time (IVRT) are important variables of diastolic function derived from the transmitral flow waveform (**Fig. 5-2**).

# ■ STRESS ECHOCARDIOGRAPHY

Recognizing abnormal regional wall-motion abnormalities (hypokinesia, akinesia, dyskinesia) is essential in the evaluation of patients with coronary artery disease. Because wall motion at rest can be normal in a patient with significant coronary artery disease, echocardiographic imaging during provoked ischemia (stress echocardiography) is needed for diagnosis. In a vessel with a flow-limiting stenosis, the increased oxygen demands of the stressed myocardium cannot be met by an increase in flow, and ischemia with impairment of diastolic function, myocardial thickening, and endocardial motion results. Stress or provoked ischemia can be induced by increasing myocardial oxygen demand either with exercise or by pharmacologic interventions (Table 4-3; see also Chapter 4). In addition to the technical adequacy of the accompanying echocardiographic images and their proper interpretation, key elements in the analysis of a stress test results include duration of exercise, maximum

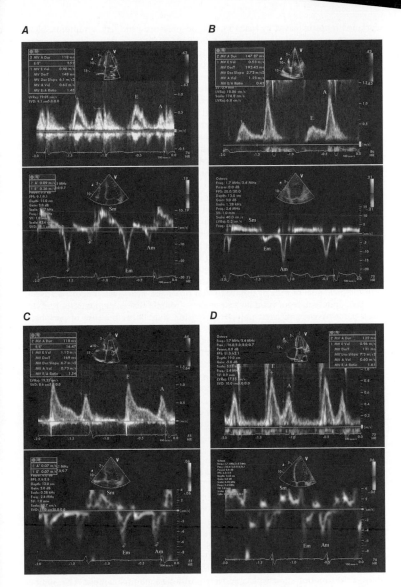

**FIGURE 5-2.** Diastolic function assessment by echocardiography using transmitral flow Doppler (*top*) and tissue Doppler (*bottom*). Annotations represent early diastolic flow velocity with LV relaxation (E) and late diastolic flow velocity with atrial contraction (A) for transmitral flow Doppler (*top panels*) and myocardial velocity during systole (Sm), early filling (Em), and late filling (Am) for tissue Doppler (bottom panels). **A** shows normal diastolic function, **B** impaired relaxation, **C** pseudonormal filling, and **D** restrictive filling, indicating a progressive impairment of LV diastolic function.

workload (approximated by heart rate–blood pressure product), symptoms, blood pressure response, arrhythmias, and ST-segment changes on the electrocardiogram (ECG). The basic principles of image acquisition for stress echocardiography (SE) are to use standard image planes and comparable views at rest and stress, ensure that all myocardial segments are visualized, and to record images in a digital cine loop format with parallel display of rest and stress images. The cine loop format is essential, as the change in heart rate between rest and stress makes interpretation of wall motion difficult. For evaluation of regional ventricular function, optimal endocardial definition is essential, which may require careful patient positioning, use of harmonic imaging, or contrast echocardiography for opacification of the LV cavity. The sensitivity of SE for detection of coronary disease depends on acquisition of stress images at the maximal cardiac workload, which declines rapidly on cessation of exercise. Three-dimensional echocardiography acquisition systems that allow simultaneous real-time imaging in multiple image planes offer the promise of faster acquisition times at peak stress, with the potential for improved diagnostic sensitivity.

The major limitations of SE are failure to achieve an adequate workload and poor endocardial definition. In patients who cannot exercise to a maximal workload due to various conditions, pharmacologic testing can be substituted using intravenous dobutamine, which is a potent β-agonist, increasing heart rate and contractility. The infusions are started at a low dose (5 mg/kg/min) and titrated up every 3 to 5 minutes until the maximum dose (30-40 mg/kg/min) or a clinical end point has been reached. Atropine can be added to achieve an appropriate increase in heart rate with a typical goal of 85% of the maximum predicted heart rate. Reported adverse effects of dobutamine infusion include anxiety, tremulousness, palpitations, arrhythmias, paresthesias, and chest pain. Hypotension may occur because of peripheral $\beta_2$-receptor–mediated vasodilation or LV outflow obstruction but is uncommon. In patients with abnormal global or regional function at rest, SE is more difficult to interpret, decreasing its specificity for the diagnosis of coronary disease. Evaluation of areas adjacent to the resting wall-motion abnormality may be problematic due to the tethering effect by the abnormal region. Tissue velocities and strain analysis have potential in this regard. In patients with suboptimal echocardiographic windows, images can be obtained using nuclear perfusion imaging. Vasodilator stress using persantine or adenosine is used less often with echocardiography than with nuclear medicine techniques (see Chapter 4).

# RADIONUCLIDE ANGIOGRAPHY

Radionuclide angiography (RNA) may be performed using equilibrium or first-pass methods; both can assess ventricular volumes, EF, and regional wall motion. With the first-pass approach, imaging is performed during the initial transit of radionuclide. Equilibrium radionuclide angiocardiography, also referred to as multiple gated acquisition (MUGA) or gated blood pool imaging, is usually regarded as the most accurate technique for measurement of LVEF. MUGA is performed by labeling the patient's red blood cell pool with a radioactive tracer and measuring radioactivity over the anterior chest with a suitably positioned gamma camera. The number of counts recorded per unit of time is proportional to the blood volume, giving a direct volumetric assessment of the cardiac chambers throughout the cardiac cycle. Blood pool labeling is routinely performed with technetium Tc-99m, which achieves high red cell labeling, has a relatively short half-life (6 hours), and has an emission photo peak (140 keV) close to the maximal sensitivity of the gamma camera crystal. Labeling can be performed in vitro by incubating a small autologous blood sample with Tc-99m or, more commonly, in vivo with the direct intravenous injection of Tc-99m pertechnetate. The in vivo labeling technique is more convenient for most patients because it involves only 1 venipuncture, is less time consuming, and is less costly. Although red blood cell labeling is generally more efficient with the in vitro techniques, more than 80% of the injected radionuclide usually binds to red blood cells with the in vivo approach. Shortly after injection, the labeled red blood cells equally distribute throughout the entire blood pool. Image acquisition is performed for 800 to 1000 heartbeats for each projection, corresponding to a time period of 5 to 10 minutes. The RR interval is divided into 16 to 32 equal phases (gating windows), and counts are recorded separately for each phase. At the end of the acquisition, the counts are summed for all cardiac cycles, and images obtained for each phase are then displayed in sequence, creating a cine loop of the entire cardiac cycle. Images are obtained in the anterior, left posterior oblique, and modified left anterior oblique projections to best visualize all cardiac chambers and provide indirect information for all left ventricular walls. The left anterior oblique projections are used for measurements of ejection fraction because the LV is free of any overlap with other cardiac chambers. Left ventricular time–volume curves are used to derive a number of indices of systolic and diastolic function.

MUGA scans are *contraindicated* in lactating and pregnant women because of the concern of ionizing radiation exposure, although quite small (620 mrem). ECG gating also becomes unreliable in patients with arrhythmias and significant variability of the RR interval, which can be corrected to an extent with modified acquisition and postprocessing protocols. Obtaining the optimum projection for separation of the ventricles and defining the ventricular contours is operator dependent and poor technique can introduce measurement errors.

# COMPUTED TOMOGRAPHY

Both *multidetector* computed tomography (MDCT) and *electron beam* computed tomography (EBCT) can provide anatomic and functional data on both ventricles using various protocols specific to the information of interest, and allow precise measurement of ventricular volumes, function, regional wall motion, and mass. MDCT is *not* a first-line method of EF measurement, but may be useful if echocardiographic images are poor and CMR is contraindicated. Evaluation by CT for ischemic heart disease includes CT angiography with intravenous contrast injection for assessment of coronary atherosclerotic burden and calcium scoring without contrast enhancement for identification and quantification of calcification within the coronary arteries, which has a high predictive value for cardiac events. The data obtained during coronary CT angiography can be further used to create multiplanar reconstruction (**Fig. 5-3**) cine images in the LV short axis from the cardiac base to the apex to evaluate LV function and calculate EF in addition to other parameters, which is likely to provide useful additional information; when compared to CMR, MDCT is an adequate alternative for functional assessment. Moreover, with dynamic contrast administration and fast scanning capability, myocardial perfusion defects can be identified at rest in regions of myocardial infarction. CT has also been used to assess myocardial infarction location and size by using delayed contrast-enhanced methods, which are performed 5 to 10 minutes after intravenous iodinated contrast injection.

The major limitations of CT include contrast-related nephropathy and radiation dose exposure. Although the radiation dose for calcium scoring is relatively low, coronary CT angiography and functional imaging methods provide a radiation dose of 8 to 10 mSv on 16-detector and 14 to 18 mSv on 64-detector systems.

# SINGLE-PHOTON EMISSION COMPUTED TOMOGRAPHY

Single-photon emission computed tomography (SPECT) is a tomographic nuclear medicine technique in which a radionuclide is injected and its distribution through

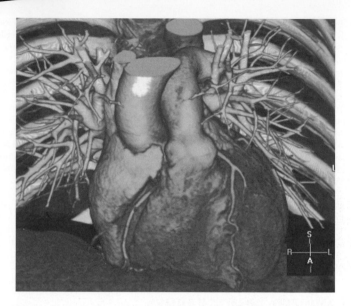

**FIGURE 5-3.** CT angiography with 3-dimensional reconstruction of a normal heart.

the body imaged using a gamma camera (see also Chapter 4). Two-dimensional projections from multiple angles are acquired and reconstructed using specific algorithms to yield 3-dimensional images. The use of ECG-gated SPECT allows simultaneous assessment of LV wall motion and myocardial perfusion with good correlation with other imaging techniques and high reproducibility. Automated methods are used to quantify global systolic and diastolic function; regional wall motion and thickening are usually assessed by semiquantitative visual analysis. LV volumes and EF by thallium Tl 201 SPECT correlate highly with Tc-99 sesta-mibi SPECT, which in turn have been validated against a number of nonnuclear methods. Gated SPECT further allows the detection of coronary artery disease and myocardial viability by combining the evaluation of regional wall motion and thickening with the assessment of perfusion (**Fig. 5-4**). Disadvantages of SPECT include the relatively low spatial resolution compared to other techniques, moderate cost, and complexity of quantification due to the presence of considerable image noise.

Myocardial perfusion imaging in conjunction with exercise or pharmacologic stress testing has been validated as an alternative modality for noninvasive assessment of coronary artery disease (see also Chapter 4). Exercise stress testing is performed using protocols similar to those for SE, followed by SPECT scan to assess regional myocardial perfusion. As an alternative, pharmacologic stress testing can be performed in those patients who cannot exercise, using vasodilating agents such as adenosine and dipyridamole, or less often, catecholamines such as dobutamine. Pharmacologic vasodilator stress imaging does not provoke ischemia, but rather induces a differential pattern of coronary blood flow (see also Chapter 4). This flow disparity translates into relative hypoperfusion of the ischemic myocardium, which can be detected on the radionuclide myocardial perfusion images.

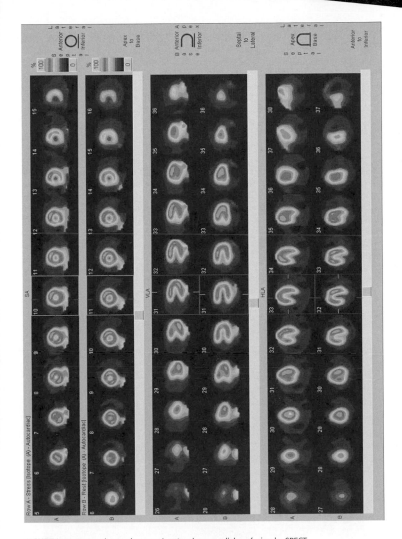

**FIGURE 5-4.** Rest and stress images of regional myocardial perfusion by SPECT.

# POSITRON EMISSION TOMOGRAPHY

Positron emission tomography (PET) images the decay of an injected radioactive tracer as it distributes in the body. Although it lacks high spatial resolution, important quantitative physiologic parameters, such as perfusion and metabolism, can be imaged, making PET the gold standard for these measurements. Major disadvantages include the limited availability of PET imaging centers, a high complexity of obtaining measurements, increased cost, and limited spatial resolution compared to other imaging techniques.

## ■ CARDIAC MAGNETIC RESONANCE IMAGING

Cardiac magnetic resonance imaging (CMR) is recognized as the most accurate noninvasive imaging modality for the assessment of LV function and is now the *gold standard* for determination of cardiac EF. ECG-gated cine images from state-of-the-art magnetic resonance imaging scanners depict LV function with high contrast and excellent spatial and temporal resolution (**Fig. 5-5**), and are readily acquired in breath-holds of 5 to 10 heartbeats. For patients in whom breath-holding and ECG gating are difficult, real-time cine imaging without ECG gating and breath-holding can be performed. ECG-gated CMR with breath-holding delivers a spatial resolution of approximately $1.5 \times 2$ mm$^2$, slice thickness of 5 to 10 mm, and temporal resolution of 30 to 50 milliseconds per frame compared to cine CMR, which has lower spatial and temporal resolution with shorter data acquisition times and typically more artifacts. Cine CMR is also suitable for quantitative analysis from multislice images covering the LV, including myocardial mass, volumes, EF, and wall thickness and thickening. These parameters are commonly computed after manual planimetry of the LV epicardial and endocardial borders at end diastole and end systole. Cardiac volumes are calculated by multiplying the blood pool area by the slice thickness and summing over slices; myocardial mass is computed as the difference between the volumes determined by the epicardial and endocardial borders multiplied by the specific gravity of myocardium.

Beyond conventional CMR, a variety of tissue-tracking methods exist for quantifying tissue displacement, velocity, strain, strain rate, twist, and torsion by measuring

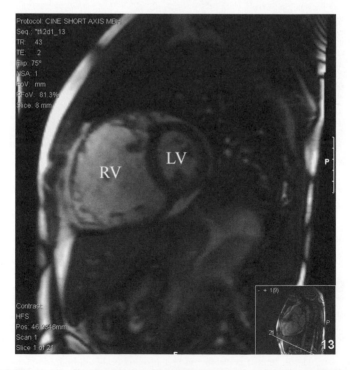

**FIGURE 5-5.** CMR with a short-axis view of the left ventricle (LV) in a patient with a grossly dilated right ventricle (RV)

motion of small regions of tissue within the myocardium. Tissue-tracking techniques include myocardial tagging, velocity-encoded phase contrast CMR, harmonic phase analysis, and displacement encoding with stimulated echoes. Phase contrast CMR can also be applied to measure early and late diastolic ventricular inflow for assessment of diastolic dysfunction (see also Chapter 4).

Cardiac magnetic resonance (CMR) imaging has a number of disadvantages, the greatest one being the exclusion of patients with pacemakers or implantable cardiac defibrillators due to the high magnetic fields, which can tamper with the function of these devices. However, CMR safe devices and CMR protocols are being developed to overcome this significant problem. Other limitations include the need for breath-holding, the gantry's claustrophobic environment, high cost, increased complexity of data analysis, and limited availability of the technology.

## SUGGESTED READINGS

DeMaria AN, Blanchard DG. Echocardiography. In: Fuster V, Walsh RA, Harrington RA, et al, eds. *Hurst's The Heart*. 13th ed. New York, NY: McGraw-Hill. 2011;18:411-489.

Berman DS, Hayes SW, Hachamovitch R, Shaw LJ, Germano G. Nuclear cardiology. In: Fuster V, Walsh RA, Harrington RA, et al, eds. *Hurst's The Heart*. 13th ed. New York, NY: McGraw-Hill. 2011;21:562-598.

Bogaert J, Dymarkowski S, Taylor AM. *Clinical Cardiac MRI*. Berlin, Germany: Springer-Verlag; 2005.

Budoff MMJ, Shinbane JS. *Cardiac CT Imaging: Diagnosis of Cardiovascular Disease*. London, UK: Springer-Verlag; 2006.

Heller GV, Hendel RC. *Nuclear Cardiology: Practical Applications*. New York, NY: McGraw-Hill; 2004.

Otto CM. *Textbook of Clinical Echocardiography*. 3rd ed. Philadelphia, PA: Elsevier Saunders; 2004.

Woodard PK, Bhalla S, Javidan-Nejad C, et al. Non-coronary cardiac CT imaging. *Semin Ultrasound CT MRI*. 2006;27:56-75.

# CHAPTER 6
# CARDIAC CT AND MRI

Melissa A. Daubert, Michael Poon, Matthew J. Budoff,
Han W. Kim, Afshin Farzaneh-Far, Igor Klem,
Wolfgang Rehwald, and Raymond J. Kim

## COMPUTED TOMOGRAPHY OF THE HEART

Although best known for its ability to noninvasively provide information about the epicardial coronary arteries, computed tomography (CT) is a technique that, in actuality, can fully evaluate both cardiac structure and function. Advances in spatial and temporal resolution and image reconstruction software have helped in the evaluation of cardiac structures, including coronary veins, pulmonary veins, atria, ventricles, aorta, and thoracic arterial and venous structures.

## ■ TECHNICAL CONSIDERATIONS

### Multirow Detector Computed Tomography

Multidetector computed tomography (MDCT) scanners produce images by rotating an x-ray tube around a circular gantry through which the patient advances on a table. By increasing the numbers of detectors, a reduction in the time to image the entire cardiac anatomy has been achieved. Additionally, the introduction of multirow spiral CT detector systems currently allows acquisition of 4 to 64 simultaneous images, with slice thickness reduced to 0.5 to 0.625 mm. Retrospective electrocardiography gating with MDCT employs acquisition of multiple images throughout each cardiac cycle. Prospective gating during either spiral or nonspiral acquisitions employs image triggering only at a specific temporal location of the cardiac cycle, thereby significantly reducing radiation exposure.

### Electron-Beam Computed Tomography

Electron-beam computed tomography (EBCT) uses an electron beam deflected via a magnetic coil and focused to strike a series of 4 tungsten targets located beneath the patient. As they pass through the patient, the x-rays are attenuated and recorded by 2 detector arrays. As there are no moving parts, the image is aquired within 50 milliseconds.

## ■ EVALUATION OF CORONARY ARTERY DISEASE

### Detection of Coronary Artery Calcification

A calcified lesion is generally defined as either 2 or 3 adjacent pixels (0.68-1.02 mm$^2$ for a 512$^2$ reconstruction matrix and camera field size of 30 cm) of >130 Hounsfield units (HU). Using the traditional Agatston method, each calcified lesion is multiplied by a density factor as follows: 1 for lesions with a maximal density between

130 and 199 HU; 2 for lesions between 200 and 299 HU; 3 for lesions between 300 and 399 HU; and 4 for lesions > 400 HU. The total coronary artery calcium score (CACS) is calculated as the sum of each calcified lesion in the 4 main coronary arteries over all the consecutive tomographic slices.

MDCT imaging protocols vary among different camera systems and manufacturers. Generally 40 consecutive 2.5- to 3-mm-thick images are acquired per cardiac study. Calcified lesions are defined as 2 or 3 adjacent pixels with a tomographic density of either > 90 or > 130 HU. Calcium scoring is usually based on the traditional Agatston method (ie, initial density of > 130 HU). As with EBCT scoring, the total CACS is calculated as the sum of each calcified plaque over all the tomographic slices.

## Coronary Artery Calcification and Atherosclerotic Plaque Burden

The presence of CAC is an indicator of coronary atherosclerosis (**Fig. 6-1**). Furthermore, its severity is directly related to the total atherosclerotic plaque burden present in the epicardial coronary arteries. Thought to begin early in life, CAC progresses more rapidly in older individuals who have advanced atherosclerotic lesions. Calcification is an active, organized, and regulated process that occurs in atherosclerotic plaques where calcium phosphate precipitates in the vessel wall in a way similar to bone mineralization. Although lack of calcification does not exclude the presence

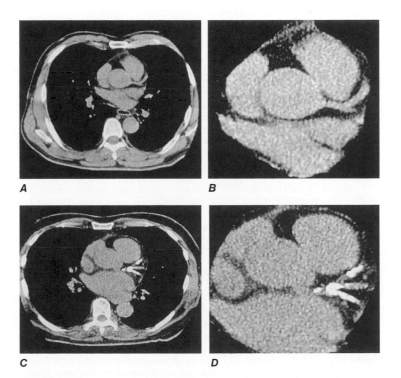

A         B

C         D

**FIGURE 6-1.** Single-level noncontrast electron-beam computed tomography (EBCT) scan of a normal subject (*top*) and an individual with severe coronary artery calcification (*bottom*). Calcium is shown as intensely white areas within the coronary arteries.

of atherosclerotic plaque, calcification occurs exclusively in atherosclerotic arteries and is not found in normal coronary arteries. The total calcium area underestimates total plaque area, with approximately *5 times as many noncalcified as calcified plaques.*

## Coronary Artery Calcification and Stenosis Severity

Significant (> 50%) coronary artery stenosis by angiography is almost universally associated with the presence of coronary artery calcium. However, the severity of angiographic coronary artery stenosis is not directly related to the total CACS. The poor *specificity of coronary calcium scanning* can be reconciled by the fact that the coronary calcification confirms the presence of atherosclerotic plaque, but it may not necessarily be obstructive. There appears to be a threshold CACS above which most patients will have significant coronary artery stenosis. The accuracy for identifying significant CAD based on CACS may be further improved by incorporating age, gender, and traditional risk-factor information. The current American College of Cardiology/American Heart Association (ACC/AHA) guidelines on coronary angiography *do not recommend coronary angiography on the basis of a positive EBCT but do suggest angiography may be avoided with the finding of a negative (zero score) study.*

## Coronary Artery Calcification: Prognostic Implications

The likelihood of plaque rupture and the development of acute cardiovascular events are related to the total atherosclerotic plaque burden. Although controversy exists as to whether calcified or noncalcified plaques are more prone to rupture, extensive calcification indicates the presence of both plaque morphologies. There is a direct relationship between the CACS severity, the extent of atherosclerotic plaque, and the presence of silent myocardial ischemia. Therefore, the CACS could be useful for risk assessment of asymptomatic individuals and potentially guide therapeutics.

Traditional risk-factor analysis is commonly used to identify individuals who are at increased risk for developing cardiovascular disease based on standard clinical criteria. Because the development of symptomatic cardiovascular disease occurs almost exclusively in patients with atherosclerosis, CAC score appears to provide complementary prognostic information to that obtained by the Framingham risk model.

Several recent trials in both symptomatic and asymptomatic patients have studied whether the extent of CAC can predict subsequent patient outcome. The calcium score seems to predict cardiovascular events independently of standard risk factors. In addition to the risk conferred by a high calcium score, an increase in CAC over time also increases risk of a major coronary event.

## ■ COMPUTED TOMOGRAPHY ANGIOGRAPHY

### Assessment of Native Coronary Arterial Disease

Noninvasive detection of CAD is one of the most interesting but most challenging applications of coronary CT angiography (**Fig. 6-2**). Invasive coronary angiography carries procedural risk as well as high procedural cost. It was estimated that approximately 20% to 27% of patients who undergo coronary angiography have normal angiograms, and many patients with significant CAD do not require revascularization procedures.

Because of its high negative predictive value, the consensus among many imaging experts is that MDCT may be used as a reliable filter before invasive coronary

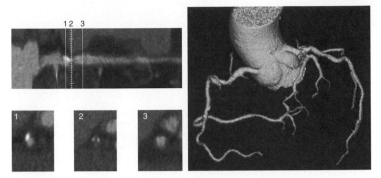

**FIGURE 6-2.** Four noncontrast EBCT images (*left*). The total CACS is moderate at 271 and highest in the RCA (176). Longitudinal maximum-intensity projection (MIP) view of RCA lesion (*top*) with 3 axial multiplanar reconstruction (MPR) views obtained at 3 sequential points (*below*): (**1**) calcified plaque, (**2**) mixed plaque, and (**3**) normal reference vessel. Coronary 3-dimensional arteriogram (*right*) demonstrates a nonobstructive plaque in the mid-RCA; the LAD and LCX coronary arteries were normal. The patient also had a normal exercise myocardial perfusion scan. EBCT, electron-beam computed tomography; LAD, left anterior descending; LCX, left circumflex; RCA, right coronary artery.

angiography in the assessment of symptomatic patients with intermediate risk of CAD and in patients with uninterpretable or equivocal stress tests. A recent scientific statement from the American Heart Association on cardiac CT concluded, "CT coronary angiography is reasonable for the assessment of obstructive disease in symptomatic patients (Class IIa, Level of Evidence B)." Use of CT angiography in asymptomatic persons as a screening test for atherosclerosis (noncalcific plaque) is not recommended (Class III, Level of Evidence C). (See Chapter 57).

Careful selection of patients is crucial to increase the diagnostic yield of coronary CTA using MDCT. Three major limitations of spiral coronary CT angiography are relatively fast heart rate (ie, more than 70 bpm), irregular heart rhythm, and extensive CAC. Heavy calcification does not affect the negative predictive value of MDCT on a segment-based analysis, and the newer generation of MDCT technology with even faster gantry rotation may further reduce the blooming artifact associated with coronary calcification. The recent appropriateness criteria for coronary CT angiography do not endorse the use of coronary CTA in the evaluation of patients with a body mass index (BMI) > 40 kg/m$^2$.

## Assessment of Coronary Bypass Grafts

Coronary CT angiography demonstrated good diagnostic accuracy for evaluating graft stenosis; however, the assessment of bypass graft stenosis has several important limitations, namely the image artifacts caused by surgical clips and the presence of extensive coronary calcification in the native coronary arteries.

Presently, coronary CTA may be used for the evaluation of coronary bypass grafts and coronary anatomy in symptomatic patients. In the case of reoperation, coronary CTA may provide critically important information on the status and anatomy of the bypass grafts. The AHA Scientific Statement on Cardiac CT states, "It might be reasonable in most cases to not only assess the patency of bypass graft but also the presence of coronary stenoses in the course of the bypass graft or at the anastomotic site as well as in the native coronary artery system (Class IIb, Level of Evidence C)."

## Assessment of In-Stent Restenosis

Despite promising results, assessment of symptomatic patients with implanted coronary stents using current CT technology is one of the uncertain areas in terms of its overall clinical utility. The problems faced by the current imaging technology relates to the partial volume effect caused by the metallic stents with or without the coexistence of coronary calcification. Such artifact limits the overall visibility of the inner lumen of a deployed stent. The expert consensus thus far does not advocate the routine use of MDCT in ruling out in-stent restenosis except for highly selected cases.

## ■ EVALUATION OF CARDIAC STRUCTURE

Although echocardiography is generally used to assess native and prosthetic valvular heart disease, CT can be an alternative for patients with poor acoustic windows who cannot undergo CMR or transesophageal echocardiography. Cardiac CT has been used to evaluate mitral and aortic valve calcification, bicuspid aortic valves, as well as other structures such as the atrial and ventricular septum. Use of MDCT to evaluate valvular flow abnormalities, however, continues to remains more challenging.

In addition to cardiac MRI, cardiac CT has been used increasingly for the assessment of congenital heart disease. Both modalities can be rendered into 3-dimensional (3D) images that are useful in clarifying the often complex anatomic relationships in patients with congenital heart disease. Additionally, the development of 4-dimensional (4D) capability has accelerated over the last few years. The heart is a dynamic organ best understood when studied throughout the cardiac cycle. Hence, the development of 4D CT cineangiography (time being the fourth dimension) is a milestone in the clinical application of this technology.

## ■ EVALUATION OF CORONARY ANOMALIES

Anomalies of the coronary arteries are reported in 0.3% to 1% of healthy individuals, and despite usually being benign, they can be hemodynamically significant and some lead to abnormalities of myocardial perfusion and/or sudden death. The coronary anomalies that may be associated with significant clinical symptoms or adverse outcomes including sudden death are those that course between the pulmonary artery and the aorta.

Until recently, invasive coronary artery angiography has been the gold standard for the detection of such anomalies. However, MDCT angiography has proven its worth in diagnosing these anomalies. Coronary CTA is considered the preferred imaging modality in patients with suspected coronary artery anomalies and in patients in whom an invasive diagnostic procedure was inconclusive.

## ■ EVALUATION OF PERICARDIAL DISEASE

CT scanning provides excellent visualization of the pericardium and associated mediastinal structures. CT is aided by the fact that epicardial and extrapericardial fat often outlines the normal pericardium. Fat, being of very low density, serves as a natural contrast agent. Therefore, even minimal pericardial thickening (4-5 mm) is well recognized by cardiac CT (**Fig. 6-3**). The high density of pericardial calcium makes its detection relatively easy. The 3D representation of anatomy by CT provides the surgeon with precise detail of the extent of calcification and the degree of myocardial invasion. CT scanning can be useful particularly when visualization of the pericardium is suboptimal with echocardiography. CT scanning can readily detect pericardial effusion and can help determine the characteristics of the fluid based on CT density. Additionally, CT scanning is useful in accurately diagnosing constrictive pericarditis and distinguishing it from similar conditions,

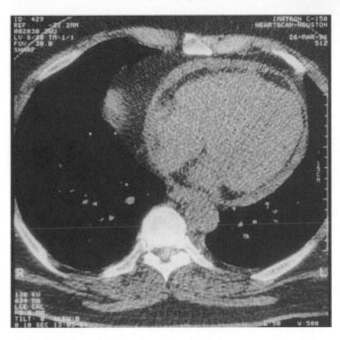

**FIGURE 6-3.** Diffuse pericardial thickening surrounding the entire heart in a patient with pericardial constriction. (Reproduced with permission from Brundage BH, Mao SS. In: Schlant RC et al, eds. *Diagnostic Atlas of the Heart*. New York, NY: McGraw-Hill; 1996:243.)

such as restrictive myopathy. Cine mode images of the right atrium and RV can also detect diastolic collapse when pericardial tamponade is present. Enlargement of the superior and inferior venae cavae can also be identified when either constriction or tamponade is present.

## ■ DISEASES OF THE GREAT VESSELS

Conventional CT scanning is widely used for diagnosing thoracic aortic aneurysms and dissections. With the introduction of MDCT scanners, hundreds of images of approximately 0.625 to 2.5 mm thickness can be acquired within a single breath-hold. A complete study of the thoracic aorta can be completed in only 10 to 15 seconds. Following scan acquisition, 3D reconstructions are readily produced, which can be rotated in multiple views.

Aortic dissection, aneurysms, and coarctation can be readily diagnosed with CT angiography. In patients undergoing *redo* coronary artery bypass surgery, CT scanning has several advantages. CT angiography may guide the surgical approach by defining the position of the sternum to the right ventricle, existing grafts, and aorta, and thereby avoid unnecessary bleeding. CT is an excellent modality to evaluate the aorta for plaque and atherosclerotic disease, allowing the surgeon to plan an arterial revascularization rather than depending on saphenous vein grafting.

Finally, CT angiography of the pulmonary arteries may be particularly useful in the diagnosis of acute pulmonary embolism, replacing the nuclear ventilation perfusion scan in many centers.

## ■ SUMMARY

CAC is helpful in risk-stratifying intermediate-risk patients as well as ruling out obstructive disease in the symptomatic patient with low probability of disease. CTA, with detection of both luminal stenosis and calcified and noncalcific plaque, should significantly aid in improving risk stratification and diagnoses. CTA is likely to become an initial test in the symptomatic patient with a low to intermediate probability of obstructive CAD. Given a consistent negative predictive power > 97% in multiple studies, CTA is unlikely to misclassify a patient at risk for CAD. It affords significant clinical information but must be used in context of other tests and in specific clinical situations, because the current radiation dose and contrast requirements preclude its use as a screening test. MDCT angiography can be a powerful tool in assessing structural abnormalities of the heart, including coronary anomalies and pulmonary veins.

# MAGNETIC RESONANCE IMAGING OF THE HEART

Advances in technical abilities and clinical utilization of cardiovascular magnetic resonance (CMR) imaging has allowed CMR to provide dynamic, rapid, and high-resolution imaging of ventricular function, valvular motion, and myocardial perfusion. Moreover, CMR is now considered the gold standard for the assessment of regional and global systolic function, myocardial infarction and viability, and the assessment of congenital heart disease.

## ■ BASIC PRINCIPLES

Magnetic resonance imaging (MRI) acquires images through the transmission and reception of energy. However, unlike other modalities, MRI offers the ability to modulate both the emitted and received signals so that a multitude of tissue characteristics can be examined and differentiated without the need to change scanner hardware. As a result, from a single imaging session, a wide variety of information about cardiac function and morphology, perfusion and viability, hemodynamics, and large vessel anatomy can be obtained. This information is gathered from multiple short acquisitions, each requiring different pulse sequences (software programs that drive the scanner) with specific operational parameters and optimal settings.

## ■ MAGNETIC RESONANCE PHYSICS

An MRI scanner is not a single device, but rather consists of multiple separate components that perform 3 basic operations: (1) the generation of a static magnetic field, (2) the transmission of energy within the radiofrequency (RF) range to the patient, and (3) the reception of the MR signal following the transmission of RF energy. When a patient is placed within the bore of the scanner, hydrogen protons within the patient's body align parallel or antiparallel to the static magnetic field. More protons align parallel to the field than against the field, leading to a small net magnetization vector. While aligned in the magnetic field, these protons rotate or precess about the field (in the same way a spinning top precesses in a gravitational field) at a rate known as the *Larmor frequency*. This frequency ($\omega_o$) depends on magnetic field strength ($B_0$) and a nuclei-specific physical constant, known as the gyromagnetic ratio ($\gamma$), by the formula, $\omega_o = \gamma B_0$.

With the absorption of the energy from the RF pulse, the net magnetization vector is tilted from its equilibrium orientation parallel to the static magnetic field (longitudinal direction) into the transverse plane. Following the RF excitation, 2 independent relaxation processes return the net magnetization vector to its thermal equilibrium (realigned with the static magnetic field). Longitudinal relaxation time (T1) results from the transfer of energy from the excited protons to surrounding molecules in the local environment. The time constant, T1, describes the exponential regrowth of longitudinal magnetization. The second process, known as *transverse* or *spin-spin relaxation*, describes the decay of the magnetization vector in the transverse (x-y) plane. The T1 and T2 are intrinsic properties of any given tissue. Pulse sequences use differences in T1 and T2 to generate image contrast between tissues.

## ■ IMAGE ACQUISITION AND SIGNAL PROCESSING

The MR signals following RF excitation are localized in 3D space by the use of magnetic fields generated by 3 sets of gradient coils. These gradient coils alter the strength of the static magnetic field as a linear function of distance from the isocenter of the magnet in each of 3 orthogonal directions (x-, y-, and z-axes). The variation in field strengths across space produces differences in proton precessional frequencies along each axis. The raw data from the scanner consists of a 2-dimensional grid of data (also known as *k-space*), which is converted to an MR image by an inverse 2-dimensional Fourier transform by the image reconstruction computer.

## ■ CREATING CONTRAST IN MAGNETIC RESONANCE IMAGES

One of the important advantages of MRI is the ability to generate substantial soft-tissue contrast by the use of pulse sequences and the administration of contrast media. In general, pulse sequences are adjusted to emphasize differences in tissue T1 and T2, which can be inherent or altered by the presence of contrast media. The administration of intravenous contrast agents can also be used to affect image contrast by altering tissue T1 and/or T2. The magnitude of T1 and/or T2 change depends on the specific relaxivities of the contrast media, the distribution characteristics (ie, intravascular, extracellular, or targeted to a specific tissue), and tissue perfusion. Gadolinium-based contrast media is commonly used in CMR imaging. When administered, it primarily shortens the T1 in the tissues where it is distributed.

## ■ CMR IMAGING SAFETY

The CMR imaging environment has the potential to pose serious risks to patients and facility staff in several ways. Injuries can result from the static magnetic field (projectile impact injuries), very rapid gradient-field switching (induction of electric currents leading to peripheral nerve stimulation), RF-energy deposition (heating of the imaged portion of the body), and acoustic noise. Patients with medical devices or implants can face additional potential hazards, including device heating, movement, or malfunction. Recently, in several small case series, it has been reported that a small subset of patients with end-stage renal disease, receiving gadolinium contrast, may be at risk for developing nephrogenic systemic fibrosis (NSF). NSF is characterized by an increased tissue deposition of collagen, often resulting in thickening and tightening of the skin and predominantly involving the distal extremities. A policy statement regarding the use of gadolinium contrast agents in the setting of renal disease has been published by the American College of Radiology.

# ■ THE CARDIOVASCULAR EXAMINATION

## Function and Volumes

The assessment of cardiac function and volumes is a fundamental component of the core examination. Cine MRI has been shown to be highly accurate and reproducible in the measurement of ejection fraction, ventricular volumes, and cardiac mass. In recent years, cine MRI has become widely accepted as the gold standard for the measurement of these parameters. Moreover, it is also increasingly used as an end point in studies of left ventricular (LV) remodeling and as a reference standard for other imaging techniques.

Cine MRI can be acquired in real-time, single-shot, free-breathing mode or by means of a segmented k-space data acquisition approach, which is performed using a breath-hold and offers substantial improvement in image quality with superior spatial and temporal resolution. Thus, in clinical practice, segmented imaging is usually preferred. In segmented acquisition, data are collected over multiple, consecutive heartbeats (typically 5-10). During each heartbeat, blocks of data (segments) are acquired with reference to ECG timing, which represent the separate phases or frames of the cardiac cycle. Following the full acquisition, data from a given phase, collected from the multiple heartbeats, are combined to form the complete image of the particular cine frame. For the core examination, a short-axis stack from the mitral-valve plane through the apex and 2-, 3-, and 4-chamber long-axis views are obtained.

## Perfusion at Stress and Rest

The goal of perfusion imaging is to create a movie of the transit of contrast media (typically gadolinium based) with the blood during its initial pass through the LV myocardium (*first-pass contrast enhancement*). After scout and cine imaging, adenosine is infused under continuous electrocardiography and blood pressure monitoring for at least 2 minutes prior to the initiation of perfusion imaging. Gadolinium contrast is then administered, followed by a saline flush. The perfusion images are observed as they are acquired, with breath-holding starting from the appearance of contrast in the RV cavity. Once the contrast bolus has transited the LV myocardium, adenosine is stopped and imaging is completed 5 to 10 seconds later. Prior to the rest perfusion scan, a waiting period of approximately 15 minutes is required for gadolinium to sufficiently clear from the blood pool. Approximately 5 minutes after rest perfusion, delayed enhancement imaging (see the following section) can be performed.

## Viability and Infarction

Myocardial viability and infarction are simultaneously examined using the technique known as delayed enhancement magnetic resonance imaging (DEMRI). In the literature, DEMRI is used interchangeably with late gadolinium-enhancement CMR imaging or delayed hyperenhancement imaging. Although, at first glance, the utility of DEMRI appears to be limited to those with coronary artery disease, new applications are steadily arising over a wide range of cardiovascular disorders. Thus, DEMRI is an essential component of the core examination.

Following an intravenous bolus, gadolinium distributes throughout the intravascular and interstitial space, while simultaneously being cleared by the kidneys. In normal myocardium, where the myocytes are densely packed, tissue volume is predominately intracellular. Because gadolinium is unable to penetrate intact sarcolemmal membranes, the volume of distribution is small, and one can consider viable myocytes as actively excluding gadolinium media. In acute myocardial infarction, myocyte membranes are ruptured, allowing gadolinium to passively diffuse into the intracellular space. This results in an increased gadolinium volume of distribution, and thus increased tissue concentration compared with normal myocardium. Similarly in chronic infarction, as necrotic tissue is replaced by collagenous scar, the interstitial space is expanded and gadolinium tissue concentration is increased. T1-weighted can depict infarcted regions as bright or *hyperenhanced* whereas viable regions appear black or *nulled*. Compared with other imaging techniques that are currently used to assess myocardial viability, an important advantage of DEMRI is the high spatial resolution.

## Flow and Velocity

Depending on the clinical question, the core examination can include velocity-encoded cine MRI (VENC MRI) to measure blood velocities and flows in arteries and veins, and across valves and shunts. Also known as phase-contrast velocity mapping, the underlying principle is that signal from moving blood or tissue will undergo a phase shift relative to stationary tissue, if a magnetic-field gradient is applied in the direction of motion.

VENC MRI allows blood flow through an orifice to be directly measured on an *en-face* image of the orifice. With echocardiography there are 2 limitations. First, the blood flow profile is not directly measured but assumed to be flat (ie, velocity in the center of the orifice is the same as near the edges) so that, hopefully, one sampling velocity would indicate average velocity. Additionally, the cross-sectional area of the orifice is estimated from a diameter measurement of the orifice at a different time from when Doppler velocity was recorded using a different examination (M-mode or 2-dimensional imaging). Conversely, VENC MRI has some disadvantages. Perhaps most importantly, VENC MRI is not performed in real time and requires breath-holding to minimize artifacts from respiratory motion. One consequence is that it is difficult to measure changes in flow that occur with respiration.

## ■ CLINICAL APPLICATIONS

### Coronary Artery Disease and Ischemia

**Dobutamine-Stress Cine MRI** Analogous to echocardiography, cine MRI during dobutamine stimulation can be used to detect ischemia-induced wall-motion abnormalities. Dobutamine cine MRI can yield higher diagnostic accuracy than dobutamine echocardiography and can be effective in patients not suited for echocardiography because of poor acoustic windows. Limitations include the need to administer dobutamine while the patient is inside the magnet, the risk of inducing ischemia with dobutamine, and the diminished diagnostic utility of the ECG as it is altered by the magnetic field.

**Adenosine Stress-Perfusion MRI** The diagnostic performance of stress-perfusion MRI has shown good correlations with radionuclide imaging and x-ray coronary angiography, although there have been some variable results. On average, the sensitivity and specificity of perfusion MRI for detecting obstructive CAD were 83% (range, 44%-93%) and 82% (range, 60%-100%), respectively. Likely on the basis of these studies, the most recent consensus report on clinical indications for CMR imaging classified perfusion imaging as a Class II indication for the assessment of CAD (provides clinically relevant information and is frequently useful).

**Coronary MR Angiography** Coronary magnetic resonance angiography (MRA) is technically demanding for several reasons. The coronary arteries are small (3-5 mm) and tortuous compared with other vascular beds that are imaged by MRA, and there is nearly constant motion during both the respiratory and cardiac cycles. Currently, the only clinical indication that is considered appropriate for coronary MRA is the evaluation of patients with suspected coronary anomalies.

**Viability and Infarction** Abundant animal model data demonstrate a nearly exact relationship between the size and shape of infarcted myocardium by DEMRI to that by histopathology. Human studies demonstrate that DEMRI is effective in identifying the presence, location, and extent of myocardial infarction in both the acute and chronic settings (**Fig. 6-4**). DEMRI can also distinguish between acute infarcts with only necrotic myocytes and acute infarcts with necrotic myocytes and damaged microvasculature. The latter, termed the *no-reflow phenomenon*, indicates the presence of compromised tissue perfusion despite epicardial artery patency. Importantly, if imaging is repeated over time, no-reflow regions can gradually become hyperenhanced, as contrast slowly accumulates in these regions.

Clinically, DEMRI is used to differentiate patients with potentially reversible ventricular dysfunction from those with irreversible dysfunction. In the setting of ischemic heart disease, it is primarily the former group that will benefit from coronary revascularization. Kim and coworkers published the initial study demonstrating that DEMRI done before coronary revascularization could be used to predict functional improvement after revascularization, as measured by improved wall motion and global function.

Prior reports have concluded that in patients with CAD and ventricular dysfunction regions with thinned myocardium represent scar tissue and cannot improve

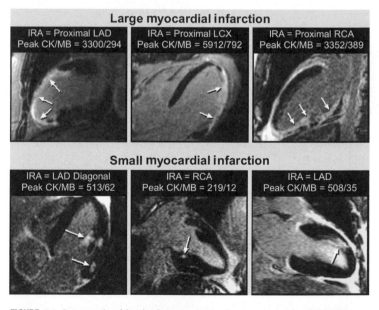

**FIGURE 6-4.** Representative delayed enhancement magnetic resonance imaging (DE-MRI) images in patients with chronic myocardial infarction. Both large (*top*) and small (*bottom*) infarcts are shown. CK, creatine kinase; IRA, infarct related artery; LAD, left anterior descending coronary artery; LCX, left circumflex coronary artery; MB, creatine kinase MB isoenzyme; MI, myocardial infarction; RCA, right coronary artery. (Modified with permission from Wu E, Judd RM, Vargas JD, et al. Visualisation of presence, location, and transmural extent of healed Q-wave and non-Q-wave myocardial infarction. *Lancet.* 2001;357:21-28.)

in contractile function after revascularization. However, data from case reports and a pilot study indicate that thinning should not be equated with the absence of viability, and that in some patients these regions can improve after revascularization. Additional studies will be needed to elucidate these provocative initial findings.

Recent work demonstrated that the presence of unrecognized myocardial scarring detected by DEMRI was associated with poor outcomes, even after accounting for common clinical, angiographic, and functional predictors. Additional investigation is needed to determine the full prognostic significance of DEMRI findings.

## Heart Failure and Cardiomyopathies

In patients with heart failure, it is important to determine the etiology of heart failure to appropriately plan therapy and provide prognostic information. The utility of DEMRI in the setting of cardiomyopathy is based on the understanding that rather than simply measuring viability, the presence and pattern of hyperenhancement (nonviable myocardium) hold additional information (**Fig. 6-5**). A stepwise algorithm has been proposed (**Fig. 6-6**):

1. The presence or absence of hyperenhancement is determined. In patients with severe cardiomyopathy but without hyperenhancement, the diagnosis of idiopathic dilated cardiomyopathy should be strongly considered.

2. If hyperenhancement is present, the location and distribution of hyperenhancement should be classified as a CAD or non-CAD pattern.

3. If hyperenhancement is present in a non-CAD pattern, further classification should be considered.

**Dilated Cardiomyopathy** The clinical presentation of ischemic and non-ischemic dilated cardiomyopathy (DCM) can be indistinguishable. However, chronic ischemic

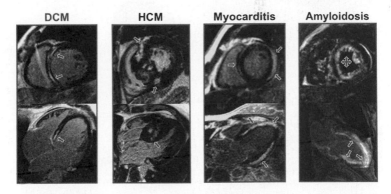

**FIGURE 6-5.** Representative delayed enhancement images in patients with various non-ischemic cardiomyopathies. The hyperenhancement patterns in all patients are distinctly non–coronary artery disease (CAD) type. Dilated cardiomyopathy (DCM): *Arrows* point to a linear stripe of hyperenhancement that is limited to the midwall of the interventricular septum. Hypertrophic cardiomyopathy (HCM): *Arrows* point to multiple foci of hyperenhancement, which are predominantly midmyocardial in location and occur in the hypertrophied septum and not in the lateral left ventricle (LV) free wall. The junctions of the right ventricle free wall and interventricular septum are commonly involved. Myocarditis: *Arrows* point to 2 separate regions of hyperenhancement: a linear midwall stripe in the interventricular septum and a large confluent region affecting the epicardial half of the LV lateral wall. Amyloidosis: *Arrows* point to hyperenhancement affecting the subendocardial half of the myocardial wall diffusely throughout the entire LV.

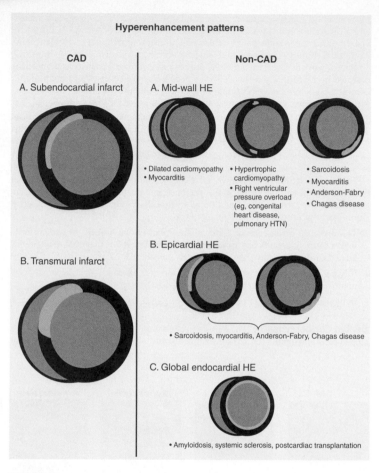

**FIGURE 6-6.** Hyperenhancement (HE) patterns that may be encountered in clinical practice. Because myocardial necrosis due to coronary artery disease (CAD) progresses as a *wavefront* from the subendocardium to the epicardium, HE (if present) should always involve the subedocardium in patients with ischemic disease. Isolated midwall or epicardial HE strongly suggests a non-ischemic etiology. Additionally, endocardial HE that occurs globally (ie, throughout the left ventricle) is uncommon, even with diffuse CAD, and therefore a non-ischemic etiology should be considered. HTN, hypertension. (Reproduced with permission from Shah DJ, Kim RJ. Magnetic resonance of myocardial viability. In: Edelman RR, ed. *Clinical Magnetic Resonance Imaging.* 3rd ed. New York, NY: Elsevier; 2005.)

cardiomyopathy demonstrates myocardial scarring consistent with prior infarcts. Conversely, prior infarction in DCM is uncommon. DEMRI hyperenhancement was the best clinical parameter in noninvasively discriminating ischemic from non-ischemic cardiomyopathy.

**Hypertrophic Cardiomyopathy**  CMR imaging is proving to be increasingly valuable in the clinical evaluation of hypertrophic cardiomyopathy (HCM). Echocardiography often underestimates the magnitude of hypertrophy in comparison with cine MRI.

This finding may be of clinical relevance since extreme hypertrophy (wall thickness ≥ 30 mm) is recognized as an important risk factor for sudden death. Because scarring is observed in the majority of patients with HCM, the clinical importance of detecting scar by DEMRI in HCM patients is currently being investigated by several groups. The presence of scarring can be helpful in distinguishing LV hypertrophy because of HCM from hypertension or physiologic hypertrophy. In the latter, unless there is coexisting CAD, scarring is usually absent (see Chapter 40).

**Anderson–Fabry Disease** Unlike patients with classic systemic Fabry disease, who present with multiple organ involvement, patients with the cardiac variant can manifest few or no symptoms and present only with idiopathic LV hypertrophy. In these patients, the cardiac phenotype is similar to that seen in HCM, and the diagnosis can be difficult. In these patients, hyperenhancement was most frequently observed in the basal inferolateral wall, and often the subendocardium was spared. Histologically, hyperenhanced regions appear to correspond to areas of replacement of viable myocardium with collagenous scar.

**Sarcoidosis** Autopsy studies have shown that cardiac involvement is found in 20% to 30% of patients with sarcoidosis. However, in vivo, cardiac involvement is recognized in < 10% of patients, as current diagnostic tools are insensitive. Underrecognition of cardiac involvement can be important clinically because sudden cardiac death is one of the most common causes of mortality in sarcoid patients. Hyperenhancement was found isolated to the mid-myocardial wall or epicardium, indicative of a non-CAD pattern. However, subendocardial or transmural hyperenhancement was also observed, mimicking the pattern of myocardial infarction.

**Amyloidosis** Cardiac amyloidosis is a common cause of restrictive cardiomyopathy and is associated with poor prognosis. DEMRI can demonstrate diffuse LV hyperenhancement in these patients. Although the subendocardium is preferentially involved, hyperenhancement is clearly in a non-CAD pattern because the distribution often is global and does not match any specific coronary artery perfusion territory. Practically speaking, it can be difficult to determine the optimal inversion time that will null normal myocardium, as there can be few areas that are completely normal. Therefore, it may be helpful to acquire multiple images using different inversion times. If a large portion of myocardium goes through the null point earlier than the blood pool, infiltrative involvement of the myocardium is highly likely.

**Myocarditis** The pattern of hyperenhancement observed in myocarditis is an evolution from a focal to a disseminated process during the first 2 weeks of symptoms. Although some investigators have interpreted this finding as evidence that hyperenhancement in the setting of acute myocarditis can represent viable myocardium, a more likely explanation is that hyperenhanced regions decrease in size because the volume of nonviable myocardium shrinks. As part of the normal healing process, necrotic regions undergo involution as they remodel and are replaced by dense collagenous scar.

**Chagas' Disease** An inflammatory disease caused by the protozoan, *Trypanosoma cruzi*, Chagas' disease starts with an acute phase. Patients then remain asymptomatic for many years, and 20% eventually develop chronic heart failure. DEMRI demonstrated that the prevalence of myocardial scarring progressively increased from 20% in asymptomatic patients without structural heart disease by echocardiography to 100% in patients with left ventricular dysfunction and ventricular tachycardia. Scarring occurred most commonly in the LV apex and inferolateral wall. Both non-CAD (isolated epicardial or midwall involvement) and CAD-type (indistinguishable from prior myocardial infarction) scar patterns were observed.

**Arrhythmogenic Right Ventricular Cardiomyopathy** Traditionally, a major focus in the evaluation of arrhythmogenic right ventricular cardiomyopathy (ARVC) by CMR has been to identify fatty infiltration of RV myocardium using spin-echo sequences. However, there is growing realization that this focus can be misplaced because of technical as well as physiologic reasons. The primary goal of the CMR-imaging examination should be to determine global and regional RV morphology and function. Cine imaging should be performed, with high spatial and temporal resolution and complete anatomic coverage including the RV outflow tract.

## Hemodynamics

**Atrial Septal Defect** CMR-imaging evaluation of atrial septal defect (ASD) has focused on hemodynamic severity as measured indirectly by VENC MRI of the pulmonary artery and aorta (ie, Qp/Qs). From the *en face* view, the rim of tissue separating the ASD from the base of the aorta (retroaortic rim), tricuspid valve, venae cavae, and coronary sinus can be viewed from a single-image plane. Flow across the ASD can also be measured directly from the *en face* view by VENC MRI. Failure to capture the optimal *en face* view, however, leads less accurate measurements than measuring flow in the pulmonary artery and aorta.

**Valvular Lesions** Measurements of aortic valve area in aortic stenosis assessed by planimetry on cine MRI agree with those values obtained by echocardiography and cardiac catheterization. Planimetry for valve area is performed on cine MRI with higher spatial and temporal resolution than usual for standard imaging. On cine MRI, regurgitant jets appear as signal voids associated with nonlaminar flow (turbulence, acceleration, etc). Similar to echocardiography, the size and extent of the regurgitant jet can be used to semiquantitatively grade the severity of regurgitation. For quantitative assessment of regurgitation, the regurgitation fraction can be calculated from data derived from VENC MRI sometimes in combination with cine MRI. For example, with MR the regurgitant volume can be obtained by subtracting the effective forward flow across the proximal ascending aorta from the diastolic inflow across the mitral valve from 2 separate through-plane VENC MRI acquisitions.

## Pericardial Disease and Cardiac Masses

**Constrictive Pericarditis** Older CMR sequences could accurately determine the thickness of the pericardium, thereby was helpful in confirming the diagnosis of constrictive pericarditis, if the pericardial thickening was found to be extreme (> 5 mm). Newer real-time cine MRI can be used to demonstrate increased ventricular interdependence, a hemodynamic hallmark of pericardial constriction. Specifically, abnormal ventricular septal motion toward the left ventricle in early diastole is seen during the onset of inspiration. Although the number of patients who have been studied is quite small, this finding appears helpful in distinguishing between constrictive pericarditis and restrictive cardiomyopathy.

**Pericardial Effusion** Both loculated and circumferential pericardial effusions are readily identified by CMR imaging. Simple (transudate) effusions typically appear bright and homogenous on T2-weighted images and dark on T1-weighted images. Complex effusions can appear heterogeneous and darker on T2 imaging.

**Masses** In the past, characterization of cardiac masses by CMR imaging focused primarily on comparing image intensities on T1-, T2-, and proton-density–weighted images. Presently, a typical protocol for the evaluation of a cardiac mass should consist of multiple pulse sequences where the aim is to assess morphology, motion, perfusion, and delayed enhancement, in addition to inherent differences in T1 and T2. For example, perfusion MRI can demonstrate increased vascularity, which can be prominent in malignancies such as angiosarcoma; DEMRI can identify areas of tissue necrosis within the core of a malignant tumor, which appear as areas of hyperenhancement.

**Left Ventricular Thrombus** Although most common in the LV apex, thrombus can occur elsewhere, with predilection for locations with stagnant blood flow such as adjacent to akinetic, infarcted myocardium. The presence of LV thrombus can be apparent on cine MRI, if the thrombus is clearly intracavitary. However, layered mural thrombus can be difficult to detect because image intensity differences between thrombus and myocardium are minimal. Recent studies suggest that DEMRI following contrast administration can be an improved method for detecting LV thrombus. The basic principle utilized is that thrombus is avascular and has essentially no contrast uptake. Thus, it should be easily distinguished as a nonenhancing defect surrounded by bright ventricular blood pool and contrast-enhanced myocardium.

## SUGGESTED READINGS

Daubert MA, Poon M, Budoff MJ. Computed tomography of the heart. In: Fuster V, Walsh RA, Harrington RA, et al, eds. *Hurst's The Heart*. 13th ed. New York, NY: McGraw-Hill. 2011;22:599-630.

Kim HW, Farzaneh-Far A, Klem I, Rehwald W, Kim RJ. Magnetic imaging resonance of the heart. In: Fuster V, Walsh RA, Harrington RA, et al, eds. *Hurst's The Heart*. 13th ed. New York, NY: McGraw-Hill. 2011;23:631-666.

Budoff MJ, Achenbach S, Blumenthal RS, et al. Assessment of coronary artery disease by cardiac computed tomography: a scientific statement from the American Heart Association Committee on Cardiovascular Imaging and Intervention, Council on Cardiovascular Radiology and Intervention, and Committee on Cardiac Imaging, Council on Clinical Cardiology. *Circulation*. 2006;114:1761-1791.

Detrano R, Guerci AD, Carr JJ, et al. Coronary calcium as a predictor of coronary events in four racial or ethnic groups. *N Engl J Med*. 2008;358:1336-1345.

Fuster V, Kim RJ. Frontiers in cardiovascular magnetic resonance. *Circulation*. 2005;112:135-144.

Hendel RC, Patel MR, Kramer CM, et al. ACCF/ACR/SCCT/SCMR/ASNC/NASCI/SCAI/SIR 2006 appropriateness criteria for cardiac computed tomography and cardiac magnetic resonance imaging: a report of the American College of Cardiology Foundation Quality Strategic Directions Committee Appropriateness Criteria Working Group, American College of Radiology, Society of Cardiovascular Computed Tomography, Society for Cardiovascular Magnetic Resonance, American Society of Nuclear Cardiology, North American Society for Cardiac Imaging, Society for Cardiovascular Angiography and Interventions, and Society of Interventional Radiology. *J Am Coll Cardiol*. 2006;48:1475-1497.

Kim RJ, Wu E, Rafael A, et al. The use of contrast-enhanced magnetic resonance imaging to identify reversible myocardial dysfunction. *N Engl J Med*. 2000;343:1445-1453.

# CHAPTER 7
# CARDIAC CATHETERIZATION AND CORONARY ANGIOGRAPHY

Morton J. Kern and Spencer B. King III

## INDICATIONS AND CONTRAINDICATIONS FOR CATHETERIZATION

The benefits need to outweigh the inherent risks of any invasive procedure, and such risk-benefit relationship must be carefully evaluated in each patient. Cardiac catheterization is an invasive testing modality used to evaluate and diagnose conditions such as coronary artery disease (CAD), cardiomyopathies, pulmonary hypertension, and valvular and congenital heart abnormalities by catheter-based hemodynamic monitoring and contrast angiography. **Table 7-1** lists the indications for coronary angiography. Given the invasive nature of cardiac catheterization, it is equally important to consider contraindications to the procedure. Patient refusal is the only absolute contraindication; however, there are a number of relative contraindications. **Table 7-2** lists the contraindications to cardiac catheterization.

## ◼ PATIENT PREPARATION

Prior to the study, a complete explanation of the risks and benefits of the procedure should be given to the patient. The risk of complications should be addressed. Overall risk of a major complication is less than 2%, the risk of death is 0.11%, myocardial infarction 0.05%, and cerebrovascular accident 0.07%. The risk of a vascular complication was found to be 0.43%, contrast reaction 0.37%, and a hemodynamic complication 0.26%. Prior to the procedure or administration of any sedation, a written consent must be signed by a competent patient or legal patient representative (if the patient is not able to sign). Some patients, such as the elderly, those requiring an urgent or emergent procedure, patients with cardiogenic shock or acute myocardial infarction, and patients with renal insufficiency or congestive heart failure, are at a higher risk of developing complications. In patients with renal insufficiency or a known allergy to iodine contrast, treatment prior to catheterization minimizes the risk associated with the procedure and medical condition. **Table 7-3** lists specific pretreatment regimens used.

## ◼ VASCULAR ACCESS

### Arterial Access

Percutaneous arterial access may be obtained from either the upper or lower extremities. In the upper extremity, radial, brachial, or even axillary arteries are utilized, while the common femoral artery is the preferred site in the lower extremity.

**TABLE 7-1.** Class I Recommendations for Coronary Angiography

|  | Level of Evidence |
|---|---|
| **Stable Angina or Asymptomatic Individuals** | |
| 1.   CCS class III and IV angina on medical treatment. | B |
| 2.   High-risk criteria on noninvasive testing regardless of anginal severity. | A |
| 3.   Patients who have been successfully resuscitated from sudden cardiac death or have sustained (> 30 s) monomorphic ventricular tachycardia or nonsustained (< 30 s) polymorphic ventricular tachycardia. | B |
| **Unstable Coronary Syndromes** | |
| 1.   High or intermediate risk for adverse outcome in patients with unstable angina refractory to initial adequate medical therapy or with recurrent symptoms after initial stabilization. Emergent catheterization is recommended. | B |
| 2.   High risk for adverse outcome in patients with unstable angina. Urgent catheterization is recommended. | B |
| 3.   High- or intermediate-risk unstable angina that stabilizes after initial treatment. | A |
| 4.   Initially low short-term risk unstable angina that is subsequently high risk on noninvasive testing. | B |
| 5.   Suspected Prinzmetal's angina. | C |
| **During Initial Management of Acute MI (MI Suspected and ST Elevation or BBB Present): Coronary Angiography Coupled With Intent to Perform Primary PTCA** | |
| 1.   As an alternative to thrombolytic therapy in patients who can undergo angioplasty of the infarct artery within 12 h of the onset of symptoms or beyond 12 h if ischemic symptoms persist, if performed in a timely fashion[a] by individuals skilled in the procedure and supported by experienced personnel in an appropriate laboratory environment. | A |
| 2.   In patients who are within 36 h of an acute ST elevation/Q-wave or new LBBB MI who develop cardiogenic shock, are < 75 years of age, and in whom revascularization can be performed within 18 h of the onset of shock. | A |
| **During Risk-Stratification Phase of MI (Patients With All Types of MI)** | |
| Isclschhemia at low levels of exercise with ECG changes (1-mm ST-segment depression or other predictors of adverse outcome) and/or imaging abnormalities. | B |
| **Perioperative Evaluation Before (or After) Noncardiac Surgery: Patients With Suspected or Known CAD** | |
| 1.   Evidence for high risk of adverse outcome based on noninvasive test results. | C |
| 2.   Angina unresponsive to adequate medical therapy. | C |
| 3.   Unstable angina, particularly when facing intermediate- or high-risk noncardiac surgery. | C |
| 4.   Equivocal noninvasive test result in a high-clinical-risk patient undergoing high-risk surgery. | C |

*(continued)*

**TABLE 7-1.** Class I Recommendations for Coronary Angiography

| | Level of Evidence |
|---|---|
| **Patients With Valvular Heart Disease** | |
| 1. Before valve surgery or balloon valvotomy in an adult with chest discomfort, ischemia by noninvasive imaging, or both. | B |
| 2. Before valve surgery in an adult free of chest pain but of substantial age and/or with multiple risk factors for coronary disease. | C |
| 3. Infective endocarditis with evidence of coronary embolization C. | C |
| **Patients With CHF** | |
| 1. CHF due to systolic dysfunction with angina or with regional wall motion abnormalities and/or scintigraphic evidence of reversible myocardial ischemia when revascularization is being considered. | B |
| 2. Before cardiac transplantation. | C |
| 3. CHF secondary to postinfarction ventricular aneurysm or other mechanical complications of MI. | C |

BBB, bundle-branch block; CAD, coronary artery disease; CCS, Canadian Cardiovascular Society; CHF, congestive heart failure; ECG, electrocardiogram; LBBB, left bundle-branch block; MI, myocardial infarction; PTCA, percutaneous transluminal coronary angioplasty.

[a]Performance standard: within 90 minutes. Individuals who perform > 75 PTCA procedures per year. Centers that perform > 200 PTCA procedures per year and have cardiac surgical capability.

Data from the American College of Cardiology: Scanlon PJ, Faxon DP, Audet AM, et al. ACC/AHA Guidelines for Coronary Angiography: A report of the American College of Cardiology/American Heart Association Task Force on Practice Guidelines (Committee on Coronary Angiography). *J Am Coll Cardiol*. 1999;33:1756-1824. (See also Chapter 59.)

**TABLE 7-2.** Relative Contraindications for Cardiac Catheterization

Acute renal failure
Chronic renal failure secondary to diabetes
Active gastrointestinal bleeding
Unexplained fever, which may be due to infection
Untreated active infection Acute stroke
Severe anemia
Severe uncontrolled hypertension
Severe symptomatic electrolyte imbalance
Severe lack of cooperation by patient due to psychologic or severe systemic illness
Severe concomitant illness that drastically shortens life expectancy or increases risk of therapeutic interventions
Refusal of patient to consider definitive therapy such as PTCA, CABG, or valve replacement
Digitalis intoxication
Documented anaphylactoid reaction to angiographic contrast media
Severe peripheral vascular disease limiting vascular access
Decompensated congestive heart failure or acute pulmonary edema
Severe coagulopathy
Aortic valve endocarditis

CABG, coronary artery bypass graft; PTCA, percutaneous transluminal coronary angioplasty.

Modified and reproduced with permission from the American College of Cardiology: Scanlon PJ, Faxon DP, Audet AM, et al. ACC/AHA Guidelines for Coronary Angiography: A Report of the American College of Cardiology/American Heart Association Task Force on Practice Guidelines (Committee on Coronary Angiography). *J Am Coll Cardiol*. 1999;33:1756-1824.

**TABLE 7-3.** Pretreatment Regimens for Patients Undergoing Cardiac Catheterization/ Coronary Angiography

**Patients With Renal Insufficiency**

Withholding nephrotoxic medications prior to the procedure and until renal function normalizes following the procedure (eg, metformin, NSAIDs).

Hydration

Isotonic solution (normal saline or sodium bicarbonate) given optimally for 12 h before the procedure and continued for 6-12 h after, with a goal of 1 L to be given before the procedure and rates of 100-150 mL/h.

N-Acetylcysteine

600-mg orally dosed BID for 2 doses prior to and after catheterization.

Other considerations

Use of iso-osmolar contrast.

Adjusting the dose of contrast received to the renal function.

MRCD (maximum radiographic contrast dose) = 5 mL × weight (kg)/serum creatinine.

**Patients With Radiographic Contrast Allergy**

Corticosteroids

Oral corticosteroids (methylprednisone 32 mg or prednisone 50 mg) given 6-24 h and 2 h prior to contrast. Two or 3 doses may be given. Two-dose regimen is given 12 and 2 h prior to contrast. Three-dose regimen is given 13, 7, and 1 h prior to contrast administration.

$H_1$ antagonists

Diphenhydramine 50 mg IV/IM/PO given 1 h prior to contrast.

Data compiled from Schweiger MJ, Chambers CE, Davidson CJ, et al. Prevention of contrast induced nephropathy: recommendations for the high-risk patient undergoing cardiovascular procedures. *Catheter Cardiovasc Interv.* 2007;69:135-140; and Tramer MR, von Elm E, Loubeyre P, et al. Pharmacological prevention of serious anaphylactic reactions due to iodinated contrast media: systemic review. *BMJ.* 2006;333:675-681.

The pulsation of the femoral artery is palpated 1 to 2 cm below the inguinal ligament. This site is proximal to the bifurcation of the superficial femoral and profunda arteries.

The inguinal ligament courses from the anterior superior iliac spine to the superior pubic ramus (**Fig. 7-1**). The inguinal ligament should be used as a landmark, not the inguinal crease, as the skin crease may be misleading especially in obese patients. The site of anticipated arterial puncture may be confirmed with fluoroscopy of the right groin with a metal clamp overlying the proposed site of puncture. The site of arterial puncture should overlie the middle of the head of the femur, as this location will allow for ideal compression of the arteriotomy site during manual compression. After administration of 10 to 20 mL of 1% lidocaine, an 18-gauge introducer needle is passed into the skin and directed at a 30-degree angle toward the palpated femoral artery pulsation. Before inserting the needle, a small skin incision may be made with a scalpel to facilitate passage of the needle through the skin. A single-wall arterial puncture should be made, with blood return through the needle being pulsatile and brisk. Then a 0.035-in J-tip guidewire is carefully advanced through the needle. If resistance is felt during this maneuver, the wire should be withdrawn, intraluminal position of the needle tip should be reconfirmed by pulsatile blood flow, and readvancement of the wire should be performed under fluoroscopic guidance. Once the wire is advanced up to the level of the iliac artery or aorta, the needle is removed and replaced, over the guidewire, with an appropriately sized vascular sheath. The size of the sheath used is determined by the size of the catheters being used. For diagnostic coronary angiography, catheters with diameters varying from 4 to 6 Fr

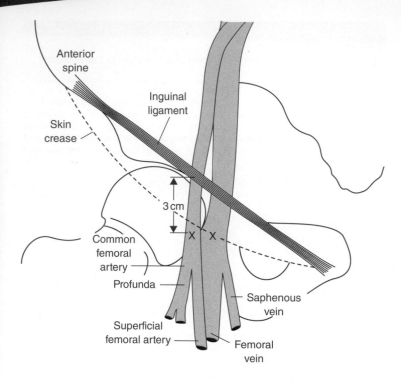

**FIGURE 7-1.** The right femoral artery and vein course underneath the inguinal ligament, which connects the anterior-superior iliac spine and pubic tubercle. The arterial skin incision (indicated by 10) should be placed approximately 3 cm below the inguinal ligament and directly over the femoral artery pulsation. The venous skin incision should be made at the same level but approximately 1 finger-breadth medial. (Reproduced with permission from Kim D, Orron DE, Skillman JJ, et al: Role of superficial femoral artery puncture in the development of pseudoaneurysm and arteriovenous fistula complicating percutaneous transfemoral cardiac catheterization, Cathet Cardiovasc Diagn 1992 Feb;25(2):91-97.)

are commonly used, although complex anatomic scenarios may require 7- or 8-Fr catheters for extra support.

Radial artery access allows for more rapid patient ambulation and is associated with fewer bleeding complications. Adoption of this technique is somewhat limited, because coronary catheterization is technically more challenging from the upper extremity. Prior to obtaining vascular access in the radial artery, patency of the palmar arch needs to be assessed, as occlusion of the radial artery during or following the procedure can lead to digit injury if the palmar arch in not intact. Patency should be assessed with a modified Allen test using a pulse oximeter. This approach places a pulse oximeter on the thumb while compressing the radial artery. The presence of an arterial waveform, even one with reduced amplitude or delayed reappearance, and a hemoglobin saturation of greater than 90% (Barbeau types A, B, C) confirm the adequacy of palmar arch blood flow. Following confirmation of the palmar arch flow, the radial artery is accessed 1 to 2 cm proximal to the radial styloid with a 4-Fr radial artery micropuncture kit. The radial artery, particularly in large males, can accommodate up to a 7- or 8-Fr vascular sheath. We recommend use of a sheath with a hydrophilic coating, and infusion of heparin and intra-arterial vasodilators immediately after access is confirmed to avoid spasm and thrombosis and facilitate removal of the sheath.

## Venous Access

Femoral vein access is obtained approximately 1 cm medial and 1 cm inferior to the site of arterial access. An 18-gauge needle is used with a syringe attached to its hub. Following a small skin incision, the needle is advanced at a 30- to 45-degree angle with slight suction applied to the syringe. Dark venous blood should be easily aspirated upon entering the vein. A 0.035-in J-tipped guidewire is the advanced, and following removal of the needle, a vascular access sheath is placed into the vein over the guidewire.

## ■ HEMOSTASIS

Hemostasis following the procedure is extremely important. The most common complications of diagnostic coronary angiography are associated with the vascular entry site.

## Manual Pressure

Manual pressure is applied to an area 3 finger-breadths above the site of skin puncture. For venous access, light manual pressure applied for 5 to 10 minutes following sheath removal is usually sufficient to effect hemostasis. For arterial access, firm manual pressure is applied following sheath removal over the area of femoral artery pulsation and arterial puncture, usually 2 finger-breadths above the site of skin puncture. Pressure should be initially firm enough to obliterate the pedal pulse and is slowly eased after 10 minutes. Duration of manual pressure is dependent on the size of the sheath and use of anticoagulant or antithrombotic medications. A useful rule of thumb is that manual pressure should be applied for 3 minutes for every French size; for example, a 6-Fr hemostasis sheath would require 18 minutes of manual compression, with longer hold times being required for patients who are anticoagulated. The application of manual pressure should not be interrupted. If bleeding is noted after releasing the pressure, the manual compression process must be restarted from time zero. Pressure may be fully released only after the predetermined amount of time has elapsed.

## Vascular Closure Devices

There are a number of devices available on the market today to facilitate arterial hemostasis following completion of a cardiac catheterization. Closure devices allow for more rapid ambulation of the patient, but have not been shown to lower bleeding or vascular complications. These devices should be used with extreme caution in patients with a low arterial puncture, below the bifurcation of the femoral artery, and in patients with peripheral arterial disease.

## ■ HEMODYNAMIC MEASUREMENTS

During a right heart catheterization, hemodynamic measurements, such as direct measurements of blood pressure, are taken from the right atrium, ventricle, and pulmonary artery and in the wedge position in a pulmonary artery. Hemodynamic measurements are important in the assessment of fluid status, evaluation of valvular lesions or shunt fractions, and calculation of cardiac output. A right heart

**TABLE 7-4.** Normal Values Associated With Right Heart Catheterization

| | |
|---|---|
| Right atrium | 8-10 mm Hg |
| Right ventricle | 25/4 mm Hg |
| Pulmonary artery | 25/9 mm Hg |
| Pulmonary capillary wedge pressure | 9 mm Hg |
| Cardiac output | 3-7 L/min |
| Cardiac index | 2.5-4 L/min/m$^2$ |
| Systemic vascular resistance | 900-1300 dyne·s/cm$^5$ |
| Pulmonary vascular resistance | 155-250 dyne·s/cm$^5$ |

catheterization is performed, by accessing a central vein, usually the femoral or internal jugular vein, advancing a balloon-tipped catheter, like a Swan-Ganz catheter, to the right atrium. Care is taken to steer the catheter from the right atrium into the right ventricle and with a clockward turn advance the catheter across the pulmonic valve and into the pulmonary artery. A 0.021-in wire may be necessary to support advancement of the catheter into the pulmonary artery. Further advancement of the catheter will allow the inflated balloon of the catheter tip to wedge into a smaller branch of the pulmonary artery, thereby transducing an approximation of the left atrial pressure via the end hole of the catheter.

**Table 7-4** lists normal values associated with a right heart catheterization.

In addition to obtaining pressure measurements, which can aid in assessing fluid status of a patient, blood samples are obtained from the superior and inferior venae cavae, right atrium and ventricle, and the pulmonary artery and in the wedge position. Hemoglobin saturation measurements obtained from the blood sample can identify and assess an intracardiac shunt, and can be used in the calculation of cardiac output and systemic and pulmonary vascular resistance.

## Cardiac Output and Vascular Resistance

Cardiac output, which is the volume of blood expelled from the heart over a period of time, may be calculated by 2 methods in the cardiac catheterization laboratory: the thermal dilution method and using the Fick calculation. The thermal dilution method uses a known volume of saline, 10 mL, at room temperature, which is rapidly injected into the proximal port of a pulmonary artery catheter. A thermistor at the distal tip of the catheter records the temperature decrease as the fluid is moved past the catheter by the pumping action of the heart. The computer in the catheterization lab, using the thermodilution equation, will calculate a cardiac output. In general, thermodilution cardiac output measurements may have an error of 5% to 10% even when performed carefully. The other common method to calculate cardiac output is the Fick equation. For the Fick equation and shunt calculations, the patient should not be receiving supplemental oxygen. The Fick equation is as follows:

$$\text{Cardiac Output} = \frac{O_2 \text{ Consumption (mL/min)}}{(\text{Arterial Saturation} - \text{Mixed Venous Saturation}) \times \text{Hgb} \times 1.35 \times 10}$$

$O_2$ consumption may be measured; however, many catheterization laboratories will assume an $O_2$ consumption of 125 mL/m$^2$ in adults and 110 mL/m$^2$ in older patients. Mixed venous saturation is calculated using the hemoglobin saturations from the superior vena cava (SVC) and inferior vena cava (IVC). IVC blood has a higher hemoglobin oxygen saturation than blood from the SVC because the kidneys use less oxygen relative to their blood flow:

$$\text{Mixed Venous Saturation} = \frac{2\,\text{SVC} + \text{IVC}}{3}$$

A normal mixed venous saturation is 60% to 80%. The cardiac output may be corrected for body size and expressed as the cardiac index:

$$\text{Cardiac Index} = \frac{\text{Cardiac Output}}{\text{Body Surface Area (m}^2)}$$

With the cardiac output calculated, systemic vascular resistance and pulmonary vascular resistance can be calculated:

$$\text{Systemic Vascular Resistance} = \frac{\text{Mean Arterial Pressure} - \text{Central Venous Pressure}}{\text{Cardiac Output}}$$

$$\text{Pulmonary Vascular Resistance} = \frac{\text{Mean Pulmonary Artery Pressure} - \text{Left Atrial Pressure}}{\text{Cardiac Output}}$$

## Shunt and Valve Area Calculations

Hemoglobin oxygen saturations are used to assess for the presence of an intracardiac shunt. A left-to-right shunt is suspected when >6% difference is noted between the mixed venous and pulmonary artery saturations. A simplified formula for the calculation of the flow ratio, between systemic and pulmonary systems, can be used to estimate the magnitude of a left-to-right shunt:

$$\frac{\text{QP}}{\text{QS}} = \frac{(\text{S}_{\text{AO}_2} - \text{M}_{\text{VO}_2})}{(\text{P}_{\text{VO}_2} - \text{P}_{\text{AO}_2})}$$

A shunt ratio less than 1.5 denotes a small left-to-right shunt. A shunt ratio greater than 2.0 denotes a large left-to-right shunt and is considered sufficient evidence to recommend repair of the defect.

Direct pressure measurements can also be used to calculate stenotic valve orifice area. By using pressure measurements proximal and distal to the stenotic valve and 1 of either 2 formulas, one can estimate the valve area of a stenotic aortic or mitral valve.

The Gorlin formula is as follows:

$$A = \frac{\text{CO}/(\text{DFP or SEP})(\text{HR})}{44.3C\sqrt{\Delta P}}$$

where A is the valve area (cm²), CO is cardiac output (cm³/min), DFP is the diastolic filling period (s/beat) for mitral valve areas, SEP is the systolic ejection period (s/beat) for aortic valve areas, HR is heart rate (beats/min), C is an empirical constant (0.85 for mitral valve calculations), and P is the pressure gradient. A simplified formula developed by Hakki and associates is also available:

$$A = \frac{\text{CO}}{\sqrt{\Delta P}}$$

# ■ CORONARY ANGIOGRAPHY

Coronary angiography remains the gold standard diagnostic modality to detect coronary artery disease. Angiography provides a visual representation of vascular structures. During a cardiac catheterization, the patient is placed in a supine position on the catheterization table. At the cranial end is the x-ray source below the table and the image intensifier, or digital flat panel detector in newer machines, above the table. These components move in tandem but in opposite directions allowing for the imaging of coronary arteries and other vascular structures in multiple views. The orientation of the view obtained is described by the detector's position relative to the patient. Cranial angulation means the detector is tilted toward the patient's head and caudal means the detector is angled toward the feet. In right anterior oblique (RAO) position, the detector is tilted to the patient's right side; in left anterior oblique (LAO) position, the detector is tilted to the patient's left side. Radiopaque contrast is used to opacify the coronary arteries. The contrast is selectively injected into the coronary arteries through specially preformed catheters. Initially, cardiac catheterization was performed via brachial cutdown using a single catheter (Sones) that was maneuvered to engage both right and left coronary artery systems as well as perform ventriculography. Subsequently, numerous preformed catheters have been developed to cannulate the left and right coronary arteries (**Fig. 7-2**). The most commonly used are the Judkins left and right catheters. Other commonly used catheters are Amplatz right or left, and multipurpose catheters. The catheters are advanced from the site of vascular access over a 0.035-in J-tipped guidewire to the ascending aorta. Basic principles of optimal coronary angiography include having a coaxial alignment of the catheter and coronary ostium, full opacification of the coronary lumen, no vessel or other structures (catheters, ECG patch, wires, etc) overlapping the coronary image, and a minimum of 2 orthogonal projections for each vessel with minimal foreshortening of the target segments.

## Left Coronary Artery

The left coronary artery originates from the left sinus of Valsalva near the sinotubular ridge. The left main coronary artery (LM) bifurcates into the left anterior descending (LAD) artery, which courses in the intraventricular groove giving off septal perforators and diagonal branches that supply the lateral wall, and the left circumflex (LCx) artery, which courses in the atrioventricular (AV) groove and gives off obtuse marginal branches supplying the lateral and posterolateral walls. The LM can be cannulated in most patients with a Judkins left catheter with a 4-cm curve (JL 4) by advancing the catheter down from just distal of the sinotubular junction, while viewing the catheter in a RAO or LAO angulation. The JL 4 catheter should advance easily and the tip will "jump" after passing the sinotubular ridge, placing the catheter tip at the ostium of the LM. In imaging the left coronary artery system, cranial images are able to visualize the mid and distal LAD segments, and caudal images are for the LM, LCx, and proximal LAD segments, with RAO and LAO angulation used to minimize overlap and better visualize specific segments of the artery. The initial image taken is in the RAO/caudal projection. This view allows for visualization of the entire LM and proximal segments of the LAD/LCx vessels, which represent >70% of the myocardium. RAO/cranial and LAO/cranial projections demonstrate the mid to distal LAD well, with a straight lateral (90-degree LAO) angulation being used to visualize an LAD that is overlapped in other traditional views. Either RAO or LAO caudal projections allow for visualization of the LCx as well as the left main and proximal LAD.

## Right Coronary Artery

The right coronary artery arises from the right sinus of Valsalva, near the sinotubular junction; however, its position of origin can be variable within the sinus. The artery

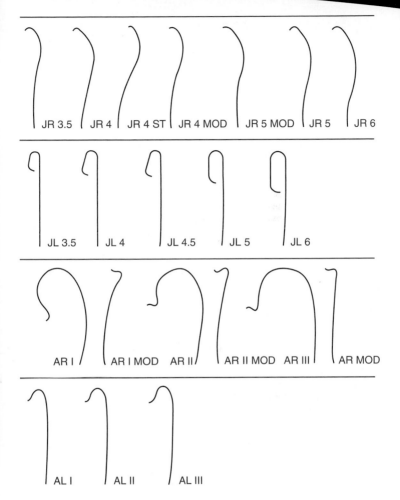

**FIGURE 7-2.** A schematic diagram demonstrating the Judkins and Amplatz variety of left and right coronary catheters, and their differing sizes.

courses along the right AV groove to the posterior LV wall, where in 85% of patients it will supply the posterior descending artery (PDA), which gives off perforating branches supplying the basal and posterior third of the septum, AV nodal artery, and posterolateral left ventricular (PLLV) branches. Dominance of the coronary arteries is ascribed to the vessel from which the PDA, PLLV, and AV nodal artery arise. In a right-dominant system, the PDA, PLLV, and AV nodal artery arise from the RCA; and in a left-dominant system they arise from the LCX. The LAO/cranial view can be used to easily determine if the LCX is dominant.

The RCA is cannulated by advancing a Judkins right catheter with a 4-cm curve (JR 4) to the cusps of the aortic valve. Gently withdrawing the catheter, while making a clockwise rotation, turns the tip of the catheter anteriorly and causes it to cannulate the right coronary artery. RAO or LAO projections demonstrate the proximal

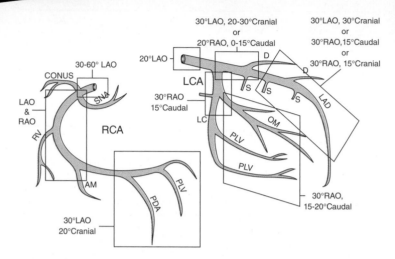

**FIGURE 7-3.** A schematic representation of the right and left coronary arteries. Approximate frontal and sagittal plane projections and angulations for visualization of various portions of the coronary arteries are indicated. (Reproduced with permission from Pepine CJ, Hill JA, Lambert CR. Coronary angiography. In: Pepine CJ, ed. *Diagnostic and Therapeutic Coronary Catheterization.* 3rd ed. Baltimore, MD: Lippincott Williams & Wilkins; 1998.)

portions of the RCA. However, the distal vessel and bifurcation of the PDA and PLLV branches are best visualized with a cranial angulation.

**Figure 7-3** demonstrates views useful in assessing specific segments of each coronary artery.

## Bypass Grafts

Saphenous vein grafts and radial artery grafts mostly originate off of the ascending aorta. Occasionally radiopaque markers are sutured near the site of implantation marking their location. The grafts can be engaged using a JR 4 catheter. Grafts are arranged, proximal to distal, on the ascending aorta in the following order: grafts to RCA, grafts to LAD, then diagonals, and then grafts to obtuse marginal branches. Grafts to the RCA or LCX branches should be imaged in an RAO caudal and LAO cranial projection. This will allow for simple identification of the native vessels supplied by the particular bypass graft. The internal mammary arteries, typically the left internal mammary artery (LIMA), are also used as bypass grafts, often to the LAD. The LIMA arises anteriorly from the caudal portion of the subclavian artery distal to the origin of the vertebral artery. It can be cannulated for selective angiography with a JR 4 catheter or with a specially formed IMA catheter. After the catheter is advanced to the distal subclavian artery over a 0.035-in J-tipped guidewire using an LAO view, the catheter is slowly withdrawn until it engages the IM artery. This maneuver is performed in the AP view. The preformed IMA catheter is frequently able to easily engage the left internal mammary artery.

## Left Ventriculography

Ventriculography is used when assessment of left ventricular wall motion or function is needed. An angled pigtail catheter is advanced to the aortic valve, and the catheter prolapsed across the valve leaflets. Occasionally a straight guidewire is needed to facilitate passage across a stenotic valve, but such a procedure should be performed by experienced operators because of the risk of coronary injury and cerebral embolic events. Once in the left ventricle, the catheter is positioned in a stable location to avoid induction of arrhythmias, including ventricular fibrillation. Contrast (at least 20 mL, optimal 30-40 mL) is injected into the ventricle by a power injector using a rate of 10 to 15 mL/s and 450 to 600 psi. A 30-degree RAO angulation will allow for visualization of the anterior and inferior walls as well as the left atrium. Mitral regurgitation is assessed by the amount of contrast visualized in the left atrium. A 60-degree LAO angulation is utilized to visualize septal and lateral walls, which are difficult to distinguish in RAO.

## Aortography

Aortography is used to visualize the aortic root, ascending aorta, and origin of the great vessels. A LAO of 30 to 45 degrees with 10-degree cranial orientation of the detector, with an injection of 40 to 60 mL of contrast injected at 20 mL/s at 600 psi, allows for opacification of the aorta to assess for aortic regurgitation, the width of the aortic root and ascending aorta, and origin of the great vessels. The use of digital subtraction might be useful. The patient should be instructed to hold his or her breath during this procedure so as to minimize motion artifact.

# FINAL REMARKS

The catheterization laboratory is a place for thoughtful, timely, and meticulous execution of procedures. Careful patient preparation and appropriate selection of devices are essential for successful outcomes. One must ensure that the catheterization laboratory is equipped with all necessary tools to treat potential complications prior to starting the procedure. Judicious manipulation of all intravascular devices and monitoring of the arterial pressure waveform and electrocardiography tracings are extremely important to avoid procedural complications. Gentle, slow, and purposeful movements of the catheter will usually engage the desired vessel. If a vessel is not engaged in the first attempt, return the catheter to a neutral position and repeat the maneuver once again. If you do not succeed in 3 or 4 attempts, exchange for a catheter with a different shape or curvature. Contrast should be restricted to the minimum necessary to obtain the diagnosis. Never inject contrast into an artery from which you see a damped waveform, as doing so could cause a dissection, or in the case of the RCA, ventricular fibrillation. The arterial sheath should be aspirated and subsequently flushed with heparinized saline following each catheter exchange, to avoid the formation of clots.

# SUGGESTED READINGS

Kern MJ, King SB III. Cardiac catheterization, cardiac angiography, and coronary blood flow and pressure measurements. In: Fuster V, Walsh R, Harrington RA, et al. *Hurst's The Heart*. 13th ed. New York, NY: McGraw-Hill; 2011;19:490-538.

Baim DS. Coronary angiography. In: Baim DS, ed. *Grossman's Cardiac Catheterization, Angiography, and Intervention*. 7th ed. Philadelphia, PA: Lippincott Williams & Wilkins; 2006.

Baim DS, Simon DI. Percutaneous approach, tncluding trans-septal and apical puncture. In: Baim DS, ed. *Grossman's Cardiac Catheterization, Angiography, and Intervention*. 7th ed. Philadelphia, PA: Lippincott Williams & Wilkins; 2006.

Barbeau GR, Arsenault F, Dugas L, et al. Evaluation of the ulnopalmar arterial arches with pulse oximetry and plethysmography: comparison with the Allen's test in 101 patients. *Am Heart J*. 2004;147:489-493.

Gorlin R, Gorlin G. Hydraulic formula for calculation of area of stenotic mitral valve, other cardiac valves and central circulatory shunts. *Am Heart J.* 1951;41:1.

Hakki AH, Iskandrian AS, Bemis CE, et al. A simplified valve formula for the calculation of stenotic cardiac valve areas. *Circulation.* 1981;63:1050-1055.

Pepine CJ, Hill JA, Lambert CR. Coronary angiography. In: Pepine CJ, ed. *Diagnostic and Therapeutic Cardiac Catheterization.* 3rd ed. Baltimore, MD: Lippincott Williams & Wilkins; 1998.

Scanlon PJ, Faxon DP, Auden AM, et al. A report of the American College of Cardiology/American Heart Association Task Force on the Practice Guideline (Committee on Coronary Angiography). Developed in collaboration with the Society for Cardiac Angiography and Interventions Committee members. ACC/AHA Guidelines for Coronary Angiography: executive summary and recommendations. *Circulation.* 1999;99:2345-2357.

Schweiger MJ, Chambers CE, Davidson CJ, et al. Prevention of contrast-induced nephropathy: recommendations for the high risk patient undergoing cardiovascular procedures. *Catheter Cardiovasc Interv.* 2007;69:135-140.

Tramer MR, von Elm E, Loubeyre P, et al. Pharmacological prevention of serious anaphylactic reactions due to iodinated contrast media: systemic review. *BMJ.* 2006;333:675-681.

# CHAPTER 8
# APPROACH TO THE PATIENT WITH CARDIAC ARRHYTHMIAS[a]

Eric N. Prystowsky and Richard I. Fogel

## HISTORY

It is imperative that a complete history of the patient's symptoms be obtained. Important elements include (1) documentation of initial onset of symptoms; (2) complete characterization of symptoms; (3) identifying conditions that appear to initiate symptoms; (4) duration of episodes; (5) frequency of episodes; (6) pattern of symptoms over time, for example, better or worse; (7) effect of any treatment; and (8) family history of a similar problem. It is also important to ascertain any pertinent past medical history. This might include history of myocardial infarction (MI), especially in a patient who presents with palpitations and syncope, or the recent initiation of an antihypertensive agent in a patient who now presents with dizzy spells.

## PHYSICAL EXAMINATION

Observations from the physical examination are helpful primarily to define whether cardiovascular disease is present. For example, in a patient who presents with dizzy spells or syncope, the presence of orthostatic hypotension, a carotid bruit, or decreased carotid pulses may be important findings that lead to a diagnosis of coronary artery disease. Most importantly, the presence of specific cardiac murmurs or an $S_3$ or $S_4$ gallop may direct the clinician toward a cardiac cause for the patient's symptoms. Also, pay attention to the patient's gender, age, and physiognomy. Paroxysmal supraventricular tachycardia (PSVT) that occurs in a 12-year-old boy is more likely caused by atrioventricular reentry tachycardia, whereas PSVT presenting in a 45-year-old woman more commonly is caused by atrioventricular (AV) node reentry.

### ■ SYNCOPE, PRESYNCOPE, DIZZINESS

Patients with syncope, presyncope, or dizziness are often referred to the electrophysiologist for evaluation for fear that the symptoms are caused by an arrhythmia. Unless an ECG rhythm strip is recorded at the time of the patient's event, it is

[a]Adapted from Chapter 36 by Eric N. Prystowsky and Richard I. Fogel in Fuster V, O'Rourke RA, Walsh RA, et al., eds. *Hurst's The Heart.* 12th ed. New York, NY: McGraw-Hill; 2008, with permission of authors and publisher.

impossible to positively eliminate an arrhythmic cause. Regardless, a detailed history typically points in the correct direction. The ECG may disclose many clues to the cause of syncope, including MI, cardiac hypertrophy, sinus node dysfunction, conduction abnormality, Wolff–Parkinson–White syndrome, long or short QT interval, or Brugada syndrome. Evaluation of the echocardiogram may lead to a variety of cardiac diagnoses (see Chapter 4).

Neurally mediated syncope is very common. Typically the patient is in an upright position, either sitting or standing, and may recount a feeling of being hot or warm with or without concomitant nausea prior to loss of consciousness. Sweating is a common feature, but the patient may state that it occurred on regaining consciousness rather than prior to syncope. Normally the patient is alert on regaining consciousness but may feel fatigued. Although patients often state that their heart was *pounding* or faster than usual on awakening, they do not give a history of a rapid regular pulse that persists for minutes after the event. This latter feature should direct one to a possible arrhythmic cause for syncope.

Cardiac syncope is often sudden in onset and frequently unaccompanied by any prodrome (eg, Stokes-Adams attack). In some circumstances patients relate a feeling of rapid palpitations prior to loss of consciousness, and these individuals should be evaluated for a cardiac arrhythmia regardless of whether heart disease is present. One should remember that rapid PSVT as well as ventricular tachycardia can cause syncope. Unfortunately, a sudden loss of consciousness without prodrome is not specific for an arrhythmia, and patients with an arrhythmia can present with some features of a vasovagal syncope.

For patients who present with dizziness or presyncope, it is important to distinguish between vertigo and true light-headedness. Ask patients whether they feel like the room is spinning or they are spinning, compared with a sensation that *the lights are going out* or they are about to lose consciousness. Cardiovascular syncope does not usually produce vertigo.

# ■ PALPITATIONS

Palpitations are described by patients in many ways, including skipped beats, a sudden thump, hard beating, fluttering in the chest, a jittery sensation, a rapid pulse, or as merely a vague feeling that their heart is irregular. The authors have noted that many patients equate a *strong heartbeat* with palpitations, and it is important to distinguish this from irregular heartbeats. A premature atrial or ventricular complex often cannot be felt by the patient, and what they experience is the strong heartbeat that follows the pause. It may be useful to tap out various cadences for the patient. For example, to distinguish between atrial fibrillation (AF) and PSVT, tap out a rapid, irregular cadence compared with a rapid regular cadence—patients often recognize one over the other. Similarly, tap out a cadence of extra beats with a pause. Palpitations are often more prominent at night, especially when patients lie on their left side.

Other historic features often tailor the initial workup. A rapid regular rhythm that occurs a few times per year and has been ongoing for many years is likely a form of PSVT. In the absence of a previous correlation with an ECG rhythm strip or 12-lead ECG, an electrophysiologic study typically is required for diagnostic and/or therapeutic reasons. Noninvasive monitoring for such infrequent arrhythmias is often futile. Implantable recorders and even electrophysiologic studies may be required to make a definitive diagnosis.

Women might present with palpitations during the week prior to menstruation. It is commonly believed that alcohol and caffeine are arrhythmogenic, and although this may be so in certain patients, it has been our experience that these agents typically play a minor role in patients who have arrhythmias. Patients with AF might have episodes during heavy alcohol intake, but such is usually not the case for PSVT and sustained ventricular tachycardia.

## ■ FATIGUE, CHEST PAIN, AND DYSPNEA

Patients may present with symptoms such as fatigue, chest pain, or dyspnea that seem unrelated to an arrhythmia. This is particularly true for those who have AF. It is surprising how many patients with AF do not experience palpitations and present with either fatigue, shortness of breath, or episodic weakness. Thus, although these symptoms typically direct the clinician down another diagnostic road, remember that they might be caused by an arrhythmia. Of particular importance are patients who present with AF and symptoms of heart failure without palpitations.

# ADJUNCTIVE TESTS

## ■ ELECTROCARDIOGRAM

The ECG is covered elsewhere (Chapter 2), but two specific findings on the 12-lead ECG during PSVT should be emphasized. A pseudo r′ in ECG lead $V_1$ is very typical for patients who present with typical AV node reentry. The r′ results from super-imposition of the P wave on the end of the QRS complex from rapid retrograde conduction over a short pathway. In contrast, the typical finding in patients with AV reentry caused by retrograde conduction over an accessory pathway (eg, Wolff–Parkinson–White syndrome) is a P wave positioned in the early ST segment due to the prolonged retrograde conduction over a longer pathway.

## ■ HEAD-UP TILT TABLE TESTING

Head-up tilt (HUT) table testing is a diagnostic technique to assess the susceptibility of an individual to neurally mediated syncope. The protocol for HUT generally involves footrest-supported head-up tilting at 70 to 80 degrees for 30 to 45 minutes (**Fig. 8-1**). If HUT is negative, the test may be repeated following pharmacologic provocation. Most laboratories use isoproterenol at a dose of 1 to 3 μg/min. Repeat tilting is generally performed for 10 minutes after a steady state has been reached. Higher doses of isoproterenol, especially when coupled with longer durations of tilt, significantly decrease the specificity of the test. In control patients with no history of syncope, 70-degree head-up tilting has a specificity of approximately 90%.

## ■ SIGNAL-AVERAGED ELECTROCARDIOGRAPHY

SAECG allows the identification of small potentials in the surface ECG that are not seen because their amplitude is less than the noise intrinsic to the ECG signal, eg, *filtered QRS complex* (**Fig. 8-2**). Late potentials, appearing at the end of the QRS complex, correspond to fragmented electrical activity generated in areas of slow con-duction within or at the border zone of infarcts. Such areas may be prone to reentry and subsequent ventricular arrhythmias. Baseline intraventricular delays generally obviate meaningful SAECG analysis.

Three parameters have been identified to describe late potentials:

1. Filtered QRS duration (abnormal QRSd >114 milliseconds).
2. Root-mean-square voltage of the terminal 40 milliseconds of the QRS complex (abnormal RMS40 <20mV).
3. The duration of the low-amplitude signal (abnormal LAS >40 mV).

Late potentials are hypothesized to be associated with an increased incidence of ventricular arrhythmias and sudden death. In some studies of patients after MI, the incidence of an arrhythmic event was 17% to 29% when late potentials were present.

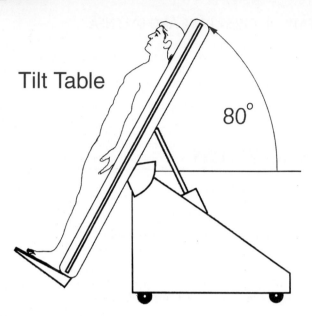

**FIGURE 8-1.** Tilt table with footboard support. (Reproduced with permission from Prystowsky EN, Klein GT. *Cardiac Arrhythmias: An Integrated Approach for the Clinician.* New York, NY: McGraw-Hill; 1994:353.)

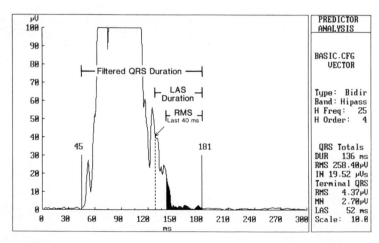

**FIGURE 8-2.** Positive signal-averaged electrocardiogram in a patient with sustained ventricular tachycardia. All three measured parameters are abnormal. Filtered QRS duration (DUR) is 136 milliseconds; and the root-mean-square (RMS) voltage of the last 40 milliseconds of the QS complex is 4.37 μV. LAS, low-amplitude signal. (Reproduced with permission from Prystowsky EN, Klein GT. *Cardiac Arrhythmias: An Integrated Approach for the Clinician.* New York, NY: McGraw-Hill; 1994:345.)

When late potentials were absent, the incidence of sudden death was 3.5% to 5%. Late potentials were an independent risk factor when assessed along with left ventricular ejection fraction (EF).

# ■ MICROVOLT T-WAVE ALTERNANS

Microvolt T-wave alternans (MTWA) is a technique that measures small changes in T-wave amplitude that occur on an alternating beat-to-beat basis. These changes have been associated with an increased risk of malignant ventricular arrhythmias and are thought to be caused by exaggerated repolarization heterogeneity. Several techniques have now been developed to detect and quantify these subtle variations in T-wave amplitude. MTWA is heart rate dependent and is generally interpreted in the context of exercise.

Exercise-induced microvolt T-wave alternans may be a predictor of arrhythmic risk. The test is considered positive if the onset of sustained MTWA occurs at <110 bpm, and negative if sustained MTWA does not occur at heart rates 105 bpm. The most common causes of an indeterminate test are failure to attain an adequate heart rate, frequent ectopy, nonsustained alternans, and excessive background electrocardiographic noise. The predictive power of MTWA appears to be independent of other risk-stratifying techniques, including heart rate variability, SAECG, baroreceptor sensitivity testing, ejection fraction, and electrophysiologic testing. In a meta-analysis of MTWA studies, positive predictive value for arrhythmic events was 19.3%. The negative predictive value was 97.2%. The RR of a positive test for an arrhythmic event was 3.77.

# ■ HEART RATE VARIABILITY

Heart rate variability (HRV) analysis is based on subtle variations in sinus cycle length and has been used to assess cardiac autonomic status (eg, parasympathetic and sympathetic tone). The time-domain methods identify the RR-interval sequences and then apply statistical techniques to express the variance. The most commonly employed measure is the standard deviation of normal-to-normal beats (SDNN), or of all RR intervals. Frequency domain methods apply the fast Fourier transform to the RR-interval sequence to develop a power spectral density that describes how the variance of the signal (ie, power) is distributed as a function of frequency.

HRV has been used for post-myocardial risk stratification. Decreased heart rate variability is associated with an increased risk of sudden death. Additionally, heart rate variability increases with β-blocker treatment and is consistent with the protective effects of β-adrenergic–blocking agents post-MI.

# ■ BAROREFLEX SENSITIVITY

Baroreflex sensitivity (BRS) testing is another technique to assess the cardiac autonomic nervous system. Typically, as carotid pressure rises, the RR interval is prolonged. The increase in carotid pressure is detected by the carotid sinus baroreceptors and results in vagal activation offsetting the rise in systemic blood pressure. Under normal circumstances there is resting vagal predominance and sympathetic inhibition. The theory underlying BRS sensitivity testing is that decreased BRS may be present post-MI and that a substantial reduction in BRS is a marker of increased risk for ventricular fibrillation.

Most commonly, BRS is assessed by measuring the heart rate response following infusion of a vasoactive agent. Usually phenylephrine is given in doses to increase systolic blood pressure 20 to 40 mm Hg. The changes in RR intervals are plotted against systolic blood pressure changes, and the slope is considered the BRS. In a group of normal controls, the average BRS was 14.8 ± 9 ms/mm Hg. Overall baroreceptor sensitivity decreases when the sympathetic nervous system is activated. An alternative technique employs neck collar suction to activate carotid baroreceptors.

## SUGGESTED READINGS

Prystowsky EN, Fogel RI. Approach to the patient with cardiac arrhythmias. In: Fuster V, Walsh R, Harrington RA, et al. *Hurst's The Heart.* 13th ed. New York, NY: McGraw-Hill; 2011; 39:949-962.

Bloomfield DM, Bigger JT, Steinman RC, et al. Microvolt T-wave alternans and the risk of death or sustained ventricular arrhythmias in patients with left ventricular dysfunction. *J Am Coll Cardiol.* 2006;47:456-463.

Chow T, Kereiakes DJ, Bartone C, et al. Prognostic utility of microvolt T wave alternans in risk stratification of patients with ischemic cardiomyopathy. *J Am Coll Cardiol.* 2006;47: 1820-1827.

Gehi AK, Stein RH, Metz LD, et al. Microvolt T-wave alternans for the risk stratification of ventricular tachyarrhythmic events. *J Am Coll Cardiol.* 2005;46:75-82.

Gomes JA, Cain ME, Buxton AE, et al. Prediction of long-term outcomes by signal-averaged electrocardiography in patients with unsustained ventricular tachycardia, coronary artery disease, and left ventricular dysfunction. *Circulation.* 2001;104: 436-441.

Narayan SM. T-wave alternans and the susceptibility to ventricular arrhythmia. *J Am Coll Cardiol.* 2006;47:269-281.

# CHAPTER 9
# ATRIAL FIBRILLATION, ATRIAL FLUTTER, AND SUPRAVENTRICULAR TACHYCARDIA[a]

## Eric N. Prystowsky and Richard I. Fogel

Atrial fibrillation, atrial flutter, and supraventricular tachycardia are common arrhythmias associated with a variety of cardiac conditions. Indeed, atrial fibrillation is the most commonly sustained cardiac arrhythmia encountered in clinical practice and is increasing in prevalence. These arrhythmias may be associated with deterioration of hemodynamics, a wide spectrum of symptoms, and significant morbidity, mortality, and medical costs. Perhaps because no single therapy has been shown to be ideal for all patients, there are a variety of treatment strategies that may be applied to these arrhythmias. These include no therapy at all, rhythm control, and rate control, and these treatment strategies have both pharmacologic and nonpharmacologic options available. This chapter describes the epidemiology, electrophysiologic mechanisms, and approach to management of patients with atrial fibrillation, atrial flutter, and atrial tachycardia.

## ATRIAL FIBRILLATION

Atrial fibrillation (AF) is characterized by disorganized atrial electrical activation and uncoordinated atrial contraction. The surface electrocardiogram characteristically demonstrates rapid fibrillatory waves with changing morphology and rate and a ventricular rhythm that is irregularly irregular (**Fig. 9-1**). Most AF originates in one or more of the pulmonary veins (PVs), and because of disparate atrial refractory periods the rapid firing focus in the left atrium (LA) cannot be conducted in a 1:1 manner to the right atrium, which leads to fibrillatory conduction. Additionally, it is thought that a driver, perhaps a reentrant focus in the LA, acts in a similar manner. Although the ECG has the characteristic appearance of disorganized atrial activation, further analysis may reveal what appears to be a regular rapid atrial rhythm, often seen best in lead $V_1$ (Fig. 9-1). Careful measurement will disclose variability in the P-P intervals, and this should not be misinterpreted as atrial flutter, or so-called *atrial fibrillation-flutter*. Atrial flutter, as discussed later, is a very regular rhythm with monotonous repetition of similar P waves with each cycle.

[a]Adapted in part from Chapter 37 by Prystowsky EN, Waldo AI. Atrial fibrillation, atrial flutter, and atrial tachycardia. In: Fuster V, O'Rourke RA, Walsh RA, et al, eds. *Hurst's The Heart.* 12th ed. New York, NY: McGraw-Hill; 2008, with permission of authors and publisher.

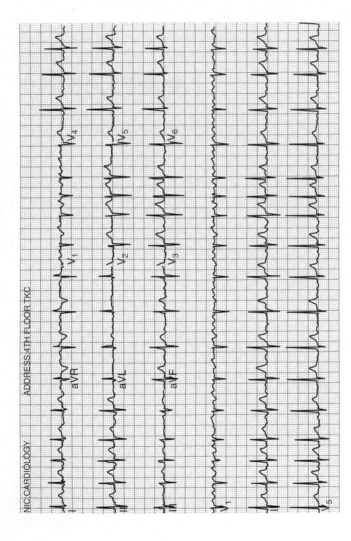

**FIGURE 9-1.** Twelve-lead electrocardiogram of atrial fibrillation. Note the rapid, irregular, changing, low-amplitude fibrillatory waves and an irregularly irregular ventricular response.

The ventricular rate during AF can be quite variable, and depends on autonomic tone, the electrophysiologic properties of the atrioventricular (AV) node, and the effects of medications that act on the AV conduction system.

The ventricular rate may be very rapid (>300 beats per min [bpm]) in patients with Wolff–Parkinson–White (WPW) syndrome, with conduction over accessory pathways (wide preexcited QRS complexes) having short antegrade refractory periods. A regular, slow ventricular rhythm during AF suggests a junctional rhythm, either as an escape mechanism with complete AV block or as an accelerated junctional pacemaker.

# ■ CLASSIFICATION

At the initial detection of AF, it may be difficult to ascertain the subsequent pattern of recurrences. Thus, a designation of *first detected* episode of AF is made on the initial diagnosis. When the patient has experienced 2 or more episodes, atrial AF is classified as *recurrent*. After the termination of an episode of AF, the rhythm can be classified as *paroxysmal* or *persistent*. Paroxysmal AF is characterized by self-terminating episodes that generally last <7 days (most <24 hours), whereas persistent AF generally lasts >7 days and often requires electrical or pharmacologic cardioversion.

AF is classified as *permanent* when it has failed cardioversion or when further attempts to terminate the arrhythmia are deemed futile. Although this classification scheme is generally useful, the pattern of AF may change in response to treatment. Thus, AF that has been persistent may become paroxysmal during pharmacologic therapy with antiarrhythmic medications.

# ■ EPIDEMIOLOGY

AF is the most common arrhythmia requiring treatment, with estimates of 2.2 to 5.0 million Americans and 4.5 million in the European Union experiencing paroxysmal or persistent AF. The incidence and prevalence of AF steadily increase with age, such that this arrhythmia occurs in <0.5% of the population <50 years of age, and increases to approximately 2% for ages 60 to 69 years, 4.6% for ages 70 to 79 years, and 8.8% for ages 80 to 89 years.

Familial AF can also occur and specific genetic defects (eg, in sodium channels) have been identified in a few families.

AF confers an increased relative risk of overall mortality ranging from 1.4 to 2.3, and is predominantly caused by stroke. In the absence of anticoagulation, the relative risk of stroke in patients with nonrheumatic AF is increased approximately 6-fold. The Framingham study demonstrated that the risk of stroke in AF is about 5% per year and is clearly related to age.

# ■ PATHOPHYSIOLOGY

AF is associated with a wide variety of predisposing factors. In the developed world, the most common clinical diagnoses associated with AF are hypertension and coronary artery disease.

AF occurs as a consequence of factors that *trigger* the onset and factors that *perpetuate* this arrhythmia. Triggering foci of rapidly firing cells within the sleeve of atrial myocytes extending into the pulmonary veins have been clearly shown to be the underlying mechanism of most paroxysmal AF. In animal models, these pulmonary vein foci manifest delayed after-potentials and triggered activity in response to catecholamine stimulation, rapid atrial pacing, or acute stretch. The pulmonary veins of patients with paroxysmal AF demonstrate abnormal properties of conduction such that there is a markedly reduced effective refractory period within the pulmonary veins, progressive conduction delay within the pulmonary veins in response to rapid pacing or programed stimulation, and often conduction block between the pulmonary veins and the LA.

For patients with pulmonary vein foci, a primary increase in adrenergic tone followed by a marked vagal predominance has been reported just prior to the onset of paroxysmal AF. A similar pattern of autonomic tone has been reported in an unselected group of patients with paroxysmal AF and a variety of cardiac conditions. Vagal stimulation shortens the refractory period of atrial myocardium but with a nonuniform distribution of effect. These factors support the importance of vagal stimulation in the induction of paroxysmal AF.

Long-standing AF ultimately results in atrial remodeling with loss of myofibrils, accumulation of glycogen granules, disruption in cell-to-cell coupling at gap junctions, and organelle aggregates at the cellular level.

In a population-based study of elderly patients without AF at baseline, Tsang and coworkers demonstrated that AF developed in direct relationship to left atrial volume. An even stronger predictor of the development of nonvalvular AF was a restrictive transmitral Doppler flow pattern, eg, diastolic dysfunction.

## ■ HEMODYNAMIC EFFECTS

AF produces several adverse hemodynamic effects, including loss of atrial contraction, a rapid ventricular rate, and an irregular ventricular rhythm. The loss of mechanical AV synchrony may have a dramatic impact on ventricular filling and cardiac output when there is reduced ventricular compliance, as with left ventricular (LV) hypertrophy from hypertension, restrictive cardiomyopathy, hypertrophic cardiomyopathy, or the increased ventricular stiffness associated with aging. In addition, patients with mitral stenosis, constrictive pericarditis, or right ventricular infarction typically experience marked hemodynamic deterioration at the onset of AF. The loss of AV synchrony results in a loss of the loading effect of atrial contraction, thereby reducing stroke volume. Although there is a reduction in the LVEDP, there is an increase in the left atrial mean diastolic pressure. Patients with significant restrictive physiology may experience pulmonary edema and/or hypotension with the onset of AF.

The irregular ventricular rhythm has adverse hemodynamic effects that are independent of the ventricular rate. Irregularity significantly reduces cardiac output and coronary blood flow compared with a regular ventricular rhythm at the same average heart rate. The effect of ventricular irregularity on coronary blood flow may explain in part why some patients with AF experience precordial pain in the presence of normal coronary arteriography.

## ■ THROMBOEMBOLISM

Stroke is the most feared consequence of AF, and its prevention is a major focus of the management of patients with this condition. Most thrombi associated with AF arise within the left atrial appendage. Flow velocity within the left atrial appendage is reduced during AF because of the loss of organized mechanical contraction. Compared with transthoracic echocardiogram, the transesophageal echocardiogram offers a much more sensitive and specific means of assessing left atrial thrombi. Several factors contribute to the enhanced thrombogenicity of AF. Nitric oxide (NO) production in the left atrial endocardium is reduced in experimental AF, with an increase in levels of the prothrombotic protein plasminogen activator inhibitor 1 (PAI-1).

In the Stroke Prevention in Atrial Fibrillation (SPAF) III study, increased plasma levels of von Willebrand factor (vWF) were strongly correlated with the clinical predictors of stroke in AF (age, prior cerebral ischemia, CHF, diabetes, and body mass index). There was a stepwise increase in vWF with increasing clinical risk of stroke in this population.

# ■ TREATMENT

## *Anticoagulation*

### Stroke Risk and Stratification Schemes for Patients With Atrial Fibrillation

The recognized risk factors for stroke are prior stroke or transient ischemic attack (TIA), hypertension, diabetes, heart failure, and age older than 75 years (**Table 9-1**). Other stroke-risk factors are mechanical prosthetic valve, mitral stenosis, coronary artery disease, thyrotoxicosis and female gender, LV dysfunction, and age older than 65 years. Not all stroke-risk factors have the same degree of association with stroke in patients with AF, which is factored in when considering indications for oral anticoagulation therapy.

The $CHADS_2$ stroke-risk stratification scheme, which is based on analysis of 1773 patients in the National Registry for Atrial Fibrillation, has gained considerable favor and is used in the ACC/AHA/ESC 2006 management guidelines to tailor therapy for stroke prevention. The *C* in CHADS stands for recent CHF, *H* for hypertension, *A* for age older than 75 years, *D* for diabetes, and *S* for prior stroke or transient ischemic attack. Each category gets 1 point except stroke, which gets 2 because it is the most serious risk factor. The adjusted stroke rate per 100 patient-years increases from 1.9 with a score of 1 to 18.2 with a score of 6 (Table 9-1). **Table 9-2** gives the new recommendations on antithrombotic therapy to prevent thromboembolism in patients with AF. There is widespread consensus that all patients with rheumatic valvular heart disease and AF require anticoagulation with warfarin unless there is an absolute contraindication.

Warfarin is remarkably effective at reducing stroke risk in patients with AF. This was clearly demonstrated by a meta-analysis by the investigators of 5 randomized, controlled clinical trials comparing warfarin versus placebo in patients with AF:

1. Copenhagen Atrial Fibrillation, Aspirin, and Anticoagulation (AFASAK) trial
2. SPAF trial
3. Boston Area Anticoagulation Trial for Atrial Fibrillation (BAATAF)
4. Canadian Atrial Fibrillation trial
5. Stroke Prevention in Nonrheumatic Atrial Fibrillation (SPINAF) trial (**Fig. 9-2**)

**TABLE 9-1.** Stroke Risk in Patients With Nonvascular Atrial Fibrillation Not Treated With Anticoagulation According to the $CHADS_2$ Index

| $CHADS_2$ Risk Criteria | Score |
|---|---|
| Prior stroke or TIA | 2 |
| Age >75 y | 1 |
| Hypertension | 1 |
| Diabetes mellitus | 1 |
| Heart failure | 1 |
| Patients ($n = 1733$) | |

**TABLE 9-2.** Antithrombotic Therapy for Patients With Atrial Fibrillation

| Risk Category | Recommended Therapy |
| --- | --- |
| No risk factors | Aspirin, 81-325 mg daily |
| One moderate-risk factor | Aspirin, 81-325 mg daily, or warfarin (INR 2.0-3.0, target 2.5) |
| Any high-risk factor or >1 moderate-risk factor | Warfarin (INR 2.0-3.0, target 2.5) |

| Less Validated or Weaker Risk Factors | Moderate-Risk Factors | High-Risk Factors |
| --- | --- | --- |
| Female gender | Age 75 y | Previous stroke, TIA, or embolism |
| Age 65-74 y | Hypertension | Mitral stenosis |
| Coronary artery disease | Heart failure | Prosthetic heart valvae |
| Thyrotoxicosis | LV ejection fraction 35% or less | |
| | Diabetes mellitus | |

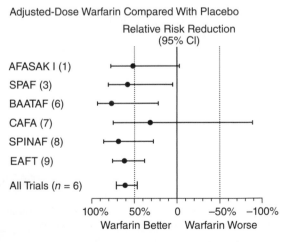

Adjusted-Dose Warfarin Compared With Placebo

Relative Risk Reduction (95% CI)

AFASAK I (1)
SPAF (3)
BAATAF (6)
CAFA (7)
SPINAF (8)
EAFT (9)
All Trials (*n* = 6)

100%    50%    0    −50%  −100%
Warfarin Better    Warfarin Worse

**FIGURE 9-2.** Effects of warfarin versus placebo on risk of stroke in 6 randomized, placebo-controlled clinical trials in nonvalvular atrial fibrillation. AFASAK I (1), the Copenhagen Atrial Fibrillation, Aspirin, and Anticoagulant Therapy Study; BAATAF (6), Boston Area Anticoagulation Trial for Atrial Fibrillation; CAFA (7), Canadian Atrial Fibrillation Anticoagulation; EAFT (9), European Atrial Fibrillation Trial; SPAF (3), Stroke Prevention in Atrial Fibrillation; and SPINAF (8), Stroke Prevention in Atrial Fibrillation. CI, confidence interval. (Data from Hart RG, Benavente O, McBride R, Pearce LA. Antithrombotic therapy to prevent stroke in patients with atrial fibrillation: a meta-analysis. *Ann Intern Med.* Oct 5, 1999;131(7):492-501.)

Using an intention-to-treat analysis that compared warfarin therapy with placebo, there was a 68% risk reduction in stroke for patients taking warfarin compared with patients taking placebo ($p<0.001$). Moreover, a subsequent on-treatment analysis demonstrated an 83% risk reduction in stroke when patients were taking warfarin compared with placebo. Warfarin should be administered to achieve an international normalized ratio (INR) between 2 and 3, with a target INR of 2.5 to provide both efficacy and safety (Figs. 9-2, **9-3**, **9-4**).

It is important that the risks of bleeding versus the benefits on stroke prevention also be weighed for each patient. However, the risk of stroke typically is greater than that of bleeding for most patients with AF at substantial risk for stroke. Thus, even though the ACC/AHA/ESC guidelines allow aspirin or warfarin therapy for patients who have 1 moderate-risk factor (see Table 9-2), we generally prefer warfarin for such patients. It is also important to remember that there is no difference in the indications for antithrombotic therapy between paroxysmal, persistent, and permanent AF.

## Cardioversion

Cardioversion can be accomplished using either antiarrhythmic drugs or the direct-current approach. In situations where urgent cardioversion is needed, such as marked hypotension, the direct-current approach is preferred. The need for anticoagulation prior to cardioversion must be considered. There is general consensus that AF that has been present for <48 hours can be cardioverted without prior anticoagulation, but there are no randomized trial data to support this practice and systemic emboli can probably occur in this situation. Because often it is impossible to time the onset of AF accurately, anticoagulation therapy is recommended for AF of uncertain duration.

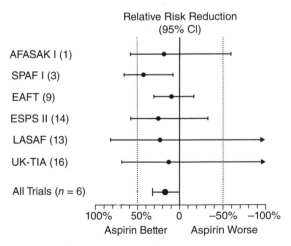

**FIGURE 9-3.** Effects of aspirin versus placebo on risk of stroke in 6 randomized, placebo-controlled trials in nonvalvular atrial fibrillation. AFASAK I (1), the Copenhagen Atrial Fibrillation, Aspirin, and Anticoagulant Therapy Study; EAFT (9), European Atrial Fibrillation Trial; ESPS II (14), European Stroke Prevention Study; LASAF (13), Alternate-Day Dosing of Aspirin in Atrial Fibrillation Pilot Study Group; SPAF I (3), Stroke Prevention in Atrial Fibrillation; and UK-TIA (16), United Kingdom Transient Ischaemic Attack Trial. CI, confidence interval. (Data from Hart RG, Benavente O, McBride R, Pearce LA. Antithrombotic therapy to prevent stroke in patients with atrial fibrillation: a meta-analysis. *Ann Intern Med.* Oct 5, 1999;131(7):492-501.)

Warfarin Compared With Aspirin

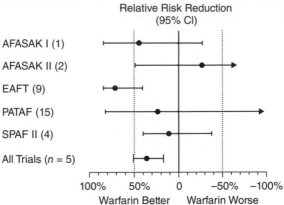

FIGURE 9-4. Effects of aspirin versus warfarin on risk of stroke in 5 randomized, controlled clinical trials in nonvalvular atrial fibrillation. AFASAK I (1) and AFASAK II (2), the Copenhagen Atrial Fibrillation, Aspirin, and Anticoagulant Therapy Study; EAFT (9) European Atrial Fibrillation Trial; PATAF (15), Primary Prevention of Arterial Thromboembolism in Nonrheumatic Atrial Fibrillation; and SPAF II (3), Stroke Prevention in Atrial Fibrillation. (Data from Hart RG, Benavente O, McBride R, Pearce LA. Antithrombotic therapy to prevent stroke in patients with atrial fibrillation: a meta-analysis. *Ann Intern Med*. Oct 5, 1999;131(7):492-501.)

There are 2 basic strategies to deal with cardioversion: (1) oral warfarin with a therapeutic INR (2-3) for 3 to 4 weeks before cardioversion followed by continued warfarin thereafter, or (2) transesophageal echocardiography (TEE) and heparin immediately before cardioversion followed by oral warfarin thereafter.

Successful electrical cardioversion requires attention to details. Always be sure the patient is adequately anticoagulated. Rather than the use of handheld paddles, adhesive gel electrodes should be placed anteriorly over the sternum (with the upper edge at the sternal angle) and posteriorly (just to the left of the spine).

The duration of AF is a major factor for cardioversion success using antiarrhythmic drugs, and AF lasting approximately 1 week has a substantial chance of cardioversion using oral flecainide, propafenone, dofetilide, and intravenous ibutilide. For longer-duration AF, only dofetilide seems to have a reasonable chance of success, but amiodarone and ibutilide may be useful. A single oral dose of propafenone (eg, 600 mg) or flecainide (eg, 300 mg) can be useful to convert recent-onset AF to sinus rhythm. A recent study demonstrated the safety of the "pill-in-the-pocket" approach to outpatient conversion of AF in some patients. Because a type 1C drug may convert AF to atrial flutter, an AV nodal-blocking agent should usually be administered concomitantly to prevent an accelerated ventricular response.

## Rate-Control Versus Rhythm-Control Strategies

Several prospective, randomized trials have been published comparing the strategies of rate control and rhythm control in patients with AF. The AFFIRM trial enrolled 4060 patients aged older than 65 years or with risk factors for stroke, randomizing them to rate versus rhythm control. Over a mean follow-up period of 3.5 years, there was no significant difference in overall mortality between the 2 groups. However, it should be noted that AFFIRM does not prove that atrial fibrillation is no different than sinus rhythm from a total mortality standpoint.

**Control of Ventricular Rate** Control of the ventricular rate involves both acute and chronic phases. In the acute phase, intravenous diltiazem, metoprolol, esmolol, and verapamil have all been demonstrated to provide slowing of AV nodal conduction within 5 minutes; these drugs are indicated for patients with severe symptoms related to a rapid ventricular rate. Intravenous digoxin requires a longer duration to achieve rate control and is less useful. For patients with only mild or moderate symptoms, oral medications that slow AV nodal conduction should be prescribed. After controlling the resting ventricular rate, attention is paid to the ambulatory heart rate.

The optimal rate control has long been debated. In the RACE II trial, 614 patients with permanent atrial fibrillation were randomized to either a lenient rate-control (resting heart rate <110 bpm) or a strict rate-control strategy (resting heart rate <80 bpm and heart rate during moderate exercise <110 bpm). The primary outcome was a composite of death from cardiovascular causes, hospitalization for heart failure, and stroke, systemic embolism, bleeding, and life-threatening arrhythmic events. There was no difference in the primary outcome, symptoms, or adverse events between the 2 arms. However, only 67% of the patients in the strict-control group achieved the target rates in contrast to 97% in the lenient-control group.

Digoxin may provide effective control of the resting heart rate (particularly in combination with another agent) but is often ineffective during exertion. β-adrenergic blockers or calcium-channel antagonists provide much better control of the ventricular rate during exercise and should be considered for most patients.

**Ablation of the Atrioventricular Node** Some patients may continue to experience significant symptoms from a rapid or irregular ventricular rhythm despite drug therapy. Chronically elevated ventricular rates (usually >120 bpm) despite adequate trials of AV nodal-blocking agents can cause a tachycardia-induced cardiomyopathy. Catheter ablation of the AV conduction system and permanent pacemaker implantation is a highly effective means of establishing permanent control of the ventricular rate during AF in selected patients. Despite the many favorable effects of this procedure, there are several limitations. First, AV nodal ablation does not change the long-term need for anticoagulation. Second, although an adequate junctional escape rhythm is typically present after ablation, patients should be considered to be permanently pacemaker dependent. Third, because this procedure does not restore AV synchrony, patients who are highly dependent on mechanical atrial contraction often do not experience as much improvement as other patients. Fourth, right ventricular pacing produces an abnormal LV contraction sequence, and acute worsening of hemodynamics has been observed in some patients. In the Post-AV Node Ablation Evaluation (PAVE) trial, patients who received biventricular versus RV apical pacing, especially those with abnormal LV ejection fractions before ablation, had longer 6-minute walking distances and higher LV ejection fractions after ablation.

**Maintenance of Sinus Rhythm** When a rhythm-control strategy is chosen for patients with paroxysmal or persistent AF, prophylactic treatment with antiarrhythmic drugs is usually needed to maintain sinus rhythm. Although the ideal of pharmacologic therapy would be to prevent all recurrences of AF, this is unrealistic for many patients. Rather, marked reduction in the frequency, duration, and symptoms of AF may be a very acceptable clinical goal. In addition, the use of pharmacologic agents to prevent AF does not change the indication for anticoagulation.

As compared with drug therapy for life-threatening arrhythmias, the choice of pharmacologic agent is largely determined by the potential side effects of a given drug in an individual patient.

**Antiarrhythmic Drug Selection** Antiarrhythmic drugs are selected on a safety-first basis (**Fig. 9-5**). The ACC/AHA/ESC guidelines suggest for patients with no

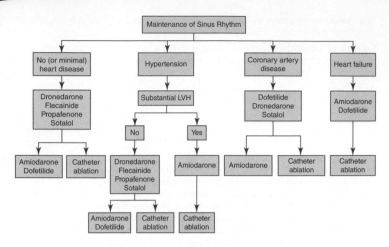

**FIGURE 9-5.** Proposed strategy for use of antiarrhythmic drugs to maintain sinus rhythm in patients with atrial fibrillation. LVH, left ventricular hypertrophy. (Modified with permission from Fuster V, Ryden LE, Cannom DS, et al. ACC/AHA/ESC 2006 guidelines for the management of patients with atrial fibrillation: a report of the American College of Cardiology/American Heart Association Task Force on Practice Guidelines and the European Society of Cardiology Committee for Practice Guidelines (Writing Committee to Revise the 2001 Guidelines for the Management of Patients With Atrial Fibrillation). Circulation. 2006; Aug 15;114(7):e257-354.)

or minimal heart disease to start with dronaderone, flecainide, propafenone, or sotalol, agents with minimal noncardiac toxicity. The second-line therapy is either amiodarone/dofetilide or catheter ablation. Patients with hypertension who do not have substantial LV hypertrophy have a similar treatment algorithm, but those with substantial LV hypertrophy are considered at increased proarrhythmia risk with most drugs other than amiodarone, which becomes first-line therapy here. Catheter ablation is second-line treatment. Safety of drugs in coronary artery disease has been demonstrated for dofetilide/sotalol/dronedarone (first-line) and amiodarone (second-line), and catheter ablation is also second-line treatment.

## Surgical Treatment

Several surgical treatments (eg, the Maze procedure) for the prevention of AF have been developed. Success rates have ranged from 70% to 95%. For patients with AF who are undergoing cardiac surgery, consideration should be given to concomitant AF surgery. Otherwise, its role is typically for patients who require sinus rhythm for symptom relief and have failed to respond to antiarrhythmic drugs and catheter ablation.

**Catheter Ablation**   Recent approaches to catheter ablation of AF, especially paroxysmal AF, have been to eliminate triggering foci, primarily within the pulmonary veins but also in the LA posterior wall, superior vena cava, crista terminalis, vein of Marshall, and coronary sinus. Various techniques have been employed to isolate the pulmonary veins, including the use of intracardiac echocardiography or an electro-anatomical mapping system to guide delivery of radiofrequency energy circumferentially outside the pulmonary veins. Current clinical trials in atrial fibrillation are comparing the efficacy and outcomes of ablative strategies versus medical therapy.

# ATRIAL FLUTTER

## ■ CLASSIFICATION AND MECHANISMS

There are several types of atrial flutter, all having rapid, regular atrial rates, generally 240 to 340 bpm, because of a reentrant mechanism in the atria. Typical atrial flutter, also called *counterclockwise atrial flutter*, is characterized by negative sawtooth flutter waves (**Fig. 9-6**). Reverse typical atrial flutter, also called *atypical* or *clockwise atrial flutter*, is characterized by positive flutter waves in ECG leads II, III, and aVF. These 2 atrial flutter types share the same right atrial reentrant circuit.

## ■ EPIDEMIOLOGY

Atrial flutter often is a persistent rhythm, but more typically it is paroxysmal, lasting for variable periods. In most patients it is spontaneously induced by a premature atrial beat or beats that produce a transitional rhythm, resembling AF. Atrial flutter commonly occurs in patients in the first week after open-heart surgery. Atrial flutter is also associated with chronic obstructive pulmonary disease, mitral or tricuspid valve disease, thyrotoxicosis, and postsurgical repair of certain congenital cardiac lesions (eg, atrial septal defect, the Mustard procedure, the Senning procedure, or the Fontan procedure), as well as enlargement of the atria for any reason, especially the right atrium.

## ■ DIAGNOSIS

Atrial flutter usually can be diagnosed from the ECG (see Fig. 9-6). The standard for the diagnosis of atrial flutter is the presence of atrial complexes of constant morphology, polarity, and cycle length. On occasion, the identification of atrial flutter complexes in the ECG may be difficult because of their temporal superimposition on other ECG deflections, such as the QRS complex or the T wave, or because of their very low amplitude. Use of vagal maneuvers or the intravenous administration of adenosine to prolong transiently AV conduction may result in AV nodal block and reveal atrial flutter complexes in the ECG if they are present.

## ■ MANAGEMENT

### Acute Treatment

The acute treatment of atrial flutter parallels the approach to acute atrial fibrillation. Control the ventricular response rate is the predominant initial strategy and urgent direct current (DC) cardioversion is reserved for poorly tolerated atrial flutter (eg, hypotension). Antiarrhythmic drug therapy can be used to acutely restore sinus rhythm; for example, intravenous ibutilide is associated with a 60% likelihood of converting recent atrial flutter to sinus rhythm. Intravenous procainamide may also be useful in converting atrial flutter to normal sinus rhythm.

Drug therapy is also used to slow the ventricular response rate as needed. Useful agents include β-blockers, verapamil, diltiazem, and digitalis, alone or in combination. It is often difficult to achieve sufficient AV nodal block to adequately slow the ventricular response during atrial flutter, and 2:1 AV conduction frequently recurs. For this reason cardioversion to sinus rhythm may be required. When using a class I antiarrhythmic drug, especially an IC agent, to treat atrial flutter, care must be taken to provide adequate AV block.

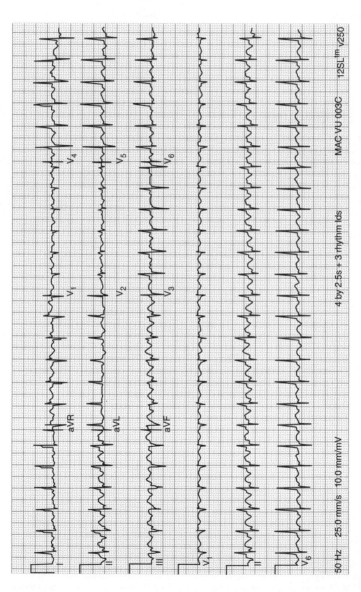

**FIGURE 9-6.** Twelve-lead electrocardiogram of typical atrial flutter. Note the negative flutter waves in leads II, III, and aVF, and the upright flutter waves in lead $V_1$. This is characteristic of counterclockwise, isthmus-dependent atrial flutter.

## Long-Term Treatment

**Catheter Ablation Therapy** Catheter ablation is highly successful in curing atrial flutter, typically >90%. Because of the inadequacy of antiarrhythmic drug therapy to maintain sinus rhythm, catheter ablation is a first-line treatment option for many patients. However, successful ablation of the atrial flutter reentrant circuit per se may not prevent subsequent AF.

**Antiarrhythmic Drug Therapy** Selection of an antiarrhythmic drug to treat atrial flutter mirrors that to treat AF. However, this form of therapy is no longer the treatment of choice for long-term therapy in most patients with atrial flutter, because catheter ablation to cure atrial flutter has superceded it.

**Anticoagulant Therapy** In patients with atrial flutter, daily warfarin therapy to achieve an INR between 2 and 3 (target 2.5) is recommended using the same criteria as for AF. In addition, several studies indicate that the incidence of stroke associated with atrial flutter is not different from AF.

# FOCAL OR ECTOPIC ATRIAL TACHYCARDIA

## ■ CLASSIFICATION

The term *atrial tachycardia* refers to rapid (usually 130-250 bpm), relatively regular rhythms that originate in the atria, do not require participation of either the sinus node or the AV node for maintenance, and are neither AF nor atrial flutter (**Fig. 9-7**). Focal atrial tachycardia is characterized by atrial activation starting rhythmically at a small area (focus). Potential mechanisms include reentry, automaticity, and triggered activity. Foci are most frequently found in the pulmonary veins in the LA and the crista terminalis in the right atrium, but can occur at various sites in both atria. When incessant, they may be associated with a dilated cardiomyopathy and CHF.

## ■ MECHANISM

An automatic focus may demonstrate progressive rate increase at tachycardia onset (warm-up) and/or progressive rate decrease before termination (cooldown), does not respond to vagal maneuvers, and often displays an incessant nature.

## ■ EPIDEMIOLOGY

The incidence of focal atrial tachycardia increases with age, reportedly occurring in up to 13% of elderly subjects. An increased incidence has been reported in patients with myocardial infarction, non-ischemic heart disease, obstructive lung disease, serum electrolyte disorders, and drug toxicity, especially caused by digitalis. However, focal atrial tachycardia may occur in normal individuals, and nonsustained episodes have been noted in 2% of healthy young adults. Most episodes of focal atrial tachycardia are paroxysmal (deemed largely caused by reentry or triggered activity), but some episodes may be incessant (considered largely caused by automaticity).

## ■ DIAGNOSIS

Ectopic atrial tachycardias are characterized by an abnormal P-wave vector, a tendency to low P-wave amplitude, and rapid atrial rates (range, 160-240 bpm). Ectopic atrial rates in excess of 200 bpm are usually accompanied by 2:1 AV conduction.

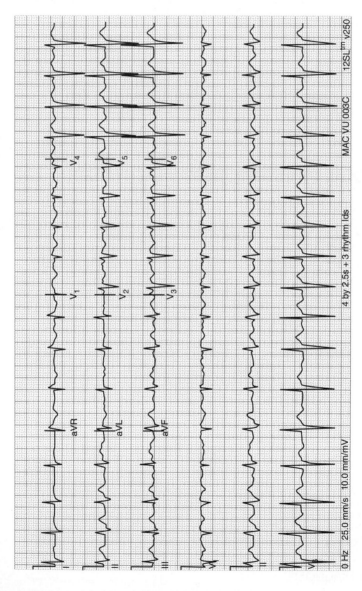

**FIGURE 9-7.** Surface electrocardiogram of an atrial tachycardia involving the right atrium. Note the discrete P waves with 2:1 AV conduction.

An ectopic atrial rhythm associated with a high-grade block and a relatively slow ventricular rate (so-called paroxysmal atrial tachycardia [PAT] with block) suggests digitalis intoxication.

A standard way to determine the presence or absence of an AV nodal independent atrial tachycardia is to demonstrate that despite the presence of conduction block at the AV node, the rhythm continues. Termination of a supraventricular tachycardia by a drug such as adenosine that causes transient AV node block generally supports the diagnosis of an underlying AV nodal-dependent reentrant tachycardia—for example, AV node reentry. However, adenosine is known to terminate some atrial tachycardias, so that termination of an atrial tachyarrhythmia after the administration of intravenous adenosine cannot be used per se to characterize the rhythm as AV nodal dependent. The same seems true for beta-blockers. A useful sign of AV nodal dependence is consistent termination of tachycardia with a P wave without conduction to the ventricles.

## ■ TREATMENT

Antiarrhythmic agents may provide effective treatment if no reversible cause can be found. Cardioversion is rarely helpful. Ectopic atrial tachycardias commonly have precipitating factors; therefore, correction of the inciting factors (eg, digitalis intoxication, decompensated chronic obstructive pulmonary disease, electrolyte imbalance, metabolic abnormalities, hypoxia, and thyrotoxicosis) is the primary therapy. In patients in whom no reversible cause can be identified, intracardiac localization of the arrhythmia's focus and subsequent radiofrequency ablation may be attempted.

In patients with symptomatic and/or incessant atrial tachycardia, catheter ablation is usually the primary therapy regardless of the underlying mechanism. Reports of catheter ablation therapy for reentrant atrial tachycardia demonstrate a success rate >75%.

# MULTIFOCAL ATRIAL TACHYCARDIA

Multifocal atrial tachycardia (MAT) remains largely a descriptive entity. MAT is diagnosed by ECG criteria that include an atrial rate greater than 100 bpm with P waves of at least 3 distinct morphologies. The diagnosis of MAT can be difficult. The chaotic nature of the P-wave morphology with varying AV and RR intervals makes confusion with AF common.

## ■ MECHANISM

The mechanism underlying MAT is unknown. Several reports have noted that MAT cannot be induced or initiated by programmed stimulation. Thus, reentry seems an unlikely mechanism. Anecdotal reports of successful treatment of MAT with calcium-channel blockers or β-blockers are consistent with both automatic and triggered mechanisms.

## ■ EPIDEMIOLOGY

MAT is often observed in patients with acute pulmonary disorders and associated hypoxia. Patients with MAT are usually acutely ill and often are receiving agonists or theophylline preparations. As such, both agonists and theophylline have been causally implicated.

## ■ TREATMENT

The therapeutic goal is to slow the rapid ventricular response rate during MAT if the patient's condition is affected. If the ventricular response is controlled (usually difficult), MAT per se probably shouldn't affect the patient's clinical course.

The cornerstone of therapy should be directed at correction of any underlying pulmonary problem. DC cardioversion has not provided successful therapy in patients with MAT. There is limited experience reported with the use of standard antiarrhythmic drugs. β-blockers have been used with variable success in selected patients, but precipitation of bronchospasm may occur in these patients with tenuous respiratory status. Thus, short-acting 1-specific agents like esmolol seem most appropriate for initial use. In selected patients, calcium channel blockers may have a role in the treatment of patients with MAT. Mortality with this arrhythmia is ultimately related to the comorbidities associated with MAT.

# SUPRAVENTRICULAR ARRHYTHMIAS

## ■ SINUS RHYTHM AND SINUS TACHYCARDIA

Normal sinus rhythm is defined as a rate of 60 to 100 bpm, originating in the sinus node; the rhythm is regular. Sinus arrhythmia is present when the variation between the longest and the shortest cycle on a resting tracing is above 0.12 second. This is a normal variant occuring most commonly in the young.

Sinus tachycardia is characterized by normal sinus P waves at a rate greater than 100 per minute. It usually does not exceed 130 to 140 bpm under resting conditions, but can be as high as 180 to 200 bpm, particularly during exercise. Sinus tachycardia is a normal physiologic response to exercise or emotional stress or may be pharmacologically induced by such drugs as epinephrine, ephedrine, or atropine. Exposure to alcohol, caffeine, or nicotine can also cause sinus tachycardia. Vagotonic maneuvers, such as carotid sinus massage or Valsalva maneuver, may help differentiate sinus tachycardia from other supraventricular tachycardias (SVTs). Gradual slowing of the rapid rate followed by gradual return to that rate is typical for sinus tachycardia. In contrast, vagal maneuvers may abruptly terminate other SVTs by blocking conduction in the AV node. Sinus tachycardia usually requires no specific treatment; management should be directed toward the underlying disorder.

## ■ PREMATURE ATRIAL CONTRACTIONS

Atrial extrasystoles or premature atrial contractions (PACs) are impulses that arise in an ectopic atrial focus and are premature in relation to the prevailing sinus rate. The early P wave has a different vector from the sinus P wave, and the PR interval of the conducted PAC may be normal or prolonged. If the coupling interval of the PAC to the previous sinus P wave is short, aberrant intraventricular conduction may occur, making the diagnosis dependent on recognition of the P wave distorting the previous T wave. The hallmark of the timing of PACs is the less than fully compensatory pause; however, this may not always occur. The significance of atrial extrasystoles depends on the clinical setting in which they occur. Often, they are found in completely normal individuals.

## ■ SUPRAVENTRICULAR TACHYARRHYTHMIAS

All tachyarrhythmias that originate above the bifurcation of the bundle of His are classified as supraventricular arrhythmias. The atrial rate must be 100 or more bpm for a diagnosis, but the ventricular rate may be less when AV conduction is incomplete. SVTs usually have narrow QRS configurations, but they may be wide because of aberrant conduction through the intraventricular conduction tissue, preexisting bundle-branch block, or conduction via an accessory pathway. Atrial activity may be identified by using a long rhythm strip with multiple leads. Recording the rhythm strip at a rapid paper speed (eg, 50 mm/s) may be helpful. Other diagnostic aids include vagal maneuvers or drug therapy to slow the AV conduction rate or an esophageal lead to identify atrial activity. Dissociating the atrial activity from the ventricular response on a rhythm strip is usually necessary to elucidate the nature of the atrial arrhythmia. Intra-atrial electrograms are occasionally required.

SVTs may be classified as *paroxysmal* (lasting seconds to hours), *persistent* (lasting days to weeks), or *chronic* (lasting weeks to years). The duration and the electrophysiologic mechanism of the tachyarrhythmia are essential for appropriate management. Paroxysmal SVT (PSVT) may occur in the presence or absence of heart disease and in patients of all ages. It is most often due to reentry involving the AV node or an accessory pathway; infrequently, sinus node reentry or intra-atrial reentry is the mechanism.

## ■ SUPRAVENTRICULAR TACHYCARDIA DUE TO ATRIOVENTRICULAR NODAL REENTRY

AV nodal reentry is the most common mechanism of SVT and is characterized by 2 functionally distinct pathways within or near the AV node. In the common form of AV nodal reentrant tachycardia, antegrade conduction occurs over the slow pathway and retrograde conduction over the fast pathway, resulting in almost simultaneous activation of the atria and ventricles. Retrograde P waves are hidden within the QRS complex or appear immediately after it (eg, r' in $V_1$). In the uncommon form, in which antegrade conduction occurs over the fast pathway, the retrograde P wave occurs well after the end of the QRS complex and is characterized by a long RP interval and a short PR interval with an inverted P wave in II, III, and aVF (**Fig. 9-8**). In the absence of structural heart disease, PSVT due

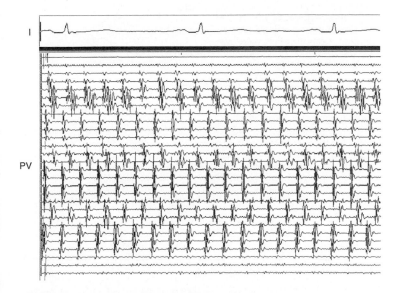

**FIGURE 9-8.** Surface electrocardiogram of an AVNRT.

to AV nodal reentry is a benign rhythm and may be treated acutely with rest, sedation, and vagotonic maneuvers. If these physiologic interventions are unsuccessful, intravenous adenosine, intravenous calcium antagonists, digoxin, or β-adrenergic blockers may be used. Adenosine, 6 mg intravenously, followed by one or two 12-mg boluses if necessary, has an extremely short half-life (10 s), causes no hemodynamic complications, and is the *first choice* for treatment of PSVT (**Table 9-3**).

Long-term therapy for control of recurrent SVT due to AV nodal reentry is most frequently achieved today with catheter ablation. No specific chronic therapy may be necessary in patients who have infrequent, short-lived, well-tolerated attacks and/or who respond to physiologic maneuvers. Patients who have more frequent attacks, who are intolerant to medications, and/or whose SVTs cause hemodynamic compromise should consider *radiofrequency catheter ablation*. Ablation of AV nodal reentry is achieved by selective ablation of the slow pathway to abolish the reentrant loop. Less commonly, ablation of the fast pathway will be performed, but the risk of iatrogenic heart block is higher. In either case, experience has demonstrated that this is a safe and effective technique for the management of AV nodal reentry (**Table 9-4**).

Pharmacologic therapy is an alternative for patients who do not desire radiofrequency ablation or who have few, well-tolerated occurrences. β-adrenergic blocking agents, verapamil, or digoxin in standard doses may be used. In patients with no structural heart disease, class IC agents may be used (**Table 9-5**).

---

**TABLE 9-3.** Differentiation of Various Narrow-QRS-Complex Tachycardias Using ECG[a] and Response to Carotid Sinus Pressure (CSP) or IV Adenosine (A)

1. Irregular tachycardia
   a. Atrial fibrillation: ventricular rate transiently slows with CSP or A
   b. Atrial flutter with varying AV conduction: ventricular rate slows with CSP or A, and flutter waves seen at ≥240/min
   c. Multifocal atrial tachycardia: different P-wave morphologies
2. Regular tachycardia with no visible P waves
   AVNRT: rate 140-250/min. No change or terminates with CSP or A
3. Regular tachycardia, atrial rate greater than ventricular (baseline, CSP or A)
   a. Atrial flutter: regular flutter waves at ≥240/min
   b. Atrial tachycardia with block: abnormal P waves at 100-240/min
4. Regular tachycardia with RP shorter than PR
   a. AVNRT: P at the end of QRS, with RP <70 msec. No change or terminates with CSP or A
   b. Orthodromic AVRT: RP >70 msec; no change or terminates with CSP or A
   c. Atrial tachycardia with first-degree AV block: RP >70 msec; AV block worsens with CSP or A
5. Regular tachycardia with RP longer than PR
   a. Ectopic atrial tachycardia: abnormal P waves, AV block with CSP or A
   b. Atypical AVNRT: abnormal P wave, no change or terminates with CSP or A
   c. Sinus node reentry: paroxysmal P wave similar to sinus, terminates with premature atrial beats, CSP or A
   d. Sinus tachycardia: normal P waves, transient slowing with CSP or A
6. AV dissociation present
   Paroxysmal junctional tachycardia

---

AVNRT, AV nodal reciprocating tachycardia; AVRT, AV reciprocating tachycardia; CSP, carotid sinus pressure.
[a]Twelve-lead ECG is necessary to identify P waves.

**TABLE 9-4.** Drugs for Acute Management of Supraventricular Tachycardia

| Drug | Dosage |
|------|--------|
| Adenosine | IV: 6 mg rapidly; if unsuccessful within 1-2 min, 12 mg rapidly |
| Diltiazem | IV: 0.25 mg/kg body wt over 2 min; if response inadequate, wait 15 min, then 0.35 mg/kg over 2 min; maintenance of 10-15 mg/h |
| Digoxin[a] | IV: 0.5 mg over 10 min; if response inadequate, 0.25 mg q4h to a maximum of 1.5 mg in 24 h |
| Esmolol | IV: 500 µg/kg/min × 1 min followed by 50 µg/kg/min × 4 min, repeat with 50-µg increments to maintenance dose of 200 µg/kg/min |
| Procainamide | IV: 10-15 mg/kg at 25 mg/min as loading dose, then 1-4 mg/min |
| Propranolol | IV: 0.1 mg/kg in divided 1-mg doses |
| Verapamil | IV: 5 mg over 1 min; if unsuccessful, one to two 5-mg boluses 10 min apart |

[a]Contraindicated in patients with Wolff–Parkinson–White syndrome.

# ■ SUPRAVENTRICULAR TACHYCARDIA DUE TO WOLFF–PARKINSON–WHITE SYNDROME

This is the second most common form of reentrant SVT. When conduction during an SVT occurs antegrade through the AV node and retrograde through the accessory pathway, it is referred to as an *orthodromic* reciprocating tachycardia. This is the common form of SVT in Wolff–Parkinson–White (WPW) syndrome; the ECG pattern is a narrow-QRS tachycardia at rates ranging from 160 to 240 bpm. *Antidromic* SVT, referring to antegrade conduction using an accessory pathway and retrograde conduction through the normal pathway, is uncommon; the QRS complexes are wide and are similar to fully preexcited impulses during sinus rhythm or premature atrial contractions.

Intracardiac EP studies permit characterization of the accessory pathway and its associated tachyarrhythmias. Electrophysiologic testing is recommended for patients who have frequent or poorly tolerated tachyarrhythmias or a history of atrial fibrillation or atrial flutter (particularly with antegrade bypass tract conduction). *Radiofrequency catheter ablation* of the accessory pathway (usually left lateral in location) is the preferred treatment. Medical therapy with class IC agents may be used temporarily in patients without structural heart disease while the patient awaits ablative therapy or in patients who do not desire ablation. Care has to be exercised with pharmacologic therapy to avoid selective antegrade conduction through the accessory pathway.

# ATRIOVENTRICULAR JUNCTIONAL AND ACCELERATED VENTRICULAR RHYTHMS

AV junctional rhythms originate within or just distal to the immediate vicinity of the AV node and may be automatic or reentrant. In AV junctional rhythm, the impulse travels antegrade and retrograde at the same time from the AV junction and is characterized by a normal QRS complex (unless coexistent BBB or aberrancy is present) and a retrograde P wave. Depending on the site of origin and the rate of conduction in each direction, the P wave may occur shortly before the QRS complex, follow the

**TABLE 9-5. Antiarrhythmic Drugs: Dosage and Kinetics**

| Drug | | Usual Dosing Range[a] | Half-Life | Therapeutic Range (μg/mL) | Plasma Protein Binding (%) | Major Route of Excretion |
|---|---|---|---|---|---|---|
| Class IA | Quinidine | Oral sulfate: 200-600 mg q6h<br>Oral long-acting: 330-60 mg, q8h or q6h | 5-7 h | 2.3-5 | 80 | H |
| | Procainamide | Oral: 250-750 mg, q4h or q6h<br>Oral long-acting: 500-1500 mg, q8h or q6h<br>IV: 10-15 mg/kg at 25 mg/min, then 1-6 mg/min | 3-5 h | 4-10 | 15 | R[b] |
| | Disopyramide | Oral: 100-200 mg q8h or q6h | 8-9 h | 2-5 | 35-95 | H/R |
| | Moricizine[c] | Oral: 150-300 mg q12h to q8h | 6-13 h | – | 95 | H |
| Class IB | Lidocaine | IV: 1-3 mg/kg at 20-50 mg/min, then 1-4 mg/min | 1-2 h | 1-5 | 60 | H |
| | Tocainide | Oral: 400-600 mg 8-12 h | 15 h | 4-10 | 10 | H |
| | Mexiletine | Oral: 200-400 mg q8h | 10-12 h | 0.5-2.0 | 55 | H |
| Class IC | Flecainide | Oral: 100-200 mg q12h | 20 h | 0.4-1.0 | 40 | H |
| | Encainide | Oral: 25-50 mg q8h | 3-4+ h | 0.5-1.0[d] | 80 | H |
| | Propafenone[a] | Oral: 150-300 mg q8h | 2-10 h | 0.5-1.5[d] | 95 | H |
| Class II | Propranolol | Oral: 10-100 mg q6h<br>IV: 0.1 mg/kg in divided 1 mg doses | 4-6 h | 0.04-0.10 | 95 | H |
| | Esmolol | IV: 500 μ/kg/min × 1 min followed by 50 μg/kg/min × 4 min, repeat with 50-μg increments to maintenance dose to 200 μ/kg/min | 9 min | – | 55 | H |
| | Acebutolol | Oral: 200-600 mg bid | 3-4 h | – | 26 | H/R |
| Class III | Amiodarone | Oral: 600-1600 mg/d × 1-3 wk, then 200-400 mg/d<br>IV: 5 mg/min × min, then 1 mg/min × 6 h, then maintenance at 0.5 mg/min | 50 d<br>? | 1-2.5<br>? | 96 | H |

| | Dose | | | | |
|---|---|---|---|---|---|
| Bretylium | IV: 5-10 mg/kg at 1-2 mg/kg, then 0.5-2.0 mg/min | 8-14 h | 0.5-1.5 | — | R |
| Sotalol[d] | Oral: 80-320 mg q12h | 10-15 h | — | 0 | R |
| Ibutilide | IV: (for >60 kg): 1 mg over 10 min, may repeat × 1.10 min after completion of initial dose[c] | 2-12 h | — | 40 | H |
| Class IV | | | | | |
| Verapamil | Oral: 80-32 mg q6-8h; IV: 5-10 mg in 1-2 min | 3-8 h | 0.1-0.15 | 90 | H |
| Diltiazem | IV: 0.25 mg/kg body wt over 2 min; if response inadequate, wait 15 min, then 0.35 mg/kg over 2 min; maintenance 10-15 mg/h | 3.5-5.0 h | 0.1-3.0 | 70-80 | H |
| Other | | | | | |
| Digoxin | Oral: 1.25-1.5 mg in divided doses over 24 h followed by 0.125-0.375 mg/d IV: Approximately 70% of oral dose | 36 h | 0.8-1.4 mg/mL | 30 | R |
| Dronedarone | Oral: 400 mg q12h | 13-19 h | — | >98 | H |
| Adenosine | IV: 6 mg rapidly; if unsuccessful within 1-2 min, 12 mg rapidly | 10 s | — | — | — |

H, hepatic; R, renal.

[a]All dosing should follow FDA-approved guidelines as outlined in package insert or Physicians' Desk Reference. (See also Chapter 43.) Does not include pediatric use in infants and young children.

[b]Parent compound metabolized to active metabolite (NAPA) in liver; both active metabolite and unmetabolized parent compound excreted by kidneys.

[c]Shares classes IB, IC activities.

[d]Active metabolite limits significance of these measurements.

**APPENDIX 9-1.** Class I (Positive) and Class III (Negative) Recommendations for Management of Atrial Fibrillation[a]

## Pharmacologic Rate Control During Atrial Fibrillation

### Class I

1. Measurement of the heart rate at rest and control of the rate using pharmacologic agents (either a β-blocker or nondihydropyridine calcium-channel antagonist, in most cases) are recommended for patients with persistent or permanent AF. (*Level of Evidence: B*)
2. In the absence of preexcitation, IV administration of β-blockers (esmolol, metoprolol, or propranolol) or nondihydropyridine calcium-channel antagonists (verapamil, diltiazem) is recommended to slow the ventricular response to AF in the acute setting, exercising caution in patients with hypotension or heart failure (HF). (*Level of Evidence: B*)
3. IV administration of digoxin or amiodarone is recommended to control the heart rate in patients with AF and HF who do not have an accessory pathway. (*Level of Evidence: B*)
4. In patients who experience symptoms related to AF during activity, the adequacy of heart rate control should be assessed during exercise, adjusting pharmacologic treatment as necessary to keep the rate in the physiologic range. (*Level of Evidence: C*)
5. Digoxin is effective following oral administration to control the heart rate at rest in patients with AF, and is indicated for patients with HF, left ventricular (LV) dysfunction, or for sedentary individuals. (*Level of Evidence: C*)

### Class III

1. Digitalis should not be used as the sole agent to control the rate of ventricular response in patients with paroxysmal AF. (*Level of Evidence: B*)
2. Catheter ablation of the AV node should not be attempted without a prior trial of medication to control the ventricular rate in patients with AF. (*Level of Evidence: C*)
3. In patients with decompensated HF and AF, intravenous administration of a nondihydropyridine calcium-channel antagonist may exacerbate hemodynamic compromise and is not recommended. (*Level of Evidence: C*)
4. IV administration of digitalis glycosides or nondihydropyridine calcium-channel antagonists to patients with AF and a preexcitation syndrome may paradoxically accelerate the ventricular response and is not recommended. (*Level of Evidence: C*)

## Preventing Thromboembolism

### Class I

1. Antithrombotic therapy to prevent thromboembolism is recommended for all patients with AF, except those with lone AF or contraindications. (*Level of Evidence: A*)
2. The selection of the antithrombotic agent should be based on the absolute risks of stroke and bleeding and the relative risk and benefit for a given patient. (*Level of Evidence: A*)
3. For patients without mechanical heart valves at high risk of stroke, chronic oral anticoagulant therapy with a vitamin K antagonist is recommended in a dose adjusted to achieve the target intensity international normalized ratio (INR) of 2.0-3.0, unless contraindicated. Factors associated with highest risk for stroke in patients with AF are prior thromboembolism (stroke, transient ischemic attack [TIA], or systemic embolism) and rheumatic mitral stenosis. (*Level of Evidence: A*)
4. Anticoagulation with a vitamin K antagonist is recommended for patients with more than 1 moderate risk factor. Such factors include age 75 years or greater, hypertension, HF, impaired LV systolic function (ejection fraction ≤ 35% or fractional shortening < 25%), and diabetes mellitus. (*Level of Evidence: A*)
5. INR should be determined at least weekly during initiation of therapy and monthly when anticoagulation is stable. (*Level of Evidence: A*)
6. Aspirin, 81-325 mg daily, is recommended as an alternative to vitamin K antagonists in low-risk patients or in those with contraindications to oral anticoagulation. (*Level of Evidence: A*)

*(continued)*

**APPENDIX 9-1.** Class I (Positive) and Class III (Negative) Recommendations for Management of Atrial Fibrillation*a* (continued)

7. For patients with AF who have mechanical heart valves, the target intensity of anticoagulation should be based on the type of prosthesis, maintaining an INR of at least 2.5. (*Level of Evidence: B*)
8. Antithrombotic therapy is recommended for patients with atrial flutter as for those with AF. (*Level of Evidence: C*)

**Class III**

Long-term anticoagulation with a vitamin K antagonist is not recommended for primary prevention of stroke in patients below the age of 60 years without heart disease (lone AF) or any risk factors for thromboembolism. (*Level of Evidence: C*)

### Cardioversion of Atrial Fibrillation

*Pharmacologic Cardioversion*
**Class I**
Administration of flecainide, dofetilide, propafenone, or ibutilide is recommended for pharmacologic cardioversion of AF. (*Level of Evidence: A*)

**Class III**
1. Digoxin and sotalol may be harmful when used for pharmacologic cardioversion of AF and are not recommended. (*Level of Evidence: A*)
2. Quinidine, procainamide, disopyramide, and dofetilide should not be started out of hospital for conversion of AF to sinus rhythm. (*Level of Evidence: B*)

*Direct-Current Cardioversion*
**Class I**
1. When a rapid ventricular response does not respond promptly to pharmacologic measures for patients with AF with ongoing myocardial ischemia, symptomatic hypotension, angina, or HF, immediate R-wave synchronized direct-current cardioversion is recommended. (*Level of Evidence: C*)
2. Immediate direct-current cardioversion is recommended for patients with AF involving preexcitation when very rapid tachycardia or hemodynamic instability occurs. (*Level of Evidence: B*)
3. Cardioversion is recommended in patients without hemodynamic instability when symptoms of AF are unacceptable to the patient. In case of early relapse of AF after cardioversion, repeated direct-current cardioversion attempts may be made following administration of antiarrhythmic medication. (*Level of Evidence: C*)

**Class III**
1. Frequent repetition of direct-current cardioversion is not recommended for patients who have relatively short periods of sinus rhythm between relapses of AF after multiple cardioversion procedures despite prophylactic antiarrhythmic drug therapy. (*Level of Evidence: C*)
2. Electrical cardioversion is contraindicated in patients with digitalis toxicity or hypokalemia. (*Level of Evidence: C*)

*Pharmacologic Enhancement of Direct-Current Cardioversion*
**Class I**
1. For patients with AF of 48-h duration of longer, or when the duration of AF is unknown, anticoagulation (INR 2.0-3.0) is recommended for at least 3 wk prior to and 4 wk after cardioversion, regardless of the method (electrical or pharmacologic) used to restore sinus rhythm. (*Level of Evidence: B*)

(continued)

**APPENDIX 9-1.** Class I (Positive) and Class III (Negative) Recommendations for Management of Atrial Fibrillation*a* (continued)

2. For patients with AF or more than 48-h duration requiring immediate cardioversion because of hemodynamic instability, heparin should be administered concurrently (unless contraindicated) by an initial intravenous bolus injection followed by a continuous infusion in a dose adjusted to prolong the activated partial thromboplastin time to 1.5-2 times the reference control value. Thereafter, oral anticoagulation (INR 2.0-3.0) should be provided for at least 4 wk, as for patients undergoing elective cardioversion. Limited data support subcutaneous administration of low-molecular-weight heparin in this indication.(*Level of Evidence: C*)

3. For patients with AF of less than 48-h duration associated with hemodynamic instability (angina pectoris, myocardial infarction [MI], shock, or pulmonary edema), cardioversion should be performed immediately without delay for prior initiation of anticoagulation. (*Level of Evidence: C*)

### Maintenance of Sinus Rhythm

**Class I**

Before initiating antiarrhythmic drug therapy, treatment of precipitating or reversible causes of AF is recommended. (*Level of Evidence: C*)

**Class III**

1. Antiarrhythmic therapy with a particular drug is not recommended for maintenance of sinus rhythm in patients with AF who have well-defined risk factors for proarrhythmia with that agent. (*Level of Evidence: A*)

2. Pharmacologic therapy is not recommended for maintenance of sinus rhythm in patients with advanced sinus node disease or atrioventricular (AV) node dysfunction unless they have a functioning electronic cardiac pacemaker. (*Level of Evidence: C*)

### Special Considerations

*Postoperative Atrial Fibrillation*

**Class I**

1. Unless contraindicated, treatment with an oral β-blocker to prevent postoperative AF is recommended for patients undergoing cardiac surgery. (*Level of Evidence: A*)

2. Administration of AV nodal blocking agents is recommended to achieve rate control in patients who develop postoperative AF. (*Level of Evidence: B*)

### Acute Myocardial Infarction

**Class I**

1. Direct-current cardioversion is recommended for patients with severe hemodynamic compromise or intractable ischemia, or when adequate rate control cannot be achieved with pharmacologic agents in patients with acute MI and AF. (*Level of Evidence: C*)

2. Intravenous administration of amiodarone is recommended to slow a rapid ventricular response to AF and improve LV function in patients with acute MI. (*Level of Evidence: C*)

3. Intravenous β-blockers and nondihydropyridine calcium antagonists are recommended to slow a rapid ventricular response to AF in patients with acute MI who do not display clinical LV dysfunction, bronchospasm, or AV block. (*Level of Evidence: C*)

4. For patients with AF and acute MI, administration of unfractionated heparin by either continuous intravenous infusion of intermittent subcutaneous injection is recommended in a dose sufficient to prolong the activated partial thromboplastin time to 1.5-2 times the control value, unless contraindications to anticoagulation exist. (*Level of Evidence: C*)

**Class III**

The administration of class IC antiarrhythmic drugs is not recommended in patients with AF in the setting of acute MI. (*Level of Evidence: C*)

*(continued)*

**APPENDIX 9-1.** Class I (Positive) and Class III (Negative) Recommendations for Management of Atrial Fibrillation$^a$ (continued)

*Management of Atrial Fibrillation Associated With Wolff–Parkinson–White (WPW) Preexcitation Syndrome*
Class I
1. Catheter ablation of the accessory pathway is recommended in symptomatic patients with AF who have WPW syndrome, particularly those with syncope due to rapid heart rate or those with a short bypass tract refractory period. *(Level of Evidence: B)*
2. Immediate direct-current cardioversion is recommended to prevent ventricular fibrillation in patients with a short anterograde bypass tract refractory period in whom AF occurs with a rapid ventricular response associated with hemodynamic instability. *(Level of Evidence: B)*
3. IV procainamide or ibutilide is recommended to restore sinus rhythm in patients with WPW in whom AF occurs without hemodynamic instability in association with a wide QRS complex on the ECG ($\geq$ 120-msec duration) or with a rapid preexcited ventricular response. *(Level of Evidence: C)*
Class III
IV administration of digitalis glycosides or nondihydropyridine calcium-channel antagonists is not recommended in patients with WPW syndrome who have preexcited ventricular activation during AF. *(Level of Evidence: B)*

*Hyperthyroidism*
Class I
1. Administration of a β-blocker is recommended to control the rate of a ventricular response in patients with AF complicating thyrotoxicosis, unless contraindicated. *(Level of Evidence: B)*
2. In circumstances when a β-blocker cannot be used, administration of a nondihydropyridine calcium-channel antagonist (diltiazem or verapamil) is recommended to control the ventricular rate in patients with AF and thyrotoxicosis. *(Level of Evidence: B)*
3. In patients with AF associated with thyrotoxicosis, oral anticoagulation (INR 2.0-3.0) is recommended to prevent thromboembolism, as recommended for AF patients with other risk factors for stroke. *(Level of Evidence: C)*
4. Once a euthyroid state is restored, recommendations for antithrombotic prophylaxis are the same as for patients without hyperthyroidism. *(Level of Evidence: C)*

*Management of Atrial Fibrillation During Pregnancy*
Class I
1. Digoxin, a β-blocker, or a nondihydropyridine calcium-channel antagonist, is recommended to control the rate of ventricular response in pregnant patients with AF. *(Level of Evidence: C)*
2. Direct-current cardioversion is recommended in pregnant patients who become hemodynamically unstable due to AF *(Level of Evidence: C)*
3. Protection against thromboembolism is recommended throughout pregnancy for all patients with AF (except for those with lone AF and/or low thromboembolic risk). Therapy (anticoagulant or aspirin) should be chosen according to stage of pregnancy. *(Level of Evidence: C)*

*Management of Atrial Fibrillation in Patients With Hypertrophic Cardiomyopathy (HCM)*
Class I
Oral anticoagulation (INR 2.0-3.0) is recommended in patients with HCM who develop AF, as for other patients at high risk of thromboembolism. *(Level of Evidence: B)*

*(continued)*

**APPENDIX 9-1.** Class I (Positive) and Class III (Negative) Recommendations for Management of Atrial Fibrillation[a] (continued)

*Management of Atrial Fibrillation in Patients With Pulmonary Disease*
Class I
1. Correction of hypoxemia and acidosis is the recommended primary therapeutic measure for patients who develop AF during an acute pulmonary illness or exacerbation of chronic pulmonary disease. *(Level of Evidence: C)*
2. A nondihydropyridine calcium-channel antagonist (diltiazem or verapamil) is recommended to control the ventricular rate in patients with obstructive pulmonary disease who develop AF. *(Level of Evidence: C)*
3. Direct-current cardioversion should be attempted in patients with pulmonary disease who become hemodynamically unstable as a consequence of AF. *(Level of Evidence: C)*
Class III
1. Theophylline and β-adrenergic agonist agents are not recommended in patients with bronchospastic lung disease who develop AF. *(Level of Evidence: C)*
2. β-blockers, sotalol, propafenone, and adenosine are not recommended in patients with obstructive lung disease who develop AF. *(Level of Evidence: C)*

[a]See also Chapter 59.

Reproduced with permission from Fuster V, Ryden LE. ACC/AHA/ESC 2006 guidelines for the management of patients with atrial fibrillation: a report of the American College of Cardiology/American Heart Association Task Force on Practice Guidelines and the European Society of Cardiology Committee for Practice Guidelines (Writing Committee to Revise the 2001 Guidelines for the Management of Patients With Atrial Fibrillation). *Circulation.* 2006;114:e257-e354.

QRS complex, or be lost within it. The rates of AV junctional escape rhythms are usually in the range of 40 to 60 bpm; therefore, these rhythms become manifest only when the sinus impulse fails to reach the AV node within physiologic ranges of rate. These rhythms are secondary, occurring as a result of sinus depression or sinoatrial block, and are a normal physiologic phenomenon. Failure of these escape rhythms can result in significant bradycardia. This is discussed in the section on bradyarrhythmias later in this chapter.

Another type of secondary rhythm is an *accelerated ventricular rhythm.* This occurs because the sinus and junctional rates are slow enough to permit an ectopic ventricular rhythm to escape. The ectopic pacemaker is accelerated above its normal physiologic rate of 20 to 40 bpm and overrides the sinus rate, which may be relatively depressed. The rate of an accelerated ventricular rhythm is usually between 50 and 100 bpm, and the QRS complexes are wide. The rhythm commonly begins with 1 or 2 fusion beats and then is regular; however, it may show progressive acceleration or deceleration until it terminates spontaneously.

If the AV junctional rate exceeds 60 bpm but is less than 100 bpm, it is referred to as an *accelerated junctional rhythm.* These rhythms are seen commonly in patients with acute myocardial infarction (MI), particularly when the inferior wall is involved. They have also been associated with digitalis intoxication, electrolyte abnormalities, hypertensive heart disease, cardiomyopathy, and congenital and rheumatic heart disease. This rhythm usually requires no specific treatment; in fact, the use of antiarrhythmic agents may suppress the subordinate pacemaker required for the maintenance of an adequate rate.

Occasionally, the rate of accelerated AV junctional rhythm increases abruptly to the tachycardia range (ie, ≥100 bpm). This phenomenon probably represents an autonomic focus firing at the faster rate, often with AV dissociation. Usually no treatment is needed except in ischemia, when faster heart rates are unacceptable. Persistent AV junctional tachycardia (sometimes referred to as *nonparoxysmal* junctional tachycardia) occasionally occurs in patients with chronic heart disease. In infants and children, this rhythm can be a cause of tachycardia-induced cardiomyopathy.

## SUGGESTED READINGS

Prystowsky EN, Padanilam BJ, Waldo AL. Atrial fibrillation, atrial flutter, and atrial tachycardia. In: Fuster V, O'Rourke RA, Walsh RA, et al, eds. *Hurst's The Heart.* 13th ed. New York, NY: McGraw-Hill; 2011;40:963-986.

AFFIRM investigators. A comparison of rate control and rhythm control in patients with atrial fibrillation. *N Engl J Med.* 2002;347:1825-1833.

Blomstrom-Lundqvist C, Scheinman MM, Aliot EM. ACC/AHA/ESC guidelines for the management of patients with supraventricular arrhythmias. *Circulation.* 2003;108:1871-1909.

Cox JL. Cardiac surgery for arrhythmias. *J Cardiovasc Electrophysiol.* 2004;15:250-262.

DiMarco JP. Implantable cardioverter-defibrillators. *N Engl J Med.* 2003;349:1836-1847.

2011 ACCF/AHA/HRS Focused Update on the Management of Patients With Atrial Fibrillation (Updating the 2006 Guideline): a report of the American College of Cardiology Foundation/American Heart Association Task Force on Practice Guidelines. *Circulation.* 2011;123:104-123.

Fuster V, Rydén LE, Cannom DS, et al. ACC/AHA/ESC 2006 guidelines for the management of patients with atrial fibrillation: a report of the American College of Cardiology/American Heart Association Task Force on Practice Guidelines and the European Society of Cardiology Committee for Practice Guidelines (Writing Committee to Revise the 2001 Guidelines for the Management of Patients With Atrial Fibrillation). *Eur Heart J.* 2006;27:1979-2030.

Hohnloser SH, Crijns H, Eickels M, et al. Effect of Dronedarone on Cardiovascular Events in Atrial Fibrillation. *N Engl J Med.* 2009;360:668-678.

Hsu LF, Jais P, Sanders P, et al. Catheter ablation for atrial fibrillation in congestive heart failure. *N Engl J Med.* 2004;351:2373-2383.

Kober L, Torp-Pedersen C, McMurray JJV, et al. Increased mortality after Dronedarone Therapy for Severe Heart Failure. *N Engl J Med.* 2008;358:2678-2687.

Myerburg RJ, Kloosterman EM, Castellanos A. Recognition, clinical assessment, and management of arrhythmias and conduction disturbances. In: Fuster V, Alexander RW, O'Rourke RA, et al, eds. *Hurst's The Heart.* 11th ed. New York, NY: McGraw-Hill; 2004:797-873.

Oral H, Scharf C, Chugh A, et al. Catheter ablation for paroxysmal atrial fibrillation: segmental pulmonary vein ostial ablation versus left atrial ablation. *Circulation.* 2003;108:2355-2360.

Van Gelder IC, Groenveld HF, Crijns HJ, et al. Lenient versus strict rate control in patients with atrial fibrillation. *N Engl J Med.* 2010;362:1363-1373.

Yu CM, Chan JY, Zhang Q, et al. Biventricular pacing in patients with bradycardia and normal ejection fraction. *N Engl J Med.* 2009;361:2123-2134.

# CHAPTER 10
# VENTRICULAR ARRHYTHMIAS

## Robert W. Rho and Richard L. Page

Ventricular arrhythmias occur commonly in clinical practice and range from benign asymptomatic premature ventricular complexes (PVCs) to ventricular fibrillation (VF) resulting in sudden death (**Table 10-1**). The presence or absence of structural heart disease and left ventricular function (ejection fraction) play a major role in risk stratification; however, it is important to recognize that potentially lethal arrhythmias may occur in structurally normal-appearing hearts. Management depends on the associated symptoms, hemodynamic consequences, and long-term prognosis. The electrocardiographic (ECG) pattern of the ventricular arrhythmia provides important guidance in selecting appropriate management strategies.

## PREMATURE VENTRICULAR COMPLEXES

Premature ventricular complexes are frequent in clinical practice. The significance of PVCs depends on their frequency, the presence and severity of structural heart disease, and the presence of associated symptoms.

In general, PVCs that occur in patients without structural heart disease are not associated with excess risk of sudden death and generally require no therapy, unless significant symptoms are present. Therapy is directed toward removal of precipitating factors; occasionally, low-dose β-adrenergic receptor blockers can offer symptomatic benefit.

The relationship between PVCs following myocardial infarction (MI) and sudden death has been studied extensively. In general, the presence of PVCs after an MI is associated with an increased risk of sudden death when the frequency of PVCs exceeds 10 per hour. Patients with larger MIs and lower left ventricular ejection fractions (LVEFs) are at the greatest risk of sudden death.

Despite the risk associated with postinfarct ectopy, the routine use of antiarrhythmic agents in the acute or more remote postinfarct period does not convey benefit, and in some cases increases risk. Thus, the routine prophylactic use of antiarrhythmics following an MI *is not recommended*. Likewise, *treatment of PVCs and nonsustained ventricular tachycardia (VT) with antiarrhythmics is also not recommended* unless they are associated with hemodynamic compromise. If frequent and persistent ventricular ectopy results in hemodynamic instability, a β-blocker or amiodarone is the preferred agent. Lidocaine may be considered temporarily when hemodynamically significant ventricular arrhythmias occur in the setting of acute MI. In all cases, electrolyte and acid–base imbalance should be vigilantly corrected.

The use of amiodarone in patients during and following an acute MI has increased but is still controversial. In this acute setting, prospective randomized trials have shown that amiodarone use for the treatment of hemodynamically significant ventricular arrhythmias or other arrhythmias, such as atrial fibrillation, appears to be safe but does not confer survival benefit.

**TABLE 10-1.** Ventricular Arrhythmias: Mechanisms and Clinical Features

| Ventricular Arrhythmia | ECG Features | Mechanism | Clinical Features |
|---|---|---|---|
| Premature ventricular complexes (PVCs) | Variable: CAD: RBBB morphology RVOT: LBBB morphology | Reentry focal triggered | Significance depends on structural heart disease |
| Ischemic ventricular tachycardia | Variable: usually RBBB morphology | Reentry most common | Significance depends on etiology/hemodynamic consequences/EF |
| VT in ARVD | LBBB VT morphology | Reentry most common | Multiple morphologies progressive disease |
| VT in cardiac sarcoid | Usually RBBB VT morphology | Reentry most common | Associated with conduction abnormalities |
| VT in Chagas disease | Variable: usually RBBB VT morphology | Reentry most common often epicardial | LV dysfunction/aneurysm South American protozoa: *Trypanosoma cruzi* |
| Bundle branch reentry VT | Usually LBBB pattern but may be RBBB pattern (in ischemic cardiomyopathy) | Reentry | A sustained monomophic VT in dilated cardiomyopathy Amenable to RF ablation |
| RVOT VT | LBBB VT with left Inferior axis | Triggered activity Increased automaticity | Benign. Treat symptoms or tachycardia |
| Idiopathic left VT | RBBB VT with left superior axis | Probably reentry involving left ant/post fascicles | Benign. Treat symptoms or tachycardia; sensitive to verapamil |
| Ventricular fibrillation | Rapid and irregular; no discernable QRS complex | Functional reentry | Fatal unless immediate defibrillation associated with ischemia |
| Torsade de Pointes | Polymorphic VT twisting around central axis | Triggered activity initiates and functional reentry maintains VT | Associated with Long QT syndrome drugs prolonging QT must be identified and discontinued |

The association between PVCs in non-ischemic cardiomyopathy and sudden death is less clear. Prospective clinical trials have found that nonsustained VT (NSVT) is a risk factor for sudden death in this population. In general, sudden and total cardiac death rates are increased in patients with high-grade PVCs (>10/h) and non-ischemic dilated cardiomyopathy, hypertensive heart disease, and hypertrophic cardiomyopathy.

# VENTRICULAR TACHYCARDIA

Sustained VT is a series of continuous ventricular impulses >100 beats per minute that lasts for longer than 30 seconds or results in hemodynamic instability (if <30 s). Nonsustained VT (NSVT) is defined by at least 3 consecutive ventricular complexes that are not sustained. Ventricular storm occurs when there are 3 sustained episodes of VT within a 24-hour period. Ventricular fibrillation is generally a reflection of acute ischemia and is not scar related.

Wide complex tachycardias may either be VT or an SVT with aberrancy. If there is a history of heart disease, the likelihood of VT is generally greater than 80%. By ECG, differentiating VT from a supraventricular tachycardia (SVT) with aberrant intraventricular conduction can be difficult. The presence of atrioventricular dissociation (with clearly discernible P waves unrelated to ventricular activity), fusion beats (single QRS complexes that are usually narrower than the VT complexes and represent "fusion" between a ventricular complex and a conducted supraventricular impulse), QRS duration >140 milliseconds, and concordantly positive or negative QRS complexes across the precordium favor VT over an SVT with aberrant conduction (**Table 10-2**).

## ■ VENTRICULAR TACHYCARDIA ASSOCIATED WITH CORONARY ARTERY DISEASE

NSVTs or sustained VTs are generally markers of increased sudden death risk when they are associated with CAD and may or may not be otherwise symptomatic. Treatment is generally considered when there is hemodynamic compromise and/or to decrease the risk of sudden death. The anatomic substrate supporting sustained monomorphic

---

**TABLE 10-2.** Electrocardiographic Features That Favor Ventricular Tachycardia in Comparison to Supraventricular Tachycardia With Aberrant Conduction

Atrioventricular (AV) dissociation
Fusion and capture beats
Positive or negative concordance of QRS morphology across the precordial leads ($V_1$-$V_6$)
Superiorly directed QRS axis, especially if directed toward right upper quadrant between − 90 degrees and +180 degrees
RBBB pattern with QRS duration longer than 140 msec, or LBBB pattern with QRS duration longer than 160 msec
RBBB pattern QRS with monophasic R wave in $V_1$
LBBB pattern QRS with one of the following:
1. Notching in S-wave downstroke in $V_1$ or $V_2$
2. Any Q wave in $V_{6/}$
3. QRS onset to nadir of S wave in $V_1$ greater than 60 msec polymorphic tachycardias

Adapted from Simmons JD, Chakko SC, Myerburg RJ. Arrhythmias and conduction disturbances. In: O'Rourke RA, Fuster V, Alexander W, eds. *Hurst's The Heart Manual of Cardiology.* 11th ed. New York, NY: McGraw-Hill; 2005:93

VT usually involves healthy and damaged myocardium interlaced with fibrous scar primarily at the border zone of a myocardial scar. The risk of VT is thought to be highest during the first year after an MI, but new onset of VT may occur many years later. In general, patients with larger infarctions and lower EFs are at highest risk of fatal ventricular arrhythmias.

Patients with VT and hemodynamic compromise, congestive heart failure, and/or ischemia should be treated promptly with DC cardioversion. In patients with stable sustained VT, intravenous procainamide is a reasonable first choice; however, it may cause hemodynamic instability because of its negative inotropic effects. In the setting of VT associated with hemodynamic instability, amiodarone is the treatment of choice over lidocaine or procainamide. All patients with VT should be treated with a β-blocker unless precluded by hypotension, bradycardia, or other clinical factors. Reversible factors contributing to VT should be corrected. Potential ischemic precipitants should be addressed as well.

Long-term management in patients with sustained VT is directed to preventing recurrent VT and sudden death, and usually involves a combination of antiarrhythmic therapy and implantation of an internal cardioverter-defibrillator (ICD) (**Table 10-3**). Patients who present with sustained VT, an LVEF <35%, on chronic optimal medical management and have a reasonable expectation for

---

**TABLE 10-3.** ACC/AHA/HRS 2008 Guidelines for Device-Based Therapy of Cardiac Rhythm Abnormalities

**Class I**

1. ICD therapy is recommended for secondary prevention of SCD in patients who are survivors of cardiac arrest due to ventricular fibrillation or hemodynamically unstable sustained VT after evaluation to define the cause of the event and to exclude any completely reversible causes. *(Level of Evidence: A)*
2. ICD therapy is indicated in patients with structural heart disease and spontaneous sustained VT, whether hemodynamically stable or unstable. *(Level of Evidence: B)*
3. ICD therapy is indicated in patients with syncope of undetermined origin with clinically relevant, hemodynamically significant sustained VT or ventricular fibrillation induced at electrophysiologic study. *(Level of Evidence: B)*
4. ICD therapy is recommended in patients with LVEF <35% due to prior myocardial infarction who are at least 40 days post–myocardial infarction and are in NYHA functional class II or III. *(Level of Evidence: A)*
5. ICD therapy is recommended in patients with non-ischemic dilated cardiomyopathy who have an LVEF ≤35% and who are in NYHA functional class II or III. *(Level of Evidence: B)*
6. ICD therapy is indicated in patients with LV dysfunction due to prior myocardial infarction who are at least 40 days post–myocardial infarction, have an LVEF <30%, and are in NYHA functional class I. *(Level of Evidence A)*
7. ICD therapy is indicated in patients with nonsustained VT due to prior myocardial infarction, LVEF <40%, and inducible ventricular fibrillation or sustained VT at electrophysiologic study. *(Level of Evidence: B)*

**Class IIa**

1. ICD implantation is reasonable for patients with unexplained syncope, significant LV dysfunction, and non-ischemic dilated cardiomyopathy. *(Level of Evidence: C)*
2. Implantation of an ICD is reasonable in patients with sustained VT and normal or near-normal ventricular function. *(Level of Evidence: C)*
3. ICD implantation is reasonable for patients with hypertrophic cardiomyopathy who have one or more major risk factors for SCD. *(Level of Evidence: C)*

*(continued)*

**TABLE 10-3.** ACC/AHA/HRS 2008 Guidelines for Device-Based Therapy of Cardiac Rhythm Abnormalities (continued)

4. ICD implantation is reasonable for the prevention of SCD in patients with arrhythmogenic right ventricular dysplasia/cardiomyopathy who have one or more risk factors for SCD. *(Level of Evidence: C)*
5. ICD implantation is reasonable to reduce SCD in patients with long QT syndrome who are experiencing syncope and/or VT while receiving β-blockers. *(Level of Evidence: B)*
6. ICD implantation is reasonable for nonhospitalized patients awaiting transplantation. *(Level of Evidence: C)*
7. ICD implantation is reasonable for patients with Brugada syndrome who have had syncope. *(Level of Evidence: C)*
8. ICD implantation is reasonable for patients with Brugada syndrome who have documented VT that has not resulted in cardiac arrest. *(Level of Evidence: C)*
9. ICD implantation is reasonable for patients with catecholaminergic polymorphic VT who have syncope and/or documented sustained VT while receiving β-blockers. *(Level of Evidence: C)*
10. ICD implantation is reasonable for patients with cardiac sarcoidosis, giant-cell myocarditis, or Chagas disease. *(Level of Evidence: C)*

**Class IIb**

1. ICD therapy may be considered in patients with non-ischemic heart disease who have an LVEF of ≤35% and who are in NYHA functional class I. *(Level of Evidence: C)*
2. ICD therapy may be considered for patients with long QT syndrome and risk factors for SCD. *(Level of Evidence: B)*
3. ICD therapy may be considered in patients with syncope and advanced structural heart disease in whom thorough invasive and noninvasive investigations have failed to define a cause. *(Level of Evidence: C)*
4. ICD therapy may be considered in patients with a familial cardiomyopathy associated with sudden death. *(Level of Evidence: C)*
5. ICD therapy may be considered in patients with LV noncompaction. *(Level of Evidence: C)*

**Class III**

1. ICD therapy is not indicated for patients who do not have a reasonable expectation of survival with an acceptable functional status for at least 1 year, even if they meet ICD implantation criteria specified in the classes I, IIa, and IIb recommendations previously. *(Level of Evidence: C)*
2. ICD therapy is not indicated for patients with incessant VT or ventricular fibrillation *(Level of Evidence: C)*
3. ICD therapy is not indicated in patients with significant psychiatric illnesses that may be aggravated by device implantation or that may preclude systematic follow-up. *(Level of Evidence: C)*
4. ICD therapy is not indicated for NYHA class IV patients with drug-refractory congestive heart failure who are not candidates for cardiac transplantation or implantation of a CRT device that incorporates both pacing and defibrillation capabilities. *(Level of Evidence: C)*
5. ICD therapy is not indicated for syncope of undetermined cause in a patient without inducible ventricular tachyarrhythmias and without structural heart disease. *(Level of Evidence: C)*
6. ICD therapy is not indicated when ventricular fibrillation or VT is amenable to surgical or catheter ablation (eg, atrial arrhythmias associated with Wolff–Parkinson–White syndrome, right ventricular or LV outflow tract VT, idiopathic VT, or fascicular VT in the absence of structural heart disease). *(Level of Evidence: C)*
7. ICD therapy is not indicated for patients with ventricular tachyarrhythmias due to a completely reversible disorder in the absence of structural heart disease (eg, electrolyte imbalance, drugs, or trauma). *(Level of Evidence: B)*

CRT, cardiac resynchronization therapy; ICD, implantable cardioverter-defibrillator; LV, left ventricular; LVEF, left ventricular ejection fraction; NYHA, New York Heart Association; SCD, sudden cardiac death; VT, ventricular tachycardia.

Reproduced with permission from Epstein AE, DiMarco JP, Ellenbogen KA, et al. ACC/AHA/HRS 2008 guidelines for device-based therapy of cardiac rhythm abnormalities, J Am Coll Cardiol 2008; May 27:51(21):e1-e62 survival with a good functional status for at least a year generally should receive an ICD. In patients with preserved LV function, amiodarone is a reasonable alternative in selected individuals. It is important that VT be clinically well-controlled in order to prevent multiple shocks from the ICD; this is often achieved with a combination of β-blockers and antiarrhythmic medications. Ventricular tachycardia that is refractory to medications may be successfully treated with *radiofrequency catheter ablation* techniques, but ablation may only be palliative (**Table 10-4**).

Patients with preserved LV function and NSVT are generally at lower risk and require no further treatment, but patients with low EF and NSVT are at high risk of sudden death. Based on recent randomized studies, those who are post-MI and have an LVEF <35% should *be considered* for ICD implantation for primary prevention of sudden death regardless of whether they have clinically documented NSVT.

---

**TABLE 10-4.** ACC/AHA/ESC 2006 Guidelines for the Role of Ablation in the Management of Ventricular Arrhythmias

**Class I**
1. Ablation is indicated in patients who are otherwise at low risk for SCD and have sustained predominantly monomorphic VT that is drug resistant, are drug intolerant, or do not wish long-term drug therapy. *(Level of Evidence: C)*
2. Ablation is indicated in patients with BBR VT. *(Level of Evidence: C)*
3. Ablation is indicated as adjunctive therapy in patients with an ICD who are receiving multiple shocks as a result of sustained VT that is not manageable by reprogramming or changing drug therapy or do not wish long-term drug therapy. *(Level of Evidence: C)*
4. Ablation is indicated in patients with Wolff–Parkinson–White syndrome resuscitated from sudden cardiac arrest caused by atrial fibrillation and rapid conduction over the accessory pathway causing VF. *(Level of Evidence: B)*

**Class IIa**
1. Ablation can be useful therapy in patients who are otherwise at low risk for SCD and have symptomatic nonsustained monomorphic VT that is drug resistant, are drug intolerant, or do not wish long-term drug therapy. *(Level of Evidence: C)*
2. Ablation can be useful therapy in patients who are otherwise at low risk for SCD and have frequent symptomatic predominantly monomorphic PVCs that are drug resistant, are drug intolerant, or do not wish long-term drug therapy. *(Level of Evidence: C)*
3. Ablation can be useful in symptomatic patients with Wolff–Parkinson–White syndrome who have accessory pathways with refractory periods <240 msec in duration. *(Level of Evidence: B)*

**Class IIb**
1. Ablation of asymptomatic PVCs may be considered when the PVCs are very frequent to avoid or treat tachycardia-induced cardiomyopathy. *(Level of Evidence: C)*
2. Curative catheter ablation or amiodarone may be considered in lieu of ICD therapy to improve symptoms in patients with LV dysfunction caused by prior MI and recurrent hemodynamically stable VT whose LVEF is >40%. *(Level of Evidence: B)*

**Class III**
1. Ablation of asymptomatic relatively infrequent PVCs is not indicated. *(Level of Evidence: C)*

---

BBR, bundle-branch reentrant; ICD, implantable cardioverter-defibrillator; LV, left ventricular; LVEF, left ventricular ejection fraction; MI, myocardial infarction; PVC, premature ventricular complexes; SCD, sudden cardiac death; VT, ventricular tachycardia.

(Data from Zipes DP, Camm AJ, Borggrefe M, et al: ACC/AHA/ESC 2006 Guidelines for the Role of Ablation in the Management of Ventricular Arrhythmias, European Heart Journal 2006: Sep;27(17):2099-140.)

# VENTRICULAR TACHYCARDIA ASSOCIATED WITH NON-ISCHEMIC CARDIOMYOPATHY

Sustained VT or VF is thought to be the most common cause of death in dilated cardiomyopathy. Nonsustained VT is relatively common and can be seen in up to 50% to 60% of these patients. The mechanisms underlying VT in this setting include myocardial scar or bundle-branch reentry (BBR, where the left and right bundle branches are part of the VT circuit), increased automaticity, or triggered activity. Clinical recognition of BBR is important as this arrhythmia may be treated successfully with radiofrequency catheter ablation. Sustained VT can also be seen in cardiac sarcoidosis and in Chagas' disease, 2 less frequent causes of non-ischemic cardiomyopathy. As in patients with ischemic cardiomyopathy, patients with nonischemic cardiomyopathy, an LVEF <35%, and NYHA class II to III heart failure symptoms should receive an ICD for primary prevention of sudden cardiac death. The role of amiodarone therapy in these individuals is unclear.

# VENTRICULAR TACHYCARDIA IN ARRHYTHMOGENIC RIGHT VENTRICULAR DYSPLASIA

Arrhythmogenic right ventricular dysplasia (ARVD) is characterized by fatty infiltration, fibrosis, and thinning of the right ventricle and is associated with ventricular arrhythmias and sudden death. Magnetic resonance imaging, echocardiography, endomyocardial biopsy, and signal-averaged electrocardiography may be helpful in the diagnosis. On ECG, T-wave inversion may be present in leads $V_1$ to $V_3$, and an increased QRS duration >140 milliseconds can be seen, as well as epsilon waves, small deflections found in the terminal portion of the QRS complex. There is a paucity of clinical data on the efficacy of antiarrhythmic therapy for sustained VT in ARVD; however, amiodarone, β-blockers, and/or sotalol are first-line agents for treatment. Patients who have had sustained VT or have suffered a cardiac arrest should receive an ICD.

# IDIOPATHIC VENTRICULAR TACHYCARDIA

Idiopathic VT occurs in patients with structurally normal hearts, and may represent approximately 10% of patients referred for evaluation of VT. The 2 main clinical entities of idiopathic VT include repetitive monomorphic VT arising from the right ventricular outflow tract (named RMVT or RVOT VT) and idiopathic left VT (fascicular VT or verapamil-sensitive VT). RMVT has a characteristic ECG pattern with a left bundle-branch block morphology and inferior axis and usually a single VT morphology. The fascicular VTs usually have a right bundle-branch block-morphology and have a QRS width <140 milliseconds. The differentiation of these VTs from VTs associated with structural heart disease is important because they often respond well to drug therapies, are associated with an excellent prognosis, and can be cured with catheter ablation.

# POLYMORPHIC VENTRICULAR TACHYCARDIA

Polymorphic VT is characterized by a tachycardia with continuously varying QRS morphology that is often seen in acute ischemic states, or in the setting of catecholamine excess. A specific variant of polymorphic VT is torsade de pointes (TdP), a rapid polymorphic VT that constantly changes (cycle length, axis, and morphology) in a pattern that appears to "twist" around a central axis. TdP is defined as occurring in the setting of a prolonged QT interval and can be precipitated by bradycardia, heart block, hypokalemia, and drugs known to prolong the QT interval. Treatment includes correcting the precipitating factors, intravenous magnesium, and rapid defibrillation for hemodynamically unstable TdP. In select patients with bradycardia, cautious use of temporary cardiac pacing may be indicated.

TdP may also be caused by congenital long QT syndromes, a heterogeneous group of genetic disorders resulting from defects in ion channels that are involved in membrane repolarization. The acquired (especially drug-induced) causes are much more common than congenital long QT syndromes. β-blockade is indicated to prevent ventricular arrhythmias and ICD placement should be considered in those who have survived sudden death and high-risk individuals with long QT syndrome.

# VENTRICULAR FIBRILLATION

VF is associated with rapid hemodynamic collapse and is the most common arrhythmia, resulting in out-of-hospital cardiac arrest. Ventricular fibrillation requires immediate defibrillation, as minimizing the delay to defibrillation is critical to survival. After successful defibrillation, underlying causes should be addressed and management is aimed at preventing recurrences of VF. In most individuals, initial workup should include an assessment of LV function and coronary angiography with revascularization in selected cases. Based on clinical trial data, almost all cardiac arrest survivors should be considered for ICD implantation after the initial workup is completed and underlying causes have been identified.

# SUGGESTED READINGS

Rho RW, Page RL. Ventricular Arrhythmias. In: Fuster V, Walsh R, Harrington RA, et al. *Hurst's The Heart*. 13th ed, New York, NY: McGraw-Hill; 2011, 42:1006-1024.

ACC/AHA/ESC 2006 Guidelines for Management of Patients With Ventricular Arrhythmias and the Prevention of Sudden Cardiac Death. *J Am Coll Cardiol*. 2006;48:e247-e346. Available at www.content.onlinejacc.org/cgi/content.

Antiarrhythmics Versus Implantable Defibrillators (AVID) investigators. A comparison of anti-arrhythmic-drug therapy with implantable defibrillators in patients resuscitated from near-fatal ventricular arrhythmias. *N Engl J Med*. 1997;337:1576-1584.

Bardy GH, Lee KL, Mark DB, et al. Amiodarone or an implantable cardioverter defibrillator for congestive heart failure. *N Engl J Med*. 2005;352:225-237.

Brugada P, Brugada J, Mont L, Smeets J, Andries EW. A new approach to the differential diagnosis of a regular tachycardia with a wide QRS complex. *Circulation*. 1991;83:1649-1659.

Buxton AE, Lee KL, Fisher JD, et al. A randomized study of the prevention of sudden death in patients with coronary artery disease. *N Engl J Med*. 1999;341:1882-1890.

Moss AJ, Zareba W, Hall WJ, et al. Prophylactic implantation of defibrillators in patients with myocardial infarction and reduced ejection fraction. *N Engl J Med*. 2002;346:877-883.

Reddy VY, Reynolds MR, Neuzil P, et al. Prophylactic catheter ablation for the prevention of defibrillator therapy. *N Engl J Med*. 2007;357:2657-2665.

# CHAPTER 11
# BRADYARRHYTHMIAS AND PACING

## Pugazhendhi Vijayaraman and Kenneth A. Ellenbogen

Bradyarrhythmias are generally caused by abnormalities of impulse formation in the sinus node or by atrioventricular (AV) conduction abnormalities. The bradyarrhythmias may be persistent or intermittent. These abnormalities may be secondary to extrinsic factors, such as drugs with negative chronotropic or dromotropic properties, or may be secondary to intrinsic factors such as fibrosis and disease in the sinus node, AV node, or bundle branch/His–Purkinje conduction system. The indications for permanent pacing depend on the underlying cause as well as the presence of associated symptoms (**Table 11-1**).

## ACUTE TREATMENT OF BRADYARRHYTHMIAS

Acute treatment of bradyarrhythmias depends on the patient's blood pressure and symptoms such as syncope, near-syncope, dizziness, and light-headedness. The hemodynamic response to bradyarrhythmias is complex and dependent on ventricular function, systemic vascular resistance, and the onset as well as duration of the bradyarrhythmia. Some patients with heart block and rates in the high 20s may be asymptomatic, whereas other patients with rates in the 40s could have symptoms of hypoperfusion. The decision to acutely intervene should not be solely based on the actual heart rate.

Atropine 1 mg intravenously, with repeat doses up to 3 mg, may be administered for acute treatment and is most useful in patients with sinus node (SN) dysfunction. In patients with second-degree or high-degree AV block, atropine may have the potential of increasing the sinus rate and increasing the level of block, which may paradoxically *lower* the heart rate. For persistent bradyarrhythmias, particularly arrhythmias associated with SN dysfunction, a sympathomimetic amine such as isoproterenol 0.5 to 2 μg/min, or dobutamine 1 to 5 μg/kg/min, may be used carefully to increase the heart rate on a temporary basis. These drugs should be avoided in patients with acute coronary syndromes, ischemic symptoms, hypertrophic cardiomyopathy, or other conditions where excess sympathetic tone is contraindicated.

Temporary pacing is used when patients experience intermittent or persistent hemodynamically relevant bradyarrhythmias or to provide standby backup pacing for patients at increased risk for sudden asystole or heart block. The end point for temporary pacing is either resolution of a temporary indication for pacing or implantation of a permanent pacemaker for a persisting bradyarrhythmia.

Transcutaneous pacing is a common rapid method for noninvasively pacing patients who require a prophylactic temporary pacer or require emergent pacing. The unit incorporates 2 large pads placed in an anterior and posterior position. However, its main drawback is the high energy requirement (50–100 mA at 20–40 ms), which may cause skeletal muscle stimulation and pain.

**TABLE 11-1.** Indications for Pacing

| | Class I | Class II | Class III |
|---|---|---|---|
| Acquired AV block | Advanced second- or third-degree AV block with:<br><br>• Bradycardia and symptoms, or exercise induced<br><br>• Requirement of drugs that result in symptomatic bradycardia<br><br>• Catheter ablation of the AV junction or postoperative AV block not expected to resolve<br><br>• Neuromuscular diseases<br><br>• Escape rhythm <40 bpm or asystole >3 s or pauses >5 s during atrial fibrillation in awake symptom-free patients, or escape >40 bpm with left ventricular dysfunction<br><br>• Second-degree AV block, permanent or intermittent, with symptomatic bradycardia | Class IIa<br>Asymptomatic complete AV block with average awake ventricular rate >40 bpm<br>Asymptomatic type II second-degree AV block (permanent or intermittent)<br>Asymptomatic second-degree AV block at or below the bundle of His (documented by electrophysiology study)<br>First- or second-degree AV block with associated symptoms<br><br>Class IIb<br>AV block in the setting of drug use or toxicity when the block is expected to recur after drug withdrawal<br>Neuromuscular disease with any degree of AV block where there is concern for progression of AV block | Asymptomatic first-degree AV block<br>Asymptomatic type I second-degree AV block above the level of the bundle of His<br><br>AV block expected to resolve |

*(continued)*

**TABLE 11-1.** Indications for Pacing (continued)

| | Class I | Class II | Class III |
|---|---|---|---|
| After myocardial infarction | Persistent second- or third-degree AV block in the His–Purkinje system<br>Transient advanced infranodal AV block and associated bundle-branch block<br>Symptomatic second- or third-degree AV block at any level | **Class IIb**<br>Persistent advanced AV block at the AV node level | Transient AV conduction disturbances without intraventricular conduction defects or with isolated left anterior fascicular block<br>New bundle-branch block in absence of AV block<br>Persistent first-degree AV block in the presence of bundle-branch or fascicular block<br>Fascicular block without AV block or symptoms<br>Fascicular block with first-degree AV block without symptoms |
| Bifascicular or trifascicular block | Intermittent complete heart block associated with symptoms<br>Type II second-degree AV block<br>Alternating bundle-branch block | **Class IIa**<br>Bifascicular or trifascicular block with syncope not proven to be due to AV block but other causes of syncope not identifiable<br>HV interval >100 msec or pacing-induced infra-His block<br>**Class IIb**<br>Neuromuscular diseases with or without symptoms | |

| Sinus node dysfunction | Sinus node dysfunction with documented symptomatic bradycardia (in somepatients, this will occur as a result of long-term essential drug therapy of a type and dose for which there is no acceptable alternative) | **Class IIa**<br>Sinus node dysfunction, occurring spontaneously or as a result of necessary drug therapy, with heart rates <40 bpm without clear association between symptoms and bradycardia | Sinus node dysfunction in asymptomatic patients |
| | | | Sinus node dysfunction in patients in whom symptoms suggestive of bradycardia are clearly documented not to be associated with a slow heart rate |
| | Symptomatic chronotropic incompetence | Syncope of undetermined etiology with sinus node dysfunction during electrophysiology study | Sinus node dysfunction with symptomatic bradycardia due to nonessential drug therapy |
| | | **Class IIb**<br>In minimally symptomatic patients, awake heart rate <40 bpm | |
| Hypersensitive carotid sinus and neurocardiac syndromes | Recurrent syncope associated with clear, spontaneous events provoked by carotid sinus stimulation; minimal carotid sinus pressure induces asystole >3 s duration in the absence of any medication that depresses the sinus node or AV conduction | **Class IIa**<br>Recurrent syncope without clear, provocative events and with a hypersensitive cardioinhibitory response | A hyperactive cardioinhibitory response to carotid sinus stimulation in the absence of symptoms or with vague symptoms |
| | | **Class IIb**<br>Recurrent syncope with sportaneous or tilt-test-induced bradycardia | Vasovagal syncope where avoidance therapy is effective |

Class I refers to conditions where there is agreement that pacer therapy is beneficial, useful, and effective. Class II refers to conditions where there is conflicting evidence and/or divergence of opinion about usefulness of pacer therapy. Class IIa refers to conditions where opinion is in favor of usefulness, and class IIb indicates conditions where evidence and opinion are less well established. Class III refers to conditions for which there is evidence and agreement that a pacer is not indicated and could possibly be harmful.

# TYPES OF BRADYARRHYTHMIAS AND INDICATIONS FOR PACEMAKERS

## ■ SINUS BRADYCARDIA

Sinus bradycardia (SB) is a rhythm in which atrial depolarization initiates from the SN at a rate less than 60/min. The P-wave morphology is similar to that observed in normal sinus rhythm. Resting sinus bradycardia due to high vagal tone is normal in otherwise healthy well-conditioned adults. Other etiologies of SB include medication with negative chronotropic properties, hypothyroidism, inferior ischemia or infarction, hypothermia, hyperkalemia, or autonomic disorders producing increased vagal tone relative to sympathetic tone. Patients are often asymptomatic and require no therapy. However, those who are unable to increase the sinus rate during exercise are generally considered abnormal, and may require permanent pacing.

## ■ SICK SINUS SYNDROME AND SINUS NODE DYSFUNCTION

Sick sinus syndrome and SN dysfunction encompass a group of disorders that have in common the presence of abnormally slow sinus rate, and may have associated intermittent atrial tachyarrhythmias such as atrial fibrillation. *This is the most common indication for pacing in the United States.* Some patients exhibit fixed or intermittent SB; others have SB alternating with normal sinus rhythm and/or supraventricular tachyarrhythmias such as atrial fibrillation (the "tachy/brady syndrome"). Many patients are at risk of periods of asystole or marked bradyarrhythmias following cessation of the tachyarrhythmia.

The guidelines for pacing therapy generally require correlation of symptoms to bradyarrhythmias. However, some symptoms are nonspecific, such as fatigue and dyspnea. *After appropriate evaluation*, pacing is indicated for symptomatic SN dysfunction or when bradycardia or pauses are documented that may be secondary to essential long-term drug therapy.

## ■ FIRST-DEGREE ATRIOVENTRICULAR BLOCK

Isolated first-degree AV block is characterized electrocardiographically (ECG) by a PR interval exceeding 200 milliseconds. It may occur as the result of increased vagal tone, vagotonic drugs, digitalis, β-adrenergic receptor blockade, hypokalemia, acute carditis, tricuspid stenosis, Chagas disease, and some forms of congenital heart disease. Isolated first-degree AV block is rarely symptomatic and therefore rarely requires therapy.

## ■ SECOND-DEGREE ATRIOVENTRICULAR BLOCK

Mobitz type I AV block, or the Wenckebach phenomenon, is characterized electrocardiographically by consecutively conducted impulses with progressively increasing PR intervals until an impulse is blocked and the P wave is not followed by a QRS complex. This is the most common form of second-degree AV block and is usually not symptomatic. *It usually does not progress to high-grade AV block*; therefore, pacing is not necessary.

In contrast, the less common Mobitz type II block is generally associated with significant distal or infrahisian conduction system disease. It is characterized by consecutively conducted impulses with fixed PR intervals and a sudden block of impulse conduction. Paroxysmal AV block, characterized by a series of nonconducted P waves, is considered a variant of the Mobitz type II pattern. The QRS complex is typically wide in Mobitz type II block, and is almost always associated with organic heart disease, including disease in the AV conduction system distal to the AV node. It may progress to complete AV block. For this reason, permanent pacing is often indicated. In some cases an electrophysiology study may be necessary to define the level of block and guide the decision for pacing therapy.

Pacing is indicated for either type of second-degree AV block in symptomatic patients.

## ■ COMPLETE ATRIOVENTRICULAR BLOCK

Complete heart block, or third-degree AV block, is characterized by a complete interruption of antegrade AV conduction; supraventricular impulses are unable to propagate to and activate the ventricles. The ventricles are subsequently activated by a subsidiary junctional or idioventricular pacemaker at a rate of 20 to 50 bpm. Two independent pacemakers then control the rhythm of the heart: one for the atria and one for the ventricles. The 2 rhythms are independent. *In general, complete heart block*, permanent or intermittent, at any anatomic level associated with symptoms such as dizziness, light-headedness, congestive heart failure, and confusion is *an indication for a permanent pacemaker*. Pacing should also be considered for complete or advanced AV block in asymptomatic patients in the absence of reversible causes. In the presence of bifascicular or trifascicular block, intermittent third-degree or type II second-degree AV block usually indicates the need for a permanent pacemaker. Patients who present with syncope and bifascicular or trifascicular block may require a pacemaker; however, further evaluation of the syncope, including electrophysiology study, may be required.

In the setting of inferior infarction, AV block typically occurs at the level of the AV node and may be due to reversible injury and/or autonomic tone; thus, AV block usually subsides if one waits for a sufficient time. In contrast, complete or intermittent AV block in association with acute anterior wall myocardial infraction (MI) may be permanent and require permanent pacing. Transient advanced infranodal AV block with associated bundle-branch block is also an indication for pacing; however, electrophysiology studies may be required to determine the level of block.

## ■ CONGENITAL AV BLOCK

The site of AV block in congenital heart block is usually at the level of the AV node. However, congenital AV block is often associated with serious complications, including syncope and sudden death. Some develop a cardiomyopathy over time in the absence of permanent pacing. Cardiac pacing is indicated in all symptomatic patients as well as in patients with associated wide QRS escape rhythm, complex ventricular ectopy, ventricular dysfunction, or other cardiac structural abnormalities. Pacing is indicated in most asymptomatic adult patients because of an increased mortality risk from persistent bradycardia and/or cardiomyopathy.

## ■ ATRIOVENTRICULAR DISSOCIATION

AV dissociation is characterized by the absence of a fixed temporal relationship between atrial and ventricular activation. The causes of AV dissociation include marked slowing of normal pacemaker activity such that the normal escape rhythm of a subsidiary focus predominates, acceleration of a subordinate focus, or third-degree AV block. The diagnosis of *AV dissociation,* however, is *not synonymous with complete AV block.* The ECG diagnosis is made when the P waves of sinus rhythm are dissociated from the QRS complexes of an ectopic junctional or idioventricular rhythm. Fortuitously timed P waves may "capture" the ventricles when AV block is not the mechanism for dissociation. If a patient with AV dissociation is symptomatic, the underlying rhythm disturbance that is responsible for the symptoms must be identified and treatment directed toward that rhythm disturbance.

# OTHER INDICATIONS FOR PACING

## ■ PACING FOR CAROTID SINUS SYNDROME AND NEUROCARDIOGENIC SYNCOPE

The diagnosis of carotid sinus syndrome is typically made by demonstrating asystolic pauses >3 seconds with carotid sinus massage or a vasodepressor response >50 mm Hg associated with clear symptoms provoked by carotid sinus stimulation, such as wearing a tight shirt or turning one's head. Improvement of symptoms and prevention of syncope has been demonstrated by treating patients with dual-chamber pacing. *Pacing* is indicated in patients with syncope associated with hypersensitive carotid sinus responses in the absence of an alternative cause, *but is not indicated in asymptomatic patients with hypersensitive carotid sinus responses.*

For patients with neurocardiogenic syncope, cardiac pacing is limited to recurrent syncope with clear associated bradycardias/asystole. However, pacing is rarely used in these patients because even with pacing, many patients still experience vasodepressor responses with hypotension and persistent symptoms.

## ■ CARDIAC RESYNCHRONIZATION THERAPY

Biventricular pacing is being used to resynchronize ventricular contraction in patients with NYHA class III or IV heart failure, ejection fraction <35%, and wide QRS complex ≥130 milliseconds. Left ventricular (LV) stimulation can be achieved by placing a transvenous pacing lead into a branch of the coronary sinus or through direct placement on the LV epicardial surface. Resynchronization of LV activation leads to improved ventricular structure and function, decreased symptoms of heart failure (CHF), and a reduction in total mortality. In practice, many of these patients also have standard indications for implantable defibrillators and usually receive both cardiac resynchronization therapy and implantable cardiac defibrillator (CRT/ICD) in a single device if they meet QRS, EF, and symptomatic criteria.

# PACEMAKERS

Pacemakers are coded by a specific abbreviation according to the *type of pacemaker* and *mode of pacing.* The first letter refers to the chamber(s) being paced and the second to the chamber(s) being sensed. The letters A and V indicate atrial or ventricular pacing and/or sensing. If both atrial and ventricular chambers are paced and/or sensed, the designation D is used. The third letter refers to the response to a sensed event. The pacemaker inhibits (I) pacing output from one or both of its leads, or triggers (T) pacing at a programmable interval after the sensed event. If a pacer can inhibit atrial output and trigger a ventricular paced complex after a sensed atrial complex, then the designation D is used for the third letter. A fourth letter R denotes rate responsiveness, that is, changes in paced rate in response to changing levels of activity.

To stimulate myocardial tissue, a minimal threshold of current is necessary. The current delivered is a function of the pacemaker voltage and pulse width, which is generally programmed to deliver 2 to 4 times the threshold current in order to have an adequate safety margin. Some pacers can automatically check thresholds, and therefore can adjust outputs to deliver less current, thereby prolonging battery longevity while preserving safety.

A pacemaker senses intrinsic cardiac activity by the intracardiac electrograms. The range for atrial and ventricular electrograms is 0.5 to 5 mV and 5 to 20 mV, respectively; therefore pacemaker sensitivities are programmed at 0.25 to 2 mV in the atrial channel and 2 to 4 mV in the ventricular channel in order to provide an adequate safety margin for sensing.

# ■ HARDWARE

Pacemaker leads can be unipolar or bipolar. Unipolar leads use a distal electrode in the catheter as the cathode and the shell of the pacemaker generator as the anode. Therefore, the myocardium and adjacent tissue complete the circuit. Because the unipolar lead uses body tissue to complete the circuit, there is the possibility of causing muscle stimulation. Unipolar sensing is also far more likely to detect extracardiac signals, including myopotentials, remote cardiac potentials (far field sensing), and electromagnetic interference. A bipolar lead consists of 2 separate conductors and electrodes within the lead. Since the electrodes for sensing in a bipolar lead are much closer together, bipolar signals are sharper and subject to less extraneous interference. Most new pacer systems use bipolar leads; *however, unipolar leads are occasionally used for LV pacing through the coronary sinus due to their smaller diameter.*

# ■ FUNCTION AND MODES

## Magnet Mode

Magnets cause asynchronous pacing in virtually all pacemakers. The specific magnet rate and response varies according to manufacturer, pacemaker model, and battery voltage. In patients who are pacemaker-dependent and experiencing oversensing, thereby inhibiting pacemaker output, a magnet is a convenient short-term method of ensuring pacing.

## VVI Mode

VVI mode ensures that a minimum ventricular rate is maintained by ventricular pacing at the pacemaker rate unless there is an intrinsic ventricular rate greater than the pacemaker's lower rate. This is useful in patients with atrial fibrillation or for those who need backup pacing.

Hysteresis is a programmable function in which the ventricular escape interval is longer after a sensed ventricular event than after a paced ventricular event. This feature is intended to conserve battery life and maintain an intrinsic rhythm, *because the effective rate at which a pacer begins to pace is lower than the actual lower rate of the pacemaker.*

## DDD Pacing

DDD pacing is the most common pacing mode for dual-chamber pacemakers. This mode is used for patients with AV node and/or sinus node dysfunction

1. *Patients with AV block and normal sinus node function.* In the DDD mode, if the lower rate of the pacer is programmed at a sufficiently low value to permit atrial tracking, the pacemaker stimulates the ventricle synchronously in response to intrinsic P waves with a programmed AV interval. If the pacer's programmed lower rate exceeds the patient's intrinsic atrial rate, then AV sequential pacing occurs.

2. *DDD pacing in patients with sinus node dysfunction.* These patients may have intermittent or chronic sinus bradycardia requiring intermittent or continuous atrial pacing. If patients have intact AV conduction, the pacemaker functions as an AAI pacer, since intrinsic conduction would inhibit pacer ventricular output. However, because patients with sinus node dysfunction may also have AV conduction system disease, DDD pacemakers frequently can pace the ventricles. Depending on intrinsic conduction and the programmed AV interval, there may be a paced ventricular complex, a fused ventricular complex combining ventricular stimulation with intrinsic AV conduction system, or a pacing spike in the middle of the QRS complex, termed "pseudofusion" (consistent with normal pacemaker function).

## AAI Pacing

AAI pacing is similar to VVI pacing except that the pacemaker is stimulating the atrium. AAIR is a useful pacing mode in a patient with sinus node dysfunction and normal AV conduction. Some pacers may automatically switch from AAI mode to DDD mode if second- or third-degree AV block develops.

## DDI Pacing

DDI pacing is a useful mode for patients with a tachycardia–bradycardia pattern of sick sinus syndrome who have intact AV conduction. During atrial tachyarrhythmias, a pacer in the DDI mode will pace the ventricles at the lower rate. During episodes of bradyarrhythmia, the pacer functions in an atrial or AV pacing mode. DDI pacing is inappropriate for patients with permanent or intermittent AV block.

## ■ USE OF PACEMAKERS IN DIFFERENT CLINICAL SITUATIONS

### Paroxysmal Atria Fibrillation, Flutter, or Other Tachycarrhythmias

In order to prevent inappropriate upper tracking behavior during atrial tachyarrhythmias, a pacer can be reprogrammed to AAI[R] or DDI[R] if the patient has intact AV conduction. Alternatively, pacers have a programmable feature, an *automatic mode switch*, that changes the pacer mode from DDD[R] to VVI[R] or DDI[R] during episodes of atrial tachyarrhythmias.

Some studies have demonstrated that atrial-based pacing (DDD, DDI, AAI) may reduce the frequency of atrial fibrillation compared with ventricular-based pacing (VVI).

### Patients With Complete or Intermittent Third-Degree AV Block

Patients with complete or intermittent third-degree AV block generally receive a dual-chamber pacemaker programmed in the DDD mode. *Occasionally, some patients have a single-lead VDD pacer that paces the ventricle but senses and tracks the atrial activity.*

**TABLE 11-2.** Strategies to Minimize Ventricular Pacing

| Strategy | Advantage | Disadvantage |
|---|---|---|
| Program long AV intervals | Available in all pacers | Pacing may occur at long AV intervals |
| DDI mode | No tracking of atrial rhythm when rate above lower rate | No tracking mode if patient goes into second- or third-degree AV block |
| AV search hysteresis | Pacing occurs with physiologic AV interval | May not minimize RV pacing |
| AAI pacing (with backup DDD) | No ventricular pacing unless second- or third-degree AV block | Excessively long PR intervals may result |

## Patients With Carotid Sinus Syndrome and Vasovagal Syncope

Patients with the neurally mediated syncope syndromes require only intermittent AV pacing unless they have concomitant sinus node dysfunction. In the absence of sinus node dysfunction, the pacing strategy involves an algorithm that tracks a drop in instrinsic heart rate to a programmable lower rate (eg, 40-50 bpm), at which time an interventional pacing rate of 75 to 100 bpm is activated for 1 to 5 minutes. This interventional rate is intended to overcome the vagal effects and prevent syncope.

### Avoiding Right Ventricular Pacing

Right ventricular pacing may cause dyssynchrony that may lead to systolic dysfunction and heart failure. **Table 11-2** shows programmable strategies to avoid or minimize ventricular pacing.

## ■ COMPLICATIONS

Early infections related to pacemaker implantation occur in approximately 1% of implants. Early infections may be caused by *Staphylococcus aureus* and can be aggressive. Late infections are commonly related to *Staphylococcus epidermidis* and may have a more indolent course. Signs of infection include local inflammation and abscess formation, erosion of the pacer, and fever with positive blood culture but without an identifiable focus of infection. Transesophageal echocardiography may help to determine whether vegetations are present on the pacemaker lead. If the pacemaker is infected, removal of the pacemaker leads and generator is usually required.

The insulation of pacer leads may break or leads may fracture, leading to problems with oversensing (due to electrical noise), undersensing, and failure to capture (due to current leak). This problem often manifests itself intermittently and may be difficult to detect during a routine pacer check. The patient may complain of pectoral muscle stimulation due to current leak around an insulation break.

### Pacemaker Syndrome

The pacemaker syndrome is a constellation of signs and symptoms representing adverse reaction to VVI pacing or dual-chamber pacing with very long AV intervals.

The basis for pacemaker syndrome involves loss of AV synchrony and inappropriate timing of the atrial complex, which follows rather than precedes the ventricular complex. Symptoms include orthostatic hypotension, near syncope, fatigue, exercise intolerance, malaise, awareness of heartbeat, chest fullness, headache, chest pain, and other nonspecific symptoms. Strategies to minimize ventricular pacing (Table 11-2) can infrequently lead to these symptoms. Restoration and optimization of AV synchrony often clears the symptoms.

### Electromagnetic Interference With Pacemaker Function

Unipolar pacemakers are usually more susceptible to electromagnetic interference (EMI) than bipolar pacemakers because the sensing circuit encompasses a larger area. Most magnetic resonance imaging (MRI) is contraindicated in patients with pacers. However, there are recent data demonstrating safe MRI scanning using 1.5-T MR systems in non–pacer-dependent patients with cardiac monitoring during their procedure. Cellular phones can rarely adversely affect pacemaker function. It is therefore recommended that patients keep cellular phones at least 20 cm away from their pacemakers.

## ◼ PACEMAKER MALFUNCTION

Pacemaker malfunction can be categorized as loss of capture, abnormal pacing rate, undersensing, oversensing, or other erratic behavior. The approach to diagnosing pacemaker malfunction is to carefully inspect the ECG; interrogate the pacemaker; check pacing and sensing thresholds, lead impedances, and battery voltage/magnet rate; and perform a chest x-ray.

Abnormal pacing rates can be due to normal or abnormal pacing function. Failure of the pacemaker output is usually due to oversensing (**Fig. 11-1**). Occasionally, the pacemaker output is not visible because bipolar pacing produces pacing artifacts of very low amplitude. Conversely, absence of pacing stimuli may be due to interruption of current flow from a lead fracture, an insulation break, or a loose set screw.

Abnormally fast pacing rates usually occur in the context of normal pacing function. They may occur in response to rate-adaptive sensors. In DDD pacing,

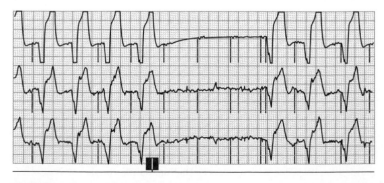

**FIGURE 11-1.** Three consecutive complexes with absent QRS complexes. In the first 2 of these complexes, there is no ventricular pacing artifact, suggesting that oversensing inhibited ventricular pacing output. However, in the third complex with absent QRS complex, there is a ventricular pacing artifact without QRS complex. This suggests lead failure (insulation break or conductor fracture that could account for either oversensing and/or failure to capture).

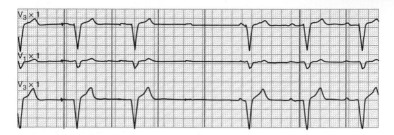

**FIGURE 11-2.** AV pacing with a single complex showing lack of ventricular output. This is a normal function of a pacer that has an algorithm that periodically checks for AV conduction to determine whether it should pace DDD versus AAI, and therefore allows one atrial paced complex to have an absent QRS complex.

upper-rate pacing may be due to sinus tachycardia, atrial tachyarrhythmias, or pacemaker-mediated tachycardia. Application of a magnet can terminate pacemaker-mediated tachycardia.

Loss of pacemaker capture occurs when there is a visible pacing stimulus and no atrial or ventricular depolarization (Fig. 11-1). This may be intermittent or persistent. Etiologies include elevation of pacing threshold, lead dislodgment, lead fracture or insulation break, and loose set screws. Battery depletion also leads to pacing failure. Oversensing leads to inappropriate pauses. The cause can be intracardiac or extracardiac or due to EMI. Analysis of the ECG, especially with pacemaker interrogation and pacemaker marker channels, may help to determine the cause. Oversensing due to lead fracture, insulation break, or other electrode problems will be random and erratic.

Oversensing can occasionally be solved by reprograming pacer sensitivity. Application of a magnet to a pacer may ensure continuous pacing in pacer-dependent patients who demonstrate inappropriate pauses. Occasionally, newer algorithms can cause the appearance of abnormal pacer function (**Fig. 11-2**).

Undersensing an intracardiac signal can lead to inappropriate pacing. Etiologies include inflammation or scar formation at the tissue–lead interface, drugs, electrolyte abnormalities, infarction, ischemia, lead fracture or insulation breaks, and cardiac defibrillation. Usually, undersensing is a greater problem in the atrium than in the ventricle. The optimal solution is to program an enhanced sensitivity (decrease the sensing level).

Other etiologies for undersensing arise when intrinsic atrial or ventricular complexes fall within one of the programmed refractory periods. Undersensing can also result when a pacer functions in an asynchronous mode (as occasionally happens with battery depletion or resetting of the pacemaker generator).

# SUGGESTED READINGS

Vijayaraman P, Ellenbogen KA. Bradyarrhythmias and pacemakers. In: Fuster V, O'Rourke RA, Walsh RA, et al. eds. *Hurst's The Heart*. 13th ed. New York, NY: McGraw-Hill; 2011; 43: 1025-1057.

Cleland JDF, Daubert JC, Erdmann E, et al. The effect of cardiac resynchronization on morbidity and mortality in heart failure. *N Engl J Med*. 2005;352:1539-1549.

Epstein AE, DiMarco JP, Ellenbogen KA, et al. ACC/AHA/HRS guidelines for device-based therapy of cardiac rhythm abnormalities. A report of the ACC/AHA Task Force on Practice Guidelines (Writing Committee to Revise the ACC/AHA/NASPE 2002 Guidelines Update for Implantation of Cardiac Pacemakers and Antiarrhythmia Devices). *Circulation*. Published online May 15, 2008.

# CHAPTER 12
# AMBULATORY ELECTROCARDIOGRAPHIC MONITORING[a]

## Eric N. Prystowsky and Richard I. Fogel

Ambulatory electrocardiographic monitoring is now possible with a variety of systems due to technological advances in telemetric recording with excellent fidelity, reliability, and a wide range of durations.

## INDICATIONS

Ambulatory ECG recording may be helpful in diagnosing and quantitating cardiac arrhythmias. The recording of an arrhythmia during a patient's symptoms may be the only means of diagnosis, particularly when the two are relatively infrequent (**Fig. 12-1**). The recording of a normal rhythm during symptoms may prove equally valuable in excluding an arrhythmia as the cause for the symptoms.

Detection of asymptomatic arrhythmias using ambulatory ECG recordings (eg, nonsustained ventricular tachycardia) may be indicated in certain patients for assessing risk for future cardiac events. These may include patients with hypertrophic cardiomyopathy and those postmyocardial infarction with left ventricular (LV) dysfunction. Patients who are treated for arrhythmias, such as atrial fibrillation or ventricular tachycardia, may benefit from ambulatory ECG recordings for assessing the efficacy of therapy. Other potential uses of ambulatory ECG are detection of myocardial ischemia from ST-segment or T-wave changes and measurement of heart rate variability and QT dispersion.

The American College of Cardiology/American Heart Association (ACC/AHA) clinical practice *Guidelines for Ambulatory Electrocardiography* provides a more complete consideration of clinical indications for ambulatory ECG recordings.

## RECORDING TECHNIQUES

Four general types of devices are currently available: continuous recorders, intermittent or event recorders, instruments for real-time recording and transmission of ECGs, and implantable recorders (**Table 12-1**).

---

[a]Adapted from Chapter 41 by Prystowsky EN, Padanilam BJ. In: Fuster V, O'Rourke RA, Walsh RA, et al, eds. *Hurst's The Heart*. 12th ed. New York, NY: McGraw-Hill; 2008, with permission of authors and publisher.

## Rapid Heartbeat Symptom

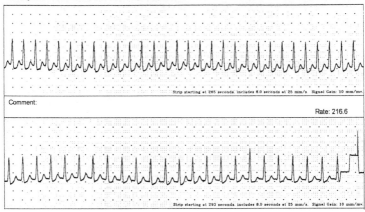

Strip starting at 285 seconds. includes 8.0 seconds at 25 mm/s.   Signal Gain: 10 mm/mv.

Comment:

Rate: 216.6

Strip starting at 293 seconds. includes 8.0 seconds at 25 mm/s.   Signal Gain: 10 mm/mv.

**FIGURE 12-1.** An episode of rapid paroxysmal supraventricular tachycardia captured with a handheld event recorder during a typical period of symptoms.

## ■ CONTINUOUS RECORDERS

The ECG can be recorded continuously (commonly known as "Holters") on cassette tape or digitally in solid-state memory. The tape recorder is a battery-powered, miniature device with a very slow tape speed that is small enough to be suspended by a strap over the shoulder or around the waist. The leads are usually attached to the patient's precordial skin using adhesive patches.

All digital recording systems amplify, digitize, and store the ECG in solid-state memory. Two types of digital recorders are available. In the first, each QRS complex is recorded, similar in this sense to the continuous tape recording. "Full disclosure" of the ECG is provided by enhanced storage capacity on a memory card the size of a credit card. With the second, microcomputers and microelectronic circuits sample the cardiac rhythm in real time as it is being recorded, convert the analog signal into a digital signal, and analyze the data in terms of maximal and minimal rates, RR intervals, and changes in RR intervals. This instrument differs in that the actual ECG has not been recorded on tape; only the histogram has been stored. However, selected brief segments of the patient's ECG can also be stored. Microcomputers are available that can analyze electronic data over periods of up to several days.

## ■ EVENT RECORDERS

This alternative method records not continuously, but only when the patient activates the device. There are 2 basic types of event recorders, which differ on the basis of their memory—post-event recorders and pre-event recorders. In the *post-event recorder*, without memory, the patient usually wears the recorder continuously, activating it when symptoms appear. The device does not record the ECG until it is activated. Alternatively, the patient may carry a miniature solid-state recorder with which the symptomatic rhythm can be recorded simply by placing the unit on the precordium or, in some cases, on the wrist. The recorded data are stored in memory until the patient submits the information either directly or transtelephonically to an ECG recorder. With a *pre-event recorder*, employing a memory loop,

**APPENDIX 12-1.** ACC/AHA Guidelines for Ambulatory Electrocardiography[a]

### A. Indications for Ambulatory ECG (AECG) to Assess Symptoms Possibly Related to Rhythm Disturbances

**Class I**
1. Patients with unexplained syncope, near syncope, or episodic dizziness in whom the cause is not obvious.
2. Patients with unexplained recurrent palpitation.

**Class IIb**
3. Patients with episodic shortness of breath, chest pain, or fatigue that is not otherwise explained.
4. Patients with neurologic events when transient atrial fibrillation or flutter is suspected.
5. Patients with symptoms such as syncope, near syncope, episodic dizziness, or palpitation in whom a probable cause other than an arrhythmia has been identified but in whom symptoms persist despite treatment of this other cause.

**Class III**
6. Patients with symptoms such as syncope, near syncope, episodic dizziness, or palpitation in whom other causes have been identified by history, physical examination, or laboratory tests.
7. Patients with cerebrovascular accidents, without other evidence of arrhythmia

### B. Indications for AECG Arrhythmia Detection to Assess Risk for Future Cardiac Events in Patients Without Symptoms From Arrhythmia

**Class IIb**
1. Post–myocardial infarction (MI) patients with LV dysfunction (ejection fraction <40%).
2. Patients with congestive heart failure (CHF).
3. Patients with hypertrophic cardiomyopathy.

**Class III**
4. Patients who have sustained myocardial contusion.
5. Diabetic subjects to evaluate for diabetic neuropathy.
6. Patients with rhythm disturbances that preclude HRV analysis (eg, atria fibrillation).

### D. Indications for AECG to Assess Antiarrhythmic Therapy

**Class I**
1. To assess antiarrhythmic drug response in individuals in whom baseline frequency of arrhythmia has been characterized as reproducible and of sufficient frequency to permit analysis.

**Class IIa**
2. To detect proarrhythmic responses to antiarrhythmic therapy in patients at high risk.

**Class IIb**
3. To assess rate control during atrial fibrillation.
4. To document recurrent or asymptomatic nonsustained arrhythmias during therapy in the outpatient setting.

### E. Indications for AECG to Assess Pacemaker and Intracardiac Cardioverter-Defibrillator (ICD) Function

**Class I**
1. Evaluation of frequent symptoms of palpitation, syncope, or near syncope to assess device function to exclude myopotential inhibition and pacemaker-mediated tachycardia and to assist in the programming of enhanced features such as rate responsivity and automatic mode switching.
2. Evaluation of suspected component failure or malfunction when device interrogation is not definitive in establishing a diagnosis.
3. To assess the response to adjunctive pharmacologic therapy in patients receiving frequent ICD therapy.

**Class IIb**
4. Evaluation of immediate postoperative pacemaker function after pacemaker or ICD implantation as an alternative or adjunct to continuous telemetric monitoring.
5. Evaluation of the rate of supraventricular arrhythmias in patients with implanted defibrillators.

*(continued)*

**APPENDIX 12-1.** ACC/AHA Guidelines for Ambulatory Electrocardiography[a] (continued)

### Class III

6. Assessment of ICD/pacemaker malfunction when device interrogation, ECG, or other available data (chest radiograph and so forth) are sufficient to establish an underlying cause/diagnosis.
7. Routine follow-up in asymptomatic patients.

### F. Indications for AECG for Ischemia Monitoring

#### Class IIa

1. Patients with suspected variant angina.

#### Class IIb

2. Evaluation of patients with chest pain who cannot exercise.
3. Preoperative evaluation for vascular surgery of patient who cannot exercise.
4. Patients with known coronary artery disease (CAD) and atypical chest pain syndrome.

#### Class III

5. Initial evaluation of patients with chest pain who are able to exercise.
6. Routine screening of asymptomatic subjects.

### G. Indications for AECG Monitoring in Pediatric Patients

#### Class I (Chapter 59)

1. Syncope, near syncope, or dizziness in patients with recognized cardiac disease, previously documented arrhythmia, or pacemaker dependency.
2. Syncope or near syncope associated with exertion when the cause is not established by other methods
3. Evaluation of patients with hypertrophic or dilated cardiomyopathies.
4. Evaluation of possible or documented long QT syndromes.
5. Palpitations in the patient with prior surgery for congenital heart disease and significant residual hemodynamic abnormalities.
6. Evaluation of antiarrhythmic drug efficacy during rapid somatic growth.
7. Asymptomatic congenital complete AV block, nonpaced.

#### Class IIa

8. Syncope, near syncope, or sustained palpitation in the absence of a reasonable explanation and where there is not overt clinical evidence of heart disease.
9. Evaluation of cardiac rhythm after initiation of an antiarrhythmic therapy, particularly when associated with a significant proarrhythmic potential.
10. Evaluation of cardiac rhythm after transient AV block associated with heart surgery or catheter ablation.
11. Evaluation of rate-responsive or physiologic pacing function in symptomatic patients.

#### Class IIb

12. Evaluation of asymptomatic patients with prior surgery for congenital heart disease, particularly when there are either significant or residual hemodynamic abnormalities, or a significant incidence of late postoperative arrhythmias.
13. Evaluation of the young patient (<3-year-old) with a prior tachyarrhythmia to determine if unrecognized episodes of the arrhythmia recur.
14. Evaluation of the patient with a suspected incessant atrial tachycardia.
15. Complex ventricular ectopy on ECG or exercise test.

#### Class III

16. Syncope, near syncope, or dizziness when a noncardiac cause is present.
17. Chest pain without clinical evidence of heart disease.
18. Routine evaluation of asymptomatic individuals for athletic clearance.
19. Brief palpitation in the absence of heart disease.
20. Asymptomatic Wolff–Parkinson–White syndrome.

[a]See also Chapter 59.

Data from Crawford MH, Berstein SJ, Deedwania PC, et al. ACC/AHA Guidelines for Ambulatory Electrocardiography. A report of the American College of Cardiology/American Heart Association Task Force on Practice Guidelines (Committee to Revise the Guidelines for Ambulatory Electrocardiography). Developed in collaboration with the North American Society for Pacing and Electrophysiology. *J Am Coll Cardiol*. Sept 1999;34(3):912-948.

**TABLE 12-1.** Types of Electrocardiographic Recording Instruments

| Type | Recording | Scanning | Transmitting |
|---|---|---|---|
| **Continuous** | | | |
| Analog | All ECG complexes, "full disclosure" | Technician with computer assistance, templating, area determination, and superimposition | None |
| Digital–continuous recording | All ECG complexes, "full disclosure" | Technician with computer assistance, templating, area determination, and superimposition | Transtelephonic |
| Digital–real-time analysis | Computer analysis of ECG and selected ECG printouts | Real time by microprocessor with retrospective technician editing | None |
| **Event Recorder** | | | |
| "Post-event," nonlooping, without memory, handheld or worn | ECG, selected by patient activation | Direct visualization | Transtelephonic |
| "Pre-event," looping, with memory, monitor worn with attached electrodes | ECG, selected by patient activation, with memory of pre-event | Direct visualization | Transtelephonic |
| Continuous mobile outpatient telemetry system | ECG, selected by patient or automatic | Direct visualization; technician with computer assistance | Transtelephonic |
| **Implantable Devices** | | | |
| Subcutaneous, implanted digital recorder | ECG, selected by patient activation with memory of pre-event or automatic | Direct visualization | Direct telemetry |
| Automatic electronic sensor in ICD or pacemaker | ECG, when activated by ICD discharge or recognized by sensor in pacemaker, with memory | Direct visualization of analysis or ECG | Direct telemetry |
| **Real Time** | | | |
| Real-time transtelephonic monitoring | ECG at central monitoring station—no recording at device | Direct visualization | Transtelephonic |

the rhythm is monitored continuously. Patients activate the unit when they experience symptoms and the loop recorder is capable of recording an ECG several seconds or minutes before and after a recognized event; the number of events that can be recorded and the allotment of recording time prior to and after activation of the unit are programmable.

The limitations of traditional event recorders include their inability to record asymptomatic arrhythmias, inability for the patient to transmit specific symptoms with each event, and missed events because of patient error in activating the device. A newer mobile cardiac outpatient telemetry system consists of a 3-electrode, 2-channel sensor transmitting wirelessly to a portable monitor, which analyzes and stores ECG data. Significant arrhythmias, whether symptomatic or asymptomatic, are transmitted automatically by the wireless network to a central monitoring station and analyzed by trained personnel.

## ■ IMPLANTABLE RECORDERS

A miniaturized event recorder can be implanted subcutaneously on the precordium. It can be manually activated by the patient to record an ECG when symptoms occur, and high and low heart rate limit parameters can be programed for the device to record events automatically. These devices are particularly useful to capture events that occur relatively infrequently—for example, a few times per year. Event recording is also provided by some newer-generation pacemakers and implantable cardioverter-defibrillators that automatically recognize and record abnormal rhythms.

## ■ REAL-TIME MONITORING

Real-time monitoring devices acquire data and transmit the ECG information directly and transtelephonically, in real time, without recording the data in the unit. The patient's ECG can be transmitted daily, or even multiple times each day, to a recording station. Routine transtelephonic pacemaker evaluations use such systems.

# SELECTION OF DEVICE AND DURATION OF RECORDING

The selection of a long-term ECG recording system depends on the individual patient's needs. If a precise count of ectopy is required, a continuous recorder with computer-based analysis is essential. If the purpose of the recording is to detect episodic arrhythmic events such as ventricular tachycardia or atrial fibrillation, an event recorder would be an excellent choice. An event recorder provides an opportunity to monitor over prolonged periods of time and is of benefit to the patient whose symptoms do not occur on a daily basis. When the goal is to correlate the patient's ECG pattern with symptoms that are very infrequent (eg, every few months), an implantable loop recorder may be the best choice. A pre-event loop recorder is needed for evaluation of symptoms of brief duration (such as syncope without warning), and allows the patient to activate the recorder after the event. The monitoring period must be extended sufficiently to incorporate a symptomatic period, which may be hours to months. For assessment of ventricular rate control for a patient with atrial fibrillation, a 24-hour ECG monitoring period is usually sufficient. However, continuous outpatient telemetry monitoring, performed for 1 to 2 weeks, may be advantageous in the titration of oral medications (eg, β-blockers, calcium-channel blockers, digoxin) in patients with atrial fibrillation and uncontrolled ventricular rates.

# ARTIFACTS AND ERRORS

Artifacts registered during prolonged ECG recording have mimicked virtually every variety of cardiac arrhythmias and have led to misdiagnosis and inappropriate treatment. Artifacts can occur at different levels of the recording process. *Patient-related* artifacts may result from involuntary muscle contractions (eg, tremors, rigors, hiccoughs) and body movements (eg, changing body position, brushing teeth, combing hair). The Parkinson disease tremor often has a frequency of 4 to 5 per second, and when captured on an ECG, it can be mistaken for atrial flutter or ventricular tachycardia.

A second type of artifact may occur during *data recording and processing*. Recording system artifacts can occur for a variety of reasons, including loose skin–electrode contact, lead fractures, processing errors, altered tape speed in the recorder, and incomplete erasure of a previous recording. The most common artifact probably is that resulting from a loose electrode or mechanical "stimulation" of the electrode. High-frequency signal dropout or generation of a high-frequency signal mimicking pacing artifacts can occur from processing errors, especially in digital systems. Failure of either the battery or the motor of the recorder generally results in a slowing of the tape speed as the ECG is recorded.

*External interferences* also offer a very common cause for ECG artifacts. "Noise" can occur in the recordings because of external sources, such as 60 Hz from alternating current or electromagnetic interference from mechanical devices. Simultaneous use of a variety of medical equipment (eg, infusion pumps, transcutaneous or implanted nerve stimulators) may result in ECG artifacts mimicking atrial or ventricular arrhythmias. Implanted or external nerve stimulators in some patients can result in an atrial flutter-like appearance, but can be distinguished by its rate, "spike-like" nature of the artifacts, and appearance of sinus P waves in some recording leads.

Most of these artifacts are readily identifiable from their characteristic appearance. One should "look through" the artifacts for normal background ECG appearance. Quite often, QRS complexes can be identified and "marched out" at cycle lengths similar to the sinus rhythm cycle lengths before the beginning of the artifacts. Look for high-frequency (spike-like activity) or low-frequency signals inconsistent with the normal PQRST waves. Nonphysiologic (eg, <140 milliseconds) coupling intervals between QRS complexes and unstable ECG baselines are sometimes more apparent at the beginning or the ending of the recorded artifacts. Lack of clinical correlation to an identified "arrhythmia" may be a useful feature, but beware that some serious cardiac arrhythmias can be asymptomatic. Ultimately, the keys to identifying artifacts are the clinician's familiarity with the various types of artifacts and the careful analysis of the ECG.

# SUGGESTED READINGS

Prystowsky EN, Fogel RI. Approach to the Patient With Cardiac Arrhythmias. In: Fuster V, O'Rourke RA, Walsh RA, et al. eds. *Hurst's The Heart*. 13th ed. New York, NY: McGraw-Hill; 2011;39:949-962.

Holter NJ. New method for heart studies: continuous electrocardiography of active subjects over long periods is now practical. *Science*. 1961;134:1214-1220.

Joshi AK, Kowey PR, Prystowsky EN, et al. First experience with a mobile cardiac out-patient telemetry (MCOT) system for the diagnosis and management of cardiac arrhythmias. *Am J Cardiol*. 2005;95:878-881.

Krahn A, Klein G, Yee R, et al. Use of an extended monitoring strategy in patients with problematic syncope. *Circulation*. 1999;99:406-410.

Myerburg JR, Chaitman BR, Ewy GA, et al. Training in electrocardiography, ambulatory electrocardiography, and exercise testing *J Am Coll Cardiol*. 2008;51:384.

Prystowsky EN. Assessment of rhythm and rate control in patients with atrial fibrillation. *J Cardiovasc Electrophysiol*. 2006;17:S7-S10.

# CHAPTER 13
# TECHNIQUES OF ELECTROPHYSIOLOGIC EVALUATION

## Eric N. Prystowsky and Richard I. Fogel

The regular, surface 12-lead electrocardiogram (ECG) provides extensive information about the heart's rhythm and its abnormalities. However, it cannot determine the exact diagnosis, mechanism, or location of a dysrhythmia to direct appropriate management. For the past few decades, the recording of intracavitary electrocardiographic signals and various forms of pacing programs have experienced enormous growth.

# TECHNIQUES OF INTRACARDIAC ELECTROPHYSIOLOGIC STUDIES

The exact type of electrical signal recordings, specific equipment used, and pacing protocol depend on the nature of the clinical problem, type of electrophysiologic assessment, and anticipated course of action. Routine cardiac electrophysiology studies (EPS) are performed while patients are in a nonsedated postabsorptive state.

The typical electrode catheters used for both recording and cardiac stimulation are multipolar, inserted via peripheral veins. They are placed under fluoroscopic guidance in the high right atrium, at the His bundle, in the right ventricular, and sometimes in the region of the coronary sinus (**Fig. 13-1**). Transseptal catheterization is invaluable when accessing the pulmonary veins via the right atrium during ablation of atrial fibrillation (AF). Left-sided heart catheterization is seldom necessary, but used therapeutically in ablating ventricular tachycardia (VT) or left-sided accessory pathway. Heparin may be given as needed, unless left-heart catheterization is desirable; then continuous heparinization is required to avoid thromboembolic complications.

## ■ ELECTROPHYSIOLOGIC RECORDINGS

Once the electrode catheters are placed appropriately, the connections are made via a junction box. Electrograms are displayed simultaneously on a multichannel oscilloscopic recorder. Filter settings between 30-40 and 500 Hz are best suited for sharp intracardiac signals. In addition to the intracardiac signals, several surface electrocardiographic leads are recorded. All equipment is reliably grounded.

Catheters have evolved into different shapes. Some of them have multiple electrodes that help localize special areas, mainly during AF ablation (eg, Basket and Lasso catheters used in isolating the pulmonary veins, Pentarrays used to locate fractionated recordings in the left atrium, and balloon catheters used in noncontact mapping).

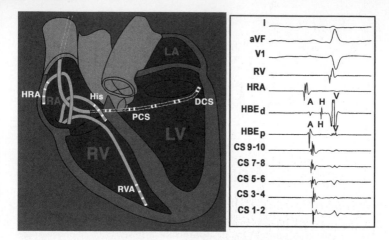

**FIGURE 13-1.** Standard catheter position for a "4-wire" diagnostic EP study (*left panel*). Electrograms display during standard 4-wire study in sinus rhythm (*right panel*). Although all 12 surface ECG leads are recorded, only 3 approximately orthogonal leads are shown, for clarity. The right ventricular apex (RV) and high right atrium (HRA) leads show sharp single-chamber electrograms. The His bundle catheter records activity adjacent to the AV node; the distal bipole (HBE$_d$) favoring the His bundle electrogram (H) and the adjacent ventricular myocardium (V), while the proximal bipole (HBE$_p$) shows a large atrial electrogram (A). The electrograms recorded by the bipoles of the decapolar coronary sinus catheter are labeled *CS 9-10* (proximal) to *CS 1-2* (distal); each shows a sharp atrial electrogram followed by a smaller ventricular electrogram. (Murgatroyd FD, Krahn AD, Yee R, et al. *Handbook of Cardiac Electrophysiology*. London, UK: ReMEDICA; 2002:8–9. Reproduced with permission from the publisher and authors.)

# ■ ELECTROPHYSIOLOGIC MAPPING

More recently, several mapping/recording systems have emerged that facilitate more accurate location of the arrhythmia. They create 3-dimensional (3D) color-coded activation and/or voltage maps, making it possible to manipulate the ablation catheter without the use of fluoroscopy.

## *Intracardiac Ultrasound*

Intracardiac ultrasound is useful in locating the fosa ovalis to perform transseptal puncture; in visualizing the mitral valve annulus, left atrial appendage, and pulmonary veins; in guiding the catheter position and its tip-to-tissue contact; and finally, in monitoring lesion formation to prevent microbubbles. Recently, it has been used with other mapping systems (eg, CARTOSOUND) to create more accurate anatomical images.

## *Computed Tomography and Magnetic Resonance Imaging*

Both computed tomography (CT) and magnetic resonance imaging (MRI) can reproduce and segment a 3D model of a specific heart chamber. This model can then be used as a reference, or can even be imported directly into the mapping application and synchronized or registered for real-time catheter location and tracking in a

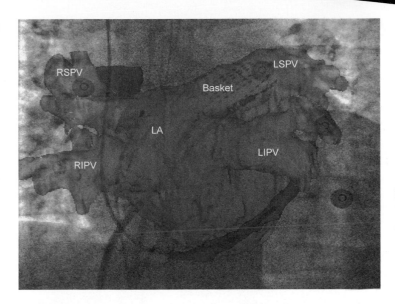

**FIGURE 13-2.** Real-time CT-fluoroscopy registration image. Anterior-posterior fluoroscopy view of the cardiac silhouette with ablation catheter and basket recording catheter in the left superior pulmonary vein. The coronary sinus, high atrial, and His bundle catheters are in their designated locations. The CT image is posterior-anterior overlapping the fluoroscopy image with sophisticated ECG-gated registration technique. LA, left atrium; LIPV, left inferior pulmonary vein; LSPV, left superior pulmonary vein; RIPV, right inferior pulmonary vein; RSPV, right superior pulmonary vein.

patient-specific anatomic model of the cardiac chamber (eg, CARTO-Merge, EnSite Fusion, and CT-fluoroscopy registration) (**Fig. 13-2**).

## ■ PROGRAMED ELECTRICAL STIMULATION

Two formats of pacing protocol are common. The first is incremental atrial or ventricular pacing, which is pacing at a constant cycle length with gradual shortening until the occurrence of a desirable event, such as induction of a tachycardia or production of atrioventricular (AV) or ventriculoatrial (VA) block. Bursts of pacing at a constant cycle length are also used.

The second pacing format is premature (or extra) stimulation from atrial or ventricular sites. For induction of supraventricular tachycardias (SVTs), single, double, or more extra stimuli may be delivered (**Fig. 13-3**). For the induction of VT, up to 3 ventricular extra stimuli are employed. The sensitivity of pacing protocols seems to be directly related to the number of extrastimuli used. This occurs, however, at the expense of specificity, when polymorphic VT/VF can be induced at very short coupling intervals by using multiple extra stimuli.

During routine EPS studies, a variety of electrophysiologic parameters are measured, including sinus node function and intra-atrial, AV nodal, and His–Purkinje system conduction. Initiation of SVT and VT is attempted to determine the mechanisms, site of origin, prognostication, and potential of overdrive termination as a therapy option. After baseline studies, intravenous drugs may be administered to

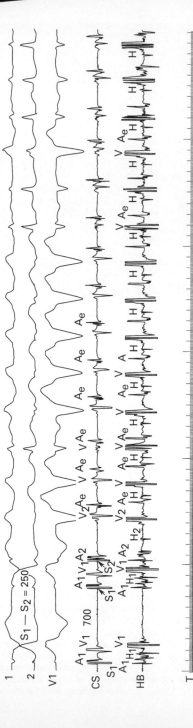

**FIGURE 13-3.** Induction of supraventricular tachycardia (SVT) in Wolff-Parkinson–White syndrome. The tracings are labeled. Atrial pacing from coronary sinus (CS) is done at a 700-millisecond basic cycle. During the basic drive pacing, left free-wall accessory pathway conduction to the ventricle produces ventricular preexcitation. A single premature beat (S₂) blocks in the accessory pathway (AP) and conducts over the normal pathway with a left bundle-branch block morphology, and the SVT is initiated. Note the intermittent normalization of the QRS complex during this SVT. (Jazayeri M, Caceres J, Tchou P, et al. Electrophysiologic characteristics of sudden QRS axis deviation during orthodromic tachycardia. *J Clin Invest.* 1989;83:952-959. Reproduced with permission from the publisher and authors.)

facilitate induction of tachycardias, aggravation of sinus node function, or production of AV block.

# INVASIVE ELECTROPHYSIOLOGIC STUDIES FOR DIAGNOSIS

## ■ SINUS NODE DYSFUNCTION

Electrophysiologic studies are performed to detect suspected sinus node dysfunction in patients with dizziness, presyncope, and/or syncope, in which the diagnosis cannot be made noninvasively. The most frequently performed test is that of sinus node suppression, using overdrive atrial pacing for approximately 30 seconds or longer. The resultant escape interval, which is called *sinus node recovery time,* is measured. By deducting the predominant sinus cycle length from this interval, one can obtain the so-called *corrected sinus node recovery time.* A value of corrected sinus node recovery time of more than 525 milliseconds is found in patients with overt sinus node dysfunction.

In the vast majority of patients with true sinus node disease, sinoatrial conduction abnormalities are the predominant reason for sinus node dysfunction. It is measured by atrial extrastimuli maneuvers, with normal conduction time of less than 100 milliseconds. It is important to test AV conduction in patients with sinus node dysfunction, as the former is also frequently abnormal.

## ■ ATRIOVENTRICULAR BLOCK

In asymptomatic individuals with second-degree AV block (Mobitz I and/or Mobitz II), electrophysiologic assessment is used to find the site of the block by discernible His bundle recording. Patients with intra- or infra-Hisian block tend to have a more unpredictable course, and permanent pacing is desirable. In symptomatic patients with second-degree AV block, the role of EPS is limited because permanent pacing is the appropriate intervention. On the other hand, if the patient's symptoms cannot be explained on the basis of AV block but may be related to another arrhythmia, such as VT, EPS should be considered. EPS are rarely required for the other types of AV block.

If 1:1 AV conduction is noted during EPS in patients suspected of intermittent AV block, incremental atrial pacing should be done to see whether AV block can be reproduced.

## ■ NARROW QRS TACHYCARDIA

Narrow QRS tachycardia is supraventricular in origin. It includes sinus and atrial tachycardia, atrial flutter, AF, AV nodal reentrant tachycardia, junctional tachycardia, and orthodromic AV reentrant tachycardia via an accessory pathway. Baseline characteristics (eg, intracardiac activation sequence, and the initiation and termination of the tachycardia) may help in identifying the etiology of the tachycardia. To confirm the diagnosis, pacing maneuvers (eg, entrainment and/or extrastimuli during His refractory period) are required most of the time.

## ■ WIDE QRS TACHYCARDIA

Wide QRS tachycardia occurs as a consequence of a variety of electrophysiologic mechanisms, both from supraventricular and ventricular origins in the presence or

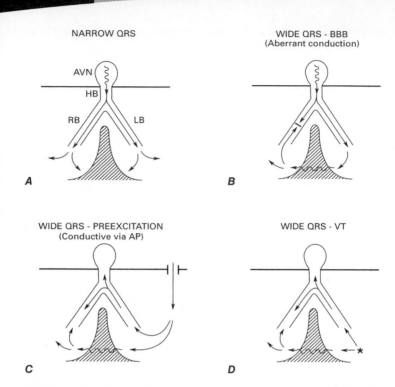

**FIGURE 13-4.** Wide QRS tachycardia. Routes of impulse propagation during a wide QRS tachycardia in various settings are depicted. It should be noted that only in **A** and **B** is His bundle activation expected to precede ventricular activation. This helps the delineation from other causes of wide QRS tachycardia shown in **C** and **D**.

absence of accessory pathways (**Fig. 13-4**). Defining the underlying nature of the wide QRS tachycardia is critical for both prognosis and therapy. With few exceptions, when the nature of the arrhythmic problem is not known and the direction of therapy is not clear, patients with wide QRS tachycardia should undergo EPS.

## ■ UNEXPLAINED SYNCOPE

Syncope may be caused by cardiovascular mechanisms. Electrophysiologic evaluation constitutes an integral part of the evaluation of patients with unexplained syncope, especially those with heart disease. Neurocardiogenic mechanisms constitute the most common cause of syncope in patients without structural heart disease, especially in younger patients (<50 years of age) with syncope and documented bradycardia (sinus arrest or AV block) and can be unmasked on a tilt table. The triage of patients toward one or the other—that is, electrophysiologic testing versus head-up tilt—is a fairly simple choice, determined by the clinical history and the presence or absence of structural heart disease.

## ■ RISK STRATIFICATION FOR SUDDEN CARDIAC ARREST

Within the last decade, implantable cardioverter defibrillators (ICDs) have been approved for primary and secondary prevention of sudden cardiac arrest (SCA). Therefore, use of EPS for justification of ICD implantation has been abandoned, except in a few scenarios where risk stratification for SCA is required.

EPS can be considered in patients

1. With left ventricular (LV) dysfunction (LV ejection fraction ≤40%) and recorded nonsustained VT occurring during the waiting period for ICD implantation

2. With symptoms suggestive of VT/VF (eg, palpitation, presyncope, or syncope)

3. With high risk of sudden cardiac death (SCD), such as those with hypertrophic obstructive cardiomyopathy or Brugada syndrome, where an ICD implant may be beneficial

In a few cases, EPS may be useful to reduce the frequency of ICD shocks by defining a strategy for mapping and ablating the cause (SVT, bundle-branch reentry VT, or ischemic VT).

# INVASIVE CARDIAC ELECTROPHYSIOLOGIC STUDIES FOR THERAPEUTIC INTERVENTION

## ■ SUPRAVENTRICULAR TACHYCARDIA

Therapeutic intervention for most SVT is very successful. In this instance, EPS and transvenous catheter-based ablation are first-line therapy. On the other hand, this is considered a second-line therapy after pharmacologic therapy fails in some SVT (eg, atrial tachycardia, atypical atrial flutter, and AF). Three-dimensional mapping aids in locating the foci in atrial tachycardia, the macroreentrant circuit in atrial flutter, and the anatomic model or electrical fractionation of the left atrium in the AF.

The introduction of catheter ablation techniques has made it rare for patients to undergo surgery for SVT. Some individuals with resistant atrial fibrillation and flutter, and those who fail catheter ablative therapy, may still be considered candidates for a surgical approach.

## ■ VENTRICULAR TACHYCARDIA

In patients with an ICD, electrophysiologic evaluation and therapy can be accomplished through the permanent leads of the ICD. Pacing, antitachycardia function, low-energy cardioversion, and cardiac defibrillation can all be programed through the device. When problems are encountered following discharge of a patient with an ICD, electrophysiologic reassessment via ICD is frequently necessary, and sometimes transvenous catheterization may be required.

EPS is essential in all patients undergoing therapeutic intervention (ablation) for VT, regardless of the etiology (normal heart structure VT, scar-related VT, or even idiopathic VF). Conventional electrical mapping (eg, pace mapping or entrainment mapping) and 3D mapping are tools to facilitate successful outcome. Catheter-based ablation is performed mainly via a percutaneous transvascular approach; if that fails, a nonsurgical transthoracic epicardial catheter ablation approach may be necessary to eliminate ventricular dysarrhythmia.

Patients with coronary artery disease and VT that can be mapped are also candidates for VT surgery if the VT cannot be managed with an ICD, antiarrhythmic drugs, and/or catheter ablation. Preoperative EPS for this eventuality is important.

## CATHETER ABLATION TECHNIQUES

The realization that the origin of VT and SVT can be effectively mapped (pace map, entrainment, or 3D map) has made the catheter ablation technique a rational approach. The radiofrequency or cryoablation forms of energy delivered through a catheter permit controlled trauma to cardiac tissue to abolish or modify reentrant circuits in both SVT and VT. Unifocal atrial tachycardia, isthmus-dependent atrial flutter, AV nodal reentry of all varieties, and accessory pathways, including atriofascicular fibers, can be cured in over 95% of patients with radiofrequency catheter ablation. The success rate of AF and atypical atrial flutter ablation ranges between 60% and 80%. Patients with monomorphic VT, associated with normal heart structure, can also be considered candidates, particularly when they fail drug therapy. Bundle-branch reentrant VT is an ideal substrate for catheter ablation in patients with abnormal heart structure. Additionally, in patients with incessant VT or frequent VT with inadequate control despite antiarrhythmic and ICD therapy, VT ablation should be considered.

## RISK AND COMPLICATIONS

The complication rate of EPS is relatively low, with almost negligible mortality. Complications include deep venous thrombosis, intracavitary thrombosis, pulmonary or systemic embolism, infection at catheter sites, systemic infection, pneumothorax, hemothorax perforation of a cardiac chamber or coronary sinus, pericardial effusion, and tamponade.

## SUGGESTED READINGS

Prystowsky EN, Fogel RI. Approach to the Patient With Cardiac Arrhythmias. In: Fuster V, O'Rourke RA, Walsh RA, et al. eds. *Hurst's The Heart.* 13th ed. New York, NY: McGraw-Hill; 2011;39:949-962.

Knight B, Ebinger M, Oral H, et al. Diagnostic value of tachycardia features and pacing maneuvers during paroxysmal supraventricular tachycardia. *J Am Coll Cardiol.* 2000;36:574-582.

Lee KW, Badhwar N, Scheinman MM. Supraventricular tachycardia. *Curr Probl Cardiol.* 2008;33:553-662.

Sra J, Akhtar M. Mapping techniques for atrial fibrillation ablation. *Curr Probl Cardiol.* 2007;32:669-767.

Stevenson WG, Friedman PL, Kocovic D, et al. Radiofrequency catheter ablation of ventricular tachycardia after myocardial infarction. *Circulation.* 1998;98:308-314.

2006 ACC/AHA Guidelines for the Management of Patients With Ventricular Tachycardia and the Prevention of Sudden Cardiac Death. *Circulation.* 2006;114:1088-1132.

# CHAPTER 14
# TREATMENT OF CARDIAC ARRHYTHMIAS WITH ABLATION THERAPY

Usha B. Tedrow, Samuel J. Asirvatham, and William G. Stevenson

Successful catheter ablation requires precise localization of the source of the arrhythmia, accurate placement of the ablation catheter, and achievement of an adequate ablation lesion. Catheter positioning is assisted primarily by fluoroscopy. Sophisticated mapping systems can also display catheter position and a three-dimensional (3D) depiction of the anatomy. Magnetic resonance imaging (MRI), computed tomography (CT), and echocardiographic data can also be integrated with these systems. Radiofrequency (RF) energy is most commonly used, but freezing with cryoablation catheters is a potential alternative. Serious complications of catheter ablation are infrequent and most often related to the catheterization procedure, usually including vascular injury and cardiac perforation with tamponade.

## REENTRANT SUPRAVENTRICULAR TACHYCARDIA

### ■ ATRIOVENTRICULAR NODAL REENTRANT TACHYCARDIA

Ablation for atrioventricular nodal reentrant tachycardia (AVNRT) is recommended when episodes are poorly tolerated, resistant to medical therapy, or if the patient cannot tolerate medications. The atrioventricular (AV) node consists of a compact portion and adjoining lobes. In patients with AVNRT, the lobe extending toward the coronary sinus likely forms a functional pathway for slow conduction between the os of the coronary sinus and the septal leaflet of the tricuspid valve that can be ablated safely. Success is achieved in more than 95% of patients. Heart block is the major risk, occurring in approximately 0.8% of patients and requiring permanent pacemaker implantation. Cryoablation may be associated with a lower risk of heart block, but has lower long-term success rates.

## ATRIOVENTRICULAR RECIPROCATING TACHYCARDIA

Patients with atrioventricular reciprocating tachycardia (AVRT) have an accessory pathway connecting atrium and ventricle and bypassing the His–Purkinje system. If the pathway has manifest antegrade conduction, the electrocardiogram (ECG) shows preexcitation, a hallmark of the Wolff–Parkinson–White syndrome. Accessory pathways conducting only from ventricle to atrium are termed *concealed* because during sinus rhythm preexcitation is absent, but AVRT still can occur. Catheter ablation is the standard of care for symptomatic Wolff–Parkinson–White syndrome, or for concealed accessory pathways causing symptomatic tachycardias when pharmacologic therapy is ineffective or not desirable.

Pathway location along the mitral or tricuspid annulus determines whether an arterial, venous, or transseptal approach is required (**Fig. 14-1**). Success rates are 95%,

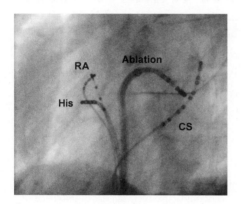

*A*

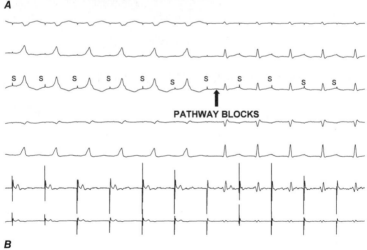

*B*

**FIGURE 14-1. A**. Ablation of a left-sided accessory pathway in a patient with Wolff–Parkinson–White syndrome. A left anterior oblique fluoroscopic image is shown depicting catheter position for catheter ablation of a left-sided accessory pathway by a transeptal approach. A decapolar catheter is seen in the coronary sinus (CS). The ablation catheter (Ablation) is passed through a sheath that crosses the fossa ovalis into the left atrium for mapping along the tricuspid valve annulus. **B**. Five surface ECG leads and two intracardiac leads depict ablation of a left lateral accessory pathway during atrial pacing. The right atrium is being paced (pacing stimuli indicated by S). Pacing stimuli initially conduct from the atrium to the ventricles over the AV node and an accessory pathway producing a pattern of ventricular preexcitation with a wide QRS with a slurred initial delta wave. The pathway blocks within seconds of the application of radiofrequency energy with sudden narrowing of the QRS complex indicating that conduction to the ventricles is occurring only over the normal conduction system of AV node and His bundle.

and serious complications are uncommon. Heart block can occur with ablation of septal pathways located close to the AV node.

# REGULAR ATRIAL ARRHYTHMIAS

## ■ FOCAL ATRIAL TACHYCARDIA

Focal atrial tachycardia (AT) tends to occur in specific anatomic locations: along the crista terminalis, tricuspid or mitral annulus, coronary sinus musculature, atrial appendages, and in the pulmonary veins. The tachycardia must be present or provocable to be successfully localized for ablation. Ablation is successful in more than 80% of patients. Significant complications occur in 1% to 2% of patients.

## ■ SINUS NODE MODIFICATION FOR INAPPROPRIATE SINUS TACHYCARDIA

Patients with inappropriate sinus tachycardia have sinus tachycardia without a discernible cause. Catheter ablation can be a last resort when severe symptoms do not respond to pharmacologic therapy. Ablation of the rapidly firing regions along the crista terminalis can slow the sinus rate. Ablation of the entire sinus node, with permanent pacemaker implantation, can require epicardial ablation, but long-term success is limited, as many patients have recurrent symptoms, some despite improvement in heart rate. Potential complications include narrowing of the superior vena cava, right phrenic nerve paralysis, and the need for chronic pacing.

## ■ ATRIAL FLUTTER AND OTHER MACROREENTRANT ATRIAL TACHYCARDIAS

Common atrial flutter is caused by a large macroreentrant circuit with a wavefront revolving around the tricuspid annulus. In typical counterclockwise atrial flutter, the wavefront proceeds up the atrial septum and down the right atrial free wall. Reentry is dependent on conduction through the cavotricuspid isthmus bounded by the tricuspid valve, inferior vena cava, eustachian ridge, and coronary sinus os. Once the diagnosis is confirmed by entrainment and activation mapping, a series of ablation lesions is placed across the cavotricuspid isthmus, creating a line of conduction block (**Fig. 14-2**). Success is achieved in more than 95% of patients. Approximately 20% to 30% of patients also have atrial disease that leads to atrial fibrillation in the next 20 months.

Other macroreentrant circuits can occur in the left or right atrium not involving the cavotricuspid isthmus. Arrhythmias from reentry occurring around atrial scars from prior heart surgery, such as atrial septal defect repair, are referred to as "scar-related" macroreentrant ATs. Catheter ablation is more difficult, with success rates of 80% to 85%, and more frequent late recurrences than are observed for common flutter.

# ATRIAL FIBRILLATION

## ■ ATRIOVENTRICULAR JUNCTION ABLATION FOR RATE CONTROL

In patients with atrial fibrillation (AF), catheter ablation of the AV junction to produce complete heart block with implantation of a permanent pacemaker can be used to control the ventricular rate. The strategy is generally reserved for older patients who may already have an implanted pacemaker or defibrillator, who cannot tolerate

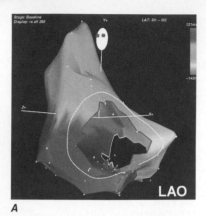

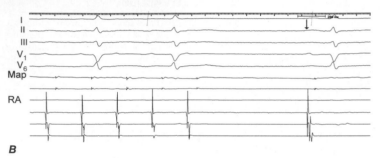

**FIGURE 14-2.** Mapping and ablation of typical counterclockwise atrial flutter. **A.** It is an activation map of the right atrium during counterclockwise atrial flutter as viewed in a left anterior oblique projection. Activation circulates up the interatrial septum, across the roof, down the free wall, and through the cavotricuspid isthmus. A line of RF lesions was placed across this isthmus, which blocked conduction in the isthmus terminating atrial flutter. **B.** The tracing shows surface ECG leads and intracardiac recordings from the mapping catheter (Map) and lateral right atrium (RA) during RF ablation. Atrial flutter terminates and is followed by sinus rhythm (*arrow*).

rate-control medications, and who are not candidates for other rhythm-control strategies. Anticoagulation for thromboembolic risk is still required. For patients with previously uncontrolled ventricular rates, quality of life, exercise tolerance, and ejection fraction can improve. However, following the abrupt decrease in heart rate, cases of sudden death have occurred, likely as a result of polymorphic ventricular tachycardia. Pacing the ventricle at 90 beats per minute for the first several weeks and then gradually reducing the rate over time reduces the risk. Right ventricular (RV) pacing can have adverse hemodynamic consequences in some patients with poor left ventricular (LV) function. Biventricular pacing likely reduces this risk.

## ■ ATRIAL FIBRILLATION ABLATION FOR MAINTAINING SINUS RHYTHM

The majority of focal triggers that initiate paroxysmal AF originate in the pulmonary veins. Although ablation strategies vary, most target areas within the atrium that encircle the pulmonary veins, often with the goal of electrically isolating these regions without ablating in the veins themselves. Extensive series of lesions are usually placed in the left atrium. Intracardiac echocardiography and 3D mapping systems that incorporate anatomy from MRI or CT images are helpful adjuncts to facilitate ablation strategies.

Success varies with the type of AF and severity of underlying heart disease. Successful maintenance of sinus rhythm after the initial healing phase is achieved in more than 70% to 80% of young patients with paroxysmal AF without structural heart disease, but reported follow-ups are still relatively short, with few studies reporting data beyond 1 year. Success rates are lower for patients with persistent or permanent AF.

For several weeks following ablation, atrial arrhythmias can occur as ablation lesions heal and the atrium remodels, but these often subsequently resolve. A second procedure is required in 20% to 50% of patients. Antiarrhythmic medications are often continued for 1 to 3 months after ablation. Anticoagulation with warfarin is required.

Major procedural complications include myocardial perforation with tamponade (1%-2%) and stroke (0.5%-1%). Severe pulmonary vein stenosis has been reported in 2% to 6% of patients. Death from atrioesophageal fistulae, presenting days to a few weeks after the procedure with endocarditis, septic emboli, or gastrointestinal bleeding, has been reported (<0.1% estimated). Appropriate patient selection requires adequate assessment of risks and benefits for each individual patient. The risks and benefits can be expected to improve as this relatively new procedure continues to evolve.

# VENTRICULAR TACHYCARDIA

## ■ IDIOPATHIC VENTRICULAR TACHYCARDIA

Idiopathic ventricular tachycardia (VT) occurs in the absence of structural heart disease and is often amenable to catheter ablation. The most common form originates from a focus in the RV outflow tract, beneath the pulmonary valve and may cause exercise-induced VT, repetitive bursts of monomorphic VT, or symptomatic premature ventricular contractions. The VT has a pattern of left bundle-branch block in $V_1$ with an inferiorly directed axis. Ablation is performed at the area of earliest activation in the outflow tract, with successful elimination of tachycardia in more than 80% of patients. Occasionally idiopathic outflow tract VT originates from sites adjacent to the aortic annulus, the LV outflow tract, or in the epicardium.

The most common form of left-sided idiopathic VT originates from the LV apical septum. This arrhythmia is characterized on surface ECG by a pattern of right bundle-branch block in lead $V_1$, usually with a superiorly directed axis. It often responds to verapamil. It appears to be caused by reentry involving the Purkinje system. Ablation targeting characteristic electrograms in the reentry region is successful in more than 80% of patients.

## ■ SCAR-RELATED REENTRY CAUSING VENTRICULAR TACHYCARDIA

Sustained VT associated with structural heart disease is associated with a risk of sudden death. Most patients receive an implanted cardioverter-defibrillator (ICD) that can terminate VT when it occurs. Catheter ablation is an important alternative to antiarrhythmic drug therapy for reducing the frequency of symptomatic VT and can be lifesaving if VT becomes incessant.

Any ventricular scar can cause reentry due to the anatomic barrier created by portions of the scar and slow conduction in areas with surviving myocytes dispersed in the scar. Myocardial infarction is the most common cause of scar, but idiopathic dilated cardiomyopathy, sarcoidosis, arrhythmogenic right ventricular dysplasia, and Chagas disease can also result in VT substrate. Prior cardiac surgery with ventriculotomy or patch repairs is a common culprit. The ECG morphology of the VT suggests the location of the scar and the VT exit.

During mapping, areas of scar are identified and highlighted on 3D anatomic maps, allowing some VT that is hemodynamically unstable to be targeted. Pacing from the mapping catheter during sinus rhythm also helps identify the exit region. Ablation then targets conducting channels or the border of the scar region that contains the VT exit. Some epicardial VT can be approached by a subxiphoid percutaneous puncture into the pericardial space for mapping and ablation. Success rates are approximately 70% due to multiple potential reentry circuits. Procedure-related mortality is approximately 3%, some from uncontrollable VT when the procedure fails.

Bundle-branch reentry VT is a type of VT that is particularly susceptible to ablation and is found in approximately 6% of patients with VT and structural heart disease. A diseased Purkinje system supports a reentry circuit revolving up 1 bundle branch and down the contralateral bundle branch. These patients often have intraventricular conduction delay or a pattern of left bundle-branch block during sinus rhythm and advanced ventricular dysfunction. Catheter ablation of the right bundle branch eliminates this VT, though other types of VT are often inducible.

## ■ ABLATION FOR ELECTRICAL STORM AND VENTRICULAR FIBRILLATION

Repetitive episodes of ventricular fibrillation causing *electrical storm* can be initiated by ectopic foci in the Purkinje system. Such cases are rare, but ablation targeting the initiating foci during periods of electrical storm with a strategy similar to that used for idiopathic VT can be lifesaving.

## CONCLUSION

Ablation is a reasonable first-line therapy for most symptomatic supraventricular tachycardias caused by accessory pathways, atrial flutter, AV node reentrant tachycardia, and idiopathic VT. Its use for atrial fibrillation is increasing and further studies will continue to define the risks and benefits. Catheter ablation is an important adjunctive therapy to an implanted defibrillator for patients with recurrent VT associated with structural heart disease and can be lifesaving for patients with incessant VT or electrical storms.

## SUGGESTED READINGS

Tedrow UB, Asirvatham SJ, Stevenson WG. Elecrophysiology and catheter-ablative technicians. In: Fuster V, Walsh R, Harrington RA, et al, eds. *Hurst's The Heart*. 13th ed. New York, NY: McGraw-Hill; 2011; 44:1058-1070.

Blomstrom-Lundqvist C, Scheinman MM, Aliot EM, et al. ACC/AHA/ESC guidelines for the management of patients with supraventricular arrhythmias—executive summary: a report of the American College of Cardiology/American Heart Association Task Force on Practice Guidelines and the European Society of Cardiology Committee for Practice Guidelines (Writing Committee to Develop Guidelines for the Management of Patients With Supraventricular Arrhythmias). *Circulation*. 2003;108:1871-1909.

Haissaguerre M, Extramiana F, Hocini M, et al. Mapping and ablation of ventricular fibrillation associated with long-QT and Brugada syndromes. *Circulation*. 2003;108:925-928.

Haissaguerre M, Jais P, Shah DC, et al. Spontaneous initiation of atrial fibrillation by ectopic beats originating in the pulmonary veins. *N Engl J Med*. 1998;339:659-666.

Joshi S, Wilber DJ. Ablation of idiopathic right ventricular outflow tract tachycardia: current perspectives. *J Cardiovasc Electrophysiol*. 2005;16(suppl 1):S52-S58.

Natale A, Newby KH, Pisano E, et al. Prospective randomized comparison of antiar-rhythmic therapy versus first-line radiofrequency ablation in patients with atrial flutter. *J Am Coll Cardiol*. 2000;35:1898-1904.

Reddy VY, Reynolds MR., Neuzil P, et al. Prophylactic Catheter Ablation for the Prevention of Defibrillator Therapy. *N Engl J Med*. 2007;357:2657-2665.

2006 ACC/AHA Guidelines for the Management of Patients With Ventricular Tachycardia and the Prevention of Sudden Cardiac Death. *Circulation*. 2006;114:1088-1132.

CHAPTER 15

# INDICATIONS AND TECHNIQUES OF ELECTRICAL DEFIBRILLATION AND CARDIOVERSION

Richard E. Kerber

## HISTORY OF DEFIBRILLATION AND CARDIOVERSION

The deleterious effects of uncontrolled electrical current on cardiac rhythm were first recognized early in the 20th century. Concerned by accidental electrocutions of its line workers, the Consolidated Edison Company of New York supported research on the mechanisms and treatment of electrical accidents. Investigators at Johns Hopkins Hospital developed techniques of defibrillation—the termination of ventricular fibrillation—by an electrical shock in the 1930s. The first human defibrillation, in the operating room, was performed by Claude Beck in 1947. Transchest defibrillation using alternating current became a clinical reality when introduced by Paul Zoll in 1956, and direct current defibrillation was pioneered by Bernard Lown in 1962. The work of Zoll and Lown in combination with the description of closed-chest cardiac massage by Jude and colleagues in 1960 has formed the foundation of cardiopulmonary resuscitation from cardiac arrest for over 40 years.

In this chapter, the term *defibrillation* refers to the electrical termination of ventricular fibrillation (VF); *cardioversion* refers to the electrical termination of atrial fibrillation, atrial flutter, and supraventricular and ventricular tachycardias.

## MECHANISMS OF DEFIBRILLATION AND CARDIOVERSION

How does an electric shock terminate a cardiac arrhythmia? There are 3 principal hypotheses. The critical mass hypothesis suggests that some proportion of the myocardium (not necessarily all) must be depolarized, so that the remaining muscle is inadequate to maintain the arrhythmia. The upper limit of vulnerability hypothesis argues that a sufficient current density throughout the ventricle must be achieved lest fibrillation be reinitiated by a subthreshold current density. Jones' group states that defibrillating shocks must prolong refractoriness in sufficient myocardium to terminate VF. These concepts are not mutually exclusive, and all 3 hypotheses may be applicable. Whether they also apply to the atrial myocardium for the termination of atrial fibrillation by electrical shock is not known. More organized arrhythmias, such as ventricular tachycardia and atrial flutter, terminate with lower energy than VF and atrial fibrillation, likely because only regional depolarization in the path of an advancing wavefront is required.

## SHOULD DEFIBRILLATION BE PERFORMED IMMEDIATELY UPON DISCOVERY OF VF, OR SHOULD IT BE PRECEDED BY A PERIOD OF CPR?

Ventricular fibrillation is a lethal arrhythmia and demands instant termination as a lifesaving maneuver. The American Heart Association has encouraged immediate defibrillation of a victim of VF upon the availability of a defibrillator. However, 2 recent investigations by Cobb, Wik, and their coworkers have shown that if the initial application of shock is delayed (usually due to late arrival of rescuers at the scene of the cardiac arrest), a brief period of cardiopulmonary resuscitation (CPR) (ventilation, closed-chest compression) *prior* to the first shock will favorably enhance outcome. However, a third clinical trial, by Jacobs and associates, did not find that a period of CPR before defibrillation facilitates resuscitation. These observations led Weisfeldt and Becker to propose a 3-phase model of VF-induced cardiac arrest: (1) the *electrical* phase consists of the first 4 minutes of VF. Shocks administered during this period have a high likelihood of achieving VF termination and resumption of spontaneous circulation. (2) The *circulatory* phase lasts from 4 to 10 minutes during VF. Shocks should be delayed in favor of a period of 1 to 3 minutes of CPR, including administration of epinephrine or vasopressin, to restore a more favorable milieu for defibrillation. (3) The *metabolic* phase begins after 10 minutes of VF. In this phase, changes in myocardial metabolism after prolonged VF require aggressive and invasive measures for reversal, such as cardiopulmonary bypass and/or hypothermia. Shocks given during this period without such preparatory measures are likely to result in pulseless electrical activity or asystole—conditions associated with a very low likelihood of survival.

The phases of VF/cardiac arrest outlined above are time-based. Could we achieve a more sophisticated insight into the myocardial milieu and thereby determine whether immediate electrical shock or preshock pharmacologic therapy or other resuscitative maneuvers should be employed in each particular case? Such insight might be afforded by a detailed analysis of the electrocardiographic VF signal itself. Experimental and clinical studies have shown that changes in VF frequency and amplitude occur over time. Such changes may be modulated pharmacologically, may correlate with coronary perfusion pressure (the difference between aortic and right atrial pressure during cardiac arrest), and may predict the response to a defibrillating shock. With better understanding of the VF signal and its relationship to the state of the myocardium, the optimal timing of the electrical shock could be guided by a microprocessor-based analysis of the VF signal integrated into the defibrillator, which would instantly instruct the operator whether to deliver a shock or employ other supportive measures, such as continuing CPR and administering vasopressors. Defibrillators employing such sophisticated techniques of VF analysis are now commercially available.

# WHO SHOULD BE CARDIOVERTED FROM ATRIAL FIBRILLATION/ATRIAL FLUTTER, AND WHEN SHOULD THIS BE PERFORMED?

Sinus rhythm improves cardiac performance, especially in patients with mitral stenosis, left ventricular hypertrophy (aortic stenosis, hypertension, idiopathic hypertrophic subaortic stenosis), and/or diminished myocardial reserve (congestive heart failure, myocardial ischemia, and infarction). The coordinated atrial contraction of sinus rhythm improves ventricular filling and the associated cardiac rate is usually slower. Patients with these conditions are thus candidates for *elective* cardioversion. *Urgent* cardioversion may be required for patients with atrial or ventricular arrhythmias who have evidence of end-organ hypoperfusion and/or pulmonary edema.

In some cases, treatment of an underlying or causative condition may restore sinus rhythm without the necessity of electrical cardioversion. Common causes of atrial arrhythmias include hyperthyroidism, pulmonary embolism, congestive heart failure, and mitral stenosis. Postoperative cardiac patients frequently experience transient rhythm disturbances that may spontaneously revert to sinus rhythm.

Important factors that determine the immediate and long-term success of cardioversion of atrial arrhythmias include the duration of the arrhythmia, the extent of atrial fibrosis, and the size of the left atrium. High success rates have been reported for cardioversion of atrial fibrillation and atrial flutter, especially when the new biphasic waveforms are used. High transthoracic impedance (TTI)—the resistance of the chest to the flow of electrical current—will degrade current flow. Because current across the heart is what accomplishes the termination of the arrhythmia, high TTI may reduce the success of defibrillation or cardioversion, especially if the operator has selected a low shock energy.

# THROMBOEMBOLISM

There is a significant risk of thromboembolism after cardioversion. Three factors contribute to this risk:

1. If there is a preexisting thrombus in the fibrillating atrium (especially likely in the left atrial appendage), the electrical shock and/or the resumption of atrial contraction may dislodge the thrombus.

2. The shock itself may have thrombogenic effects.

3. With prolonged atrial fibrillation an atrial myopathy develops, which results in a slow return to normal atrial contraction following cardioversion (see Chapter 10, which discusses this phenomenon in detail).

To prevent thromboembolism, therapeutic anticoagulation (INR 2.0-3.0) for 3 weeks prior to cardioversion and 4 weeks afterward is traditionally recommended.

The risk of thromboembolism associated with atrial fibrillation and cardioversion is higher in patients with mitral stenosis, a large left atrium from any cause, chronic atrial fibrillation, congestive heart failure, age greater than 75 years, previous thromboembolic events, diabetes, or hypertension. Although transthoracic echocardiography is able to image the left atrial cavity well, it is usually unsatisfactory for visualization of the left atrial appendage, the site of most atrial thrombi. However, transesophageal echocardiography (TEE) images the left atrial appendage well and is highly sensitive to the presence of thrombi. Manning and colleagues reported no embolic events during the cardioversion of atrial fibrillation when transesophageal echocardiography showed that no thrombi were present in the atrial appendage and the patient received intravenous heparin for 2 days before cardioversion. This approach is known as TEE-guided cardioversion. If a thrombus in the left atrial appendage is seen by TEE, cardioversion should be delayed and anticoagulation for 3 weeks should be undertaken. Some clinicians repeat the TEE to ensure that the thrombus has lysed. Although thromboembolism after cardioversion of atrial flutter is less common, it has been reported to have conditions associated with thromboembolism, such as left atrial "smoke" (spontaneous ultrasound contrast) on transesophageal echocardiography. Thus, anticoagulation before cardioversion of atrial flutter should be undertaken if persisting longer than 48 hours, similar to atrial fibrillation.

At present, TEE and cardioversion are generally carried out as 2 separate procedures, both requiring conscious sedation or anesthesia. Recently the 2 procedures have been combined by adding an electrode to the external surface of the transesophageal echo probe. Another electrode is placed on the anterior chest wall using a self-adhesive electrode pad. This allows a cardioverting direct current shock to be delivered, using the esophageal-chest pathway. Because the esophageal electrode is close to the heart and the pathway is shortened, less energy—typically 20 to 50 J—is required to terminate atrial fibrillation using this esophageal cardioversion technique. Initial clinical experience with this combined TEE/cardioversion approach has been reported and appears efficacious.

Whether the traditional or TEE-guided anticoagulation scheme is utilized, it is considered mandatory to maintain anticoagulation for at least 4 weeks after cardioversion, since in the absence of anticoagulation thrombi may form postcardioversion and embolism may occur despite a negative TEE precardioversion. Patients with paroxysmal atrial fibrillation, or those considered at high risk of recurrence of atrial fibrillation after cardioversion, may require permanent anticoagulation.

Antiarrhythmic drugs, such as amiodarone and ibutilide, may facilitate cardioversion and maintenance of sinus rhythm after cardioversion. It is customary to withhold digitalis on the day of cardioversion (although this practice is not consistent with the long half-life of this drug). Digitalis-toxic rhythms should not be cardioverted, as the enhanced automaticity of such arrhythmias, combined with the shock, could result in ventricular fibrillation or bidirectional ventricular tachycardia.

# TECHNIQUES OF CARDIOVERSION AND DEFIBRILLATION

## ■ ANESTHESIA

Because the electrical current passing across the thorax causes a painful tetanic contraction so anesthesia is required. Deep conscious sedation is most commonly employed to facilitate electrical cardioversion and typically requires an anesthesiologist to administer, eg, propofol. General anesthesia can also be used and is more effective in pain management and producing an amnestic response. Bag-valve ventilation without endotracheal intubation is usually sufficient, but the presence of an anesthesiologist ensures the ability to perform rapid endotracheal intubation if this becomes necessary.

## ■ SYNCHRONIZATION

It is essential to synchronize the electrical discharge on the R wave of the QRS complex; if the shock falls in the vulnerable period of the cardiac cycle, VF may be induced. This is the most frequent serious complication of elective cardioversion of atrial arrhythmias and usually results from the operator's failure to enable properly the synchronizing device or to verify that the R wave of the electrocardiogram (ECG) lead chosen is sufficiently tall to be recognized by the synchronizer. Recognition of the R wave of ventricular tachycardia is sometimes difficult owing to the morphology of the arrhythmia. If the patient is hemodynamically unstable owing to rapid ventricular tachycardia, unsynchronized shocks may be necessary.

# ■ ELECTRODES

Electrode placement on the chest is important to maximize current flow through the heart, which is what actually terminates the arrhythmia. Only a small proportion—as low as 4%—of the total transchest current flow actually traverses the heart. Numerous pathways have been used successfully, including apex–high right parasternal, anteroposterior, and apex–right infrascapular. The apex–high right parasternal is most frequently used. Although it has been difficult to demonstrate the superiority of any one pathway over others in clinical studies, one pathway might prove superior in the individual patient. Thus, it is the authors' practice to move the electrodes to an alternative pathway when a patient whose atrial arrhythmia is expected to respond to elective cardioversion fails to convert with the initial shocks.

Electrodes should not be placed directly over the site of implanted pacemaker or defibrillator generators. Although manufacturers commonly mark electrodes to indicate the location of chest placement, electrode polarity does not seem to influence shock success, either for monophasic or biphasic waveforms.

Electrode size influences the impedance of the chest; larger electrodes yield lower impedance and thereby improve current flow, increasing the likelihood of arrhythmia termination. For adult humans, the optimal paddle size appears to be 8 to 12 cm in diameter. The Association for the Advancement of Medical Instrumentation recommends a minimum electrode contact area of 50 cm$^2$ for each electrode. The total area of both electrodes should be at least 150 cm$^2$. Smaller pediatric paddles have been manufactured for children, but adult-size paddles should be used for children weighing more than 10 kg (approximately 1 year old). This minimizes transthoracic impedance.

Gels or pastes should not be smeared across the chest between paddle electrodes; the electrical current may follow the low-impedance pathway created by the paste, deflecting current away from the heart. In women, the apex electrode should be placed adjacent to or under the breast; placement on the breast results in a high transthoracic impedance and degrades current flow.

Cutaneous erythema after shocks is often noted at the location of the electrode placement. We have shown by skin biopsies that these are first-degree burns. Because there is preferential current flow at the edges of these electrodes, the erythema typically is most intense at the edges of the electrode location, outlining the electrode shape. Self-adhesive electrode pads constructed to have increased impedance at the pad edges allow more homogeneous current flow and may minimize these burns.

Self-adhesive electrode pads for defibrillation have other advantages. They allow continuous monitoring of cardiac rhythm before and after the shock as well as more physical separation of the generator from the patient (thus reducing the chance of the operator inadvertently receiving a shock); they also facilitate arrhythmia documentation. These pads are universally used in the new automated external defibrillators (AEDs), which are discussed later in this chapter.

# NEW WAVEFORMS FOR DEFIBRILLATION AND CARDIOVERSION

For many years, truncated exponential biphasic waveforms have been used instead of damped sinusoidal monophasic waveforms for implantable cardioverter defibrillators. Their superiority for *transthoracic* defibrillation and cardioversion has been demonstrated, initially in the operating room and the electrophysiology laboratory, where VF is deliberately induced, and subsequently during out-of-hospital cardiac arrest. They are also superior for the electrical cardioversion of atrial arrhythmias. At any energy level, these biphasic waveforms yield higher rates of arrhythmia termination than damped sinusoidal monophasic waveforms. This has resulted in lower energy recommendations for biphasic defibrillation and cardioversion; however, clinical considerations (left atrial size, duration of arrhythmia) may suggest higher or lower energies. The American Heart Association has stated that biphasic waveform shocks ≤200 J are safe and effective for defibrillation, and similar biphasic shock energies are highly effective for cardioversion. Whether biphasic shocks >200 J for defibrillation will be necessary for a significant number of VF patients is not known at present.

"Smart" biphasic waveform defibrillators incorporate technology to measure transthoracic impedance during the shock and instantaneously alter the waveform duration and/or voltage to compensate for impedance. Still other available defibrillators use a rectilinear near-rectangular fixed-pulse-duration waveform. Any of these biphasic waveform variants will be superior to the traditional damped sinusoidal monophasic waveform; whether any one biphasic waveform is superior to another for human defibrillation and cardioversion has yet to be established.

New waveforms for defibrillation have been investigated in animal models. These include sawtooth-shaped biphasic waveforms and multipulse multipathway shocks. These have not yet been used for transthoracic defibrillation in humans. Triphasic and quadriphasic waveforms do not require additional capacitors or elaborate circuitry; these have shown superiority in animal studies.

Although a lifesaving technique, direct current shocks may cause myocardial damage, especially when repeated high-energy discharges are administered. Shocks cause mitochondrial dysfunction and free radical generation in the myocardium proportional to the energy used. Reducing shock energy/current as well as minimizing the number of shocks delivered will limit shock-induced myocardial damage. Biphasic waveforms seem to be less toxic, perhaps simply by requiring less energy to achieve defibrillation.

# AUTOMATED EXTERNAL DEFIBRILLATORS AND PUBLIC ACCESS DEFIBRILLATION

In the 1980s, efforts to reduce the mortality associated with out-of-hospital cardiac arrest emphasized training of emergency medical technicians to recognize VF and to defibrillate using traditional manual defibrillators. Subsequently, automated external defibrillators (AEDs) were introduced; these small, light, and relatively inexpensive devices acquire an ECG via self-adhesive monitor-defibrillator pads applied to the cardiac arrest victim's thorax. A microprocessor in the defibrillator analyzes the ECG thus acquired; if the algorithm for VF is satisfied, the device sounds a warning and then delivers a shock. The ease of application and use of these devices make training requirements minimal, and biphasic waveforms in presently available units enhance the effectiveness of these AEDS. Requirements for AED algorithm performance and safety have been published. Initial experience with AEDs has been reported from aircraft, airports, and gambling casinos, and all reports have been highly favorable. Many communities are now equipping "first responders," such as police officers, firefighters, and security guards, with AEDs. Placement of AEDs in areas known to have a high rate of cardiac arrest—airports, prisons, gyms—is an appropriate and cost-effective strategy. Controlled trials of this strategy have shown its effectiveness.

The American Heart Association strongly supports these efforts under the rubric of *public access defibrillation*.

# AUTOMATIC IMPLANTABLE CARDIOVERTER DEFIBRILLATORS

Automatic implantable cardioverter-defibrillators (ICDs) have revolutionized the treatment of patients at risk of life-threatening ventricular arrhythmias causing sudden cardiac death. ICD pulse generators are implanted in the right or left upper chest and, in certain circumstances, they are implanted in the abdomen. Either a single-chamber device is implanted as a right ventricular lead with shock coils placed in the right ventricular apex or septum. A dual-chamber system includes a right atrial lead placed in the atrial appendage in addition to a right ventricular lead. The Food and Drug Administration first approved the use of ICDs in 1985. Initial clinical research was tailored toward secondary prevention of sudden cardiac death. Several secondary prevention clinical trials were performed to assess the utility of ICDs in cardiac arrest survivors. The Antiarrhythmics Versus Implantable Defibrillators (AVID) trial, Cardiac Arrest Study Hamburg (CASH) trial, and the Canadian Implantable Defibrillator Study (CIDS) all proved the usefulness of implantation of defibrillators in patients who already had a history of cardiac arrest or hemodynamically significant VT. Ad hoc analyses of these studies confirmed that patients with the lowest ejection fraction had the greatest benefit. Primary prevention studies including the Multicenter Automatic Defibrillator Implantation trial (MADIT), Multicenter Automatic Defibrillator Implantation trial II (MADIT II), Multicenter Unsustained Tachycardia trial (MUSTT), and the Sudden Cardiac Death in Heart Failure trial (SCD-HeFT) all demonstrated that ICDs can reduce mortality in patients at risk for sudden cardiac death due to ventricular arrhythmias. Based on these studies, ICDs are indicated for patients who present with VT and sudden cardiac death. They are also indicated for patients with NYHA class II and class III heart failure, ejection fraction < 35%, and have either ischemic or non-ischemic cardiomyopathy (based on CMS guidelines derived from the SCD-HeFT trial).

ICDs are also indicated for patients presenting with a prior infarction, with an ejection fraction <40%, who have spontaneous nonsustained VT and have also had an electrophysiology study showing inducible VT based on the MADIT and MUSTT studies. Patients who fulfill MADIT II criteria (at least 1 month post-infarction with EF ≤ 30%) are candidates for ICD implant. Several other patients at high risk for life-threatening ventricular arrhythmias due to long QT syndrome, Brugada syndrome, or hypertrophic obstructive cardiomyopathy and who usually have a normal ejection fraction may still benefit from ICD implantation.

# HOME DEFIBRILLATORS

Although widespread placement of AEDs in public spaces will improve survival after cardiac arrest, it is known that over two-thirds of cardiac arrests occur at home. Should AEDs be placed in homes of patients with known heart disease who have an increased risk of cardiac arrest? (Patients at the highest risk—eg, those with ischemic heart disease with ejection fractions less than 35%—should receive an implanted cardioverter defibrillator.) For an AED to be effective when used to treat a cardiac arrest at home, the following must happen: (1) a spouse (or family member/friend)

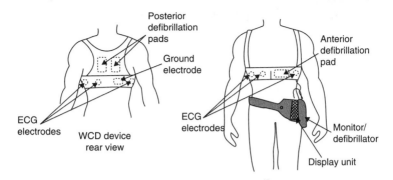

**FIGURE 15-1.** A wearable, fully automatic defibrillator. The patient wears electrodes in a vest; the ECG is continuously analyzed. If the algorithm for VF is satisfied, the device initiates an audible and tactile alarm; this allows the device to be disabled by the patient if the "arrhythmia" was artifactual (eg, a loose or faulty lead). If the device is not disabled within 20 to 30 seconds, a shock is delivered automatically. (Reprinted from Aurrichio A, Klein H, Geller C, et al. Clinical efficacy of the wearable cardioverter defibrillator in acutely terminating episodes of ventricular fibrillation. *Am J Cardiol.* 1998;81:1253-1257, with permission from Excerpta Medica, Inc.)

previously trained in AED use must be at home; (2) the spouse must witness the arrest; (3) the spouse must retrieve the AED; (4) the spouse must correctly apply and turn on the AED; and (5) the AED must be in proper operating condition. These requirements are not trivial, and initial experience with AED use at home suggested that in an emergency, spouses, often elderly, may forget to retrieve their AED and/or be unable to apply and use it correctly.

One potential solution to this problem is the recent development of a wearable defibrillator. The patient wears a vest in which electrodes are incorporated and an ECG is fed to a defibrillator that is worn in a holster-like device (**Fig. 15-1**). The ECG is continuously analyzed; if the VF algorithm is satisfied, the device initially delivers an audible and tactile alarm. If VF is not actually present (eg, if one of the ECG leads in the vest loses skin contact and the resultant artifact simulates VF), the patient has about 30 seconds to disable the device; if it is not disabled during the alert period, the defibrillator charges and then automatically delivers a biphasic shock. Initial clinical experience has been favorable.

# HYPOTHERMIA

Two recent multicenter trials have shown that the deliberate induction of hypothermia by application of external cooling devices affords protection to the brains of patients who have been defibrillated and resuscitated from VF/VT but who remain comatose after resuscitation (ie, anoxic encephalopathy). By cooling such patients to about 33°C for 24 to 36 hours, neurologic outcome improved. This strategy has been endorsed by the American Heart Association. Could hypothermia applied before or during VF/VT (intra-arrest hypothermia) facilitate defibrillation and resuscitation? A major challenge is to develop methods to lower core temperature in patients to about 33°C rapidly—within a few minutes—in order to render this a feasible strategy for intra-arrest application, because external cooling in patients requires several hours to reach 33°C. Experimental methods currently being evaluated include intravenous iced saline, chemical slurries, and intrapulmonary cold perfluorocarbons.

# SUGGESTED READINGS

Kerber RE. Indications and techniques of electrical defibrillation and cardioversion. In: Fuster V, Walsh R, Harrington RA, et al. *Hurst's The Heart*. 13th ed. New York, NY: McGraw-Hill; 2011; 46:1088-1093.

American Heart Association. Guidelines 2005 for cardiopulmonary resuscitation and emergency cardiac care. *Circulation*. 2005;112:IV1-IV41.

Barnard SA, Gray TW, Brist MD, et al. Treatment of comatose survivors of out-of-hospital cardiac arrest with induced hypothermia. *N Engl J Med*. 2002;346:557-563.

Boddicker K, Zhang Y, Zimmerman MB, et al. Hypothermia improves defibrillation success and resuscitation outcomes from ventricular fibrillation. *Circulation*. 2005;111:3195-3201.

Caffrey SL, Willoughy P, Pepe PE, et al. Public use of automated external defibrillators. *N Engl J Med*. 2002;347:1242-1247.

Moss AJ, Zareba W, Hall WJ. Prophylactic implantation of a defibrillator in patients with myocardial infarction and reduced ejection fraction (MADIT II). *N Engl J Med*. 2002;346:877-883.

Weisfeldt M, Becker L. Resuscitation after cardiac arrest: a three-phase time-sensitive model. *JAMA*. 2002;288:3035-3038.

# CHAPTER 16
# DIAGNOSIS AND MANAGEMENT OF SYNCOPE

## Mark D. Carlson and Blair P. Grubb

*Syncope* is a sudden loss of consciousness and postural tone caused by transient decreased cerebral blood flow and is associated with spontaneous recovery. Syncope can occur suddenly, without warning, or be preceded by light-headedness, dizziness, nausea, diaphoresis, and blurred vision. The incidence of syncope increases with age and its causes include cardiovascular disorders, disorders of vascular tone or blood volume, and cerebrovascular disorders. The cause is often multifactorial and cannot be determined in up to 50% of cases. Syncope caused by cardiovascular disorders is associated with the highest risk for mortality, approaching 50% over 5 years and 30% in the first year after diagnosis. Syncope that is not associated with cardiac disease or is of undetermined cause is associated with the lowest mortality risk (6%-10% over 3 years and 24% over 5 years). It is important to distinguish syncope from other causes of loss of consciousness, including seizures, hypoglycemia, and trauma.

## CARDIOVASCULAR DISORDERS

Cardiovascular disorders cause syncope due to severe obstruction or cardiac rhythm disturbances that decrease cardiac output (**Table 16-1**). Obstructive lesions and arrhythmias frequently coexist; one may accentuate the effects of the other. Loss of consciousness during or immediately after exertion is common and may be the presenting symptom in patients with obstructive lesions.

Both sinus node disease and atrioventricular conduction disorders may cause syncope. In the *bradycardia–tachycardia syndrome* (sick sinus syndrome accompanied by atrial tachyarrhythmias), syncope often occurs with asystole at the termination of tachycardia.

Supraventricular tachyarrhythmias rarely cause syncope unless other abnormalities are present (obstructive cardiovascular disease, neurocardiogenic reaction, or a rapid ventricular rate in patients with Wolff–Parkinson–White [WPW] syndrome who experience atrial fibrillation). Ventricular tachycardia is the most common arrhythmic cause of syncope and often occurs in the setting of structural heart disease; torsade de pointes can cause syncope in patients with long QT syndrome. The most common causes of acquired long QT syndrome are antiarrhythmic drugs (types Ia and III) and electrolyte disorders (hypokalemia and hypomagnesemia).

**TABLE 16-1.** Cardiovascular Disorders Associated With Syncope

**Obstructive**
Aortic stenosis
Hypertrophic cardiomyopathy
Mitral stenosis
Prosthetic mitral or aortic valve malfunction
Atrial myxoma
Pulmonary embolism
Pulmonary hypertension
Tetralogy of Fallot
Cardiac tamponade

**Arrhythmic**
Sinoatrial disease
Atrioventricular block
Supraventricular tachyarrhythmias
Ventricular tachycardia
Pacemaker disorders

# DISORDERS OF VASCULAR CONTROL OR BLOOD VOLUME

Disorders of vascular control or blood volume that cause syncope include the reflex syncopes and a number of causes for orthostatic intolerance (**Table 16-2**).

# REFLEX SYNCOPE

Reflex syncopes are caused by sudden failure of the autonomic nervous system to maintain sufficient vascular tone, resulting in hypotension (and sometimes bradycardia). The 2 most common causes are neurocardiogenic (vasodepressor or vasovagal) and the carotid sinus syndrome. The other forms are termed situational because they occur in association with specific activities or conditions (such as micturition, defecation, swallowing, coughing, or postprandial). Neurocardiogenic syncope is often provoked by standing, warm environments, emotional distress, and pain. It is usually preceded by nausea, sweating, light-headedness, or visual alterations but can occur suddenly. The reflexes responsible for neurocardiogenic syncope are normal. Gravity-mediated displacement of blood and venous pooling decreases venous return to the heart, resulting in increased myocardial contractility that activates ventricular mechanoreceptors. The increased afferent neural traffic mimics hypertension, paradoxically decreasing efferent sympathetic activity, resulting in hypotension (vasodepressor response) and, in some cases, increasing vagal efferent activity resulting in bradycardia.

## ■ CAROTID SINUS HYPERSENSITIVITY

Carotid sinus hypersensitivity is most common in men ≥50 years old and is precipitated by pressure on the carotid sinus baroreceptors that leads to sinus arrest or arteriovenous (AV) block (cardioinhibitory response), vasodilatation (a vasodepressor response), or both (mixed response).

**TABLE 16-2.** Disorders of Vascular Control and Blood Volume

**Reflex Syncope**
  Neurocardiogenic
  Situational
  Carotid sinus hypersensitivity

**Orthostatic Intolerance**
  Autonomic nervous system disorders
    Primary autonomic failure
      Pure autonomic failure
      Multiple system atrophy
      Postural orthostatic tachycardia syndrome
        Peripheral or partial dysautonomia
        Hyperadrenergic
      Acute autonomic failure
    Secondary autonomic failure
      Amyloidosis
      Diabetes
      Sarcoidosis
      Renal failure
      Cancer
      Nerve growth factor deficiency
      $\beta$-hydroxylase deficiency
    Pharmacologic agents
    Certain heavy metals
      Mercury
      Lead
      Arsenic
      Iron

**Intravascular Volume Depletion**
  Anemia
  Blood loss
  Dehydration
  Diuretics

**Venous Pooling/Vasodilation**
  Prolonged bed rest
  Prolonged weightlessness
  Pregnancy
  Venous varicosities
  Pharmacologic agents
  Hyperbradykininism
  Mastocytosis
  Carcinoid syndrome

# ■ SYNDROMES OF ORTHOSTATIC INTOLERANCE

Orthostatic hypotension may occur due to hypovolemia or disturbances in vascular control. Primary autonomic disorders that affect vascular control are often idiopathic and may follow either an acute or chronic course. The secondary forms occur in conjunction with another illness (such as amyloidosis or diabetes), in the setting of a known biochemical or structural alteration, or following exposure to various drugs or toxins (heavy metals, alcohol, and some chemotherapeutic agents) (**Table 16-3**).

**TABLE 16-3.** Pharmacologic Agents That May Cause or Worsen Orthostatic Intolerance

Angiotensin-converting enzyme inhibitors
α-receptor blockers
Calcium-channel blockers
β-blockers
Phenothiazines
Tricyclic antidepressants
Bromocriptine
Opiates
Diuretics
Hydralazine
Ganglionic-blocking agents
Nitrates
Sildenafil citrate
Monoamine oxidase inhibitors
Chemotherapeutic agents
  Vincristine
  Vinblastine

## ■ PRIMARY CAUSES OF AUTONOMIC FAILURE

Primary autonomic failure (PAF) and multiple system atrophy (MSA) are manifested by orthostatic hypotension, syncope, and varying degrees of autonomic nervous system dysfunction. MSA involves the somatic system as well. The syndromes affect twice as many men as women; symptoms usually begin between the fifth and sixth decades of life. In the postural orthostatic tachycardia syndrome (POTS), heart rate increases excessively in response to upright posture. The more common type, peripheral (or partial) dysautonomia, is associated with inability to increase peripheral vascular resistance when upright, leading to blood pooling followed by tachycardia and enhanced myocardial contraction. The hyperadrenergic form is associated with tremor, hyperhidrosis, diarrhea, panic attacks, and severe migraine headaches. Although supine catecholamine levels are normal, upright levels are often elevated (over 600 mg/dL) in patients and the response to isoproterenol is excessive (>30 bpm increase in response to 1 μg/min).

Acute autonomic failure is characterized by rapid widespread failure of both the parasympathetic and sympathetic, but not the somatic nervous systems. Merely attempting to sit up in bed may cause syncope. Many patients suffer from anhidrosis and disturbances in bowel and bladder function that result in abdominal pain, cramping, bloating, nausea, and vomiting.

A variety of systemic disorders or environmental and pharmacologic agents may cause syncope by impacting blood volume or vascular control (Tables 16-2 and 16-3).

## CEREBROVASCULAR DISORDERS

Patients with cerebrovascular occlusive disease may require higher-than-normal arterial blood pressure to maintain consciousness. Syncope can occur in patients with occluded brachiocephalic vessels, as occurs in pulseless disease (eg, aortic arch syndrome and Takayasu arteritis). Syncope associated with changing positions of the head can occur due to narrowing of the vertebral arteries by skeletal deformities of the cervical spine in patients with Klippel–Feil deformity, cervical spondylosis, and cervical osteoarthritis. In patients with the *subclavian steal syndrome,* syncope occurs during upper extremity exercise when blood flow is shunted retrograde, by the circle of Willis, to the distal subclavian artery. These patients exhibit diminished brachial arterial pressure on the affected side, a bruit that is maximal over the supraclavicular area adjacent to the origin of the vertebral artery, and symptoms during exercise of the involved extremity. Syncope can be a presenting symptom of cerebral emboli or atherosclerotic disease of the vertebrobasilar system.

## ■ APPROACH TO THE PATIENT

One of the most important goals is to determine if the patient has a cause for syncope that is life threatening. In addition, effective therapy often depends on a precise and accurate diagnosis.

## ■ HISTORY AND PHYSICAL EXAMINATION

The history and physical examination may alone diagnose the etiology or distinguish syncope from other causes of loss of consciousness. The history should include questions about the first event, how often and in what settings syncope occurred, observations of bystanders, prescription and nonprescription remedies, and family history of cardiovascular disease, neurologic disorders, and early sudden death.

Blood pressure and heart rate should be measured in the supine, sitting, and upright positions immediately and 3 to 5 minutes after standing. Orthostatic hypotension is present if systolic blood pressure falls by 20 mm Hg or diastolic blood pressure falls by 10 mm Hg during the first 2 minutes of standing. A Valsalva maneuver may reproduce cough syncope; hyperventilation for 2 to 3 minutes may reproduce episodes that are related to anxiety. Carotid sinus massage may induce bradycardia, but is not recommended for those who may have carotid atherosclerotic disease. A pause of longer than 3 seconds during massage suggests that carotid sinus hypersensitivity caused syncope.

Blood tests that contribute to diagnosis include a complete blood count, serum electrolytes, supine and upright serum catecholamine levels, and drug levels. All patients should undergo a 12-lead surface electrocardiogram (ECG). A transthoracic echocardiogram should be performed whenever heart disease is suspected. Patients at risk for coronary artery disease should undergo a stress test. Continuous ECG monitoring (Holter monitor) is used for suspected arrhythmic syncope; an event recorder may prove efficacious, particularly if the episodes are infrequent. Patients with very infrequent episodes may benefit from an implantable loop recorder. When noninvasive testing does not diagnose arrhythmic causes, an electrophysiologic study may be indicated in high-risk patients, including those with coronary artery disease and those with bundle-branch or bifascicular block.

Tilt-table testing is based on the principle that orthostatic stress provokes reflex syncope in susceptible individuals (**Table 16-4**). A positive test is one that provokes a hypotensive episode (or in the case of POTS, a tachycardic episode) that reproduces the patient's symptoms. The specificity of tilt-table testing is reported to be near 90% and the sensitivity between 20% and 74%.

## TREATMENT

Patients should minimize exposure to factors that provoke syncope, situations in which they or others could be injured were they to lose consciousness, and should take measures to avoid syncope (lie down) should they experience prodromal symptoms.

**TABLE 16-4.** Head-up Tilt-Table Testing

Indications for Head-up Tilt-Table Testing
1. Unexplained recurrent syncope or single syncopal episode associated with injury (or significant risk of injury) in absence of organic heart disease.
2. Unexplained recurrent syncopal episodes or single syncopal episode associated with injury (or significant risk of injury) in setting of organic heart disease after exclusion of potential cardiac cause of syncope.
3. After identification of a cause of recurrent syncope in situations in which determination of an increased predisposition to neurocardiogenic syncope could alter treatment.

Conditions in Which Tilt-Table Testing May Be Useful
1. Differentiating conclusive syncope from epilepsy.
2. Evaluation of recurrent near syncope or dizziness.
3. Evaluation of syncope in autonomic failure syndromes.
4. Exercise-induced or postexercise-induced syncope in absence of organic heart disease in patients in whom exercise stress testing cannot reproduce an episode.
5. Evaluation of recurrent unexplained falls.

Unconsciousness individuals should be placed supine with the head turned to the side. Clothing that fits tightly around the neck or waist should be loosened.

# ■ SYNDROMES OF ORTHOSTATIC INTOLERANCE

Patients with orthostatic hypotension should be instructed to move their legs prior to rising slowly from the bed or a chair (**Table 16-5**). If possible, medications that aggravate the problem should be discontinued. Physical maneuvers and salt and water loading have benefited some patients. Biofeedback therapy has been useful when neurocardiogenic syncope is provoked by psychogenic stimuli. β-adrenoceptor antagonists were among the first drugs used to prevent neurocardiogenic syncope. Several vasoconstrictive agents, including the α-receptor stimulants dexedrine, methylphenidate, and midodrine, have been used. Midodrine is used to treat orthostatic hypotension and has been shown to prevent neurocardiogenic syncope in 2 randomized trials. The α-2-receptor agonist clonidine may be most useful in patients with both hypertensive and hypotensive episodes. Other vasoconstrictive substances, such as theophylline, ephedrine, and yohimbine, are reported to be effective, but tolerance of these agents is often poor. Bupropion tends to have fewer sexual side effects but may aggravate hypertension.

The acetylcholinesterase inhibitor pyridostigmine may be an effective agent for both orthostatic hypotension and POTS. The agent is safe and effective and seems to be able to prevent falls in blood pressure without exacerbating supine hypertension. The serotonin reuptake inhibitors have been shown to prevent recurrent neurocardiogenic syncope. In patients with orthostatic hypotension or autonomic failure syndromes who have anemia, erythropoietin not only raises red cell counts but has vasoconstrictive effects. Octreotide, a synthetic somatostatin analogue, causes splanchnic mesenteric vasoconstriction, thus enhancing venous return to the heart.

Patients with asystole during tilt testing or syncope and those with the cardioinhibitory or mixed forms of carotid sinus hypersensitivity may benefit from permanent pacing. Pacing reduces recurrent syncope and injuries in elderly patients with frequent falls and cardioinhibitory carotid sinus hypersensitivity. Pacing may

**TABLE 16-5.** Orthostatic Intolerance Syndrome Therapies

| Treatment | Application | NCS | PD | HA | OH | Problems |
|---|---|---|---|---|---|---|
| | | Form Effective in | | | | |
| Reconditioning | Aerobic exercise 20 min 3 times/wk | X | X | X | X | If done too vigorously, may worsen symptoms |
| Physical maneuvers (tilt training, etc) | 30 min 3 times/d | X | | | | Noncompliance is common |
| Sleeping with head tilted upright | During sleep | X | | X | X | |
| Hydration | 2 L PO/d | X | X | | X | Edema |
| Salt | 2-4 g/d | X | X | | X | Edema |
| Fludrocortisone | 0.1-0.2 mg PO qd | X | X | | X | Hypokalemia, hypomagnesemia, edema |
| Metoprolol | 25-100 mg bid | X | | | | Fatigue |
| Labetalol | 100-200 mg PO bid | | | X | | Fatigue |
| Midodrine | 5-10 mg PO tid | X | X | | X | Nausea, scalp itching, supine hypertension |
| Methylphenidate | 5-10 mg PO tid | X | X | X | | Anorexia, insomnia, dependency |
| Bupropion | 150-300 mg XL/qd | | X | X | X | Tremor, agitation, insomnia |
| Clonidine | 0.1-0.3 mg PO bid 0.1-0.3 mg patch qwk | | | X | | Dry mouth, blurred vision |
| Pyridostigmine | 30-60 mg PO/d | | X | | X | Nausea, diarrhea |
| SSRI-escitalopram | 10 mg PO/d | X | X | | X | Tremor, agitation, sexual problems |
| Erythropoietin | 10 000-20 000 µg sq q/wk | X | X | | X | Pain at injection site, expensive |
| Octreotide | 50-200 µg SC tid | | X | X | X | Nausea, diarrhea, gallstone |
| Permanent pacing | | X | | | | |

HA, hyperadrenergic; NCS, neurocardiogenic syncope; OH, orthostatic hypotension; PD, peripheral dysautonomia; SSRI, selective serotonin reuptake inhibitor.

prolong the duration of prodromal symptoms, allowing patients sufficient time to take evasive action and avoid syncope.

# ■ CEREBROVASCULAR DISORDERS

Anticoagulants and/or platelet antiaggregant agents are recommended for the prevention of embolic disease from the heart or central vessels. Endarterectomy or percutaneous dilatation should be considered in carotid arterial occlusive disease.

# ■ CARDIOVASCULAR DISORDERS

Cardiac surgery is often the treatment of choice for patients with syncope caused by obstructive heart disease. Patients with hypertrophic cardiomyopathy and syncope may respond well to pharmacologic therapy, but certain patients may benefit from AV sequential pacing, sugery, or an implantable cardioverter-defibrillator. The treatment of arrhythmias that cause syncope is discussed in detail elsewhere (see Chapters 9-11). Bradyarrhythmias usually require the implantation of a permanent pacemaker but may respond to withdrawal of a drug. Implantable cardioverter-defibrillators are the first-line therapy for most ventricular tachycardias, although some patients may require antiarrhythmic drugs or catheter ablation to reduce symptoms or shocks from the ICD.

In patients with polymorphic ventricular tachycardia in the setting of a long QT interval (torsade de pointes), the potential offending drug(s) (usually an antiarrhythmic drug) should be stopped. Acute therapy includes intravenous magnesium and measures to increase the heart rate and shorten electrical diastole (eg, cardiac pacing). Long-term therapy for congenital long QT syndrome may include β-blockers, permanent pacing, an implantable defibrillator, and lifestyle changes.

Patients with syncope should be hospitalized with continuous ECG monitoring if it is reasonably likely that the episode resulted from a life-threatening abnormality or if recurrence with significant injury seems likely. Patients who are known to have a normal heart and for whom the history strongly suggests vasovagal or situational syncope may be treated as outpatients if the episodes are neither frequent nor severe. When the cause is unknown, treatment must be targeted to the most likely cause and to prolong life. Certain high-risk patients may benefit from a pacemaker or an implantable cardioverter-defibrillator even when it is not clear that bradycardia or a ventricular arrhythmia caused syncope.

# SUGGESTED READINGS

Carlson MD, Grubb BP. Diagnosis and management of syncope. *Hurst's The Heart.* 13th ed. New York, NY: McGraw-Hill; 2011;48:1123-1138.

Grubb BP. Neurocardiogenic syncope and related disorders of orthostatic intolerance. *Circulation.* 2005;111:2997-3006.

Grubb BP, Kosinski D. Orthostatic hypotension: causes, classification and treatment. *Pacing Clin Electrophysiol.* 2003;26:892-901.

Kapoor WN. Current evaluation and management of syncope. *Circulation.* 2002;106:1606-1609.

Mathias C, Bannister R, eds. *Autonomic Failure: A Textbook of Clinical Disorders of the Autonomic Nervous System.* 45th ed. Oxford, UK: Oxford University Press; 1999:307-320.

Soteriades ES, Evans JC, Larson MG, et al. Incidence and prognosis of syncope. *N Engl J Med.* 2002;347:878.

Strickberger SA, Benson DW, Biaggioni I, et al. AHA/ACCF scientific statement on the evaluation of syncope. From the American Heart Association Councils on Clinical Cardiology, Cardiovascular Nursing, Cardiovascular Disease in the Young, and Stroke, and the Quality of Care and Outcomes Research Interdisciplinary Working Group; and the American College of Cardiology Foundation; in collaboration with the Heart Rhythm Society; endorsed by the American Autonomic Society. *Circulation.* 2006;113:316-327.

# CHAPTER 17
# SUDDEN CARDIAC DEATH

Matthew R. Reynolds, Amit J. Thosani,
Duane S. Pinto, and Mark E. Josephson

## DEFINITION

*Sudden cardiac death* (SCD) is the unexpected natural death from a cardiac cause within a short time period from the onset of symptoms in a person without any prior condition that would appear lethal. SCD most commonly results from cardiac arrest due to a fatal arrhythmia and may or may not occur in the background of structural heart disease or coronary artery disease (CAD).

## EPIDEMIOLOGY

SCD accounts for almost half a million deaths each year in the United States, with exact totals depending on the definition used. Worldwide, SCD comprises 50% of overall cardiac mortality in developed countries. When the definition of SCD is restricted to death less than 2 hours from onset of symptoms, 12% of all natural deaths are sudden and 88% of these are a result of cardiac disease. SCD is also the most common and often the first manifestation of CAD. In autopsy-based studies, a cardiac etiology of sudden death has been reported in 60% to 70% of sudden death victims. Approximately 60% of SCDs occur outside the hospital setting. First-known arrhythmic events account for approximately 85% to 90% of SCDs, while the remaining 10% to 15% are due to recurrent events.

The incidence of SCD increases with age, largely in part to higher incidence and prevalence of coronary disease and left ventricular dysfunction. Among sudden natural deaths, the proportion with cardiac causes also increases with advancing age. Still, SCD accounts for approximately 20% of all sudden deaths in patients younger than age 20 years. Overall, SCD in infants, children, adolescents, and young adults is rare.

In parallel with higher incidence of CAD, SCD has a much higher incidence in men than in women. Seventy to ninety percent of SCDs occur in men. However, women are more likely than men to suffer SCD without prior evidence of coronary heart disease, and a greater percentage of sudden deaths occur outside the hospital in women. Blacks have higher age-adjusted mortality rates for SCD than nonblacks.

## RISK FACTORS

The major risk factors for SCD are established CAD or high risk for CAD, previous myocardial infarction (MI), decreased ejection fraction (EF), and a history of ventricular arrhythmias. These are potent risk factors that increase the *relative* risk of SCD, but the contribution of SCD in those with such risk factors to the cumulative rate of SCD is relatively low. Most cases of SCD occur in the general population without a known history of heart disease, followed by patients who are high risk for CAD or have established CAD. Despite the fact that numerous population-based studies have shown a strong relationship between risk factors for coronary heart disease (CHD) and SCD, no study has identified a single set of risk factors specific for SCD. Cigarette smoking is one of the few behavioral risk factors that is associated with a disproportionate number of sudden deaths. There are many reports linking stress, particularly emotional stress, to ventricular arrhythmias and SCD.

Twenty to thirty-five percent of sudden deaths in young adults occur in the absence of identifiable cardiac structural abnormalities. Among infants, up to 10% of cases of crib deaths or sudden infant death syndrome may be due to cardiac arrhythmias, including QT syndromes. Overall, sudden death is rare in young athletes, but in the United States one-third of these cases have hypertrophic cardiomyopathy on autopsy.

# PATHOPHYSIOLOGY

Ventricular tachycardia (VT) degenerating into ventricular fibrillation (VF) is the most common electrical sequence of events in SCD. Polymorphic VT or torsade de pointes may be the initial arrhythmia in patients with acute ischemia or genetic syndromes. In advanced heart failure or in the elderly, bradyarrhythmias or electromechanical dissociation may be the primary electrical event. The bradyarrhythmias may be secondary to pump or hemodynamic failure. *Commotio cordis* is an extremely rare phenomenon where a critically timed mechanical blow to the chest results in VF.

In acute ischemia, rapid polymorphic VT and VF are the predominant malignant arrhythmias. Ventricular arrhythmias can also be a sign of reperfusion after thrombolysis, percutaneous revascularization, or spontaneous reperfusion. In the subacute phase of MI (within the first 3 days), SCD may occur, but the predominant arrhythmias are accelerated idioventricular rhythm and idioventricular tachycardia, which subside after 2 or 3 days and have no prognostic significance. In the late phases, when the infarction is healed, monomorphic VT is the predominant arrhythmia. Critical areas of the reentrant circuits are formed by surviving myocardial fibers in the border zone of a healed infarction. The transition from organized VT to VF or the development of primary VF is usually from simultaneous ventricular activation by multiple localized areas of microreentry circuits.

Atrial flutter (AFL) or atrial fibrillation (AF) with very rapid ventricular responses may also be the primary electrical event preceding VT/VF, particularly in patients with CAD or advanced heart disease. SCD can also occur in patients with the Wolf–Parkinson–White (WPW) syndrome, in which very rapid ventricular response in AF degenerates into VF due to rapidly conducting accessory pathways.

# ETIOLOGY

**Table 17-1** lists cardiac abnormalities associated with sudden cardiac death.

## ◼ CORONARY ATHEROSCLEROSIS

CHD is present in 40% to 86% of SCD survivors, depending on age and gender. SCD can occur in the absence of infarction but usually happens in the presence of diffuse coronary disease. Although the majority of patients who suffer SCD have severe

**TABLE 17-1.** Cardiac Abnormalities Associated With Sudden Cardiac Death

**Ischemic Heart Disease**

Coronary atherosclerosis
  Acute MI
  Chronic ischemic cardiomyopathy
Anomalous origin of coronary arteries
Hypoplastic coronary artery

Coronary artery spasm
Coronary artery dissection
Coronary arteritis
Small vessel disease

**Non-ischemic Heart Disease**

Cardiomyopathies
  Idiopathic dilated cardiomyopathy
  Hypertrophic cardiomyopathy
  Hypertensive cardiomyopathy
  Arrhythmogenic right ventricular
    cardiomyopathy
Infiltrative and inflammatory heart disease
  Sarcoidosis
  Amyloidosis
  Hemochromatosis
  Myocarditis

Valvular heart disease
Aortic stenosis
  Aortic regurgitation
  Mitral valve prolapse
  Infective endocarditis
  Congenital heart disease
Tetralogy of Fallot
  Transposition of the great vessels
    (post–Mustard-Senning)
  Ebstein anomaly
  Pulmonary vascular obstructive disease
  Congenital aortic stenosis
  Primary electrical abnormalities
  Long QT syndrome
  Short QT syndrome
  WPW syndrome
  Congenital atrioventricular block
  Idiopathic ventricular tachycardia
  Idiopathic ventricular fibrillation
    Syndrome of right bundle-branch
      block, ST elevation, and sudden
      death (Brugada syndrome)
    Catecholaminergic polymorphic
      ventricular tachycardia
Nocturnal death in Southeast Asian men

Drug-induced and other toxic agents
  Antiarrhythmic drugs (class Ia, Ic, and III)
  Erythromycin
  Clarithromycin
  Astemizole

  Terfenadine
  Pentamidine
  Ketoconazole
  Trimethoprim-sulfamethoxazole
  Psychotropic drugs (tricyclic antidepressants,
    haloperidol, phenothiazines, chloral
    hydrate)

  Probucol
  Cisapride
  Cocaine
  Chloroquine
  Alcohol
  Phosphodiesterase inhibitors
  Organophosphates

Electrolyte abnormalities
  Hypokalemia
  Hypomagnesemia
  Hypocalcemia
  Anorexia nervosa and bulimia
  Liquid protein dieting
  Diuretics

multivessel coronary disease, fewer than half of the patients resuscitated from VF exhibit evidence of MI in the form of elevated cardiac enzymes, and fewer than 20% have Q-wave MI. Following recovery from acute MI, patients remain at chronically increased risk for SCD. Ejection fraction is the most important predictor of sudden death in this group.

# ■ NONATHEROSCLEROTIC DISEASE OF THE CORONARY ARTERIES

Congenital coronary artery anomalies, found in approximately 1% of all patients undergoing angiography and in 0.3% of those undergoing autopsy, can be complicated by SCD, often exercise related, in up to 30% of patients. The highest-risk anomalies are origin of the left main coronary artery from the right aortic sinus or origin of the right coronary artery from the left coronary sinus. Life-threatening ventricular arrhythmias and SCD have been described in patients with coronary artery spasm.

Acquired and inherited disease of the connective tissue and blood vessels may also affect the coronary arteries, leading to ischemia and SCD, including Marfan syndrome, after labor and delivery, and infections and inflammatory vasculitides. Myocardial bridges have been reported in association with SCD during exercise, but they are also an incidental finding at autopsy in up to 25% of patients dying of other causes.

# ■ CARDIOMYOPATHIES

## Idiopathic Dilated Cardiomyopathy

*Idiopathic dilated cardiomyopathy* is the substrate for approximately 10% of SCDs in the adult population. Mortality in idiopathic dilated cardiomyopathy is high, reaching 10% to 50% annually, and seems most closely tied to the severity of pump dysfunction. SCD in idiopathic dilated cardiomyopathy is usually attributed to both polymorphic and monomorphic ventricular tachyarrhythmias. The terminal event can, however, also be asystole or electromechanical dissociation, especially in patients with advanced left ventricular dysfunction.

## Hypertrophic Cardiomyopathy

The incidence of SCD in patients with *hypertrophic cardiomyopathy* (HCM) is 2% to 4% per year in adults and 4% to 6% per year in children and adolescents. There are few reliable predictors of SCD in patients with HCM. A clinical history of spontaneous, sustained monomorphic VT or sudden death in family members with HCM indicates a worse prognosis, as does onset of symptoms in childhood. The magnitude of outflow tract gradient does not appear to predict the risk of sudden death, but an association between extreme hypertrophy and SCD has been reported. Patients with wall thicknesses >30 mm had a 20-year risk of sudden death approaching 40% in 1 series. Genotypic analysis is considered less reliable in risk assessment than family history. (See also Chapter 39.)

## Hypertensive Cardiomyopathy

Left ventricular hypertrophy (LVH) has been identified as one of the strongest blood pressure-independent risk factors for sudden death. In the Framingham study, electrocardiogram (ECG) evidence of LVH doubled the risk of SCD. Hypertensive patients with LVH also have a significantly greater prevalence of premature ventricular contractions and complex ventricular arrhythmias than do patients without LVH or normotensive patients.

# ■ INFLAMMATORY OR INFILTRATIVE MYOCARDIAL DISEASE

Myocardial scar, regardless of etiology, may lead to ventricular arrhythmias and sudden death due to tissue electrical heterogeneity. Myocarditis, which can lead to minimal scarring, is responsible for 11% to 22% of SCD, according to one autopsy study. Primary amyloidosis may involve the heart in one-third of cases. Amyloid deposition in the ventricular myocardium leads to electrical heterogeneity and delayed activation, which are risk factors for sudden death. *Arrhythmogenic right ventricular dysplasia* (ARVD) is a rare, usually inherited cardiomyopathy characterized by fatty or fibrofatty replacement of myocardium associated with recurrent ventricular tachycardia with left bundle-branch block morphologies. In the early stages of the disease, VT is often precipitated by exercise. The course and prognosis of ARVD are highly variable.

# ■ CONGENITAL HEART DISEASE

An increased risk of SCD has been found predominantly in 4 congenital conditions: *tetralogy of Fallot, transposition of the great vessels, aortic stenosis,* and *pulmonary vascular obstruction.* Patients who have undergone reparative surgery for *tetralogy of Fallot* have a reported risk of sudden cardiac death of 6% before age 20. A QRS duration ≥180 milliseconds has been found to be the most sensitive predictor of SCD, and ventricular tachyarrhythmias in adults after repair of tetralogy of Fallot and correlates with other parameters of right ventricular volume overload.

# ■ PRIMARY ELECTRICAL ABNORMALITIES

## Long QT Syndrome

Sudden cardiac death is one of the hallmarks of the idiopathic long QT syndrome (LQTS), a group of genetically distinct disorders resulting from an ion channel or auxillary subunit mutation. Congenital LQTS accounts for 3000 to 4000 sudden childhood deaths per year in the United States.

The long QT interval reflects abnormal prolongation of repolarization. Other characteristics of this disorder, in addition to the prolonged (>440 milliseconds for males or >460 milliseconds for females, corrected for heart rate) QT interval, include abnormal T-wave contours, relative sinus bradycardia, a family history of early sudden death, and a propensity for recurrent syncope and SCD due to polymorphic VT (torsade de pointes) and VF. Mutations in 7 genes have been identified so far. Most cases are caused by 3 mutations: LQT1 (42%), LQT2 (45%), and LQT3 (8%). The rare autosomal recessive Jervell–Lange–Nielsen syndrome is also associated with congenital deafness. Cases of SCD and abnormally short QT interval have also been recently described and attributed to a potassium channel mutation.

Over 90% of the congenital forms of LQTS have been linked to specific chromosomal defects, resulting in a genetically based classification (LQT1 through LQT6) with important functional and prognostic implications. The risk of sudden death in LQTS is influenced by the duration of the QT interval, corrected for heart rate (QTc), the specific genetic defect, gender, family history, and possibly other factors. Torsade de pointes can be triggered by different stimuli, typically involving high adrenergic states (eg, exercise).

## Brugada Syndrome

The syndrome of SCD associated with complete or incomplete right bundle-branch block and persistent ST-segment elevation in leads $V_1$ through $V_3$ in patients without demonstrable structural heart disease is known as the Brugada syndrome. Patients with this ECG pattern and prior cardiac arrest or syncope have high rates of sudden death during follow-up. Mutations in the sodium channel gene SCN5A have been implicated as the cause of Brugada syndrome in some families; different mutations of the same gene are also responsible for LQTS type 3. The significance of Brugada-type ECG findings in individuals with no personal or family history of arrhythmias remains unclear.

## Idiopathic Ventricular Fibrillation

Several types of idiopathic polymorphic VT have been described that are associated with an unfavorable prognosis. These include idiopathic VF, torsade de pointes with a short coupling interval, and catecholaminergic polymorphic VT. They can occur in sporadic or familial forms and are frequently associated with catecholamine release during physical or emotional stress. In survivors of cardiac arrest, the diagnosis of idiopathic VF is made by exclusion. Catecholaminergic or familial polymorphic VT is an exceptionally rare form of bidirectional or polymorphic VT due to mutations in the cardiac ryanodine receptor (RyR2) and calsequestrin (CASQ2) genes.

# ■ DRUGS AND OTHER TOXIC AGENTS

## Proarrhythmia

Classes I and III antiarrhythmic drugs exhibit a dose-dependent antiarrhythmic effect in structurally normal and abnormal hearts. Many other agents with diverse actions have been implicated in the induction of tachyarrhythmias, including erythromycin, terfenadine, pentamidine, and certain psychotropic drugs. Most of these drugs produce toxicity by prolonging repolarization and QTc, leading to torsade de pointes. In other patients, drug-induced LQTS may actually make a background mutation or polymorphism(s) in a congenital LQTS gene clinically apparent. The list of drugs implicated in LQTS is vast and rapidly expanding, and online sites such as www.torsades.org can provide comprehensive, timely information.

## Cocaine

Cocaine can precipitate life-threatening cardiac events, including SCD. Cocaine causes coronary vasoconstriction, increases cardiac sympathetic effects, and precipitates cardiac arrhythmias irrespective of the amount ingested, prior use, or whether there is an underlying cardiac abnormality.

## Electrolyte Abnormalities

There is an almost linear inverse relationship between serum potassium concentration and the probability of VT in patients with acute MI. *Hypokalemia* is often found in patients during and following resuscitation from a cardiac arrest. Many of the electrophysiologic effects of hypokalemia are similar to those caused by digitalis and catecholamine stimulation, explaining the high risk of ventricular arrhythmias when a combination of these factors is present. An association between *magnesium deficiency* and SCD has been reported in humans, especially as a cofactor in drug-induced torsade de pointes. Hypomagnesemia in humans is generally associated with CHF, digitalis use, chronic diuretic use, hypokalemia, and hypocalcemia, making it difficult to establish whether the hypomagnesemia alone precipitates arrhythmias. Acute administration of magnesium has been successfully used in the treatment of drug-induced torsade de pointes, although hypomagnesemia is not usually documented in this situation.

# MANAGEMENT

## ■ ESTABLISHING THE UNDERLYING CARDIAC PATHOLOGY

After successful resuscitation from cardiac arrest and a period of hemodynamic and respiratory stabilization, every effort should be made to establish the cause of cardiac arrest and the likelihood of recurrence. It is important to determine if cardiac arrest was the result and not cause of acute circulatory or respiratory collapse.

Underlying cardiac disease should first be investigated. Myocardial ischemia and infarction should be excluded. Echocardiography can help determine left ventricular function, regional wall-motion abnormalities, valvular heart disease, or cardiomyopathies. Cardiac catheterization is often recommended to evaluate the coronary anatomy and hemodynamics. Other tests—such as radionuclide studies, magnetic resonance imaging, or cardiac biopsy—may be necessary in selected patients. An underlying cardiac disease can be found in most patients.

At the same time, every effort should be made to exclude potentially reversible causes of SCD, including transient ischemic episodes in patients who are candidates for complete revascularization and in whom the onset of the arrhythmia is clearly preceded by ischemic ECG changes or symptoms.

## ■ RISK STRATIFICATION FOR SUDDEN CARDIAC DEATH

Current parameters used to risk-stratify patients with CAD for SCD include medical history (presence of nonsustained VT, syncope), EF, ECG (QRS duration, QT interval, QT dispersion), signal-averaged electrocardiogram (SAECG), heart rate variability, and baroreflex sensitivity. Unfortunately, each of these individual parameters lacks very high sensitivity and specificity for identifying vulnerable patients. Measurement of microvolt T-wave alternans, which assess beat to beat changes in ventricular repolarization, has been shown to have strong negative predictive value in some select patient groups.

Even invasive electrophysiologic testing showed that patients with ischemic cardiomyopathy who had no inducible for ventricular tachyarrhythmias had essentially the same risk of SCD as those who had inducible ventricular arrythmias. Moreover, the positive predictive accuracy of inducibility of ventricular tachycardia has been relatively low in consecutive series of patients with recent MI. Therefore, at present, only LV dysfunction reliably defines "high risk" for SCD in patients with ischemic cardiomyopathy.

*Invasive electrophysiologic studies* (EPS) may be useful in select patient groups (see Chapter 13). Electrode-tipped catheters are typically placed via the femoral or internal jugular veins to right atrium, right ventricle, and His bundle, and repeated programed electrical stimulation is administered to pace the heart in an attempt to induce arrhythmias. Induction of sustained monomorphic VT is the generally accepted end point for programmed ventricular stimulation. Inducible VT on EPS has been demonstrated to strongly predict recurrent ventricular arrhythmias and sudden death. EP testing is also useful in patients with structural heart disease who present with unexplained syncope. VT is the most common abnormal finding in these patients, but demonstration of His–Purkinje conduction disease or hemodynamically unstable supraventricular tachycardia can also be important. In survivors of cardiac arrest due to VF, the value of electrophysiologic testing is less clear, but it may be of diagnostic utility in selected circumstances. However, EP testing is not used in selecting non-ischemic patients for ICDs because of its poor sensitivity and specificity.

# TREATMENT OPTIONS FOR PATIENTS AT RISK FOR SUDDEN CARDIAC DEATH

## ■ PHARMACOLOGIC THERAPY

### β-Blockers

Of all the therapies currently available for the prevention of SCD, none is more established or effective in patients with CHD than β-blockers. Large randomized studies have repeatedly and compellingly demonstrated marked reductions in total mortality and SCD by nonselective β-blockers (propranolol) and cardioselective agents such as metoprolol. The benefits of β-blockade are additive to standard treatment for CHF. β-blockers are effective in the setting of ventricular arrhythmias provoked by a high sympathetic tone, as in patients with congenital long-QT syndrome, arrhythmogenic right ventricular dysplasia, or CHF. Importantly, the beneficial effects of β-blockers on cardiac mortality are most pronounced in patients who are at higher risk for SCD, such as those with CHF, atrial and ventricular arrhythmias, post-MI, and diabetes.

### Angiotensin-Converting Enzyme Inhibitors

Although the mortality benefit from angiotensin-converting enzyme (ACE) inhibitors in heart failure patients is thought to stem primarily from a reduction in pump failure, a specific reduction in the incidence of sudden death may be present as well. Although data from individual trials have been conflicting on this issue, a meta-analysis of trials including over 15 000 post-MI patients reported a 20% reduction in SCD in ACE-inhibitor-treated subjects (HR 0.80; 95% confidence interval [CI] 0.70-0.92). Whether these results also pertain to angiotensin receptor blockers is not known.

### Antiarrhythmic Drugs

The efficacy and safety of antiarrhythmic drugs in preventing sudden death has been disappointing. Amiodarone is widely considered the most effective antiarrhythmic agent for treating a variety of arrhythmias, including AF and VT. It is a class III antiarrhythmic agent with additional Vaughan–Williams class I, II, and IV properties and has unusual pharmacokinetics, with a delayed onset of action and an elimination half-life of up to 53 days after chronic therapy.

Amiodarone has been shown to reduce SCD rates significantly following MI in several placebo-controlled randomized studies, but its effects on total mortality are inconsistent. Intravenous amiodarone remains a powerful parenteral drug for the acute treatment of patients with life-threatening ventricular arrhythmias. The efficacy of intravenous amiodarone in patients with recurrent, hemodynamically unstable VT refractory to lidocaine, procainamide, and bretylium is approximately 40% in prospective studies, and about 80% of the arrhythmias are suppressed within the first 48 hours. For out of hospital cardiac arrest, intravenous amiodarone has been shown to be more effective than intravenous lidocaine.

## ■ NONPHARMACOLOGIC THERAPY

### Implantable Cardioverter-Defibrillators

In patients with ischemic cardiomyopathy, implantable cardioverter-defibrillators (ICDs) have demonstrated remarkable effectiveness in prevention of SCD, with an overall 1-year survival rate of 92% in patients with documented life-threatening ventricular tachyarrhythmias (see also Chapter 16). Three randomized, controlled trials have demonstrated ICDs to be superior to antiarrhythmic medications in the secondary prevention of SCD. Recent primary prevention studies have also demonstrated improved survival of *high-risk* patients with ischemic cardiomyopathy who have had ICDs implanted as compared to conventional drug therapy. ICDs are effective in detecting and terminating ventricular tachyarrhythmias and can prevent bradycardia with pacing. Because their mode of action is therapeutic rather than preventive, ICD therapy must often be combined with other antiarrhythmic strategies, such as drugs or catheter ablation, to prevent frequent recurrences of tachyarrhythmias.

Several ICD primary prevention trials in patients with non-ischemic cardiomyopathy and heart failure have also been conducted, but the results have not been as consistently positive as in the post-MI population. The largest of these is the SCD-HeFT, in which the benefit of ICDs in the trial was highly statistically significant and appeared similar for the ischemic and non-ischemic subgroups. The most compelling data may come from a pooled analysis of 5 primary prevention trials enrolling 1854 patients. ICD therapy led to a 31% relative risk reduction in mortality. The absolute risk reduction was estimated at 2% per year.

ICDs are also used in less common conditions associated with a high risk of sudden cardiac death, including hypertrophic cardiomyopathy, long QT syndrome, and the Brugada syndrome.

## SUGGESTED READINGS

Reynolds MR, Thosani MJ, Pinto DS, Josephson ME. Sudden cardiac death. In: Fuster V, Alexander RW, O'Rourke RA, et al, eds. *Hurst's The Heart*. 13th ed. New York, NY: McGraw-Hill; 2011; 49:1139-1162.

Bardy GH, Lee KL, Mark DB, et al. Amiodarone or an implantable cardioverter-defibrillator for congestive heart failure. *N Engl J Med*. 2005;352:225-237.

Moss AJ, Hall WJ, Cannom DS, et al. Improved survival with an implanted defibrillator in patients with coronary disease at high risk for ventricular arrhythmia. Multicenter Automatic Defibrillator Implantation Trial investigators. *N Engl J Med*. 1996;335:1933-1940.

Moss AJ, Zareba W, Hall WJ, et al. Prophylactic implantation of a defibrillator in patients with myocardial infarction and reduced ejection fraction. *N Engl J Med*. 2002;346:877-883.

Priori SG, Schwartz PJ, Napolitano C, et al. Risk stratification in the long-QT syndrome. *N Engl J Med*. 2003;348:1866-1874.

Solomon SD, Zelenkofske S, McMurray JJ, et al. Sudden death in patients with myocardial infarction and left ventricular dysfunction, heart failure, or both. *N Engl J Med*. 2005;352:2581-2588.

Weaver EF, Robles de Medina EO. Sudden death in patients without structural heart disease. *J Am Coll Cardiol*. 2004;43:1137-1144.

Zipes DP, Camm AJ, Borggrefe M, et al. ACC/AHA/ESC 2006 guidelines for management of patients with ventricular arrhythmias and the prevention of sudden cardiac death: a report of the American College of Cardiology/American Heart Association Task Force and the European Society of Cardiology Committee for Practice Guidelines (Writing Committee to Develop Guidelines for Management of Patients With Ventricular Arrhythmias and the Prevention of Sudden Cardiac Death). *J Am Coll Cardiol*. 2006;48:e247-e346.

# CHAPTER 18
# CPR AND POST-RESUSCITATION MANAGEMENT

Jooby John and Gordon A. Ewy

Sudden death, primarily due to out-of-hospital cardiac arrest (OHCA), remains the single leading cause of death in the United States, with more than a thousand deaths daily. Cardiac arrest itself is the abrupt termination of organized cardiac activity resulting in circulatory collapse, due to either electrical or mechanical malfunction. Its consequences are immediate and devastating with rapid development of end-organ damage. Permanent neurologic damage sets in within 4 minutes of circulatory arrest. The gravest of these consequences include hypoxic encephalopathy, permanent neurologic damage, and death. Cardiac arrest is clinically suspected when sudden collapse occurs and is confirmed by the absence of a discernible pulse or cardiac sounds. An electrocardiogram (ECG), if performed, will show the patient to have a rhythm consistent with ventricular tachycardia (VT), ventricular fibrillation (VF), asystole, or an organized nonperfusing rhythm. The latter is referred to as *pulseless electrical activity* (PEA) or electromechanical dissociation (EMD).

This chapter summarizes our current state of knowledge regarding the pathophysiology, as well as recommendations for treatment, of this near-lethal disease. It will also serve to introduce the concept of cardiocerebral resuscitation (CCR), a new approach that has been shown to dramatically improve survival in patients with OHCA.

OHCA survival rates hover close to 1% to 7% in major cities in the United States, with in-hospital rates being around 10% to 15%. Despite 5 decades of guidelines advocating cardiopulmonary resuscitation (CPR) as a treatment for cardiac arrest, survival rates have remained stagnant. As it stands today, CPR is advocated for 2 distinct diseases, primary arrhythmogenic cardiac arrest (typically pulseless VT or VF), and respiratory arrest with consequent hypoxia and *secondary* precipitation of global cardiac ischemia and arrest (usually PEA or asystole).

## PATHOPHYSIOLOGY OF CARDIAC ARREST

Cardiac arrest in adults secondary to VF is a consequence of uncoordinated myocardial activity. One minute into persistent VF, coronary blood flow declines to zero, and by 4 minutes carotid blood flow is also at zero. In the absence of resuscitative efforts, progressive equalization of arterial and venous pressures occurs, leading to circulatory standstill. The end result is a distension of the right ventricle and progressive impairment in left ventricular diastolic function and a final agonal contraction terminating in the "stone heart" (**Fig. 18-1**).

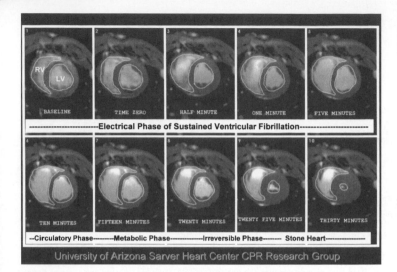

**FIGURE 18-1.** MRI depiction of changes in right ventricular (RV) and left ventricular (LV) volumes with untreated ventricular fibrillation in the swine VF model. Notice how initially LV and RV are both enlarged. However, with time, the LV undergoes agonal ischemic contracture leading to a "stone heart." (Reprinted with permission from Sorrell VL, Bhatt RD, Berg RA, et al. Cardiac magnetic resonance imaging investigation of sustained ventricular fibrillation in a swine model–with a focus on the electrical phase. *Resuscitation*. 2007; May;73(2):279-286. Copyright © Elsevier.)

# ■ RESPIRATORY ARREST

Alternatively, respiratory arrest leads to a predictable drop in arterial oxygen tension, ensuing myocardial hypoxia, and secondary cardiac arrest. These usually present as PEA or asystole. Logically, the appropriate management of this disease would involve mitigation of the precipitating cause. Examples of this form of cardiac arrest, in adults, include drug overdose, choking ("café coronary"), catastrophic neurologic events, suffocation, drowning, and carbon monoxide poisoning. A ready application of this doctrine, in the café coronary setting, is the utility of the Heimlich maneuver in relieving respiratory arrest secondary to choking.

## Cardiac Arrest in the Pediatric Population

Respiratory arrests encompass the majority of cardiac arrests in children. This is an important subgroup to recognize, as children rarely have underlying primary cardiac or coronary artery disease (CAD). Consequently, they are far more likely to have had a respiratory arrest and secondary cardiac arrest, and in them the restoration of oxygenation and ventilatory function is of overriding importance. It is in this population that reestablishment of arterial oxygen tension is crucial for successful resuscitation and survival. Therefore, the emphasis in children has to be on the *reestablishment of alveolar gas exchange*, while simultaneously supporting circulation with chest compressions and vasoactive medications. Nonetheless, it is sobering to note that once cardiac arrest has set in for a prolonged period of time, it becomes the determining factor in the patient's survival. It is important to restore circulation while simultaneously working on correcting the primary etiology of the respiratory arrest.

## Cardiac Arrest in Adults

Conversely in adults, most cardiac arrests are of primary cardiac origin with VF, as a consequence of myocardial ischemia secondary to CAD. In these patients, the pulmonary alveoli and the entire left heart, intrinsically untouched from the primary arrhythmogenic process, are flush with oxygenated blood and require no immediate replenishment. Moreover, these patients continue to breathe for a brief period of time, postarrest, as the medullary respiratory center is still active and continues to fire. This is responsible for the gasping and agonal breathing phenomenon seen in up to 40% of individuals with OHCA. They stop spontaneous respiratory efforts when the respiratory center finally succumbs to hypoxic injury and shuts down its phasic discharge activity. However, the lack of blood flow ensures that the alveoli remain replete with oxygen. This is the essential logic behind *prioritizing circulatory support over respiratory support* in the case of adults with cardiac arrest.

Circulatory support is, of course, established by precordial chest compressions. Chest compressions halt the progression of circulatory arrest and its downstream consequences by providing phasic arterial blood flow. When chest compressions are accurately executed, pressure on the cardiac chambers during the "compression phase" ejects blood out of the left ventricle (LV) and into the peripheral circulation and from the right ventricle into the pulmonary capillary system. This physiology dominates in the early phase of cardiac arrest and is similar to the mechanism of open cardiac massage. However, there is also a "thoracic pump" mechanism that predominates in the later components of cardiac arrest. In this process, the chest compression causes passive inflow and outflow of blood from the thoracic cage with the heart acting as a flaccid conduit. This theory comes from the observation that patients in cardiac arrest were able to stay awake by repetitively coughing and thereby moving blood through the circulation simply based on their intrathoracic pressure fluctuations. Case reports in the cardiac catheterization laboratory have shown patients able to maintain hemodynamically significant blood pressures during malignant ventricular arrhythmias by coughing forcefully 30 to 60 times a minute. Obviously this is not a strategy that can be widely advocated because of its unpredictable outcome. The consensus opinion is that both mechanisms play a role in reestablishing circulatory flow, "cardiac compression" in the early phase and "thoracic pump" in the later phase. Nevertheless, it is sobering to remember that total coronary flow with precordial compressions is only around 20% to 40% of pre-arrest values. With the increasing duration of cardiac arrest, LV relaxation is first affected. The LV continues to progressively thicken. Magnetic resonance imaging (MRI) studies have shown that ischemic contracture finally sets in after about 20 to 30 minutes of untreated VF, the so called "stone heart." At this point, reversion to a perfusing rhythm is highly improbable.

## ■ CORONARY PERFUSION PRESSURE

*Coronary perfusion pressure* (CPP) is defined as the difference between the aortic and right atrial pressure during the release phase of external cardiac compression. It is the "driving pressure" that causes blood to flow into the coronary tree. This pressure is built up slowly with chest compressions, such that first compressions do not generate a significant CPP, but the last compressions (prior to stopping compressions for the rescue breaths) generate significant CPP (**Figs. 18-2 and 18-3**). The CPP has been shown to be the *central* determinant of survival in prolonged VF. When chest compressions are interrupted (for so-called rescue breathing, tracheal intubation, placement of an intravenous line, or even rhythm and pulse analysis), the CPP falls, and with it the chances for survival. This is the theoretical rationale for continuous chest compression (CCC), wherein the essential determinant for cardiac survival, the CPP, is constantly preserved. The same principle applies for cerebral perfusion where near-continuous chest compressions are essential for cerebral perfusion.

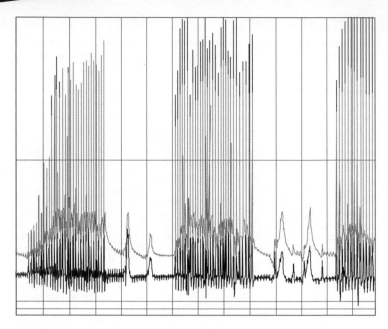

**FIGURE 18-2.** Coronary perfusion pressures with interrupted chest compressions (30:2 compression-to-breaths ratio). Aortic pressure is in dark blue and right atrial pressure is in light blue. The CPP is the difference between these 2 pressures. Notice how the coronary perfusion pressure takes time to build up. It drops once chest compressions are interrupted and has to be reestablished with the next round of chest compressions. (Reprinted with permission from Ewy GA, Zuercher M, Hilwig RW, et al. Improved neurological outcome with continuous chest compressions compared with 30:2 compressions-to-ventilations cardiopulmonary resuscitation in a realistic swine model of out-of-hospital cardiac arrest. *Circulation.* 2007; Nov 27;116(22):2525-2530. Copyright © Lippincott Williams & Wilkins.)

## ■ PHASES OF VENTRICULAR FIBRILLATION

Survival rates decrease by about 7% to 10% for every *1 minute* that a person remains in ventricular fibrillation. VF is a common arrhythmia associated with cardiac arrest in adults, and is the one associated with the best prognosis. The time-sensitive, 3-phase concept for VF was put forth in 2002 by Weisfeldt and Becker. This elegant model divides VF into an electrical phase (0-5 minutes), circulatory/mechanical phase (5-15 minutes), and metabolic phase (after 15 minutes). The appropriate management for VF has to be tailored to the phase during which it will be delivered.

### Electrical Phase (0-5 Minutes)

In the *electrical phase*, there is enough myocardial energy reserve that defibrillation alone (without chest compression) is sufficient to restore a perfusing rhythm. The most well-known application of this is the implantable cardiac defibrillators (ICDs) that deliver therapy within seconds of an unstable VT or VF and are consequently highly effective. Automated external defibrillators (AEDs) are also extremely useful in this phase. Public access AEDs have demonstrated dramatic improvements in survival in patients who have collapsed in casinos or airports. These patients are

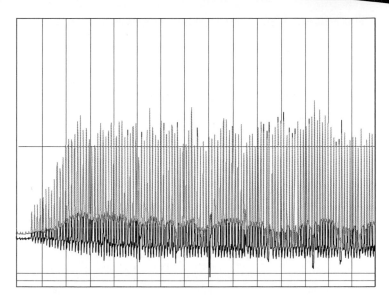

**FIGURE 18-3.** Coronary perfusion pressures with continuous chest compressions. Here the coronary perfusion pressures are established, and secondary to the uninterrupted nature of the chest compressions, they remain constant. (Reprinted with permission from Ewy GA, Zuercher M, Hilwig RW, et al. Improved neurological outcome with continuous chest compressions compared with 30:2 compressions-to-ventilations cardiopulmonary resuscitation in a realistic swine model of out-of-hospital cardiac arrest. *Circulation.* 2007; Nov 7;116(22):2525-2530. Copyright © Lippincott Williams & Wilkins.)

defibrillated within minutes because of their proximity to an AED and, since they are in the electrical phase, they do often return to a perfusing hemodynamically stable rhythm.

## Circulatory/Mechanical Phase (5-15 Minutes)

In the *circulatory phase* of VF, the incessant myocardial contractions coupled with the now-prolonged lack of coronary blood flow will have resulted in depletion of myocardial high-energy phosphate stores as well as cellular acidosis. Electrocardiographically, this is manifested by the decreasing amplitude of the VF waveform with a transition to the "fine" fibrillatory waves on the ECG. Defibrillation in the absence of chest compressions is rarely successful in this phase, as even if the VF is terminated, the patient ends up in a PEA rhythm. Successful resuscitation here requires the restoration of myocardial energy stores. It is here that chest compressions play a pivotal role in restoring some degree of coronary (and cerebral) perfusion. Postcompression VF waveforms show an increase in amplitude, higher median frequency, and a "coarser" rhythm, and are associated with higher likelihood of successful defibrillation and neurologically intact survival.

## Metabolic Phase (After 15 Minutes)

The third phase, the *metabolic phase*, is universally associated with diminishing odds of successful defibrillation. End-organ damage has already set in, with irreversible cellular impairment. Strategies that may delay the onset of this *phase of irremediable damage* are being investigated. Therapeutic hypothermia may be useful even in this late stage. However, very few patients survive following >15 minutes of untreated cardiac arrest.

# PULSELESS ELECTRICAL ACTIVITY AND ASYSTOLE

PEA and asystole are important to recognize because they are not amenable to *electrical defibrillation therapy*. When VF is the initial rhythm, the chance of survival is significantly higher than when PEA or asystole is the presenting rhythm. Although VF in an adult is very strongly associated with CAD, PEA and asystole are usually not. The exception is when they are seen in the terminal phase of VF arrests. When VF is defibrillated in the circulatory/mechanical phase without pre-defibrillatory chest compressions, these postdefibrillation rhythms are usually PEA. Predefibrillatory *and* postdefibrillatory chest compressions have been shown to be effective in preventing the emergence of PEA.

One has to consider secondary causes of cardiac arrest when PEA is otherwise the primary rhythm; the **5 Hs** (**H**ypovolemia, **H**ypoxia, **H**ydrogen ion = acidosis, **H**yperkalemia or **H**ypokalemia, and **H**ypothermia) and the **5 Ts** (**T**ension pneumothorax, **T**amponade, **T**ablets = drug overdose, **T**hrombosis coronary, and **T**hrombosis pulmonary). Identifying and remedying the underlying cause is of vital importance in the successful resuscitation of these patients.

Asystole is often a secondary and invariably terminal rhythm, and is the inevitable result of both nonintervened PEA and VF. Patients are often later in time and have consequently poorer prognosis. However, the same etiologies of PEA can also sometimes be present with asystole and should therefore be investigated, and treated if found. One of the pitfalls in diagnosing and treating asystole is when very fine VF is interpreted as asystole. In these cases, it would be prudent to make sure that the cables are connected and the gain is turned up, and to look at other ECG leads (especially perpendicular leads) to see if the VF pattern can be discerned. If the ECG leads are not available and fine VF is suspected, the defibrillatory paddles can be turned by 90 degrees to confirm that it is not VF. If fine VF is suspected, the arrhythmia should be defibrillated. There is no convincing evidence that a mistake here (ie, defibrillation of asystole) adversely affects the patient's chances of survival.

It should be noted that in a recent North American prospective epidemiologic study, about 20% of adult cardiac arrest patients who initially presented as PEA/asystole had subsequent conversion to VF.

*Recognition of life extinct* (ROLE) guidelines in England deem 20 minutes of asystole, despite advanced resuscitative measures, as grounds for termination of resuscitative efforts.

# GUIDELINES FOR CPR AND ECC

Evidence-based guidelines for CPR and emergency cardiac care (ECC) have been hampered by the relative paucity of controlled clinical trials in humans. CPR was first introduced as a treatment for cardiac arrest in 1960, when Kouwenhoven and coworkers developed the technique of external chest compression in the supine position. This practice was quickly adopted and standardized. Subsequently periodic guidelines (most recently in 2010) are regularly published by the American Heart Association (AHA) in collaboration with the International Liaison Committee on Resuscitation (ILCOR), with an emphasis on CPR and ECC.

The 2010 guidelines continue to emphasize the central role of uninterrupted chest compressions and the limited role of ventilation since *overventilation and interruptions in chest compressions* are independent predictors of adverse outcomes. Thus, the current recommendation maintains the chest compression to ventilation ratio from the previous 15:1 to 30:2. Quality of compressions with downward displacement of at least 2 in of the sternum has also been emphasized. "Look, Listen, and Feel" has also been removed from the BLS algorithm due to the delay in initiating compressions in a cardiac arrest situation. Most importantly, the 2010 guidelines formally recommend a change in the traditional sequence of BLS from "A (airway)-B (breathing)-C (chest compressions)" to "C-A-B".

# CARDIOCEREBRAL RESUSCITATION

CCR is an innovative approach to the management of cardiac arrest that specifically capitalizes on the fact that the CPP is the most important determinant of survival in an adult cardiac arrest. Chest compression is the only realistic means by which coronary and cerebral perfusion pressures can be maintained in the presence of circulatory arrest. Thus, one may attempt continuous chest compressions (CCC) in cardiac arrest.

The AHA "chain of survival" has bystander-administered CPR as an integral link. However, various clinical studies have shown bystander CPR to be present in only about 20% to 30% of witnessed arrests. Anonymous surveys have indicated that bystanders are more likely to do chest compressions if they do not have to perform mouth-to-mouth rescue breathing. "Hands-only (compression-only)" CPR is now encouraged by the AHA/ACC because it can be more easily accomplished by the untrained lay rescuer and more readily guided by emergency dispatchers. The other major hindrance is that, even when following guidelines, EMS (emergency medical services) providers are rarely able to deliver the *recommended 80 to 100 compressions a minute* because of the interruption for rescue breaths. Motivated basic life support (BLS)–trained medical students at the University of Arizona were able to deliver only an average of 43 compressions a minute when following the old 15:2 AHA guidelines, as opposed to 133 compressions per minute while doing CCC. As a final point, CCC is easier to learn and teach and is much more likely to be implemented in an out-of-hospital witnessed cardiac arrest.

The effectiveness of CCC has now been tested in several clinical studies. Two large randomized trials in 2010 confirmed that in fact compression-only CPR was as effective as traditional CPR with rescue breathing. Thus, CCR with CCC is easier to perform, more likely to be performed, and is as effective (if not more) as traditional CPR.

# COMPONENTS OF CCR

CCR is a comprehensive approach to resuscitation with 3 vital interrelated components for each level of the disease (**Fig. 18-4**):

1. The bystander who witnesses the arrest.
2. Emergency medical services (EMS) personnel.
3. Post-resuscitation hospital care.

Bystanders respond after calling EMS with continuous chest compressions at an approximate rate of 100 per minute. They are then told to continue compression till EMS personnel arrive or until an AED is found and deployed.

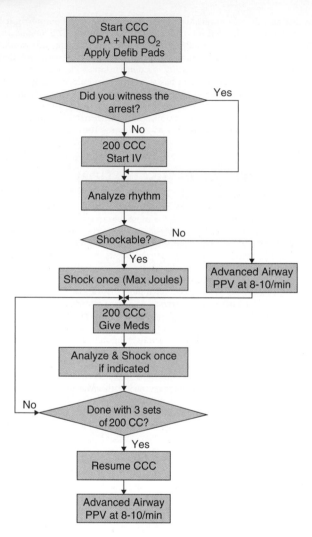

**FIGURE 18-4.** Cardiocerebral resuscitation improves neurologically intact survival of patients with witnessed out-of-hospital cardiac arrest and a shockable rhythm. CCC, continuous chest compressions; NRB, non-rebreather OPA oropharyngeal airway; PPV positive-pressure ventilation. (This figure is based on data presented in the publication by Kellum MJ, Kennedy KW, Barney R, et al. Cardiocerebral resuscitation improves neurologically intact survival of patients with out-of-hospital cardiac arrest. *Ann Emerg Med.* 2008;52:244-252.)

EMS personnel are specifically instructed to defibrillate VF only if the patient has been receiving chest compressions by a bystander or if they have personally witnessed the arrest. If not, they are to give CCC for 2 minutes *before* analysis to determine if a patient has shockable rhythm. *Even if the patient is in a shockable VF/VT rhythm on arrival* and there are no chest compressions performed, EMS personnel are instructed to give CCC for 2 minutes. If they witness the collapse, the patient is now in the electrical phase of VF and can safely be defibrillated first without initiating CCC. Even if they arrive in the electrical phase of an unwitnessed arrest, EMS personnel do no harm by initiating CCC prior to defibrillation. However, if the patient is in the circulatory phase, defibrillation without CCC can be detrimental to survival. However, in a randomized experience from the Resuscitation Outcome Consortium, the timing of rhythm analysis (after 30-60 seconds vs 180 seconds of CCC) did not make an impact on outcome.

One of the aspects of CCR that has been incorporated into the 2005 guidelines is the approach to patients who revert back to a normal rhythm after defibrillation of VF. Despite restoration of a postdefibrillation organized electrical rhythm, these hearts are still mechanically sluggish, and thus will most likely present as PEA instead of a hemodynamically stable rhythm. Immediate postdefibrillation chest compressions will restore coronary flow, replenish high-energy myocardial phosphate stores, and ultimately increase the likelihood that these patients will reach neurologically intact hospital discharge end points.

## ■ VENTILATION

Notwithstanding these differences, the paradigm change in CCR as opposed to traditional CPR is the role of ventilation. The fundamental precept of ABC (airway, breathing, and circulation) is not applicable in the setting of cardiac arrest, for the simple reason that establishing an airway or breathing for the patient does not address the primary reason for the collapse—that is, a malignant arrhythmia that has precipitated cardiac arrest. In fact, (1) interruption of chest compressions for intubation or even establishment of an airway diminishes CPP; and (2) positive-pressure ventilation that increases intrathoracic pressures decreases passive venous return, which further compromises an already feeble cardiac output. In the primary cardiac arrest patient, CCC does appear to provide passive ventilatory efforts that occur during chest compressions. The 2010 resuscitation guidelines incorporate these principles and now recommend a "C (chest compressions)-A (airway)-B (breathing)" sequence for basic life support (BLS).

## POST-RESUSCITATION CARE

The effectiveness of resuscitative efforts is not just linked to return of spontaneous circulation (ROSC). Neurologically intact survival is the ultimate goal of resuscitation treatment strategies and is reflected in the inclusion of "cerebral" in "cardiocerebral resuscitation." Even after successful ROSC, more than 60% of patients do not survive to hospital discharge. Following ROSC these patients are subject to a vicious and global reperfusion injury, mediated through lipolysis, proteolysis, inflammation, coagulation, and ultimately cellular death and apoptosis. Promising data suggest that by intermittently supplying blood flow at reduced rates, chest compression may condition organs (so-called ischemic preconditioning) to reperfusion injury and thus attenuate eventual cellular death and end-organ damage.

About 50% of adult patients with VF arrest have an acute myocardial infarction as the underlying etiology. If a myocardial infarction (confirmed by an ECG or cardiac biomarkers) is suspected, prompt revascularization of the target vessel by percutaneous techniques is usually the preferred therapy. More aggressive approaches envision routine cardiac catheterization for all patients who have had a cardiac arrest as significant CAD and occlusion have been demonstrated even in the absence of diagnostic ECG changes.

Post-resuscitation disease refers to the multisystem damage sustained as a result of ischemic and reperfusion organ injury. This permutation of post-resuscitation ischemic and reperfusion injury combined with a systemic inflammatory response and multiorgan dysfunction has been defined as the *post-cardiac arrest syndrome*. This manifests as hypoxic encephalopathy, myocardial dysfunction, aspiration pneumonia, ischemic gut injury, ischemic hepatopathy, renal dysfunction, and peripheral limb ischemia. Myocardial dysfunction manifests as depressed biventricular function immediately post-resuscitation that improves over the next few days (in the absence of significant myocardial infarction). Post-ischemic stunning, as well as free radical endotoxin- and cytotoxin-mediated injury, is thought to be instrumental in this usually transient myocardial depression.

One of the more exciting treatments for post-resuscitation care is therapeutic hypothermia. Early studies of moderate (28°C-32°C) and severe induced hypothermia (28°C) showed worse outcomes compared to standard treatment. However, *mild therapeutic induced hypothermia* (32°C-34°C for 12-24 hours) has been shown to be beneficial. The data come from 3 randomized controlled trials and a meta-analysis that all show improved outcomes with the use of *mild* therapeutic hypothermia. It is now a recommendation advocated by the 2010 AHA Guidelines and ILCOR for patients with VF arrest who have ROSC, but remain in a coma. However, rates of use remain low (30%-40%) both in the United States and Europe. Another strategy that might possibly improve outcomes is the establishment of euglycemia, though the results from clinical studies were less compelling. Hyperventilation is preferably avoided as low $Pco_2$ levels in head-injury patient have been shown to be associated with worse outcomes. Seizures/myoclonus, consequent to hypoxic brain injury are seen in up to 40% of resuscitated patients and should be treated promptly with anticonvulsants. There is, however, no evidence that prophylactic anticonvulsants are useful.

Predictors of poor outcomes for OHCA include (1) advanced age, (2) severe comorbidities including cancer or stroke, (3) preexisting cardiac disease and/or LV systolic dysfunction, (4) CPR greater than 5 minutes duration, (5) development of sepsis, (6) recurrence of arrhythmias, (7) PEA or asystole on presentation, (8) persistent coma, and (9) unwitnessed arrest and/or lack of bystander CPR. Most in-hospital deaths are secondary to noncardiac causes, usually respiratory complications or anoxic encephalopathy. Bilateral absence of cortical response *to median nerve somatosensory*–evoked potentials predicted poor outcome with 100% specificity when used in normothermic patients who were comatose for at least 72 hours after cardiac arrest. The best prognostic sign post-resuscitation recovery is the return of consciousness.

# THE PHARMACOLOGY OF RESUSCITATION

The most significant determinant of drug effectiveness in cardiac arrest is the early use of the drug in the resuscitative efforts. No placebo-controlled clinical trials have ever been done testing the use of vasopressors in cardiac arrest. Their use is entirely based on animal studies, observational data, and consensus opinion. Epinephrine has stood the test of time as first-line agent for a cardiac arrest and is used in all forms of cardiac arrest. Epinephrine causes immediate peripheral vasoconstriction by its α-adrenergic effect, and thereby increases coronary and cerebral perfusion. Of lesser importance (and possibly harmful) are the positive cardiac inotropic and chronotropic effects secondary to its β-adrenergic effects. Epinephrine can cause resolution of asystole and make the VF waveform coarser and more susceptible to defibrillation. Epinephrine 0.5 to 1 mg IV is administered every 3 to 5 minutes till ROSC is achieved.

There are several case reports describing the use of β-blockers in VF/pulseless VT. Animal studies indicate that β-blockers might improve myocardial oxygen requirements and attenuate ischemic myocardial damage. Nevertheless, concerns remain about their negative inotropic effects as well as iatrogenic hypotension. Because high-quality human clinical data are lacking, β-blockers currently have no proven role in the acute management of cardiac arrest. However, they can be still considered if multiple doses of epinephrine have been given and the patient exhibits recurrent ventricular tachyarrhythmia.

Vasopressin, which causes peripheral vasoconstriction through AVPR1 receptors on vascular smooth muscle, is a more controversial drug. Two large randomized trials subsequently have shown no benefit for vasopressin over epinephrine. *Since the half-life of vasopressin is 10 to 20 minutes*, it is administered as a 1-time 40-U IV dose.

Amiodarone, developed originally as an antianginal agent in 1961, and to a lesser extent, lidocaine are antiarrhythmic drugs of choice for pulseless VT/VF, especially of presumed ischemic etiology. Amiodarone was superior to lidocaine in the ALIVE trial and is the recommended first-line antiarrhythmic agent for VF/VT arrest. Amiodarone is administered as a single 300-mg IV push, followed if necessary by another 150-mg IV push. Lidocaine is given as a 1- to 1.5-mg/kg IV push up to a maximum of 3 mg/kg. Procainamide is no longer recommended as an antiarrhythmic agent.

Sodium bicarbonate (1 mEq/kg every 15 minute) is currently *not recommended* in cardiac arrests. Even though cardiac arrest is associated with both metabolic and respiratory acidosis, exogenous bicarbonate has not been shown to improve outcomes. Furthermore, it has been associated with post-resuscitation hypernatremia, volume overload, worsened intracellular acidosis and cardiac contractility, and downstream metabolic alkalosis. Specific situations in which it might be useful include hyperkalemia and prearrest severe metabolic acidosis, as in aspirin or tricyclic antidepressant overdose.

Magnesium sulfate (1-4 mg IV) can be given in suspected cases of torsade de pointes and polymorphic VT with suspected hypomagenesmia. However, it is not recommended as a routine strategy for cardiac arrest.

Atropine (1-mg IV every 3-5 minutes) is helpful when PEA is secondary to severe bradycardia though infra-His and advanced heart blocks do not typically respond to atropine. Atropine has no role in VF/VT arrests. Severe bradycardia may also respond to *transcutaneous pacing* (TCP). However, asystole usually does not, and routine TCP is *not recommended for asystolic patients*.

*Routine fibrinolysis in cardiac arrest patients was not associated with improved survival in clinical studies and is not at present recommended.*

# ■ ROUTE OF ADMINISTRATION

As soon as feasible, IV access should be established in a patient with cardiac arrest (without interruption of chest compressions!). The upper extremity is preferred, as lower extremity circulation is feeble in the setting of a cardiac arrest. One particular advantage of epinephrine, vasopressin, atropine, naloxone, and lidocaine is their ability to be delivered through the endotracheal tube into the bronchial tree. The IV dose is typically diluted in 5 to 10 mL of water or normal saline and squirted deep into the bronchial tree. Endotracheal instillation should be followed sequentially by insufflations of the Ambu bag to facilitate drug delivery. The optimal endotracheal doses of these drugs are, however, unknown, and so the recommendation is to deliver them endotracheally only if IV access is not available and cannot be obtained in a timely manner. Lately in adults, direct intraosseus injections of these medications are frequently used by EMS personnel. *In animal studies, this route has been shown to be comparable to central venous administration.*

# SUGGESTED READINGS

John J, Ewy GA. Cardiopulmonary and cardiocerebral resuscitation. In: Fuster V, Walsh R, Harrington RA, et al. *Hurst's The Heart.* 13th ed. New York, NY: McGraw-Hill; 2011;50: 1163-1180.

Bobrow BJ, Clark LL, Ewy GA, et al. Minimally interrupted cardiac resuscitation by emergency medical services for out-of-hospital cardiac arrest. *JAMA.* 2008;299:1158-1165.

Ewy GA. Cardiology patient page. New concepts of cardiopulmonary resuscitation for the lay public: continuous-chest-compression CPR. *Circulation.* 2007;116:e566-e568.

Ewy GA. Continuous-chest-compression cardiopulmonary resuscitation for cardiac arrest. *Circulation.* 2007;116:2894-2896.

Ewy GA, Zuercher M, Hilwig RW, et al. Improved neurological outcome with continuous chest compressions compared with 30:2 compressions-to-ventilations cardiopulmonary resuscitation in a realistic swine model of out-of-hospital cardiac arrest. *Circulation.* 2007;116:2525-2530.

Rea TD, Fahrenbruch C, Culley L, et al. CPR with chest compression alone or with rescue breathing. *N Engl J Med.* 2010;363:423-433.

Svensson L, Bohm K, Castrèn M, et al. Compression-only CPR or standard CPR in out-of-hospital cardiac arrest. *N Engl J Med.* 2010;363:434-442.

2010 AHA Guidelines for cardiopulmonary resuscitation and emergency cardiovascular care. *Circulation.* 2010;122:S640-S656.

Weisfeldt ML, Becker LB. Resuscitation after cardiac arrest: a 3-phase time-sensitive model. *JAMA.* 2002;288:3035-3038.

Weisfeldt ML, Everson-Stewart S, Sitlani C, et al. Ventricular tachyarrhythmias after cardiac arrest in public versus at home. *New Engl J Med.* 2011;364:313-321.

# CHAPTER 19
# DIAGNOSIS AND MANAGEMENT OF HEART FAILURE

## William T. Abraham and Ayesha Hasan

Chronic heart failure is a complex clinical syndrome that has multiple causes and etiologies. The core lesion involves structural and functional changes in the heart and peripheral vasculature that lead to impaired systolic and diastolic function. The resultant clinical manifestations are variable, but the most common symptoms include exertional dypsnea, orthopnea, and nocturnal dypsnea. Other common signs and symptoms include edema, fatigue, and chest congestion.

## PATHOPHYSIOLOGY

In heart failure there is always an index event that occurs in the heart leading to structural and functional changes. The index event may be clinically obvious, such as an acute myocardial infarction, or it may be more insidious, such as genetic mutations that over time lead to structural and functional abnormalities. When there is left ventricular (LV) damage or abnormal loading conditions, the myocardium responds with chronic myocyte hypertrophic and fibrotic adaptation. The LV diameter can enlarge, thereby temporarily maintaining stroke volume. LV performance can remain adequate in the face of a low stroke volume to meet metabolic needs and symptoms can be minimal. However, with progressive dilation of the LV, the capacity of the heart to eject blood is impaired and LV filling pressure rises, leading to dypsnea, fatigue, and tissue congestion. In the late stages of systolic heart failure, further dilation of the LV and left atrial chambers leads to mitral regurgitation and replacement of normal myocardial architecture with elongated myocytes and extensive fibrosis.

Systolic heart failure can be due to many causes, including hypertension, valvular heart disease, coronary artery disease, chemotherapy, myocarditis, infiltrative processes, and endocrine disorders. In every patient, a specific etiology should be sought out and treated according to etiology when possible. The central feature of systolic heart failure is a large heart with a dilated LV chamber and impaired ejection of blood. The process of LV remodeling or dilation can take years to occur. In many cases, the progression can be attenuated, eliminated, or even reversed with appropriate medical therapy. The term "cure," however, is rarely applied.

Diastolic heart failure or heart failure with a preserved ejection fraction (EF) often coincides with systolic heart failure. However, certain features of diastolic heart failure are distinct, including impaired ventricular filling, increased chamber stiffness, and increased LV end-diastolic pressure relative to end-diastolic volume. The LV chamber is often small with hypertrophy of the LV myocardium being common but not invariable. The epidemiology of heart failure with preserved EF and the natural history of this syndrome are also somewhat different than what is observed with systolic heart failure.

**TABLE 19-1.** RAAS Blocking Drugs Commonly Used to Treat Heart Failure in the United States

| Generic | Brand | Dose |
|---------|-------|------|
| **ACE Inhibitors** | | |
| Captopril | Capoten | 6.25-150 mg tid |
| Enalapril | Vasotec | 2.5-20 mg bid |
| Fosinopril | Monopril | 10-80 mg qd |
| Lisinopril | Prinvil, Zestril | 5-20 mg qd |
| Quinapril | Accupril | 5-20 mg bid |
| Ramipril | Altace | 2.5-20 mg qd |
| **ARBs** | | |
| Candesartan | Atacand | 8-32 mg qd/bid |
| Losartan[a] | Cozaar | 50-100 mg qd/bid |
| Valsartan | Diovan | 80-320 mg qd |
| Irbesartan[a] | Avapro | 150-300 mg qd |
| Telmisartan[a] | Micardis | 40-80 mg qd |
| Olmesartan[a] | Benicar | 20-40 mg qd |
| **Aldosterone Antagonists** | | |
| Spironolactone | Aldactone | 25-50 mg qd |
| Eplerenone[b] | Inspra | 25-50 mg qd |

[a]Currently not approved by the US Food and Drug Administration for heart failure.

[b]Approved for post–myocardial infarction.

Diastolic heart failure tends to occur in older patients, particularly women, and there are no well-established guidelines for treatment. However, once a patient is hospitalized with overt heart failure and a preserved EF, the prognosis is equally severe as that of systolic heart failure. Dyspnea, tissue congestion, and renal insufficiency occur similarly in diastolic and systolic heart failure.

Heart failure is characterized by neurohormonal activation, presumably in an attempt to maintain perfusion pressure. However, excessive chronic activation of the sympathetic nervous system and the renin–angiotensin–aldosterone system (RAAS) eventually facilitates LV remodeling at the cellular level, thus contributing to the progression of the syndrome. Other neurohormones and cytokines also contribute to the pathophysiology, promoting fibrosis, hypertrophy, and impaired LV function. Specific molecular abnormalities can be identified in the myocytes of the failing heart. The recognition that neurohormonal activation leads to a progression of heart failure has laid the framework for drugs designed to block the sympathetic nervous system (β-adrenergic blockers) and the RAAS (angiotensin-converting enzyme [ACE] inhibitors, angiotensin receptor blockers [ARBs], and aldosterone receptor blockers) (**Tables 19-1** and **19-2**).

# DIAGNOSIS

The diagnosis of heart failure is made by performing a careful history and physical examination. It should be verified by imaging of the heart, typically echocardiography.

**TABLE 19-2.** β-Blockers Commonly Used to Treat Heart Failure in the United States

| Generic | Brand | Dose |
| --- | --- | --- |
| Carvedilol | Coreg | 3.125-25 mg bid |
| Metoprolol succinate | Toprol XL | 25-200 mg qd |
| Bisoprolol[a] | Zebeta | 1.25-10 mg qd |

[a]Currently not approved by the US Food and Drug Administration for heart failure.

In acute heart failure when there is doubt about the diagnosis, plasma B-type natriuretic peptide (BNP or NT-proBNP) levels are helpful for verification. In patients with advanced heart failure, there is often increased jugular venous pressure and pulmonary rales, and in some cases ascites and peripheral edema. A murmur of mitral and tricuspid regurgitation may be evident and an $S_3$ gallop can sometimes be heard at the apex of the heart. The severity of the symptoms does not always parallel the magnitude of LV dysfunction as reflected by the LV EF. The target of therapy depends on the extent of symptoms. For example, lung congestion, worsening shortness of breath, and edema are most responsive to loop diuretics. Progressive remodeling is most responsive to long-term β-blockers and drugs designed to block the RAAS.

# MANAGEMENT OF HEART FAILURE

## ■ STAGE I: AT RISK FOR HEART FAILURE

Stage I does not represent true heart failure, but rather indicates the presence of risk factors that are known to precede the onset of heart failure. Structural changes in the heart have not yet developed and cardiac function is normal. However, conditions such as hypertension, diabetes mellitus, and hyperlipidemia need to be vigorously treated to prevent heart failure.

## ■ STAGE II: STRUCTURAL ABNORMALITIES PRESENT IN THE ABSENCE OF SIGNS AND SYMPTOMS OF HEART FAILURE

Patients with stage II heart failure have demonstrable cardiac pathology, such as left ventricular hypertrophy (LVH), coronary disease, or valvular heart disease, but signs and symptoms of heart failure are absent. A low EF in the absence of heart failure symptoms is not uncommon. As with stage I, in the absence of symptoms there is no heart failure, but the patient is at even greater risk to develop heart failure than in stage I, and now has underlying structural heart disease. Such patients should be aggressively treated. Blood pressure must be well-controlled, and ACE inhibitors or ARBs along with β-blockers are indicated. Therapy with β-blockers and RAAS blockers can slow the progression of LV remodeling, including LVH and LV dilation. Loop diuretics to relieve congestion may not always be necessary, but thiazides might be employed to control high blood pressure. Concomitant risk factors, such as diabetes mellitus, obstructive sleep apnea, and hyperlipidemia should be vigorously controlled.

# ■ STAGE III: SIGNS AND SYMPTOMS OF HEART FAILURE WITH DEMONSTRABLE STRUCTURAL HEART DISEASE

These patients make up the bulk of the heart failure population. They are often stable and ambulatory, but may be hospitalized with acute decompensation. Nearly all of these patients will benefit from a loop diuretic, though perhaps not on a daily basis. They must be followed with careful monitoring of their volume status and have their therapy adjusted accordingly. β-blockers, ACE inhibitors, or ARBs—and in advanced cases aldosterone antagonism with spironolactone or eplerenone—should be used to control progressive LV remodeling. Intolerance of β-blockers and/or RAAS blockers is predictive of a very poor prognosis. The need for hospitalization also predicts a much worse prognosis. A low-sodium diet is usually necessary, typically less than 2 g/d. Moderate exercise is encouraged for ambulatory patients.

# ■ STAGE IV: HIGHLY SYMPTOMATIC HEART FAILURE

The highly symptomatic heart failure of stage IV requires special measures, such as hospitalization for intra-aortic balloon pump (IABP), left ventricular assist devices (LVAD), ultrafiltration or dialysis, heart transplantation, heart failure surgery, or palliative care.

These patients are said to have "end-stage heart failure," and have special needs that are sometimes uniquely available at large academic health centers. They are often cared for by teams of heart failure specialists experienced in the complex care of critically ill patients.

# ■ RAAS BLOCKERS

ACE inhibitors or ARBs are almost always indicated in patients with symptomatic heart failure and are also indicated in pre-heart failure (stage II). These drugs should be titrated slowly over days to weeks to maximal doses used in the large clinical trials. Patients who are intolerant of ACE inhibitors should be given a trial of ARBs. In some cases, ACE inhibitors and ARBs are used together, but hypotension, hyperkalemia, and renal insufficiency are more frequent. Patients with antecedent renal insufficiency and diabetes mellitus must be monitored very carefully when using RAAS blockers to avoid serious hyperkalemia and worsening renal function. It is not unexpected that some patients will have about a 20% increase in serum creatinine and/or develop modest, asymptomatic hypotension while taking RAAS blockers, but these changes are not typically an indication to stop the RAAS inhibitor. Aldosterone receptor blockers (spironolactone) are usually initiated for patients with New York Heart Association (NYHA) class IV heart failure, or patients who were class IV but have become class III. When symptomatic hypotension occurs with RAAS blockers, it may be related to volume depletion from loop diuretics. Temporarily withdrawing loop diuretics and resuming them at lower doses often alleviates symptomatic hypotension. Intolerance to RAAS blockers is associated with a very poor prognosis.

# ■ β-ADRENERGIC BLOCKERS

As with RAAS blockers, patients should be started on a β-blocker if LV dilation or reduced LV EF is detected by echocardiogram, even in the absence of signs and symptoms of heart failure. These drugs should be continued indefinitely, along with RAAS blockers, even if LV dilation and EF return to normal following treatment. There are few contraindications to β-blockers in patients with heart failure, but these might include high-grade AV block, severe hypotension or shock, or severe decompensated heart failure with a very low cardiac index (ie, <2.0 L/min/m$^2$). When patients are hospitalized with acute heart failure, β-blockers are often temporarily discontinued, but can usually be restarted in the hospital prior to discharge when the patient is hemodynamically stable. Thus severe but stable NYHA class IV heart failure is not a contraindication for β-blockers; tolerability remains very high in patients with advanced heart failure. Patients who do not tolerate beta-blockers usually have a very poor prognosis.

## ■ DIURETICS

Most patients with stage III and IV heart failure will require loop diuretics. Patients hospitalized with volume overload will usually require intravenous loop diuretics, often given as a continuous drip. The aim of therapy in acute heart failure is to effect a diuresis with a weight loss of 3 to 5 lb/d. Low blood pressure is not usually a contraindication to use of loop diuretics in patients with overt pulmonary congestion. Often, potassium must be replenished in order to maintain a serum potassium level of at least 4 mEq/L. For hospitalized patients who are refractory to intravenous loop diuretics, oral metolazone, and in some cases intravenous thiazide, should be added. In the absence of pulmonary congestion, especially when there is a poor diuretic response, there may be no compelling need for high-dose diuretics, and one might consider stopping the medication or lowering the dose.

## ■ DIGITALIS GLYCOSIDES

Digitalis is sometimes symptomatically helpful in patients with NYHA class III and class IV heart failure with persistent signs and symptoms. Smaller doses are recommended with an aim toward serum digoxin levels around 1 ng/mL. Digitalis reduces sympathetic tone, increases parasympathetic activity, and is useful in controlling heart rate when atrial fibrillation is present. There is only modest improvement in inotropic state. Current trials indicate that use of digoxin in patients with symptomatic heart failure reduces the severity of symptoms and the frequency of hospitalization for decompensated heart failure. However, there are no data indicating a significant survival benefit.

## ■ SPECIAL CONSIDERATIONS

In many patients, drug and dietary noncompliance are an important cause of acute heart failure exacerbations. Patients with heart failure tend to be older and have multiple comorbidities. Therapy should be continuous with all comorbidities considered while treating the patient. Uncontrolled hypertension, myocardial ischemia, rapid atrial fibrillation, nonsteroidal anti-inflammatory drugs, chemotherapy, and thiazolidinediones can each precipitate decompensation of stable heart failure. Infection and uncontrolled diabetes should be vigorously treated.

## ■ HEART TRANSPLANT AND ASSIST DEVICES

Patients who are stage IV or late stage III are potentially candidates for heart transplantation. The primary indication for heart transplantation is severe, very symptomatic heart failure despite optimal medical therapy when there are no alternative options or contraindications. It is expected that following heart transplantation the patient will be able to lead a full life, have excellent psychological and social support systems, and that other organs will remain in good working order. The decision to do heart transplantation is very complex and beyond the scope of this synopsis.

Because of severe organ shortages, heart transplantation is essentially rationed to those patients who have the greatest chance of durable benefit. The follow-up of patients is also complex, and is usually carried out by teams of health care workers with expertise and experience in this area. In general, patients are referred to a heart transplant center for complete evaluation.

When it is likely that the patient will die within 24 to 48 hours without a new heart, various strategies have been devised to temporarily sustain cardiac function using a left ventricular assist device (LVAD) until a new heart becomes available. Right ventricular, biventricular, and total artificial hearts are also available, depending on need. The new specialty of device therapy is rapidly changing, and busy heart transplant centers now have teams of health care workers who are expert in formulating the decision to implant a mechanical device, choosing which device to implant, the actual implantation of the device itself (which can entail open heart surgery), and the post-op care of device patients. Cardiologists and heart transplant surgeons usually work closely together. An LVAD may be used as a "bridge to transplant" until a new heart becomes available, usually for 1 to 3 months, or even as "destination therapy" where there is no intent to ever do heart transplantation, but the goal is to basically alleviate signs and symptoms of heart failure and extend life if possible. The destination therapy strategy is under intensive study, and device therapy in general is now being carefully monitored. Data are being systematically collected and entered into a national registry so we can learn more about these evolving treatments. Device therapy and heart transplantation are expensive, labor intensive, and aimed at a relatively narrow spectrum or patients with severe heart failure. Only through the systematic collection and analysis of longitudinal data can we learn how to use these emerging tools.

# ■ UNRESOLVED ISSUES

There are several vexing problems regarding the treatment of patients with heart failure:

1. So-called diastolic heart failure or heart failure with preserved LV systolic function is poorly defined and proper treatment is unclear. There are currently no large clinical trials to guide therapy. As with systolic heart failure, β-blockers, RAAS blockers, and diuretics are commonly used.

2. The treatment of acute decompensated heart failure is an area of intense research, but proof of a survival benefit with commonly used therapies has been elusive. Treatment is largely empirical. As with diastolic heart failure, there are no large clinical trials to guide therapy. Positive inotropic agents tend to increase mortality, but they may have some role in patients who are in a state of low cardiac output with a systolic blood pressure less than 90 mm Hg. Intravenous diuretics are commonly used to relieve acute congestion. Intravenous vasodilators such as nitroglycerin and nitroprusside can be employed to reduce congestion and improve forward flow, provided that the mean BP is greater than 65 mm Hg.

3. Selecting patients who will most likely benefit from an implantable cardiodefibrillator (ICD) has been a difficult problem, as sudden cardiac death is not a clearly predictable event in an individual patient. Moreover, NYHA class II patients have a somewhat greater chance of sudden cardiac death, but have fewer symptoms and often a more preserved EF. There is an inverse relationship between the EF and incidence of sudden death, so that patients with an EF less than or equal to 30% are more likely to benefit from an ICD. However, the implanted ICD is unlikely to be used to terminate ventricular tachycardia and/or ventricular fibrillation in many patients with a low EF, leading to a tendency to overprescribe ICDs, an expensive form of treatment that is not without inherent risk. Better predictors of which patient will benefit from ICD placement are needed.

# SUGGESTED READINGS

Abraham WT, Hasan A. Diagnosis and management of heart failure. In: Fuster V, Walsh RA, Harrington RA, et al, eds. *Hurst's The Heart*. 13th ed. New York, NY: McGraw-Hill; 2011;28:748-780.

Francis GS, Tang WHW. Angiotensin converting enzyme inhibitors, angiotensin II receptor blockers and aldosterone receptor blockers. In: Manson JA, Buring J, Ridker P, et al, eds. *Clinical Trials in Heart Disease. A Companion to Braunwald's Heart Disease*. Philadelphia, PA: Saunders; 2004:227-241.

Francis GS, Tang WHW. Clinical evaluation of heart failure. In: Mann D, ed. *Heart Failure: A Companion to Braunwald's Heart Disease*. Philadelphia, PA: Saunders. 2004:507-526.

Francis GS, Tang WHW, Walsh, RA, et al. Pathophysiology of heart failure. In: Fuster V, Walsh RA, Harrington RA, et al. *Hurst's The Heart*. 13th ed. New York, NY: McGraw-Hill; 2011;26:719-738.

Hunt SA, Abraham WT, Chin MH, et al. ACC/AHA 2005 guideline update for the diagnosis and management of chronic heart failure in the adult: summary article. *J Am Coll Cardiol*. 2005;46:1116-1143.

# CHAPTER 20
# DYSLIPIDEMIA AND OTHER CARDIAC RISK FACTORS

Michael J. Blaha, Kerunne S. Ketlogetswe, Chiadi E. Ndumele, Ty J. Gluckman, and Roger S. Blumenthal

Prevention of coronary heart disease (CHD) requires identification and treatment of risk factors. *Primary prevention* refers to strategies to prevent clinical manifestation of disease in asymptomatic individuals. *Secondary prevention* refers to efforts to prevent recurrent clinical events in patients with established disease. *Risk factor management prevents and treats coronary atherosclerosis, and should be included as an integral part of any management plan for the many acute and chronic manifestations of this disease.* The intensity of preventive interventions should correspond to the patient's level of absolute risk.

## RISK ASSESSMENT AND RISK FACTOR EVALUATION

### ■ CATEGORIES OF ABSOLUTE RISK

Most risk algorithms divide absolute risk into 3 categories: high, intermediate, and low. Patients at high risk deserve the most intense risk-reduction therapy. Those at intermediate risk are candidates for preventive interventions to the extent that therapy is safe, efficacious, and cost-effective. Finally, low-risk patients should follow public health recommendations for primary prevention of CHD and may benefit from risk-reducing drug therapy.

Each category of absolute risk can be expressed quantitatively (**Table 20-1**). Patients without CHD whose absolute 10-year risk for CHD equals that of patients who already manifest clinical CHD (such as those with diabetes mellitus) are said to have a *CHD risk equivalent*. It is recognized that there are limitations to this approach, as these risk estimates are highly dependent on age. Lifetime risk may be more appropriate than 10-year risk in several prevention settings.

### ■ IDENTIFICATION OF VERY-HIGH-RISK PATIENTS

An update to the National Cholesterol Education Program (NCEP) Adult Treatment Panel III (ATP III) guidelines proposed a new classification of patients as very high risk who deserve especially aggressive low-density lipoprotein cholesterol (LDL-C) lowering. These individuals are those with established CHD plus (1) multiple major risk factors (especially diabetes), (2) severe and poorly controlled risk factors (especially continued cigarette smoking), (3) the metabolic syndrome (especially triglycerides ≥200 mg/dL plus non–high-density lipoprotein cholesterol ≥130 mg/dL with high-density lipoprotein cholesterol [HDL-C] <40 mg/dL), and (4) patients

**TABLE 20-1.** Risk Categories

| Risk Category | 10-Year Absolute Risk for Myocardial Infarction (%) (Nonfatal + Fatal) |
| --- | --- |
| High | >20 |
| Intermediate | 10-20 |
| Low | <10 |

Adapted from *Third Report of the National Cholesterol Education Program (NCEP) Expert Panel on Detection, Evaluation, and Treatment of High Blood Cholesterol in Adults (Adult Treatment Panel III). Final Report.* National Heart, Lung, and Blood Institute National Institutes of Health NIH pub. no. 02-5215 September 2002, or http://www.nhlbi.nih.gov/guidelines/cholesterol/atp3full.pdf. Accessed March 3, 2008.

with acute coronary syndromes. Patients with established CHD and elevated levels of C-reactive protein (CRP) also are classified as a very-high-risk group.

# ■ IDENTIFICATION OF HIGH-RISK PATIENTS WITH CORONARY HEART DISEASE RISK EQUIVALENTS

## Clinical Coronary Heart Disease

In the category of clinical CHD, patients with a history of acute coronary syndromes, stable angina, and coronary revascularization procedures are included. Patients with a prior history of myocardial infarction (MI) have a 10-year risk for recurrent nonfatal or fatal MI of about 26%. Stable angina pectoris confers a 10-year risk for acute MI of approximately 20%.

## Noncoronary Atherosclerosis

Patients in this group include those with peripheral arterial disease, abdominal aortic aneurysm, and symptomatic carotid artery disease or asymptomatic disease with >50% stenosis. The absolute risk for MI in patients with noncoronary atherosclerosis is equal to recurrent MI in patients with established CHD.

## Diabetes

Patients with diabetes, particularly middle-age and older patients with type 2 diabetes, who do not manifest CHD, carry a risk for major coronary events equivalent to that of nondiabetic patients with established CHD. Moreover, many patients with type 2 diabetes have had a silent MI, and many others have silent ischemia. Thus, patients with diabetes are at high risk, and ATP III has designated *diabetes as a CHD equivalent.*

# ■ MULTIPLE RISK FACTORS WITHOUT CLINICAL CORONARY HEART DISEASE

Patients without known atherosclerosis often have multiple risk factors (**Table 20-2**) that contribute to CHD risk. Absolute risk for development of CHD over the next

**TABLE 20-2.** Major Risk Factors Other Than LDL Cholesterol[a]

Cigarette smoking
Hypertension (blood pressure ≥140/90 mm Hg or on antihypertensive medication)
Low HDL cholesterol (<40 mg/dL)
Family history of premature CHD (CHD in male first-degree relative <55 y; CHD in female
first-degree relative <65 y)
Age (men ≥45 y; women ≥55 y)

[a]Diabetes is regarded as a CHD risk equivalent.

Adapted from *Third Report of the National Cholesterol Education Program (NCEP) Expert Panel on Detection,
Evaluation, and Treatment of High Blood Cholesterol in Adults (Adult Treatment Panel III). Final Report.*
National Heart, Lung, and Blood Institute National Institutes of Health NIH pub. no. 02-5215 September 2002,
or http://www.nhlbi.nih.gov/guidelines/cholesterol/atp3full.pdf. Accessed March 3, 2008.

decade can be estimated by Framingham risk tables (**Tables 20-3** and **20-4**). These
tables calculate absolute risk for the development of *hard CHD* (nonfatal and fatal MI)
over the next 10 years but exclude *soft CHD* (stable and unstable angina). Using
this method, asymptomatic patients with multiple risk factors can be stratified into
high-risk and intermediate-risk categories. *A CHD risk equivalent is defined when the
absolute 10-year risk for hard CHD events exceeds 20%.*

## High-Risk Patients Identified by Major Risk Factors Plus Emerging Risk Factors

Some intermediate-risk patients (10-year CHD risk of 10%-20%) determined by the
Framingham risk score are at higher risk because of advanced subclinical coronary
atherosclerosis. These individuals can be identified by screening for "emerging risk
factors" defined by the NCEP ATP III guidelines (**Table 20-5**). *Noninvasive testing
in asymptomatic patients should be used for risk assessment (prognosis) and not for
diagnosis of coronary artery disease.* Noninvasive tests with the most evidence to
improve risk prediction beyond the Framingham risk score include high-sensitivity
CRP, coronary artery calcium scanning, exercise treadmill testing, and carotid ultrasound. Currently, the American Heart Association (AHA) and Centers for Disease
Control and Prevention (CDC) recommend the optional use of CRP in intermediate-
risk patients to direct further evaluation and therapy.

## ■ IDENTIFICATION OF INTERMEDIATE-RISK AND LOW-RISK PATIENTS

Patients at intermediate risk are those without known atherosclerosis but with 2 or
more conventional risk factors whose 10-year risk for CHD is 10% to 20%. Patients
with no more than 1 risk factor are low risk and have a 10-year risk for CHD of less
than 10%.

An important question is how to manage patients who have a single, treatable categorical risk factor but are otherwise at low risk. A fundamental principle of primary
prevention is that *all categorical risk factors must be treated, regardless of absolute
risk.* Although a person with only 1 risk factor—such as hypertension, smoking, or
hypercholesterolemia—has less than a 10% 10-year risk of CHD, the presence of a
single major risk factor at 50 years of age is associated with a substantially increased

**TABLE 20-3.** Estimate of 10-Year Risk for Men (Framingham Point Scores)

| Age (years) | Points |
|---|---|
| 20-34 | −9 |
| 35-39 | −4 |
| 40-44 | 0 |
| 45-49 | 3 |
| 50-54 | 6 |
| 55-59 | 8 |
| 60-64 | 10 |
| 65-69 | 11 |
| 70-74 | 12 |
| 75-79 | 13 |

| | Points | | | | |
|---|---|---|---|---|---|
| Total Cholesterol (mg/dL) | Age 20-39 years | Age 40-49 years | Age 50-59 years | Age 60-69 years | Age 70-79 years |
| <160 | 0 | 0 | 0 | 0 | 0 |
| 160-199 | 4 | 3 | 2 | 1 | 0 |
| 200-239 | 7 | 5 | 3 | 1 | 0 |
| 240-279 | 9 | 6 | 4 | 2 | 1 |
| ≥280 | 11 | 8 | 5 | 3 | 1 |

| | Points | | | | |
|---|---|---|---|---|---|
| | Age 20-39 years | Age 40-49 years | Age 50-59 years | Age 60-69 years | Age 70-79 years |
| Nonsmoker | 0 | 0 | 0 | 0 | 0 |
| Smoker | 8 | 5 | 3 | 1 | 1 |

| HDL (mg/dL) | Points |
|---|---|
| ≥60 | −1 |
| 50-59 | 0 |
| 40-49 | 1 |
| <40 | 2 |

| Systolic BP (mm Hg) | If Untreated | If Treated |
|---|---|---|
| <120 | 0 | 0 |
| 120-129 | 0 | 1 |
| 130-139 | 1 | 2 |
| 140-159 | 1 | 2 |
| ≥160 | 2 | 3 |

| Point Total | 10-Year Risk (%) |
|---|---|
| <0 | <1 |
| 0 | 1 |
| 1 | 1 |
| 2 | 1 |
| 3 | 1 |

(continued)

**TABLE 20-3.** Estimate of 10-Year Risk for Men (Framingham Point Scores) (continued)

| Point Total | 10-Year Risk (%) |
| --- | --- |
| 4 | 1 |
| 5 | 2 |
| 6 | 2 |
| 7 | 3 |
| 8 | 4 |
| 9 | 5 |
| 10 | 6 |
| 11 | 8 |
| 12 | 10 |
| 13 | 12 |
| 14 | 16 |
| 15 | 20 |
| 16 | 25 |
| ≥17 | ≥30 |

Adapted from *Third Report of the National Cholesterol Education Program (NCEP) Expert Panel on Detection, Evaluation, and Treatment of High Blood Cholesterol in Adults (Adult Treatment Panel III). Final Report.* National Heart, Lung, and Blood Institute National Institutes of Health NIH pub. no. 02-5215 September 2002, or http://www.nhlbi.nih.gov/guidelines/cholesterol/atp3full.pdf. Accessed March 3, 2008.

lifetime risk for CHD and markedly shorter survival. Therefore, patients with even 1 categorical risk factor should not be ignored even if found to have a low absolute risk by Framingham scoring (Tables 20-3 and 20-4).

# PRACTICE RECOMMENDATIONS

The remainder of this chapter provides specific practice recommendations in accordance with national guidelines for primary and secondary prevention of CHD (**Tables 20-6** and **20-7**).

## ▇ LOWERING LOW-DENSITY LIPOPROTEIN CHOLESTEROL

**Table 20-8** shows the LDL cholesterol goals and cutpoints for therapy classified by risk category. For patients at very high risk, it is <70 mg/dL. LDL lowering can be achieved with nondrug and drug therapies. *The importance of nondrug therapies must not be minimized.* Reducing the intake of cholesterol-raising fatty acids (saturated and *trans* fatty acids) and dietary cholesterol is a key component of nondrug therapy. Major sources of dietary saturated fatty acids are dairy fats (eg, milk, butter, cream, cheese, and ice cream) and animal fats (eg, fatty cuts of meat [especially hamburger], fatty processed meats, lard, and tallow). *Trans* fatty acids are present in shortening and hard margarine, and often in processed foods. Rich sources of dietary cholesterol are eggs, dairy fats, and other animal products. For patients on cholesterol-lowering therapies, their daily intake of cholesterol-raising fatty acids should be less than 7% of total calories. Dietary cholesterol intake should be lowered to less than 200 mg/d.

**TABLE 20-4.** Estimate of 10-Year Risk for Women (Framingham Point Scores)

| Age (years) | Points |
|---|---|
| 20-34 | −7 |
| 35-39 | −3 |
| 40-44 | 0 |
| 45-49 | 3 |
| 50-54 | 6 |
| 55-59 | 8 |
| 60-64 | 10 |
| 65-69 | 12 |
| 70-74 | 14 |
| 75-79 | 16 |

| Total Cholesterol (mg/dL) | Points | | | | |
|---|---|---|---|---|---|
| | Age 20-39 years | Age 40-49 years | Age 50-59 years | Age 60-69 years | Age 70-79 years |
| <160 | 0 | 0 | 0 | 0 | 0 |
| 160-199 | 4 | 3 | 2 | 1 | 1 |
| 200-239 | 8 | 6 | 4 | 2 | 1 |
| 240-279 | 11 | 8 | 5 | 3 | 2 |
| ≥280 | 13 | 10 | 7 | 4 | 2 |

| | Points | | | | |
|---|---|---|---|---|---|
| | Age 20-39 years | Age 40-49 years | Age 50-59 years | Age 60-69 years | Age 70-79 years |
| Nonsmoker | 0 | 0 | | 0 | 0 |
| Smoker | 9 | 7 | 4 | 2 | 1 |

| HDL (mg/dL) | Points |
|---|---|
| ≥60 | −1 |
| 50-59 | 0 |
| 40-49 | 1 |
| <40 | 2 |

| Systolic BP (mm Hg) | If Untreated | If Treated |
|---|---|---|
| <120 | 0 | 0 |
| 120-129 | 1 | 3 |
| 130-139 | 2 | 4 |
| 140-159 | 3 | 5 |
| ≥160 | 4 | 6 |

| Point Total | 10-Year Risk (%) |
|---|---|
| <9 | <1 |
| 9 | 1 |
| 10 | 1 |
| 11 | 1 |
| 12 | 1 |

(continued)

**TABLE 20-4.** Estimate of 10-Year Risk for Women (Framingham Point Scores) (continued)

| Point Total | 10-Year Risk (%) |
|---|---|
| 13 | 2 |
| 14 | 2 |
| 15 | 3 |
| 16 | 4 |
| 17 | 5 |
| 18 | 6 |
| 19 | 8 |
| 20 | 11 |
| 21 | 14 |
| 22 | 17 |
| 23 | 22 |
| 24 | 27 |
| ≥25 | ≥30 |

Adapted from *Third Report of the National Cholesterol Education Program (NCEP) Expert Panel on Detection, Evaluation, and Treatment of High Blood Cholesterol in Adults (Adult Treatment Panel III). Final Report.* National Heart, Lung, and Blood Institute National Institutes of Health NIH pub. no. 02-5215 September 2002, or http://www.nhlbi.nih.gov/guidelines/cholesterol/atp3full.pdf. Accessed March 3, 2008.

**TABLE 20-5.** Emerging Risk Factors

**Lipid**
- Triglycerides
- Lipoprotein remnant particles
- Lipoprotein(a)
- Small LDL particles
- HDL subspecies
- Apolipoprotein B
- Apolipoprotein AI
- Total cholesterol/HDL cholesterol ratio

**Nonlipid**
- Homocysteine
- Thrombogenic/hemostatic factors
- Inflammatory markers
- Impaired fasting glucose

**Detection of Subclinical Atherosclerosis**
- Ankle brachial index
- Tests for myocardial ischemia
- Tests for atherosclerotic plaque burden (eg, coronary calcium scanning, carotid sonography)

HDL, high-density lipoprotein; LDL, low-density lipoprotein.

Adapted from *Third Report of the National Cholesterol Education Program (NCEP) Expert Panel on Detection, Evaluation, and Treatment of High Blood Cholesterol in Adults (Adult Treatment Panel III). Final Report.* National Heart, Lung, and Blood Institute National Institutes of Health NIH pub. no. 02-5215 September 2002, or http://www.nhlbi.nih.gov/guidelines/cholesterol/atp3full.pdf. Accessed March 3, 2008.

**TABLE 20-6.** Guide to Primary Prevention of Cardiovascular Disease

| Risk Intervention and Goals | Recommendations |
| --- | --- |
| Smoking<br>Goal: Complete cessation. No exposure to environmental tobacco smoke | Ask about tobacco use status at every visit. In a clear, strong, and personalized manner, advise every tobacco user to quit. Assess the tobacco user's willingness to quit. Assist by counseling and developing a plan for quitting. Arrange follow-up, referral to special programs, or pharmacotherapy. Urge avoidance of exposure to second-hand smoke at work or home. |
| BP control<br>Goal: <140/90 mm Hg; <130/85 mm Hg if renal insufficiency or heart failure is present; or <130/80 mm Hg if diabetes is present | Promote healthy lifestyle modification. Advocate weight reduction; reduction of sodium intake; consumption of fruits, vegetables, and low-fat dairy products; moderation of alcohol intake; and physical activity in persons with BP ≥130 mm Hg systolic or 80 mm Hg diastolic. For persons with renal insufficiency or heart failure, initiate drug therapy if BP ≥130 mm Hg systolic or 85 mm Hg diastolic (≥80 mm Hg diastolic for patients with diabetes). Initiate drug therapy for those with BP ≥140/90 mm Hg if 6-12 mo of lifestyle modification is not effective, depending on the number of risk factors present. Add BP medications, individualized to other patient requirements and characteristics (eg, age, race, need for drugs with specific benefits). |
| Dietary intake<br>Goal: An overall healthy eating pattern | Advocate consumption of a variety of fruits, vegetables, grains, low-fat or nonfat dairy products, fish, legumes, poultry, and lean meats. Match energy intake with energy needs and make appropriate changes to achieve weight loss when indicated. Modify food choices to reduce saturated fats (<10% of calories), cholesterol (<300 mg/d), and *trans* fatty acids by substituting grains and unsaturated fatty acids from fish, vegetables, legumes, and nuts. Limit salt intake to <6 g/d. Limit alcohol intake (≤2 drinks/d in men, ≤1 drink/d in women) among those who drink. |

(continued)

**TABLE 20-6.** Guide to Primary Prevention of Cardiovascular Disease (continued)

| Risk Intervention and Goals | Recommendations |
| --- | --- |
| **Aspirin**<br>Goal: Low-dose aspirin in persons at higher CHD risk (especially those with 10-y risk of CHD ≥10%) | Do not recommend for patients with aspirin intolerance. Low-dose aspirin increases risk for gastrointestinal bleeding and hemorrhagic stroke. Do not use in persons at increased risk for these diseases. Benefits of cardiovascular risk reduction outweigh these risks in most patients at higher coronary risk. Doses of 75-160 mg/d are as effective as higher doses. Therefore, consider 75-160 mg aspirin per day for persons at higher risk (especially those with 10-y risk of CHD ≥10%). |
| **Blood lipid management**<br>Primary goal: LDL-C <160 mg/dL. If ≤1 risk factor is present, LDL-C <130 mg/dL; if ≥2 risk factors are present and 10-y CHD risk is <20%; or LDL-C <100 mg/dL if ≥2 risk factors are present and 10-y CHD risk is ≥20% or if patient has diabetes<br><br>Secondary goals (if LDL-C triglycerides >200 mg/dL, then use non–HDL-C as a secondary goal: non–HDL-C <190 mg/dL for ≤1 risk factor; non–HDL-C <160 mg/dL for ≥2 risk factors and 10-y CHD risk ≤20%; non–HDL-C <130 mg/dL for diabetics or for ≥2 risk factors and 10-y CHD risk >20% is at goal range)<br><br>Other targets for therapy: Triglycerides >150 mg/dL; HDL-C <40 mg/dL in men and <50 mg/dL in women | If LDL-C is above goal range, initiate additional therapeutic lifestyle changes consisting of dietary modifications to lower LDL-C: <7% of calories from saturated fat, cholesterol <200 mg/d, and, if further LDL-C lowering is required, dietary options (plant stanols/sterols not to exceed 2 g/d and/or increased viscous [soluble] fiber [10-25 g/dl), and additional emphasis on weight reduction and physical activity. If LDL-C is above goal range, rule out secondary causes (liver function test, thyroid-stimulating hormone level, urinalysis). After 12 wk of therapeutic lifestyle change, consider LDL-lowering drug therapy if ≥2 risk factors are present, 10-y risk >10%, and LDL-C ≥130 mg/dL; ≥2 risk factors are present, 10-y risk <10%, and LDL-C ≥160 mg/dL; or ≤1 risk factor is present and LDL-C is ≥190 mg/dL. Start drugs and advance dose to bring LDL-C to goal range, usually a statin but also consider bile acid–binding resin or niacin. If LDL-C goal is not achieved, consider combination therapy (statin + resin, statin + niacin). After LDL-C goal has been reached, consider triglyceride level: if 150-199 mg/dL, treat with therapeutic lifestyle changes. If 200-499 mg/dL, treat elevated non–HDL-C with therapeutic lifestyle changes and, if necessary, consider higher doses of statin or adding niacin or fibrate. If >500 mg/dL, treat with fibrate or niacin to reduce risk of pancreatitis. If HDL-C <40 mg/dL in men and <50 mg/dL in women, initiate or intensify therapeutic lifestyle changes. For higher-risk patients, consider drugs that raise HDL-C (eg, niacin, fibrates, statins). |

Physical activity
Goal: At least 30 min of moderate-intensity physical activity on most (and preferably all) days of the week

If cardiovascular, respiratory, metabolic, orthopedic, or neurologic disorders are suspected, or if patient is middle-aged or older and is sedentary, consult physician before initiating vigorous exercise program. Moderate-intensity activities (40%–60% of maximum capacity) are equivalent to a brisk walk (15-20 min/mile). Additional benefits are gained from vigorous-intensity activity (>60% of maximum capacity) for 20-40 min on 3-5 d/wk. Recommend resistance training with 8-10 different exercises 1-2 sets per exercise, and 10-15 repetitions at moderate intensity ≥2 d/wk. Flexibility training and an increase in daily lifestyle activities should complement this regimen.

Weight management
Goal: Achieve and maintain desirable weight (body mass index 18.5-24.9 kg/m²). When body mass index is ≥25 kg/m², waist circumference at iliac crest level ≤40 in men, ≤35 in women

Initiate weight-management program through caloric restriction and increased caloric expenditure as appropriate. For overweight/obese persons, reduce body weight by 10% in first year of therapy.

Diabetes management
Goals: Normal fasting plasma glucose (<110 mg/dL) and near normal HbA$_{1c}$ (<7%)

Initiate appropriate hypoglycemic therapy to achieve near-normal fasting plasma glucose or as indicated by near-normal HbA$_{1c}$. First step is diet and exercise. Second step is usually oral hypoglycemic drugs: sulfonylureas and/or metformin with ancillary use of acarbose and thiazolidinediones. Third step in the therapy is insulin. Treat other risk factors more aggressively (eg, change BP goal to <130/80 mm Hg and LDL-C goal to <100 mg/dL).

BP, blood pressure; CHD, coronary heart disease; HD–C, high-density lipoprotein cholesterol; INR, international normalized ratio; LDL–C, low-density lipoprotein cholesterol.

Reproduced with permission from Pearson TA, Blair SN, Daniels SR, et al. AHA guidelines for primary prevention of cardiovascular disease and stroke: 2002 update. Consensus panel guide to comprehensive risk reduction for adult patients without coronary or other atherosclerotic vascular diseases. *Circulation.* 2002;106:388-391.

**TABLE 20-7.** Secondary Prevention for Patients With Coronary and Other Vascular Disease (See Chapter 57 for ACC/AHA Classification)

| Goals | Intervention Recommendations and Level of Evidence |
|---|---|
| **Smoking**<br>Goal<br>Complete cessation; no exposure to environmental tobacco smoke | • Ask about tobacco use status at every visit. I (B)<br>• Advise every tobacco user to quit. I (B)<br>• Assess the tobacco user's willingness to quit. I (B)<br>• Assist by counseling and developing a plan for quitting. I (B)<br>• Arrange follow-up, referral to special programs, or pharmacotherapy (including nicotine replacement and bupropion). I (B)<br>• Urge avoidance of exposure to environmental tobacco smoke at work and home. I (B) |
| **Blood Pressure Control** | **For All Patients** |
| Goal<br><140/90 mm Hg<br>Or<br><130/80 mm Hg if patient has diabetes or chronic kidney disease | • Initiate or maintain lifestyle modification—weight control; increased physical activity; alcohol moderation; sodium reduction; and emphasis on increased consumption of fresh fruits, vegetables, and low-fat dairy products. I (B)<br>For Patients With BP >140/90 mm Hg (or >130/80 mm Hg for Individuals With Chronic Kidney Disease or Diabetes)<br>• As tolerated, add BP medication, treating initially with β-blockers and/or ACE inhibitors, with addition of other drugs such as thiazides as needed to achieve goal BP. I (A)<br>(For compelling indications for individual drug classes in specific vascular diseases, see Seventh Report of the Joint National Committee on Prevention, Detection, Evaluation, and Treatment of High Blood Pressure [JNC 7].) |
| **Lipid Management** | **For All Patients** |
| Goal<br>LDL-C <100 mg/dL<br>If TGs are ≥200 mg/dL, non–HDL-C should be <130 mg/dL[b] | • Start dietary therapy. Reduce intake of saturated fats (to <7% of total calories), *trans* fatty acids, and cholesterol (to <200 mg/d). I (B)<br>• Adding plant stanol/sterols (2 g/d) and viscous fiber (>10 g/d) will further lower LDL-C.<br>• Promote daily physical activity and weight management. I (B)<br>• Encourage increased consumption of omega-3 fatty acids in the form of fish or in capsule form (1 g/d) for risk reduction. For treatment of elevated TGs, higher doses are usually necessary for risk reduction. IIb (B) |

**For Lipid Management**

Assess fasting lipid profile in all patients, and within 24 h of hospitalization for those with an acute cardiovascular or coronary event. For hospitalized patients, initiate lipid lowering medication as recommended below before discharge according to the following schedule:

- LDL-C should be <100 mg/dL **I (A)**, and
- Further reduction of LDL-C to <70 mg/dL is reasonable. **IIa (A)**
- If baseline LDL-C is ≥100 mg/dL, initiate LDL-lowering drug therapy.[d] **I (A)**
- If on-treatment LDL-C ≥100 mg/dL, intensify LDL-lowering drug therapy (may require LDL-lowering drug combination[e]). **I (A)**
- If baseline LDL-C is 70–100 mg/dL, it is reasonable to treat to LDL-C <70 mg/dL. **IIa (B)**
- If TGs are 200–499 mg/dL, non–HDL-C should be <130 mg/dL. **I (B)**
- Further reduction of non–HDL-C to <100 mg/dL is reasonable. **IIa (B)**
- Therapeutic options to reduce non–HDL-C are
  - More intense LDL-C-lowering therapy **I (B)**, or
  - Niacin[f] (after LDL-C-lowering therapy) **IIa (B)**, or
  - Fibrate therapy[f] (after LDL-C-lowering therapy) **IIa (B)**
- If TGs ≥500 mg/dL,[g] therapeutic options to prevent pancreatitis are fibrate[f] or niacin[f] before LDL-lowering therapy, and treat LDL-C to goal after TG-lowering therapy. Achieve non–HDL-C ≤130 mg/dL if possible. **I (C)**

| | |
|---|---|
| **Physical Activity**<br>Goal<br>30 min, 7 d/wk (minimum 5 d/wk) | - For all patients, assess risk with a physical activity history and/or an exercise test, to guide prescription. **I (B)**<br>- For all patients, encourage 30-60 min of moderate-intensity aerobic activity, such as brisk walking, on most, preferably all, days of the week, supplemented by an increase in daily lifestyle activities (eg, walking breaks at work, gardening, house-hold work). **I (B)**<br>- Encourage resistance training 2 d/wk. **IIb (C)** |
|  | - Advise medically supervised programs for high-risk patients (eg, recent acute coronary syndrome or revascularization, heart failure). **I (B)**<br>- Encourage resistance training 2 d/wk. **IIb (C)**<br>- Advise medically supervised programs for high-risk patients (eg, recent acute coronary syndrome or revascularization, heart failure). **I (B)** |

*(continued)*

**TABLE 20-7.** Secondary Prevention for Patients With Coronary and Other Vascular Disease$^a$ (See Chapter 57 for ACC/AHA Classification) (continued)

| Goals | Intervention Recommendations and Level of Evidence |
| --- | --- |
| **Weight Management**<br>Goal<br>BMI: 18.5–24.9 kg/m$^2$<br>Waist circumference: men <40 in, women <35 in | • Assess BMI and/or waist circumference on each visit and consistently encourage weight maintenance/reduction through an appropriate balance of physical activity, caloric intake, and formal behavioral programs when indicated to maintain/achieve a BMI between 18.5 and 24.9 kg/m$^2$. **I (B)**<br>• If waist circumference (measured horizontally at the iliac crest) is ≥35 in in women and ≥40 in in men, initiate lifestyle changes and consider treatment strategies for metabolic syndrome as indicated. **I (B)**<br>• The initial goal of weight loss therapy should be to reduce body weight by approximately 10% from baseline. With success, further weight loss can be attempted if indicated through further assessment. **I (B)** |
| **Diabetes Management**<br>Goal<br>HbA$_{1c}$ <7% | • Initiate lifestyle and pharmacotherapy to achieve near-normal HbA$_{1c}$. **I (B)**<br>• Begin vigorous modification of other risk factors (eg, physical activity, weight management, BP control, and cholesterol management as recommended above). **I (B)**<br>• Coordinate diabetic care with patient's primary care physician or endocrinologist. **I (C)** |
| **Antiplatelet Agents/Anticoagulants** | • Start aspirin 75–162 mg/d and continue indefinitely in all patients unless contraindicated. **I (A)**<br>• For patients undergoing coronary artery bypass grafting, aspirin should be started within 48 h after surgery to reduce saphenous vein graft closure. Dosing regimens ranging from 100 to 325 mg/d appear to be efficacious. Doses higher than 162 mg/d can be continued for up to 1 y. **I (B)**<br>• Start and continue clopidogrel 75 mg/d in combination with aspirin for up to 12 mo in patients after acute coronary syndrome or percutaneous coronary intervention with stent placement (≥1 mo for bare metal stent, ≥3 mo for sirolimus-eluting stent, and ≥6 mo for paclitaxel-eluting stent). **I (B)** |

- Patients who have undergone percutaneous coronary intervention with stent placement should initially receive higher-dose aspirin at 325 mg/d for 1 mo for bare metal stent, 3 mo for sirolimus-eluting stent, and 6 mo for paclitaxel-eluting stent. **I (B)**
- Manage warfarin to international normalized ratio = 2.0–3.0 for paroxysmal or chronic atrial fibrillation or flutter, and in post-MI patients when clinically indicated (eg, atrial fibrillation, left ventricular thrombus). **I (A)**
- Use of warfarin in conjunction with aspirin and/or clopidogrel is associated with increased risk of bleeding and should be monitored closely. **I (B)**

**ACE Inhibitors**

- Start and continue indefinitely in all patients with left ventricular ejection fraction ≤40% and in those with hypertension, diabetes, or chronic kidney disease, unless contraindicated. **I (A)**
- Consider for all other patients. **I (B)**
- Among lower-risk patients with normal left ventricular ejection fraction in whom cardiovascular risk factors are well controlled and revascularization has been performed, use of ACE inhibitors may be considered optional. **IIa (B)**

**Angiotensin Receptor Blockers**

- Use in patients who are intolerant of ACE inhibitors and have heart failure or have had an MI with left ventricular ejection fraction ≤40%. **I (A)**
- Consider in other patients who are ACE inhibitor intolerant. **I (B)**
- Consider use in combination with ACE inhibitors in systolic-dysfunction heart failure. **IIb (B)**

**Aldosterone Blockade**

- Use in post-MI patients, without significant renal dysfunction[h] or hyperkalemia,[i] who are already receiving therapeutic doses of an ACE inhibitor and β-blocker, have a left ventricular ejection fraction ≤40%, and have either diabetes or heart failure. **I (A)**

Renin–Angiotensin–Aldosterone System Blockers

*(continued)*

**TABLE 20-7.** Secondary Prevention for Patients With Coronary and Other Vascular Disease[a] (See Chapter 57 for ACC/AHA Classification) (continued)

| Goals | Intervention Recommendations and Level of Evidence |
|---|---|
| β-Blockers | • Start and continue indefinitely in all patients who have had MI, acute coronary syndrome, or left ventricular dysfunction with or without heart failure symptoms, unless contraindicated. I (A) |
| | • Consider chronic therapy for all other patients with coronary or other vascular disease or diabetes unless contraindicated. IIa (C) |
| Influenza Vaccination | • Patients with cardiovascular disease should have an influenza vaccination. I (B) |

ACE, angiotensin-converting enzyme; BMI, body mass index; BP, blood pressure; CHF, congestive heart failure; HbA$_{1c}$, major fraction of adult hemoglobin; MI, myocardial infarction; TG, triglyceride.

[a]Patients covered by these guidelines include those with established coronary and other atherosclerotic vascular disease, including peripheral arterial disease, atherosclerotic aortic disease, and carotid artery disease. Treatment of patients whose only manifestation of cardiovascular risk is diabetes will be the topic of a separate AHA scientific statement.

[b]Non–HDL-C total cholesterol minus HDL-C.

[c]Pregnant and lactating women should limit their intake of fish to minimize exposure to methylmercury.

[d]When LDL-lowering medications are used, obtain at least a 30%–40% reduction in LDL-C levels. If LDL-C <70 mg/dL is the chosen target, consider drug titration to achieve this level to minimize side effects and cost. When LDL-C <70 mg/dL is not achievable because of high baseline LDL-C levels, it generally is possible to achieve reductions >50% in LDL-C levels by either statins or LDL-C–lowering drug combinations.

[e]Standard dose of statin with ezetimibe, bile acid sequestrant, or niacin.

[f]The combination of high-dose statin and fibrate can increase risk for severe myopathy. Statin doses should be kept relatively low with this combination. Dietary supplement niacin must not be used as a substitute for prescription niacin.

[g]Patients with very high TGs should not consume alcohol. The use of bile acid sequestrant is relatively contraindicated when TGs >200 mg/dL.

[h]Creatinine should be <2.5 mg/dL in men and <2.0 mg/dL in women.

[i]Potassium should be <5.0 mEq/L.

Reproduced with permission from Smith SC, Allen J, Blair SN, et al. AHA/ACC guidelines for secondary prevention for patients with coronary and other atherosclerotic disease: 2006 update. *J Am Coll Cardiol.* 2006;47:2130-2139.

**TABLE 20-8.** LDL Cholesterol Goals and Cutpoints for Initiating Therapy Classified by Risk Category

| Risk Category | LDL Goal (mg/dL) | LDL Level at Which to Initiate Therapeutic Lifestyle Changes (mg/dL) | LDL Level at Which to Consider Drug Therapy (mg/dL) |
|---|---|---|---|
| CHD or CHD risk equivalents (10-y risk >20%) | <100 | ≥100 | ≥130 (100-129: drug optional) |
| 2+ risk factors (10-y risk 20%) | <130 | ≥130 | 10-y risk 10%-20%: ≥130 10-y risk <10%: ≥160 |
| 0-1 risk factor | <160 | ≥160 | ≥190 (160-189: LDL-lowering drug optional) |

Adapted from *Third Report of the National Cholesterol Education Program (NCEP) Expert Panel on Detection, Evaluation, and Treatment of High Blood Cholesterol in Adults (Adult Treatment Panel III). Final Report.* National Heart, Lung, and Blood Institute National Institutes of Health NIH pub. no. 02-5215 September 2002, or http://www.nhlbi.nih.gov/guidelines/cholesterol/atp3full.pdf. Accessed March 3, 2008.

LDL-C may also be lowered by the addition of certain foods. A daily intake of 2 to 3 g/d of plant stanols or sterol esters can reduce LDL-cholesterol by 6% to 15%. High intakes (5-10 g) of viscous dietary fiber can decrease LDL levels to another 3% to 5%. Monounsaturated and polyunsaturated fatty acids will lower LDL and may reduce global risk for CHD via other mechanisms. When combined with a low-saturated-fat, low-*trans*-fat diet, the addition of plant sterols, viscous fibers, and nuts can reduce LDL-C comparable to the effect of a low-dose statin.

**Table 20-9** shows drugs used for lipid therapy. Statins are the most effective LDL-lowering drugs. Most patients tolerate statins with few side effects. Occasional patients (0.5%-2%) may have a mild rise in liver transaminases, but this change is not believed to be an indication of hepatotoxicity. Statin-induced myopathy, defined as a serum creatinine kinase level of more than 10 times the upper limit of normal, has been observed in 0.1% to 0.5% of patients treated with statins during randomized controlled trials. Some patients have biopsy-proven myopathy but normal creatinine kinase levels; thus, normal creatinine kinase levels do not rule out myopathy. **Table 20-10** lists risk factors for severe myopathy.

For every doubling of the dose of a statin, the LDL level will fall by about 6%. A more efficacious way to enhance LDL lowering is to combine statins with ezetimibe or bile acid sequestrants.

# ■ IDENTIFICATION AND TREATMENT OF METABOLIC SYNDROME

Patients with the metabolic syndrome should be counseled to make intensive lifestyle changes, especially weight reduction and increased physical activity.

Furthermore, in higher-risk patients with the metabolic syndrome, drug therapies directed toward metabolic risk factors are indicated, such as lipid-lowering drugs,

**TABLE 20-9.** Drugs Used for Lipid Therapy

| Drug Class | Agents and Daily Doses | Lipid/Lipoprotein | Effects | Side Effects | Contraindications |
|---|---|---|---|---|---|
| Statins | Lovastatin (20-80 mg)<br>Pravastatin (20-80 mg)<br>Simvastatin (20-80 mg)<br>Fluvastatin (20-80 mg)<br>Atorvastatin (10-80 mg)<br>Rosuvastatin (5-40 mg) | LDL-C<br>HDL-C<br>TG | ↓18%-63%<br>↑5%-15%<br>↓7%-30% | Myopathy<br>Increased liver enzymes | Absolute:<br>Active or chronic liver disease<br>Relative:<br>Concomitant use of certain drugs (see Table 20-10) |
| Cholesterol absorption inhibitors | Ezetimibe (10 mg) | LDL-C<br>HDL-C<br>TG | ↓18%[a]<br>↑1%-2%<br>↓7%-9% | Rare increase in liver enzymes | None established; statin should not be added to ezetimibe in patients with active or chronic liver disease |
| Bile acid sequestrants | Cholestyramine (4-16 g)<br>Colestipol (5-20 g)<br>Colesevelam (2.6-3.8 g) | LDL-C<br>HDL-C<br>TG | ↓15%-30%<br>↑3%-5%<br>No change or increase | GI distress<br>Constipation<br>Decreased absorption of other drugs | Absolute:<br>Dysbetalipoproteinemia TG >400 mg/dL<br>Relative:<br>TG >200 mg/dL |
| Nicotinic acid | Immediate-release nicotinic acid (1.5-3 g), extended-release nicotinic acid (1-2 g), sustained-release hepatotoxicity nicotinic acid (1-2 g) | LDL-C<br>HDL-C<br>TG | ↓5%-25%<br>↑15%-35%<br>↓20%-50% | Flushing<br>Hyperglycemia<br>Hyperuricemia (or gout)<br>Upper GI distress | Absolute:<br>Chronic liver disease<br>Severe gout<br>Relative:<br>Diabetes<br>Hyperuricemia<br>Peptic ulcer disease |

| Fibric acids | Gemfibrozil (600 mg bid) | LDL-C (may increase in patients with high TG) ↓5%-20% | Dyspepsia Gallstones | Absolute: Severe renal disease |
| | Fenofibrate (160 mg) | HDL-C ↑10%-20% TG ↓20%-50% | Myopathy | Severe hepatic disease |

[a]LDL reduction is as great as 25% when combined with a statin.

Adapted from *Third Report of the National Cholesterol Education Program (NCEP) Expert Panel on Detection, Evaluation, and Treatment of High Blood Cholesterol in Adults (Adult Treatment Panel III). Final Report.* National Heart, Lung, and Blood Institute National Institutes of Health NIH pub. no. 02-5215 September 2002, or http://www.nhlbi.nih.gov/guidelines/cholesterol/atp3full.pdf. Accessed March 3, 2008.

**TABLE 20-10.** Risk Factors for Severe Myopathy From Statin Therapy

- Age >80 y
- Small body frame and frailty
- Multisystem disease (eg, chronic renal insufficiency, especially as a result of diabetes)
- Multiple medications
- Specific concomitant medications or consumptions (with various statins, check package insert for warnings)
  - Fibrates (especially gemfibrozil, but other fibrates too)
  - Nicotinic acid (rarely)
  - Cyclosporine
  - Azole antifungals
  - Itraconazole and ketoconazole
  - Macrolide antibiotics
  - Erythromycin and clarithromycin
  - HIV protease inhibitors
  - Nefazodone (antidepressant)
  - Verapamil
  - Large quantities of grapefruit juice (>1 quart per day)
  - Alcohol abuse (independently predisposes to myopathy)
- Perioperative periods[a]
- Acute illnesses[a]

[a]In most patients admitted to the hospital for acute illnesses or surgery, statin therapy should be temporarily discontinued.

Data from Pasternak RC, Smith SC Jr, Bairey-Merz CN, et al. ACC/AHA/NHLBI clinical advisory on the use and safety of statins. *Circulation.* 2002;106;1024-1028.

anti-hypertensives, and low-dose aspirin. Insulin-sensitizing agents may be helpful; however, there is insufficient evidence from controlled clinical trials that they will reduce risk. See Chapter 47 for a discussion of the metabolic syndrome.

# ■ ATHEROGENIC DYSLIPIDEMIA: HYPERTRIGLYCERIDEMIA, LOW HIGH-DENSITY LIPOPROTEIN, AND SMALL, DENSE LOW-DENSITY LIPOPROTEIN

Although high LDL-C is the primary lipid risk factor, other lipid parameters increase the risk of CHD in persons with or without an elevated LDL-C. Specifically, the combination of elevated concentrations of triglycerides, small, dense LDL-C, and low levels of HDL-C is referred to as *atherogenic dyslipidemia*. This is a complex dyslipidemia that usually results from a generalized metabolic disorder related to *insulin resistance*. Patients with insulin resistance often have the metabolic syndrome. Atherogenic dyslipidemia is an increasingly common contributor to CHD because of the growing prevalence of obesity, diabetes, and the metabolic syndrome. Patients with atherogenic dyslipidemia often have concomitant abnormalities of inflammation (elevated CRP) and hypofibrinolysis (elevated plasminogen activator inhibitor-1).

The drugs that most effectively modify atherogenic dyslipidemia are fibrates and niacin. Several trials with fibrates have shown a significant reduction of major coronary events. The role of fibrates as add-on therapy to statins is being evaluated in ongoing clinical trials. The risk for severe myopathy is increased in patients treated with statins and fibrates; hence it is prudent to limit the use of a statin and fibrate combination to higher-risk patients. Niacin lowers the concentration of triglycerides and small, dense LDL particles, and raises HDL-C. Niacin has more side effects than fibrates. Omega-3 fatty acids (fish oil) in doses of 2 to 4 g are effective in reducing triglycerides by 20% to 30% associated with small increases in HDL-C and LDL-C. Novel therapies for raising HDL-C are under development. Pharmacologic inhibition of cholesteryl ester transfer protein is capable of raising HDL-C by 50% to 100%; however, their efficacy in decreasing CHD outcomes has recently come into question.

## ■ CIGARETTE SMOKING

Patients and their family members may be especially receptive to a smoking cessation intervention after an acute event (ie, a teachable moment). The goal is *complete cessation and no exposure to environmental tobacco smoke.*

Intervention for smoking cessation includes asking about tobacco use status at every visit; advising to quit smoking; assessing willingness to quit; assisting by counseling and developing a plan to quit; and arranging follow-up, referral to special programs, or pharmacotherapy (nicotine replacement, buproprion, or varenicline). Even brief interventions may be effective and should, at a minimum, be provided to every patient who uses tobacco (**Table 20-11**). In primary prevention of CHD events, *a previous smoker's relative risk declines nearly to that of a nonsmoker in a year or less.* In patients with CHD, *achieving complete abstinence from smoking compares favorably with the health benefits of any intervention in modern cardiology.*

## ■ HYPERTENSION

Normal blood pressure is <120/80 mm Hg. The Joint National Committee (JNC) on Detection, Evaluation, and Treatment of High Blood Pressure recommends a treatment goal of <140/90 mm Hg. Lower goals are recommended for patients with renal

**TABLE 20-11.** Strategies for Successful Cessation of Cigarette Smoking: The 5 A's

| | |
|---|---|
| Ask | Systematically identify all tobacco users at every visit (eg, include tobacco as a vital sign). Determine exposure to environmental tobacco smoke at home or at work. |
| Advise | Provide a clear, strong, and personalized message, urging every tobacco user to quit. Review benefits of quitting and risk of continuing. |
| Assess | Assess patient's willingness to quit at each visit. |
| Assist | Have the patient develop a quit plan, including setting a quit date, identifying sources of support for cessation for family and friends, removing tobacco and other cues from the home and work environment. |
| | Provide counseling, information materials, and other behavioral interventions. |
| | Recommend use of pharmacotherapy, including varenicline, bupropion SR, nicotine gum, nicotine inhaler, nicotine nasal spray, or nicotine patch. |
| Arrange | Provide a reminder on the quit date. |
| | See the patient shortly after the quit date to assess success. |
| | If unsuccessful, identify barriers and solutions to their removal. |

Adapted from Fiore MC. *Treating Tobacco Use and Dependence.* Rockville, MD: U.S. Department of Health and Human Services, Public Health Service; 2000; or http://www.ncbi.nlm.nih.gov/books/bv.fcgi?rid=hstat2.section.7741. Accessed March 18, 2008.

insufficiency, heart failure, or diabetes (Tables 20-6 and 20-7). The reader is referred to Chapter 28 for a discussion of the treatment of hypertension.

# ■ DIABETES

Diabetes mellitus is an independent risk factor for CHD, increasing risk for type 1 as well as type 2 patients by 2 to 4 times. At least 65% of people with diabetes die from cardiovascular disease. Approximately 25% of MI survivors have diabetes. *Diabetic patients without a history of MI have as high a risk of coronary mortality as do nondiabetic patients with a history of MI.* Once patients with type 2 diabetes suffer an MI, their prognosis for recurrent MI and survival is much worse than that for CHD patients without diabetes. See Chapter 48 for a complete discussion of diabetes and CHD.

*Diabetes abolishes the usual protection from CHD afforded a premenopausal woman. Diabetic women have twice the risk of recurrent MI compared with diabetic men.*

Weight loss and exercise are key lifestyle modifications because they improve the constellation of metabolic abnormalities that accompany diabetes. Although the optimal proportion of dietary fat and carbohydrate is controversial, calorie restriction for obesity and avoidance of sugar and saturated fat are recommended. *β-blockers should not be withheld from diabetic patients following MI unless strong contraindications exist, because diabetic MI survivors have fewer deaths if treated with beta-blockers. Although there is no consistent evidence to support intensive glycemic control as a strategy to reduce macrovascular complications, aggressive lipid and blood pressure management in patients with diabetes lowers CHD risk.* Hemoglobin $A_{1C}$ of <7% is the treatment goal for patients with diabetes.

# ■ PHYSICAL INACTIVITY

*Physical inactivity is an independent risk factor for CHD and roughly doubles the risk.* There is an inverse dose-response relation between the amount of exercise performed weekly, from 700 to 2000 kcal of energy, and death from cardiovascular disease and all causes. Walking 1 mile burns approximately 100 kcal. For primary and secondary prevention, 30 minutes or more of moderate-intensity physical activity on most, and preferably all, days is recommended. Only about 20% of US adults meet this goal. Exercise testing should be recommended to apparently healthy men over 45 and women over 55 who are sedentary, as well as to younger adults with coronary risk factors, before starting a *vigorous* physical activity program (intensity >60% individual maximum oxygen consumption). For secondary prevention, exercise testing is recommended to guide exercise prescription, and high-risk patients should exercise in a medically supervised setting.

# ■ OBESITY

Body mass index (BMI) should be calculated for all patients, and waist circumference measured in patients with a BMI ≥25. *Overweight* is defined as a BMI of 25 to 29.9, and *obesity* as BMI ≥30. In adults with BMI ≥25, increased relative risk is indicated with a waist circumference >102 cm (>40 in) in men and >88 cm (>35 in) in women. See Chapter 52 for a discussion on obesity.

Treatment should focus on diet and exercise to prevent weight gain and to produce moderate weight loss over years. Lost weight is usually regained unless a program consisting of dietary therapy, physical activity, and behavior therapy is continued indefinitely. There is no effective pharmacologic therapy for long-term weight loss.

# RISK FACTORS FOR WHICH INTERVENTIONS HAVE NOT BEEN SHOWN TO LOWER RISK OF CORONARY HEART DISEASE

## ■ LIPOPROTEIN(A)

Several retrospective case-control studies support the view that lipoprotein(a), or Lp(a), is an independent risk factor for thromboembolic disease. However, results of the major prospective studies evaluating baseline Lp(a) concentration and future risks of MI and stroke are inconsistent. It is unclear whether Lp(a) provides information incremental to the conventional lipid profile, and no recommendation for screening can be made. If elevated levels prove to increase risk among hypercholesterolemic individuals, it may be prudent to lower levels of LDL-C even more aggressively in such individuals than the current guidelines dictate. Knowledge of Lp(a) levels may also be useful in the selection of agents to lower LDL-C (eg, niacin) and may identify a possible treatable cause in the occasional patient with CHD and none of the major risk factors.

## ■ HYPERHOMOCYSTEINEMIA

Hyperhomocysteinemia is an independent marker for cardiovascular disease in several groups of high-risk subjects. Hyperhomocysteinemia may be classified as moderate (16-30 μmol/L), intermediate (31-100 μmol/L), or severe (>100 μmol/L). The most important factor affecting plasma concentration is dietary intake of folate and vitamins $B_6$ and $B_{12}$. Lowering homocysteine has not been shown to be effective in reducing CHD risk; therefore its routine measurement and treatment is not recommended.

## ■ OXIDATIVE STRESS

Evidence from randomized controlled trials indicates that supplementation with β-carotene, vitamin C, and vitamin E offers no benefit for CHD prevention. Observational evidence supports the consumption of diets rich in fruits and vegetables.

# UNMODIFIABLE RISK FACTORS

## ■ AGE AND SEX AS RISK FACTORS FOR ATHEROSCLEROTIC DISEASE

The incidence and prevalence of CHD increase sharply with age, so that age might be considered one of the most potent cardiovascular risk factors. CHD incidence rates in men are similar to those in women 10 years older. Persons at an advanced age (eg, 75+ years) should have the risks and benefits of preventive cardiology interventions weighed on an individual basis, but typically derive the greatest benefit because they have the highest risk.

## ■ POSTMENOPAUSAL STATUS

Postmenopausal women with or without CHD who have not been on estrogen replacement therapy should not be started on hormonal therapy for the purpose of primary or secondary prevention. The decision to continue or discontinue hormone therapy should be based on established noncardiovascular benefits and risks, and on patient preference. In chronic users of hormone therapy, medication should be discontinued, at least temporarily, if a woman develops an acute coronary syndrome or is immobilized. Oral estrogen therapy is contraindicated in women with moderately severe hypertriglyceridemia (eg, serum triglycerides >400 mg/dL), but in such women transdermal estrogen might be an appropriate substitute for noncardiovascular indications.

## ■ FAMILY HISTORY OF EARLY-ONSET CHD

*More than 35 case-control and prospective studies have consistently identified an association between CHD and a history of first-degree relatives with early-onset CHD.* Although CHD in a male relative with onset at age 55 years or less, or in a female relative with onset at age 65 years or less, is defined as a positive family history, the larger the number of relatives with early-onset CHD or the younger the age of CHD onset in the relative, the stronger is the predictive value. *Although considered a nonmodifiable risk factor, a positive family history should result in the careful screening of individual risk factors known to aggregate in families. Such familial aggregations may represent monogenic factors with known phenotypic expressions and inheritance patterns, polygenic factors with less clear modes of expression and inheritance, or shared environments.* Thus, family members of patients with CHD at a younger age represent fruitful targets for risk factor assessment. *Risk factor screening should extend to the siblings and children of early-CHD patients.*

# OTHER PHARMACOLOGIC THERAPY

## ■ ANTIPLATELET AND ANTICOAGULANT THERAPY

Low-dose aspirin, 75 to 160 mg/d, is recommended for primary and secondary prevention among individuals with a 10-year risk of CHD ≥10%. Treatment should be continued indefinitely. If aspirin is contraindicated in a CHD patient, clopidogrel 75 mg daily is recommended. If neither antiplatelet agent can be taken, warfarin (international normalized ratio [INR] goal of 2.0-3.0) is recommended for secondary prevention.

## ■ β-BLOCKERS

For primary prevention, β-blockers are recommended as first-line therapy for hypertension. For secondary prevention, β-blockers are recommended for all patients who have had MI, an acute coronary syndrome, or left ventricular dysfunction with or without heart failure symptoms, and continued indefinitely unless contraindicated. β-blockers should be considered as chronic therapy for all patients with CHD, other vascular disease, or diabetes unless contraindicated.

## ■ RENIN–ANGIOTENSIN–ALDOSTERONE SYSTEM BLOCKERS

Angiotensin-converting enzyme (ACE) inhibitors are at least as effective as diuretics in the primary prevention of CHD death or nonfatal MI, although national guidelines continue to recommend diuretics as first-line agents for the treatment of hypertension. ACE inhibitors are appropriate first-line antihypertensive therapy in patients with diabetes, and they are an excellent second step after diuretic therapy in most hypertensive patients. For secondary prevention, ACE inhibitors should be prescribed indefinitely to all patients following MI and to patients with clinical evidence of congestive heart failure. ACE inhibitors should be considered as chronic therapy for all other patients with coronary or other atherosclerotic vascular disease.

Angiotensin-receptor blockers (ARBs) should be prescribed for patients who are intolerant of ACE inhibitors and have heart failure or have had an MI with left ventricular ejection fraction ≤40%. ARBs should be considered in other patients with CHD or other atherosclerotic disease who are ACE inhibitor intolerant.

# THE PRACTICE OF PREVENTIVE CARDIOLOGY

## ■ IMPLEMENTATION OF PREVENTIVE CARDIOLOGY SERVICES

Improved application of proven interventions for prevention requires a variety of strategies targeted to patients, health care providers, inpatient care settings, ambulatory care settings, and health systems. *Professional societies strongly recommend that risk-factor management be part of the optimal care of patients at high risk for cardiovascular disease, and therefore the responsibility of all health care providers.*

# SUGGESTED READINGS

Blaha MJ, Ketlogetswe KS, Ndumele CE, Gluckman TJ, Blumenthal RS. Preventive strategies for coronary heart disease. In: Fuster V, Walsh RA, Harrington RA, et al. *Hurst's The Heart*. 13th ed. New York, NY: McGraw-Hill; 2011;51:1183-1224.

Pearson TA, Blair SN, Daniels SR, et al. AHA guidelines for primary prevention of cardiovascular disease and stroke: 2002 update. Consensus panel guide to comprehensive risk reduction for adult patients without coronary or other atherosclerotic vascular diseases. *Circulation*. 2002;106:388-391.

Smith SC, Allen J, Blair SN, et al. AHA/ACC guidelines for secondary prevention for patients with coronary and other atherosclerotic disease: 2006 update. Endorsed by the National Heart, Lung, and Blood Institute. *J Am Coll Cardiol*. 2006;47:2130-2139.

*Third Report of the National Cholesterol Education Program (NCEP) Expert Panel on Detection, Evaluation, and Treatment of High Blood Cholesterol in Adults (Adult Treatment Panel III). Final Report*. National Heart, Lung, and Blood Institute National Institutes of Health NIH pub. no. 02-5215 September 2002, or http://www.nhlbi.nih.gov/guidelines/cholesterol/atp3full.pdf. Accessed March 3, 2008.

# CHAPTER 21
# MANAGEMENT OF PATIENTS WITH CHRONIC ISCHEMIC HEART DISEASE

## Richard A. Walsh and Robert A. O'Rourke[†]

Chronic stable angina is the first presentation of ischemic heart disease in about 50% of patients. The number of patients with stable angina in the United States approximates 17 million people, excluding patients who do not seek medical attention for their chest pain or who are shown to have a noncardiac cause of chest discomfort. Angina pectoris is a clinical syndrome that consists of recurrent discomfort or pain in the chest, jaw, shoulder, back, or arm associated with myocardial ischemia, but without myocardial necrosis. It is typically precipitated or aggravated by exertion or emotional stress and relieved by nitroglycerin. Angina usually occurs in patients with coronary artery disease (CAD) affecting one or more large epicardial arteries. However, angina often is present in individuals with valvular heart disease, hypertrophic cardiomyopathy, and uncontrolled hypertension. It also occurs in patients with normal coronary arteries and myocardial ischemia due to coronary artery spasm or endothelial dysfunction. The symptom of "angina" is often observed in patients with noncardiac disorders affecting the esophagus, chest wall, or lungs.

## ETIOLOGY

Coronary atherosclerosis is the cause of angina pectoris in most patients. Other causes include congenital artery abnormalities, coronary artery spasm, coronary thromboembolism, coronary vasculitis, aortic stenosis, mitral stenosis with resulting severe right ventricular hypertension, severe pulmonary hypertension, pulmonic stenosis, hypertrophic cardiomyopathy, and systemic arterial hypertension. Disorders in which angina occurs less frequently include aortic regurgitation, idiopathic dilated cardiomyopathy, and syphilitic heart disease. Mitral valve prolapse rarely causes true angina pectoris. Certain conditions may alter the balance between myocardial oxygen supply and demand and precipitate or aggravate angina pectoris, including severe anemia, tachycardia, fever, and hyperthyroidism.

## CLASSIFICATION

The Canadian Cardiovascular Society Grading Scale is commonly used to classify the severity of angina pectoris, with the most severe symptoms occurring at rest and the least severe only with excessive exercise.

[†]Deceased.

# DIAGNOSIS OF ANGINA PECTORIS

## ■ HISTORY AND PHYSICAL EXAMINATION

After a description of the chest discomfort is obtained, the physician makes an integrated assessment of the location, quality, and duration of discomfort; inciting factors; and factors relieving the pain. The most commonly used classification scheme for chest pain divides patients into three groups: *typical angina, atypical angina,* and *noncardiac chest pain* (**Table 21-1**). Angina is further labeled as *stable* when its characteristics have been unchanged over the preceding 60 days. The presence of unstable angina predicts a much higher short-term risk of an acute coronary event. *Unstable angina* is defined as angina that presents in one of three major ways: rest angina, severe new-onset angina, or prior angina increasing in severity (see Chapter 23).

Usually, the discomfort of chronic stable angina pectoris is precipitated by physical activity, emotions, eating, or cold weather. Certain patients are able to describe accurately the extent and type of exercise at which they reproducibly experience their chest pain. Emotions—particularly anger, excitement, and frustration—often precipitate angina in patients with coronary CAD. Cigarette smoking induces chest discomfort or lowers the exertion threshold for angina in some patients. In most patients, anginal discomfort has a characteristic crescendo nature. It develops and increases to a plateau over 10 to 30 s and disappears within minutes if the exertion is discontinued. The discomfort usually lasts only a few minutes, occasionally 10 to 15 minutes. Very rarely, it may last up to 30 minutes. The discomfort of angina is most often located substernally or just to the left of the sternum. In describing the discomfort, some patients clench their fists over their upper sternum (Levine's sign), a sign of high diagnostic accuracy. Radiation of the pain down the left arm or to the neck or jaw is common. The pain often radiates down the arms or to the neck, jaw, teeth, shoulders, or back. In addition to exertion drugs such as cocaine that increase heart rate and blood pressure can precipitate angina

Patients with stable angina may have many asymptomatic or silent episodes of myocardial ischemia. Also, myocardial ischemia may result in symptoms from either systolic or diastolic left ventricular (LV) dysfunction without the characteristic chest discomfort. Exertional dyspnea and fatigue are two common manifestations equivalent to angina that are usually also relieved with rest and nitroglycerin.

During an anginal attack, many patients appear pale and quiet. Diaphoresis and alterations in blood pressure and heart rate are common. A fourth (most common) or third heart sound, mitral regurgitant systolic murmur, bibasilar pulmonary rates, or palpable systolic impulse at the apex may be present. Evidence of noncoronary

---

**TABLE 21-1.** Clinical Classification of Angina

Typical angina (definite)
(1) Substernal chest discomfort with a characteristic quality and duration that is (2) provoked by exertion or emotional stress and (3) relieved by rest or NTG.
Atypical angina (probable)
    Meets two of the above characteristics.
Noncardiac chest pain
    Meets one or none of the typical anginal characteristics.

Data complied from Diamond GA, Staniloff HM, Forrester JS, et al. Computer-assisted diagnosis in the noninvasive evaluation of patients with suspected coronary disease. *J Am Coll Cardiol.* 1983;1:444-455.

atherosclerotic disease such as a carotid bruit, diminished pedal pulse, or abdominal aneurysm increases the likelihood of CAD.

# ■ CLINICAL EVALUATION OF THE LIKELIHOOD OF CORONARY ARTERY DISEASE

Clinicopathologic studies have demonstrated that it is possible to predict the probability of CAD on the basis of the history and the physical examination. The most powerful predictors of the probability of CAD are pain type, age, and sex (**Table 21-2**).

# ■ DIAGNOSTIC TESTS

For further information on diagnostic tests, see Chapter 4.

## Electrocardiogram and Chest Roentgenogram

A resting 12-lead electrocardiogram (ECG) should be recorded in all patients with symptoms suggestive of angina; however, it will be normal in 50% of patients with chronic angina. Evidence of prior Q-wave myocardial infarction (MI) on the ECG makes CAD very likely. An ECG obtained during chest pain is abnormal in about 50% of patients with angina and a normal resting ECG. ST-segment elevation or depression establishes a high likelihood of angina and indicates ischemia at a low workload, suggesting an unfavorable prognosis. The chest roentgenogram is often normal in patients with stable angina pectoris and is more useful in diagnosing noncardiac causes of chest pain.

## Electrocardiographic Exercise Stress Testing

The ECG exercise stress test is the test that is most frequently used to obtain objective evidence of myocardial ischemia as well as prognostic information in patients with known CAD (see also Chapter 4). Although wide variations are seen, the mean sensitivity is 68% and the mean specificity about 77%. The modest sensitivity of the exercise ECG is generally lower than that of imaging procedures. The diagnostic value of the test is significantly decreased by the presence of abnormalities such as

**TABLE 21-2.** Pretest Likelihood of Cad in Symptomatic Patients According to Age and Sex[a]

| Age (years) | Nonanginal Chest Pain | | Atypical Angina | | Typical Angina | |
|---|---|---|---|---|---|---|
| | Men | Women | Men | Women | Men | Women |
| 30–39 | 4 | 2 | 34 | 12 | 76 | 26 |
| 40–49 | 13 | 3 | 51 | 22 | 87 | 55 |
| 50–59 | 20 | 7 | 65 | 31 | 93 | 73 |
| 60–69 | 27 | 14 | 72 | 51 | 94 | 86 |

[a]Each value represents the percent with significant CAD on catheterization.

Data from Diamond GA, Forester JS. Analysis of probability as an aid in the clinical diagnosis of coronary-artery disease. N Engl J Med. 1979;300:1350-1358 and Chaitman BR, Bourassa MG, Davis K, Rogers WJ, Tyras DH, Berger R, Kennedy JW, Fisher L, Judkins MP, Mock MB, Killip T. Angiographic prevalence of high-risk coronary artery disease in patient subsets (CASS). Circulation. 1981;64:360-367.

bundle-branch block, ST-T-wave changes, or left ventricular hypertrophy (LVH) on the resting ECG. Diagnostic testing is most valuable when the pretest probability of obstructive CAD is intermediate. In these conditions, the test result has the largest effect on the post-test probability of disease and thus on clinical decisions.

## Rest Echocardiography

Assessment of global systolic function and the presence of regional systolic wall-motion abnormalities may help establish the diagnosis of chronic ischemic heart disease and estimate prognosis. The extent and severity of regional and global abnormalities are important considerations in choosing appropriate medical or surgical therapy.

## Myocardial Perfusion Imaging

Patients who should undergo cardiac stress testing with imaging, as opposed to exercise ECG alone, for the diagnosis of CAD include those in the following categories: (1) complete left bundle-branch block (LBBB), electronically paced ventricular rhythm, and preexcitation syndromes; (2) patients who have >1 mm of resting ST-segment depression, including those with LVH or who are taking drugs such as digitalis; (3) patients who are unable to exercise to a level high enough to give meaningful results on routine stress ECG (pharmacologic stress imaging should be considered); and (4) patients with angina who have undergone prior revascularization, in whom localization of ischemia, establishing the functional significance of lesions, and demonstrating myocardial viability are important considerations. Several methods can be used to induce stress, including (1) exercise (treadmill or bicycle) and (2) pharmacologic techniques (dipyridamole, adenosine, or dobutamine). When the patient can exercise to an appropriate level of cardiovascular stress for 6 to 12 minutes, exercise stress testing generally is preferred to pharmacologic stress. Myocardial perfusion imaging (MPI) is more expensive than exercise ECG testing, but it provides higher sensitivity and specificity. MPI plays a major role in risk stratification of patients with CAD. A normal perfusion scan in patients with CAD indicates a rate of cardiac death and MI of 0.9% per year, nearly as low as that of the general population. Incremental prognostic information will be gained from the number, size, and location of perfusion defects in combination with the amount of thallium 201 lung uptake on poststress images (see also Chapter 4).

## Stress Echocardiography

Stress echocardiography relies on imaging LV segmental wall motion and thickening during stress compared with baseline. It has a reported sensitivity and specificity similar to those of MPI (see also Chapter 4). If a patient is unable to exercise, pharmacologic stress is achieved most commonly by using dobutamine. To help enhance endocardial border definition, intravenous (IV) contrast agents are frequently used. The choice of stress echocardiography or MPI depends on the available facilities, local expertise, and considerations of cost-effectiveness.

## Coronary Angiography

Coronary angiography (also discussed in Chapter 7) is considered the "gold standard" for the diagnosis of CAD, although it is invasive and moderately expensive. Direct referral for diagnostic coronary angiography in patients with chest pain possibly due to myocardial ischemia is appropriate when noninvasive tests are contraindicated or likely to be inadequate. Patients with noninvasive tests that are abnormal but not clearly diagnostic often require clarification of an uncertain diagnosis by coronary angiography. In certain cases a second noninvasive test (imaging modality) may be recommended for a patient with a low likelihood of CAD but an intermediate-risk exercise treadmill result. Coronary angiography is likely to be most appropriate for patients with typical anginal symptoms and a high clinical probability of severe CAD or for individuals with *high-risk noninvasive tests*. In diabetic patients, the diagnosis of chronic stable angina can be particularly difficult because of the absence of characteristic symptoms of myocardial ischemia as a result of autonomic and sensory neuropathy. Thus, a lower threshold for coronary angiography is appropriate. The American College of Cardiology/American Heart Association (ACC/AHA) recommendations concerning the value of coronary angiography are listed in **Table 21-3**. Coronary luminal contrast angiography may underestimate coronary artery stenosis because of coronary artery remodeling in areas of atheroma, which demonstrate much more disease by intravascular ultrasound.

**TABLE 21-3.** Invasive Testing–Coronary Angiography Recommendations for Coronary Angiography to Establish a Diagnosis in Patients with Suspected Angina, Including Those with Known CAD Who have a Significant Change in Anginal Symptoms

**Class I[a]**
1. Patients with known or possible angina pectoris who have survived sudden cardiac death.

**Class IIa[b]**
1. Patients with an uncertain diagnosis after noninvasive testing in whom the benefit of a more certain diagnosis outweighs the risk and cost of coronary angiography.
2. Patients who cannot undergo noninvasive testing due to disability, illness, or morbid obesity.
3. Patients with an occupational requirement for a definitive diagnosis.
4. Patients who by virtue of young age at onset of symptoms, noninvasive imaging, or other clinical parameters are suspected of having a nonatherosclerotic cause of myocardial ischemia (coronary artery anomaly, Kawasaki disease, primary coronary artery dissection, radiation-induced vasculoplasty).
5. Patients in whom coronary artery spasm is suspected and provocative testing may be necessary.
6. Patients with a high pretest probability of left main or three-vessel CAD.

**Class IIb**
1. Patients with recurrent hospitalization for chest pain in whom a definite diagnosis is judged necessary.
2. Patients with an overriding desire for a definitive diagnosis and a greater than low probability of CAD.

**Class III[c]**
1. Patients with significant comorbidity in whom the risk of coronary arteriography outweighs the benefits of the procedure.
2. Patients with an overriding personal desire for a definitive diagnosis and a low probability of CAD.

[a]*Class I:* Conditions for which there is evidence and/or general agreement that a given procedure or treatment is useful and effective.

[b]*Class II:* Conditions for which there is conflicting evidence and/or a divergence of opinion about the usefulness/efficacy of a procedure or treatment.

*IIa:* Weight of evidence/opinion is in favor of usefulness/efficacy.

*IIb:* Usefulness/efficacy is less well established by evidence/opinion.

[c]*Class III:* Conditions for which there is evidence and/or general agreement that the procedure/treatment is not useful and in some cases may be harmful.

Data compiled from Gibbons RJ, Abrams J, Chatterjee K, et al., Guidelines for the management of patients with chronic stable angina: a report of the ACC/AHA Task Force on Practice Guidelines. *J Am Coll Cardiol*. 2007;50(23):2264-2274.

Fast computed tomography with calcium scoring is being used with increasing frequency for diagnosis and prognosis of coronary artery disease. The most recent ACCF/AHA guidelines suggest that calcium scoring may be useful in asymptomatic individuals found to be at low (6%-10 % risk of a cardiovascular event in 10 years) or intermediate (10%-20%) risk for coronary artery disease by the Framingham Score (level of evidence 2b and 2a, respectively)

## ■ PATHOPHYSIOLOGY

A disparity between the supply of coronary blood flow (CBF) and the metabolic demands of the myocardium ($MVO_2$) is the primary factor in ischemic heart disease. This imbalance may result in clinical manifestations of ischemia when myocardial demand exceeds the capacity of the coronary arteries to deliver an adequate supply of oxygen. In normal hearts there is an excess CBF reserve, so that ischemia does not occur even with very vigorous exercise. Atherosclerosis in the epicardial coronary arteries or in the coronary microvasculature may cause an imbalance between supply and demand at even modest levels of exercise. Heart rate, myocardial contractility, and systolic wall tension—which is related to LV systolic pressure and volume—are the major determinants of myocardial oxygen demand. Oxygen supply to the myocardium is dependent upon the oxygen-carrying capacity of blood and the CBF. Narrowing of the large coronary arteries transiently by vasospasm or permanently by obstructive lesions may increase the coronary resistance sufficiently to reduce CBF. Patients with coronary atherosclerosis also have endothelial dysfunction, which may manifest itself by a failure of the coronary vasculature to dilate in response to normal vasodilatory stimuli such as increased flow, exercise, tachycardia, acetylcholine, or cold pressor testing. Most patients with angina pectoris due to coronary atherosclerosis have *myocardial ischemia caused by both epicardial coronary obstruction and endothelial dysfunction* of both large and small vessels.

## ■ CIRCADIAN RHYTHM OF MYOCARDIAL ISCHEMIA

The prevalence of MI, unstable angina, variant angina, and silent ischemia is greatest in the morning, during the first few hours after awakening; the threshold for precipitating anginal attacks in patients with stable angina also appears to be lowest in the morning. The diurnal variation in ischemic threshold is attributed to the endogenous rhythms of catecholamine secretion and to the sensitivity to coronary vasoconstrictors, both of which appear to be highest in the morning. The increase in sympathetic nervous system activity is associated with increase in heart rate, blood pressure, contractility, and $MVO_2$. The lowered morning anginal threshold and the higher morning systolic blood pressure mandate early-morning use of antianginal and antihypertensive medications.

# RISK STRATIFICATION OF PATIENTS WITH CHRONIC ISCHEMIC HEART DISEASE

The prognosis for the patient with chronic artery disease is usually related to four patient factors. First, LV performance is the strongest predictor of long-term survival in patients with CAD, and the ejection fraction (EF) is the most often used measure of the presence and the degree of LV dysfunction. The second predictive factor is the anatomic extent and severity of atherosclerotic involvement of the coronary arteries. The number of stenosed coronary arteries is the most common measure of this factor. The third patient factor affecting prognosis is evidence of a recent coronary plaque rupture, indicating a much higher short-term risk for cardiac death or

**TABLE 21-4.** Noninvasive Risk Stratification

*High risk* (greater than 3% annual mortality rate)
1. Severe resting left ventricular dysfunction (LVEF < 35%).
2. High-risk treadmill score (score ≤ 11).[a]
3. Severe exercise left ventricular dysfunction (exercise LVEF < 35%).
4. Stress-induced large perfusion defects (particularly if anterior).
5. Stress-induced multiple perfusion defects of moderate size.
6. Large, fixed perfusion defect with LV dilation or increased lung uptake (thallium 201).
7. Stress-induced moderate perfusion defect with LV dilation or increased lung uptake (thallium 201).
8. Echocardiographic wall-motion abnormality (involving more than two segments) developing at low dose of dobutamine (≤ 10 mg/kg/min) or at a low heart rate (< 120 beats per minute).
9. Stress echocardiographic evidence of extensive ischemia.

*Intermediate risk* (1%-3% annual mortality rate)
1. Mild/moderate resting left ventricular dysfunction (LVEF = 35%-49%).
2. Intermediate-risk treadmill score (−11 < score < 5).
3. Stress-induced moderate perfusion defect without LV dilation or increased lung intake (thallium 201).
4. Limited stress echocardiographic ischemia with a wall motion abnormality only at higher doses of dobutamine involving less than or equal to two segments.

*Low risk* (less than 1% annual mortality rate)
1. Low-risk treadmill score (score ≥ 5).
2. Normal or small myocardial perfusion defect at rest or with stress.
3. Normal stress echocardiographic wall motion or no change of limited resting wall-motion abnormalities during stress.

[a]Duke Treadmill Score.

Data compiled from Gibbons RJ, Abrams J, Chatterjee K, et al., Guidelines for the management of patients with chronic stable angina: a report of the ACC/AHA Task Force on Practice Guidelines. *J Am Coll Cardiol*. 2007;50(23):2264-2274.

nonfatal MI. Worsening clinical symptoms with unstable features is an important clinical marker of a complicated plaque. The fourth prognostic factor is the patient's general health and noncoronary comorbidity. Risk stratification of patients with chronic stable angina by stress testing with exercise or pharmacologic agents has been shown to permit identification of groups of patients with low, intermediate, or high risk for subsequent cardiac events. Noninvasive test findings that identify high-risk patients are listed in **Table 21-4**. Patients identified as high risk are generally referred for coronary arteriography independent of their symptomatic status. The ACC/AHA Guidelines for Risk Stratification using Coronary Angiography in Patients with Stable Angina are listed in **Table 21-5**.

# ■ TREATMENT OF CHRONIC STABLE ANGINA

There are two major purposes in the treatment of stable angina. The first is to prevent MI and death and thereby *increase the quantity of life*. The second is to reduce symptoms of angina and the frequency and severity of ischemia, which should *improve the quality of life*. The choice of therapy often depends on the clinical response to initial medical therapy, although some patients (and many physicians) prefer coronary revascularization in situations where either may be successful.

**TABLE 21-5.** Recommendations for Coronary Angiography for Risk Stratification in Patients with Chronic Stable Angina

*Class I*
1. Patients with disabling (Canadian Cardiovascular Society [CCS] classes III and V) chronic stable angina despite medical therapy.
2. Patients with high-risk criteria on noninvasive testing regardless of anginal severity.
3. Patients with angina who have survived sudden cardiac death or serious ventricular arrhythmia.
4. Patients with angina and symptoms and signs of congestive heart failure.
5. Patients with clinical characteristics that indicate a high likelihood of severe CAD.

*Class IIa*
1. Patients with significant LV dysfunction (EF < 45%), CCS class I or II angina, and demonstrable ischemia but less than high-risk criteria on noninvasive testing.
2. Patients with inadequate prognostic information after noninvasive testing.

*Class IIb*
1. Patients with disabling CCS class I or II angina, preserved LV function (EF > 45%), and less than high-risk criteria on noninvasive testing.

*Class III*
1. Patients with disabling CCS classes I or II angina who respond to medical therapy and have no evidence of ischemia on noninvasive testing.
2. Patients who prefer to avoid revascularization.

See classes I to III as described in Table 22–4.

Data compiled from Gibbons RJ, Abrams J, Chatterjee K, et al., Guidelines for the management of patients with chronic stable angina: a report of the ACC/AHA Task Force on Practice Guidelines. *J Am Coll Cardiol*. 2007;50(23):2264-2274.

Patient education, cost-effectiveness, and patient preference are important components in this decision-making process.

# ■ GENERAL

Patients with angina pectoris due to coronary atherosclerosis should be evaluated for risk factors for coronary disease; whenever possible, these risk factors should be corrected. Tobacco in all forms should be avoided. Hypertension and diabetes should be well controlled. Ideal body weight should be achieved. A low-fat, low-cholesterol diet should be instituted, and a lipid profile determined.

# ■ ANTIPLATELET AGENTS

Aspirin, 80 to 325 mg/day, should be used routinely by all patients with acute and chronic ischemic heart disease with and without clinical symptoms in the absence of contraindications. In those who are unable to take aspirin, clopidogrel may be used. The efficacy of newer antiplatelet agents, such as glycoprotein IIb/IIIA inhibitors in the management of chronic stable angina has not been established.

# ■ LIPID-LOWERING AGENTS

Recent clinical studies have consistently demonstrated that lowering of low-density-lipoprotein (LDL) cholesterol with HMG-CoA reductase inhibitors (statins) can decrease the risk of adverse ischemic events in patients with established CAD. Thus, lipid-lowering therapy should be recommended even in the presence of mild to moderate elevations of LDL cholesterol in patients with chronic stable angina. Patients with ischemic heart disease should have LDL cholesterol levels below 100 mg/dL (2.6 mmol/L). It is now known that the statins have many favorable effects on endothelial function beyond decreasing LDL cholesterol levels and may reverse the endothelial response to chemical or physical stresses causing coronary vasoconstriction. Lowering of LDL cholesterol with statins has been shown by intravascular ultrasound to cause regression of atherosclerotic plaques in many coronary stenotic lesions.

## ■ NITROGLYCERIN AND NITRATES

The standard first-line therapy of angina remains sublingual nitroglycerin (NTG), which usually relieves the symptoms within 1 to 5 minutes NTG may be taken acutely either as a sublingual tablet (0.3-0.6 mg) or as an oral spray, each puff of which is calculated to deliver 0.4 mg. Monotherapy with sublingual or oral spray NTG is usually not satisfactory unless the episodes are rare.

The American College of Cardiology/AHA–ASIM Guidelines for chronic stable angina recommend long-acting beta-blockers and/or calcium antagonists in preference to long-acting nitrates in patients with recurrent angina (see Chapter 59). Nevertheless, long-acting nitrates are used prophylactically in many patients who have frequent episodes of angina. The many forms of nitrates include a slowly absorbed buccal capsule, a transdermal ointment or patch, and sublingual or oral forms that are absorbed more slowly. In general, it is important to start with a low dosage and to increase the dose progressively. The most common side effects are headache, dizziness, and postural hypotension. It should also be noted that the coadministration of long-acting nitrates and sildenafil (Viagra) significantly increases the risk of potentially life-threatening hypotension.

The *major problem* with long-term use of nitroglycerin and long-acting nitrates is the development of *nitrate tolerance*. For practical purposes, the administration of nitrates with an adequate nitrate-free interval (8-12 hours) appears to be the most effective method of preventing nitrate tolerance. For many patients, this can be from about 9 PM to 7 AM. Nitroglycerin ointments should be removed about 8 or 9 PM. Isosorbide dinitrate (ISDN; 10-60 mg) can be given orally in doses of 30 mg twice a day at 8 AM and 5 PM or three times a day at 8 AM, 1 PM, and 5 PM. Isosorbide mononitrate (ISMO), a metabolite of ISDN, is administered orally in 20-mg doses at 7 AM and 2 PM. An extended-release form of isosorbide mononitrate (IMDUR) can be taken orally as a single 60-mg dose at 7 or 8 AM. Patients who have angina at night may need either to plan the nitrate-free period for another time or to use a beta-blocker or calcium-channel blocker concurrently.

Patients should be instructed that if an anginal episode persists for more than 10 minutes despite their having taken three sublingual NTG tablets or an equivalent dose of NTG spray, they should report promptly to the nearest medical facility for further evaluation and management.

## ■ β-BLOCKERS

Beta-adrenergic blocking agents, which reduce heart rate and myocardial contractility both at rest and during exertion, are very effective in the management of patients with angina pectoris. Many beta-blockers are available. In general, long-acting cardioselective agents (eg, metoprolol) are preferred in patients who have a history of bronchospastic disease, diabetes mellitus, or peripheral vascular disease. However, it should be noted that even cardioselective beta-blockers can produce bronchospasm in some patients. All beta-blockers can worsen heart block or depress LV function and worsen heart failure. Fatigue, inability to perform exercise, lethargy, insomnia, nightmares, worsening claudication, and erectile dysfunction are other possible side effects.

In treating stable angina, it is essential that the dose of beta-blockers be adjusted to *lower the resting heart rate to 55 to 60* beats per minute. If discontinued, beta-blockers should be tapered over 3 to 10 days, when possible, to avoid a rebound worsening of angina pectoris.

## ■ CALCIUM ANTAGONISTS

Calcium-channel blockers decrease myocardial oxygen requirements by producing arterial dilation and often by reducing myocardial contractility. In addition, calcium-channel blockers produce coronary vasodilation and prevent coronary artery spasm. Drugs, such as verapamil and diltiazem also tend to reduce heart rate. Clinical trials comparing calcium antagonists and beta-blockers have demonstrated that calcium antagonists are as effective as beta-blockers in relieving angina and improving exercise time to onset of angina or ischemia. The calcium antagonists are also effective in reducing the incidence of angina in patients with vasospastic angina. In the International Multicenter Angina Exercises (Image Trial), combination therapy with metoprolol and nifedipine increased the exercise time to ischemia compared to either drug alone.

Thus, long-acting calcium antagonists, including slow-release and long-acting dihydropyridines (nifedipine and amlodipine) and nondihydropyridines (verapamil and diltiazem), should be used in combination with beta-blockers when initial treatment with beta-blockers is not successful or as a substitute for beta-blockers when initial treatment leads to unacceptable side effects. Calcium-channel blockers are the preferred agents in patients with a history of asthma, chronic obstructive pulmonary disease, or severe peripheral vascular disease. Combined therapy with a long-acting cardioselective beta-blocker and a long-acting dihydropyridine calcium-channel blocker is particularly beneficial. Some patients may benefit from triple therapy with a long-acting nitrate, a beta-blocker, and a calcium-channel blocker.

## ■ ANGIOTENSIN-CONVERTING ENZYME INHIBITORS

The potential cardiovascular protective effects of angiotensin-converting enzyme (ACE) inhibitors have been suspected for some time. As early as 1990, results from the Survival and Ventricular Enlargement (SAVE) and Studies of Left Ventricular Dysfunction (SOLVD) trials showed that ACE inhibitors reduced the incidence of recurrent MI and that this effect could not be attributed to the effect on blood pressure alone. At the same time, Alderman demonstrated that a high plasma renin level was associated with a significantly higher incidence of death from MI in patients with moderate hypertension and that this effect was independent of blood pressure level.

The results of the Heart Outcomes Prevention Evaluation (HOPE) trial now confirm that the use of the ACE inhibitor ramipril (10 mg/day) reduced cardiovascular death, MI, and stroke in patients who were at high risk for, or had, vascular disease in the absence of heart failure. The primary outcome in HOPE was a composite of cardiovascular death, MI, and stroke. However, the results of HOPE were so definitive that each of the components of the primary outcome by itself also showed statistical significance.

The Microalbuminuria, Cardiovascular, and Renal Outcomes (MICRO)-HOPE, a substudy of the HOPE study, has provided new clinical data on the cardiorenal therapeutic benefits of ACE inhibitor intervention in a broad range of middle-aged patients with diabetes mellitus who are at high risk for cardiovascular events.

ACE inhibitors should be used as routine secondary prevention for patients with known CAD, particularly in diabetics without severe renal disease.

## ■ POTENTIAL NEW ANTIANGINAL THERAPIES

Ranolazine is the first member of a new class of drugs believed to reduce angina by partially inhibiting fatty acid oxidation, thereby increasing glucose oxidation and generating more adenosine triphosphate (ATP) per molecule of oxygen consumed. In the Monotherapy Assessment of Ranolazine, a well-designed, well-conducted clinical trial in which patients were randomized to receive one of two doses of ranolazine or placebo showed that both doses of ranolazine were more effective than placebo at reducing symptoms and improving exercise capacity when added to conventional doses of atenolol, diltiazem, or amlodipine. This drug has been approved by the U.S. Food and Drug Administration for the treatment of angina refractory to other medical therapy.

# ■ MYOCARDIAL REVASCULARIZATION

Some patients with stable angina pectoris are candidates for revascularization, either with coronary artery bypass graft (CABG) surgery or with percutaneous coronary intervention (PCI). The two general indications for revascularization are (1) the presence of symptoms that are not acceptable to the patient, either because of restriction of physical activity and lifestyle or because of side effects from medications; or (2) the presence of coronary arteriographic findings indicating clearly that the patient would have a significantly better prognosis with revascularization than with medical therapy. In general, patients with stable angina should have objective evidence of myocardial ischemia prior to revascularization. Additional major considerations include the age of the patient, presence of other comorbid conditions, grade or class of angina experienced by the patient on maximal therapy, extent and severity of myocardial ischemia on noninvasive testing, degree of LV dysfunction, and distribution and severity of CAD.

In a recent clinical trial using revascularization and aggressive drug evaluation, which randomized 2287 patients to optimal medical therapy (OMT) versus OMT and PCI and which followed patients 4.6 years on average, there was no difference in the primary end point of MI, death, and stroke in these patients with moderate angina in these two treatment arms. These patients had stable angina, abnormal coronary arteriography, and rest- or stress-induced myocardial ischemia. They *did not* have acute coronary syndrome. Thus, patients with stable angina can be treated initially with modifiable risk factor reduction and antianginal medication for up to 3 years following OMT alone and later if necessary; about 30% will eventually require revascularization.

CABG provides good symptomatic relief for most patients who have suitable vessels. It is the treatment of choice for patients with severe CAD, including greater than 50% left main stenosis or three-vessel disease with impaired LV function. It is also indicated in severely symptomatic patients with two-vessel disease that includes a high-grade stenosis of the proximal left anterior descending artery and in patients in whom revascularization is indicated, but who have a lesion that is not amenable to PCI. Vein grafts have a failure rate that approaches 50% at 10 years. In contrast, internal mammary grafts have a superior patency and thus should be used whenever possible during the CABG. CABG plus optimal medical therapy in patients with chronic ischemic heart disease and heart failure has been shown to be of marginal incremental benefit to optimal medical therapy alone.

With the proliferation of various new debulking techniques, intracoronary stents, and drug-eluting stents, PCI can be successfully performed on a wide variety of native vessel and graft lesions. The advantages of PCI for the treatment of CAD include a low level of procedure-related morbidity and mortality, a short hospital stay, early return to activity, and the feasibility of multiple procedures. However, PCI is not possible for all patients; it is accompanied by a significant incidence of restenoses; and there is an occasional need for emergency CABG surgery. The recommendations of the ACC/AHA/ACP–ASIM Chronic Stable Angina Guidelines for revascularization with PCI or CABG in patients with stable angina are listed in **Table 21-6**.

It is important to remember that most patients with chronic angina have not been shown to have an increased survival rate with invasive treatment, but require invasive treatment mainly to control their symptoms.

**TABLE 21-6.** Revascularization for Chronic Stable Angina[a]

*Class I*
1. CABG for patients with significant left main coronary disease.
2. CABG for patients with three-vessel disease. The survival benefit is greater in patients with abnormal LV function (EF < 50%).
3. CABG for patients with two-vessel disease with significant proximal left anterior descending CAD and either abnormal LV function (EF < 50%) or demonstrable ischemia on noninvasive testing.
4. PCI for patients with two- or three-vessel disease with significant proximal left anterior descending CAD, who have anatomy suitable for catheter-based therapy, normal LV function, and no treated diabetes.
5. PCI or CABG for patients with one- or two-vessel disease CAD without significant proximal left anterior descending CAD but with a large area of viable myocardium and high-risk criteria on noninvasive testing.
6. CABG for patients with one- or two-vessel CAD without significant proximal left anterior descending CAD who have survived sudden cardiac death or sustained ventricular tachycardia.
7. In patients with prior PCI, CABG, or PCI for recurrent stenosis associated with a large area of viable myocardium or high-risk criteria on noninvasive testing.
8. PTCA[b] or CABG for patients who have not been successfully treated by medical therapy and can undergo revascularization with acceptable risk.

*Class IIa*
1. Repeat CABG for patients with multiple saphenous vein graft stenoses; especially when there is significant stenosis of a graft supplying the LAD, it may be appropriate to use PTCA for local saphenous vein graft lesions or multiple stenoses in poor candidates for reoperative surgery.
2. Use of PCI or CABG for patients with one- or two-vessel CAD without significant proximal LAD disease but with a moderate area of viable myocardium and demonstrable ischemia on noninvasive testing.
3. Use of PCI or CABG for patients with one-vessel disease with significant proximal LAD disease.

*Class IIb*
1. Compared with CABG, PCI for patients with two- or three-vessel disease with significant proximal left anterior descending CAD, who have anatomy suitable for catheter-based therapy, and who have treated diabetes or abnormal LV function.
2. Use of PCI for patients with significant left main coronary disease who are not candidates for CABG.
3. PCI for patients with one- or two-vessel disease CAD without significant proximal left anterior descending CAD who have survived sudden cardiac death or sustained ventricular tachycardia.

*Class III*
1. Use of PCI or CABG for patients with one- or two-vessel CAD without significant proximal left anterior descending CAD, who have mild symptoms that are unlikely due to myocardial ischemia or who have not received an adequate trial of medical therapy and (a) have only a small area of viable myocardium or (b) have no demonstrable ischemia on noninvasive testing.
2. Use of PCI or CABG for patients with borderline coronary stenoses (50%–60% diameter in locations other than the left main coronary artery) and no demonstrable ischemia on noninvasive testing.
3. Use of PCI or CABG for patients with insignificant coronary stenosis (< 50% diameter).
4. Use of PCI in patients with significant left main coronary disease who are candidates for CABG.

See classes I to III as described at bottom of Table 22-4 and Chapter 59.

CABG, coronary artery bypass graft; CAD, coronary artery disease; EF, ejection fraction; LAD, left anterior descending (coronary artery); LV, left ventricular; PCI, percutaneous coronary intervention; PTCA, percutaneous transluminal coronary angioplasty.

[a]Recommendations for revascularization with PTCA (or other catheter-based techniques) and CABG in patients with stable angina.

[b]PTCA is used in these recommendations to indicate PTCA or other catheter-based techniques, such as stents, atherectomy, and laser therapy.

# OTHER THERAPIES IN PATIENTS WITH REFRACTORY ANGINA

Evidence has emerged regarding the relative efficacy, or lack thereof, of a number of techniques for the management of refractory chronic angina pectoris. These techniques should be used only in patients who cannot be managed adequately by medical therapy and who are not candidates for revascularization (interventional and/or surgical) (see *Hurst's The Heart*, 13th Edition 2011).

## SUGGESTED READINGS

Maron BA, O'Gara PT. The evaluation and management of chronic ischemic heart disease. In: Fuster V, Walsh RA, Harrington RA, et al. *Hurst's The Heart*. 13th ed. New York, NY: McGraw-Hill; 2011;64:1472-1489.

Eagle KA, Guyton RA, Davidoff R, et al. ACC/AHA 2004 guideline update for coronary artery bypass graft surgery: a report of the American College of Cardiology/American Heart Association Task Force on Practice Guidelines (Committee to Update the 1999 Guidelines for Coronary Artery Bypass Graft Surgery). *J Am Coll Cardiol*. In press.

Gibbons RJ, Chatterjee K, Daley J, et al. American College of Cardiology/American Heart Association, American College of Physicians–American Society of Internal Medicine (ACC/AHA/ACP–ASIM) guidelines for the management of patients with chronic stable angina: a report of the ACC/AHA Task Force on Practice Guidelines (Committee on the Management of Patients with Chronic Stable Angina). *J Am Coll Cardiol*. 2003;41:160–168.

King SB, III, Smith SC, Hirshfeld JW, Jr, et al. 2007 Focused update of the ACC/AHA/SCAI 2005 guideline update for percutaneous coronary intervention: a report of the American College of Cardiology/American Heart Association Task Force on Practice Guidelines. *J Am Coll Cardiol*. 2008;51:172–209.

# CHAPTER 22
# DEFINITIONS AND PATHOGENESIS OF ACUTE CORONARY SYNDROMES

Michael C. Kim, Annapoorna S. Kini, and Valentin Fuster

Atherosclerosis represents a systemic disease involving the intima of large- and medium-sized arteries, including the aorta, carotid, coronary, and peripheral arterial systems. Now considered a chronic immunoinflammatory, fibroproliferative, lipid-driven, progressive process, atherosclerosis is the leading underlying mechanism for coronary heart disease (CHD). Widely accepted as the most common cause of death and disability in the United States, it is estimated that 40 million individuals live with CHD in the world today. CHD represents a continuum of disease pathologies and has been classified as chronic CHD, acute coronary syndromes, and sudden cardiac death. Acute coronary syndromes are a spectrum of ischemic myocardial events that range from unstable angina (UA) to non–ST-elevation myocardial infarction (NSTEMI) and ST-elevation myocardial infarction (STEMI). Although distinct in clinical presentation, they all share a similar pathophysiologic mechanism of vulnerable atherosclerotic plaque disruption with superimposed thrombus formation and subsequent degrees of antegrade coronary blood flow cessation with reduced myocardial oxygen supply. The thrombotic sequelae underlying this response are mainly the consequences of a multifactorial disease process triggered by endothelial injury followed then by a cascade of events that include a complex interplay of inflammation, cell signaling, immunomodulation, cellular proliferation, angiogenesis, vasoconstriction, and cell death. A comprehensive understanding of the pathogenesis of atherosclerosis and thrombosis as well as the clinical manifestations of acute coronary syndromes will ultimately assist the clinician in preventing, diagnosing, and treating this common and potentially fatal disease.

## PATHOGENESIS OF ATHEROTHROMBOSIS AND ACUTE CORONARY SYNDROMES

### ■ INFLAMMATION

Studies have indicated that there are certain vascular sites of predilection for atherosclerosis. These sites are classically characterized by areas of low sheer stress frequently found in arterial branches, bifurcations, and curvatures that predispose to turbulent blood flow. Interestingly, these changes in blood flow dynamics have been shown to locally upregulate the genetic expression of specific cellular adhesion molecules such as intercellular adhesion molecule (ICAM-1) and vascular cell adhesion molecule (VCAM-1) on the endothelium and circulating leukocytes. This process leads to the adherence, migration, and accumulation of monocytes

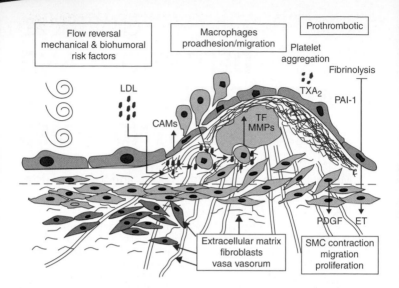

**FIGURE 22-1.** Schematic representation of atherosclerotic lesion progression. Initial blood flow dynamics in vulnerable areas of circulation promote upregulation of genes that promote cell adhesion. Endothelial activation by inflammatory cell response mediates LDL cholesterol migration through a more permeable endothelial surface. Macrophage foam cells and activated T cells release proteolytic enzymes, which soften the lipid core and increase the vulnerability for rupture. CAM, cell adhesion molecules; ET, endothelin; LDL, low-density lipoprotein; MMP, metalloproteinase; PAI-1, plasminogen activator inhibitor-1; PDGF, platelet-derived growth factor; SMC, smooth muscle cells; TF, tissue factor; TXA2, thromboxane $A_2$. (Reproduced with permission from Fuster V, Moreno PR, Fayad ZA, et al. Atherothrombosis and high-risk plaque. pt1: evolving concepts. *J Am Coll Cardiol.* 2005;46:937-954. Fig. 7. Elsevier, Inc.)

and T cells to the endothelium. Chemoattractants, such as monocyte chemotactic protein-1 (MCP-1), osteopontin, and modified low-density lipoprotein (LDL), are produced by the endothelium as well as monocytes and vascular smooth muscle cells and attract monocytes, macrophages, and T cells into the endothelium, which migrate through to the vessel wall. Further upregulation of cell adhesion molecules and receptors facilitates subendothelial recruitment of mononuclear cells within the arterial wall, which eventually helps to delineate a focal region of inflammation (**Fig. 22-1**).

# ■ ENDOTHELIAL ACTIVATION AND INFLAMMATION

Endothelial activation refers to a specific change in endothelial phenotype, characterized by an increase in endothelial–leukocyte-platelet adhesiveness and interactions, increased cell–cell permeability, a shift from an anticoagulant to a procoagulant milieu, and a change from a growth-inhibiting state to a growth-promoting state mediated through an elaborate cytokine release. An increasing body of evidence indicates an important role for reactive oxygen species (ROS)–mediated modulation of signal-transduction pathways in many of the processes involved in endothelial activation, and various factors have been found to contribute to ROS formation and endothelial activation, including many well-described cardiovascular risk factors (**Table 22-1**). Specifically, elevated LDL cholesterol, elevated very-low-density

**TABLE 22-1.** Endothelial Activation/Dysfunction in Atherosclerosis

Phenotypic features
1. Reduced vasodilator and increased vasoconstrictor capacity
2. Enhanced oxidant stress with increased inactivation of nitric oxide
3. Increased expression of endothelin
Enhanced leukocyte molecule expression (ICAM, VCAM)
Increased chemotactic molecule expression (MCP-11, IL-8)
Increased prothrombotic and reduced fibrinolytic phenotype
Increased growth-promoting phenotype
Factors contributing to endothelial activation/dysfunction
1. Dyslipidemia and atherogenic lipoprotein modification, elevated LDL, VLDL, Lp(a)
2. LDL modification (oxidation, glycation)
3. Reduced HDL
4. Increased angiotensin II and hypertension
5. Insulin resistance
6. Estrogen deficiency
7. Smoking
8. Hyperhomocysteninemia
9. Advancing age
10. Infection

lipoprotein (VLDL), low concentrations of high-density lipoprotein (HDL), and reactive oxygen species caused by hypertension, cigarette smoking, diabetes mellitus, estrogen deficiency, and advancing age have all been linked to endothelial activation and injury.

In a nonathrogenic state, locally produced nitric oxide (NO) normally acts as a local vasodilator through the vascular smooth muscle cells (VSMC) and can additionally inhibit platelet aggregation. However, in the setting of endothelial dysfunction, a paradoxical response to NO is observed in large vessels and the microcirculation, leading instead to a vasoconstrictive response. This paradoxical response and an actual reduction in NO release and prostaglandin (PGI2) synthesis together act to facilitate the permeability of lipids into subendothelial spaces.

Oxidized LDL cholesterol is a major contributor to endothelial dysfunction. Influx and retention of these and other athrogenic lipoproteins in the arterial intima constitutes the central pathogenic process in atherogenesis. Once LDL cholesterol becomes internalized through the activated vascular endothelium and into the vessel wall, it is taken up by resident macrophages and activated foam cells. Modified LDL cholesterol is also chemotactic for other monocytes through a monocyte-derived chemotactic protein (MCP-1), thereby expanding the inflammatory response and precipitating proliferation of smooth muscle cells and fibroblasts—a process that results in thickening of the arterial wall.

By continually multiplying in the focal lesion, monocyte-derived activated macrophages and lymphocytes release proteolytic enzymes, metalloproteinases, hydrolytic enzymes, cytokines, and growth factors that can cause focal necrosis, thereby slowly creating an enlarging necrotic lipid core surrounded by a fibrous cap. T-cell activation that follows antigen presentation by macrophages further enhances the inflammatory response by releasing interferon-$\gamma$ and TNF-$\alpha$ and -$\beta$. It has been suggested that the intricate inflammatory regulation and maladaptive functions of the resident macrophages in atheromatous plaques is orchestrated by CD40 ligand that is expressed on macrophages, T cells, endothelial cells, and smooth muscle cells.

In fact, the central role of CD40 ligand in atherosclerosis is further supported by the observation of antiathrogenic effects CD40-blocking antibodies have in murine models of atherosclerosis.

Angiogenesis or neovascularization also plays a pivotal role in the atheroma-forming process and may further contribute to plaque progression. By providing a direct conduit and source for inflammatory cell recruitment into the vessel wall, extracellular cholesterol deposits into the lipid core and a potential source for intraplaque hemorrhage, neovascularization contributes to plaque destabilization increased vulnerability.

# ■ PLAQUE RUPTURE AND THROMBOSIS

Uneven thinning, weakening, and rupture of the fibrous cap usually occur at the shoulder regions of lesions, as this is an area that is the site of T-cell and macrophage accumulation, activation, and apoptosis. The release of matrix-degrading proteinases such as the matrix metalloproteinases (MMPs) weakens the vulnerable, already thinned fibrous cap. This in combination with apoptosis of vascular smooth muscle cells eventually exposes tissue factor (TF) that is abundant in the atheroma in macrophages to circulating blood. Upon contact of TF with the circulating blood, the extrinsic coagulation cascade is initiated and the formation of prothrombin (factor II) and thrombin (factor IIa) ensues. A potent platelet activator, thrombin formation along with fibrin creates the obstruction that ultimately diminishes antegrade blood flow (**Fig. 22-2**).

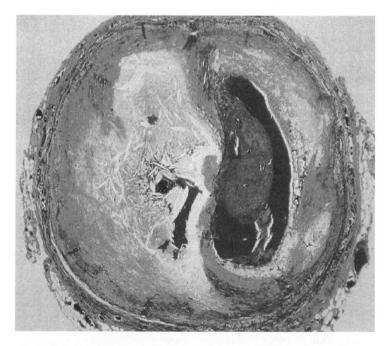

**FIGURE 22-2.** Plaque rupture. Cross-section of a coronary artery delineating atherosclerotic plaue rupture with a nonocclusive intracoronary thrombus.

# ■ CELLULAR MECHANISMS OF THROMBUS FORMATION

As a consequence of plaque rupture, platelets progress through a sequence of stages leading to adhesion, activation, and aggregation all in a fashion to contain the damaged endothelium via a platelet plug. Platelets adhere to the ruptured plaque core through interactions with exposed TF. TF, in turn, has a potent effect on further activating platelets. The circulating von Willebrand factor (vWF) is capable of binding exposed collagen in the plaque and glycoprotein (GP) receptors in the platelet membrane. Platelet activation results from the action of numerous agonists that bind to the platelet membrane and initiate intracellular signaling. These platelet agonists include 5-hydroxytryptamine (5-HT), epinephrine, adenosine diphosphate (ADP), and arachadonic acid (AA). Once activated, platelets continue to secrete agonists from dense granules, prompting further activation of platelets and culminating in the formation of a platelet plug that provides a surface for coagulation cascades. At the same time, activated platelets synthesize thromboxane ($TXA_2$), which is a potent platelet activator and vasoconstrictor. These processes occur in the environment of the atherosclerotic plaque lesion as a developing thrombus if formed.

The efficiency of the platelet response and recruitment is largely dependent on both local as well as systemic factors that mediate the magnitude of thrombus formation. Local factors include the severity of the arterial wall damage. It is believed that when the initial injury is limited, the thrombogenic response is limited when compared to a deep ulcerated plaque rupture that precipitates a more robust thrombus formation. In addition, the platelet response depends in part on the geometric changes the ruptured plaque assumes.

Systemic influences associated with an increased blood thrombogenicity include cardiovascular risk factors (diabetes mellitus, smoking, catecholamines, elevated LDL, decreased HDL). This is supported by the observation that in approximately one-third of cases of acute coronary syndrome (ACS), there is no disruption of lipid-rich plaque, but only superficial erosion of small nonstenosis plaque. It is interesting to note that these plaques usually go undetected by standard angiography.

In addition to platelet aggregation on the injured endothelium, the clotting mechanism is similarly activated by expose of the plaque components to flowing blood. Through various pathways, the coagulation cascade generates thrombin, which catalyzes the formation of fibrin from fibrinogen. As well as possessing potent platelet agonist properties, fibrin acts to stabilize the platelet thrombus by forming a mesh network across the injured area.

Increased knowledge of both the complex platelet activation and aggregation pathways as well as the coagulation cascades has created numerous targets for potential pharmacologic therapies aimed at diminishing or eliminating the response to endothelial injury. These therapies are categorized as fibrinolytic agents, intrinsic coagulation cascade inhibitors (warfarin, direct thrombin inhibitors), and antiplatelet agents (aspirin and clopidogrel).

# DEFINITIONS OF ACUTE CORONARY SYNDROMES

The clinical manifestation of a platelet-rich thrombus in a coronary artery is the development of an acute coronary syndrome (ACS). Acute coronary syndromes have a common end result: acute myocardial ischemia that has been shown to be associated with an increased risk of cardiac death and myonecrosis. The term ACS encompasses acute myocardial infarction with resultant ST-segment elevation or non–ST-segment elevation and unstable angina (**Fig. 22-3**). Efficient and timely triage of patients with ACS is essential given the life-threatening nature of the disease processes and the proven benefit that both medical and mechanical therapies provide. In the setting of more sensitive and specific serologic markers, imaging techniques, and pathologic

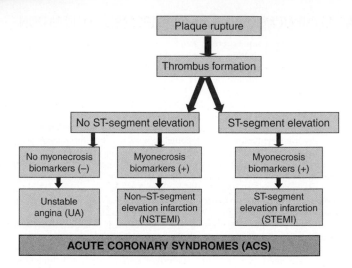

**FIGURE 22-3.** The development of atherosclerotic plaque rupture and the consequent clinical manifestations of acute coronary syndromes (ACS).

characteristics, the European Society of Cardiology (ESC) and the American College of Cardiology (ACC) in 2000 reexamined the definition of myocardial infarction to provide for a more universal definition. A recently published revision in 2008 further qualified infarct size, circumstances leading up to the infarct, and the timing of the necrosis relative to the time of the observation (**Table 22-2**).

# ■ UNSTABLE ANGINA

Unstable angina (UA) characteristically originates from a nonocclusive thrombus without any evidence of myocardial necrosis. Given the subjective nature of angina pectoris, many classification schemes have been developed for unstable angina. For example, the Canadian Cardiovascular Society (CCS) rates anginal symptoms with level of activity. By categorizing the severity and clinical circumstances in which angina occurs, Braunwald further classified unstable angina in 1989 as a means of providing a more uniform working definition of the syndrome in addition to obtaining valuable prognostic and diagnostic information of this common and potentially fatal symptom.

Braunwald's classification of angina has been linked to risk of death or myocardial infarction at 1 year. The Agency for Health Care Policy and Research (AHCPR) has published guidelines that assess short-term risks of death or nonfatal myocardial infarction in patients with unstable angina.

There are other causes that may lead to acute coronary ischemia. For example, dynamic obstruction of Printzmetal's angina occurs in epicardial arteries commonly in the setting of endothelial dysfunction with an imbalance of vasoconstrictive properties. Coronary restenosis after percutaneous coronary intervention is also a mechanism of myocardial ischemia. This process is largely due to cellular proliferation and does not involve thrombus formation or spasm. Lastly, any condition that worsens cardiac myocardial oxygen supply in the setting of high demands such as fever or anemia in a patient with chronic coronary artery disease can also be a mechanism of myocardial ischemia.

**TABLE 22-2.** Clinical Classification of Different Types of Myocardial Infarction

Type 1
Spontaneous myocardial infarction related to ischemia due to a primary coronary event such as plaque erosion and/or rupture, fissuring, or dissection.

Type 2
Myocardial infarction secondary to ischemia due to either increased oxygen demand or decreased supply—eg, coronary spasm, coronary embolism, anemia, arrhythmias, hypertension, or hypotension.

Type 3
Sudden unexpected cardiac death, including cardiac arrest, often with symptoms suggestive of myocardial ischemia, accompanied by presumably new ST elevation, or new LBBB, or evidence of fresh thrombus in a coronary artery by angiography and/or autopsy, but death occurring before blood samples could be obtained, or at a time before the appearance of cardiac biomarkers in the blood.

Type 4a
Myocardial infarction associated with PCI.

Type 4b
Myocardial infarction associated with stent thrombosis as documented by angiography at autopsy.

Type 5
Myocardial infarction associated with CABG.

Adapted from ESC/ACCF/AHA/WHF Expert Consensus Document. Reproduced with permission from Thygesen K, Alpert J, White HD. Universal definition of myocardial infarction. *J Am Coll Cardiol.* 2007;50:2173-2195.

# ■ NON–ST-SEGMENT ELEVATION MYOCARDIAL INFARCTION

Those patients with acute ischemic chest pain without electrocardiographic evidence of ST-segment elevation or Q waves, but with ischemia severe enough to cause significant myocardial damage by evidence of myocardial necrosis, represent non–ST-segment elevation myocardial infarction. Current markers for myocardial injury include creatinine kinase (CK), CK-MB isoforms, and troponin (**Fig. 22-4**). CK is very sensitive for detecting myocardial damage and has been shown to be related to the degree of infracted myocardium. Initially elevated 4 to 8 hours after myocardial insult, CK measurement provides a valuable tool for assessing acute or subacute angina. However, noncardiac elevation of CK precludes the sole utilization of this enzyme.

Methods to increase the specificity of CK include measurements of CK-MB levels by immunoassay. CK-MB isoforms exist as only 1 form in cardiac muscle (CK-MB2), but do exist as different forms in the blood (CK-MB1). A ratio of CK-MB2 to CK-MB1 of greater than 2.5 has significantly improved the sensitivity of detecting myonecrosis within 6 hours.

The troponin complex consists of 3 subunits (TnI, TnT, and TnC) that act to regulate cardiac muscle contraction. Monoclonal antibody-based immunoassays have been developed to specifically detect cardiac TnT and TnI. As a consequence of the heightened sensitivity and specificity of cardiac troponins when compared to CK, it has been shown that up to 30% of patients with negative CK-MB levels are reclassified as having a NSTEMI with a positive troponin.

The level of troponin release has been linked to prognosis, and the higher the level, the higher risk for death or nonfatal myocardial infarction at 30 days. Regardless of

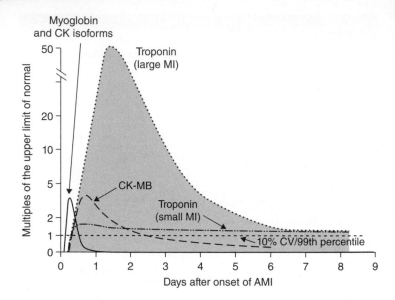

**FIGURE 22-4.** Timing and release of various biomarkers after acute ischemic myocardial infarction. (Reproduced with permission from Anderson JL, Adams CD, Antman EM, et al: ACC/AHA 2007 guidelines for the management of patients with unstable angina/non ST-elevation myocardial infarction: a report of the American College of Cardiology/American Heart Association Task Force on Practice Guidelines (Writing Committee to Revise the 2002 Guidelines for the Management of Patients With Unstable Angina/Non ST-Elevation Myocardial Infarction): developed in collaboration with the American College of Emergency Physicians, the Society for Cardiovascular Angiography and Interventions, and the Society of Thoracic Surgeons: endorsed by the American Association of Cardiovascular and Pulmonary Rehabilitation and the Society for Academic Emergency Medicine, Circulation 2007:Aug 14;116(7):e148-304.)

the cause of elevation, it has been shown that troponin elevation represents an increased risk of death when compared to those patients without troponin elevation.

Troponin measurement early in the evaluation of a patient with angina is essential as there is evidence from randomized controlled trials showing the benefit of administration of glycoprotein IIb/IIIa inhibition to those patients with elevated troponin levels. Furthermore, early angiography with mechanical revascularization has been shown to be superior to medical therapy in patients with NSTEMI and troponin release. Within the first 6 hours of symptom onset, CK-MB isoforms and myoglobin were most efficient for the diagnosis of NSTEMI, and troponin elevation was most useful for the late diagnosis of myocardial infarction as troponin levels remain elevated for 7 days.

# ■ ST-SEGMENT ELEVATION MYOCARDIAL INFARCTION

Considered the form of ACS with the highest mortality, ST-elevation myocardial infarction is manifested as an occlusive atherothrombosis followed by complete cessation of antegrade myocardial blood flow with subsequent ST-segment elevation on the surface electrocardiogram (ECG). Approximately 500 000 STEMIs occur each year in the United States, but there has been a steady decline in the mortality rates of this disease largely due to decreased a fatality with early reperfusion. The accurate diagnosis of STEMI is important, as its presence mandates immediate consideration for reperfusion therapy via thrombolytic agents or mechanically with percutaneous intervention. The World Health Organization criteria for an acute myocardial infarction require that 2 of the following 3 elements be present: (1) a history suggestive of coronary ischemia for a prolonged period of time (>30 minutes), (2) evolutionary changes on serial ECGs suggestive of myocardial infarction, and (3) a rise and fall in serum cardiac markers that is consistent with myonecrosis. The 2004 ACC/AHA STEMI guidelines emphasize the importance of establishing regionalization of STEMI care facilities in an effort to reduce both the mortality and morbidity of this disease.

## CONCLUSION

Atherosclerosis is a systemic disease that is initiated by endothelial injury by various mechanisms that produce a cascade of localized inflammation, lipid influx, and cellular proliferation that culminates in weakening of the atherosclerotic plaque. Platelet adherence, activation, and aggregation begin the process of localized hemostasis, but this soon develops into a maladaptive response with the formation of intraluminal thrombus and obstruction of coronary blood flow. ACS is the clinical manifestation of a platelet-rich thrombus developing in a coronary artery. By accurately diagnosing each patient as having unstable angina, NSTEMI, or STEMI with clinical acumen, ECG, and serum biomarkers, clinicians are now able to rapidly treat this potentially fatal disease.

## SUGGESTED READINGS

Kim M, Kini A, Fuster V. Definitions of acute coronary syndromes. In: Fuster V, Walsh RA, Harrington RA, et al. *Hurst's The Heart*. 13th ed. New York, NY: McGraw-Hill; 2011;56: 1287-1295.

Braunwald E. Application of current guidelines to the management of unstable angina and non-ST-elevation myocardial infarction. *Circulation*. 2003;108(suppl 1):III28-III37.

Falk E, Fuster V. Atherothrombosis: disease burden, activity, and vulnerability. In: Fuster V, Walsh RA, Harrington RA, et al. *Hurst's The Heart*. 13th ed. New York, NY: McGraw-Hill; 2011;52:1215-1223.

Fuster V, Badimon L, Badimon JJ, et al. The pathogenesis of coronary artery disease and the acute coronary syndromes. Part 1. *N Engl J Med*. 1992;326:242-250.

Fuster V, Moreno PR, Fayad ZA, et al. Atherothrombosis and high-risk plaque. Part 1: evolving concepts. *J Am Coll Cardiol*. 2005;46:937-954.

Libby P. Inflammation in atherosclerosis. *Nature*. 2002;420:868-874.

Thygesen K, Alpert J, White HD. Universal definition of myocardial infarction. *J Am Coll Cardiol*. 2007;50:2173-2195.

# CHAPTER 23
# DIAGNOSIS AND MANAGEMENT OF PATIENTS WITH ST-SEGMENT ELEVATION MYOCARDIAL INFARCTION

Emily E. Hass, Eric H. Yang, Bernard J. Gersh, and Robert A. O'Rourke[†]

## EPIDEMIOLOGY

Approximately 935 000 Americans suffer from an acute myocardial infarction (AMI) per year, one-third of whom are caused by an acute ST-segment elevation myocardial infarction (STEMI). The incidence of AMI declined from 244 per 100 000 population in 1975 to 162 per 100 000 population in 2006. The in-hospital mortality rate also declined from 18% in 1975 to 10% in 2006. Nonetheless, AMI continues to be a serious public health problem. It has been estimated that 15-year period of life is lost secondary to an AMI, and the cost to American society (both direct and indirect) is $165.4 billion per year.

## DIAGNOSIS AND SYMPTOMS

The classic symptom of AMI is precordial or retrosternal discomfort that is commonly described as a pressure, crushing, aching, or burning sensation. Radiation of the discomfort to the neck, back, or arms frequently occurs, and the pain is usually persistent. The discomfort typically achieves maximum intensity over several minutes and can be associated with nausea, diaphoresis, generalized weakness, and a fear of impending death. Some patients, particularly the elderly, may also present with syncope, unexplained nausea and vomiting, acute confusion, agitation, or palpitations.

Approximately 20% of AMI patients are asymptomatic or have atypical symptoms. Painless myocardial infarction (MI) occurs more frequently in the elderly, women, diabetics, and postoperative patients. These patients tend to present with dyspnea or frank congestive heart failure as their initial symptom.

---

[†]Deceased.

# PHYSICAL EXAMINATION

Patients can appear anxious and uncomfortable. Those with substantial left ventricular (LV) dysfunction at presentation may have tachycardia, pulmonary rales, tachypnea, and a third heart sound. The presence of a mitral regurgitant murmur suggests ischemic dysfunction of the mitral valve apparatus, rupture, or ventricular remodeling.

In patients with right ventricular infarction, increased jugular venous pressure, Kussmaul sign, and a right ventricular third sound may be present. Such patients virtually always have inferior infarctions, usually without evidence of left-heart failure. They are exquisitely sensitive to hypovolemiia and venodilation. Nitrates are contraindicated in such patients. In patients with extensive left ventricular dysfunction, shock is indicated by hypotension, diaphoresis, cool skin and extremities, pallor, oliguria, and possible confusion.

## ■ ELECTROCARDIOGRAM

All patients presenting with chest pain should have an electrocardiogram (ECG) performed within 10 minutes of arrival to the emergency department. The classic initial ECG manifestations of STEMI, discussed in Chapter 2, involve an increase in the amplitude of the T wave (peaking), followed within minutes by ST-segment elevation. The R wave may initially increase in height but soon decreases, and often Q waves form. If the jeopardized myocardium is reperfused, the ST segment may promptly revert to normal, although T waves can remain inverted, and Q waves may or may not regress. Persistent ST-segment elevation after restoration of flow in the epicardial coronary artery is a marker of failed myocardial perfusion and associated with an adverse prognosis. In the absence of reperfusion, the ST segment gradually returns to baseline in several hours to days, and T waves become symmetrically inverted. Failure of the T wave to invert in 24 to 48 hours suggest regional pericarditis.

*New-onset left bundle-branch block (LBBB) in the setting of chest pain is considered STEMI.* The diagnosis of STEMI in the setting of old LBBB can be difficult. Findings suggesting STEMI include (1) ST-segment elevation ≥1 mm concordant with the QRS complex; (2) ST-segment depression ≥1 mm in leads $V_1$, $V_2$, or $V_3$; and (3) ST-segment elevation ≥5 mm discordant with the QRS.

The ECG has several limitations (Chapter 2), which relate to specificity and sensitivity.

# LABORATORY STUDIES

## Myoglobin

Myoglobin is a 17.8-kd protein that is released from injured myocardial cells. As shown in **Fig. 23-1**, myoglobin release occurs within hours after the onset of infarction, reaches peak levels at 1 to 4 hours, and remains elevated for about 24 hours. Although the rapid rise allows for its use as an early marker for STEMI, myoglobin is not specific to myocardial cells and should not be used in isolation as a method for diagnosing MI.

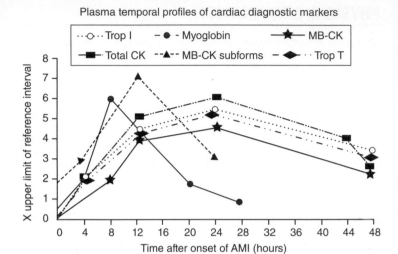

**FIGURE 23-1.** Temporal profile of the diagnostic biomarkers used for detecting MI. The plasma temporal profile for early detection is illustrated for myoglobin and CK-MB subforms. The markers CK-MB, total CK, and cardiac troponins I and T are all released with a similar initial time profile. However, troponins I and T remain elevated for 10 to 14 days and thus are better markers for late diagnosis than CK-MB.

## CK-MB

The MB isoenzyme of creatine kinase is present in the largest concentration in the myocardium, although small amounts (1%-2%) can be found in skeletal muscle, tongue, small intestine, and diaphragm. Creatinine kinase-MB (CK-MB) appears in serum within 3 hours after the onset of infarction, reaches peak levels at 12 to 24 hours, and has a mean duration of activity of 1 to 3 days. Other cardiac but non-AMI etiologies of increased CK-MB levels can occur after cardioversion, cardiac surgery, myopericarditis, percutaneous coronary intervention (PCI), and occasionally after rapid tachycardia. Noncardiac causes of increased CK-MB levels may occur with hypothyroidism, extensive skeletal muscle trauma, rhabdomyolysis, and muscular dystrophy.

Occasionally, the concentration of creatinine kinase-MB (CK-MB) isoenzyme may be increased in the presence of normal total levels of CK enzyme. This finding usually indicates a small amount of myocardial necrosis in a patient whose baseline total CK enzyme level is at the low-normal end of the range (see Chapter 24).

## Troponins

The cardiac troponins regulate the interaction of actin and myosin and are more cardiac specific than CK-MB. Two isoforms of cardiac troponin: T and I are used as biomarkers. Their levels start to rise 3 to 12 hours after the onset of ischemia, peak at 12 to 24 hours, and may remain elevated for 8 to 21 days (troponin T) or 7 to 14 days (troponin I). Elevated troponin levels correlate with pathologically proven myocardial necrosis and indicate poor prognosis in patients with suspected acute coronary syndromes (see Chapter 24).

# INITIAL MANAGEMENT

## ■ EVALUATION IN THE EMERGENCY DEPARTMENT

The cornerstone of STEMI therapy is a rapid and accurate evaluation in the emergency department. All patients presenting with complaints of chest discomfort should be rapidly triaged and allowed to bypass the emergency department waiting room. *An ECG should be obtained within the first 10 minutes of arrival and a focused history and physical examination assessing the symptoms and signs described in the diagnosis section of this chapter should be quickly performed.*

The physical examination also provides a method for the risk stratification of STEMI patients. As shown in **Table 23-1**, the Killip classification can be used as method to stratify patients and predict clinical outcomes.

# INITIAL THERAPY

The initial management of patients in the emergency department includes the use of oxygen, aspirin, β-blockers, analgesia, nitroglycerin, and anticoagulation with heparin (**Table 23-2**).

## Oxygen

Although routine use of supplemental oxygen is common practice, hard evidence supporting its use is lacking. Low-flow oxygen therapy delivered by nasal cannula should be routinely given during the first 24 to 48 hours in most STEMI patients. Mild hypoxemia is not uncommon, even in the absence of apparent pulmonary congestion. Additionally, some patients may have dyspnea related to acute changes in left ventricular compliance and secondarily increased pulmonary interstitial fluid.

## Aspirin

Aspirin is an antiplatelet agent that has been shown to decrease mortality in AMI patients by about 20%. It should be administered as early as possible and continued indefinitely in patients with acute coronary syndromes. Chewable aspirin 160 to 325 mg should be given to patients at presentation, with a subsequent dose of 75 to 325 mg daily. For those with a history of a documented significant adverse reaction to aspirin, 300 mg of clopidogrel can be used as an alternative.

**TABLE 23-1.** Killip Classification for Patients With STEMI

| Killip Class | Hospital Mortality (%) |
|---|---|
| I. No CHF | 6 |
| II. Mild CHF, rales, $S_3$, congestion on chest radiograph | 17 |
| III. Pulmonary edema | 38 |
| IV. Cardiogenic shock | 81[a] |

CHF, congestive heart failure.

[a]Has improved to about 60% with current therapy.

**TABLE 23-2.** Initial Management of STEMI

| Treatment | Dose | Notes |
|---|---|---|
| Oxygen | 1-2 L | Use for first 24-48 h |
| Aspirin | 160-325 mg chewable | If aspirin allergy exists, use clopidogrel 300 mg |
| β-blockers | Metoprolol 5 mg IV every 5 min for max 15 mg, then oral | Do not use if there are signs of heart failure of cardiogenic shock |
| Morphine | 1-2 mg IV | Do not oversedate patient |
| Nitroglycerin | Start drip at 5-10 μg/min and titrate to pain and blood pressure | Do not use in patients with recent use of a phosphodi esterase type 5 inhibitor (Viagara, etc) or suspected RV infarct |
| Heparin | Unfractionated: 60 U/kg IV bolus (4000 U max) followed by 12 U/kg/h drip (max 100 U/h) Low molecular weight: enoxaparin 30 mg IV bolus then 1 mg/kg SQ every 12 h | Unfractionated heparin should be favored in patients undergoing primary PCI and those with severe renal dysfunction |

## β-Blockers

The efficacy of β-blockers in acute coronary syndromes has been documented with a decrease in early and late mortality. In pooled data from 28 trials of β-blockers, the average mortality decrease was 28% at 1 week, with the majority of benefit occurring in the first 48 hours. Specifically, reinfarction was reduced by 18% and cardiac arrest by 15%. The long-term effects of β-blockade for the secondary prevention of death after MI have also been established by large-scale randomized trials.

Traditionally, metoprolol has been the agent of choice and is initially administered intravenously as 5-mg boluses at 10-minute intervals for 3 doses followed by an oral dose. However, in patients with clinical evidence of heart failure, there is a 30% relative increase in the risk of cardiogenic shock. *Therefore, the use of β-blockade in patients with evidence of hemodynamic instability should be delayed until the patients become stable.* Also, the routine initial intravenous dose should be reconsidered as standard therapy. Finally, the benefits of β-blockade in patients undergoing primary PCI remain unclear and there have been no randomized prospective studies.

## Analgesia

Morphine is frequently used for pain relief and is best administered intravenously in boluses of 1 to 2 mg, to a maximum of 10 to 15 mg for a normal adult. Respiratory depression can occur and care must be taken not to oversedate patients. Morphine should be used with caution in patients with hemodynamic instability because of its effects on reducing cardiac preload.

## Nitrates

Nitroglycerin causes a nonendothelium-dependent coronary vasodilatation, systemic venodilatation, reduced cardiac preload, and enhanced perfusion of ischemic myocardial zones. Intravenous nitroglycerin is effective in relieving chest pain and should be initiated at 5 to 10 μg/min and gradually increased with a goal of a 10%

to 30% reduction in systolic blood pressure and symptomatic pain relief. In most patients, use of this agent will be tapered within 24 to 36 hours. Nitrates should not be administered to patients with recent sildenafil use. In addition, nitrates should be used with caution in RV infarct patients in order to avoid profound hypotension.

## Heparin

Anticoagulation with heparin is essential in the management of STEMI. Currently 2 forms of heparin are utilized: unfractionated heparin and low-molecular-weight heparin (LMWH).

Unfractionated heparin, when bound to antithrombin III, inactivates factor Xa and thrombin. Its use has been widely studied and unfractionated heparin is considered a class I (see Chapter 57) indication for patients with STEMI undergoing primary PCI or receiving fibrin-specific thrombolytic agents. An initial bolus of 60 U/kg (4000 U maximum) followed by a 12-U/kg/h (1000 U/h maximum) infusion should be administered promptly. A goal aPTT of 1.5 to 2.0 times normal should be achieved. The LMWHs are glycosaminoglycans consisting of chains of alternating residues of D-glucosamine and uronic acid. When compared to unfractionated heparin, they have a more predictable anticoagulation effect due to a longer half-life, better bioavailability, and dose-independent clearance. The LMWHs have a greater activity against Xa than thrombin and their anticoagulation effect cannot be measured with standard laboratory tests.

The use of the LMWH enoxaparin in conjunction with thrombolysis has been studied in the ASSENT 3 (Assessment of the Safety and Efficacy of a New Thrombolytic regimen) and TIMI-25 EXTRACT (Enoxaparin and Thrombolysis Reperfusion for Acute Myocardial Infarction Treatment) trials. In the ASSENT 3 trial, patients treated with enoxaparin plus tenecteplase had a lower combined end point of 30-day mortality, in-hospital reinfarction, and in-hospital refractory ischemia than those treated with unfractionated heparin plus tenecteplase (11.4% vs 15.4 %, $p = 0.0002$). The TIMI 25 EXTRACT trial randomized 20 506 patients undergoing thrombolytic therapy for STEMI to anticoagulation with enoxaparin through the entire index hospitalization or unfractionated heparin for the initial 48 hours. The combined primary end point of death or recurrent MI at 30 days occurred in 9.9% of patients in the enoxaparin group and in 12% of those in the heparin group ($p < 0.001$).

Because of the delay in the onset of action of subcutaneous administration, an initial intravenous loading dose of 30 mg of enoxaparin followed by the traditional 1 mg/kg subcutaneous dose every 12 hours was used in both trials for patients younger than 75 years.

## Direct Thrombin Inhibitors

*Direct thrombin inhibitors bind directly to thrombin and should be used as an alternative to heparin in patients with known or suspected heparin-induced thrombocytopenia.* A recent meta-analysis of 11 randomized trials demonstrated that compared with heparin, direct thrombin inhibitors were associated with a lower risk of death or MI both at the end of treatment (4.3% vs 5.1%, $p = 0.001$) and at 30 days (7.4% vs 8.2%, $p = 0.02$). This difference was primarily due to a reduction in the incidence of reinfarction (2.8% vs 3.5%, $p <0.001$) with *no difference in mortality*. There was no excess in intracranial hemorrhage with any direct thrombin inhibitor.

# REPERFUSION STRATEGIES

Rapid reperfusion of ischemic myocardium is the main goal of STEMI management. Currently, the 3 main reperfusion strategies for STEMI are thrombolytic therapy, primary PCI, and thrombolytic facilitated PCI.

# ■ THROMBOLYTICS

Thrombolytic therapy for STEMI has been shown to be effective in reducing mortality in numerous randomized trials involving over 100 000 patients. It is widely available, easily administered, and is relatively inexpensive. However, only approximately 50% of STEMI patients are eligible for thrombolytic therapy (**Table 23-3**), and only 50% to 60% of patients treated with thrombolytics will achieve complete reperfusion. In addition, 10% to 20% of patients will experience reocclusion and 1% will suffer from a stroke caused by intracranial hemorrhage. Thrombolytic therapy is most effective when given within 3 hours from onset of chest pain.

Although streptokinase is still widely used around the world, fibrin-specific agents are almost exclusively used in the United States. Clinical trials of these agents have shown TIMI-3 flow rates in excess of 60%; however, there was no significant reduction in mortality or in the incidence of stroke when compared to nonfibrin-specific agents.

# ■ PRIMARY PCI

Approximately 95% of patients treated with primary PCI obtain complete reperfusion versus 50% to 60% of patients treated with thrombolytics. Primary PCI is also associated with a lower risk of stroke, and diagnostic angiography quickly defines coronary anatomy, LV function, and mechanical complications. However, invasive cardiovascular services are only available at <20% of hospitals in the United States and require a significant investment in infrastructure, personnel, and training as well as maintenance in case volume and expertise.

A meta-analysis by Keeley and colleagues of 23 trials including 3872 patients treated with primary PCI and 3867 patients treated with thrombolytics showed that

**TABLE 23-3.** Absolute and Relative Contraindications for Thrombolytic Therapy in Patients With ST-Segment Elevation Myocardial Infarction

**Absolute Contraindications**

Any prior intracranial hemorrhage
Known structural cerebral vascular lesion
Known intracranial neoplasm
Ischemic stroke within the past 3 mo (except for acute stroke within 3 h)
Suspected aortic dissection
Active bleeding or bleeding diathesis (excluding menses)
Significant closed-head or facial trauma within 3 mo

**Relative Contraindications**

History of chronic, sever, poorly controlled hypertension
Systolic pressure >180 mm Hg or diastolic 110 mm Hg
History of prior ischemic stroke >3 mo previously, dementia, or known intracranial pathology not covered in absolute contraindications
Recent (within 2-4 wk) internal bleeding
Noncompressible vascular punctures
Pregnancy
Active peptic ulcer
Current use of anticoagulants: the higher the INR, the higher the risk of bleeding
For streptokinase/anistreplase: prior exposure (more than 5 d previously) or prior allergic reaction to these agents

PCI was superior to thrombolytic therapy. Primary PCI was associated with a lower mortality rate (7% vs 9%, $p = 0.0002$), less reinfarction (3% vs 7%, $p = 0.0001$), and fewer strokes (1% vs 2%, $p = 0.0004$) at 30 days when compared to thrombolysis. PCI capability, however, is only available at <20% of hospitals in the United States, and each 30-minute delay from symptom onset to balloon inflation during primary PCI is associated with a 7.5% relative increase in mortality at 1 year. In addition, a meta-analysis of data from 23 trials containing 7739 patients comparing thrombolytic therapy to primary PCI by Nallamothu and Bates demonstrated that the mortality advantage of primary PCI is lost if the door-to-balloon time is 60 minutes greater than the door-to-needle time for thrombolytic therapy.

Three large-scale randomized trials have compared thrombolysis to transfer for primary PCI in STEMI patients. The combined end point of death, reinfarction, and disabling stroke at 30 days was significantly lower in the patients treated with primary PCI. Although transfer for primary PCI appears to be the treatment of choice, 2 important points need emphasizing. First, the transport time in these trials was extremely short (median time in the DANAMI2 trial was 32 minutes), and these times may not be achievable outside a clinical trial and in areas in which longer distances and weather may play a substantial role in transit time. Second, thrombolytic therapy still has a critically important role during the "golden hour" of MI or when there is a delay in transfer. The mortality rates and infarct size in patients treated with thrombolytic therapy within the first 60 to 90 minutes of symptoms are extremely low, suggesting that thromoblytic therapy still plays a vital role in the management of patients presenting to hospitals without primary PCI capability.

## ■ THROMBOLYTIC FACILITATED PCI

Thrombolytic-facilitated PCI refers to the pretreatment with thrombolytics in STEMI patients as a bridge to immediate PCI. This pretreatment has been proposed as a method to initiate earlier reperfusion and reduce ischemic time and infarct size in patients who experience a delay before the onset of PCI. Thrombolytic-facilitated therapy, however, can also expose patients to a higher risk of bleeding. Thrombolytic-facilitated PCI showed no survival benefit compared to primary PCI. In addition, thrombolytic-facilitated PCI is associated with a higher risk of major and minor bleeding compared to primary PCI. *Thus, thrombolytic-facilitated PCI should not be considered as a first-line reperfusion strategy for STEMI patients.*

## ■ SELECTION OF THE OPTIMAL REPERFUSION STRATEGY

STEMI patients presenting to a hospital with PCI capabilities should undergo primary PCI. Selection of a reperfusion strategy in patients who present to a hospital without PCI facilities is more complex. Patients who are not eligible for thrombolytic therapy should be immediately transferred to a tertiary care hospital for primary PCI. For those who are eligible for thrombolytic therapy, the clinician must consider 2 important factors: duration from onset of symptoms ("fixed" ischemia time) and transport time to the nearest PCI facility ("incurred" ischemia time). These 2 factors can be incorporated into a 2 × 3 table to select a reperfusion strategy (**Fig. 23-2**).

*Patients facing a transport time <30 minutes should be transferred for primary PCI. Thrombolytic-eligible patients who present <2 to 3 hours from onset of symptoms and have >60 minutes transport time should receive thrombolytic therapy. Patients presenting >2 to 3 hours after the onset of chest pain and have a transport time of 60 minutes or less should be promptly transported for primary PCI. If the anticipated transport time is >60 minutes for a patient presenting >3 hours from the onset of chest pain, either thrombolytic therapy or primary PCI can be considered. The choice of*

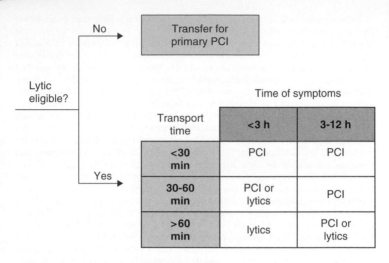

**FIGURE 23-2.** Reperfussion strategy for STEMI patients who present to hospitals without primary PCI. Lytics, thrombolysis and transfer; PCI, transfer for percutaneous coronary intervention.

*using thrombolytic therapy should always be considered along with the risk of bleeding in each individual patient.*

*All patients receiving thrombolytic therapy should also be transferred to a PCI facility for potential failure to reperfuse (ongoing chest pain or <50% resolution of ST-segment elevation at 90 minutes) and rescue PCI.* Recent randomized data suggest that all STEMI patients treated with thrombolytic therapy benefited from routine coronary angiography during the index hospitalization.

# ADJUVANT ANTIPLATELET THERAPY

## ■ CLOPIDOGREL

Clopidogrel is an oral thienopyridine prodrug whose active metabolite inhibits the activation of platelets by adenosine diphosphate. Its antiplatelet effects are more potent than aspirin and less potent than the glycoprotein IIb/IIIa inhibitors.

### Use With Thrombolytic Therapy

Clopidogrel, in combination with thrombolytic therapy, has been studied in the CLARITY-TIMI 28 trial. A total of 3491 STEMI patients 75 years of age or younger treated with thrombolytics were randomized to therapy with aspirin plus placebo or aspirin plus clopidogrel. Clopidogrel was given as a 300-mg loading dose within minutes of thrombolysis and 75 mg daily thereafter. The composite primary end point of death, reinfarction prior to angiography, or occluded infarct-related artery at angiography occurred in 15% of patients in the clopidogrel group and 22% of patients in the placebo group ($p$ <0.001). The use of clopidogrel was not associated with a higher rate of major or minor bleeding.

Patients older than 75 years were included in COMMIT (Randomized, Placebo-Controlled trial of adding clopidogrel to aspirin in 46 000 AMI patients), which randomized 45 849 STEMI patients treated with thrombolysis to therapy with aspirin plus placebo or aspirin plus clopidogrel. In this trial, patients randomized to the clopidogrel arm received 75 mg of clopidogrel at the time of thrombolysis and then 75 mg daily for the duration of hospitalization. Patients in the clopidogrel arm had a lower rate of the composite end point of death, reinfarction, or stroke (9.3% vs 10.1%, $p = 0.002$) and no increase in major or minor bleeding.

*The data from these 2 trials suggest that patients treated with thrombolytics should receive clopidogrel.* For patients older than 75 years, 75 mg of clopidogrel without a loading dose should be used. In patients 75 years of age or younger, the current data suggest that a 300-mg loading dose followed by 75 mg daily of clopidogrel is beneficial and safe.

## Use With Primary PCI

The benefit of aspirin plus clopidogrel in the setting of primary PCI for STEMI is unknown. No studies have compared early administration of clopidogrel to the early use of glycoprotein IIb/IIIa inhibitors in STEMI patients. *Therefore, clopidogrel should not be used in STEMI patients prior to visualization of the coronary anatomy at the time of coronary angiography.*

# ■ GLYCOPROTEIN IIB/IIIA INHIBITORS

Glycoprotein IIb/IIIa inhibitors are potent agents that inhibit the final common pathway for platelet aggregation. There are currently 3 intravenous agents available in the United States: abciximab, tirofiban, and eptifibatide.

## Use With Thrombolytic Therapy

Thrombolysis has been shown to be a potent activator of platelets and the concomitant use of aspirin along with thrombolysis has been shown to be of benefit. Two dose-finding studies have shown that the glycoprotein IIb/IIIa inhibitor abciximab, when used in combination with half-dose thromoblytics, improves coronary artery blood flow in STEMI patients. Three subsequent randomized trials have investigated combination therapy with a glycoprotein IIb/IIIa inhibitor and half-dose thrombolytic therapy. These studies showed that combination therapy increases risk of bleeding and does not improve mortality. *Thus, glycoprotein IIb/IIIa inhibitors should not be used in combination with thrombolytic therapy.*

## Use with Primary PCI

The early (prior to arrival in the catherization laboratory) versus delayed (at the time of catherization) use of glycoprotein IIb/IIIa inhibitors in STEMI patients has been investigated in 8 randomized trials involving abciximab, tirofiban, and eptifibatide. A meta-analysis of 6 of these trials by Montalescot and colleagues showed that early administration of glycoprotein IIb/IIIa inhibitors in STEMI patients was associated with a greater prevalence of TIMI 2 or 3 flow (41.7 % vs 29.8 %, $p <0.001$) in the infarct-related artery prior to PCI. Since prior studies have shown that better coronary artery flow after PCI is associated with fewer in-hospital and 1-year adverse outcomes, early administration of glycoprotein IIb/IIIa inhibitors should be *considered* in STEMI patients undergoing primary PCI.

# PHARMACOTHERAPY AFTER REPERFUSION

## ◼ ANGIOTENSIN-CONVERTING ENZYME INHIBITORS

Treatment with angiotensin-converting enzyme (ACE) inhibitors within the first 24 hours of reperfusion is reasonable as long as no contraindications exist and the patient is hemodynamically stable. Patients with an ejection fraction of more than 45% and no clinical evidence of heart failure, significant mitral regurgitation, or hypertension can have therapy discontinued after determination of risk status while still hospitalized. Since captopril has the shortest half-life, overdosing and inadvertent hypotension may be most easily correctable with the use of this agent. In addition, the short half-life allows for more rapid titration. Intravenous administration is unnecessary unless the patient is unable to take oral medication. Duration of treatment is uncertain; however, many patients will be treated indefinitely.

## ◼ β-BLOCKERS

Initiation of β-blockade therapy in the CCU is essential in the management of STEMI patients. *β-blockers* have been shown to have both *acute and long-term benefits in STEMI patients* treated with either lysis or primary PCI. Short-acting β-blockade with metoprolol should be initiated as early as possible and rapidly titrated to the maximally tolerated dose. In patients who present with shock or heart failure, the initiation of β-blockers should be delayed until patients become hemodynamically stable.

## ◼ ASPIRIN

The use of aspirin in the initial management of STEMI patients was previously discussed. Once initiated, patients should remain on aspirin indefinitely. A dose between 75 and 162 mg a day is recommended. Patients who are allergic to aspirin should be given 75 mg of clopidogrel daily.

## ◼ THIENOPYRIDINES

A thienopyridine, ticlopidine, or clopidogrel, should be given in addition to aspirin to patients receiving *coronary artery stenting*. The minimal duration of therapy depends on the type of stent implanted. Patients with bare metal stents should be treated for a minimum of 30 days, while those with a drug-eluting stent should receive at least 1 year of therapy.

## ◼ STATINS

Several trials have demonstrated that statins should be used in the secondary prevention of patients with coronary artery disease. In addition to lowering LDL cholesterol, statins have also been demonstrated to improve endothelial function, have antiplatelet effects, and reduce inflammation.

# SECONDARY PREVENTION

Aggressive secondary prevention measures should be instituted during the initial hospitalization. These include smoking cessation, weight reduction, dietary modifications, glucose control, and enrollment in a cardiac rehab program.

# SUGGESTED READINGS

Hass EE, Yang EH, Gersh BJ, O'Rourke RA. ST-segment elevation myocardial infarction. In: Fuster V, Walsh RA, Harrington RA, et al. *Hurst's The Heart*. 13th ed. New York, NY: McGraw-Hill. 2011;60:1354-1385.

Angiolillo DJ, Giugliano GR, Simon DI. Pharmacologic therapy for acute coronary syndromes. In: Fuster V, Walsh RA, Harrington RA, et al. *Hurst's The Heart*. 13th ed. New York, NY: McGraw-Hill. 2011;61:1386-1429.

Antman EM, Anbe DT, Armstrong PW, et al. ACC/AHA guidelines for the management of patients with ST-elevation myocardial infarction: a report of the American College of Cardiology/American Heart Association Task Force on Practice Guidelines (Committee to Revise the 1999 Guidelines for the Management of Patients With Acute Myocardial Infarction). *J Am Coll Cardiol*. 2004;44:e1-e211.

Ting H, Yang EH, Rihal CS. Reperfusion strategies for ST-segment elevation myocardial infarction. *Ann Intern Med*. 2006;145:610-617.

CHAPTER 24

# DIAGNOSIS AND MANAGEMENT OF PATIENTS WITH UNSTABLE ANGINA AND NON– ST-SEGMENT ELEVATION MYOCARDIAL INFARCTION

James A. de Lemos, Robert A. O'Rourke[†],
and Robert A. Harrington

Unstable angina (UA) and non–ST-elevation myocardial infarction (NSTEMI) are 2 related forms of acute coronary syndrome (ACS) caused by rupture or erosion of an atherosclerotic plaque with platelet-thrombus formation and subsequent obstruction to coronary artery blood flow. They are differentiated from ST-elevation MI (STEMI; see Chapter 23) by the absence of ST elevation or a new left bundle-branch block on the presenting electrocardiogram (ECG). NSTEMI is further differentiated from UA by the detection of bloodstream markers of myocardial injury, including troponin I, troponin T, or creatinine kinase myocardial band (CK-MB). In 2004, the National Center for Health Statistics reported 1 565 000 discharges for ACS, of which 896 000 were for MI (both STEMI and NSTEMI), and 669 000 were for UA. Treatment of UA and NSTEMI is essentially identical, depending on level of risk.

Serum biomarkers, such as troponins I and T, C-reactive protein (CRP), brain natriuretic peptide (BNP), and N-terminal pro-BNP (NT pro-BNP) aid in more accurate risk stratification in patients with ACS. Newer therapies, including low-molecular-weight heparins (LMWH), factor Xa inhibitors and direct anti-thrombins, platelet glycoprotein (GP) IIb/IIIa receptor antagonists, thienopyridines (clopidogrel), early use of high-dose statins, and percutaneous revascularization with drug-eluting stents for *higher-risk* patients have improved outcomes in patients with UA/NSTEMI.

## DEFINITION AND CLASSIFICATION

UA/NSTEMI is a clinical syndrome usually caused by atherosclerotic plaque rupture and thrombosis within a coronary artery, resulting in an imbalance in myocardial oxygen supply and demand, and associated with an increased risk of subsequent cardiac death and new or recurrent myocardial infarction. UA is defined as angina

[†]Deceased.

that is new-onset or abruptly increased in intensity, duration, or frequency within the past 60 days. NSTEMI is identified by clinical symptoms as UA plus myocardial injury as evidenced by elevated serum cardiac biomarkers.

# ETIOLOGY

There are several potential causes for the imbalance between myocardial oxygen supply and demand seen in UA/NSTEMI, including the following:

1. Coronary artery luminal narrowing due to a nonocclusive thrombus that develops following rupture or erosion of an atherothrombotic plaque.

2. Severe coronary artery narrowing without spasm or thrombosis, which typically occurs in patients with progressive atherosclerosis or with restenosis within 6 months after percutaneous coronary intervention (PCI).

3. Intense focal spasm of a segment of an epicardial coronary artery (Prinzmetal or variant angina) causing dynamic obstruction of the coronary artery lumen.

4. Coronary artery dissection (a cause of ACS in women in the peripartum period).

5. Precipitating factors extrinsic to the coronary arterial bed that limit myocardial perfusion, including sudden increases in myocardial oxygen demand (sepsis, fever, tachycardia), reductions in coronary blood flow (hypotension), or decreased myocardial oxygen delivery (hypoxia, severe anemia).

# DIAGNOSIS AND RISK STRATIFICATION

Expeditious evaluation of ACS patients is paramount to providing timely and appropriate therapies (**Fig. 24-1**). Initial evaluation of chest pain should triage patients into 1 of 4 categories: (1) noncardiac chest pain, (2) chronic stable angina, (3) possible ACS, or (4) definite ACS. Patients with symptoms suggesting ACS should be referred to a facility that can perform a thorough history and physical, ECG, and biomarker determination. Any chest pain lasting longer than 20 minutes, hemodynamic instability, or recent syncope or presyncope should be referred to a hospital emergency department and ideally should be transported by emergency medical services. Once it has been determined that a patient has a probable cardiac source of their symptoms, risk stratification into low-, intermediate-, or high-risk categories should be performed.

The American College of Cardiology/American Heart Association (ACC/AHA) 2007 Guideline Update for the Management of Patients With UA and NSTEMI uses features of the clinical history (advanced age, accelerating angina in last 48 hours, prior MI, coronary artery bypass grafting [CABG], cerebrovascular or peripheral arterial disease, aspirin use); pain characteristics (intensity, duration, provocation of angina); clinical findings (pulmonary edema or other signs of heart failure); ECG findings; and levels of cardiac biomarkers to determine an individual's risk (**Table 24-1**). Transient ST-segment changes (>0.05 mV) during a symptomatic episode at rest that resolve when the patient becomes asymptomatic strongly suggest acute ischemia and a high likelihood of underlying severe coronary artery disease (CAD). This early risk assessment is critical, as it establishes the intensity of future therapies. A patient with a low risk may be discharged home with aspirin and β-blockers, often with an early outpatient stress test (within 72 hours of admission). High-risk patients may be admitted to a coronary care unit, treated with multiple drugs, and undergo coronary angiography and revascularization urgently. The risk assessment should be updated during hospitalization if a patient's clinical status, ECG, or cardiac biomarkers change, and as new data become available. Clinical risk predictor models, such as the TIMI and GRACE prediction tools, can help determine an individual's short-term and long-term risk and the need for aggressive therapy (**Fig. 24-2**).

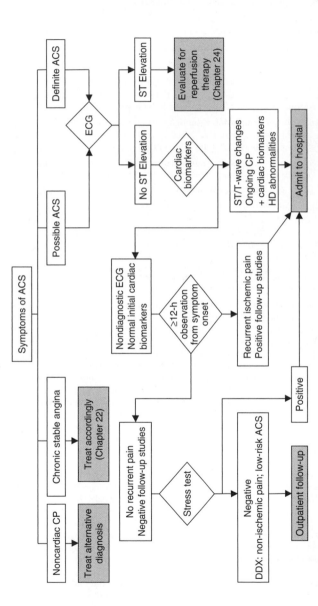

**FIGURE 24-1.** Algorithm for evaluation and management of patients suspected of having ACS. ACS, acute coronary syndrome; CP, chest pain; DDX, differential diagnosis; ECG, electrocardiogram; HD, heart disease. (Adapted with permission from Anderson JL, Adams, CD, Antman EM: ACC/AHA 2007 guidelines for the management of patients with unstable angina/non-ST-Elevation myocardial infarction: a report of the American College of Cardiology/American Heart Association Task Force on Practice Guidelines (Writing Committee to Revise the 2002 Guidelines for the Management of Patients With Unstable Angina/Non-ST-Elevation Myocardial Infarction) developed in collaboration with the American College of Emergency Physicians, the Society for Cardiovascular Angiography and Interventions, and the Society of Thoracic Surgeons endorsed by the American Association of Cardiovascular and Pulmonary Rehabilitation and the Society for Academic Emergency Medicine, J. Am. Coll. Cardiol  2007; Aug 14;50(7):e1-e157.)

**TABLE 24-1.** Short-Term Risk of Death or Nonfatal Myocardial Infarction in Patients With UA/NSTEMI[a]

| Feature | High Risk (≥2 Features) | Intermediate Risk (No High-Risk Features, ≥1 of the Following Features) | Low Risk (No High- or Intermediate-Risk Features, but Following Features May Be Present) |
|---|---|---|---|
| History | ↑ Ischemic symptoms over last 48 h | Prior MI, PVD, CVD, disease, or CABG; prior ASA use | |
| Character of pain | >20 min of ongoing rest pain | >20 min rest pain, now resolved, with moderate or high likelihood of CAD<br>Rest pain relieved with rest or SL NTG *or* lasting <20 min<br>Nighttime chest pain<br>New or progressive CCS class II or IV chest pain in the past 2 wk without >20 min of rest pain with moderate or high likelihood of CAD | New-onset chest pain within 2 wk to 2 mo |
| Clinical findings | Age >75 y<br>Pulmonary edema, rales<br>New or worsening MR murmur, S₃ ↓ BP, ↓ HR, ↑ HR | Age >70 y | |
| ECG findings | Rest pain with transient ST-segment changes >0.05 mV<br>New bundle-branch block<br>Sustained VT | T-wave changes<br>Pathologic Q waves<br>Resting ST depressions <1 mm in multiple leads | Normal or unchanged ECG |
| Cardiac markers | TnT or TnI >0.1 ng/mL | 0.01 ng/mL < TnT <0.1 ng/mL | Normal |

ASA, aspirin; CABG, coronary artery bypass grafting; CAD, coronary artery disease; CCS, Canadian Cardiovascular Society; CVD, cerebrovascular disease; ECG, electrocardiogram; MR, mitral regurgitation; PVD, peripheral vascular disease; SL NTG, sublingual nitroglycerin; TnT, troponin T; TnI, troponin I.

[a]Estimation of the short-term risk of death and nonfatal cardiac ischemic events in UA is a complex multivariable problem that cannot be fully specified in a table; therefore, this table is meant to offer general guidance and illustration rather than rigid algorithms.

Adapted from Braunwald E, Mark CB, Jones RH, et al. *AHCPR Clinical Practice Guideline no. 10. Unstable Angina: Diagnosis and Management.* Rockville, MD: Agency for Health Care Policy and Research and the National Heart, Lung, and Blood Institute, U.S. Public Health Service, U.S. Department of Health and Human Services; 1994; AHCPR pub. no. 94-0602.

# ■ INITIAL EVALUATION

UA/NSTEMI may present as rest angina, new-onset severe angina, or increasing angina as graded by the Canadian Cardiovascular Society Classifications. In patients with known underlying CAD, symptoms similar to prior episodes of angina or MI suggest ischemia and should be managed aggressively. Patients with known CABG may have atherothrombosis of venous bypass grafts and patients with PCI within

| GRACE Risk Predictors: | | Points | GRACE Risk Predictors: | | Points |
|---|---|---|---|---|---|
| Age (y): | ≤39 | 0 | SBP (mm Hg): | ≤79.9 | 24 |
| | 40-49 | 18 | | 80-99.9 | 22 |
| | 50-59 | 36 | | 100-119.9 | 18 |
| | 60-69 | 55 | | 120-139.9 | 14 |
| | 70-79 | 78 | | 140-159.9 | 10 |
| | 80-89 | 91 | | 160-199.9 | 4 |
| | ≥90 | 100 | | ≥200 | 0 |
| Positive CHF Hx | | 24 | ST segment depression | | 11 |
| Positive MI Hx | | 12 | Cr (mg/dL): | ≤0.39 | 1 |
| Rest HR (bpm): | ≤49.9 | 0 | | 0.4-0.79 | 3 |
| | 50-69.9 | 3 | | 0.8-1.19 | 5 |
| | 70-89.9 | 9 | | 1.2-1.59 | 7 |
| | 90-109.9 | 14 | | 1.6-1.99 | 9 |
| | 110-149.9 | 23 | | 2-3.99 | 15 |
| | 150-199.9 | 35 | | ≥4.0 | 20 |
| | ≥200 | 43 | Positive cardiac markers | | 15 |
| | | | No in-house PCI | | 14 |

**TOTAL SCORE:**

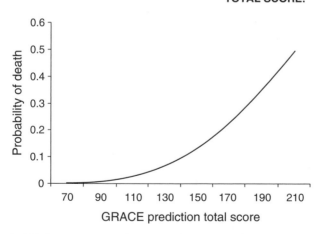

**FIGURE 24-2.** Clinical risk prediction tools. The GRACE scorecard and nomogram predict mortality 6 months postdischarge, and the TIMI risk score predicts risk of death, MI, or recurrent ischemia within 14 days of randomization. (Data compiled from Antman EM, Cohen M, Bernink PJ, et al. The TIMI risk score for unstable angina/non-ST elevation MI: a method of prognostication and therapeutic decision making. *JAMA.* 2000;284:835-842; and Eagle KA, Lim MJ, Dabbous OH, et al. A validated prediction model for all forms of acute coronary syndrome: estimating the risk of 6-month post-discharge death in an international registry. *JAMA.* 2004;291:2727-2733.)

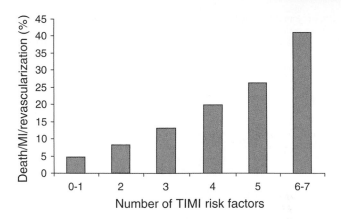

**TIMI Risk Predictors**

- Age ≥65 y
- ≥3 CAD risk factors
  (hypertension, diabetes, high
  cholesterol, family history,
  smoking)
- Prior coronary stenosis ≥50%
- ST deviation
- ≥2 anginal events in 24 h
- Elevated troponin or CK-MB
- ASA use within last 7 d

**FIGURE 24-2.** (*Continued*)

the past 6 months may have restenosis and benefit from an early invasive treatment strategy.

"Atypical" symptoms such as acute dyspnea, indigestion, unusual locations of pain, agitation, altered mental status, profound weakness, or syncope may be the presenting manifestations of ACS particularly in women, the elderly, and patients with long-standing diabetes mellitus. Atypical symptoms, especially within these patient subgroups, are associated with a higher risk of death and major complications.

## ■ HISTORY AND PHYSICAL EXAMINATION

Myocardial ischemia is commonly experienced as a pressure-like sensation in the retrosternal area; however, "anginal equivalents" may present as epigatric, arm, jaw, or back discomfort. Patients may describe the discomfort as *burning, squeezing, pressure-like*, or *heavy*, but less commonly *sharp, jabbing*, or *knife-like*. However, atypical features do not reliably exclude the possibility of UA/NSTEMI.

In a patient younger than 50 years who presents with symptoms of UA/NSTEMI, cocaine use should be considered as a potential trigger.

Once a complete history and physical have been performed, the physician caring for the patient with suspected UA/NSTEMI should classify the likelihood of the patient's symptoms being due to myocardial ischemia as being high, intermediate, or low. The history should take into account the nature of the anginal symptoms, prior CAD history, age, sex, and the number of traditional risk factors for CAD.

# ■ THE ELECTROCARDIOGRAM

A 12-lead ECG should be performed and shown to a physician within 10 minutes of arrival to the emergency room or other facility for all patients presenting with symptoms suggesting UA/NSTEMI. If the initial ECG is not diagnostic but there is a high clinical suspicion for ACS, serial ECGs should be performed to detect the development of ST depressions or elevations over the next 24 to 48 hours. A normal ECG during an episode of chest pain does not rule out ACS. Transient ST-segment depressions of at least 0.5 mm during chest discomfort that disappear with relief of the chest pain provide objective evidence of transient myocardial ischemia. Persistent T-wave inversions over the involved territory are common in patients with UA. Deep, symmetric T-wave inversions across the precordial leads suggest proximal, severe left anterior descending (LAD) coronary artery stenosis. An ECG with Q waves from a previous infarction or an old left bundle-branch block, signifying prior LV damage, may be seen in patients with UA/NSTEMI and is associated with a higher risk.

# ■ CARDIAC BIOMARKERS

Cardiac biomarkers are both diagnostic and prognostic in UA/NSTEMI. Traditionally, elevated serum levels of creatinine kinase (CK) or CK-MB were used to distinguish between UA and NSTEMI. However, the widespread use of the more sensitive cardiac biomarker, troponin, has improved the ability to diagnosis lesser degrees of myocardial necrosis. As a result, the proportion of patients classified as NSTEMI has increased markedly in recent years. Elevated levels of troponin T or I are independent predictors of adverse events in patients with clinical symptoms consistent with ACS, even when levels of CK and CK-MB are normal. Patients with elevated troponin have a NSTEMI by definition and should be treated as being at high risk compared with UA patients with normal troponin levels. Patients with symptoms consistent with ACS and an initial set of enzymes that are negative within 6 hours of onset of symptoms should have serial enzymes drawn 8 to 12 hours after symptom onset to ensure that no myocardial damage has occurred.

Other biomarkers that provide important risk information in patients with UA/NSTEMI include BNP and NT-proBNP. Even when troponin levels are normal and no evidence of heart failure is present, higher levels of these neurohormones identify patients at increased risk for death and heart failure after an ACS presentation. Unlike the troponins, however, the therapeutic implications of BNP or NT-proBNP elevation in ACS are not entirely clear. Thus, it is recommended that these tests be ordered selectively rather than routinely in ACS.

# ■ ACUTE MYOCARDIAL PERFUSION IMAGING

In patients with normal cardiac biomarkers and nondiagnostic ECGs but a high suspicion of UA, acute rest myocardial perfusion imaging with technetium 99 sestamibi can be beneficial in diagnosing myocardial ischemia. Since imaging can be delayed for several hours after injection, sestamibi is more useful than thallium for rest myocardial imaging. ECG-gated imaging provides an assessment of myocardial wall motion in addition to perfusion information (Chapter 4). The sensitivity and negative predictive value of acute rest perfusion imaging are extremely high if sestamibi is injected during an episode of acute chest pain. The sensitivity decreases if the injection is done after the chest pain has resolved.

# FOLLOW-UP TESTING

## ■ STRESS TESTING

Stress testing is often used for risk assessment in low- to intermediate-risk patients with UA/NSTEMI. If the purpose of the stress test is risk assessment in a patient with confirmed ACS, the testing should be performed with the patient on appropriate precautionary pharmacotherapy (aspirin, β-blocker). However, in low-risk patients in whom the suspicion of ACS is low and the purpose is to *diagnose* CAD, it is reasonable to withhold β-blockers to improve the diagnostic yield.

If the stress test shows high-risk findings, such as ST-segment depression at low exercise levels or large reversible perfusion defects on perfusion imaging, the patient should be referred urgently for coronary angiography since high-risk stress test abnormalities are correlated with higher event rates and more commonly with 3-vessel CAD. If the stress test is negative or has low-risk results, the patient can be treated medically. In patients with baseline ECG abnormalities, exercise stress testing should be performed in conjunction with echocardiographic or nuclear imaging. In patients who are unable to exercise, pharmacologic stress testing should be performed with adenosine, dipyridamole, or dobutamine and nuclear or echocardiographic imaging.

## ■ CORONARY CT ANGIOGRAPHY

The ACC/AHA 2007 Guideline Update for the Management of Patients With UA and NSTEMI now states that noninvasive coronary CT imaging is a reasonable alternative to stress testing in low-risk to intermediate-risk patients (level of evidence B, class IIa). Since coronary CT angiography provides only diagnostic information, patients with *high-risk clinical features should not undergo coronary CT angiography* but should instead proceed to traditional coronary angiography and potential revascularization.

## ■ CORONARY ANGIOGRAPHY

In chronic CAD patients, the risk of future cardiovascular events is proportional to the number of vessels with >50% diameter stenosis and the presence and severity of left ventricular (LV) systolic dysfunction. However, the risk of short-term events in UA/NSTEMI is dominated by features of the *culprit lesion* (ECG changes, troponin elevation).

Among patients with UA/NSTEMI who undergo coronary angiography, approximately 85% will have significant CAD. CABG confers a survival benefit in patients with ≥50% left main stenosis or 3-vessel disease with LV dysfunction. Importantly, patients with *no* significant lesions at angiography benefit from a reorientation of their management. Alternative causes of chest pain should be considered in patients with no significant coronary lesions on angiography, including pulmonary embolism, "syndrome X," and variant angina. If the coronaries are completely normal, antithrombotic and antiplatelet drugs can often be discontinued, and the need for antianginal medication reassessed. Symptomatic patients with "normal" coronary arteries may have significant atherosclerosis by intravascular ultrasound secondary to coronary artery remodeling.

# PROGNOSIS

Prognosis in UA/NSTEMI depends on the morbidity and mortality expected from the extent of coronary disease, LV systolic function, and the short-term risk associated with the stability of the culprit lesion. Short-term risk is highest soon after the onset of symptoms due to risk from MI and its complications and the recurrence of ACS. Long-term risk is more difficult to quantify. However, the Global Registry of Acute Coronary Events (GRACE) study, a multinational observational study of 5209 NSTEMI patients and 6149 UA patients, found a 6-month mortality rate of 6.2% in patients with NSTEMI and 3.6% in those with UA.

# TREATMENT

The goals of therapy for UA/NSTEMI patients are 3-fold: (1) control/alleviate symptoms; (2) improve ischemia; and (3) prevent death, MI, or reinfarction.

## ◼ IN-HOSPITAL TREATMENT

Suspected ACS patients should be treated with an aspirin (ASA), clopidogrel or a GP IIb/IIIa inhibitor, and either unfractionated heparin (UFH) or low-molecular-weight heparin (LMWH). If a patient has recurrent ischemia on ASA and clopidogrel, a GP IIb/IIIa inhibitor should be added prior to proceeding to coronary angiography. Statins and β-blockers should be administered orally within the first 24 hours provided that the patient does not have any contraindications. Bed rest for the early phase of hospitalization and supplemental oxygen to keep arterial oxygen saturation >90% should be ordered. All nonsteroidal anti-inflammatory drugs should be discontinued.

## ◼ EARLY INVASIVE VERSUS EARLY CONSERVATIVE INITIAL MANAGEMENT

The ACC/AHA 2007 UA/NSTEMI Guideline Update advocates 2 main strategies with regard to early catheterization and revascularization, "early invasive" and "early conservative" (**Fig. 24-3**). Low-risk patients or patients who prefer to avoid angiography and do not have high-risk features can be managed with intensive medical therapy in the early conservative strategy. These patients will only undergo coronary angiography if they experience recurrent ischemia (angina or ST-segment changes at rest or with minimal activity) or heart failure, or have a strongly positive stress test following completion of 48 to 72 hours of antithrombotic therapy. This strategy is better termed a "selective invasive" strategy, as 30% to 50% of patients managed with this strategy will cross over and undergo catheterization during or shortly following admission. In the early invasive strategy, patients who have no contraindications to cardiac catheterization undergo coronary angiography within 24 to 48 hours and PCI or surgical revascularization if suitable coronary anatomy is present.

A meta-analysis of the 7 large, prospective, randomized trials that have evaluated the risks and benefits of each approach found that the relative risk (RR) of all-cause mortality (RR 0.75, 95% CI 0.63-0.90), nonfatal MI (RR 0.83, 95% CI 0.72-0.96), and recurrent UA (RR 0.69, 95% CI 0.65-0.74) were all reduced with an early invasive strategy. However, one of these 7 trials, the Invasive versus Conservative Treatment in Unstable coronary Syndromes (ICTUS) trial, found no difference in the composite ischemic end point of MI and unstable angina requiring revascularization in the early conservative versus early invasive strategies at 1 year and 3-year follow-up in 1200 UA/NSTEMI patients who were troponin positive. Because of this trial, the

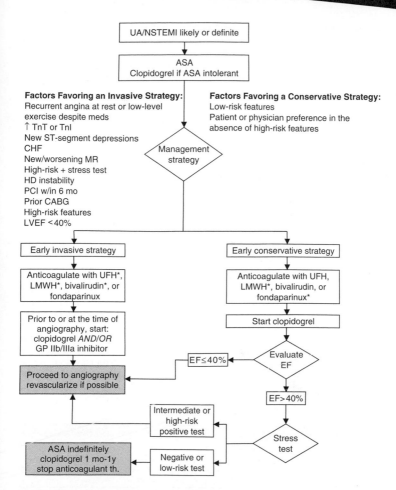

**FIGURE 24-3.** The ACC/AHA 2007 Guideline Update for the Management of Patients With UA and NSTEMI describes 2 different treatment strategies, termed "early conservative" and "early invasive." (*Preferred anticoagulant therapy.) ASA, aspirin; CABG, coronary artery bypass grafting; CHF, congestive heart failure; GP IIb/IIIa inhibitor, glycoprotein IIb/IIIa inhibitor; HD, hemodynamic; LMWH, low-molecular-weight heparin; LVEF, left ventricular ejection fraction; MR, mitral regurgitation; PCI, percutaneous coronary intervention; TnI, troponin-I; TnT, troponin-T; UA/NSTEMI, unstable angina/non–ST-elevation myocardial infarction; UFH, unfractionated heparin.

ACC/AHA 2007 Guideline Update for the Management of Patients With UA and NSTEMI recognizes that an early invasive strategy may be an appropriate strategy for *some* cases of UA/NSTEMI.

The 2007 Guideline update recognizes important interactions between patient risk and the benefit of the invasive treatment strategy. The benefits of the early invasive approach are accentuated in high-risk patient prediction tools (see Table 24-1 and Fig. 24-2). In contrast, no benefit of a routine invasive approach is observed in low-risk UA patients.

Additional advantages of the early invasive strategy include earlier and more definitive risk stratification with early identification of the 10% to 15% of patients with no significant coronary stenoses and the approximately 20% of patients with 3-vessel or left main CAD. This strategy reduces the need for antianginal medications and rehospitalization for myocardial ischemia among those who can have PCI performed on their culprit lesion.

Advantages of the early conservative strategy are the avoidance of the potential risks of invasive procedures, such as catheterization and the identification of high-risk patients with noninvasive stress testing.

# ■ ANTI-ISCHEMIC DRUGS

An overview of anti-ischemic and antithrombotic drugs is given in **Table 24-2**.

## Nitrates

Nitroglycerin (NTG) reduces myocardial oxygen demand while enhancing myocardial oxygen delivery by vasodilating coronary vascular beds. NTG decreases preload via venous pooling, thereby decreasing LV wall tension and decreasing myocardial oxygen demand. Epicardial and collateral coronary vasodilation by NTG can improve the redistribution of blood flow to ischemic myocardial regions.

Patients whose symptoms are not relieved with three 0.4-mg sublingual NTG tablets or sprays taken 5 minutes apart may benefit from intravenous NTG. The use of sildenafil (Viagra) within the previous 24 hours, tadalafil (Cialis) within the previous 48 hours, or the presence of hypotension (SBP <90 mm Hg or >30 mm Hg below baseline) are contraindications to NTG administration. The time between nitrate use and use of vardenafil (Levitra) has not been studied; therefore until further data are available, vardenafil should not be prescribed to patients who may need nitrate therapy. Intravenous NTG may be initiated at a rate of 10 µg/min as a continuous

**TABLE 24-2.** Anti-ischemic and Antithrombotic Drugs in UA/NSTEMI

| Medications | Route | Dose |
|---|---|---|
| NTG and nitrates | | |
|   NTG | Sublingual tablets | 0.3-0.6 mg, up to 1.5 mg |
| | Spray | 0.4 mg as needed |
| | Transdermal | 0.2-0.8 mg/h every 12 h |
| | Intravenous | 5-200 µg/min |
|   Isosorbide dinitrate | Oral | 5-80 mg 2 or 3 times daily |
| | Oral, slow release | 40 mg 1 or 2 times daily |
|   Isosorbide mononitrate | Oral | 20 mg twice daily |
| | Oral, slow release | 60-240 mg once daily |
| β-blockers | | |
|   Metoprolol | Oral | 25-100 mg twice daily |
|   Atenolol | Oral | 25-100 mg once daily |
|   Esmolol | Intravenous | 50-200 µg/kg/min |
| Calcium-channel blockers[a] | | |
|   Diltiazem | Oral | 30-90 mg 4 times daily |
|   Verapamil | Oral | 80-120 mg 3 times daily |

*(continued)*

**TABLE 24-2.** Anti-ischemic and Antithrombotic Drugs in UA/NSTEMI (continued)

| Medications | Route | Dose |
|---|---|---|
| Amlodipine | Oral | 2.5-10 mg once daily |
| Nisoldipine | Oral | 10-60 mg once daily |
| Felodipine | Oral | 2.5-10 mg once daily |
| ACE inhibitors[b] | | |
| Ramipril | Oral | 2.5-5 mg twice daily |
| Captopril | Oral | 25-100 mg 2 or 3 times daily |
| Enalapril | Oral | 5-20 mg 2 twice daily |
| Perindopril | Oral | 4-8 mg once daily |
| Angiotensin receptor blockers | | |
| Candesartan | Oral | 4-32 mg once daily |
| Losartan | Oral | 25-100 mg once or twice daily |
| Valsartan | Oral | 40-160 mg twice daily |
| Aldosterone receptor blockers | | |
| Eplerenone | Oral | 25-50 mg once daily |
| Spironolactone | Oral | 25 mg once daily |
| Antiplatelets | | |
| Aspirin | Oral | Initial dose of 325 mg followed by 81-325 mg daily |
| Clopidogrel | Oral | Initial dose of 300-600 mg followed by 75 mg daily |
| Anticoagulant therapy | | |
| UFH | Intravenous | Initial dose 60 U/kg (max 4000 U) bolus then 12 U/kg/h (max 1000 U/h) for goal aPTT 50-70 s |
| Enoxaparin | Subcutaneous/ intravenous | 1 mg/kg twice a day (first dose may be preceded by 30-mg U IV bolus); if CrCl <30 mL/min then 1 mg/kg once daily |
| Bivalirudin[c] | Intravenous | 0.1 mg/kg bolus followed by infusion of 0.25 mg/kg/h |
| Fondaparinux | Subcutaneous | 2.5 mg, once daily |
| Glycoprotein IIb/IIIa inhibitors | | |
| Abciximab | Intravenous | 0.25 mg/kg bolus followed by infusion of 0.125 µg/kg/min (maximum 10 µg/min) for 12-24 h |
| Eptifibatide | Intravenous | 180 µg/kg bolus × 2 (10 min apart) followed by infusion of 2.0 µg/kg/min for 72-96 h |
| Tirofiban | Intravenous | 0.4 µg/kg/min for 30 min followed by infusion of 0.1 µg/kg/min for 48-96 h |

ACE, angiotensin-converting enzyme; aPTT, activated partial thromboplastin time; CrCl, creatinine clearance; UFH, unfractionated heparin.

infusion and increased by 10 µg/min every 3 to 5 minutes until symptom relief or blood pressure response is noted. IV NTG can be administered as needed for the first 48 hours after UA/NSTEMI for persistent ischemia, heart failure, or hypertension as long as it does not preclude the use of other evidence-based cardioprotective medicines such as angiotensin-converting enzyme (ACE) inhibitors or β-blockers. An upper limit of 200 µg/min of IV NTG is commonly used. After 48 hours, the patient should be transitioned to oral nitrate therapy for medical management of residual angina.

## Morphine Sulfate

Morphine sulfate relieves pain through the opioid pain receptor as well as by diminishing the sympathetic nervous system's pain response, thereby decreasing catecholamine secretion and oxygen demand. Morphine also is a venodilator and decreases preload. Morphine sulfate is recommended (1-5 mg IV) for patients whose symptoms are not relieved despite NTG therapy.

## β-Adrenergic Blockers

β-blockers reduce myocardial oxygen demand by slowing the heart rate, decreasing myocardial contractility, decreasing afterload, and prolonging the duration of diastole, thereby improving coronary and collateral blood flow. In the absence of contraindications, β-blockers should be started *orally* within the first 24 hours of UA/NSTEMI. *Routine early intravenous β-blocker therapy is no longer recommended.* Intravenous use should be reserved for specific indications such as hypertension or atrial arrhythmias and should not be administered to hemodynamically unstable patients or patients with signs of heart failure or a low output state.

Patients with significant sinus bradycardia (heart rate <50 bpm) or hypotension (SBP <90 mm Hg) generally should not receive β-blockers until these issues are resolved. Short-acting cardioselective β-blockers should be used in patients with reactive airways disease and uptitrated to obtain a heart rate of *50 to 60 bpm* as tolerated.

## Calcium-Channel Blockers

Calcium-channel blockers inhibit both myocardial and vascular smooth muscle contraction, thereby reducing myocardial oxygen demand and improving myocardial blood flow. Nifedipine and amlodipine have the greatest peripheral arterial dilatory effect but little chronotropic effect, whereas verapamil and diltiazem have chronotropic and inotropic as well as some peripheral arterial dilatory effects.

Calcium-channel blockers may be useful for ongoing or recurring angina in patients receiving adequate doses of nitrates and β-blockers, in those who are intolerant to either or both of these agents, or in patients with variant angina. Rapid-release short-acting dihydropyridines (eg, nifedipine) must be avoided in ACS because of risk for adverse outcomes. Verapamil and diltiazem should be avoided in patient with pulmonary edema or severe LV systolic dysfunction and should be used with caution when combined with beta-blockers.

## Angiotensin-Converting Enzyme Inhibitors/Angiotensin Receptor Blockers

ACE inhibitors reduce mortality and CV events in patients with MI and LV systolic dysfunction (LVEF <40%), in patients with diabetes and CAD, and in patients with high-risk chronic CAD despite normal LV systolic function. Accordingly,

ACE inhibitors should be used in most patients following UA/NSTEMI, unless contraindicated or blood pressure is borderline. Angiotensin receptor blockers (ARBs) may be useful in patients post-MI or with ischemic heart failure (HF) who are intolerant to ACE inhibitors.

## Aldosterone Receptor Blockers

Eplerenone, a selective aldosterone receptor blocker, has been shown to have a mortality and morbidity benefit in patients who have had an MI with LV systolic dysfunction (LVEF <40%) and HF or diabetes. Spironolactone has been shown to have a mortality and morbidity benefit in both ischemic and non-ischemic severe HF patients (NHYA class III and IV). Aldosterone receptor blockers should be administered to patients with HF or diabetes and an EF less than or equal to 40% who do not have significant renal dysfunction or hyperkalemia and are already on a therapeutic dose of an ACE inhibitor.

## ■ ANTIPLATELET THERAPY

### Aspirin

ASA irreversibly inhibits cyclooxygenase-1 within the platelet, preventing the formation of thromboxane $A_2$ and thereby diminishing platelet aggregation, a critical contributor to thrombus formation after plaque rupture. In UA/NSTEMI patients, ASA therapy should be initiated immediately at a dose of 162 to 325 mg. The first dose should be chewed, and preferably a nonenteric coated ASA because it has faster buccal absorption. Subsequent doses may be swallowed. Thereafter, daily doses of 75 to 325 mg are prescribed. In patients who undergo PCI, higher initial dosages of 162 to 325 mg daily of ASA for 1 month after a bare-metal stent and 3 to 6 months after DES are recommended, which can then be decreased to 81 mg daily indefinitely (level of evidence A, class I recommendation [Chapter 57]). For patients not undergoing stenting, the patient may be discharged on an 81-mg daily dose.

### Adenosine Diphosphate Receptor Antagonists

Ticlopidine and clopidogrel are thienopyridine derivatives that block the binding of ADP to the $P_2Y_{12}$ receptor on the platelet surface, inhibiting ADP-mediated platelet activation. Because of potential safety concerns with ticlopidine (neutropenia, thrombotic thrombocytopenia [TTP]), clopidogrel has replaced ticlopidine for essentially all indications. The Clopidogrel versus Aspirin in Patients at Risk of Ischaemic Events (CAPRIE) trial compared 325 mg of ASA to 75 mg of clopidogrel and found that there was a slight reduction in the composite end point of ischemic stroke, MI, or symptomatic peripheral arterial disease in the clopidogrel arm in 1 to 3 years of follow-up. Because of the excess expense of clopidogrel and the lack of substantial improvement in risk, *clopidogrel monotherapy is indicated only for patients with a true allergy or serious intolerance to ASA*; otherwise ASA is the first-line antiplatelet medicine in patients with ACS.

The Clopidogrel in Unstable Angina to Prevent Recurrent Ischemic Events (CURE) trial evaluated the effects of combination therapy with ASA and clopidogrel versus ASA alone in UA/NSTEMI, since the drugs inhibit platelet aggregation through different pathways. The composite end point of CV death, MI, or stroke was significantly reduced from 11.5% of patients assigned to ASA alone to 9.3% of patients assigned to clopidogrel and ASA therapy; this difference persisted in both medical therapy and revascularization patients. *This is why dual antiplatelet therapy with both clopidogrel and ASA is recommended for at least 1 month and up to 1 year after UA/NSTEMI in medically treated patients.* Because of the risk of late in-stent thrombosis with drug-eluting stents (DES), clopidogrel is recommended for at least 1 year in patients who undergo PCI with DES. *For patients undergoing PCI with bare-metal stents, the preferred duration of clopidogrel therapy is 1 year.*

Excess bleeding was seen in the clopidogrel and ASA groups in clinical trials; however, this mostly occurred in patients who underwent CABG within 5 days of receiving clopidogrel. Therefore administering a loading dose of clopidogrel (300-600 mg) prior to catheterization presents logistic challenges because a given patient may require CABG and would likely have surgery delayed if he or she had received clopidogrel. Many hospitals will delay clopidogrel loading until the need for CABG has been ruled out after angiography and then give a loading dose (300-600 mg) on the catheterization table if PCI is to be carried out immediately.

## Platelet Glycoprotein IIb/IIIa Receptor Inhibitors

The GP IIb/IIIa receptor is a platelet surface receptor that undergoes a configurational change when activated that results in the binding of fibrinogen to platelet receptors, leading to platelet aggregation. The platelet GP IIb/IIIa receptor antagonists occupy these receptor sites and inhibit fibrinogen binding.

The GP IIb/IIIa receptor inhibitors are IV agents that are monoclonal antibodies to the $\beta$-3 integrin of the IIb/IIIa receptor (abciximab) or synthetic molecules that mimic the fibrinogen receptor glycoprotein-binding sequence, either as peptidomimetics (eptifibatide) or as small inhibitory molecules (tirofiban).

There are 2 broad strategies for GP IIb/IIIa inhibitor use in ACS: (1) an "upstream" strategy in which either eptifibatide or tirofiban is administered in the emergency department or hospital for medical stabilization, usually in anticipation of an early invasive approach to PCI; or (2) use of eptifibatide or abciximab as adjunctive therapy in the cardiac catheterization laboratory immediately prior to PCI.

Because of cost and because cardiac catheterization is increasingly performed early after presentation, GP IIb/IIIa inhibitor administration may be deferred until the time of PCI. In the c7E3 Fab Anti-Platelet Therapy in Unstable Refractory Angina (CAPTURE) study, abciximab was associated with a 68% relative risk reduction in death or MI in troponin-positive patients but had no observable benefit in troponin-negative patients. The Intracoronary Stenting and Anti-thrombotic Regimen: Rapid Early Action for Coronary Treatment (ISAR-REACT)-2 study found that in UA/NSTEMI patients treated with ASA and clopidogrel, abciximab reduced the primary end point of death or MI by 25% in patients who were troponin-positive, but was ineffective in troponin-negative patients.

In general, antiplatelet therapy with ASA and antithrombotic therapy with either UFH or LMWH (see below) are administered to all patients with UA/NSTEMI. Additional antiplatelet therapy with clopidogrel is usually given (300-600 mg loading dose, then 75 mg daily) prior to or at the time of PCI. The GP IIb/IIIa inhibitors are usually reserved for high-risk patients who are likely to undergo early PCI and may be administered either upstream or at the time of PCI.

## ■ ANTITHROMBIN THERAPY

### Indirect Thrombin Inhibitors: UFH and LMWH

UFH is a heterogeneous mixture of polysaccharides that inactivates factor IIa (thrombin), factor IXa, and factor Xa by accelerating the action of circulating antithrombin and preventing thrombus generation. LMWH is a mixture of smaller-molecular-weight chains of heparin that more preferentially inactivate factor Xa. Both UFH and LMWH help to prevent thrombus generation but do not lyse clot-bound thrombin.

Several trials have shown benefit to using UFH over placebo in ACS. In a meta-analysis of 6 trials comparing UFH and ASA therapy to ASA therapy alone, death, nonfatal MI, and recurrent angina were reduced by 33% in UFH-treated patients ($p = 0.06$).

UFH has poor bioavailability, with marked variability in anticoagulation response. UFH anticoagulant effects must be closely monitored by the activated partial thromboplastin time (aPTT). Dosing should be adjusted for weight (Table 24-2) and the aPTT should be measured every 6 hours until it has stabilized between 60 and 80 seconds and then every 12 to 24 hours to ensure stability of the anticoagulant effects. Heparin-induced thrombocytopenia (HIT) is a potential adverse effect of heparin (incidence, 1%-5%), and therefore requires serial platelet monitoring. There are 2 forms of HIT: (1) a mild form in which there is a slight decrease in platelet counts (rarely <100 000/μL) that occurs early (1-4 days) after initiation of therapy, reverses quickly after discontinuation of heparin, and is of little clinical consequence; and (2) a more severe form that is an immune-mediated thrombocytopenia that typically occurs more than 5 days from therapy in heparin-naïve patients (earlier in patients who have received heparin within the previous 3-4 months), which can lead to thrombosis and significant morbidity and mortality. Heparin should be discontinued immediately when HIT is suspected, the patient's blood should be screened for antiplatelet antibodies, and direct thrombin inhibitors should be initiated for anticoagulation.

Compared to UFH, LMWH offers the advantages of more predictable anticoagulation, no need for routine laboratory monitoring, and once- or twice-daily subcutaneous dosing due to LMWH decreased nonspecific binding. LMWH also has a lower incidence of HIT than UFH.

Nine large randomized trials have directly compared LMWH with UFH. In 5 of 6 trials that used enoxaparin, enoxaparin versus UFH was associated with a pooled odds ratio of 0.91 (95% CI 0.83-0.99) for the composite end point of death, MI, or recurrent angina. However, 3 other trials evaluating 2 other LMWHs, nadroparin and dalteparin, showed no significant difference in death or nonfatal MI compared to UFH-treated patients. Enoxaparin has been shown to be superior to UFH in trials utilizing an early conservative strategy but not when an early invasive strategy was employed. Both UFH and enoxaparin have class I recommendations for use in UA/NSTEMI according to the ACC/AHA 2007 Guideline Update (Chapter 57).

## Direct Thrombin Inhibitors

Two direct thrombin inhibitors, hirudin and bivalirudin, have been tested in patients with UA/NSTEMI. Only bivalirudin has adequate data to support a class I (Chapter 57) recommendation in the updated guideline. Lepirudin, the recombinant form of hirudin, is only indicated to treat patients with HIT.

Two studies have compared bivalirudin, a semisynthetic direct thrombin inhibitor, to heparin-based therapy. Bivalirudin offered no advantage to heparin in terms of 30-day rates of ischemia, major bleeding, and clinical outcomes. Given its higher cost, bivalirudin is not an attractive option for patients receiving GP IIb/IIIa inhibitors. In contrast, bivalirudin alone was comparable to heparin and a GP IIb/IIIa inhibitor with regard to efficacy and was associated with lower bleeding in patients who had received a thienopyridine prior to catheterization, but inferior to heparin and a GP IIb/IIIa if no thienopyridine had been administered.

## Factor Xa Inhibitors

Factor Xa inhibitors act early in the coagulation cascade in order to prevent downstream reactions that promote thrombin generation. Fondaparinux is a pentasaccharide factor Xa inhibitor with a dose-independent clearance, a longer half-life than UFH, and less protein and endothelial binding, leading to predictable anticoagulation that only requires once-daily subcutaneous administration.

The Organization to Assess Strategies for Ischemic Syndromes (OASIS)-5 study evaluated fondaparinux versus LMWH in the treatment of UA/NSTEMI patients and found that compared to LMWH, fondaparinux was associated with identical short-term efficacy but less major bleeding at 9 days; moreover, rates of death, MI, and stroke at 6 months were reduced compared to UFH (11.3% vs 12.5%, $p < 0.001$). There was, however, an increased incidence of catheter-associated thrombus in the fondaparinux group, leading the ACC/AHA to recommend that supplemental UFH would be needed during angiography/PCI in patients treated with fondaparinux. Because of its long half-life, lack of reversibility, and the potential risk for catheter-associated thrombi, fondaparinux *is not* an attractive agent for invasively managed patients.

# ◾ FIBRINOLYTIC THERAPY

Fibrinolytics are contraindicated for the treatment of UA/NSTEMI because of an increased risk of MI and bleeding with their use.

# ◾ INTRA-AORTIC BALLOON PUMP

Although randomized data are limited for evaluating the use of intra-aortic coun-terpulsation for the treatment of refractory ischemia, it has been used effectively to improve myocardial blood flow by increasing coronary filling during diastole and to reduce myocardial oxygen demand by decreasing afterload in early systole. Balloon pumps are particularly useful when UA/NSTEMI is complicated by cardiogenic shock.

# ◾ LIPID-LOWERING THERAPY

The major clinical trials of lipid management post-ACS have supported aggressive LDL lowering. In the Myocardial Ischemia Reduction with Aggressive Cholesterol Lowering (MIRACL) study, atorvastatin 80 mg/d versus placebo started 24 to 96 hours after ACS was associated with an absolute risk reduction of 2.6% in the primary end point of death, MI, resuscitated cardiac arrest, or recurrent myocardial ischemia ($p = 0.048$) 16 weeks after therapy initiation.

The Zocor (Z) phase of the A to Z trial compared an early intensive statin regimen (simvastatin 40 mg followed by 80 mg) with a delayed and less-intensive regimen (placebo for 4 months followed by simvastatin 20 mg) for up to 24 months in patients with ACS. The primary end point of cardiovascular death, MI, readmission for ACS, or stroke was reduced in the early intensive statin arm compared to the delayed, less-intensive arm (HR 0.89; 95% CI 0.76-1.04), and cardiovascular death was reduced by 25% in the early intensive statin arm ($p = 0.05$).

In the Pravastatin or Atorvastatin Evaluation and Infection Therapy (PROVE IT)-TIMI 22 trial an intensive statin regimen of atorvastatin 80 mg was compared with a standard statin regimen of pravastatin 40 mg/d among 4162 patients with ACS. The atorvastatin arm achieved an average LDL cholesterol of 62 mg/dL versus an average of 95 mg/dL in the pravastatin arm. The primary end point of death, MI, UA, or revascularization after 30 days was reduced by 16% in the atorvastatin arm ($p <0.0001$).

The ACC/AHA 2007 Guideline Update for the Management of Patients With UA and NSTEMI (Chapter 57) recommends that all UA/NSTEMI patients have a fasting lipid profile drawn within 24 hours of hospitalization and that statins be given to all UA/NSTEMI patients, regardless of baseline LDL-C. LDL-C should be reduced to at least less than 100 mg/dL and ideally to less than 70 mg/dL, as endorsed by the National Cholesterol Education Panel.

# ■ CORONARY REVASCULARIZATION

Coronary angiography is useful for defining the coronary artery anatomy in patients with UA/NSTEMI as well as identifying the subset of high-risk patients who will benefit from early revascularization. The goals of revascularization (surgical or percutaneous) are 4-fold: (1) to improve prognosis, (2) to relieve symptoms, (3) to prevent ischemic complications, and (4) to improve functional capacity. The decision to revascularize a given lesion is based on the coronary anatomy, quantity of myocardium at risk, LV systolic function, and individual patient characteristics (comorbidities, life expectancy, symptom severity, functional status). The decision to perform revascularization must take all of these issues into account (**Fig. 24-4**).

# ■ PERCUTANEOUS CORONARY INTERVENTION

Given continued technical advances, widespread antiplatelet and anticoagulant therapy, as well as the use of stents, PCI provides a safe and durable option for revascularization in UA/NSTEMI patients. Stenting has reduced the incidence of both acute

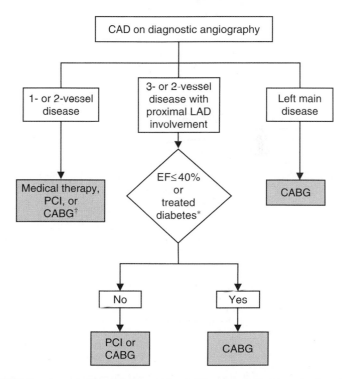

**FIGURE 24-4.** Revascularization strategy in UA/NSTEMI. (*There is conflicting information about these patients; most consider CABG to be preferable to PCI.) (†Therapeutic decision based on patient and lesion characteristics including comorbid conditions, severity of symptoms, lesion amenability to PCI, patient and physician preference.) CABG, coronary artery bypass grafting; CAD, coronary artery disease; LAD, left anterior descending artery; PCI, percutaneous intervention. (Data compiled from ACC/AHA 2007 guidelines.)

vessel closure and late restenosis. The use of DES has improved the restenosis rates but has modestly increased the risk of late coronary thrombosis. In select patients who have a high surgical risk and amenable coronary anatomy, multivessel PCI can offer complete revascularization without surgical intervention.

Given recent concerns about late stent thrombosis with DES, particularly when ASA or clopidogrel are prematurely discontinued, it is imperative to ensure that a patient will be able to take ASA and clopidogrel uninterrupted for at least 1 year before placing a DES in a patient with UA/NSTEMI. Alternatives for patients at risk for premature antiplatelet therapy discontinuation—including those who are noncompliant, at increased bleeding risk, or who have upcoming surgery—include bare-metal stents, PTCA alone, CABG (if anatomy is suitable), or medical therapy.

# ■ SURGICAL REVASCULARIZATION

Because of dramatic changes in surgical, medical, and percutaneous therapy, there are very few data from trials using current PCI and surgical techniques to guide selection between PCI and CABG in patients with ACS and multivessel CAD (see Chapter 25).

CABG should be considered in high-risk patients with LV systolic dysfunction, patients with diabetes mellitus and multivessel CAD, and patients with 2-vessel disease with severe proximal left anterior descending artery involvement, severe 3-vessel CAD, or left main disease. In patients with multivessel disease and normal systolic function, multivessel PCI may be performed if the coronary lesion anatomy is amenable to PCI, the likelihood of complete revascularization with PCI is high, and the patient prefers a nonsurgical approach to revascularization.

# SUGGESTED READINGS

de Lemos JA, O'Rourke RA, Harrington RA. Unstable angina and non–ST-segment elevation myocardial infarction. In: Fuster V, Walsh RA, Harrington RA, et al. *Hurst's The Heart*. 13th ed. New York, NY: McGraw-Hill. 2011;59:1328-1353.

Angiolillo DJ, Giugliano GR, Simon DI. Pharmacologic therapy for acute coronary syndromes. In: Fuster V, Walsh RA, Harrington RA, et al. *Hurst's The Heart*. 13th ed. New York, NY: McGraw-Hill. 2011;61:1386-1429.

Anderson J, Adams C, Antman E, et al. ACC/AHA 2007 guidelines for the management of patients with unstable angina/non-ST-elevation myocardial infarction: a report of the American College of Cardiology/American Heart Association Task Force on Practice Guidelines (Writing Committee to Revise the 2002 Guidelines for the Management of Patients With Unstable Angina/Non-ST-Elevation Myocardial Infarction) developed in collaboration with the American College of Emergency Physicians, the Society for Cardiovascular Angiography and Interventions, and the Society of Thoracic Surgeons endorsed by the American Association of Cardiovascular and Pulmonary Rehabilitation and the Society for Academic Emergency Medicine. *J Am Coll Cardiol.* 2007;50:e1-e157.

Antman EM, Cohen M, Bernink PJ, et al. The TIMI risk score for unstable angina/non-ST elevation MI: a method of prognostication and therapeutic decision making. *JAMA.* 2000;284: 835-842.

Bavry AA, Kumbhani DJ, Rassi AN, et al. Benefit of early invasive therapy in acute coronary syndromes: a meta-analysis of contemporary randomized clinical trials. *J Am Coll Cardiol.* 2006;48:1319-1325.

Boersma E, Harrington RA, Moliterno DJ, et al. Platelet glycoprotein IIb/IIIa inhibitors in acute coronary syndromes: a meta-analysis of all major randomized clinical trials. *Lancet.* 2002;359:189-198.

Eagle KA, Lim MJ, Dabbous OH, et al. A validated prediction model for all forms of acute coronary syndrome: estimating the risk of 6-month post-discharge death in an international registry. *JAMA.* 2004;291:2727-2733.

Hayden M, Pignone M, Phillips C, et al. Aspirin for the primary prevention of cardiovascular events: a summary of the evidence for the U.S. Preventive Service Task Force. *Ann Intern Med.* 2002;136:161-172.

Hirsh J, Raschke R. Heparin and low-molecular-weight heparin: the seventh ACCP conference on antithrombotic and thrombolytic therapy. *Chest.* 2004;126:188S-203S.

Lichtenstein AH, Appel LJ, Brands M, et al. Diet and lifestyle recommendations revision 2006: a scientific statement from the American Heart Association Nutrition Committee. *Circulation.* 2006;114:82-96.

Shapiro BP, Jaffe AS. Cardiac biomarkers. In: Murphy JG, Lloyd MA, eds. *Mayo Clinic Cardiology: Concise Textbook.* 3rd ed. Rochester, MN: Mayo Clinic Scientific Press; 2007:773-780.

# CHAPTER 25
# PERCUTANEOUS CORONARY INTERVENTION

John S. Douglas, Jr and Spencer B. King III

## DEVELOPMENT OF BALLOON ANGIOPLASTY

Percutaneous transluminal coronary angioplasty (PTCA) was conceived and shepherded into worldwide acceptance and application by Andreas R. Gruentzig; this technique has now eclipsed coronary bypass surgery as the most frequently performed revascularization procedure. Initially, coronary balloon angioplasty was performed for discrete, proximal, noncalcified subtotal lesions located in 1 coronary artery. A 10-year follow-up of Gruentzig's early Zurich series revealed an overall survival rate of 90%, and of 95% for those with single-vessel disease. Reintervention rates for patients undergoing percutaneous coronary intervention (PCI) have fallen steadily from the PTCA period to the stent period, and are now even lower with the drug-eluting stent (DES). Although PCI for stable angina does not impact myocardial infarction (MI) or death, PCI reduces these end points in high-risk acute coronary syndromes (ACS).

## RANDOMIZED TRIALS OF PERCUTANEOUS CORONARY INTERVENTION

The Angioplasty Compared to Medical Therapy Evaluation (ACME), involving 212 patients with single-vessel disease and abnormal stress tests, revealed greater freedom from angina in the angioplasty group at 6 months, but there was no difference in rates of death or MI. The second Randomized Intervention Treatment of Angina (RITA-2) trial randomized 1018 patients with stable angina and predominantly single-vessel disease to PTCA or medical therapy. Angina relief and treadmill performance were significantly better in the PTCA patients, but survival was not different after 7 years of follow-up. The Clinical Outcomes Utilizing Revascularization and Aggressive Drug Evaluation (COURAGE) trial randomized 2287 patients with stable angina and 1-, 2-, or 3-vessel disease to PCI (predominantly using bare-metal stents) or aggressive medical therapy. There was no reduction in death or MI in the PCI arm; however, there was greater improvement in angina at 1 year, which was not sustained over 5 years. A similar improvement in symptoms but not death or MI was found with revascularization compared with medical therapy in the Atorvastatin Versus Revascularization Treatment (AVERT) trial and the Medicine, Angioplasty, or Surgery Studies (MASS) I and II. Taken together, these data indicate that for patients with stable coronary syndromes, PCI reduces anginal symptoms but does not reduce death or MI rates.

In contrast, patients with ACS derive both symptomatic benefit and a reduction in death and recurrent MI with PCI compared with medical therapy. The Fast Revascularization During Instability in Coronary Disease (FRISC II) study strongly

**TABLE 25-1.** Early Invasive Strategy Recommended in Unstable Angina or Non–ST-Elevation Myocardial Infarction

Class I Indication
Any of the high-risk indications:
- Recurrent angina at rest or minimal activity despite therapy
- Elevated troponin
- New ST-segment depression
- Recurrent angina/ischemia with symptoms or signs of congestive heart failure or new or worsening mitral regurgitation
- Positive stress test
- Ejection fraction <40%
- Hemodynamic instability
- Sustained ventricular tachycardia
- Percutaneous coronary intervention within 6 mo or prior coronary artery bypass grafting
- Depressed LV systolic function
- High-risk score (eg, TIMI, GRACE)

Reproduced with permission from King SB, Smith SC Jr, Hirshfeld JW Jr, et al. 2007 focused update of the ACC/AHA/SCAI 2005 guideline update for percutaneous coronary intervention: a report of the American College of Cardiology/American Heart Association Task Force on Practice guidelines. *J Am Coll Cardiol*. Jan15;2008;51(2):172-209.

supported an invasive approach in patients with ACS randomized after 5 days of dalteparin (Fragmin) therapy. Among men, the invasive strategy in FRISC II resulted in a 34% reduction in death or MI at 6 months and a 52% reduction in mortality. The invasive approach to ACS was further supported by the results of the Treat Angina with Aggrastat and Determine Cost of Therapy with Invasive and Conservative Strategy (TACTICS-TIMI 18) and has been incorporated as a class I recommendation in the ACC/AHA Guideline (**Table 25-1**).

# PERCUTANEOUS CORONARY INTERVENTION VERSUS CORONARY ARTERY BYPASS GRAFTING

Two trials of patients with multivessel coronary artery disease were sponsored by the National Heart, Lung, and Blood Institute and performed in the United States. The first, the Emory Angioplasty versus Surgery Trial (EAST), was a single-center study; while the larger Bypass Angioplasty Revascularization Investigation (BARI) involved 18 centers. In-hospital mortality was similar for angioplasty and bypass surgery. Survival for 7 to 8 years was similar in both studies. The difference favoring surgery is completely explained by a striking advantage of surgery for the diabetic patients. The Arterial Revascularization Therapy Study (ARTS), Stent or Surgery (SOS) study, and Argentine Randomized Study of Stents Versus CABG in Multivessel Disease (ERACI-2) have shown reduced reintervention rates with stents but have not established that PCI is comparable to surgery in multivessel diabetic patients. ARTS II was a comparison of patients with multivessel disease treated with DES with the surgical and bare-metal stent arm of ARTS I. At 1 year, 89.5% of DES-treated patients with MACE-free had a better outcome than ARTS I CABG patients. However, repeat intervention was performed in 8.5% of ARTS II DES patients compared with 4.1% of ARTS I CABG patients, showing a narrowing of the reintervention gap of PCI versus CABG. The New York state registry allowed comparison of 59 314 patients treated for multivessel disease with bare-metal stents and CABG. After adjusting for baseline differences between groups, the CABG patients had significantly better outcomes at 3 years. The SYNTAX Trial (Synergy Between Percutaneous Coronary Intervention with Taxus and Cardiac Surgery)—comparing DES to CABG in multivessel coronary disease demonstrated less need for subsequent revascularization but a higher stroke rate in the surgical group.

# DEVICES AND STRATEGIES FOR CORONARY INTERVENTION

Directional atherectomy, rotational ablation, cutting balloons, and intravascular laser therapy have been used for debulking coronary lesions. Although each has niche applications, their use has declined in recent years. Directional atherectomy is sometimes used in bulky bifurcation lesions, laser therapy, and cutting balloons for in-stent restenosis, and rotational atherectomy for heavily calcified lesions.

## ■ STENTS: THE DOMINANT STRATEGY

Stents were developed for 2 indications: to reduce restenosis and to solve acute vessel closure after angioplasty; they were first implanted in 1986. Stents were approved in 1994 for the elective treatment of de novo lesions in native coronary arteries. Stenting became firmly established when it was found that antiplatelet therapy with thieno-pyridines and aspirin was effective in preventing stent thrombosis.

## ■ DRUG-ELUTING STENTING

Prevention of restenosis postintervention was first documented with endovascular brachytherapy for in-stent restenosis. The inhibition of cell division by radiation has now been replicated with drugs delivered locally from a polymer coating on stents. Rapamycin (sirolimus)- and paclitaxel-eluting stents have been shown to reduce angiographic restenosis from 20% to 30% with the control stents to 5% to 10% with the drug-eluting stents. The Sirolimus-Eluting Balloon Expandable Stent in the Treatment of Patients with de Novo Native Coronary Artery Lesions (SIRIUS) and Paclitaxel Eluting Stent (TAXUS) trials showed marked inhibition of neointima formation over the stents and therefore a reduction in angiographic restenosis. Recently, a third DES, the Medtronic AVE ABT-578 eluting Driver stent, was approved by the Food and Drug Administration (FDA) for clinical use in the United States based on the ENDEAVOR 1, 2, and 3 trials demonstrating safety and efficacy. Preliminary data from SPIRIT II comparing the everolimus-eluting stent with the Taxus stent revealed similar late lumen loss, restenosis, and MACE. The Xience everolimus-eluting stent is currently under consideration by the FDA for approval. It should be noted that *the trial results overestimate the restenosis impact because of the routine angiograms required. In real-world practice, where routine angiograms are not performed in asymptomatic patients, the impact on reintervention has been less* and a reduction in MI or death rates has not yet been demonstrated.

The cost-effectiveness of DES compared with bare-metal stents is a balance between their higher up-front costs and the avoidance of repeat revascularization. Subgroups in which DES are most likely to be cost-effective compared with bare-metal stents include diabetics, long lesions, small vessels, perhaps left main or proximal left anterior descending (LAD) locations, saphenous vein grafts, or other lesions with high restenosis rates with bare-metal stents.

## Emerging Concerns With Drug-Eluting Stents

Although drug-eluting stents have clearly become the dominant PCI strategy in the United States, recent reports of coronary endothelial dysfunction, coronary vasospasm, hypersensitivity reactions, delayed vessel healing, delayed endothelialization, and latestent thrombosis have emerged. The clinical presentation of stent thrombosis is often ST-elevation MI, with mortality rates of 30% to 50%. The data regarding the incidence of late stent thrombosis with DES compared with bare-metal stents are conflicting. Some studies suggest nonsignificantly higher rates of late stent thrombosis with DES (**Fig. 25-1**), while other studies suggest that when stenting is performed in "off-label" locations (eg, bifurcation disease, left main disease, ostial or diffuse disease), there may be a mortality advantage of DES over bare-metal stenting (NHLBI Dynamic Registry). What is clear is that there is consensus on the need for adequate patient counseling against the premature discontinuation of dual antiplatelet therapy and the need for its prolonged use in patients receiving DES. Risk factors for stent thrombosis include performance of complex PCI, inadequate stent expansion or strut apposition, and premature discontinuation of dual antiplatelet therapy.

# ADJUNCTIVE STRATEGIES

## ■ THIENOPYRIDINES

Clopidogrel inhibits platelet activation by irreversibly blocking the ADP (P2Y12) receptor. In stable angina and troponin-negative ACS patients, a 600-mg clopidogrel loading dose administered 2 hours prior to PCI is as effective as clopidogrel plus abciximab. However, in troponin-positive patients the combination of clopidogrel and abciximab is superior to clopidogrel alone. Recent guidelines recommend (1) for patients receiving bare-metal stents, at least 4 weeks of dual antiplatelet therapy and ideally up to 12 months unless patients are at increased risk of bleeding, in which case it should be given for 2 weeks; and (2) for patients receiving DES, at least 12 months of dual antiplatelet therapy with DES implantation, if patients are not at high risk of bleeding. Dual antiplatelet therapy for long term (beyond 12 months) may be considered for patients receiving DES. Patients taking daily aspirin prior to PCI should take 75 to 325 mg before PCI is performed. For patients not previously on aspirin, 300 to 325 mg should be taken at least 2 hours prior to PCI. After PCI, 162 to 325 mg of aspirin should be given for at least 1 month in patients receiving bare-metal stents, 3 months for patients receiving sirulomus-eluting stents, and 6 months for patients receiving pacletaxileluting stents, after which all patients should receive 75 to 162 mg of aspirin daily lifelong. Reports of 10% to 15% of aspirin resistance and up to 25% clopidogrel resistance potentially contributing to higher stent thrombosis risk have emerged. The use of reliable, standardized, simple tests of platelet activity would facilitate the diagnosis of aspirin and clopidogrel resistance.

## ■ IIB/IIIA PLATELET RECEPTOR INHIBITORS

These platelet receptor blockers have been used as an adjunct to coronary intervention. The antibody fragment, abciximab; the peptide, eptifibatide; and the nonpeptide small-molecule agent, tirofiban, have each reduced periprocedural events, most commonly CK-MB elevation. Meta-analysis has suggested a small survival benefit. Other studies have shown no benefit on cardiac events in stable patients who have been given high-dose clopidogrel several hours before the procedure. These agents are recommended for PCI in the ACC/AHA unstable angina and non–ST-segment elevation MI guidelines.

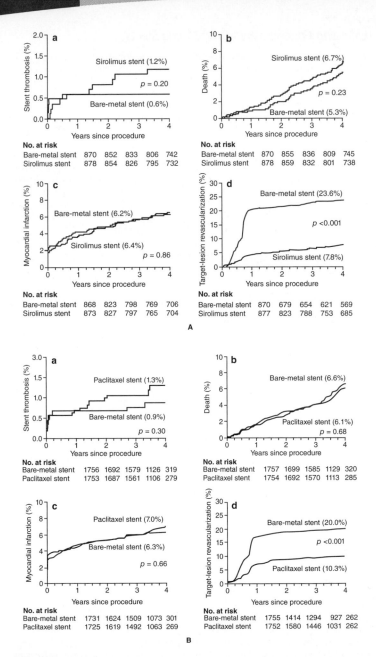

**FIGURE 25-1. A.** Analysis of randomized trials of sirolimus versus bare-metal stents on stent thrombosis, death, myocardial infarction, and target-lesion revascularization. **B.** Analysis of randomized trials of paclitaxel versus bare-metal stents on stent thrombosis, death, myocardial infarction, and target-lesion revascularization.

# ■ THROMBIN INHIBITORS

Unfractionated heparin has been the primary thrombin inhibitor used during PCI over the last 2 decades. An activated clotting time of 300 seconds is targeted (or 200-250 seconds with concomitant IIb/IIIa inhibitor use). Low-molecular-weight heparin (LMWH) has advantages over unfractionated heparin (UFH) in being more bioavailable; being less inhibited by platelet factor 4; causing less thrombocytopenia; and having more predictable anticoagulant effects, eliminating the need for activated clotting time monitoring in the cath lab. Therefore, LMWH use for PCI is currently a class IIa indication. Achieving a factor Xa level >0.5 IU/mL has been a suggested target that was achieved by a 0.5-mg/kg bolus of intravenous enoxaparin. In the absence of factor Xa level monitoring, if PCI is performed within 8 hours of LMWH, no further LMWH is recommended. If the PCI is performed between 8 and 12 hours, a 0.3-mg/kg bolus of enoxaparin is recommended intravenously. The direct thrombin inhibitor Hirulog (bivalirudin) is also FDA approved for use during PCI. Advantages of these agents for PCI include the ease of monitoring their action with ACT measurement, their ability to inactivate clot-bound thrombin, and a favorable safety profile. In the latest guideline statement, bivalirudin has a class IIa indication for use in low-risk patients who are undergoing elective PCI. It has been suggested that optimal antithrombin therapy for PCI in certain complex patient subgroups, such as those with a high risk of bleeding, renal failure, and heparin-induced thrombocytopenia, is perhaps best accomplished with a direct thrombin inhibitor, whereas those with troponin positivity, diabetes, thrombus-containing lesions, and ST-elevation infarction are probably best managed with an indirect thrombin inhibitor and IIb/IIIa platelet receptor inhibitor.

# ■ INTRAVASCULAR ULTRASOUND

Although coronary angiography is the reference standard for the diagnosis of coronary artery disease, it has major limitations. Assessment of the significance of intermediate or indeterminant lesions, plaque characterization, recognition of diffuse intimal thickening, and accurate assessment of vessel dimensions and lesion extent are important pre-PCI determinations in which intravascular ultrasound (IVUS) greatly surpasses angiography. A minimal lumen cross-sectional area of 3.0 to 4.0 mm$^2$ in major epicardial vessels and a left main minimal lumen diameter of 2.8 mm or minimal lumen area of 5.9 mm$^2$ indicates physiologic significance. Unopposed stent struts and stent underexpansion are thought to contribute to DES thrombosis and restenosis. It has been suggested that routine IVUS imaging during DES implantation is indicated in a number of high-risk patient subsets (renal failure, limitations to dual antiplatelet use, diabetes, poor LV function) and in high-risk lesion subsets (left main, bifurcations, ostial site, small vessels, long lesions, instent restenoses). Newly developed virtual histology IVUS, permitting plaque characterization into 1 of 4 phenotypes (fibrous, fibrofatty, necrotic core, or calcium) is a potentially useful addition to the diagnostic armamentarium of the interventionalist and is currently being studied.

# ■ FRACTIONAL FLOW RESERVE

Even experienced angiographers cannot adequately assess the physiologic significance of moderate coronary lesions. Fractional flow reserve (FFR) has emerged as a simple, reliable, and reproducible guidewire-based physiologic assessment of lesion severity and is defined as the ratio of distal coronary and aortic pressure during maximal hyperemia. An FFR <0.75 has been shown to be accurate in predicting ischemia, and it is safe to defer PCI when FFR is ≥0.75. When microvascular disease is suspected, an FFR value of <0.80 is indicative of ischemia. This adjunctive tool, which can be safely performed in a few minutes, brings substantial value to the patient and is cost-effective in many applications.

## ■ EMBOLIC PROTECTION AND THROMBECTOMY DEVICES

A variety of occlusion–aspiration and filter-based strategies have evolved for embolic protection during saphenous vein graft interventions, which reduce atheroembolic MI by approximately 50% and constitute a class I indication in PCI guidelines. There has been limited application of embolic protection in native vessel PCI. A rheolytic thrombectomy device known as the AngioJet (POSSIS Medical, Minneapolis, MN) has become available for treatment of intracoronary thrombus, and it has proved useful in the setting of ACS associated with large thrombi and in treatment of stent thrombosis. The Export (Medtronic-AVE, Santa Rosa, CA) and PRONTO (Vascular Solutions, Minneapolis, MN) catheters are much simpler aspiration catheters that have proved useful in removing intracoronary thrombus.

# HYBRID REVASCULARIZATION

The hybrid approach incorporates DES implantation and minimally invasive coronary surgery, the combination of these adjunctive strategies permitting complete revascularization. Most commonly, the left internal mammary artery (LIMA) is used to bypass the LAD coronary artery, and non-LAD coronary artery targets are stented. This approach is thought to be ideal for patients with complex LAD coronary artery disease (ostial, bifurcation, or diffuse proximal involvement), significant but noncritical left main disease, and diabetes where LIMA-to-LAD coronary artery may have a mortality advantage. Avoidance of a sternotomy and cardiopulmonary bypass shortens hospitalization and hastens recovery. However, specialized surgical skills are necessary and long-term follow-up is not yet available.

# HEMODYNAMICALLY SUPPORTED PCI

Intra-aortic balloon pump counterpulsation is widely available for hemodynamic support of high-risk PCI but provides limited support. The Tandem Heart Percutaneous Ventricular Assist device (CardiacAssist, Pittsburgh, PA) is a relatively simple centrifugal pump that provides sufficient hemodynamic support (up to 5.5 L/min) to sustain patients who are transiently without cardiac output, and has been used to provide circulatory protection during high-risk PCI or bridging to another therapy such as cardiac surgery, a left ventricular assist device, or transplantation. Complications such as bleeding, infection, thrombocytopenia, and anemia have been described with this device.

# CLOSURE DEVICES

A variety of devices are currently available to close common femoral artery access sites following PCI. They permit earlier ambulation, enhance patient comfort, increase costs, and do not significantly alter overall access site complication rates. Rarely, infection or vascular compromise may occur and necessitate surgery.

# INDICATIONS FOR CORONARY INTERVENTION

In general, when one is selecting PCI, there should be assurance that the operator can treat, with a high probability of success, the coronary lesion(s) accounting for the symptoms or signs of myocardial ischemia. Further, the associated risk and durability of the revascularization should be acceptable—as compared with bypass surgery or medical therapy—during both early and long-term follow-up. The latter estimate requires consideration of the likelihood and consequences of acute, subacute, late, and very late stent thrombosis, restenosis, and incomplete revascularization. Additional factors to be considered include the use of DES versus bare-metal stents, and the tolerability, cost, and risks associated with long-term dual antiplatelet therapy. The American College of Cardiology/American Heart Association Guidelines for Percutaneous Transluminal Coronary Angioplasty and Coronary Bypass Surgery provide a detailed analysis of many of these issues. **Table 25-2** summarizes the Guideline recommendations for patients with asymptomatic ischemia or classes I to III angina.

# SELECTION OF PATIENTS

## ■ SINGLE-VESSEL DISEASE

Percutaneous revascularization is an attractive option for many symptomatic patients who fail medical therapy and who have anatomically suitable lesions. For patients with complex bifurcation proximal LAD disease, consideration should be given to surgical revascularization. In experienced hands, endoscopic LIMA to LAD may be an attractive approach. It is important, however, to remember that there is no survival benefit of angioplasty compared with medical therapy.

**TABLE 25-2.** Recommendations for PCI Adopted From the ACC/AHA/SCAI 2005 Guideline Update in Patients With Asymptomatic Ischemia or Class I to III Angina

| | |
|---|---|
| Class IIa | 1 or more lesions in 1 or more vessels with high likelihood of success and low risk; vessels subtend large area of viable myocardium or produce moderate to severe ischemia (*level of evidence: B*); or a recurrent stenosis following PCI (*level of evidence: C*); or left main stenosis >50% in CABG-ineligible patient (*level of evidence: B*); or SVG lesions in poor candidate for reoperation (*level of evidence: C*). |
| Class IIb | Efficacy of PCI in multivessel disease patients with proximal LAD stenosis and diabetes or an abnormal left ventricle is less well established (*level of evidence: B*); PCI may be considered in non-LAD sites producing ischemia (*level of evidence: C*). |
| Class III | Small amount of myocardium at risk, absence of ischemia, low PCI success, mild symptoms unlikely to be ischemia, increased PCI risk, left main stenosis and eligible for CABG, <50% stenosis (*level of evidence: C*). |

ACC, American College of Cardiology; AHA, American Heart Association; CABG, coronary artery bypass grafting; LAD, left anterior descending artery; PCI, percutaneous coronary intervention; SCAI, Society of Cardiac Angiography and Intervention; SVG, saphenous vein graft.

# ■ MULTIVESSEL DISEASE

Rational selection of patients requires a careful analysis of multiple issues, including a risk-benefit assessment of each ischemia-producing lesion, a projection of the possible completeness and durability of the physiologic revascularization, and an estimate of resource consumption compared with surgery and medical therapy. In the experience of the Emory Angioplasty Versus Surgery Trial (EAST), 71% of index segments were revascularized in PTCA patients; while in the Bypass Angioplasty Revascularization Investigation (BARI 2D), 90% of the segments were revascularized by PCI or CABG. Culprit-lesion angioplasty is clearly an accepted strategy, but care must be taken to avoid significant residual ischemia after intervention. A strategy of physiologic (FFR)-guided PCI for multivessel disease may ensure complete revascularization of ischemic territories without subjecting patients to the short- and long-term risk of unnecessary revascularization of angiographically stenotic but non-ischemic lesions. Retrospective analyses have shown that compared to the standard angiographic-guided approach, this strategy results in fewer stents deployed, lower costs, and improved outcomes. A randomized trial of physiologic (FFR) versus angiographic-guided revascularization in multivessel disease is currently under way. The risks of PCI are increased in the presence of unstable angina, advanced age, poor left ventricular function, extensive coronary disease, comorbid conditions, and female gender.

# SELECTION OF LESIONS

## ■ LESION CHARACTERISTICS

In the ACC/AHA/SCAI 2005 Guideline Update for PCI, 6 high-risk lesion characteristics (type C) were recognized as important in the stent era. Four lesion classifications were suggested by considering the presence or absence of a type-C lesion and whether the vessel was patent or occluded (**Table 25-3**). This classification was shown to provide improved prediction of success and complications compared to the old ACC/AHA lesion classification. Interestingly, thrombus, bifurcation, and left main lesions do not appear but remain important predictors of adverse outcome in the experience of the authors (see "Left Main Coronary Lesions" and "Bifurcation Lesions" as follows).

# LEFT MAIN CORONARY LESIONS

The early experience with PTCA of left main lesions was unfavorable. Although acute results were more favorable with bare-metal stents, late outcomes remained poor (restenosis rate of 21%, late death 7.4%). With DES, 6- to 12-month mortality of left main PCI is approximately 2% to 4% in experienced hands. This is comparable to in-hospital mortality for CABG. Angiographic restenosis for the ostial and mid left main coronary artery is ≤5%, but much higher for distal left main stenosis, particularly when it involves the bifurcation. With 2-stent approaches, there is an approximately 2% stent thrombosis rate and a 20% to 40% restenosis rate. This mandates angiographic surveillance at 3 months, and probably at 9 months, in order to detect and treat restenosis. Even for ostial or mid left main disease, longer-term follow-up will be required before this strategy is recommendable to all comers. The ACC/AHA/SCAI guidelines recommend CABG for patients with left main disease who are surgical candidates. However, for patients who are not candidates for CABG, PCI is an option, but prolonged dual antiplatelet therapy and angiographic surveillance should be mandated.

**TABLE 25-3.** Society of Cardiac Angiography and Intervention Lesion Classification System: Characteristics of Class I to IV Lesions[a]

Type I lesions (highest success expected, lowest risk)
1. Does not meet criteria for C lesion
2. Patent vessel

Type II lesions
1. Meets any of these criteria for ACC/AHA C lesion:diffuse (>2 cm length); excessive tortuosity of proximal segment; extremely angulated segments, >90 degrees; inability to protect major side branches; degenerated vein grafts with friable lesions
2. Patent vessel

Type III lesions
1. Does not meet criteria for C lesion
2. Occluded vessel

Type IV lesions
1. Meets any of these criteria for ACC/AHA C lesion: diffuse (>2 cm length); excessive tortuosity of proximal segment; extremely angulated segments, >90 degrees; inability to protect major side branches; degenerated vein grafts with friable lesions; occluded for more than 3 mo
2. Occluded vessel

[a]See Chapter 57.

ACC, American College of Cardiology; AHA, American Heart Association.

Adapted from Krone RJ, Shaw RE, Klein LW, et al. Evaluation of the American College of Cardiology/American Heart Association and the Society for Coronary Angiography and Interventions lesion classification system in the current "stent era" of coronary interventions (from the ACC-National Cardiovascular Data Registry). *Am J Cardiol.* 2003;92:389-394.

# ■ CHRONIC TOTAL OCCLUSIONS

Chronic total occlusions (CTO) are found in up to 30% of diagnostic angiograms, but accounted for only 5.7% of coronary interventions in the NHLBI Dynamic Registry in 2004. Unrevascularized CTOs in multivessel disease patients may portend worse prognosis at 3-year follow-up. However, PCI of CTOs remains technically challenging and has lower success rates (50%-70%) even with experienced operators. Stiffer guidewires, the Safe Cross guidewire (IntraLuminal Therapeutics, Carlsbad, CA), coupling guidance with radiofrequency energy, and a helical screw-in microcatheter are examples of new technology to assist the PCI operator in successfully crossing the CTO. Drug-eluting stent implantation significantly improves outcomes compared with bare-metal stents.

# ■ BIFURCATION LESIONS

Bifurcation lesions remain difficult to treat effectively in the cath lab. Compared to nonbifurcation lesions, bifurcations were found to be more complex (angulated, eccentric, ostial, tortuous) and have a higher need for repeat intervention. To protect the side branch, many bifurcation techniques were developed (T-stenting, modified T-stenting, provisional T-stenting, Y- and V-stenting, culotte stenting, and crush stenting). None, however, proved superior to a single stent if side-branch patency was achieved with balloon dilation. The simple approach of stenting the main branch and provisional stenting of the side branch is currently recommended for most situations. If there is uncertainty regarding the need to stent the side branch, measurement of FFR is both safe and feasible. Koo and associates found that no side branch with <75% stenosis had FFR <0.75, and of 73 lesions with ≥75% stenosis, only 27% were functionally significant. Dedicated bifurcation stents are under development.

# ■ IN-STENT RESTENOSIS

The clinical presentation of in-stent restenosis includes exertional angina (64%), unstable angina (26%), and acute MI in 10% of 1186 cases. The treatment options included balloon angioplasty, cutting balloon angioplasty, rotational atherectomy, and repeat bare-metal stent deployment. The use of intracoronary brachytherapy was shown to reduce restenosis, but brachytherapy was cumbersome, resulted in delayed healing, and raised concerns regarding late stent thrombosis and aneurysm formation. Drug-eluting stents have become the dominant strategy for treatment of bare-metal stent restenosis. When DES restenosis occurs, performing IVUS may be particularly important to rule out stent underexpansion or strut malapposition, both of which could be treated with high-pressure inflations. If the stent appears well deployed, repeat DES placement, medical therapy, or surgical revascularization should be considered, although there are very few data to guide therapy in this situation.

# ■ AORTOCORONARY GRAFT LESIONS

PCI of distal anastomotic stenoses of saphenous vein grafts (SVGs) and LIMA grafts occurring within 1 year of CABG is safe and effective. Proximal SVG anastomotic and midgraft lesions have high restenosis rates, especially when long lesions are present. Atheromatous SVG lesions begin to appear about 3 years after CABG, and PCI is frequently associated with periprocedural MI caused by atheroembolization, a complication *not* prevented by IIb/IIIa platelet receptor inhibitors. Stent implantation is more effective than balloon angioplasty in SVG PCI. Distal and proximal embolic protection devices result in approximately 50% reduction in 30-day MACE. Proximal embolic protection are used when there is insufficient room beyond the target lesion for distal protection. Use of embolic protection during PCI of de novo SVG lesions is a class I indication in the ACC/AHA Guideline Statement and is cost-effective. Treatment of no-reflow after stenting includes aspiration of the stagnant dye column, hemodynamic support if needed, and administration of microvascular dilators distally (nitroprusside, calcium-channel blocker, or adenosine). Drug-eluting stents yield superior outcomes to bare-metal stents for SVG PCI. A high late cardiac event rate following SVG PCI relates largely to progression of atherosclerosis outside the stented segments. Consideration of native vessel intervention, including CTO recanalization whenever possible, careful surveillance, and aggressive risk factor modification, is warranted for these patients.

# LESION CHARACTERISTICS

The importance of coronary stenosis angiographic morphology in predicting the outcome of coronary angioplasty is reflected in the ACC/AHA PTCA guidelines. In an effort to update this classification based on the results of contemporary coronary intervention using stents and IIb/IIIa platelet inhibitors, Ellis and colleagues analyzed results from 10 907 lesions and proposed a new classification scheme for risk stratification (**Table 25-4**). Nine preintervention variables were independently correlated with adverse outcome. Recent predictive models have been developed

**TABLE 25-4.** New Risk-Assessment Schema[a]

| | |
|---|---|
| Strongest correlates | Nonchronic total occlusion |
| | Degenerated saphenous vein graft (SVG) |
| Moderately strong correlates | Length ≥10 mm |
| | Lumen irregularity |
| | Large filling defect |
| | Calcium + angle ≥45 degrees |
| | Eccentric |
| | Severe calcification |
| | SVG age ≥10 y |
| Highest risk | Either of strongest correlates |
| High risk | ≥3 moderate correlates and the absence of strong correlates |
| Moderate risk | 1-2 moderate correlates and the absence of strong correlates |
| Low risk | No risk factors |

[a]Based on analysis of 10 907 lesions treated in the stent and IIb/IIIa era.

Adapted from Ellis SG, Guetta V, Miller D, et al. Relation between lesion characteristics and risk with percutaneous intervention in the stent and glycoprotein IIb/IIIa era: an analysis of results from 10 907 lesions and proposal for new classification scheme. *Circulation.* 1999;100:1971-1976.

in the New York State Registry, in the Northern New England Registry, and at the Cleveland Clinic.

# SELECTION OF DEVICES

**Table 25-5** outlines the various technologies compared with balloon dilation. In the United States, stents are selected for primary treatment of almost all lesions in vessels ≥2.5 mm in diameter in patients who can tolerate at least short-term dual antiplatelet therapy. However, balloon angioplasty remains a useful option in persistently symptomatic patients with critical lesions in vessels <2.5 mm or in selected patients who cannot tolerate dual antiplatelet therapy. Rotational atherectomy or cutting balloon angioplasty is reserved for heavily calcified lesions and for debulking instent restenosis. Suitable lesions for directional atherectomy are generally ostial or bifurcation lesions in vessels ≥3 mm in diameter.

# PERFORMANCE OF CORONARY INTERVENTION

Current guidelines recommend that cardiologists who wish to become competent in coronary intervention receive special training in diagnostic and therapeutic catheterization during an additional year after the standard fellowship training program, and maintain skills by performance of a minimum of 75 procedures per year. Ideally, operators with an annual procedural volume <75 should only work at active centers (>600 procedures per year) with on-site cardiac surgery. The Accreditation Council for Graduate Medical Education (ACGME) has defined the curriculum for the fourth year of training in interventional cardiology, and the American Board of Internal Medicine (ABIM) has established a subspecialty cardiac examination to certify

**TABLE 25-5.** New Coronary Interventional Strategies Compared With Balloon Angioplasty

| Technique | Indications | Contraindications | Advantages and Limitations |
|---|---|---|---|
| Balloon angioplasty | Focal stenosis | Insignificant narrowing, no ischemia, unimportant artery | Broad applicability, lower cost; poor outcome in thrombotic, calcified lesions; significant restenosis |
| Stents | Focal stenosis | Heavy calcification or thrombus, vessel diameter <2.5 mm | Reduced emergency CABG and restenosis; more expensive, rare stent thrombosis |
| Directional atherectomy | Focal noncalcified | Diffuse disease, severe tortuosity or bend | Debulks, reduced restenosis; more expensive, frequent non–Q-wave MI, more expensive, technically diffcult |
| Rotational atherectomy | Focal calcified stenosis, ostial site | Thrombus, large plaque burden, severe tortuosity or bend | Effective in calcified lesions, reduced elastic recoil; more expensive, similar restenosis, transient left ventricular dysfunction |
| Laser | Ostial lesion, SVG, in-stent restenosis | Severe calcification, tortuosity or bend | Debulks effectively; increased cost, similar restenosis |
| Transluminal extraction atherectomy | Thrombotic lesion, bulky SVG lesion | Severe tortuosity or bend, calcification | Thrombus and plaque removed; high complication rate in native vessels, distal embolization |
| Rheolytic thrombectomy | Thrombus | No thrombus | Effective thrombus removal; no plaque removal |

CABG, coronary artery bypass grafting; MI, myocardial infarction; SVG, saphenous vein graft.

properly trained cardiologists in interventional cardiology. Laboratory procedural volume is important and inversely related to adverse procedural outcomes.

# ■ CORONARY INTERVENTIONAL PROCEDURE

Prior to coronary intervention, patients receive an explanation of the procedure, including the operator's estimate of success, possible complications, risks, and benefits. Antiplatelet therapy is used routinely. The therapy most widely used is aspirin, 160 to 325 mg daily. Patients in whom stenting is planned also receive clopidogrel, usually in a 300- to 600-mg loading dose, unless pretreatment for several days has been performed. The platelet glycoprotein (GP) IIb/IIIa receptor blockers are frequently used in patients with a high risk of thrombotic events.

# RESULTS OF CORONARY INTERVENTION

The technical performance of balloon angioplasty, atherectomy, and stenting is beyond the scope of this manual. Experienced interventional cardiologists should offer the best insight into the performance of the procedure and should be valuable consultants in the process of determining which patients are expected to benefit from interventions. Experienced operators should achieve primary success rates in excess of 95% in ideal proximal lesions, compared with a reduced success rate in recent (<3 months) total occlusions or in attempts to treat fibrotic, calcified, eccentric stenoses located distally in tortuous coronary arteries. In all techniques, including stenting, lesion characteristics are a major determinant of the outcome of the procedure. Selection for interventional procedures should always consider the expected long-term as well as the acute outcomes.

# COMPLICATIONS

Patients undergoing PCI are subject to the same complications encountered with the performance of coronary arteriography. In addition, because instrumentation of the atherosclerotic lesion takes place, coronary artery dissection, perforation, thrombus formation, and coronary artery spasm may occur, leading to acute occlusion of the coronary artery or of side branches arising from it. Atheroembolism may occur and lead to MI in an otherwise successful procedure. Occlusion of the treated artery is the most common serious complication of coronary angioplasty and accounts for most of the morbidity and mortality related to the procedure.

The use of stents has significantly reduced the risk of urgent bypass surgery and Q-wave MI. New complications specifically related to the use of nonballoon devices include coronary perforation, distal atheroembolization, arterial access complications increased by the use of GP IIb/IIIa blockers, and "domino stenting" (additional stents to treat end-of-stent dissections). The progression of disease at sites that are not treated should also be considered a late complication of PCI. Aggressive lipid management in the Lescol Intervention Prevention Study (LIPS) trial has been shown to reduce post-PCI events. Other prevention measures are critical and must be part of the management of all patients undergoing interventional procedures (see also Chapter 20).

# FUTURE DIRECTIONS

The future of coronary intervention is bright indeed. Restenosis is becoming a small, manageable problem; however, progression of disease remains a challenge that is currently being addressed on multiple fronts, with good prospects for meaningful solutions.

# SUGGESTED READINGS

Douglas JS Jr, King SB III. Percutaneous coronary intervention. In: Fuster V, Walsh RA, Harrington RA, et al. *Hurst's The Heart.* 13th ed. New York, NY: McGraw-Hill; 2011;62:1430-1456.

Braunwald E, Antman EM, Beasley JW, et al. ACC/AHA 2002 guidelines for the management of patients with unstable angina and non-ST-segment elevation myocardial infarction—summary article: a report of the American College of Cardiology/American Heart Association task force on practice guidelines (Committee on the Management of Patients With Unstable Angina). *J Am Coll Cardiol.* 2002;40:1366-1374.

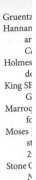

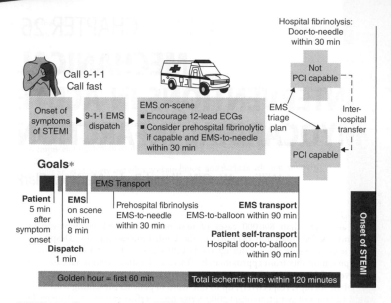

**FIGURE 26-1.** Transport scheme for STEMI. (Reproduced with permission from Antman EM, anbe DT, Armstrong PW: ACC/AHA guidelines for the management of patients with ST-elevation myocardial infarction–executive summary: a report of the American College of Cardiology/American Heart Association Task Force on Practice Guidelines (Writing Committee to Revise the 1999 Guidelines for the Management of Patients With Acute Myocardial Infarction), Circulation 2004 Aug 3;110(5):588-636.)

In a previous meta-analysis of 23 randomized STEMI trials comparing primary PCI with fibrinolytic therapy (**Fig. 26-2**), there were significant reductions in short-term mortality, nonfatal MI, and stroke. Additionally, based on the 5 studies (**Table 26-1**) that compared emergent hospital transfer for primary PCI (with additional transfer-related delay averaging 39 minutes) with on-site fibrinolysis, PCI was still associated with significantly better outcomes; however, the difference was mainly driven by less reinfarction in the setting of low rates of rescue and early angiography. As noted previously, the greatest absolute benefit of primary PCI occurs among patients at highest risk, as reported in several randomized trials. The Should We Emergently Revascularize Occluded Coronaries for Cardiogenic Shock (SHOCK) trial randomized 302 patients with cardiogenic shock to emergency revascularization versus medical stabilization and showed that mortality at 6 months was 50% versus 63%, respectively ($p = 0.03$). This important observation has been corroborated in other smaller studies of STEMI patients presenting in cardiogenic shock.

# BENEFITS OF EARLY REPERFUSION: THE EARLY-OPEN-ARTERY THEORY

The early-open-artery theory suggests that benefits of reperfusion in patients with STEMI are directly related to the speed and completeness with which patency of the infarct-related coronary artery is reestablished, and may be more important than whether pharmacologic or mechanical intervention is used. Mortality is lower among patients in whom TIMI grade 2 to 3 flow, compared with TIMI grade 0 to 1 flow, was achieved within 90 minutes after acute MI. This is strongly supported by clinical

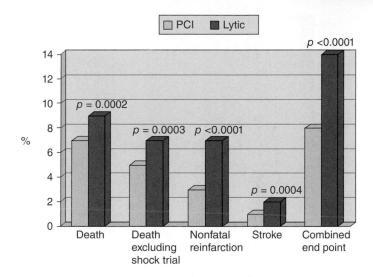

**FIGURE 26-2.** Meta-analysis of 23 randomized trials of PCI versus lysis ($n = 7739$).

studies confirming the important relationship between achieving prompt antegrade coronary flow of the infarct artery and improved clinical outcomes, both for primary PCI and fibrinolysis. An analysis by Boersma and associates indicated that the 35-day mortality benefit associated with early treatment equated to 1.6 lives per 1000 patients per hour of delay from symptom onset to treatment, with even more of an impact of time in the early hours (**Fig. 26-3**). Achieving normal (TIMI-3) antegrade flow in the infarct artery is critical to optimizing clinical outcomes with both thrombolytic therapy and primary PCI. Primary PCI typically achieves TIMI-3 flow in 90% to 95% of patients, versus 50% to 55% in patients treated with new-generation thrombolytic agents. ACC guidelines recommend a target door-to-balloon time <90 minutes. Newer combination therapy with low-dose thrombolytic and platelet glycoprotein IIb/IIIa inhibitors may further improve TIMI-3 flow rate (to 70%-75%), but this is still well below the TIMI-3 flow rates achieved with primary PCI.

# MECHANICAL REPERFUSION AND ADJUNCTIVE THERAPIES

## ■ STENTS AND ADJUNCTIVE MECHANICAL DEVICES

The continued evolution in the development and use of stents—particularly over the last decade—has revolutionized the treatment of coronary artery disease (CAD) and has proven to diminish mortality and immediately alleviate anginal symptoms in STEMI patients. Studies have established the superiority of the drug-eluting stent (DES) in the reduction of target-vessel revascularization (TVR) and restenosis when compared to the bare-metal stent (BMS) (Taxus IV, SIRIUS, and RAVEL trials). There are only a handful of noteworthy randomized clinical trials directly evaluating the efficacy of DES in acute MI to date. These studies include the Paclitaxel Eluting Stent Versus Conventional Stent in Myocardial Infarction with ST-segment Elevation (PASSION) trial, the Trial to Assess the Use of the Cypher Stent in

**TABLE 26-1.** Randomized Trials Comparing 30-day Outcomes in Patients Transferred for Primary PCI Versus Fibrinolytic

| | Death | Reinfarction | Stroke | Composite | p-value | Delay (minutes) |
|---|---|---|---|---|---|---|
| **Vermeer** (n = 150) | | | | | | |
| PCI | 6.7 | 1.3 | 2.7 | 10.7 | 0.25 | 90 |
| Alteplase | 6.7 | 9.3 | 2.7 | 18.7 | | |
| **PRAQUE-1** (n = 200) | | | | | | |
| PCI | 6.9 | 1.0 | 0 | 7.9 | 0.005 | 88 |
| Alteplase | 14.1 | 10.1 | 1.0 | 23.2 | | |
| **AIR PAMI** (n = 137) | | | | | | |
| PCI | 8.4 | 1.4 | 0 | 8.5 | 0.33 | 104 |
| Alteplase | 12.1 | 0 | 4.5 | 13.6 | | |
| **DANAMI-2** (n = 1572) | | | | | | |
| PCI | 6.6 | 1.6 | 1.1 | 8.0 | 0.0004 | 61 |
| Alteplase | 7.5 | 6.3 | 2.0 | 13.5 | | |
| **PRAQUE-2** (n = 850) | | | | | | |
| PCI | 6.8 | NA | NA | 8.4 | 0.003 | 92 |
| Streptokinase | 10.0 | | | 15.2 | | |

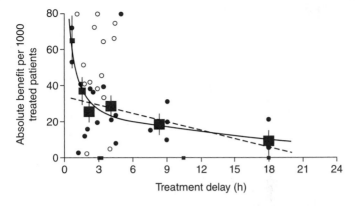

**FIGURE 26-3.** Absolute 35-day mortality versus fibrinolytic treatment delay. Solid circle, information from trials included in Fibrinolytic Therapy Trialists' Collaborative Group Analysis. Open circles, information from additional trials. *Small squares*, data beyond scales of x/y cross. The linear and nonlinear regression lines are fitted within these data, weighted by inverse of the variance of the absolute benefit in each data point. *Solid squares*, average effects in 6 time-to-treat groups (areas of squares inversely proportional to variance of absolute benefit described). (Reproduced with permission from Boersma E, Maas AC, Deckers JW, et al. Early thrombolytic treatment in acute myocardial infarction: reappraisal of the golden hour. *Lancet*. 1996;348:771-775.)

Acute Myocardial Infarction Treated with Balloon Angioplasty (TYPHOON), the Sirolimus Eluting Stent Versus Bare Metal Stent in Acute Myocardial Infarction (SESAMI) trial, and the Comparison of Angioplasty with Infusion of Tirofiban or Abciximab and with Implantation of Sirolimus Eluting or Uncoated Stents for Acute Myocardial Infarction (MULTISTRATEGY) trial. These trials are summarized in **Table 26-2**. Despite the many differences in trial design and primary study end points, these trial data generally support the safety of using DES in patients with acute MI. It has been consistently observed that DES significantly reduces restenosis without major short-term risk, as compared with BMS implantation. These findings are important, as there was historical concern regarding the increased risk of subacute stent thrombosis in acute MI due to significant thrombus burden.

A meta-analysis from 7 pivotal randomized trials evaluating DES versus BMS in STEMI concluded that DES significantly reduces the need for revascularization in patients with acute MI, without changes in incidence of subsequent death or MI (**Fig. 26-4**).

# ■ INTRACORONARY ASPIRATION/THROMBECTOMY DEVICES

Significant clot burden may complicate acute STEMI management. Prospective clinical studies have shown that intracoronary thrombectomy and thrombus aspiration may improve TIMI-3 flow, hasten ST-segment elevation resolution, and enhance myocardial tissue perfusion and reduce MI. The Thrombus Aspiration During Percutaneous Coronary Intervention in Acute Myocardial Infarction (TAPAS) trial showed that patients with STEMI benefit from aspiration thrombectomy. At 1-year follow-up, the study demonstrated a significant correlation between myocardial blush grade and death ($p = 0.001$) and a reduction in mortality ($p = 0.04$). Rheolytic thrombectomy, which employs a more sophisticated mechanism, has greater efficacy toward the removal of large thrombus burden compared to manual aspiration, but in

**TABLE 26-2. Combined Analysis of Randomized Control Trials of Drug-Eluting Stents in Myocardial Infarction**

| | Death | | | TLR/TVR | | | Stent Thrombosis | | | Restenosis | | |
|---|---|---|---|---|---|---|---|---|---|---|---|---|
| | DES | BMS | p | DES | BMS | p | DES | BMS | p | DES | BMS | p |
| TYPHOON[a] (n = 712) | 1.9% | 1.4% | 0.55 | 5.6% | 13.4% | 0.0004 | 3.3% | 3.6% | 0.80 | 7% | 20% | NA |
| PASSION[a] (n = 605) | 4% | 6.3% | 0.20 | 5.3% | 7.6% | 0.23 | 1% | 1% | 0.99 | — | — | — |
| SESAMI[a] (n = 307) | 1.8% | 4.3% | 0.36 | 5.0% | 13.1% | 0.015 | 3.1% | 3.7% | 0.43 | 9% | 21% | NA |
| MULTISTRATEGY[b] (n = 745) | 3% | 4% | 0.42 | 3.2% | 10.2% | <0.001 | 0.8% | 1.1% | 0.71 | — | — | — |

BMS, bare-metal stent; DES, drug-eluting stent; TLR, target-lesion revascularization; TVR, target-vessel revascularization.

[a] 1 year follow-up.

[b] 8 months follow-up.

Modified from Anderson HV, Smalling RW, Henry TD. Drug-eluting stents for acute myocardial infarction. *J Am Coll Cardiol.* 2007;49:1931-1933.

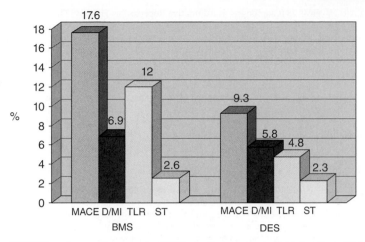

*MACE: major cardiac events; D/MI: death or myocardial infarction; TLR: target-vessel revascularization; ST: stent thrombosis; BMS: bare-metal stent; DES: drug-eluting stent

**FIGURE 26-4.** Meta-analysis of clinical trials on use of DES for treatment of acute MI.

a clinical trial of 480 STEMI patients (including those without visible clot) randomly assigned to PCI alone or PCI with AngioJet catheter thrombectomy, there was a greater infarct size measured by sestamibi imaging at 14 to 28 days with thrombectomy compared to PCI alone (12.5% vs 9.8%).

## ■ EMBOLIZATION PROTECTION DEVICES

Embolization protection devices, including the Percusurge (balloon-occluding device) and FilterWire (filter basket device), were designed to enhance myocardial tissue perfusion by reducing distal embolization of atherothrombotic debris. Both the Saphenous Vein Graft Angioplasty Free of Emboli Randomized (SAFER) and FilterWire EX Randomized Evaluation (FIRE) studies demonstrated selective protection in saphenous vein graft interventions only. Several other studies have also failed to illustrate any benefits of these devices in native coronary artery interventions. Although the explanation for such a discrepancy is unclear, smaller thrombus burden in native coronary arteries, embolization due to the crossing a stenotic lesion with the device, delayed reperfusion due to the occlusive nature of the device, and difficulty in protecting vulnerable side branches are thought to be several possibilities.

# ADJUNCTIVE ANTICOAGULANT AND ANTIPLATELET AGENTS

Regardless of the reperfusion strategy, the ACC guidelines recommend the inclusion of unfractionated or low-molecular-weight heparin (LMWH) as a class Ia indication. The ExTRACT-TIMI 25 (Enoxaparin and Thrombolysis Reperfusion for Acute Myocardial Infarction Treatment—Thrombolysis in Myocardial Infarction 25) and

CLARITY-TIMI 28 (Clopidogrel as Adjunctive Reperfusion Therapy–Thrombolysis in Myocardial Infarction 28) trials demonstrated that LMWH improved clinical outcomes, including a reduction in the rate of composite end point of death and nonfatal reinfarction but associated with modestly increased bleeding when compared with unfractionated heparin (ExTRACT-TIMI 25). The factor Xa inhibitor, fondaparinux, demonstrated improved clinical outcomes in patients who received fibrinolysis or no reperfusion therapy, but not with primary PCI, in contrast to unfractionated heparin or placebo, in the OASIS-6 (Organization for the Assessment of Strategies for Ischemic Syndromes-6) trial, although fondaparinux did not show benefit in STEMI patients undergoing PCI compared to heparin, and was associated with catheter thrombus in 1.6% of patients.

## ■ GLYCOPROTEIN IIB/IIIA INHIBITORS

Abciximab remains the best-studied glycoprotein IIb/IIIa inhibitor in STEMI patients. In the Controlled Abciximab and Device Investigation to Lower Late Angioplasty Complications (CADILLAC) trial, one of the largest studies available, stent implantation resulted in significantly lower rates of death, MI, TVR, or stroke at 30 days and 6 months when compared to balloon angioplasty, regardless of the use of abciximab. Subacute stent thrombosis and recurrent ischemia in index vessels were significantly reduced by the use of abciximab (0% vs 1.0%, $p = 0.03$). The Direct Angioplasty and Stenting in Myocardial Infarction Regarding Acute and Long-Term Follow-up (ADMIRAL) trial evaluated the timing of abciximab administration in STEMI patients, and showed that the greatest benefit of early abciximab administration was improving vessel patency and preserving left ventricular function. While there was no significant different in mortality at 30 days (3.4% vs 6.6%, $p = 0.19$) and 6 months (3.4% vs 7.3%, $p = 0.13$) when compared to placebo, abciximab significantly reduced the combined end point of death, reinfarction, and TVR at 30 days (6.0% vs 14.6%, $p = 0.01$) and 6 months (7.4% vs 15.9%, $p = 0.02$). There was no significant excess in major bleeding with abciximab, but there was an increased rate of minor bleeding (12.1% vs 3.3%, $p = 0.004$).

A meta-analysis of 6 major randomized clinical trials utilizing glycoprotein IIb/IIIa inhibitors (tirofiban, eptifibatide, lamifiban, and abciximab) in ACS, comprising both STEMI and non-STEMI patients, indicated that the use of glycoprotein IIb/IIIa inhibitors reduce death or MI in patients presenting with ACS (**Fig. 26-5**).

## ■ DIRECT THROMBIN INHIBITORS

The benefit of bivalirudin in both low- and high-risk patients was elucidated in ACS patients enrolled in the Randomized Evaluation in PCI Linking Angiomax to Reduced Clinical Events (REPLACE-2) and Acute Catheterization and Urgent Intervention Triage Strategy (ACUITY) trials, respectively. Significant protection of bivalirudin against major bleeding without a significant benefit on ischemic outcomes was demonstrated in the ACUITY trial. The Intracoronary Stenting and Antithrombotic Regimen-Rapid Early Action for Coronary Treatment 3 (ISAR-React-3) trial evaluated the efficacy of bivalirudin versus unfractionated heparin in patients pretreated with clopidogrel and, like REPLACE-2, showed less bleeding without any significant overall ischemic end point benefit, when compared to patients treated with unfractionated heparin after preloading with clopidogrel.

## ■ ANTIPLATELET THERAPY

Dual antiplatelet therapy using clopidogrel and aspirin has been shown to be effective in preventing a composite end point of death, MI, and stroke in patients who

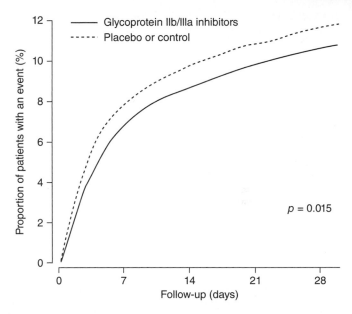

**FIGURE 26-5.** Kaplan–Meier estimates of cumulative occurrence of death of MI within 30 days with platelet glycoprotein IIB/IIIa. (Reproduced with permission from Boersma E, Harrington RA, Moliterno DJ, et al. Platelet glycoprotein IIb/IIIa inhibitors in acute coronary syndromes: a meta-analysis of all major randomised clinical trials. *Lancet*. Jan 19; 2002;359(9302):189-198.

have ACS without ST-segment elevation or who have undergone PCI. Recently, 2 major studies have examined whether aggressive antiplatelet therapy with clopidogrel in combination with aspirin would be beneficial in STEMI patients. The Clopidogrel as Adjunctive Reperfusion Therapy–Thrombolysis in Myocardial Infarction (CLARITY-TIMI 28) trial, conducted in 3491 patients presenting within 12 hours of onset of STEMI, compared the effects of adding clopidogrel (300 mg loading dose, then 75 mg once daily) or placebo to an aspirin- and heparin-based fibrinolytic regimen. The primary composite end point (occluded infarct-related artery [IRA] upon angiography or recurrent MI/death from any cause before angiography) occurred in 21.7% of placebo-treated patients versus 15% in the clopidogrel group ($p$ <0.001). This 36% improvement was driven largely by a lower incidence of IRA occlusion with clopidogrel than placebo (11.7% vs 18.4%, $p$ <0.001). At 30 days, addition of clopidogrel to aspirin/fibrinolytic therapy produced a 20% relative risk reduction in cardiovascular mortality, recurrent MI, and recurrent ischemia leading requiring urgent revascularization (from 14.1% to 11.6%, $p$ = 0.03). The rates of bleeding and other safety outcomes were similar in both treatment groups. A prospectively planned subanalysis of patients who underwent PCI showed that pretreatment with clopidogrel plus aspirin significantly reduced the rate of cardiovascular death, MI, or stroke after PCI to 30 days after randomization (odds ratio 0.54, 95% CI 0.35-0.85, $p$ = 0.008).

While the CLARITY trial was not powered to show a survival benefit in STEMI patients, this question was addressed in a separate study, the COMMIT/CCS-2 trial (Clopidogrel and Metoprolol in Myocardial Infarction Trial/Second Chinese Cardiac Study—The Clopidogrel Arm). This randomized, placebo-controlled trial, conducted in 46 000 patients in China, investigated the effects of dual antiplatelet therapy on mortality rates in STEMI patients presenting within 24 hours, who were randomized to ≤4 weeks of clopidogrel (75 mg/d) treatment or placebo; all patients received aspirin 162 mg/d for the duration of the study. Clopidogrel treatment produced a 9% reduction in the coprimary composite end point of death, MI, or stroke, compared with placebo (95% CI 3-14, $p$ = 0.002). At hospital discharge or day 28 (whichever came first), clopidogrel-treated patients had significantly lower rates of all-cause mortality (7.5% vs 8.1%, $p$ = 0.03). Although a loading dose was not used in this trial, the survival curves began to diverge as early as day 1. The benefits appeared to be greatest where clopidogrel was administered early (within 6 hours) after symptom onset. Major bleeding was similar in both groups, but minor bleeding was more common with clopidogrel.

More recently, prasugrel, a new and more powerful $P_2Y_{12}$ inhibitor, has been evaluated in a large ACS trial in which both STEMI and non-STEMI patients were randomized to either prasugrel + aspirin or clopidogrel + aspirin where patients underwent early coronary angiography and either PCI or CABG surgery. Compared to clopidogrel, there was a 20% incremental reduction in the composite of cardiac death, MI, or stroke during long-term follow-up, but with an increased signal of both fatal and major bleeding. This agent is not yet FDA approved for use in ACS patients.

# RESCUE AND FACILITATED ANGIOPLASTY

Rescue angioplasty, the mechanical reopening of an occluded infarct artery after failed thrombolysis, has been used as adjunctive therapy in STEMI patients with failed thrombolysis, but has been associated with inconsistent results. Despite the intuitive benefit of rescue PCI and the well-recognized improvement in procedural results with stenting, the role of rescue PCI for STEMI, based on evidence from multiple randomized trials, remains controversial. However, even in the absence of conclusive clinical benefit, it does appear reasonable to consider acute angiography with rescue angioplasty in patients with anterior or large STEMI who are thought to have failed thrombolysis, as evidenced by persistent chest pain, lack of resolution of ST-segment elevation, or hemodynamic compromise at greater than 90 minutes following treatment.

Similarly, a number of recent studies have evaluated so-called facilitated PCI, where pharmacologic therapy is followed immediately by PCI, but at present the data suggest that it is not beneficial and may be harmful. Worse outcomes were seen with facilitated PCI versus primary PCI in a recent meta-analysis—driven largely by the largest trial to date, the ASSENT-4 PCI (Assessment of the Safety and Efficacy of a New Treatment Strategy with Percutaneous Coronary Intervention) trial, which showed that routine immediate PCI following full-dose fibrinolytic therapy was associated with higher rates of abrupt vessel closure, reinfarction, and death versus primary PCI alone in patients with only modest treatment delays and treated with low-dose heparin. One implication of this trial is that patients receiving full-dose fibrinolytic therapy, together with signs of presumptive reperfusion (eg, resolution of chest pain and/or ST-segment elevation), should not undergo routine immediate PCI, as there may be an early prothrombotic state following fibrinolytic therapy. Most recently, the Facilitated Intervention with Enhanced Reperfusion Speed to Stop Events (FINESSE) trial results were published, in which STEMI patients were randomized in a 1:1:1 fashion to primary PCI with in-lab abciximab, up-front abciximab-facilitated primary PCI, or half-dose reteplase/abciximab-facilitated PCI. At 90 days, there was no difference among treatment arms for the primary composite end point (all-cause mortality, readmission for heart failure, ventricular fibrillation, or cardiogenic shock). The rates for TIMI non-intracranial major bleeding and minor bleeding were significantly higher for the abciximab/lytic-facilitated PCI strategy as compared with the primary PCI or the abciximab-only group, as were major and minor bleeding combined. Current evidence does not justify the facilitated PCI approach.

In summary, the acute interventional approach to STEMI management has continued to undergo important and profound changes, both in terms of catheter-based treatment approaches and the evolving role of adjunctive pharmacotherapies.

# SUGGESTED READINGS

O'Neill W, Martinez-Clark P. Mechanical interventions in acute myocardial infarction. In: Fuster V, Walsh RA, Harrington RA, et al. *Hurst's The Heart*. 13th ed. New York, NY: McGraw-Hill; 2011;63:1457-1471.

Ali A, Cox D, Dib N, et al. Rheolytic thrombectomy with percutaneous coronary intervention for infarct size reduction in acute myocardial infarction: 30-day results from multicenter randomized study. *J Am Coll Cardiol*. 2006;48:244-252.

American College of Cardiology. *Clinical Statement and Guidelines*. http://www. acc.org/qualityandscience/clinical/guidelines/stemi. 2005.

Anderson HV, Smalling RW, Henry TD. Drug eluting stents for acute myocardial infarction. *J Am Coll Cardiol*. 2007;49:1931-1933.

Brodie BR, Hansen C, Stuckey TD, et al. Door-to-balloon time with primary percutaneous coronary intervention for acute myocardial infarction impacts late cardiac mortality in high-risk patients and patients presenting early after the onset of symptoms. *J Am Coll Cardiol*. 2006;47:289-295.

Hochman JS, Sleeper LA, Webb JG, et al. Early revascularization in acute myocardial infarction complicated by cardiogenic shock. *N Engl J Med*. 1999;341:625-634.

Kastrati A, Dibra A, Spaulding C, et al. Meta-analysis of randomized trials on drug eluting stents vs. bare-metal stents in patients with acute myocardial infarction. *Eur Heart J*. 2007;28:2706-2713.

Smith SC Jr, Feldman TE, Hirshfeld JW Jr, et al. ACC/AHA/SCAI 2005 Guideline Update for Percutaneous Coronary Intervention. A report of the American College of Cardiology/American Heart Association Task Force on Practice Guidelines (ACC/AHA/SCAI Writing Committee to Update the 2001 Guidelines for Percutaneous Coronary Intervention). *J Am Coll Cardiol*. 2006;47:1-121.

Valgimigli M, Campo G, Percoco G, et al. Comparison of angioplasty with infusion of tirofiban or abciximab and with implantation of sirolimus-eluting or uncoated stents for acute myocardial infarction: the MULTISTRATEGY randomized trial. *JAMA*. 2008;299:1788-1799.

Welsh RC, Gordon P, Westerhout CM, et al. A novel enoxaparin regime for ST elevation myocardial infarction patients undergoing primary percutaneous coronary intervention: a West substudy. *Catheter Cardiovasc Interv*. 2007;70:341-348.

# CHAPTER 27
# SYSTEMIC HYPERTENSION: PATHOGENESIS AND ETIOLOGY

## Gbenga Ogedegbe and Thomas G. Pickering†

A direct positive relationship between blood pressure (BP) and cardiovascular disease (CVD) risk has been observed in men and women of all ages, races, ethnic groups, and countries, regardless of other risk factors for CVD. Observational studies indicate that death from CVD increases linearly as BP rises above 115 mm Hg systolic and 75 mm Hg diastolic pressure. For every 20 mm Hg systolic or 10 mm Hg diastolic increase in BP, there is a doubling of mortality from both ischemic heart disease and stroke in all age groups from 40 to 89 years old. Despite major advances in our understanding of its pathophysiology and the availability of many drugs that can effectively reduce BP in most hypertensive subjects, hypertension continues to be the most important modifiable risk factor for CVD.

## BASIC PRINCIPLES OF BLOOD PRESSURE REGULATION

Adequate BP is critical to provide the driving force for tissue blood flow. Consequently, the regulation of BP is a complex physiologic function that depends on the integrated actions of multiple cardiovascular, renal, neural, endocrine, and local tissue control systems.

The multiple local control, hormonal, neural, and renal systems that regulate BP are often discussed in terms of how they influence cardiac pumping or vascular resistance because of the well-known formula: *mean arterial pressure = cardiac output × total peripheral resistance*. This conceptual framework (with the addition of factors that influence vascular capacity and transcapillary exchange) adequately explains short-term BP regulation, but is inadequate when discussing abnormalities of long-term BP regulation, such as hypertension. To explain long-term BP regulation, we must introduce 2 other concepts: (1) time dependency of BP control mechanisms and (2) the necessity of maintaining balance between intake and output of water and electrolytes, and the role of BP in maintaining this balance.

## ■ FEEDBACK CONTROL SYSTEMS

Feedback control systems for BP are time dependent. Three important neural control systems begin to function within seconds after a disturbance of BP (**Fig. 27-1**):

---

†Deceased.

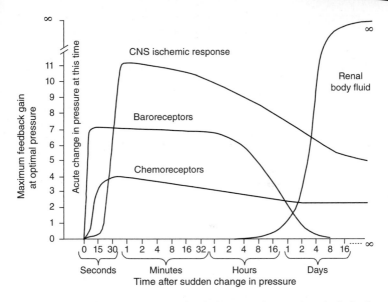

**FIGURE 27-1.** Time dependency of BP control mechanisms. Approximate maximum feedback gains of various BP control mechanisms at different time intervals after the onset of a disturbance to arterial pressure. (Redrawn with permission from Guyton AC, Hall JE. *Textbook of Medical Physiology*. 11th ed. Philadelphia, PA: Elsevier; 2006:230.)

(1) the arterial baroreceptors, which detect changes in BP and send appropriate autonomic reflex signals back to the heart and blood vessels to return the BP toward normal; (2) the chemoreceptors, which detect changes in oxygen or carbon dioxide in the blood and initiate autonomic feedback responses that influence BP; and (3) the central nervous system, which responds within a few seconds to ischemia of the vasomotor centers in the medulla, especially when BP falls below about 50 mm Hg. Within a few minutes or hours after a BP disturbance, several additional control systems react, including (1) a shift of fluid from the interstitial spaces into the bloodstream in response to decreased BP (or a shift of fluid out of the blood into the interstitial spaces in response to increased BP); (2) the renin–angiotensin system (RAS), which is activated when BP falls too low and suppressed when BP increases above normal; and (3) multiple vasodilator systems that are suppressed when BP decreases and stimulated when BP rises above normal.

Most of the BP regulators are *proportional* control systems. This means that they will correct a BP abnormality only part of the way back to the normal level. However, there is one BP control system, the renal–body fluid feedback system, that has *near-infinite feedback gain* if it is given enough time to operate. Thus, the renal–body fluid feedback control mechanism does not stop functioning until the arterial pressure returns all the way back to its original control level, discussed as follows.

# ■ RENAL-BODY FLUID FEEDBACK

Renal-body fluid feedback is a dominant mechanism for long-term BP regulation. **Figure 27-2** shows the conceptual framework for understanding long-term control of BP by the renal-body fluid feedback mechanism. Extracellular fluid volume is determined by the balance between intake and excretion of salt and water by the kidneys.

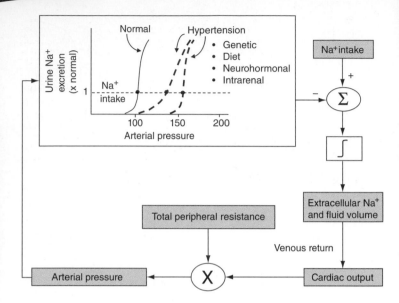

**FIGURE 27-2.** Block diagram showing the basic elements of the renal-body fluid feedback mechanism for long-term regulation of arterial pressure.

Under steady-state conditions there must always be a precise balance between intake and output of salt and water; otherwise, there would be continued accumulation or loss of fluid leading to complete circulatory collapse within a few days. In fact, it is more critical to maintain salt and water balance than to maintain a normal level of BP and, as discussed in the following text, increased BP is a means of regulating these balances in the face of impaired kidney function.

A key mechanism for regulating salt and water balance is pressure natriuresis and diuresis, the effect of increased BP to raise sodium and water excretion. Under most conditions this mechanism stabilizes BP and body fluid volumes. For example, when BP increases above the renal set point, because of increased TPR or increased cardiac pumping ability, this also increases sodium and water excretion via pressure natriuresis if kidney function is not impaired. As long as fluid excretion exceeds fluid intake, extracellular fluid volume will continue to decrease, reducing venous return and cardiac output, until BP returns to normal and fluid balance is reestablished.

An important feature of pressure natriuresis is that various hormonal and neural control systems can greatly amplify or blunt the basic effects of BP on sodium and water excretion. For example, during chronic increases in sodium intake only small changes in BP are needed to maintain sodium balance in most people. One reason for this insensitivity of BP to changes in salt intake is decreased formation of antinatriuretic hormones, such as angiotensin II (ANG II) and aldosterone, which enhance the effectiveness of pressure natriuresis and allow sodium balance to be maintained with minimal increases in BP. On the other hand, excessive activation of these antinatriuretic systems can reduce the effectiveness of pressure natriuresis, thereby necessitating greater increases in BP to maintain sodium balance.

Another important feature of pressure natriuresis is that it continues to operate until BP returns to the original set point. In other words, it acts as part of an *infinite gain* feedback control system. As far as we know, it is the only infinite gain feedback system for BP regulation in the body, and it is this property which makes it a dominant long-term controller of BP.

Therefore, in all forms of human or experimental hypertension studied thus far, there is impaired pressure natriuresis that appears to initiate and sustain the hypertension. In some cases, abnormal kidney function is caused by intrarenal disturbances that impair renal hemodynamics or increase tubular reabsorption. In other cases, impaired kidney function is caused by extrarenal disturbances, such as increased SNS activity or excessive formation of antinatriuretic hormones that reduce the kidney's ability to excrete sodium and water and eventually raise BP. *Consequently, effective treatment of hypertension requires interventions that reset pressure natriuresis toward normal levels of BP either by directly increasing renal excretory capability (eg, with diuretics) or by reducing extrarenal antinatriuretic influences (eg, with RAS blockers) on the kidneys.*

# RENAL MECHANISMS OF HYPERTENSION

An observation that points toward abnormal kidney function as a key factor in hypertension is that almost all forms of experimental hypertension, as well as all monogenic forms of human hypertension thus far discovered, are caused by obvious insults to the kidneys that alter renal hemodynamics or tubular reabsorption. For example, constriction of the renal arteries (eg, Goldblatt hypertension), compression of the kidneys (eg, perinephritic hypertension), or administration of sodium-retaining hormones (eg, mineralocorticoids or ANG II) are all associated with either initial reductions in renal blood flow and glomerular filtration rate (GFR) or increases in tubular reabsorption prior to development of hypertension. Likewise, in all known monogenic forms of human hypertension, the common pathway to hypertension appears to be increased renal tubular sodium reabsorption caused by mutations that directly increase renal electrolyte transport or the synthesis and/or activity of antinatriuretic hormones. As BP rises, the initial renal changes are often obscured by compensations that restore kidney function toward normal. The rise in BP then initiates a cascade of cardiovascular changes, including increased TPR that may be more striking than the initial disturbance of kidney function. The general types of renal abnormalities that can cause chronic hypertension include (1) increased preglomerular resistance, (2) decreased glomerular capillary filtration coefficient, (3) reduced numbers of functional nephrons, and (4) increased tubular reabsorption.

# NEUROHUMORAL MECHANISMS OF HYPERTENSION

Although impaired renal pressure natriuresis plays a central role in all forms of experimental and human hypertension studied thus far, not all disorders of pressure natriuresis originate within the kidneys. Inappropriate activation of antinatriuretic hormone systems (eg, ANG II, aldosterone) that normally regulate sodium excretion or a deficiency of natriuretic influences (eg, atrial natriuretic peptide, nitric oxide) on the kidneys can impair renal pressure natriuresis and cause chronic hypertension. Likewise, excessive activation of the SNS plays a major role in elevating BP in many hypertensive patients.

## ■ SYMPATHETIC NERVOUS SYSTEM

The SNS is a major short-term and long-term controller of BP. Sympathetic vasoconstrictor fibers are distributed to almost all of regions of the vasculature, as well as to the heart, and activation of the SNS can raise BP within a few seconds by causing vasoconstriction, increased cardiac pumping capability, and increased heart rate. Conversely, sudden inhibition of SNS activity can decrease BP to as low as half normal within less than a minute. Therefore, changes in SNS activity, caused by various reflex mechanisms, central nervous system ischemia, or by activation of higher centers in the brain, provide powerful and rapid, moment-to-moment regulation of BP.

The SNS also is important in long-term regulation of BP and in the pathogenesis of hypertension, in large part by activation of the renal sympathetic nerves. There is extensive innervation of the renal blood vessels, the juxtaglomerular apparatus, and the renal tubules, and excessive activation of these nerves causes sodium retention, increased renin secretion, and impaired renal pressure natriuresis. Evidence for a role of the renal nerves in hypertension comes from multiple studies showing that renal denervation reduces BP in several models of experimental hypertension. Human primary hypertension, especially when associated with obesity, is often associated with increased renal sympathetic activity. Although the mechanisms that cause activation of renal sympathetic nerves in primary hypertension are still unclear, excess weight gain contributes to increased SNS activity in many patients with primary (essential) hypertension, as discussed later.

# ■ RENIN–ANGIOTENSIN SYSTEM

The renin–angiotensin system (RAS) is perhaps the most powerful hormone system for regulating body fluid volumes and BP as evidenced by the effectiveness of various RAS blockers in reducing BP in normotensive and hypertensive subjects. Although the RAS has many components, its most important effects on BP regulation are exerted by angiotensin II (ANG II), which participates in both short-term and long-term control of BP. ANG II is a powerful vasoconstrictor and helps maintain BP in conditions associated with acute volume depletion (eg, hemorrhage), sodium depletion, or circulatory depression (eg, heart failure). The long-term effects of ANG II on BP, however, are closely intertwined with volume homeostasis through direct and indirect effects on the kidneys.

Blockade of the RAS, with ANG II receptor blockers (ARBs) or angiotensin-converting enzyme (ACE) inhibitors, increases renal excretory capability so that sodium balance can be maintained at reduced BP. However, blockade of the RAS also reduces the slope of pressure natriuresis and makes BP salt sensitive. Thus, the effectiveness of RAS blockers in lowering BP is greatly diminished by high-salt intake and improved by the reduction in sodium intake or addition of a diuretic.

Inappropriately high levels of ANG II impair pressure natriuresis, thereby necessitating increased BP to maintain sodium balance. The mechanisms mediating the potent antinatriuretic effects of ANG II include renal hemodynamic effects (eg, constriction of efferent arterioles) as well as direct and indirect effects to increase sodium reabsorption in proximal, loop of Henle, and distal tubules.

When renal perfusion pressure is reduced to low levels or when other disturbances such as sodium depletion are superimposed on low BP, the vasoconstrictor effect of ANG II on efferent arterioles is important in preventing excessive decreases in GFR. This effect is especially important in patients with renal artery stenosis and/or sodium depletion or with heart failure who may have substantial decreases in GFR when treated with RAS blockers. On the other hand, RAS blockade may be beneficial when nephrons are hyperfiltering, especially if ANG II is not appropriately suppressed. For example, in diabetes mellitus and in certain forms of hypertension associated with glomerulosclerosis and nephron loss, ANG II blockade, by decreasing efferent arteriolar resistance and arterial pressure, lowers glomerular hydrostatic pressure and attenuates glomerular hyperfiltration and progression of renal injury.

# ■ ALDOSTERONE

Aldosterone is a powerful sodium-retaining hormone and consequently has important effects on renal pressure natriuresis and BP regulation. The primary sites of actions of aldosterone on sodium reabsorption are the principal cells of the distal tubules, cortical collecting tubules, and collecting ducts where aldosterone stimulates sodium reabsorption and potassium secretion. Aldosterone binds to intracellular mineralocorticoid receptors (MRs) and activates transcription by target genes which, in turn, stimulate synthesis or activation of the $Na^+$-$K^+$-ATPase pump on the basolateral epithelial membrane and activation of amiloride-sensitive sodium channels on the luminal side of the epithelial membrane. These effects are termed *genomic* because they are mediated by activation of gene transcription and require 60 to 90 minutes to occur after administration of aldosterone. Aldosterone also appears to exert rapid *nongenomic* effects on the cardiovascular and renal systems, although the importance of these actions on renal function and BP regulation is still unclear.

Some investigators suggest that hyperaldosteronism may be more common than previously believed, especially in patients with hypertension that is resistant to treatment with the usual antihypertensive medications. For example, the prevalence of primary aldosteronism is reported to be almost 20% among patients referred to specialty clinics for resistant hypertension. Many of these patients, however, are overweight or obese. Regardless of the prevalence of primary aldosteronism, antagonism of MRs may provide an important therapeutic tool for preventing target-organ injury and reducing BP in patients with resistant hypertension.

# ■ ENDOTHELIN

Endothelin-1 (ET-1), a powerful vasoconstrictor, has receptor-binding sites throughout the body, with the greatest numbers in the kidneys and lungs. ET-1 causes vasoconstriction and hypertension by activation of type A ($ET_A$) receptors but also has antihypertensive effects through activation of type B ($ET_B$) receptors which cause vasodilation and inhibit sodium reabsorption in the kidneys. Although $ET_A$ receptor activation may play a role in certain forms of hypertension, this effect does not appear to have a major influence on cardiovascular and renal function under normal physiologic conditions.

# ■ NITRIC OXIDE (NO)

Tonic release of NO by the vascular endothelium plays a major role in regulating vascular function, and impairment of NO formation causes impaired renal pressure natriuresis and sustained hypertension. The magnitude of the increase in BP during NO inhibition is greater with high-sodium intake. Reductions in NO synthesis may decrease renal sodium excretory function by increasing renal vascular resistance directly or by enhancing the renal vascular responsiveness to vasoconstrictors such as ANG II or norepinephrine. Reductions in NO synthesis also increase renal tubular sodium reabsorption via direct effects on renal tubular transport and through changes in intrarenal physical factors, such as renal interstitial hydrostatic pressure and medullary blood flow.

# ■ OXIDATIVE STRESS

Oxidative stress occurs when total oxidant production exceeds antioxidant capacity. Recent studies suggest that reactive oxygen species (ROS) may play a role in the initiation and progression of cardiovascular dysfunction associated with hyperlipidemia, diabetes mellitus, and hypertension. In many forms of hypertension, increased ROS appear to be derived mainly from nicotinamide adenine dinucleotide phosphate oxidases, which could serve as a triggering mechanism for uncoupling endothelial nitric oxide synthase (NOS) by oxidants. ROS produced by migrating inflammatory cells and/or vascular cells have distinct effects on different cell types. These effects include endothelial dysfunction, increased renal tubule sodium transport, cell growth and migration, inflammatory gene expression, and stimulation of extracellular matrix formation. ROS, by affecting vascular and renal tubule function, can also impair renal pressure natriuresis, alter systemic hemodynamics, and raise BP.

## ■ ATRIAL NATRIURETIC PEPTIDE

Atrial natriuretic peptide (ANP) is a peptide synthesized and released from atrial cardiocytes in noresponse to stretch. ANP reduces vascular resistance while enhancing sodium excretion through extrarenal and intrarenal mechanisms. ANP increases GFR but has little effect on renal blood flow. ANP may also inhibit renal tubular sodium reabsorption either directly by inhibiting active tubular transport of sodium or indirectly via alterations in medullary blood flow, physical factors, and intrarenal hormones. ANP reduces renin secretion and reductions in intrarenal ANG II levels likely contribute to ANP-induced natriuresis. ANP also decreases aldosterone release either by direct effects on the adrenal gland or by reducing ANG II secondary to suppression of renin. Long-term physiologic elevations in plasma ANP enhance renal pressure natriuresis and reduce BP.

# SECONDARY CAUSES OF HYPERTENSION

In a small percentage of patients, the clinical features, history, and physical examination point to a specific cause of increased BP and the hypertension is therefore said to be *secondary*. Some types of secondary hypertension have a definite genetic basis, whereas others are caused by CVD and target-organ injury associated with various disorders, such as diabetes and kidney disease. In some instances, hypertension can be caused by drugs or treatments that the patient receives. Nearly all forms of secondary hypertension, however, are characterized by impaired renal function or altered activity of the SNS or hormones that, in turn, impair the ability of the kidneys to excrete salt and water.

**Table 27-1** lists some of the most frequent causes of secondary hypertension, including those caused by drugs that either themselves raise BP or exacerbate underlying disorders that contribute to hypertension. These drugs include nonsteroidal anti-inflammatory drugs, oral contraceptive agents, glucocorticoids, and sympathomimetics that are used as cold remedies. This chapter discusses only a few of the more common causes of secondary hypertension.

## ■ RENOVASCULAR HYPERTENSION

Renovascular hypertension, although accounting for only 2% to 3% of all hypertension, is one of the most common causes of secondary hypertension. The pathophysiology of renovascular hypertension is related directly to the reduction in renal perfusion that occurs as a result of stenosis of the main renal artery, one of its branches, or stenosis/injury of other smaller preglomerular blood vessels and glomeruli. The majority of renal vascular lesions reflect either fibromuscular dysplasia or atherosclerosis. The predominant lesion found in the main renal artery or its branches in patients older than 50 years is atherosclerotic disease. More subtle functional (constriction) or structural changes in smaller blood vessels (eg, afferent arterioles, glomeruli), however, are difficult to detect clinically and can also contribute

**TABLE 27-1.** Some Secondary Causes of Hypertension

A. Renal parenchymal disease
  • Acute and chronic glomerulonephritis
  • Chronic nephritis (eg, pyelonephritis, radiation)
  • Polycystic disease
  • Diabetic nephropathy
  • Hydronephrosis
  • Neoplasms
B. Renovascular
  • Renal artery stenosis/compression
  • Intrarenal vasculitis
  • Suprarenal aortic coarctation
C. Renoprival (renal failure, loss of kidney tissue)
D. Endocrine disorders
  • Renin-producing tumors
  • Cushing syndrome
  • Primary aldosteronism
  • Pheochromocytoma (adrenal or extra-adrenal chromaffin tumors)
  • Acromegaly
E. Pregnancy-induced hypertension
F. Sleep apnea
G. Increased intracranial pressure (brain tumors, encephalitis)
H. Exogenous hormones and drugs (partial list)
  • Glucocorticoids
  • Mineralocorticoids
  • Sympathomimetics
  • Tyramine-containing foods and monoamine oxidase inhibitors
  • Estrogen (eg, oral contraceptive pills)
  • Apparent mineralocorticoid excess (eg, licorice)
  • Nonsteroidal anti-inflammatory drugs
  • Cyclosporine
  • Excess alcohol use
  • Drug abuse (eg, amphetamines, cocaine)

to increased BP. Renal artery stenosis produces a rise in BP that is proportional to the severity of the constriction. Renovascular hypertension can be unilateral, involving only 1 kidney, or bilateral and can result in a homogeneous or a nonhomogeneous ischemia of nephrons. However, there are some important differences in the pathophysiology of homogeneous compared to nonhomogenous impairment of renal perfusion.

## ◼ ADRENAL CORTEX HYPERTENSION

Aldosterone normally exerts nearly 90% of the mineralocorticoid activity of adrenocortical secretions. However, cortisol, the major glucocorticoid secreted by the adrenal cortex, can also provide significant mineralocorticoid activity in some conditions. Aldosterone's mineralocorticoid activity is about 3000 times greater than that of cortisol, but the plasma concentration of cortisol is nearly 2000 times that of aldosterone. The renal MR is normally protected from activation by cortisol as a result of the effects of 11β–HSD2, which converts active cortisol into inactive cortisone, but when activity of this enzyme is reduced or when cortisol levels are very high, the MR can be activated by cortisol.

*Primary aldosteronism* (PA) is the syndrome that results from hypersecretion of aldosterone in the absence of a known stimulus. The excess aldosterone secretion almost always comes from the adrenal cortex and is usually associated with a solitary adenoma or bilateral hyperplasia of the adrenal cortex. Secondary aldosteronism refers to increased aldosterone secretion that occurs secondary to a known stimulus, such as activation of the RAS. This is the most common form of aldosteronism and occurs in various conditions associated with increased renin secretion, such as congestive heart failure, sodium depletion, or renal artery stenosis.

Excess aldosterone increases sodium reabsorption and potassium secretion by the principal cells of the renal tubules leading to an expansion of extracellular fluid volume, hypertension, suppression of renin secretion, hypokalemia, and metabolic alkalosis, hallmarks of primary aldosteronism. Most of these effects are highly salt sensitive, and low-sodium intake can greatly attenuate the hypertension and hypokalemia associated with primary aldosteronism.

Adrenal adenomas and bilateral adrenal hyperplasia account for more than 95% of PA. However, this is a rare form of hypertension, and in most studies of unselected patients, the classic form of PA was found in fewer than 1% of hypertensive patients. Some adrenal glands in patients with PA may have varying degrees of hyperplasticity, and the term *idiopathic hyperaldosteronism* (IHA) was coined to describe this condition. Clinically, PA and IHA are difficult to distinguish, although patients with PA often have more severe hypertension and hypokalemia compared to those with IHA.

# ■ CUSHING SYNDROME (GLUCOCORTICOID EXCESS)

Cushing syndrome is a serious disorder. Hypertension occurs in approximately 80% of patients with Cushing syndrome and is difficult to control. Cushing syndrome can be caused by either administration of excess cortisol (eg, for treatment of various inflammatory disorders) or by excess endogenous cortisol secretion. The most common cause of endogenous cortisol excess is overproduction of adrenocorticotrophic hormone (ACTH) from a pituitary adenoma, a condition referred to as *Cushing disease*. The increased ACTH causes adrenal hyperplasia and stimulates cortisol secretion. Cushing disease can also occur as a result of ectopic secretion of ACTH by tumors outside the pituitary, such as an abdominal carcinoma.

# ■ PHEOCHROMOCYTOMA

This is a rare form of secondary hypertension occurring in approximately 0.05% of hypertensive patients. Although rare, pheochromocytoma can provoke fatal hypertensive crises if unrecognized and untreated. Pheochromocytoma can arise from neuroectodermal chromaffin cells, which are part of the sympathoadrenal system. The chromaffin cells have the capacity to synthesize and store catecholamines and are normally found mainly in the adrenal medulla. The symptoms and severity of hypertension associated with pheochromocytoma are highly variable, depending on the secretory pattern and amount of catecholamines released. Tumors that continuously release large amounts of catecholamines may cause sustained hypertension with few paroxysms, or sudden bursts of very high levels of BP. Tumors that are less active may have cyclical release of catecholamines stores that induce paroxysms of hypertension. The periodic bursts of catecholamine release may cause moderate to severe hypertension and lead to target-organ injury. Consequently, diagnosis and effective treatment of pheochromocytoma are essential.

# ■ PREECLAMPSIA

Preeclampsia in women is characterized by hypertension and proteinuria after 20 weeks gestation and is associated with significantly increased risk for fetal and maternal morbidity and mortality. Although numerous factors—including genetic, immunologic, behavioral, and environmental factors—have been implicated in the pathogenesis of preeclampsia, reduced uteroplacental perfusion as a result of abnormal cytotrophoblast invasion of spiral arterioles appears to play a key role. Placental ischemia is thought to cause widespread activation/dysfunction of the maternal vascular endothelium, which results in enhanced formation of endothelin, thromboxane, and superoxide, increased vascular sensitivity to ANG II, and decreased formation of vasodilators such as nitric oxide and prostacyclin. These endothelial abnormalities, in turn, cause hypertension by impairing renal function and increasing total peripheral vascular resistance.

# GENETIC CAUSES OF HYPERTENSION

With the development of superb tools for genetic studies, there has been great enthusiasm for the possibility that genetic causes of primary hypertension can be identified. However, there have been no clear successes in identifying genes that cause human primary hypertension. On the other hand, at least 10 monogenic disorders have been identified that have either high BP or low BP as part of the phenotype (**Table 27-2** shows some of these that are associated with high BP). In all monogenic hypertensive disorders thus far, the final common pathway to hypertension is increased sodium reabsorption and volume expansion. Monogenic hypertension, however, is rare, and all of the known forms together account for less than 1% of human hypertension.

# PATHOPHYSIOLOGY OF PRIMARY (ESSENTIAL) HYPERTENSION

Widespread human primary (essential) hypertension appears to be a relatively modern disorder associated with industrialization and ready availability of food. Studies of industrialized populations have demonstrated that BP, and therefore the prevalence of hypertension, rises with age. Hunter-gatherers living in nonindustrialized societies, however, rarely develop hypertension or progressive increases in BP that occur in the majority of individuals living in industrialized societies. This suggests that environmental factors play a major role in raising BP in many patients with primary hypertension. However, genetic variation almost certainly is responsible for differences in baseline BP that result in normal distribution of BP in a population. When hypertension-producing environmental factors are added to the population baseline BP, the normal distribution is shifted toward higher BP. Experimental, clinical, and population studies suggest some of the key environmental factors that affect BP include excess weight gain, excess sodium intake, and excess alcohol consumption.

# ■ OBESITY

Obesity is a major cause of primary hypertension. Current estimates indicate that more than 1 *billion* people in the world are overweight or obese. In the United States, 64% of adults are overweight, and almost one-third of the adult population is

**TABLE 27-2. Known Genetic Causes of Hypertension**

| Genetic Disorder | Age of Onset | Pattern of Inheritance | Aldosterone Level | Serum Potassium Level | Treatment[a] |
|---|---|---|---|---|---|
| FH-I (GRA)[b] | 2nd or 3rd decade | Autosomal dominant | High | Decreased in 50% of cases; marked decrease with thiazides | Glucocorticoids |
| FH-II[c] | Middle age | Autosomal dominant | High | Low to normal | Spironolactone, eplerenone |
| DOC oversecretion due to CAH[d] | Childhood | Autosomal recessive | Low | Low to normal | Glucocorticoids |
| Activating MR mutation exacerbated by pregnancy[e] | 2nd or 3rd decade | Unknown | Low | Low to normal | Delivery of fetus |
| AME2[f] | Childhood | Autosomal recessive | Low | Low to normal | Spironolactone, dexamethasone |
| Liddle syndrome[g] | 3rd decade | Autosomal dominant | Low | Low to normal | Amiloride, triamterene |
| Gordon syndrome[h] | 2nd or 3rd decade | Autosomal dominant | Low | High | Thiazide diuretic, low-sodium diet |

ACTH, adrenocorticotropic hormone; AME, apparent mineralocorticoid excess; CAH, congenital adrenal hyperplasia; DOC, deoxycorticosterone; FH-I, familial hyperaldosteronism type I; FH-II, familial hyperaldosteronism type II; GRA, glucocorticoid-remediable aldosteronism; MCR, mineralocorticoid receptor.

[a]Treatment for underlying mechanisms; other forms of treatment, including different antihypertensive medications, might be needed to adequately control BP.

[b]Familial hyperaldosteronism.

[c]Excess production of nonaldosterone mineralocorticoids.

[d]Congenital adrenal hyperplasia, DOC-producing tumors.

[e]Because of increased activity of MCRs.

[f]Apparent mineralocorticoid excess caused by either licorice ingestion or ectopic ACTH secretion.

[g]Increased activity of sodium channels.

[h]Increased activity of Na–Cl cotransporter in the distal tubule.

Data from Garovic VD, Hilliard AA, Turner ST. Monogenic forms of low-renin hypertension. *Nat Clin Pract Nephrol.* 2006;2:624-630.

obese with a body mass index (BMI) greater than 30. Population studies show that excess weight gain is the best predictor we have for the development of hypertension, and the relationship between BMI and BP appears to be nearly linear in diverse populations throughout the world. Clinical studies also indicate that weight loss is effective in reducing BP in most hypertensive subjects and in primary prevention of hypertension.

## Mechanisms of Impaired Renal Pressure Natriuresis in Obesity Hypertension

Three mechanisms appear to be especially important in mediating impaired pressure natriuresis in obesity hypertension: (1) increased SNS activity, (2) activation of the RAS, and (3) physical compression of the kidneys by fat accumulation within and around the kidneys.

**Hyperleptinemia and SNS Activation**  Leptin is released from adipocytes and acts on the hypothalamus and brainstem to reduce appetite and increase SNS activity. In rodents, increasing plasma leptin concentration to levels comparable to those found in severe obesity not only increases SNS activity but also raises BP. Moreover, the hypertensive effects of leptin are enhanced when NO synthesis is inhibited, as often occurs in obese subjects with endothelial dysfunction. Leptin's stimulatory effect on SNS activity appears to be mediated by interaction with other hypothalamic factors, especially the proopiomelanocortin pathway. Antagonism of the melanocortin 3/4 receptors (MC3/4-R) completely abolished leptin's chronic BP effects.

**Renin–Angiotensin–Aldosterone System Activation in Obesity**  Obese individuals, especially those with visceral obesity, often have mild to moderate increases in plasma renin activity, angiotensinogen, ACE activity, ANG II, and aldosterone despite sodium retention, volume expansion, and hypertension, all of which would normally tend to suppress renin secretion and ANG II formation. RAS blockade blunts sodium retention, volume expansion, and increased BP during the development of obesity in experimental studies. Small clinical trials have also shown that ARBs, ACE inhibitors, and MR receptor antagonists are all effective in lowering BP in obese hypertensive patients.

**Renal Compression Caused by Visceral Obesity**  Visceral obesity also leads to physical compression of the kidneys, which impairs renal pressure natriuresis and causes hypertension. Although this cannot account for the initial increase in BP that occurs with rapid weight gain, it may help to explain why abdominal obesity is much more closely associated with hypertension than subcutaneous obesity.

## Kidney Injury in Obesity Hypertension

Obese patients often develop proteinuria that is followed by progressive loss of kidney function. The most common types of renal lesions observed in renal biopsies of obese subjects are focal and segmental glomerular sclerosis and glomerulomegaly. The gradual loss of kidney function, as well as the hypertension and diabetes that commonly coexist with obesity, lead to progressive impairment of pressure natriuresis, increasing salt sensitivity, and greater increases in BP. Thus, renal injury in obese subjects makes the hypertension more severe and more difficult to control with antihypertensive drugs.

Effective control of BP is essential in treating patients with obesity and metabolic syndrome, and for preventing CVD. Weight reduction is an essential first step in the effective management of most patients with metabolic syndrome and hypertension, and more emphasis should be placed on lifestyle modifications that help patients to maintain a healthier weight and prevent CVD.

# SUGGESTED READINGS

Ogedegbe G, Pickering TG. Epidemiology of hypertension. In: Fuster V, Walsh RA, Harrington RA, et al, eds. *Hurst's The Heart*. 13th ed. New York, NY: McGraw-Hill; 2011;68:1533-1548.

Hall JE, Granger JP, Jones DW, et al. Pathophysiology of hypertension. In: Fuster V, Walsh RA, Harrington RA, et al, eds. *Hurst's The Heart*. 13th ed. New York, NY: McGraw-Hill; 2011;69: 1549-1584.

Chobanian AV, Bakris GL, Black HR, et al. Seventh report of the Joint National Committee on Prevention, Detection, Evaluation, and Treatment of High Blood Pressure. *Hypertension*. 2003;42:1206-1252.

Guyton AC, Hall J E. *Textbook of Medical Physiology*. 11th ed. Philadelphia, PA: Elsevier; 2006.

Hall JE. The kidney, hypertension, and obesity. *Hypertension*. 2003;41:625-633.

Hall JE, Brands MW, Henegar JR. Angiotensin II and long-term arterial pressure regulation: the overriding dominance of the kidney. *Kidney Int*. 1999;10:s258-s265.

Hall JE, Granger JP. Regulation of fluid and electrolyte balance in hypertension: role of hormones and peptides. In: Battegay EJ, Lip GHY, Bakris GL, eds. *Hypertension: Principles and Practice*. Boca Raton, FL: Taylor & Francis; 2005:121-142.

Hall JE, Guyton AC, Brands MW. Pressure-volume regulation in hypertension. *Kidney Int*. 1996;49(suppl 55):S35-S41.

Kaplan NM. *Clinical Hypertension*. 8th ed. Philadelphia, PA: Lippincott William & Wilkins; 2002:89-92.

Lifton RP. Molecular genetics of human blood pressure variation. *Science*. 1996;272:676-680.

# CHAPTER 28
# DIAGNOSIS AND TREATMENT OF HYPERTENSION

G. Brandon Atkins, Mahboob Rahman,
and Jackson T. Wright, Jr

## EVALUATION OF THE HYPERTENSIVE PATIENT

### ■ BLOOD PRESSURE MEASUREMENT

The seventh report of the Joint National Committee on prevention, detection, evaluation, and treatment of High Blood Pressure (JNC 7) classifies hypertension 1 into 4 categories (**Table 28-1**). Accurate measurement of blood pressure requires a trained health care provider using a mercury or *calibrated* alternative sphygmomanometer under standardized conditions. These include the removal of tight clothing, 5 minutes of rest in a chair (not an examination table), back supported with feet on the floor, the arm supported at heart level, and avoidance of talking during the measurement. The bladder of the cuff should encircle at least 80% of the upper arm and be a width that is at least 40% of arm circumference such that the distal margin is at least 3 cm proximal to the antecubital fossa. The cuff should be inflated to a pressure about 30 mm Hg above the point where the palpable pulse disappears, and then deflated at 2 to 3 mm Hg per second. The onset of phase I of the Korotkoff sounds (tapping sounds corresponding to the appearance of a palpable pulse) corresponds to systolic pressure. The disappearance of sounds (phase V) corresponds to diastolic pressure. The fifth phase should be used, except in situations in which the disappearance of sounds cannot reliably be determined because sounds are audible even after complete deflation of the cuff, as in pregnant women. In this case the fourth phase (muffling) may be used to define the diastolic pressure. At least 2 measurements spaced by 1 to 2 minutes apart should be taken. Blood pressure should be measured in both arms at the first visit to detect possible differences because of peripheral vascular disease, and, if present, the higher value should be used. In those at risk for orthostatic hypotension (eg, the elderly, diabetics, autonomic instability), blood pressure should be measured after 2 minutes of standing.

### ■ HISTORY, PHYSICAL EXAMINATION, AND LABORATORY EVALUATION

The 3 main goals of the initial evaluation of the hypertensive patient are to (1) assess the presence of target-organ damage related to hypertension, especially those that might influence choice of therapy; (2) determine the presence of other cardiovascular risk factors and disease; and (3) evaluate for possible underlying secondary causes of hypertension.

**TABLE 28-1.** Classification of Blood Pressure for Adults

| Blood Pressure Classification | Systolic Blood Pressure (mm Hg) | Diastolic Blood Pressure (mm Hg) |
|---|---|---|
| Normal | <120 | <80 |
| Prehypertension | 120-139 | 80-89 |
| Stage 1 hypertension | 140-159 | 90-99 |
| Stage 2 hypertension | ≥160 | ≥100 |

Adapted from Chobanian AV, Bakris GL, Black HR, et al. *Seventh Report of the Joint National Committee on Prevention, Detection, Evaluation, and Treatment of High Blood Pressure*. NIH pub. no. 04-5230. Available at: http://www.nhlbi.nih.gov/guidelines/hypertension/jnc7full.htm.

The key issues that need to be addressed in the history include the following:

- Age of onset, duration, levels of high blood pressure, as well as the impact and adverse effects of previous antihypertensive therapy
- Symptoms suggestive of secondary causes of hypertension (**Table 28-2**)
- Lifestyle factors including diet (fat, salt, alcohol), smoking, physical activity, and weight gain since early adult life

**TABLE 28-2.** Important Findings in Physical Examination That Might Help to Diagnose Secondary Hypertension or Find End-Organ Damage

| | Finding | Significance |
|---|---|---|
| Vital sign | Pulse pressure >60 mm Hg | ↑ CVD risk |
| | Tachycardia | Hyperthyroid, pheochromocytoma, HF |
| Body habitus | Cushingoid | Cushing syndrome |
| Skin | Oral-facial tumors | MEN2A/2B (pheochromocytoma) |
| | Neurofibromas, café-au-lait spots | Pheochromocytoma |
| Eyes | AV nicking, hemorrhages, exudates | Hypertensive retinopathy |
| Neck | Bruits | Carotid disease |
| | Thyroid | Hypothyroid MEN2A |
| Chest wall | Rib bruits | Coarctation of aorta |
| | Renal bruits heard over the Kidneys | Renal artery stenosis |
| Lungs | Crackles, wheezes | Heart failure |
| Cardiac | Gallops, LVH, murmur | Heart failure, valvular disease |
| Abdomen | Palpable kidneys, bruit, epigastric and post | Polycystic kidneys, renal artery stenosis |
| Extremities | Diminished pulses, femoral pulse delay | Coarctation of aorta |
| | Bruits | Vascular damage |

AV, atrioventricular; CVD, cardiovascular disease; HF heart failure; LVH, left ventricular hypertrophy; MEN, multiple endocrine neoplasia.

Data compiled from 2003 European Society of Hypertension-European Society of Cardiology guidelines for the management of arterial hypertension. *J Hypertens*. 2003;21:1011-1053.

- Symptoms of target-organ damage, including neurologic dysfunction, heart failure, coronary heart disease, or peripheral arterial disease
- Use of medications that influence blood pressure, such as oral contraceptives, licorice, nasal decongestants, cocaine, amphetamines, steroids, nonsteroidal anti-inflammatory drugs, erythropoietin, and cyclosporine
- Presence of other cardiovascular risk factors

Routine laboratory investigations before initiation of therapy include urine for protein and blood, serum creatinine (estimated glomerular filtration rate [GFR]) and electrolytes, fasting blood glucose, fasting lipid profile, and electrocardiogram (ECG). Additional workup is guided by the clinical presentation in an individual patient and the need to evaluate possible causes of secondary hypertension.

# ■ SECONDARY CAUSES OF HYPERTENSION

Secondary hypertension is defined by identifying a specific cause of hypertension, in contrast to the more common essential hypertension, where no direct cause is evident. The most common causes of secondary hypertension are renal artery stenosis, renal parenchymal disease, sleep apnea, primary hyperaldosteronism, Cushing syndrome, and pheochromocytoma (see Tables 28-2 and 28-3).

# ■ RENAL ARTERY STENOSIS

Renovascular hypertension occurs in 1% to 2% of the overall hypertensive population, but the prevalence may be as high as 10% in patients with resistant hypertension, and even higher in patients with accelerated or malignant hypertension. Renovascular disease may be due to 2 distinct pathophysiologic processes: fibromuscular dysplasia in younger patients, especially women 15 to 50 years of age,

**TABLE 28-3.** Clinical and Laboratory Clues for Diagnosis of Secondary Hypertension

| Cause | Clues |
|---|---|
| Renovascular hypertension | Abrupt onset before age 30 y or worsening after age 55 y; renal artery diastolic or lateralizing abominal bruit; resistance to therapy; sustained rise in creatinine after initiation of angiotensin-converting enzyme inhibitor, renal failure of uncertain etiology; retinal hemorrhages, exudates, or papilledema; recurrent "flash" pulmonary edema; coexisting diffuse atherosclerotic vascular disease |
| Renoparenchymal disease | Abnormal urinalysis (proteinuria, hematuria); elevated serum creatinine; abnormal renal ultrasonography |
| Sleep apnea | Obesity; gaspy nocturnal breathing with prominent snoring |
| Primary aldosteronism | Unexplained hypokalemia, metabolic alkalosis |
| Cushing syndrome | Truncal obesity, acne, plethora, fat pads, striae, and bruising; hyperglycemia |
| Pheochromocytoma | Labile blood pressure, paroxysms of, palpitations, pallor, perspiration, headache (pain) |

Adapted from Hall WD. Resistant hypertension, secondary hypertension, and hypertensive crises. *Cardiol Clin.* 2002;20:281-289.

and atherosclerotic renal artery stenosis in older persons often associated with other peripheral vascular disease. Duplex ultrasonography is a useful and noninvasive technique to evaluate for renal artery stenosis. However, the sensitivity and specificity of this measurement are operator dependent. Renal angiography remains the gold standard for diagnosis and provides information about the site and severity of stenoses, thereby suggesting appropriate revascularization strategies. Therapeutic options include renal artery angioplasty with stent placement and surgical revascularization; however, not all patients benefit from renal revascularization. The presence of urinary protein excretion of at least 1 g/d; estimated GFR of <40 mL/min; age older than 65 years the presence of coronary artery disease, arterial occlusive disease of the legs, or cerebrovascular disease; and a resistance index >80 in the segmental arteries of both kidneys are useful in identifying patients who are less likely to benefit from vascular intervention. Appropriate management of renal artery stenosis requires close collaboration between the internist, interventional radiologist, and vascular surgeon.

# ■ SLEEP APNEA

Obstructive sleep apnea is a common medical condition characterized by abnormal collapse of the pharyngeal airway during sleep causing repetitive arousals from sleep. It may occur in up to 50% of patients with hypertension. The most common clinical presentation of obstructive sleep apnea is loud snoring or breathing pauses observed by the bed partner, nightmares or abrupt awakening from sleep, and excessive daytime sleepiness. There are several questionnaires that can be used in screening for this disorder, although a formal sleep study usually is needed for diagnosis of obstructive sleep apnea and the determination of corrective interventions. Continuous positive airway pressure can reduce nocturnal blood pressure in patients with obstructive sleep apnea.

# ■ PRIMARY HYPERALDOSTERONISM

Screening for hyperaldosteronism should be considered for at least the following patients: hypertensive patients with spontaneous hypokalemia ($K^+$ <3.5 mmol/L); hypertensive patients with marked diuretic-induced hypokalemia ($K^+$ <3.0 mmol/L); patients with hypertension refractory to treatment with 3 or more drugs; and hypertensive patients found to have an incidental adrenal adenoma. Screening for hyperaldosteronism includes assessment of plasma aldosterone and plasma renin activity measured under standardized conditions, (the collection of morning samples taken from patients in a sitting position after resting at least 15 minutes and after restoration of normokalemia). Antihypertensive drugs, with the exception of aldosterone antagonists, may be continued before initial testing. The screening test is considered positive if the plasma aldosterone/renin activity ratio is greater than 30 pmol/L/ng/mL or 550 SI units. The diagnosis of primary aldosteronism is established by demonstrating inappropriate autonomous hypersecretion of aldosterone after oral or IV saline loading. Imaging with adrenal computed tomography scan or magnetic resonance imaging may help differentiate between adrenal adenoma and bilateral adrenal hyperplasia, although selective adrenal venous sampling may be needed. The treatment of confirmed unilateral aldosterone-producing adenoma is surgical removal of the affected adrenal gland, usually by laparoscopic adrenalectomy. Prior to surgery, patients should be treated medically for 8 to 10 weeks to correct metabolic abnormalities and to control blood pressure. Aldosterone antagonists (spironolactone or eplerenone) should be considered for patients with adrenal hyperplasia, bilateral adenoma, or increased risk of perioperative complications. Amiloride is another alternative for the patient who is intolerant to spironolactone.

# ■ CUSHING SYNDROME

Cushing syndrome is more common in women and results from excessive concentrations of circulating free glucocorticoids, which is corticotropin-dependent in approximately 80% to 85% of cases ( see Chapter 27). The 24-hour urinary free cortisol (>90 mg/d; sensitivity = 100%; specificity = 98%) is a useful screening test; however, the single-dose (1-mg) overnight dexamethasone suppression test is equally sensitive but less specific. Treatment of Cushing syndrome is either medical or surgical. Metyrapone, ketoconazole, and mitotane can all be used to lower cortisol by directly inhibiting synthesis and secretion in the adrenal gland.

# ■ PHEOCHROMOCYTOMA

Patients with paroxysmal and/or severe sustained hypertension that is refractory to the usual antihypertensive therapy should be evaluated for pheochromocytoma. Hypertension triggered by β-blockers, anesthesia induction, monoamine oxidase inhibitors, micturition, or changes in abdominal pressure should increase suspicion for pheochromocytoma. It may also be present with other conditions such as multiple endocrine neoplasias (MEN2A/2B), von Recklinghausen neurofibromatosis, or von Hippel–Lindau disease. A 24-hour urinary metanephrine is highly sensitive and specific with a cutoff point >3.70 nmol/d. Plasma metanephrines are easy to obtain, and may represent a good screening test for pheochromocytoma, especially if the patient is symptomatic or blood pressure is elevated. Because they have limited specificity (85%) at cutoffs of metanephrine >0.66 nmol/L or normetanephrine >0.30 nmol/L, a positive plasma metanephrine should be confirmed by the 24-hour urinary metanephrine-to-creatinine ratio (cutoff point >0.354; specificity = 98%) before proceeding to anatomic localization of the tumor. Imaging studies commonly used to localize pheochromocytomas include CT scan and meta-iodobenzylguanidine (MIBG) scintigraphy; the latter is particularly useful when an extraabdominal focus is suspected. α-blockers (prazosin, doxazosin, phenoxybenzamine) should be used as first-line agents in suspected pheochromocytoma, but surgical resection is indicated for confirmed tumors. It is important not to use β-blockers alone because the unopposed α-activity will worsen the vasoconstriction, resulting in a further increase in blood pressure. Thus, β-blockers should generally be withheld until surgery is performed, unless there are arrhythmias present and adequate alpha-blockade has been achieved. Perioperative care of the patient with pheochromocytoma requires careful monitoring by an experienced anesthesiologist. For patients with inoperable or metastatic malignant pheochromocytoma, blood pressure and adrenergic symptoms may be controlled with α-adrenergic blockade plus β-blockade and/or tyrosine hydroxylase inhibition with metyrosine.

# TREATMENT OF ESSENTIAL HYPERTENSION

Hypertension is the most important preventable cause of premature death, and treatment should focus on achieving the recommended blood pressure goal. For most patients, reductions to <140 mm Hg for the systolic blood pressure and <90 mm Hg for the diastolic blood pressure are the recommended goals while lower goals (<130/80 mm Hg) are recommended for those with diabetes and chronic kidney disease.

# ■ LIFESTYLE MODIFICATION

Clear verbal and written guidance on lifestyle measures, such as eating a healthy diet and getting regular exercise, should be provided for all prehypertensive and

**TABLE 28-4.** Lifestyle Modifications to Prevent and Manage Hypertension

| Modification | Recommendation | Approximate Systolic Blood Pressure Reduction (Range) |
| --- | --- | --- |
| Weight reduction | Maintain normal body weight (body mass index 18.5-24.9 kg/m²) | 5-20 mm Hg/10 kg |
| Adopt DASH (Dietary Approaches to Stop Hypertension) eating plan | Consume a diet rich in fruits, vegetables, and low-fat dairy products with a reduced content of saturated and total fat | 8-14 mm Hg |
| Dietary sodium reduction | Reduce dietary sodium intake to no more than 100 mmol/d 2.4 g sodium or 6 g sodium chloride) | 2-8 mm Hg |
| Physical activity | Engage in regular aerobic physical activity such as brisk walking (at least 30 min/d, most days of the week). | 4-9 mm Hg |
| Moderation of alcohol consumption | Limit consumption to no more than 2 drinks (eg, 24 oz beer, 10 oz wine, or 3 oz 80-proof whiskey) per day in most men and to no more than 1 drink per day in women and lighter-weight persons | 2-4 mm Hg |

Adapted from Chobanian AV, Bakris GL, Black HR, et al. *Seventh Report of the Joint National Committee on Prevention, Detection, Evaluation, and Treatment of High Blood Pressure.* NIH pub. no. 04-5230. Available at: http://www.nhlbi.nih.gov/guidelines/hypertension/jnc7full.htm.

hypertensive patients (**Table 28-4**). Lifestyle interventions reduce the need for drug therapy, enhance the antihypertensive effects of drugs, and favorably influence overall CVD risk. Failure to adopt these measures may attenuate the response to antihypertensive drugs.

# ■ DRUG THERAPY OF HYPERTENSION

The placebo-controlled outcome trials have demonstrated a reduction in cardiovascular disease, renal disease, and stroke with nearly all classes of antihypertensive agents. With few exceptions, the benefit from the various regimens correlated with degree of blood pressure lowering rather than specific drug characteristics. Most patients will require 2 or more antihypertensives to achieve their blood pressure goal (**Table 28-5**).

Thiazide-type diuretics, introduced in the early 1950s, have been the most studied, most recommended, and most cost-effective of all the antihypertensive drug classes. As initial therapy, they remain unsurpassed by any other antihypertensive class in preventing clinical outcomes and should be included in most multidrug regimens.

## Thiazide-Type Diuretics

Thiazide-type diuretics inhibit the Na–Cl cotransporter in the distal tubule to reduce extracellular volume and cardiac output. Diuresis is essential to their antihypertensive

**TABLE 28-5.** Antihypertensive Drug Classes[a]

| Class | Drug (Trade Name) | Usual Dose Range (md/d) | Usual Daily Frequency[a] |
|---|---|---|---|
| Thiazide diuretics | | | |
| | Chlorothiazide (Diuril) | 125-500 | 1-2 |
| | Chlorthalidone (generic) | 12.5-25 | 1 |
| | Hydrochlorothiazide (Microzide, HydroDIURIL[b]) | 12.5-50 | 1 |
| | Polythiazide (Renese) | 2-4 | 1 |
| | Indapamide (Lozol[b]) | 1.25-2.5 | 1 |
| | Metolazone (Mykrox) | 0.5-1.0 | 1 |
| | Bendroflumethiazide | 2.5-5 | 1 |
| | Metolazone (Zaroxolyn) | 2.5-10 | 1-2 |
| Loop diuretics | | | |
| | Bumetanide (Bumex[b]) | 0.5-2 | 2 |
| | Furosemide (Lasix[b]) | 20-80 | 2 |
| | Torsemide (Demadex[b]) | 2.5-10 | 1 |
| Potassium-sparing diuretics | | | |
| | Amiloride (Midamor[b]) | 5-10 | 1-2 |
| | Triamterene (Dyrenium) | 50-100 | 1-2 |
| Aldosterone receptor blockers | | | |
| | Eplerenone (Inspra) | 50-100 | 1-2 |
| | Spironolactone (Aldactone[b]) | 25-50 | 1 |
| β-blockers | | | |
| | Atenolol (Tenormin[b]) | 25-100 | 1 |
| | Betaxolol (Kerlone[b]) | 5-20 | 1 |
| | Bisoprolol (Zebeta[b]) | 2.5-10 | 1 |
| | Metoprolol (Lopressor[b]) | 50-100 | 1-2 |
| | Metoprolol extended release (Toprol XL) | 50-100 | 1 |
| | Nadolol (Corgard[b]) | 40-120 | 1 |
| | Propranolol (Inderal[b]) | 40-160 | 2 |
| | Propranolol long-acting (Inderal LA[b]) | 60-180 | 1 |
| | Timolol (Blocadren[b]) | 20-40 | 2 |
| | Nebivolol (Nebilet[c]) | 5 | 1 |
| β-blockers with intrinsic sympathomimetic activity | | | |
| | Acebutolol (Sectral[b]) | 200-800 | 2 |
| | Penbutolol (Levatol) | 10-40 | 1 |
| | Pindolol (generic) | 10-40 | 2 |
| Combined α- and β-blockers | | | |
| | Carvedilol (Coreg[c]) | 12.5-50 | 2 |
| | Labetalol (Normodyne, Trandate[b]) | 200-800 | 2 |

*(continued)*

**TABLE 28-5.** Antihypertensive Drug Classes[a] (continued)

| Class | Drug (Trade Name) | Usual Dose Range (md/d) | Usual Daily Frequency[a] |
|---|---|---|---|
| ACE inhibitors | | | |
| | Benazepril (Lotensin[b]) | 10-40 | 1 |
| | Captopril (Capoten[b]) | 50-200 | 2 |
| | Enalapril (Vasotec[b]) | 50-40 | 1-2 |
| | Fosinopril (Monopril) | 10-40 | 1 |
| | Lisinopril (Prinivil, Zestril[b]) | 10-40 | 1 |
| | Moexipril (Univasc) | 7.5-30 | 1 |
| | Perindopril (Aceon) | 4-8 | 1 |
| | Quinapril (Accupril) | 10-80 | 1 |
| | Ramipril (Altace) | 2.5-20 | 1 |
| | Trandolapril (Mavik) | 1-4 | 1 |
| Angiotensin II antagonists | | | |
| | Candesartan (Atacand) | 8-32 | 1 |
| | Eprosartan (Teveten) | 400-800 | 1-2 |
| | Irbesartan (Avapro) | 150-300 | 1 |
| | Losartan (Cozaar) | 25-100 | 1-2 |
| | Olmesartan (Benicar) | 20-40 | 1 |
| | Telmisartan (Micardis) | 20-80 | 1 |
| | Valsartan (Diovan) | 80-320 | 1-2 |
| Calcium-channel blockers–nondihydropyridines | | | |
| | Diltiazem extended release (Cardizem CD, Dilacor XR, Tiazac[b]) | 180-420 | 1 |
| | Diltiazem extended-release (Cardizem LA) | 120-540 | 1 |
| | Verapamil immediate-release (Calan, Isoptin[b]) | 80-320 | 2 |
| | Verapamil long acting (Calan SR, Isoptin SR[b]) | 120-480 | 1-2 |
| | Verapamil (Covera HS, Verelan PM) | 120-360 | 1 |
| CCBs–dihydropyridines | | | |
| | Amlodipine (Norvasc) | 2.5-10 | 1 |
| | Felodipine (Plendil) | 2.5-20 | 1 |
| | Isradipine (Dynacirc CR) | 2.5-10 | 2 |
| | Nicardipine sustained-release (Cardene SR) | 6-120 | 2 |
| | Nifedipine long-acting (Adalat CC, Procardia XL) | 30-60 | 1 |
| | Nisoldipine (Sular) | 10-40 | 1 |
| α-1 blockers | | | |
| | Doxazosin (Cardura) | 1-16 | 1 |
| | Prazosin (Minipress[b]) | 2-20 | 2-3 |
| | Terazosin (Hytrin) | 1-20 | 1-2 |

*(continued)*

**TABLE 28-5.** Antihypertensive Drug Classes[a] (continued)

| Class | Drug (Trade Name) | Usual Dose Range (md/d) | Usual Daily Frequency[a] |
|---|---|---|---|
| Central α-2 agonists and other centrally acting drugs | Clonidine (Catapres[b]) | 0.1-0.8 | 2 |
| | Clonidine patch (Catapres-TTS) | 0.1-0.3 | 1 wk |
| | Methyldopa (Aldomet[b]) | 250-1000 | 2 |
| | Reserpine (generic) | 0.1-0.25 | 1 |
| | Guanfacine (Tenex[b]) | 0.5-2 | 1 |
| Direct vasodilators | Hydralazine (Apresoine[b]) | 25-100 | 2 |
| | Minoxidil (Loniten[b]) | 2.5-80 | 1-2 |
| Renin inhibitor | Aliskiren | 50-600 | 1 |

[a]In some patients treated once daily, the antihypertensive effect may diminish toward the end of the dosing interval (trough effect). Blood pressure should be measured just prior to dosing to determine if satisfactory blood pressure control is obtained. Accordingly, an increase in dosage or frequency may need to be considered. These dosages may vary from those listed in the *Physicians' Desk Reference,* 61st ed. (2007).

[b]Available in generic preparations.

[c]License may only exist in some countries.

Adapted from Chobanian AV, Bakris GL, Black HR, et al. *Seventh Report of the Joint National Committee on Prevention, Detection, Evaluation, and Treatment of High Blood Pressure.* NIH pub. no. 04-5230. Available at: http://www.nhlbi.nih.gov/guidelines/hypertension/jnc7full.htm.

action, and their antihypertensive efficacy can be antagonized by high-salt intake; however, their mechanism of action is not fully understood and may include reduction in peripheral vascular resistance. Hydrochlorothiazide is the most commonly prescribed agent of this class in the United States. Indapamide, at the recommended doses produces less hypokalemia, although at higher doses it behaves similar to other thiazides. With the exception of metolazone and indapamide, most thiazide diuretics lose their antihypertensive effectiveness when the GFR declines to <30 to 40 mL/min. Most side effects are related to fluid and electrolyte abnormalities including hypokalemia and hyponatremia, but they can also increase blood glucose and lipids (each approximately 5 mg/dL).

## Loop Diuretics

Loop diuretics inhibit Na–K–2Cl transport in the thick ascending limb of the loop of Henle and include furosemide, bumetanide, ethacrynic acid, and torsemide. Because of their short half-life, they are less effective than thiazide-type diuretics in lowering blood pressure in patients with normal renal function when prescribed once or twice daily. In those with estimated GFR <30-40 mL/min/1.73 m$^2$, their use is essential to achieve blood pressure goals. They are also usually required for volume control in those requiring vasodilators, especially minoxidil. Most adverse reactions are related to electrolyte abnormalities and extracellular volume depletion. NSAIDs and probenecid blunt the effect of loop diuretics, and thiazide diuretics have synergic effects with loop diuretics.

## Potassium-Sparing Diuretics

Potassium-sparing diuretics include triamterene and amiloride and inhibit the renal epithelial Na channels and cause small increases in NaCl excretion. They are relatively weak diuretics and rarely used as a single agent in the treatment of hypertension or edema. They are useful in preventing diuretic-induced hypokalemia when prescribed with other diuretics. The most serious side effect of this class of diuretics is hyperkalemia. Use with NSAIDs, angiotensin-converting enzyme (ACE) inhibitors, ARBs, β-blockers, and in diabetic hypertensives with or without nephropathy increases the risk of this side effect.

Mineralocorticoid receptor antagonists are another class of potassium-sparing diuretics and include spironolactone and eplerenone. Mineralocorticoids bind to the mineralocorticoid receptor to cause salt and water retention and increase the excretion of potassium and $H^+$. Mineralocorticoid antagonists, often in combination with thiazides or loop diuretics, are effective in treating hypertension, particularly resistant hypertension and hypertension associated with sleep apnea. They are particularly useful in the treatment of primary hyperaldosteronism. The major adverse effects include hyperkalemia, hypertriglyceridemia, and antiandrogen effects like breast pain, gynecomastia, and sexual dysfunction in males. Eplerenone is more selective for the mineralocorticoid receptor than the spironolactone and less likely to produce antiandrogenic effects.

## Calcium-Channel Blockers

Calcium-channel blockers (CCBs) inhibit calcium entry into vasculature smooth muscle through the voltage-sensitive L-type $Ca^{2+}$ channels, resulting in vasodilation of coronary and peripheral arteries. Two subclasses of calcium-channel blockers, dihydropyridines (DHPs; eg, nifedipine, felodipine, amlodipine) and non-dihydropyridines (non-DHPs; eg, verapamil and diltiazem) are available and have similar antihypertensive efficacy. Non-DHP CCBs substantially reduce contractility and atrioventricular nodal conduction. Thus, they are inappropriate for the patient with significant left ventricular dysfunction or >$1^0$ atrioventricular block and should be replaced by DHP-CCBs if used with β-blockers. Unlike the DHP-CCBs, they are less likely to produce headache, edema, and palpitations. Typical antihypertensive doses of diltiazem range from 180 to 540 mg/d while lower doses are used for their antianginal effect. A common side effect of verapamil is constipation because of its effect on gastrointestinal smooth muscle relaxation.

The DHP-CCBs are potent arteriolar vasodilators and especially effective in the more resistant patient as their antihypertensive action and side-effect profile complements that of β-blockers when used together. They have little effect on cardiac conduction and contractility. Both felodipine and amlodipine have demonstrated their safety in hypertensives with systolic dysfunction in heart failure trials. The most common side effect of the DHP-CCBs include headache, flushing, and dose-dependent peripheral edema. The edema results from precapillary arteriolar dilatation and transudation of fluid from the vascular compartments into dependent tissues rather than from fluid retention; it does not respond well to treatment with diuretics.

## β-Blockers

β-blockers lower blood pressure predominantly by inhibiting β1-adrenergic receptors, thereby decreasing cardiac contractility and heart rate and thus reducing

**TABLE 28-6.** Compelling Indications for Individual Drug Classes

| Compelling Indication | Recommended Drugs | | | | | |
|---|---|---|---|---|---|---|
| | Diuretic | BB | ACEI | ARB | CCB | Aldo ANT |
| Heart failure | × | × | × | × | | × |
| Postmyocardial infarction | | × | × | | | × |
| High coronary disease risk | × | × | × | | × | |
| Diabetes | × | × | × | × | × | |
| Chronic kidney disease | | | × | × | | |
| Recurrent stroke prevention | × | | × | | | |

ACEI, angiotensin-converting enzyme inhibitor; Aldo ANT, aldosterone antagonist; ARB, angiotensin-receptor blocker; BB, β-blocker; CCB, calcium-channel blocker.

Adapted from Chobanian AV, Bakris GL, Black HR, et al. *Seventh Report of the Joint National Committee on Prevention, Detection, Evaluation, and Treatment of High Blood Pressure.* NIH pub. no. 04-5230. Available at: http://www.nhlbi.nih.gov/guidelines/hypertension/jnc7full.htm.

cardiac output. Renin release and the generation of angiotensin II are also inhibited by this mechanism. Additionally, β-blockers are reported to alter baroceptor sensitivity, downregulate peripheral adrenergic receptors, and increase prostacyclin biosynthesis, thereby facilitating vasodilation. They are particularly beneficial in hypertensive patients with coronary disease and heart failure (**Table 28-6**). They are less effective in lowering blood pressure in black patients and in the elderly unless accompanied by diuretics or calcium-channel blockers.

## Inhibitors of the Renin–Angiotensin System

Inhibitors of the renin–angiotensin system (RAS) include the ACE inhibitors, angiotensin-receptor blockers (ARBs), and renin inhibitors. The ACE inhibitors and ARBs (and presumably the renin inhibitors, though outcome data are not yet available) are specifically indicated in hypertensive patients with heart failure and chronic kidney disease and useful in hypertensive patients following myocardial infarction and stroke when combined with thiazide-type diuretics. The incidence of side effects is low; however, angioedema, while rare, can occur at any time during treatment and occurs more frequently in blacks. Cough occurs in up to 25% of all treated patients but occurs more frequently in blacks. ARBs (and presumably renin inhibitors) are reasonable alternatives for patients with ACE inhibitor-associated cough. Generally, it is recommended to avoid ARBs in patients with a history of ACE inhibitor–related angioedema, although there are case reports of this substitution being done safely.

## α-Blockers

α-blockers like prazosin, terazosin, and doxazosin block the activation of the vasoconstricting α-1 adrenoreceptors and are indicated as add-on therapy for blood pressure control. They also alleviate some symptoms of benign prostatic hypertrophy. Postural hypotension is an important side effect to keep in mind while using this class of drugs.

## α-2 Agonists

α-2 agonists include methyldopa, clonidine, guanabenz, and guanfacine and stimulate central nervous system α-2 receptors to reduce central nervous system sympathetic outflow. As monotherapy, their antihypertensive efficacy diminishes with time. Their effect is enhanced with concomitant diuretic, vasodilator, or CCB administration but not with other sympatholytics or RAS inhibitors. The most common side effects include sedation, dry mouth, and fatigue. Liver dysfunction and a Coombs-positive hemolytic anemia can be seen with methyldopa.

## Vasodilators

Vasodilators, such as hydralazine and minoxidil, have been largely replaced by better-tolerated and more effective drugs such as the CCBs. However, vasodilators can be used to treat resistant hypertension. Their major side effects include fluid retention, including heart failure, and hirsuitism with minoxidil.

The findings of clinical trials to date suggest that for the patient with uncomplicated hypertension, as well as for the patient with diabetes but without nephropathy, initial therapy with "newer therapies" (eg, ACE inhibitors, CCBs, and ARBs) is effective, but not superior to thiazide-type diuretics at reducing stroke, coronary heart disease morbidity or mortality, or all-cause mortality. Recent studies indicate that β-blockers may be less effective than ARBs and CCBs in preventing cardiovascular disease outcomes. In addition, compelling indications exist for specific drug classes in those with hypertension and specific target-organ damage (see Table 28-6).

Since most hypertensive patients require multiple agents for blood pressure control, nearly all guideline panels support the initiation of treatment with 2 or more antihypertensive medications when blood pressure is more than 20/10 mm Hg above goal. Patients with indications for specific agents should obviously have these included in their regimen.

# SPECIAL POPULATIONS

## ◼ ELDERLY

The prevalence of hypertension is high, 60% to 80%, in populations older than 65 years. Systolic blood pressure rises and diastolic blood pressure declines after the age of 50 to 55 years in both normotensive and untreated hypertensive subjects. In older hypertensives, measuring standing blood pressure becomes important because of the increased risk of orthostatic hypotension and the greater need for agents that may aggravate this condition. Antihypertensive medications should be initiated at lower doses in the elderly to facilitate a more gradual reduction in blood pressure.

## ◼ DIABETES

Diabetes is highly prevalent in hypertensive patients, and increases the risk for complications of both diseases. The goal of appropriate treatment of diabetes is to minimize the effects of these disorders on the cardiovascular and renal systems. Multiple studies have demonstrated that blood pressure lowering using either an ACE inhibitor or an ARB slows the progression of both types 1 and 2 diabetic renal disease. Nearly every patient with renal insufficiency will require a diuretic to lower blood pressure, especially to the recommended goal for diabetics (<130/80 mm Hg). In the ALLHAT, one of the few renal outcome studies able to address this question, there was no loss of protection against renal disease progression when a diuretic-based regimen was compared with one containing an ACE inhibitor, even in participants with diabetes. A CCB-based regimen is less effective in preventing renal outcomes than one containing either an ACE inhibitor or ARB.

# ■ RACE/ETHNICITY

Ethnic and racial differences in hypertension prevalence, severity, and response to therapy have been reported. Hypertension is more common and severe in black populations than in white populations, and has an earlier onset. It is less common and less severe in Mexican Americans and Native Americans, but blood pressure control rates are generally lower when hypertension is present. In general, the treatment of hypertension is similar for all demographic groups. However, African Americans demonstrate somewhat reduced blood pressure lowering in response to monotherapy with β-blockers, ACE inhibitors, or ARBs, compared to diuretics or CCBs. These differential responses are largely eliminated by drug combinations that include adequate doses of a diuretic or CCB. RAS inhibitors were less effective in preventing many major clinical outcomes (including heart failure, stroke, and coronary events) than diuretics in black participants in several large studies. However, in patients with compelling indications (ie, heart failure or renal disease), RAS-blocking agents (either ACE inhibitors or ARBs) or β-blockers should be prescribed regardless of race. Because of the severity of hypertension in black patients, RAS inhibitors will usually be required as part of most multidrug therapy to achieve the blood pressure goal.

# ■ RENAL DISEASE

Hypertension is well-recognized as a risk factor for progression of renal disease. Current Kidney Disease Outcomes Quality Initiative (K/DOQI) Clinical Practice Guidelines on Hypertension and Antihypertensive Agents in Chronic Kidney Disease and the JNC 7 recommend a goal blood pressure of 130/80 mm Hg in patients with chronic kidney disease. Patients with proteinuria >1 g/d have been shown to benefit from an even lower blood pressure goal (<125/75 mm Hg). Inhibition of the renin–angiotensin axis is superior to conventional antihypertensive therapy in slowing the decline of renal function in patients with diabetic and nondiabetic nephropathy with proteinuria (total protein/ creatinine ratio of 200 mg/g or greater).

# ■ HYPERTENSION DURING PREGNANCY

Hypertension occurring during pregnancy falls into 1 of 4 major classifications:

1. Chronic hypertension is the presence of preexisting hypertension or developing within 20 weeks of gestation pregnancy.
2. Gestational hypertension (also called transient hypertension) refers to elevated blood pressure first detected after 20 weeks of gestation without proteinuria.
3. Preeclampsia-eclampsia (also called pregnancy-induced hypertension) is defined by a systolic blood pressure ≥140 mm Hg or a diastolic blood pressure ≥90 mm Hg after the 20th week of gestation in a previously normotensive woman and which is accompanied by more than 300 mg proteinuria in 24 hours.
4. Preeclampsia superimposed on underlying hypertension.

   For management and counseling purposes, chronic hypertension in pregnancy is also categorized as either low risk or high risk. Low-risk pregnant patients have mild essential hypertension without any organ involvement and can expect an outcome similar to that in the general obstetric population. Initiation of therapy is usually considered in women without end-organ damage if systolic blood pressure exceeds 160 mm Hg or diastolic pressure exceeds 110 mm Hg.

   In pregnant patients with end-organ damage, it is desirable to keep the blood pressure below 140/90 mm Hg. ACE inhibitors and ARBs are contraindicated, and should be discontinued as soon as pregnancy is detected. If drug therapy is necessary, methyldopa (250 mg twice daily orally, maximum dose 3 g/d) has a long track record of safety and efficacy in pregnant patients, and is often the initial drug of choice. Hydralazine (25 mg twice daily orally; maximum dose 300 mg/d) and β-blockers, such as labetalol (100 mg twice daily orally, maximum dose 800 mg every 8 hours) can also be used; however, β-blockers may be associated with reduced intrauterine fetal growth. For severe hypertension, >160/110 mm Hg, with end-organ damage (encephalopathy, hemorrhage, or eclampsia), IV preparations of labetalol or hydralazine are recommended.

Preeclampsia occurs in approximately 5% of pregnancies. It is associated with significant maternal and fetal risk. The major decisions in the management are obstetrical ones regarding timing of delivery. In preeclamptic hypertension, the reasonable goals for systolic and diastolic blood pressures are 140 to 155 mm Hg and 90 to 105 mm Hg, respectively.

In breastfeeding mothers, the following drugs are considered safe for control of hypertension: captopril, diltiazem, enalapril, hydralazine, HCTZ, labetalol, methyldopa, minoxidil, nadolol, nifedipine, oxprenolol, propranolol, spironolactone, timolol, and verapamil. It should be noted that diuretics may reduce milk production.

## ■ HYPERTENSION ASSOCIATED WITH SOLID-ORGAN TRANSPLANTATIONS

Hypertension is common in patients who undergo solid-organ transplantation and is associated with increased risk for cardiovascular morbidity and graft loss. Preexisting hypertension may be exacerbated by use of calcineurin inhibitors, corticosteroids, and progressive chronic kidney disease. Treatment goals are similar to the goals for the general population, including lower blood pressure goals (<130/80 mm Hg) in patients with diabetes and chronic kidney disease. Although there are few prospective clinical trials to guide choice of antihypertensive therapy in transplantation patients, dihydropyridine calcium-channel blockers are commonly used in the regimen because of their pharmacologic property to antagonize calcineurin-mediated vasoconstriction. It is important to consider any possible interactions with immunosuppressive therapy when initiating antihypertensive drug therapy in transplantation patients.

## HYPERTENSIVE EMERGENCIES AND URGENCIES

Hypertensive emergency is defined by acute and rapidly evolving end-organ damage, such as aortic dissection, heart failure, symptomatic coronary heart disease, progressive renal disease, stroke, or cerebral dysfunction associated with significant hypertension. Although there is no blood pressure threshold for the diagnosis of hypertensive emergency, most end-organ damage is noted with systolic blood pressures exceeding 220 mm Hg or diastolic blood pressures exceeding 120 mm Hg. In these patients, immediate but monitored reduction, often in a critical care setting, is accomplished with parenteral medications and is essential to prevent long-term organ damage.

Hypertensive urgency is defined by a markedly elevated blood pressure, usually in the same range seen in a hypertension emergency, but without the rapid progression of target-organ damage. If the patient is asymptomatic or clinically stable, the patient can be managed as an outpatient with close follow-up within days. In fact, there is evidence that the rapid reduction of blood pressure in asymptomatic hypertension may also precipitate adverse outcomes.

The initial assessment of hypertensive crisis is straightforward. A history and physical examination will rapidly direct further investigation to the involved organs while appropriate chemistry measurements and ECG will assess their involvement. Urine toxicology for cocaine metabolites is helpful in select populations. Plain chest radiographs are useful for assessing volume status and cardiac size and as a first screen for aortic dissection, but false-positive and false-negative results occur.

In hypertensive emergency, the goal of therapy is to lower the mean arterial pressure by approximately 25% within 2 hours, and to 160/100 mm Hg by 6 hours. Multiple medications are available for the treatment of hypertension crisis (**Table 28-7**).

**TABLE 28-7.** Medical Treatment for Management of Hypertension Crises

| Agent | Dose | Onset of Action | Precautions |
|---|---|---|---|
| **Parenteral Vasodilators** | | | |
| Sodium nitroprusside | 0.25-10 µg/kg/min IV infusion | Immediate | Thiocyanate toxicity with prolonged use |
| Nitroglycerin | 5-100 µg/min IV infusion | 2-5 min | Headache, tachycardia, tolerance Protracted hypotension after prolonged use |
| Nicardipine | 5-15 mg/h IV infusion | 1-5 min | |
| Fenoldopam mesylate | 0.1-0.3 µg/kg/min IV infusion | 1-5 min | Headache, tachycardia, increased intraocular pressure |
| Hydralazine | 5-10 mg as IV bolus or 10-40 mg IM repeat q4-6h | 10 min IV\n\n20 min IM | Unpredictable and excessive falls in pressure; tachycardia; angina exacerbation |
| Enalaprilat | 0.625-1.25 mg q6h IV bolus | 15-60 min | Unpredictable and excessive falls in pressure; acute renal failure in patients with bilateral renal artery stenosis |
| **Parenteral Adrenergic Inhibitors** | | | |
| Labetalol | 20-80 mg as slow IV injection q10min, or 0.5-2 mg/min IV as infusion | 5-10 min | Bronchospasm, heart block, orthostatic hypotension |
| Metoprolol | 5 mg IV q10mi × 3 doses | 5-10 min | Bronchospasm, heart block, heart failure, exacerbation of cocaine-induced myocardial ischemia |
| Esmolol | 500 µg/kg IV over 3 min then 25-100 mg/kg/min as IV infusion | 1-5 min | Bronchospasm, heart block, heart failure |
| Phentolamine | 5-10 mg IV bolus q5-15min | 1-2 min | Tachycardia, orthostatic hypotension |

Adapted from Victor R. Arterial hypertension. In: Goldman L, ed. *Cecil Textbook of Medicine*. 23rd ed. Philadelphia, PA: Saunders; 2008, with permission from Elsevier Company.

Sodium nitroprusside produces concomitant venous and arterial dilation, improving forward flow and cardiac output, and is the drug of choice because of its immediate onset of action and short duration of effect (1-2 minutes). Hypertension-induced acute pulmonary edema and acute aortic dissection are best treated with sodium nitroprusside. Prolonged treatment can result in accumulation of thiocyanate, particularly in patients with hepatic or renal insufficiency. Parenteral labetalol is another first-line agent for hypertensive emergency with a fast onset of action. It should be used cautiously in patients who have severe bradycardia, congestive heart failure, or bronchospasm.

## ■ RESISTANT HYPERTENSION

Resistant hypertension is the failure to reach goal blood pressure in patients who are adhering to full doses of an appropriate 3-drug regimen which includes a diuretic. Although white-coat hypertension and substandard measurement techniques, and pseudohypertension (artifactually high blood pressure measured due to a stiffened brachial artery that does not compress with the blood pressure cuff) should be considered, an important etiology of refractory hypertension is poor compliance with therapy. Other causes include dietary indiscretion, volume overload from kidney disease, or inadequate therapy. Some concomitant medications may interfere with blood pressure control, including nonsteroidal anti-inflammatory drugs, cyclooxygenase-2 inhibitors, cocaine, amphetamines, other illicit drugs, sympathomimetics (decongestants, anorectics), oral contraceptives, adrenal steroids, cyclosporine and tacrolimus, erythropoietin, licorice (including some chewing tobacco), and selected over-the-counter dietary supplements. After eliminating these contributing factors, secondary causes should be considered as discussed previously. A trial of aldosterone antagonists may be effective even in the absence of hyperaldosteronism.

# SUGGESTED READINGS

Atkins GB, Rahman M, Wright JT Jr. Diagnosis and treatment of hypertension. In: Fuster V, Walsh RA, Harrington RA, et al, eds. *Hurst's The Heart*. 13th ed. New York, NY: McGraw-Hill; 2011;70:1585-1605.

Chobanian AV, Bakris GL, Black HR, et al. Seventh report of the Joint National Committee on Prevention, Detection, Evaluation, and Treatment of High Blood Pressure. *Hypertension*. 2003;42:1206-1252.

European Society of Hypertension–European Society of Cardiology. 2003 European Society of Hypertension-European Society of Cardiology guidelines for the management of arterial hypertension. *J Hypertens*. 2003;21:1011-1053.

Ezzati M, Lopez AD, Rodgers A, et al. Selected major risk factors and global and regional burden of disease. *Lancet*. 2002;360:1347-1360.

Hemmelgarn BR, Zarnke KB, Campbell NR, et al. The 2004 Canadian Hypertension Education Program recommendations for the management of hypertension: part I—blood pressure measurement, diagnosis and assessment of risk. *Can J Cardiol*. 2004;20:31-40.

Hoffman BB. Therapy of hypertension. In: Brunton LL, Lazo JS, Parker KL, eds. *The Pharmacological Basis of Therapeutics*. New York, NY: McGraw-Hill; 2006:845-868.

K/DOQI clinical practice guidelines for chronic kidney disease: evaluation, classification, and stratification. *Am J Kidney Dis*. 2002;39(suppl 1):S1-S266.

Newell-Price J, Bertagna X, Grossman AB, et al. Cushing's syndrome. *Lancet*. 2006;367:1605-1617.

Pickering TG, Hall JE, Appel LJ, et al. Recommendations for blood pressure measurement in humans and experimental animals: part 1: blood pressure measurement in humans: a statement for professionals from the Subcommittee of Professional and Public Education of the American Heart Association Council on High Blood Pressure Research. *Hypertension*. 2005;45:142-161.

Podymow T, August, P. Update on the use of antihypertensive drugs in pregnancy. *Hypertension.* http://hyper.ahajournal.org. Accessed February 8, 2008.

Report of the National High Blood Pressure Education Program Working Group on High Blood Pressure in Pregnancy. *Am J Obstet Gynecol.* 2000;183:S1-S22.

Wright JT Jr, Dunn JK, Cutler JA, et al. Outcomes in hypertensive black and nonblack patients treated with chlorthalidone, amlodipine, and lisinopril. *JAMA.* 2005;293:1595-1608.

CHAPTER 29
# PULMONARY HYPERTENSION

Robyn J. Barst and Lewis J. Rubin

Pulmonary arterial hypertension, a hemodynamic abnormality present in a variety of conditions, is characterized by increased right ventricular afterload and work. The clinical manifestations, natural history, and reversibility of pulmonary hypertension (PH) depend on the nature of the pulmonary vascular lesions and the etiology and severity of the hemodynamic disorder. The degree of pulmonary hypertension that develops is a function of the amount of the pulmonary vascular tree that has been eliminated. PH is usually secondary to cardiac or pulmonary disease. Although idiopathic pulmonary arterial hypertension (IPAH) is uncommon, it is usually considered a distinctive clinical entity in which intrinsic pulmonary vascular disease is free of the complicating features of secondary PH contributed by diseases of the heart and/or lungs. Mild or even moderate PH can exist for a lifetime without becoming evident clinically. When pulmonary hypertension does become manifest clinically, the symptoms tend to be nonspecific.

## DEFINITIONS

This chapter deals with *chronic* pulmonary arterial hypertension. Acute pulmonary arterial hypertension is usually a result of either pulmonary embolism or the adult respiratory distress syndrome. Pulmonary *venous* hypertension is usually encountered clinically as a consequence of left ventricular failure or mitral valvular disease. Occasionally it may occur in the course of fibrosing mediastinitis. Only rarely is the entity known as pulmonary venoocclusive disease (PVOD) encountered. The hallmarks of pulmonary venous hypertension are pulmonary congestion and edema. Pulmonary venous hypertension is said to exist when pulmonary venous (or left atrial) pressure rises above 15 mm Hg.

*Cor pulmonale* signifies the presence of PH in the setting of chronic respiratory disease. The degree of pulmonary hypertension that develops in patients with chronic lung disease tends to be less severe than that in connective tissue diseases, chronic thromboembolic disease, or IPAH. Pulmonary hypertension may be severe, however, in some patients with interstitial lung disease.

## HEMODYNAMICS

At *sea level,* a cardiac output of 5 to 6 L/min is associated with a pulmonary arterial pressure of about 20/12 mm Hg, with a mean of about 15 mm Hg. At an altitude of 15 000 ft, the same level of blood flow is associated with somewhat higher pressures. Pulmonary arterial pressures also tend to increase somewhat with age.

A pressure drop of only 5 to 10 mm Hg between the pulmonary artery and left atrium accompanies the cardiac output of 5 to 6 L/min. Determination of pulmonary vascular resistance, calculated as the ratio of the difference in mean pressure at the 2 ends of the pulmonary vascular bed (pulmonary arterial minus left atrial pressure divided by the cardiac output), is a practical clinical tool for assessing the hemodynamic state of the pulmonary system. In practice, since the left atrium is not readily accessible, pulmonary wedge pressure is generally substituted for left atrial pressure.

# PULMONARY HYPERTENSION: GENERAL FEATURES

## ■ CLINICAL MANIFESTATIONS

Pulmonary hypertension is a final common hemodynamic consequence of multiple etiologies and diverse mechanisms. Most cases of PH are secondary. Among the underlying causes of pulmonary hypertension are mechanical compression and distortion of the resistance vessels of the lungs, hypoxic vasoconstriction (eg, in severe obstructive airways disease or diffuse parenchymal diseases), intravascular obstruction (eg, thromboemboli or tumor emboli), and combinations of mechanical and vasoconstrictive influences. The significance of PH, however, is that if uncontrolled, it leads to right ventricular failure. Once pulmonary arterial pressures reach systemic levels, right ventricular failure becomes inevitable.

## ■ SPECIAL STUDIES

The "gold standard" for the diagnosis of pulmonary hypertension is right-sided heart catheterization. This technique enables the direct determination of right atrial and ventricular pressures, pulmonary arterial pressure, pulmonary wedge pressure (as an approximation of pulmonary venous pressure), pulmonary blood flow (cardiac output), and the responses of these parameters to interventions (vasodilators, oxygen, exercise). From the measurements and samples obtained during cardiac catheterization, pulmonary vascular resistance can be calculated. In general, noninvasive methods are less reliable and less informative.

# CHEST RADIOGRAPHY

The characteristic findings of pulmonary hypertension are enlargement of the pulmonary trunk and hilar vessels in association with attenuation (pruning) of the peripheral pulmonary arterial tree. Right-sided heart enlargement can be best detected radiographically on the lateral view as fullness in the retrosternal air space. In secondary pulmonary hypertension, changes in the lungs (eg, hyperinflation, fibrosis) and in the position of the heart and diaphragm often mask the radiologic changes of pulmonary hypertension.

# THE ELECTROCARDIOGRAM

The electrocardiogram (ECG) can disclose hypertrophy of the right ventricle and is more reliable in respiratory disorders that do not involve the parenchyma of the lungs (eg, alveolar hypoventilation and sleep apnea) than in obstructive airways disease or parenchymal lung disease (see also Chapter 2). Since RV mass is considerably less than LV mass under normal conditions, the ECG is a specific but insensitive tool for detection of right ventricular hypertrophy.

# ECHOCARDIOGRAPHY

Echocardiographic techniques have proved useful in providing a measure of right ventricular thickness as an index of right ventricular hypertension. In most clinics, reliable estimates of the level of pulmonary hypertension have been obtained by determining regurgitant flows across the tricuspid and pulmonic valves using continuous-wave Doppler echocardiography.

# LUNG SCANS

Ventilation/perfusion scans are of most value in the diagnosis and exclusion of chronic pulmonary thromboembolic disease. In many institutions this has been replaced by high-resolution CT.

# LUNG BIOPSY

The sampling of lung tissue by open thoracotomy or video-assisted thoracoscopy is occasionally helpful in identifying the etiology of the pulmonary hypertension—for example, in the setting of suspected pulmonary vasculitis. However, the procedure carries substantial risk in these hemodynamically compromised individuals.

# SECONDARY PULMONARY HYPERTENSION

Cardiac and/or respiratory diseases are the most common causes of secondary pulmonary hypertension. Chronic thromboembolic disease ranks third. Cardiac disease leads to PH by increasing pulmonary blood flow (eg, with large left-to-right shunts) or by increasing pulmonary venous pressure (eg, with left ventricular failure). In respiratory disease, the predominant mechanism for the PH is an increase in resistance to pulmonary blood flow arising from perivascular parenchymal changes coupled with pulmonary vasoconstriction due to hypoxia. In chronic thromboembolic disease, clots in various stages of organization and affecting pulmonary vessels of different sizes increase resistance to blood flow.

## ■ ACQUIRED DISORDERS OF THE LEFT SIDE OF THE HEART

Left ventricular failure is the most common cause of pulmonary hypertension. Among the various etiologies, myocardial disorders and lesions of the mitral and aortic valves predominate. Both categories of lesions lead to an increase in pulmonary venous pressure, which in turn evokes an increase in pulmonary arterial pressure. The medical management of myocardial failure is considered elsewhere. The treatment of congenital heart disease and of mitral valvular disease is usually mechanical (eg, surgical or balloon mitral valvuloplasty). The prospect for relief of the pulmonary venous hypertension, as by mitral valve commissurotomy or replacement, depends on the reversibility of the pulmonary vascular and perivascular lesions.

# ■ CONGENITAL HEART DISEASE

Pulmonary hypertension is part of the natural history of many types of congenital heart disease and is often a major determinant of the clinical course, feasibility of surgical intervention, and outcome. Congenital defects of the heart associated with large left-to-right shunts (eg, atrial septal defect) or abnormal communication between the great vessels (eg, patent ductus arteriosus) are commonly associated with pulmonary arterial hypertension. The major cause of PH in congenital heart disease is an increase in blood flow, an increase in resistance to blood flow, or most often, a combination of the two.

Caution is required in administering vasodilator agents to patients with congenital heart disease because of their potential to increase right-to-left shunting by reducing systemic vascular resistance to a greater degree than its pulmonary counterpart. Phlebotomy, with replacement of fluid (eg, plasma or albumin), is helpful in congenital cyanotic heart disease in which severe hypoxemia has evoked a large increase in red cell mass.

# ■ THROMBOEMBOLIC DISEASE

Thromboembolic disease is a form of occlusive pulmonary vascular disease. It may be acute or chronic. Tumor emboli carried to the lungs from extrapulmonary sites (eg, the breast) can cause pulmonary hypertension by invading the adjacent minute vessels of the lungs. Intravenous drug use may be associated with talc or cotton fiber embolism to the lungs, which can result in a granulomatous pulmonary arteritis.

# CHRONIC PROXIMAL PULMONARY THROMBOEMBOLISM

In some patients who have survived large to massive pulmonary emboli, resolution fails to occur, and the clots become organized and incorporated into the walls of the major pulmonary arteries, leading to pulmonary hypertension. By the time the diagnosis is made, the obstructing lesions in the central pulmonary arteries have become an integral part of the vascular wall through the processes of endothelialization and recanalization.

The importance of recognizing *proximal* pulmonary thromboembolism as a cause of PH lies in the possibility of relieving the pulmonary hypertension by surgical intervention—that is, by pulmonary thromboendarterectomy. Ventilation/perfusion lung scanning is the critical diagnostic test. As a rule, patients with proximal pulmonary thromboembolism show 2 or more segmental perfusion defects. If the perfusion defects are segmental or larger, selective pulmonary angiography is required to define the location, extent, and number of pulmonary vascular occlusions. Cardiac catheterization for selective pulmonary angiography also enables hemodynamic assessment.

Surgery is advocated for patients with pulmonary hypertension who have persistent clotting in lobar or more proximal pulmonary arteries after at least 6 months of anticoagulation. Thromboendarterectomy is done via a median sternotomy using deep hypothermic cardiopulmonary bypass with intermittent periods of circulatory arrest. Postoperatively, hemodynamic improvement is usually quite dramatic. Reperfusion pulmonary edema can be a severe complication immediately after the obstruction has been relieved. In experienced hands, mortality is of the order of 5%. After the operation, patients are placed on lifelong anticoagulants. A filter is usually placed in the inferior vena cava to further prevent recurrence.

# RESPIRATORY DISEASES AND DISORDERS

In addition to intrinsic pulmonary diseases, disturbances in respiratory muscle function or in the control of breathing can also lead to pulmonary hypertension. Among the intrinsic lung diseases are those affecting the airways (eg, chronic bronchitis) as well as those affecting the parenchyma (ie, emphysema, pulmonary fibrosis). Among the ventilatory disorders are the syndromes of alveolar hypoventilation due to respiratory muscle weakness and sleep-disordered breathing.

## ■ INTERSTITIAL FIBROSIS

Pulmonary sarcoidosis, asbestosis, idiopathic fibrosis, and radiation-induced fibrosis are common causes of widespread pulmonary fibrosis that culminates in cor pulmonale. Dyspnea and tachypnea generally dominate the clinical picture of interstitial fibrosis; cough is rarely prominent. As a rule, severe PH occurs toward the end of the illness, when hypoxemia and hypercapnia are present at rest. Right ventricular failure is a common sequel.

Systemically administered vasodilators have no proven place in dealing with the pulmonary hypertension associated with interstitial fibrosis and may worsen intrapulmonary gas exchange. Oxygen therapy, particularly during daily activity or sleep, can be important in attenuating the hypoxic pulmonary pressor response. Glucocorticoids and other potent immunosuppressive agents are the mainstay of therapy and often result in some symptomatic relief. The advent of lung transplantation has greatly widened the therapeutic horizons for dealing with widespread interstitial fibrosis.

## ■ CHRONIC OBSTRUCTIVE AIRWAYS DISEASE

Chronic bronchitis and emphysema (chronic obstructive pulmonary disease [COPD]) are the most common causes of cor pulmonale in patients with intrinsic pulmonary disease. Cystic fibrosis is an example of a mixed airway and parenchymal lung disease in which pulmonary hypertension plays a significant role in outcome.

Cor pulmonale is encountered in 2 different settings: *acutely* in the setting of decompensation, which is often due to an acute respiratory infection; and *chronically* when progressive lung disease and worsening gas exchange lead to unremitting vascular remodeling.

In the patient with COPD with acute cor pulmonale precipitated by a bout of bronchitis or pneumonia, the goal of therapy is to maintain tolerable levels of arterial oxygenation while waiting for the upper respiratory infection to subside. Supplemental oxygen, such as 28% oxygen delivered by a Venturi mask, generally suffices to relieve arterial hypoxemia and to restore pulmonary arterial pressures toward normal. Considerable improvement may also be accomplished even in the individual who has chronic PH by sustained (>18 h/d) breathing of oxygen-enriched air.

Arterial blood gas composition is the therapeutic compass for the control of PH in COPD. The degree of hypoxia may be underestimated by blood sampling while the patient is awake and at rest, since hypoxemia is more marked during sleep and with physical activity. Determinations of the oxygen saturation during sleep or with ambulation, using pulse oximetry, are helpful in optimally prescribing supplemental oxygen.

Vasodilators have recently been tried in various types of secondary pulmonary hypertension, including that due to COPD. The agents tried are the same as those outlined for *idiopathic* pulmonary arterial hypertension. They run the risk of aggravating arterial hypoxemia by exaggerating ventilation/perfusion abnormalities.

To date, the safest and most effective approach to pulmonary vasodilatation in obstructive lung disease with arterial hypoxemia is the use of supplemental oxygen.

# CONNECTIVE TISSUE DISEASES

Pulmonary vascular disease is an important component of certain connective tissue diseases. Among these, the more common are systemic lupus erythematosus (SLE), the scleroderma spectrum of diseases, and dermatomyositis.

In progressive systemic sclerosis (scleroderma) and its variants, such as the CREST syndrome (calcinosis, Raynaud syndrome, esophageal involvement, sclerodactyly, and telangiectasis), and in overlap syndromes (eg, mixed connective tissue disease), the incidence of pulmonary vascular disease is high. In these patients, pulmonary hypertension is the cause of considerable morbidity and mortality. The pulmonary vascular disease may be independent of pulmonary or other visceral disease. As in the case of SLE, the pathology of these lesions is often indistinguishable from that of primary pulmonary hypertension. Vasodilator therapy has not proved to be highly effective; however, continuous intravenous epoprostenol and oral bosentan, an endothelin receptor antagonist, have both been shown to improve hemodynamics and exercise tolerance.

## ■ ALVEOLAR HYPOVENTILATION IN PATIENTS WITH NORMAL LUNGS

In patients who hypoventilate despite normal lungs (alveolar hypoventilation), the primary pathogenetic mechanism is alveolar hypoxia potentiated by respiratory acidosis. These abnormal alveolar and arterial blood gases play the same role in eliciting pulmonary hypertension in patients with alveolar hypoventilation as in those in whom the abnormal alveolar and blood gases are the result of ventilation/perfusion abnormalities. For the patient with alveolar hypoventilation with combined respiratory and cardiac (right ventricular) failure, the highest therapeutic priority is to improve oxygenation. Assisted ventilation, particularly during sleep, may be particularly helpful in improving oxygenation and reducing hypercapnic (eg, continuous positive airway pressure [CPAP]) breathing.

# IDIOPATHIC PULMONARY ARTERIAL HYPERTENSION

## ■ DEFINITION

Idiopathic pulmonary arterial hypertension (IPAH), a disorder intrinsic to the pulmonary vascular bed, is characterized by sustained elevations in pulmonary artery pressure and vascular resistance that generally lead to right ventricular failure and death. The diagnosis of IPAH requires the exclusion on clinical grounds of other conditions that can result in pulmonary artery hypertension. PPH is a rare disease, with an incidence of 1 to 2 per million. Its prevalence is about 0.1% to 0.2% of all patients who come to autopsy.

The clinical diagnosis of IPAH rests on 3 different types of evidence: (1) clinical, radiographic, and electrocardiographic manifestations of PH; (2) hemodynamic features, consisting of abnormally high pulmonary arterial pressures and pulmonary vascular resistance in association with normal left-sided filling pressures

**TABLE 29-1.** Nomenclature and Classification of Pulmonary Hypertension

**Diagnostic Classification**

1. Pulmonary arterial hypertension
   1.1 Idiopathic familial
   1.2 Related to
      (a) Connective tissue disease
      (b) Congenital systemic to pulmonary shunts
      (c) Portal hypertension
      (d) HIV infection
      (e) Drugs/toxins
         (1) Anorexigens
         (2) Other
      (f) Persistent pulmonary hypertension of the newborn
      (g) Other
2. Pulmonary venous hypertension
   2.1 Left-side atrial or ventricular heart disease
   2.2 Left-side valvular heart disease
   2.3 Extrinsic compression of central pulmonary veins
      (a) Fibrosing mediastinitis
      (b) Adenopathy/tumors
   2.4 Pulmonary venoocclusive disease/pulmonary capillary hemangiomatosis
   2.5 Other
3. Pulmonary hypertension associated with disorders of the respiratory system and/or hypoxemia
   3.1 Chronic obstructive pulmonary disease
   3.2 Interstitial lung disease
   3.3 Sleep-disordered breathing
   3.4 Alveolar hypoventilatory disorders
   3.5 Chronic exposure to high altitude
   3.6 Neonatal lung disease
   3.7 Alveolar-capillary dysplasia
   3.8 Other
4. Pulmonary hypertension caused by chronic thrombotic and/or embolic disease
   4.1 Thromboembolic obstruction of proximal pulmonary arteries
   4.2 Obstruction of distal pulmonary arteries
      (a) Pulmonary embolism (thrombus, tumor, ova and/or parasites, foreign material)
      (b) In situ thrombosis
      (c) Sickle-cell disease
5. Pulmonary hypertension as a consequence of disorders directly affecting the pulmonary vasculature
   5.1 Inflammatory
      (a) Schistosomiasis
      (b) Sarcoidosis
      (c) Other

and a normal or low cardiac output; and (3) exclusion of the causes of secondary PH. (**Table 29-1**).

# ■ SPECIAL TYPES

Certain associations of IPAH have attracted interest because of their prospects for shedding light on some etiologies. These include so-called anorexigen-induced pulmonary hypertension, familial pulmonary hypertension, human immunodeficiency virus (HIV)–associated pulmonary hypertension, and portal-pulmonary hypertension. In each of these, the clinical findings and the histologic appearance of the lungs at autopsy are identical to those that characterize the sporadic form of IPAH. This diversity in associations underscores the likelihood that so-called IPAH is the final common expression of heterogeneous etiologies.

As a rule, median survival of untreated patients can be predicted on the basis of the New York Heart Association functional classification: 6 months for class IV; 21/2 years for class III; and 6 years for classes I and II. Unless interrupted by sudden death, which occurs in approximately 15% of patients, the usual downhill course terminates in intractable right ventricular failure.

The combination of right-sided heart catheterization and vasodilator testing is particularly useful, not only for defining the hemodynamic state of the patient but also to provide a hemodynamic baseline for future invasive and noninvasive studies, such as serial echocardiograms.

## ■ TREATMENT

A patient with IPAH has several therapeutic options, ranging from oral calcium-channel blockers to continuous infusion of prostacyclin to lung transplantation.

In experienced centers, the trial of nifedipine or diltiazem orally is preceded by testing for acute vasoreactivity using 1 or more of 3 agents: (1) inhaled nitric oxide (NO), in concentrations of 10 to 40 ppm for 5 to 10 minutes; (2) prostacyclin ($PGI_2$; epoprostenol, Flolan), administered intravenously in increasing doses—a starting dose of 1 to 2 ng/kg/min followed by successive increments every 15 minutes of 2 ng/kg/min until a maximal dose of 12 ng/kg/min is reached or side effects preclude further increases; and (3) adenosine, 50 to 200 ng/kg/min. Only patients who manifest significant reductions in pulmonary vascular resistance (usually to a value <5-6 U), resulting from a fall in pulmonary artery pressure without systemic hypotension and accompanied by an unchanged or increased cardiac output, are considered candidates for chronic therapy with oral calcium-channel blockers.

Intravenous epoprostenol (Flolan, prostacyclin, $PGI_2$), a metabolite of arachidonic acid, and its analogues continue to be a major focus of attention as treatments for a variety of forms of pulmonary hypertension. Success in long-term management has been reported using aerosolized iloprost and subcutaneous treprostinil, stable prostacyclin analogues. The dual endothelin receptor antagonist bosentan and the selective endothelin-A receptor analogues sitaxsentan and ambrisentan have also been demonstrated to improve exercise tolerance and delay the time to clinical deterioration. Sildenafil, a phosphodiesterase-5 inhibitor used to treat male erectile dysfunction, also improves pulmonary hemodynamics and exercise capacity in pulmonary arterial hypertension.

The use of anticoagulants has been incorporated into the therapeutic regimen in patients with IPAH. The usual goal of anticoagulation is to achieve and maintain an international normalized ratio (INR) of 2 to 2.5.

## ATRIAL SEPTOSTOMY

Blade-balloon atrial septostomy has been performed in patients with severe right ventricular pressure and volume overload refractory to maximal medical therapy. The goal of this approach is to decompress the overloaded right heart and improve the systemic output of the underfilled left ventricle. Improvements in exercise function and signs of severe right heart dysfunction, such as syncope and ascites, have been observed. Since the creation of an interatrial communication results in an increased venous admixture, worsening hypoxemia is an expected outcome. The size of the septostomy that is created should be carefully monitored in order to achieve the ideal balance of optimizing systemic oxygen transport and reducing right heart filling pressures without overfilling a noncompliant left ventricle or producing extreme degrees of venous admixture.

# LUNG TRANSPLANTATION

Fewer than 20% of patients with IPAH are responsive to long-term oral vasodilator therapy. Of the remainder, approximately 65% to 75% maintain sustained clinical improvement with long-term oral therapies or continuous intravenous prostanoid therapy. When pulmonary hypertensive disease has progressed or threatens to progress to the stage of right ventricular failure, the physician and patient are left with few therapeutic options other than lung transplantation. Lung transplantation is performed at specialized centers and is almost invariably handicapped by shortage of donor lungs, which can lead to long delays. Double-lung transplantation has largely replaced heart-lung transplantation as the procedure of choice for pulmonary arterial hypertension. Rejection phenomena, notably bronchiolitis obliterans, are the major limiting factor to prolonged survival. The median survival after lung transplantation is approximately 3 to 5 years. Recurrence of IPAH after transplantation has not been reported.

# SUGGESTED READINGS

Barst RJ, Rubin LJ. Pulmonary hypertension. In: Fuster V, Walsh RA, Harrington RA, et al, eds. *Hurst's The Heart.* 13th ed. New York, NY: McGraw-Hill; 2011;71:1609-1633.

Badesch DB, Abman SH, Simonneau G, et al. Medical therapy for pulmonary arterial hypertension: updated ACCP evidence-based clinical practice guidelines. *Chest.* 2007;131:1917-1928.

Chin K, Rubin LJ. Pulmonary arterial hypertension. *J Am Coll Cardiol.* 2008;51(16):1527-1538.

Fedullo PF. Pulmonary embolism. In: Fuster V, Walsh RA, Harrington RA, et al, eds. *Hurst's The Heart.* 13th ed. New York, NY: McGraw-Hill; 2011;72:1634-1654.

Rubin LJ, Badesch DB. Evaluation and management of the patient with pulmonary arterial hypertension. *Ann Intern Med.* 2005;143:282-292.

# CHAPTER 30
# PULMONARY EMBOLISM

## Peter F. Fedullo

Despite advances in diagnostic technology, therapeutic approaches, and preventive strategies, pulmonary embolism (PE) remains directly responsible for approximately 100 000 deaths annually in the United States while contributing to an additional 100 000 deaths in patients with concomitant disease. Autopsy studies have repeatedly documented the high frequency with which PE has gone unsuspected and undetected, while clinical studies have established that prophylaxis is underutilized and that death from embolism is unusual once the diagnosis has been confirmed and effective therapy initiated, except in patients who initially present with hemodynamic compromise.

## DEEP VENOUS THROMBOSIS: RISK FACTORS AND PATHOGENESIS

Because PE arises from venous thrombosis, the 2 conditions are considered a continuum of the same condition, venous thromboembolism (VTE). Virchow proposed that the pathogenesis of venous thrombosis was based on several potential initiating events, including stasis, venous injury, and hypercoagulability. Risk factors for venous thrombosis—which may be acquired or inherited—are based on these processes (**Table 30-1**). Frequently more than 1 risk factor is present. Antecedent pulmonary thromboembolism forecasts an appreciable risk of recurrence in the hospitalized patient. Surgery, trauma, immobility, cancer, anticardiolipin antibodies or a lupus anticoagulant, and pregnancy and the postpartum period are important acquired risks. In addition, several hereditary risk factors have been identified over recent years. These include deficiencies in antithrombin III, protein C, and protein S; the factor V Leiden and the prothrombin gene (G20210A) mutations; hyperhomocysteinemia; and elevated levels of coagulation factors VIII, IX, and XI. The identification of these inherited risk factors has proved useful in providing insight into the etiologic basis for thromboembolism in many patients with idiopathic disease. However, most patients who develop venous thromboembolism do so as the consequence of some clinical predisposition. Even in those with an identified thrombophilic predisposition, interaction with a defined clinical state may be necessary to shift the normal hemostatic balance toward thrombosis.

## ACUTE PULMONARY EMBOLISM: PATHOPHYSIOLOGY

The clinical manifestations of pulmonary embolism are related to the size of the emboli and degree of occlusion of the pulmonary vasculature. Secondary neurohumoral responses may also contribute to the pathophysiologic consequences and may explain why similar degrees of vascular obstruction may result in different clinical

**TABLE 30-1.** Risk Factors for Venous Thromboembolism

**Acquired Factors**
Age >40 y
Prior history of venous thromboembolism
Prior major surgical procedure
Trauma
Hip fracture
Immobilization/paralysis
Venous stasis
Varicose veins
Congestive heart failure
Myocardial infarction
Obesity
Pregnancy/postpartum period
Oral contraceptive therapy
Cerebrovascular accident
Malignancy
Severe thrombocythemia
Paroxysmal nocturnal hemoglobinuria
Antiphospholipid antibody syndrome
   (including lupus anticoagulant)

**Inherited Factors**
Antithrombin III deficiency
Factor V Leiden (activated protein C resistance)
Prothrombin gene (G20210A) defect
Protein C deficiency
Protein S deficiency
Dysfibrinogenemia
Disorders of plasminogen

outcomes. The underlying cardiopulmonary status of the patient may have a significant impact on the physiologic response to the event.

# ■ GAS EXCHANGE ABNORMALITIES

Hypoxemia develops in the preponderance of patients with PE and has been
attributed to various mechanisms. When no previous cardiopulmonary disease is
present, a decrease in the mixed venous oxygen content related to a decrease in
cardiac output, redistribution of pulmonary blood flow to lung regions with low
ventilation/perfusion ratios, and shunting due to perfusion of atelectatic areas appear
to be the predominant mechanisms of hypoxemia.

# ■ HEMODYNAMIC ALTERATIONS

The hemodynamic sequelae of the embolic event depend on the extent of obstruction
of the pulmonary vascular bed, the presence or absence of underlying cardiovascular disease, and the effects of endothelial and platelet-derived mediators on the
pulmonary vascular bed. When no underlying cardiopulmonary disease is present,
occlusion of 25% to 30% of the vascular bed by emboli is associated with a rise in
pulmonary artery pressure. Greater than 40% to 50% obstruction of the pulmonary
arterial bed is generally present before there is substantial elevation of the mean

pulmonary artery pressure (PAP), which is associated with a rise in right atrial pressure and a decline in cardiac output. When the extent of embolic occlusion approaches 75%, a previously normal right ventricle becomes incapable of compensating for the increased afterload and subsequently dilates and fails. The maximal *mean* PAP capable of being generated by a previously normal right ventricle is in the range of 40 mm Hg. A mean PAP in excess of 40 mm Hg in the setting of acute embolism strongly suggests an element of chronic cardiopulmonary disease.

# DIAGNOSIS OF DEEP VENOUS THROMBOSIS AND PULMONARY EMBOLISM

Most clinically significant pulmonary emboli arise from venous thrombosis of the proximal deep veins (including and proximal to the popliteal veins) of the legs, although upper extremity, abdominal, and pelvic vein thrombi may also result in embolism. Patients with venous thromboembolism may present with symptoms of venous thrombosis, pulmonary embolism, or both.

## ■ HISTORY AND PHYSICAL EXAMINATION

The clinical diagnosis of both venous thrombosis and pulmonary embolism, based on the history and physical examination, is insensitive and nonspecific. Patients with lower extremity venous thrombosis may be asymptomatic or may have erythema, warmth, pain, swelling, and/or tenderness. These findings, however, while not specific for deep venous thrombosis, suggest the need for further evaluation. The differential diagnosis of venous thrombosis includes cellulitis, edema from other causes, musculoskeletal pain, or trauma (some of these may be concomitant and may or may not be related). The clinical presentation of pulmonary embolism ranges from asymptomatic incidentally discovered events to those that are massive, resulting in cardiogenic shock and death. Dyspnea and pleuritic chest pain are common in embolism, and pulmonary embolism must always be considered when these symptoms are present. Hemoptysis occurs much less frequently. Anxiety, light-headedness, and syncope may also occur but may result from a number of other entities that cause hypoxemia or hypotension. Tachypnea, rales, and tachycardia are the most common signs of PE. Syncope or sudden hypotension should suggest the possibility of massive embolism. With the exception of massive PE, in which the physical examination may disclose findings consistent with right ventricular failure (see Chapter 1), the physical examination findings are nonspecific. The differential diagnosis of embolism includes viral or bacterial pleuritis, pneumonia, pneumothorax, costochondritis, pericarditis, asthma, or an exacerbation of preexisting chronic obstructive pulmonary disease or congestive heart failure. A high clinical suspicion of the possibility of the disease, therefore, must be an integral part of the diagnostic pathway. Diagnostic efforts aimed at possible venous thromboembolism should always be considered if risk factors and the clinical setting are suggestive.

## ■ LABORATORY TESTING FOR ACUTE DEEP VENOUS THROMBOSIS AND PULMONARY EMBOLISM

Routine laboratory testing is not useful in proving the presence of venous thrombosis or pulmonary embolism, but may be helpful in confirming or excluding other diagnoses. Hypoxemia is common in acute PE, although the diagnosis of acute PE *cannot* be excluded based on a normal $Pao_2$. Some individuals, particularly young patients without underlying lung disease, may have a normal $Pao_2$ and even a normal alveolar–arterial $O_2$ gradient.

Electrocardiography (ECG) cannot be relied on to confirm or exclude the possibility of embolism, although electrocardiographic evidence of a clear alternative diagnosis, such as myocardial infarction or pericarditis, is useful when PE is among the possible diagnoses. ECG findings in acute PE are generally nonspecific and include T-wave changes, ST-segment abnormalities, and left or right axis deviation. The S1Q3T3 pattern, while commonly considered specific for PE, is seen in only a minority of patients.

The utility of plasma measurements of circulating D-dimer, a specific derivative of cross-linked fibrin, as a diagnostic aid in venous thromboembolism has been extensively evaluated. D-Dimer testing has proven to be highly sensitive but not specific; that is, elevated levels are present in nearly all patients with venous thrombosis and pulmonary embolism but also occur in a wide range of circumstances, including advancing age, pregnancy, trauma, the postoperative period, inflammatory states, and malignancy. The role of D-dimer testing, therefore, is limited to one of thrombotic exclusion. D-Dimer testing has been utilized successfully as part of a number of different diagnostic strategies, and negative results of standardized, highly sensitive enzyme-linked immunosorbent assays (ELISA) have proved to be capable of safely excluding venous thromboembolism in outpatients presenting with a low or intermediate clinical likelihood of disease. It must be emphasized that commercially available D-dimer assays vary in terms of their sensitivity, negative likelihood ratio, and variability, and that the value of D-dimer testing is enhanced when it is incorporated into a comprehensive diagnostic pathway.

# ■ CHEST RADIOGRAPHY IN SUSPECTED PULMONARY EMBOLISM

Most patients with PE have abnormal but nonspecific chest radiographic findings that are incapable of conclusively diagnosing or excluding PE. The main use of the chest radiograph in suspected embolism is to exclude diagnostic possibilities that may simulate the disease. Common radiographic findings include atelectasis, pleural effusion, pulmonary infiltrates, and mild elevation of a hemidiaphragm. Classic findings of pulmonary infarction—such as "Hampton hump" (pleural-based wedge-shaped density) or decreased vascularity (Westermark sign)—are suggestive but infrequent. A normal chest radiograph in a patient with otherwise unexplained acute dyspnea or hypoxemia is strongly suggestive of embolism.

# ■ OTHER IMAGING STUDIES FOR SUSPECTED ACUTE PULMONARY EMBOLISM

Until recently, ventilation-perfusion scanning has been the pivotal diagnostic test performed when PE is suspected. Normal and high-probability scans are considered diagnostic. A normal perfusion scan rules out the diagnosis of PE with a high enough degree of certainty that further diagnostic evaluation is unnecessary. Matching areas of decreased ventilation and perfusion in the presence of a normal chest radiograph generally represent a process other than PE. However, scans characterized as low- or intermediate-probability (nondiagnostic) scans are commonly found with PE; in such situations, further evaluation depending on the clinical circumstance may be appropriate. In the Prospective Investigation Overview of Pulmonary Embolism Diagnosis (PIOPED) study, for example, embolism was confirmed in 40% of those with low-probability scans when the clinical suspicion of the disease was considered high. The diagnosis of PE should be rigorously pursued even when the lung scan is of low or intermediate probability if the clinical scenario suggests PE. Therefore, while the scan may sometimes be diagnostic of PE or may exclude the possibility with sufficient certainty, it is often nondiagnostic.

Computed tomography has represented a major advance in the diagnosis of PE by providing the capability to directly visualize emboli as well as to detect parenchymal abnormalities that may support the diagnosis of embolism or provide an alternative basis for the patient's complaints. A wide range of sensitivities and specificities for helical CT scanning for embolism diagnosis has been reported. Factors responsible for this wide divergence relate to the proximal extent of vascular obstruction that can be detected and to rapid advances in CT technology that outpace the medical literature. The absence of detectable filling defects reduces the likelihood of embolism, but appears incapable of excluding the possibility with the same degree of certainty as a negative ventilation-perfusion scan.

In the recently published Prospective Investigation of Pulmonary Embolism Diagnosis II (PIOPED II) trial, the sensitivity of CTA alone was 83%. When coupled with simultaneous CT venography, the sensitivity increased to 90%. The positive predictive value of CTA is dependent on the proximal location of the thrombus and the pretest likelihood of the disease. Positive predictive values for CTA in PIOPED II were 97% for emboli in the main or lobar arteries, 68% for segmental vessels, and 25% for subsegmental involvement. In patients with a high or intermediate probability of disease and a positive CTA or CT venogram, the positive predictive value was in excess of 98%. Alternatively, in patients with a low clinical probability of disease and a positive CT angiogram or venogram, the positive predictive value fell to 57%.

Conventional pulmonary angiography remains the accepted "gold standard" for PE diagnosis, although it has a number of limitations as a gold standard. It requires expertise in study performance and interpretation, is invasive, and has associated risks, although published studies would suggest that the use of modern techniques and contrast materials has reduced the reality of those risks well below the lingering perception. Angiography is reserved for the small subset of patients in whom the diagnosis of embolism cannot be established or excluded by less invasive means. Even in this defined set of circumstances, angiography appears to be underutilized.

Echocardiography is not generally useful for proving the presence of PE, although it may offer compelling clues to its presence in certain clinical settings and has been suggested as a potential means by which to determine the need for thrombolytic therapy. Studies of patients with documented PE have revealed that more than 50% have imaging or Doppler abnormalities of right ventricular size or function that may suggest acute PE. Unfortunately, because patients with PE often have underlying cardiopulmonary disease, neither right ventricular dilation nor hypokinesis can be reliably used as even indirect evidence of PE in such settings.

Because the majority of pulmonary emboli arise from the deep veins of the lower extremities, the detection of lower extremity, proximal-vein thrombosis in a patient suspected of embolism, although not confirming that embolism has occurred, is strongly suggestive of that diagnosis and has an equivalent therapeutic implication. Ultrasonography has been reported to be positive in approximately 10% to 20% of patients with suspected embolism and in 50% of patients with proven embolism. A negative ultrasound finding, therefore, cannot exclude the diagnosis.

## ■ IMAGING STUDIES FOR SUSPECTED DEEP VENOUS THROMBOSIS

Doppler ultrasonography is a portable and accurate diagnostic technique for proximal lower extremity venous thrombosis. Its sensitivity and specificity for symptomatic, proximal venous thrombosis have been well above 90% in most recent clinical trials. Limitations include a lack of sensitivity for asymptomatic disease, operator dependence, the inability to accurately distinguish acute from chronic thrombi in symptomatic patients, and a decreased sensitivity for calf vein thrombosis. Compared to other technology, it is portable, noninvasive, and relatively inexpensive, and it has become the most commonly utilized initial diagnostic modality for suspected lower extremity deep venous thrombosis.

CT venography as an adjunct to helical CT scanning has been investigated, and preliminary results suggest that it is capable of detecting femoropopliteal thrombosis with the same accuracy as duplex ultrasonography, while also detecting pelvic and abdominal thrombosis.

While contrast venography remains the diagnostic "gold standard," it has been less commonly performed since the advent of Doppler ultrasonography. Venography should be performed whenever noninvasive testing is nondiagnostic or impossible to perform.

## ■ CLINICAL PREDICTION RULES

A major advance in the diagnostic approach to venous thrombosis and PE has been the derivation and validation of clinical prediction rules that are capable of stratifying patients into probability categories. By combining this derived clinical probability with the results of 1 or more noninvasive diagnostic techniques, diagnostic accuracy in terms of both the confirmation and the exclusion of venous thromboembolism can be increased well beyond that achieved by the use of either clinical probability or the noninvasive diagnostic techniques alone, and the number of patients who require invasive diagnostic testing can be substantially limited. Standardized prediction rules vary in their complexity and have not been demonstrated to be superior to empiric assessment, but can help avoid variance among practitioners with different levels of experience and training.

## ■ DIAGNOSTIC APPROACH

The recommended diagnostic pathway for outpatients with a low or intermediate probability of pulmonary embolism is to first perform a highly sensitive D-dimer assay. A negative result is capable of excluding the diagnosis of embolism in these probability categories. Lower extremity evaluation in those with an intermediate probability of disease is recommended and is a prudent and low-cost option. For those with a positive D-dimer result, CTA coupled with either CT venography or a lower extremity ultrasound is recommended. Outcome studies have demonstrated that withholding anticoagulant therapy in patients with a negative CT scan coupled with a negative lower extremity ultrasound study is a safe strategy except in those patients who present with a high clinical likelihood of embolism.

In patients with a high clinical probability of embolism, D-dimer testing is not recommended given that a negative result would not exclude the need for additional evaluation. CTA coupled with either CT venography or a lower extremity ultrasound is recommended. Negative studies will exclude embolism in the large majority of patients. It is prudent to consider additional imaging (conventional pulmonary angiography, ventilation/perfusion scanning) in cases of high clinical suspicion even if CTA is negative, especially when there is coexisting cardiopulmonary disease in which recurrent embolism would be poorly tolerated.

# PRINCIPLES OF MANAGEMENT

## ■ PROPHYLAXIS OF DEEP VENOUS THROMBOSIS

A significant reduction in the incidence of deep venous thrombosis (DVT) can be achieved when patients at risk receive appropriate prophylaxis. Such preventive measures appear to be grossly underutilized. Unfractionated heparin (UFH), low-molecular-weight heparin (LMWH), fondaparinux (a synthetic, specific anti-Xa inhibitor), warfarin, and mechanical means of prophylaxis have proven effective in various clinical settings. Surgical and medical patients can be stratified according to their risk of thrombosis, with the intensity of the prophylactic intervention being appropriate to the risk of thrombosis. The American College of Chest Physicians has published guidelines for antithrombotic therapy that offer evidence-based recommendations for the prevention and therapy of venous thromboembolism (VTE). These guidelines offer specific preventive recommendations for general, orthopedic, trauma, stroke, spinal cord injury, and medical patients.

## ■ TREATMENT OF ESTABLISHED VENOUS THROMBOEMBOLISM WITH HEPARIN AND LOW-MOLECULAR-WEIGHT HEPARIN

Anticoagulation has been proven to reduce thromboembolic recurrence and therefore mortality in acute PE. When VTE is diagnosed or strongly suspected, anticoagulation therapy should be instituted promptly unless contraindications exist. Confirmatory testing should always be planned if anticoagulation is to be continued. Heparin and LMWH exert a prompt antithrombotic effect, preventing thrombus growth. While thrombus growth can be prevented, early recurrence can develop even in the setting of therapeutic anticoagulation. With the institution of continuous intravenous heparin, the activated partial thromboplastin time (aPTT) should be followed at 6-hour intervals until it is consistently in the therapeutic range of 1.5 to 2.0 times control values. Standardized dosing regimens should be utilized, thereby decreasing the risk of subtherapeutic anticoagulation. Although supratherapeutic levels are sometimes achieved initially, bleeding complications do not appear to be increased. One such approach utilizes an intravenous bolus of 5000 U followed by a maintenance dose of 30000 or 40000 U/24 h by continuous infusion, with the lower dose being administered if the patient is considered at high risk for bleeding. Another commonly employed dosing regimen utilizes an initial intravenous bolus of 80 U/kg of heparin followed by a continuous infusion initiated at 18 U/kg/h; this approach has been demonstrated to reach therapeutic thresholds more quickly than regimens utilizing fixed dosing (**Table 30-2**). Most recently, a fixed dose regimen of

**TABLE 30-2.** Weight-Based Nomogram for Heparin Therapy in Acute Venous Thromboembolism

Initial heparin dose = 80-U/kg bolus, then 18 U/kg/h.
Subsequent modifications are shown below.

| aPTT | | Heparin Dose Adjustment |
|------|------|------|
| (s) | (Times Control) | |
| <35 | <1.2 | 80-U/kg bolus, then increase by 4 U/kg/h |
| 35-45 | 1.2-1.5 | 40-U/kg bolus, then increase by 2 U/kg/h |
| 46-70 | 1.5-2.3 | No change |
| 71-90 | 2.3-3 | Decrease infusion rate by 2 U/kg/h |
| >90 | >3 | Hold infusion 1 h, then decrease rate by 3 U/kg/h |

Data adapted from American College of Chest Physicians Guidelines. Hyers TM, Agnelli G, Hull RD, et al. Antithrombotic therapy for venous thromboembolic disease. *Chest.* 1998;114:561S-578S; and Raschke RA, Reilly BM, Guidry JR, et al. The weight-based heparin dosing nomogram compared with a "standard care" nomogram. *Ann Intern Med.* 1993;119:874.

**TABLE 30-3.** Potential Advantages of Low-Molecular-Weight Heparins Over Unfractionated Heparin

Comparable or superior efficacy
Comparable or superior safety
Superior bioavailability
Once- or twice-daily dosing
No laboratory monitoring
Less phlebotomy
Subcutaneous administration
Earlier ambulation
Home therapy in certain patient subsets

*subcutaneous* heparin administered as an initial dose of 333 U/kg followed by a 250 U/kg every 12 h was demonstrated to be as effective and safe as LMWH. Warfarin therapy may be initiated as soon as the aPTT is therapeutic, and heparin should be maintained until a therapeutic international normalized ratio (INR) of 2.0 to 3.0 has been overlapped with a therapeutic aPTT for 3 consecutive days.

Although calf-limited thrombi are rarely associated with embolism, approximately 20% may extend proximally. If untreated, calf-limited thrombi should be followed for proximal extension over 10 to 14 days with noninvasive testing.

A number of clinical trials have strongly suggested the efficacy and safety of LMWH for treatment of established acute proximal DVT, using recurrent symptomatic VTE as the primary outcome measure. There are several advantages of these drugs. They have excellent bioavailability and can be administered once or twice daily. No monitoring is required in most patients. Because of the ease of administration of these preparations, home therapy of DVT is becoming frequent. However, many patients may not be candidates for home therapy as a result of hemorrhagic risk, compliance issues, renal insufficiency, significant comorbidity, inadequate cardiopulmonary reserve, or poor likelihood of obtaining adequate outpatient care. Advantages of LMWH preparations are summarized in **Table 30-3**, and dosing guidelines are outlined in **Table 30-4**.

# ■ DURATION OF ANTICOAGULATION

Following a first episode of embolism, patients appear to be at lifelong risk for recurrence regardless of whether the event was idiopathic or related to a well-defined predisposing factor. The risk of recurrence appears to be several-fold higher following discontinuation of anticoagulation in those who have experienced an idiopathic event. Among patients with a low risk of recurrence (first episode, provoked PE), 3 to 6 months of anticoagulation is recommended. For those with a high risk of recurrence (recurrent idiopathic events, ongoing predisposition, active malignancy), longer-term or indefinite anticoagulation is recommended. The optimal duration of anticoagulation among those with an initial unprovoked event remains undefined. In all circumstances, treatment decisions should be based on the estimated benefits versus the risk of bleeding, the inconvenience of treatment, and the potential hemodynamic consequences of a recurrent event.

# ■ COMPLICATIONS OF ANTICOAGULATION

Complications of heparin include bleeding and heparin-induced thrombocytopenia (HIT). The rates of major bleeding in recent trials using heparin by continuous

**TABLE 30-4.** Use of FDA-Approved Low-Molecular-Weight Heparins and Pentasaccharides for Treatment of Deep Venous Thrombosis With or Without Pulmonary Embolism[a]

| Therapeutic Indication | Enoxaparin | Tinzaparin | Fondaparinux |
|---|---|---|---|
| Treatment of acute DVT with or without PE with transition to warfarin[b] | 1 mg/kg SC twice daily, or 1.5 mg/kg SC daily | 175 U/kg SC daily | <50 kg = 5 mg SC daily 50-100 kg = 7.5 mg SC daily >100 kg = 10 mg SC daily |
| Outpatient treatment of acute DVT without PE with transition to warfarin | 1 mg/kg SC twice daily | X | X |
| Treatment of acute PE with transition to warfarin | X | X | <50 kg = 5 mg SC daily 50-100 kg = 7.5 mg SC daily >100 kg = 10 mg SC daily |

DVT, deep venous thrombosis; PE, pulmonary embolism; SC, subcutaneously.

[a]There are inadequate data from randomized trials to treat symptomatic pulmonary embolism in the outpatient setting.

[b]Warfarin is initiated within 24 hours after the LMWH is started. At least 5 days of therapy with LMWH is appropriate; the international normalized ratio (INR) should be 2.0 or greater for 2 consecutive mornings prior to discontinuing the LMWH.

infusion or high-dose subcutaneous injection are less than 5%. When necessary, the effect of heparin can be reversed with protamine, although this intervention may be associated with hypotension or anaphylaxis. Heparin-induced thrombocytopenia (defined alternatively as a platelet count less than $150\,000$ mm$^3$ or a greater than 50% reduction in platelet count) typically develops 5 or more days after the initiation of heparin therapy and occurs in 1% to 5% of patients. Two types of thrombocytopenia are associated with heparin administration: an early-onset (1-5 days), non–immune-mediated reduction in platelet count (type I) and a late-onset (>5 days), immune-mediated thrombocytopenia (type II) that may be associated with venous and arterial thrombosis. Development of type II HIT can occur earlier if there has been prior exposure to heparin. The substitution of LMWHs for unfractionated heparin in this circumstance should *not* be considered because of the potential for cross-reactivity. The direct thrombin inhibitors, argatroban, which undergoes hepatic metabolism and excretion, and lepirudin (hirudin), which is renally cleared, are approved for use in heparin-induced thrombocytopenia.

## ■ VENA CAVA INTERRUPTION

If anticoagulation therapy cannot be administered, inferior vena cava (IVC) filter placement can be undertaken. Established indications for filter placement in the therapy of venous thromboembolism include (1) protection against PE in patients with acute venous thromboembolism in whom conventional anticoagulation is contraindicated (recent surgery, hemorrhagic cerebrovascular accident, active bleeding, heparin-associated thrombocytopenia, etc); (2) protection against PE in patients with acute venous thromboembolism in whom conventional anticoagulation has proven ineffective; and (3) protection of an already compromised pulmonary vascular bed from further thromboembolic risk (massive PE). With the increased ease of percutaneous filter placement and the introduction of retrievable devices, IVC filters have been increasingly utilized for prophylaxis in patients with a high risk of developing venous thrombosis. Prophylactic filter placement has been utilized in patients with traumatic injuries and those undergoing spinal, neurosurgical, and bariatric surgery as an alternative or adjunct to pharmacologic prophylaxis. The evidence that filter placement, whether permanent or temporary, reduces the risk of pulmonary embolism or death in these populations is not conclusive. In general, anticoagulation should be utilized following filter placement if no contraindications exist or as soon as any existing bleeding risk resolves.

## ■ THROMBOLYTIC THERAPY AND ACUTE EMBOLECTOMY

The use of thrombolytic agents in acute PE *remains controversial*. While thrombolytic therapy does appear to accelerate the rate of thrombolysis, there is no convincing evidence to suggest that it decreases mortality, increases the ultimate extent of resolution when measured at 7 days, reduces thromboembolic recurrence rates, improves symptomatic outcome, or decreases the incidence of thromboembolic pulmonary hypertension. The use of thrombolytic therapy in PE should be limited to those circumstances in which an accelerated rate of thrombolysis may be considered lifesaving—that is, in patients with PE who present with hemodynamic compromise, patients who develop hemodynamic compromise during conventional therapy with heparin, and patients with embolism associated with intracavitary right heart thrombi. Specific thrombolytic regimens are listed in **Table 30-5**. The role of thrombolytic therapy in patients with anatomically massive embolism or echocardiographic evidence of right ventricular dysfunction in the absence of systemic hypotension is less well defined. Risk stratification approaches using echocardiography and troponin or brain natriuretic peptide (BNP) levels are currently under investigation and may help resolve this area of controversy. At present, urokinase, streptokinase, and recombinant tissue plasminogen activator (rt-PA) are approved for use in the treatment of PE. The method of delivery of thrombolytic agents has also been investigated. Intrapulmonary arterial delivery of thrombolytic agents appears to offer no advantage over the intravenous route. It is reasonable to consider catheter-directed or systemic thrombolytic therapy in patients with proximal occlusive DVT associated with significant swelling and symptoms when there are no absolute or relative contraindications.

The use of systemic thrombolytic agents is associated with a substantially increased risk of bleeding, including intracranial hemorrhage, which has been reported in 1% to 2% of patients undergoing therapy for pulmonary embolism.

**TABLE 30-5.** Thrombolytic Therapy for Acute Pulmonary Embolism: Approved Regimens

Streptokinase: 250 000 U IV (loading dose over 30 min); then 100 000 U/h for 24 h[a]
Urokinase: 4400 U/kg IV (loading dose over 10 min); then 4400 U/kg/h for 12 h
Tissue-type plasminogen activator: 100 mg IV over 2 h

[a]Streptokinase administered over 24 to 72 hours at this loading dose and rate has also been approved for use in patients with extensive deep venous thrombosis.

Hemorrhagic complications due to thrombolytic therapy can be minimized when venous cut-downs, central venous catheters, and unnecessary arterial punctures are avoided. Patients with severe or refractory bleeding should be transfused with blood, cryoprecipitate, and fresh frozen plasma, and heparin can be reversed with protamine.

Pulmonary embolectomy may be performed in the setting of acute massive PE. While many patients die of PE before surgical embolectomy would be feasible, some deteriorate hours after the initial episode and in the setting of maximal medical therapy, suggesting that surgery may occasionally be appropriate. This approach is especially useful when there are contraindications to thrombolytic therapy. Transvenous embolectomy using a suction-catheter device has been utilized by some but has not achieved widespread acceptance. Catheter-directed thrombolytic therapy has been successfully employed in the setting of acute iliofemoral DVT.

## ■ HEMODYNAMIC MANAGEMENT OF MASSIVE PULMONARY EMBOLISM

Once massive PE associated with hypotension and/or severe hypoxemia is suspected, supportive treatment is immediately initiated. Intravenous saline should be infused rapidly but cautiously, since right ventricular function is often markedly compromised, and excessive preload may further distend the right ventricle and increase right ventricular wall tension, resulting in decreased coronary perfusion and right ventricular ischemia. Dopamine or norepinephrine appear to be the favored choice of vasoactive therapy in massive PE and should be administered if the blood pressure is not rapidly restored. Oxygen therapy is administered to minimize hypoxic pulmonary vasoconstriction, and thrombolytic therapy or pulmonary embolectomy should be considered, as described previously. Intubation and institution of mechanical ventilation are begun as needed to support respiratory failure.

## CHRONIC THROMBOEMBOLISM

See Chapter 29 on pulmonary hypertension.

## OTHER FORMS OF EMBOLISM

Because the blood receives all of the blood flow returned from the venous system, the pulmonary vascular bed serves as a "sieve" for all particulates entering the venous blood and is the first vascular bed to be exposed to any toxic substance injected intravenously. As a result of its strategic position, therefore, the pulmonary vascular bed is exposed to a wide variety of potentially obstructing and injurious agents. Other forms of emboli include fat embolism; air embolism; amniotic fluid embolism; tumor embolism; embolism from heroin (talc), bullets, or shotgun shot, cardiac catheters, or indwelling venous catheters; embolism from bone marrow, parasites, and cardiac vegetations; and bile thromboembolism. The acuity and severity of these entities depend on the specific embolic event and the clinical circumstances.

## SUGGESTED READINGS

Fedullo PF. Pulmonary embolism. In: Fuster V, Walsh RA, Harrington RA, et al, eds. *Hurst's The Heart*. 13th ed. New York, NY: McGraw-Hill; 2011;72:1634-1654.

Büller HR, Agnelli G, Hull RD, et al. Antithrombotic therapy for venous thromboembolic disease: the seventh ACCP conference on antithrombotic and thrombolytic therapy. *Chest*. 2004;126:401S-429S.

Chagnon I, Bounameaux H, Aujesky D, et al. Comparison of two clinical prediction rules and implicit assessment among patients with suspected pulmonary embolism. *Am J Med.* 2002;113:269-275.

Geerts WH, Pineo GF, Heit JA, et al. Prevention of venous thromboembolism: the seventh ACCP conference on antithrombotic and thrombolytic therapy. *Chest.* 2004;126:338S-400S.

Kearon C, Ginsberg JS, Julian JA, et al. Comparion of fixed-dose weight-adjusted unfractionated heparin and low-molecular-weight heparin for acute treatment of venous thromboembolism. *JAMA.* 2006;296:935-942.

Kelly J, Hunt BJ. The utility of pretest probability assessment in patients with clinically suspected venous thromboembolism. *J Thromb Haemost.* 2003;1:1888-1896.

Lutz B, Pieske B, Olschewski M, et al. N-terminal pro-brain natriuretic peptide or troponin testing followed by echocardiography for risk stratification of pulmonary embolism. *Circulation.* 2005;112:1573-1579.

Prandoni P, Noventa F, Ghirarduzzi A, et al. The risk of recurrent venous thromboembolism after discontinuing anticoagulation in patients with acute proximal deep vein thrombosis or pulmonary embolism: a prospective cohort study in 1,626 patients. *Haematologica.* 2007;92:199-205.

Stein PD, Beemath A, Matta F, et al. Clinical characteristics of patients with acute pulmonary embolism: data from PIOPED II. *Am J Med.* 2007;120: 871-879.

Stein PD, Fowler SF, Goodman LR, et al. Multidetector computed tomography for acute pulmonary embolism. *N Engl J Med.* 2006;354:2317-2327.

Stein PD, Woodard PK, Weg JG, et al. Diagnostic pathways in acute pulmonary embolism: recommendations of the PIOPED II investigators. *Am J Med.* 2006;119:1048-1055.

Tapson VF. Acute pulmonary embolism. *N Engl J Med.* 2008;358:1037-1052.

Wood KE. Major pulmonary embolism: review of a pathophysiologic approach to the golden hour of hemodynamically significant pulmonary embolism. *Chest.* 2002;121: 877-905.

# CHAPTER 31
# AORTIC VALVE DISEASE

Rosario V. Freeman and Catherine M. Otto

## AORTIC STENOSIS

### ■ DEFINITIONS, ETIOLOGY, AND PATHOLOGY

Aortic stenosis (AS) is obstruction to outflow of blood flow from the left ventricle (LV) to the aorta. The obstruction may be at the valve, above the valve (supravalvular), or below the valve (membranous or subvalvular).

The most common causes of valvular AS are congenital, rheumatic, and calcific ("degenerative"). Calcific AS occurs in patients 35 years of age or older and results from calcification of a congenital or rheumatic valve or of a normal valve. Rare causes of AS include obstructive infective vegetations, homozygous type II hyperlipoproteinemia, Paget disease of the bone, systemic lupus erythematosus, rheumatoid involvement, ochronosis, and irradiation.

Calcific AS in the older patient is the most common valve lesion requiring valve replacement. Among patients under age 70, a congenital bicuspid valve accounted for one-half of the surgical cases; degenerative changes were the cause in 18%. In contrast, over age 70, degenerative changes accounted for almost one-half of the surgical cases and a congenital bicuspid valve for approximately 25% of the cases.

Although a bicuspid aortic valve (BAV) is a congenital lesion, its clinical importance is largely in adults. The incidence of BAV varies from 0.5% to 1.39%, with a male to female ratio of 3:1. The incidence of familial recurrence of BAV is approximately 9% and is commonly associated with an aortopathy. Inheritance is most likely with an autosomal-dominant inheritance pattern with variable penetrance and screening recommended for first-degree relatives of patients with BAV. Complications associated with BAV include infective endocarditis, aortic stenosis, aortic regurgitation, aneurysm of the aortic root or the ascending thoracic aorta, and ascending aortic dissection. Congenital cardiovascular lesions associated with BAV include patent ductus arteriosus (PDA), coarctation of the aorta, coronary anatomic variants, and abnormalities involving the mitral and aortic valves. Shone complex is a constellation of vascular and valvular obstructions, including aortic stenosis, parachute mitral stenosis, and coarctation.

Supravalvular (eg, William syndrome) and membranous subvalvular AS are usually congenital. Congenital bicuspid valves can produce severe obstruction to LV outflow after the first few years of life. The valvular abnormality produces turbulent flow, traumatizes the leaflets, and eventually leads to fibrosis, rigidity, and calcification. In a congenitally abnormal tricuspid aortic valve, the cusps are of unequal size and have some degree of commissural fusion; the third cusp may be diminutive. Eventually, the abnormal structure leads to changes similar to those seen in a bicuspid valve, and significant LV outflow obstruction often results. In calcific AS, early changes show chronic inflammatory cell infiltrate (macrophages and T lymphocytes), lipid within the lesion and in adjacent fibrosa, and thickening of fibrosa with collagen and elastin. These patients also have a higher incidence of risk factors for coronary atherosclerosis.

Studies have demonstrated histologic and immunohistochemical similarities in the thoracic aorta of patients with BAV and Marfan syndrome. The dimensions of the aortic root are larger in children with BAV than in children with tricuspid

AV further suggesting a primary aortopathy which is progressive over time. The anatomy of the BAV usually includes 1 large cusp (caused by fusion of 2 cusps) and a central raphe that is identifiable in most patients with BAV. The raphe does not contain valve tissue. The calcification process that occurs in BAV is similar in its cellular and molecular mechanisms to the processes involved in calcific AS of tricuspid AV, but is accelerated.

Rheumatic AS results from adhesions and fusion of the commissures and cusps. The leaflets and the valve ring become vascularized, which leads to retraction, stiffening, and calcification. In severe forms of hypercholesterolemia, lipid deposits may occur in the aortic valve, occasionally producing AS.

The LV is concentrically hypertrophied. The hypertrophied cardiac muscle cells are increased in size. There is an increase in connective tissue and a variable amount of fibrous tissue in the interstitium. Myocardial ultrastructural changes may account for the LV systolic dysfunction that occurs late in the disease.

# ■ PATHOPHYSIOLOGY

The aortic valve must be reduced to one-fourth of its natural size before significant changes occur in the circulation. The normal aortic valve is 2.0 to 4.0 $cm^2$. In average-sized individuals, symptoms are unusual if the valve area is >1.0 $cm^2$.

Based on natural history and hemodynamic studies, AS is graded as mild when the aortic valve area (AVA) is >1.5 $cm^2$ (>0.9 $cm^2/m^2$), moderate when the AVA is >1.0 to 1.5 $cm^2$ (>0.6-0.9 $cm^2/m^2$), and severe when the AVA is ≤1.0 $cm^2$ (≤0.6 $cm^2/m^2$). The AVA must be reduced by about 50% of normal before a measurable gradient can be demonstrated in humans.

The outflow obstruction imposes a pressure overload on the LV, which compensates by an increase in wall thickness and mass. The concentric left ventricular hypertrophy (LVH) normalizes systolic wall stress and preserves normal systolic function; however, diastolic function may be abnormal. When LVH alone is inadequate to overcome outflow obstruction, the LV uses preload reserve to maintain systolic function. When the preload reserve is no longer adequate, a decrease in systolic function and LV dilation occurs.

Left atrial contraction is of considerable benefit to these patients. Loss of effective atrial contraction—either due to atrial fibrillation or an inappropriately timed atrial contraction—results in elevation of mean left atrial pressure, reduction in cardiac output, or both. This may precipitate clinical heart failure with pulmonary congestion.

In most patients with AS, cardiac output is in the normal range and initially increases normally with exercise. Later, as the severity of AS increases progressively, the cardiac output remains within the normal range at rest. On exercise, however, it either no longer increases in proportion to the amount of exercise undertaken or does not increase at all.

In severe AS, myocardial oxygen needs are increased because of an increased muscle mass, elevations in LV pressures, and prolongation of the systolic ejection time. Patients may have classic angina pectoris even in the absence of coronary artery disease. Associated obstructive CAD further increases the imbalance between myocardial oxygen needs and supply and also of the coronary flow reserve.

# ■ CLINICAL FINDINGS

## History

Patients with congenital valvular stenosis may give a history of a murmur since childhood or infancy; those with rheumatic stenosis may have a history of rheumatic fever. Most patients with valvular AS, including some with severe valvular AS, are asymptomatic.

The classic triad of symptoms of AS is *angina pectoris, syncope,* and *heart failure.* Sudden cardiac death is said to occur in 5% of patients with AS and is rarely the first manifestation of severe aortic stenosis. Symptoms are unusual unless the AS is severe.

Angina pectoris may be the initial clinical manifestation. Syncope is the result of reduced cerebral perfusion. Syncope occurring on effort is caused by systemic vasodilation in the presence of a fixed or inadequate cardiac output, an arrhythmia, or both. Syncope at rest is usually due to a transient tachyarrhythmia from which the patient recovers spontaneously. Other possible causes of syncope include transient atrial fibrillation or transient AV block.

Dyspnea on exertion, orthopnea, paroxysmal nocturnal dyspnea, and pulmonary edema result from varying degrees of pulmonary venous hypertension.

There is an increased incidence of gastrointestinal arteriovenous malformations (eg, Heyde syndrome and may be associated with abnormalities of von Willebrand anticoagulation factor). As a result, these patients are susceptible to gastrointestinal hemorrhage and anemia. Calcific systemic embolism may occur.

## Physical Findings

There is a spectrum of physical findings in patients with AS, depending on the severity of the stenosis, stroke volume, LV function, and the rigidity and calcification of the valve. The arterial pulse rises slowly, taking longer than normal to reach peak pressure; the peak is reduced (parvus et tardus) (Chapter 1); and the pulse pressure may be narrowed. A systolic thrill may be felt in the carotid arteries. The cardiac impulse is heaving and sustained in character, and there may be a palpable fourth heart sound ($S_4$). An aortic systolic thrill is often present at the base of the heart. In 80% to 90% of adult patients with severe AS, there is an $S_4$ gallop sound, a midsystolic ejection murmur that peaks late in systole, and a single second heart sound ($S_2$) because $A_2$ and $P_2$ are superimposed or $A_2$ is absent or soft. There is often a faint early diastolic murmur of minimal aortic regurgitation. The $S_2$ may be paradoxically split due to late $A_2$. In many patients, the midsystolic ejection murmur is atypical and may be heard only at the apex of the heart (Gallaverdin sign).

A functionally normal BAV may have an ejection sound (systolic ejection click) that may be followed by an early peaking systolic flow murmur. The ejection sound diminishes as the valve cusps become more immobile and stenotic and in the presence of moderate or severe AR. The differential diagnosis of an ejection sound includes a small perimembranous ventricular septal defect with a septal aneurysm, mitral/tricuspid valve prolapse, and mild valvar pulmonary stenosis.

In many patients 60 years of age or older, the clinical features may differ from those typical of younger patients. Systemic hypertension is common, being present in over 20% of the patients, half of whom have moderate or severe systolic and diastolic hypertension. Twenty percent first present in congestive heart failure. The male to female ratio is 2:1. Because of thickening of the arterial wall and its associated lack of distensibility, the arterial pulse rises normally or even rapidly and the pulse pressure is wide.

## Chest X-Ray

The characteristic finding is a normal-sized heart. Some patients have poststenotic dilation of the ascending aorta. Calcium in the aortic valve can be seen on the lateral film but is most easily recognized on 2-dimensional echocardiography. Calcium in the aortic valve is the hallmark of AS in adults 40 to 45 years of age. The presence of calcium, however, does not necessarily mean that the valve is stenotic or that the AS is severe. In patients with heart failure, the cardiac size is increased because of dilation of the LV and left atrium; the lung fields show pulmonary edema and pulmonary venous congestion, and the right ventricle and atrium may be dilated.

## Electrocardiogram

The electrocardiogram (ECG) in severe AS shows LV hypertrophy with or without secondary ST–T-wave changes. Conduction abnormalities are common and range from bundle-branch block to first-degree block; higher grades of block occur but are uncommon. The patients are usually in sinus rhythm. Atrial fibrillation indicates the presence of associated mitral valve disease, coronary artery disease (CAD), or heart failure.

## ■ LABORATORY INVESTIGATIONS

### Echocardiography/Doppler Ultrasound

Echocardiography/Doppler ultrasound is an extremely important and useful noninvasive test. The aortic valve leaflets normally are barely visible in systole, and the normal range of aortic valve opening is 1.6 to 2.6 cm. In the presence of a bicuspid aortic valve, eccentric valve leaflets may be seen. The aortic valve leaflets may appear to be thickened as a result of calcification and/or fibrosis; however, the older patient without valve stenosis may also have thickened cusps. The aortic valve may have a reduced opening, but this also occurs in other conditions in which the cardiac output is low. The LV hypertrophy often results in thickening of both the interventricular septum and the posterior LV wall. The cavity size is normal. When LV systolic function is impaired, the LV and left atrium are dilated and the percentage of dimensional shortening is reduced. When properly applied, Doppler echocardiography is extremely useful for estimating the valve gradient and AVA noninvasively. The calculated mean gradient from continuous-waveform Doppler interrogation correlates reasonably closely with that obtained at cardiac catheterization. The AVA can be calculated from the velocity of the jet across the aortic valve and from the velocity and character of the LV outflow tract. Transesophageal echocardiography/Doppler ultrasound is very useful in defining aortic valve abnormality and in assessing its severity when an adequate examination cannot be obtained with the transthoracic technique.

### Cardiac Catheterization/Angiography

Cardiac catheterization remains the *standard technique* for assessing the severity of AS "accurately." This is done by measuring simultaneous LV and ascending aortic pressures and the cardiac output by either the Fick principle or the indicator dilution technique. The AVA can be calculated. The state of LV systolic pump function can be quantitated by measuring LV end-diastolic and end-systolic volumes and ejection fraction. *It must be recognized that ejection fraction may underestimate myocardiac function in the presence of the increased afterload of severe AS.*

The presence of CAD and its site and severity can be estimated only by selective coronary angiography, which should be performed in all patients 35 years of age or older who are being considered for valve surgery and in those <35 years if they have LV systolic dysfunction, symptoms or signs suggesting CAD, or 2 or more risk factors for premature CAD (excluding gender).

### Other Laboratory Studies

MRI can also be used to assess aortic stenosis and provides excellent information regarding ventricular size and function as well as aortic structure and size.

Exercise testing should be undertaken in patients with severe AS only if there is a specific reason for such studies and there is no associated CAD. However, critical aortic stenosis (eg, AVA <0.6 cm$^2$) is a contraindication to formal stress testing. Ambulatory ECG recordings may be needed in an occasional patient suspected of having an arrhythmia or painless ischemia.

## ◼ NATURAL HISTORY AND PROGNOSIS

Valvular AS is frequently a progressive disease, with the severity increasing over time. The factors that control this progression are unknown. In 1 study, patients with "mild" stenosis (catheterization-proven AVA >1.5 cm$^2$), the rate of progression to severe stenosis was 8% in 10 years and 22% in 20 years. The duration of the asymptomatic period after the development of severe AS is also unknown; some recent data suggest that it may be less than 2 years. In patients aged 63 ± 16 years, the actuarial probability of death or aortic valve surgery was 7 ± 5% at 1 year, 38 ± 8% at 3 years, and 74 ± 10% at 5 years.

Severe disease in adults is lethal, particularly if the patient is symptomatic, with a prognosis that is worse than that for many forms of neoplastic disease. The 3-year mortality is approximately 36% to 52%, the 5-year mortality is about 52% to 80%, and the 10-year mortality is 80% to 90%; the average life expectancy is 2 to 3 years. Almost all patients with heart failure are dead in 1 to 2 years.

## ◼ MEDICAL THERAPY

Antibiotic prophylaxis is no longer formally recommended in aortic stenosis. Patients with mild or moderate stenosis rarely have symptoms or complications. In mild stenosis, the patient should be encouraged to lead a normal life. Those with moderate AS should avoid moderate to severe physical exertion and competitive sports. If atrial fibrillation should occur, it should be reverted rapidly to sinus rhythm. Although the pathogenesis of calcific aortic stenosis and atherosclerosis are related, randomized clinical trials have not demonstrated any benefit of statins to the delay the progression of AS.

Echocardiography should be recommended, and its importance emphasized, for first-degree relatives of the patients to detect BAV and/or ascending aorta dilation. Considering the similarity of pathologic findings in the ascending aorta in BAV and Marfan syndrome, it is reasonable to recommend long-term β-blocker therapy, if there are no contraindications to this use, to patients with a dilated aorta that is not yet in the range of needing surgery (**Table 31-1**).

## ◼ SURGICAL THERAPY

Operation should be advised for the symptomatic patient who has severe AS. In young patients, if the valve is pliable and mobile, simple commissurotomy or valve repair may be feasible; the operative mortality is <1%. Such a procedure will relieve outflow obstruction to a major degree. In these patients, catheter balloon valvuloplasty is the procedure of choice in experienced and skilled centers. Both of these are *palliative procedures* that postpone valve replacement. Catheter balloon valvuloplasty is a *temporary palliative procedure* for high-risk elderly patients with advanced symptoms and for emergency situations.

The natural history of symptomatic patients with severe AS is dismal—a 10-year mortality of 80% to 90%—but the outcome after surgery is good, particularly in patients without any comorbid conditions. Some recommend valve replacement in asymptomatic patients with severe AS if predicted operative mortality is <1%.

The overall operative mortality of valve replacement is generally <5%. In patients without associated CAD, heart failure, or other comorbid factors, it may be 1% to 2% in centers with experienced and skilled staff. Patients with associated CAD should

**TABLE 31-1.** Guidelines for Patients With Bicuspid Aortic Valve (BAV)

| Indication | Class | LOE[a] |
|---|---|---|
| 1. Patients with known BAV should undergo an initial transthoracic echocardiogram to assess diameter of the aortic root and ascending aorta | I | B |
| 2. Cardiac magnetic resonance or cardiac computed tomography is indicated in patients with BAV when morphology of the aortic root or ascending aorta cannot be assessed accurately by echocardiography | I | C |
| 3. Patients with BAV and dilation of the aortic root or ascending aorta (diameter >4 cm) should undergo serial evaluation of aortic root/ascending aorta size and morphology by echocardiography, cardiac magnetic resonance, or CT on a yearly basis | I | C |
| 4. Surgery to repair the aortic root or replace the ascending aorta is indicated in patients with BAV if the diameter of the aortic root or ascending aorta is >5.0 cm or if the rate of increase in diameter is ≥0.5 cm/y | I | C |
| 5. Surgery in patients with bicuspid valves undergoing AVR because of severe AS or AR, repair of the aortic root, or replacement of the ascending aorta is indicated if the diameter of the aortic root or ascending aorta is >4.5 cm | I | C |
| 6. It is reasonable to give β-adrenergic–blocking agents to patients with BAV and dilated aortic roots (diameter >4.0 cm) who are not candidates for surgical correction and who do not have moderate to severe AR | IIa | C |
| 7. Cardiac magnetic resonance or cardiac computed tomography is indicated in patients with bicuspid aortic valves when aortic root dilation is detected by echocardiography to further quantify severity of dilation and involvement of ascending aorta | IIa | B |

[a]LOE, level of evidence.

Data from ACC/AHA 2006 guidelines for the management of patients with valvular heart disease: a report of the American College of Cardiology/American Heart Association Task Force on Practice Guidelines (Writing Committee to revise the 1998 Guidelines for the Management of Patients With Valvular Heart Disease): developed in collaboration with the Society of Cardiovascular Anesthesiologists Endorsed by the Society for Cardiovascular Angiography and Interventions and the Society of Thoracic Surgeons. *J Am Coll Cardiol.* 2006;48(3):e1-e148. Available at: www.acc.org, e24.

have coronary bypass surgery at the same time as valve surgery because it results in a lower operative and late mortality. Patients with severe AS who need coronary bypass surgery should have aortic valve replacement at the same time. In severe AS, valve replacement results in an improvement in survival, even in those with normal preoperative LV function. Aortic valve replacement is not recommended for asymptomatic patients with severe AS to prevent sudden death (**Table 31-2**).

For choice(s) of prosthetic valve, see Chapter 35.

# TRANSCATHETER APPROACHES

Transcatheter aortic valve implantation (TAVI) or replacement (TAVR) was first performed by Alan Cribier in 2002 and was approved in Europe in 2007. Many systems are in development and approval of the Sapien valve (Edwards Lifesciences) is anticipated by 2012. This breakthrough technology uses a collapsible valve that

**TABLE 31-2.** Recommendations for Aortic Valve Replacement in Aortic Stenosis[a]

| Indication | Class | LOE[b] |
|---|---|---|
| 1. Symptomatic patients with severe AS | I | B |
| 2. Patients with severe AS undergoing coronary artery bypass surgery | I | B |
| 3. Patients with severe AS undergoing surgery on the aorta or other heart valves | I | B |
| 4. Severe AS and left ventricular systolic dysfunction | I | C |
| 5. Patients with moderate AS undergoing coronary artery bypass surgery or surgery on the aorta or other heart valves | IIa | B |
| 6. Asymptomatic patients with severe AS and abnormal response to exercise (eg, development of symptoms or hypotension) | IIb | C |
| 7. Adults with severe asymptomatic AS if there is a high likelihood of rapid progression (age, calcification, and CAD) or if surgery might be delayed at the time of symptom onset | IIb | C |
| 8. Patients undergoing CABG who have mild AS when there is evidence, such as moderate-severe valve calcification, that progression may be rapid | IIb | C |
| 9. Asymptomatic patients with extremely severe AS (AVR <0.6 cm$^2$, mean gradient >60 mm Hg, and jet velocity >5.0 m/s) when the patient's expected operative mortality is ≤ 1.0% | IIa | C |
| 10. Prevention of sudden death in asymptomatic patients with none of the findings listed under indication 5 | III | C |

[a]See also Chapter 38.

[b]LOE, level of evidence.

Data from ACC/AHA 2006 guidelines for the management of patients with valvular heart disease: a report of the American College of Cardiology/American Heart Association Task Force on Practice Guidelines (Writing Committee to revise the 1998 Guidelines for the Management of Patients With Valvular Heart Disease): developed in collaboration with the Society of Cardiovascular Anesthesiologists Endorsed by the Society for Cardiovascular Angiography and Interventions and the Society of Thoracic Surgeons. *J Am Coll Cardiol*. 2006; 48(3):e1-e148. Available at: www.acc.org, e24.

can be crimped onto a catheter and delivered via 18-25 French delivery systems following balloon valvuloplasty via the femoral, axillary/subclavian, or even apical approaches (**Fig. 31-1**). Although durability is not yet defined, clinical trials have clearly demonstrated the superiority of TAVI to medical therapy in nonsurgical candidates with symptomatic aortic stenosis and comparable to surgical replacement in high-risk surgical candidates. Complications include vascular injury and bleeding, heart block requiring pacing, aortic insufficiency, ostial coronary occlusion/myocardial infarction, and stroke (1%-10%). Adverse event rates have decreased with successive clinical trials and new designs.

# AORTIC REGURGITATION

## ■ DEFINITION, ETIOLOGY, AND PATHOLOGY

Aortic regurgitation (AR) is a flow of blood in diastole from the aorta into the LV due to incompetence of the aortic valve. The 2 most common causes of acute AR are infective endocarditis and prosthetic valve dysfunction. Other common causes include dissection of the aorta and trauma.

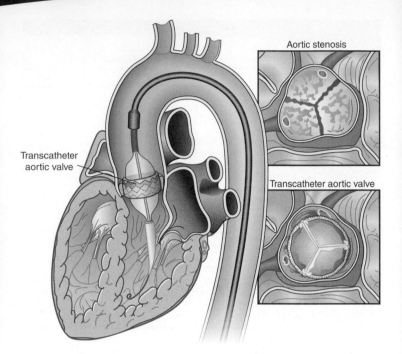

**FIGURE 31-1.** Transcatheter aortic valve replacement. The transcatheter valve is positioned at the level of the native aortic valve during the final step of valve replacement, when the balloon is inflated within the native valve during a brief period of rapid ventricular pacing. The delivery system is shown after it has traversed the aorta retrograde over a guidewire from its point of insertion in the femoral artery (transfemoral placement). Before balloon inflation, the valve and balloon are collapsed on the catheter (dark blue) and fit within the sheath (blue). After balloon inflation, the calcified native valve (upper panel) is replaced by the expanded transcatheter valve (lower panel, shown in short-axis view from the aortic side of the valve). (Reproduced with permission from Smith CR, Leon MB, Mack MJ, eds. Transcatheter versus surgical aortic-valve replacement in high-risk patients. *New Engl J Med.* 2011;364:2187.)

In North America, the most common cause of chronic, isolated severe AR is aortic root/annular dilation that is presumably the result of medial disease. Common causes include a congenital bicuspid valve, previous infective endocarditis, hypertension, and rheumatic disease. Chronic AR also occurs in association with a variety of other diseases, particularly those that result in dilation of the aortic root. Between 40% and 60% of the surgically removed valves from patients with isolated severe AR are classified as idiopathic; half show histologic criteria of myxomatous degeneration.

In AR, volume overload of the LV is the basic hemodynamic abnormality. The extent of overload depends on the volume of the regurgitant blood flow, which is determined by the area of the regurgitant orifice, the diastolic pressure gradient between the aorta and the LV, and the duration of diastole.

# ■ PATHOPHYSIOLOGY

The LV diastolic pressure–volume relationship plays a very important role in the pathophysiology of acute AR. The ability of the LV to dilate acutely is limited; as a result, the volume overload of acute AR produces a rapid increase in LV diastolic pressure. If the LV is already stiff or less compliant than normal due to an associated lesion, the LV diastolic pressure will rise more precipitously as a result of the volume overload of acute AR than if the LV were normal. On the other hand, if the LV is somewhat dilated from a previous lesion—for example, mild AR—the LV pressure will initially rise more gradually with acute AR but may subsequently rise to the same high levels as are seen with a normal or stiff LV. Acute AR that is mild produces little or no hemodynamic abnormality—for example, when associated with systemic hypertension. Increasing severity of AR produces greater degrees of hemodynamic abnormalities, and severe AR often produces the clinical picture of "heart failure."

Acute AR that is severe results in a large volume of regurgitant blood; the increased LV diastolic pressure results in an increase in mean left atrial and pulmonary venous pressures and produces varying degrees of pulmonary edema. Two compensatory mechanisms are utilized: an increase in myocardial contractility and tachycardia to maintain an adequate forward cardiac output.

In chronic AR, the AR becomes severe over a period of time; therefore, the LV diastolic pressure–volume relationships are different from those seen in acute AR. If the AR is mild to moderate, the LV end-diastolic volume is increased moderately, the LV diastolic pressure–volume curve is moved to the right of normal, and the LV diastolic pressure is usually normal. In severe AR, the LV diastolic pressure–volume curves are moved further to the right. If the LV systolic pump function is normal, the LV end-diastolic volume can be quite large without significant elevation of LV end-diastolic pressure. If the LV diastolic volume increases further, however, the LV diastolic pressures will be increased. If LV systolic pump dysfunction supervenes, the LV diastolic pressure–volume curve relationships are moved even further to the right, with quite marked LV dilation and increase in LV diastolic pressure.

In severe chronic AR, the increase in LV end-diastolic volume is a result of the regurgitant volume (and is proportional to the amount of AR) and LV systolic dysfunction. The subsequent large LV stroke volume produces LV systolic hypertension. Both of these increase LV wall stress (afterload), which can result in an impairment of LV function. The heart responds by becoming hypertrophied, and function remains normal. In time, the hemodynamic burden of the volume overload will result in depressed myocardial contractility and decreased LV compliance. Total coronary blood flow is increased, but coronary flow reserve is reduced.

# ■ CLINICAL FEATURES

## History

Patients with mild to moderate AR usually do not have symptoms that can be attributed to the heart. Even patients with severe AR may be asymptomatic for many years. The earliest symptom may be an awareness of the increased force of contraction of the dilated heart, which undergoes a large volume change in systole; patients complain of pounding of the heart or palpitations. The main symptoms of severe AR result from elevated pulmonary venous pressures and include dyspnea on exertion, orthopnea, and paroxysmal nocturnal dyspnea. Heart failure and angina occur in 20% of such patients and may be present even in the absence of CAD.

## Physical Findings

Most of the classic findings are seen in chronic, not acute AR. The arterial pulse is very characteristic and consists of an abrupt distention with a rapid rise and a quick collapse (Corrigan pulse). The arterial pulse may be bisferiens, a double impulse during systole. The systolic arterial pressure is increased, the diastolic pressure is reduced, and Korotkoff sounds persist down to 0 mm Hg. The absence of a wide pulse pressure (>50% of peak systolic pressure) or diastolic pressure greater than 70 mm Hg in a patient without heart failure makes severe, chronic aortic regurgitation unlikely. The LV dilation with severe AR displaces the apical impulse inferiorly and laterally. The AR murmur is a high-pitched, blowing, early-diastolic murmur along the left sternal border. A third heart sound ($S_3$ gallop) and low-pitched diastolic and/ or presystolic murmurs (Austin–Flint) may be heard at the apex.

Acute AR is clinically dominated by a picture of rapid pulmonary edema and shock with a narrow pulse pressure, minimal diastolic murmur, tachycardia, and tachypnea. The physical examination is rarely diagnostic in such a setting, and the diagnosis is often made by echocardiography in the absence of clinical suspicion.

## Chest X-Ray

In chronic AR, there is usually cardiomegaly, the ascending aorta may be dilated, and there is aortic valve calcium. In the later stages, heart failure will be evident.

## Electrocardiogram

The ECG shows LV hypertrophy with or without associated ST–T-wave changes. Conduction abnormalities, such as atrioventricular block or left or right bundle-branch block with or without axis deviation, may be present. The PR interval may be prolonged, particularly in patients with ankylosing spondylitis or endocarditis.

## Echocardiography/Doppler

The echocardiogram can provide information about the etiology of AR as well as LV size and function and the severity of AR. Diastolic fluttering of the anterior leaflet of the mitral valve is often present on M-mode and 2D echocardiography. Echocardiography is of particular value for excluding the presence of associated mitral stenosis in patients with an Austin Flint diastolic murmur. Three-dimensional echocardiography is also useful in defining the nature of aortic regurgitation. A dilated ascending aorta can be detected on echocardiography, as can an enlarged left atrium. Aortic valve vegetations suggest infective endocarditis. Some other conditions can easily be detected by echocardiography—for example, prolapse of the aortic leaflet into the left ventricle in diastole in the presence of a membranous VSD. Doppler ultrasound is useful for diagnosing and assessing the severity of AR and is characterized by a shortened pressure half-time reflecting a rapid equalization of the diastolic aortic pressure and the LV end-diastolic pressure. Transesophageal echocardiography is a useful technique when transthoracic echocardiography is unsatisfactory; it can be used in certain instances for identifying the anatomy of the valve leaflets and the aortic root/annulus, and it is essential for evaluating whether the valve is suitable for repair. It is also very useful for assessing disease of other valves.

## Cardiac Catheterization/Angiography

Cardiac catheterization permits the measurement of intracardiac and intravascular pressures and cardiac output, both at rest and during exercise. In addition, other valvular disease can be excluded. LV angiography demonstrates enlarged LV and allows the calculation of LV volumes and LV ejection fraction. Angiography performed with injection of contrast medium in the ascending aorta demonstrates AR and allows a semiquantitative assessment of the degree of AR. In addition, the angiogram demonstrates the dimensions of the aortic root and the state of the ascending aorta. The indications for selective coronary angiography are the same as for aortic stenosis.

## *Other Laboratory Tests*

A treadmill exercise test provides an objective assessment of the degree of functional impairment and documentation of arrhythmias related to exertion. In some patients, however, the exercise test may remain normal despite deterioration of LV function. Ambulatory ECG recording may be needed in an occasional patient suspected of having an arrhythmia. MRI can demonstrate AR but is rarely needed clinically.

## ■ NATURAL HISTORY AND PROGNOSIS

Patients with mild or moderate AR that does not progress should have normal or near-normal life expectancy. Their major risk is the development of infective endocarditis and further valve destruction.

Patients with severe AR are known to have a long asymptomatic period before the condition is discovered. In asymptomatic patients with normal LV function at rest, symptoms and/or LV dysfunction (and/or sudden death) develop at the rate of about 3% to 6% per year. The predictor of development of symptoms is LV systolic dysfunction and/or an increased LV size (LV dimension at end diastole ≥70 mm and at end systole ≥50 mm). Sudden death in asymptomatic patients appears to occur only in those with a massively dilated left ventricle (LV end-diastolic dimension ≥80 mm).

## ■ MEDICAL THERAPY

Antibiotic prophylaxis is no longer recommended in aortic regurgitation. Patients with mild to moderate AR need no specific therapy, do not need to restrict their activities, and can lead a normal life. Asymptomatic patients with severe AR and normal LV systolic function should be treated if hypertension is present, but there is little evidence that routine use of vasodilators (eg, calcium antagonist or ACE inhibitors) delays symptom onset or the need for surgery.

## ■ SURGICAL THERAPY

Most patients with severe chronic AR will eventually need valve surgery. The correct timing of surgical therapy is now better defined, but it is not fully clarified. Valve replacement should be performed before irreversible LV dysfunction occurs (**Table 31-3**).

Decisions about surgery in AR should be based on the clinical functional class and on the LV ejection fraction. Patients with chronic severe AR who are *symptomatic* (NYHA classes II to IV) need valve replacement. The benefit from valve replacement has been demonstrated even when the LV ejection fraction is 25% or less. Recent data indicate that patients with severe AR, LV end-diastolic dimension on echocardiography ≥80 mm, and mild to moderate reduction in LV ejection fraction can obtain benefit from valve replacement. Postoperatively, they are symptomatically improved, LV ejection fraction increases, and LV size is reduced; the 5- and 10-year survival rates are 87% and 71%, respectively.

Patients who are *asymptomatic* and have a reduced ejection fraction at rest should be offered aortic valve replacement. If the ejection fraction is normal at rest, one should consider valve replacement in NYHA functional class I patients if they have severe obstructive CAD and/or if they need surgery for other valve disease. Patients with associated significant CAD should have coronary bypass surgery performed at the time of valvular surgery.

Aortic valve replacement, with or without associated coronary bypass surgery for obstructive CAD, can be performed at many surgical centers with an operative mortality of 5% or less (see Chapter 35). In patients without associated CAD or reduced

**TABLE 31-3.** Recommendations for Aortic Valve Replacement in Chronic Severe Aortic Regurgitation[a]

| Indication | Class | LOE[b] |
|---|---|---|
| 1. Symptomatic patients with severe AR irrespective of LV systolic function | I | B |
| 2. Asymptomatic patients with chronic severe AR and LV systolic dysfunction (ejection fraction ≤0.50) at rest | I | B |
| 3. Patients with chronic severe AR while undergoing CABG or surgery on the aorta or other heart valves | I | C |
| 4. Asymptomatic patients with severe AR with normal LV systolic function (ejection fraction >0.50) but with severe LV dilation (end-diastolic dimension >75 mm or end-systolic dimension >55 mm) | IIa | B |
| 5. Patients with moderate AR while undergoing surgery on the ascending aorta | IIb | C |
| 6. Patients with moderate AR while undergoing CABG | IIb | C |
| 7. Asymptomatic patients with severe AR and normal LV systolic function at rest (ejection fraction >0.50) when the degree of LV dilation exceeds an end-diastolic dimension of 70 mm or end-systolic dimension of 50 mm, when there is evidence of progressive LV dilation, declining exercise tolerance, or abnormal hemodynamic responses to exercise | IIb | C |
| 8. Asymptomatic patients with mild, moderate, severe AR, and normal LV systolic function at rest (ejection fraction >0.50) when the degree of dilation is not moderate or severe (end-diastolic dimension <70 mm, end-systolic dimension <50 mm) | III | B |

[a]Lower threshold values should be considered for patients of small stature of either gender. Clinical judgment is required.

[b]LOE, level of evidence.

LV systolic function, the operative mortality may be in the range of 1% to 2%. If aortic valve replacement is successful and uncomplicated, LV volume and hypertrophy regress but do not return to normal. Impaired LV systolic pump function improves postoperatively in 50% or more of patients. The 5-year survival of patients with LV ejection fraction ≥45% is 87%, versus 54% in patients with an ejection fraction <45%. Successful valve repair is uncommon and restricted to certain centers and specific patient subgroups.

Mixed valvular lesions, eg, aortic stenosis and regurgitation, should be treated surgically if symptomatic. For the asymptomatic patient, clinical judgment and individualized recommendations for surgery are based on the predominant lesion and its associated hemodynamic consequences.

# SUGGESTED READINGS

Elmariah E, Freeman RV, Otto CM, Miller M. Aortic valve disease. In: Fuster V, Walsh R, Harrignton RA, et al, eds. *Hurst's The Heart.* 13th ed. New York, NY: McGraw-Hill; 2011;76:1692-1720.

Bonow RO, Carabello B, Chatterjee K, et al. ACC/AHA 2006 guidelines on the management of patients with valvular heart disease: a report of the ACC/AHA Task Force on Practice Guidelines 2006. Available at: www.acc.org, e24.

Braverman AC, Guven H, Beardslee MA, et al. The bicuspid aortic valve. *Curr Probl Cardiol.* 2005;30:461-522.

2008 Focused update incorporated into the ACC/AHA 2006 guidelines on the management of patients with valvular heart disease. *Circulation.* 2008;118:e523-e661.

Evangelista A. Long-term vasodilator therapy in patients with severe aortic regurgitation. *N Engl J Med.* 2005;353:1342-1349.

Leon MB, Smith CR, Mack M, et al; PARTNER Trial Investigators. Transcatheter aortic-valve implantation for aortic stenosis in patients who cannot undergo surgery. *N Engl J Med.* 2010;363:1597-1607.

Rossebø AB, Pedersen TR, Boman K, et al; SEAS Investigators. Intensive lipid lowering with simvastatin and ezetimibe in aortic stenosis. *N Engl J Med.* 2008;359:1343-1356.

Smith CR, Leon MB, Mack MJ, et al; PARTNER Trial Investigators. Transcatheter versus surgical aortic-valve replacement in high-risk patients. *N Engl J Med.* 2011;364:2187-2198.

Webb J, Cribier A. Percutaneous transarterial aortic valve implantation. *Eur Heart J.* 2011;32:140-147.

# CHAPTER 32
# MITRAL VALVE STENOSIS

Blasé A. Carabello

## DEFINITION, ETIOLOGY, AND PATHOLOGY

Mitral stenosis (MS), an obstruction to blood flow between the left atrium (LA) and the left ventricle (LV), is caused by previous rheumatic carditis in virtually all adults. About 60% of patients with rheumatic mitral valve disease do not give a history of rheumatic fever or chorea, and about 50% of patients with acute rheumatic carditis do not develop clinical valvular heart disease. Isolated MS occurs in approximately 40% of all patients with rheumatic heart disease. Other infrequent causes of obstruction to LV inflow can be congenital or due to active infective endocarditis, neoplasm, massive annular calcification, systemic lupus erythematosus, carcinoid, methysergide therapy, Hunter-Hurler syndromes, Fabry disease, Whipple disease, rheumatoid arthritis, left atrial myxoma, massive left atrial ball thrombus, and cor triatriatum.

Acute rheumatic carditis is a pancarditis involving the pericardium, myocardium, and endocardium. In temperate climates and developed countries, there is usually a long interval (10-20 years) between an episode of rheumatic carditis and the clinical presentation of symptomatic MS. In tropical and subtropical climates and in less developed countries, the latent period is often shorter, and MS may occur during childhood or adolescence.

## PATHOPHYSIOLOGY

The histopathologic hallmark of rheumatic carditis is an *Aschoff* nodule. Rheumatic valvulitis results in scarring and fusion. The combination of commissural fusion, valve leaflet contracture, and fusion of the chordae tendineae results in a narrow, funnelshaped orifice.

The pathophysiologic features of MS result from obstruction of the flow of blood between the LA and the LV. With reduction in valve area, energy is lost to friction during the transport of blood from the LA to the LV. Accordingly, a pressure gradient is present across the stenotic valve.

The pressure gradient between the LA and the LV increases markedly with increased heart rate or cardiac output (CO); this is responsible for LA hypertension. The LA gradually enlarges and hypertrophies. Pulmonary venous pressure rises with the increase in LA pressure and is passively associated with an increase in pulmonary arterial (PA) pressure. In up to 20% of patients, the pulmonary vascular resistance is also elevated, which further increases PA pressure. PA hypertension results in right ventricular (RV) hypertrophy and RV enlargement. The changes in RV function eventually result in right atrial (RA) hypertension and enlargement and systemic venous congestion; frequently, tricuspid regurgitation also occurs.

Pulmonary venous hypertension alters the distribution of blood flow in the lung, with a relative increase in flow to the upper lobes and therefore in physiologic dead space. Pulmonary compliance generally decreases with increasing pulmonary capillary pressure, increasing the work of breathing, particularly during exercise. Chronic changes in the pulmonary capillaries and pulmonary arteries include fibrosis and thickening. These changes protect the lungs from the transudation of fluid into the alveoli (alveolar pulmonary edema) yet further add to the abnormalities of ventilation and perfusion.

Long-standing MS with severe PA hypertension and resultant RV dysfunction may be accompanied by chronic systemic venous hypertension. Tricuspid regurgitation is frequently present, even in the absence of intrinsic disease of this valve (see Chapter 34).

# CLINICAL MANIFESTATIONS

## ■ HISTORY

An asymptomatic interval is usually present between the initiating event of acute rheumatic fever and the presentation of symptomatic MS. Initially, there is little or no gradient at rest, but with increased cardiac output, LA pressure rises and exertional dyspnea develops. As mitral valve obstruction increases, dyspnea occurs at lower work levels. The progression of disability is so subtle and protracted that patients may adapt by circumscribing their lifestyles. It becomes imperative, therefore, to document what activities the patient can perform without symptoms and at what activity level symptoms begin.

As obstruction progresses, patients note orthopnea and paroxysmal nocturnal dyspnea, apparently resulting from redistribution of blood to the thorax upon assuming the supine position. With severe MS and elevated pulmonary vascular resistance, fatigue rather than dyspnea may be the predominant symptom. Dependent edema, nausea, anorexia, and right-upper-quadrant pain reflect systemic venous congestion resulting from elevated systemic venous pressure and salt and water retention. Symptoms of RV failure (hepatomegaly, edema, and ascites) may predominate in patients with severe pulmonary hypertension.

Palpitations are a frequent complaint in patients with MS and may represent frequent premature atrial contractions or paroxysmal atrial fibrillation/flutter. Fifty percent of patients with severe symptomatic MS have chronic atrial fibrillation.

Systemic embolism, a frequent complication of MS, may result in stroke, occlusion of extremity arterial supply, occlusion of the aortic bifurcation, and visceral or myocardial infarction. Hemoptysis, hoarseness, and exertional chest pain are infrequent manifestations of MS.

Progression of symptoms in MS is generally slow but relentless. Thus, a sudden change in symptoms rarely reflects a change in valve obstruction. Rather, there is usually a noncardiac precipitating event causing tachycardia, which decreases diastolic flow period, or paroxysmal AF in which a loss of atrial transport function occurs.

## ■ PHYSICAL FINDINGS

During the latent, presymptomatic interval, incidental physical findings may be normal or may provide evidence of mild MS. Frequently, the only characteristic finding noted at rest will be a loud $S_1$ and a presystolic murmur. A short diastolic decrescendo rumble may be heard only with exercise. In patients with symptomatic stenosis, the findings are more obvious, and careful physical examination usually leads to the correct diagnosis (see also Chapter 1).

The jugular venous pressure may be normal or may show evidence of elevated RA pressure. A prominent A wave is a result of RV hypertension/hypertrophy or of associated tricuspid stenosis. A prominent V wave is caused by tricuspid regurgitation. Atrial fibrillation produces an irregular venous pulse with absent A waves. The chest findings may be normal or may reveal signs of pulmonary congestion with rales or pleural fluid.

On palpation, the apical impulse should feel normal or be tapping. An abnormal LV impulse suggests disease other than isolated MS. A diastolic thrill is usually appreciated only when the patient is examined in the left lateral decubitus position. When PA hypertension is present, a sustained RV lift along the left sternal border and pulmonic valve closure may be palpable.

Upon auscultation in the supine position, the only abnormality appreciated may be the accentuated $S_1$, which is caused by flexible valve leaflets and the wide closing excursion of the valve leaflets. *Failure to examine the patient in the left lateral decubitus position accounts for most of the missed diagnoses of symptomatic MS.* The diastolic rumble is heard best with the bell of the stethoscope applied at the apical impulse. Nevertheless, the murmur may be localized, and so the region around the apical impulse should also be auscultated. The *opening snap* (OS) occurs when the movement of the domed mitral valve into the LV is suddenly stopped. It is heard best with the diaphragm and is often most easily appreciated midway between the apex and the left sternal border. In this intermediate region, the $S_1$, $P_2$, and OS can be identified.

The OS occurs after the LV pressure falls below the LA pressure in early diastole. When LA pressure is high, as in severe MS, the snap occurs earlier in diastole. The OS may be absent in patients with stiff, fibrotic, or calcified leaflets. Thus, absence of the OS in severe MS suggests that mitral valve replacement rather than commissurotomy may be necessary.

The low-pitched diastolic rumble follows the OS and is best heard with the bell of the stethoscope. In some patients with low cardiac output or mild MS, brief exercise, such as sit-ups or walking, is adequate to increase flow and bring out the murmur. The murmur is low-pitched, rumbling, and decrescendo. In general, the more severe the MS, the longer the murmur. Presystolic accentuation of the murmur occurs in sinus rhythm and has been reported even in atrial fibrillation.

The 2 most important auscultatory signs of severe MS are a short $A_2$–OS interval and a pandiastolic rumble. The diastolic murmur may not be full length in severe MS if the stroke volume is low and there is no tachycardia.

Systolic murmurs also may be heard in association with the murmur of MS. A blowing murmur at the apex suggests associated mitral regurgitation, whereas a systolic blowing murmur heard best at the lower left sternal border that increases with inspiration usually signifies tricuspid regurgitation. The Graham Steell murmur is a high-pitched diastolic decrescendo murmur of pulmonic regurgitation caused by severe PA hypertension. In most patients with MS, such a murmur usually indicates aortic regurgitation.

## Chest Roentgenogram

The posteroanterior and lateral chest films are often so typical that experienced clinicians can make the tentative diagnosis from them (see also Chapter 3). The thoracic cage is normal. The lung fields show evidence of elevated pulmonary venous pressure. Blood flow is more evenly redistributed to the upper lobes, resulting in apparent prominence of upper-lobe vascularity. Increased pulmonary venous pressure results in transudation of fluid into the interstitium. Accumulation of fluid in the interlobular septa produces linear streaks in the bases, which extend to the pleura (Kerley B lines). Interstitial fluid may also be seen as perivascular or peribronchial cuffing (Kerley A lines). With transudation of fluid into the alveolar spaces, alveolar pulmonary edema is seen. These changes represent long-standing elevated

LA pressure. PA hypertension results in enlargement of the main PA and the right and left main pulmonary arteries.

The cardiac silhouette usually does not show generalized cardiomegaly, but the LA is invariably enlarged. In the posteroanterior chest film, LA enlargement is recognized by a density behind the RA border (double atrial shadow), prominence of the LA appendage on the left heart border between the main PA and LV apex, and elevation of the left main bronchus. The lateral film shows the LA bulging posteriorly. Mitral valve calcification is occasionally seen on the plain chest x-ray.

## Electrocardiogram

Patients in sinus rhythm may have a widened P wave caused by interatrial conduction delay and/or prolonged LA depolarization. Classically, the P wave is broad and notched in lead II and biphasic in lead $V_1$; it measures 0.12 seconds or more. AF is common and LV hypertrophy is not present unless there are associated lesions. RV hypertrophy may be present if PA hypertension is marked.

## ■ CLINICAL INDICATIONS OF SEVERE MITRAL STENOSIS

Some clinical features make it virtually certain that MS is severe. These include (1) moderate to severe PA hypertension, as indicated by clinical and ECG evidence of RV hypertrophy, PA hypertension, or both; and/or (2) moderate to severe elevation of LA pressure, as indicated by orthopnea, a short $P_2$–OS interval, a diastolic rumble that occupies the whole length of a long diastolic interval in patients with AF, and pulmonary edema on the chest x-ray. In both of these clinical circumstances, one must be certain that there is no other cause for elevated LA pressure and that LA hypertension is not caused mainly by a correctable transient elevation of LV diastolic pressure.

# LABORATORY TESTS

## ■ ECHOCARDIOGRAPHY/DOPPLER ULTRASOUND

Echocardiography/Doppler ultrasound has proved to be both sensitive and specific for MS when adequate studies are done. The characteristic M-mode echocardiographic features are a decreased EF slope of the anterior mitral leaflet. Two- (2D) and three-dimensional (3D) echocardiography will demonstrate the valve orifice and allow calculation of mitral valve area. Doppler echocardiography will provide estimates of the gradient across the valve and of pulmonary artery pressure.

Transesophageal echocardiography (TEE) is a useful technique to assess LA thrombus, the anatomy of the mitral valve and subvalvular apparatus, and the suitability of the patient for catheter balloon commissurotomy or surgical valve repair.

Echocardiography/Doppler ultrasound is a useful test in MS and should be performed in all patients. It is essential for determining the suitability of the valve for commissurotomy and/or repair and for determining the likely result.

Exercise echocardiography may be useful when there is diagnostic uncertainty when trying to reconcile the severity of symptoms with the degree of MS.

## ■ CARDIAC CATHETERIZATION/ANGIOGRAPHY

In most patients with disabling symptoms from presumed MS, right and left heart catheterization should be performed as part of a preoperative assessment. Simultaneous measurement of cardiac output and the gradient between the LA and the LV and calculation of valve area remain the "gold standard" for assessing the severity of MS. Aortic valve function should be evaluated in all patients. Tricuspid valve function can be assessed when there is a question of coexisting lesions. In certain circumstances, dynamic exercise in the catheterization laboratory with measurement of mitral valve gradient, CO, and LA and PA pressures can be extremely useful. Selective coronary arteriography establishes the site, severity, and extent of coronary artery disease and should be performed in patients with angina, LV dysfunction, and/or risk factors for coronary artery disease and in those 35 years of age or older.

# NATURAL HISTORY AND PROGNOSIS

The population presenting with MS is changing because of the sharp decline in the incidence of acute rheumatic fever in the past 40 years. Native-born American citizens with symptomatic MS are presenting at an older age. Young adults in the third and fourth decades with symptomatic MS are more likely to come from low socioeconomic backgrounds and from the inner city or to be immigrants, particularly from Latin America, the Middle East, Africa, or Asia. The mechanism for the progression from no symptoms to mild to severe symptoms is progressive stenosis of the mitral valve. Approximately 50% of patients develop symptoms gradually. Sudden deterioration is usually the result of AF, systemic embolization, or other conditions that result in tachycardia and/or increased cardiac output.

The 10-year survival rate of patients with MS who are asymptomatic is approximately 84%, and that of those who are mildly symptomatic is 34% to 42%. Patients in NYHA functional class IV have very poor survival without treatment: 42% at 1 year and 10% or less at 5 years. All are dead within 10 years.

# MEDICAL TREATMENT

All streptococcal infections should be diagnosed rapidly and correctly treated. All patients with known previous acute rheumatic fever/rheumatic carditis with or without obvious valve disease should receive appropriate antibiotic prophylaxis against recurrent streptococcal infection (see Chapter 37). Secondary prevention against infective endocarditis is a lifelong requirement. If AF is present, digitalis plays a critical role in controlling ventricular rate. In selected patients, β-adrenergic–blocking agents, diltiazem, or amiodarone may be added if digoxin alone is not satisfactory in controlling ventricular rate at rest or exercise. Diuretics reduce pulmonary congestion and peripheral edema, and allow most patients freedom from severe salt restriction. For the patient with mild symptoms, maintenance of sinus rhythm is desirable. Cardioversion of AF and maintenance of sinus rhythm using antiarrhythmic therapy with either digitalis and quinidine or digitalis and amiodarone should be offered to these patients. In patients who need interventional therapy, cardioversion is usually performed after completion of the procedure. Anticoagulation with warfarin is usually begun about 3 weeks in advance of cardioversion and continued for 4 weeks after the procedure. Alternatively, if left atrial thrombus is excluded by TEE, 2 to 3 days of intravenous heparin should be instituted, the patient cardioverted to sinus rhythm, and warfarin therapy continued for at least 4 weeks. Patients with chronic AF and those with a previous history of embolism should receive anticoagulation with warfarin (international normalized ratio [INR] of 2 to 3) unless there is a specific contraindication. Systemic embolization necessitates permanent anticoagulation. A single systemic embolic episode is not an *absolute* indication for mitral

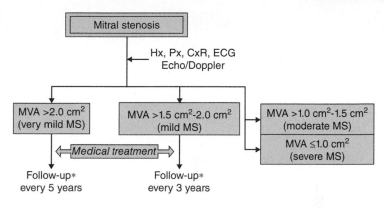

**FIGURE 32-1.** Management of mild mitral stenosis.

valve surgery, as emboli can and do occur in patients with mild mitral stenosis (see **Figs. 32-1** to **32-3**).

# INTERVENTIONAL THERAPY

Unless there is a contraindication, surgery or catheter balloon commissurotomy (CBC) should be recommended to an MS patient with functional class III or IV symptoms. For younger patients with a pliable, noncalcified valve and without

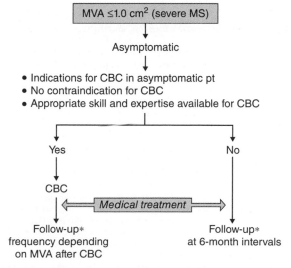

**FIGURE 32-2.** Management of asymptomatic severe mitral stenosis.

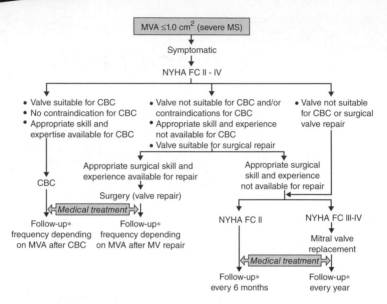

**FIGURE 32-3.** Management of symptomatic severe mitral stenosis.

important mitral regurgitation, this means valve repair or CBC. The hemodynamic results of surgical commissurotomy or CBC are excellent. Because of the low morbidity and mortality of CBC/valve repair, surgery is also offered to patients when functional class II symptoms are present (**Table 32-1**). The results of successful commissurotomy are excellent; in experienced and skilled centers, surgical mortality is less than 1%. Late mortality at 10 years is less than 5%, the thromboembolism rate is 2% per year or less, and the reoperation rate ranges from 0.5% to 4.5% per year.

For the older patient with a stiff or calcified valve, or when moderate mitral regurgitation is present, mitral valve replacement is usually performed. Valve replacement carries a higher operative mortality than does commissurotomy (up to 5%) and the morbidity associated with prostheses. Hemodynamic results of mitral valve replacement are often not ideal (see also Chapter 35). Survival at 10 years after mitral valve replacement for functional class III and IV patients is better than 60% (**Table 32-2**).

Use of the double-balloon technique or the Inoue balloon produces immediate and 3-month hemodynamic and clinical results comparable to those obtained by surgical commissurotomy. The mitral valve area increases from a mean of 1.0 to 2.0 cm². There are reductions in LA and PA pressures at rest and on exercise and an increase of exercise capacity. The immediate results of CBC are greatly influenced by the characteristics of the valve and its supporting apparatus, which are best determined by echocardiography (transthoracic and/or transesophageal) (Table 32-1). Echocardiographic scores ≤8 (MGH) or of 0 to 1 (USC) determined by the 2 different methods provide a clue to the best immediate results. Repeat CBC or mitral valve replacement is needed in 20% of patients within 5 to 7 years. Late survival is poorer in those in whom functional class IV, higher echocardiographic score, higher LV end-diastolic pressure, or higher PA systolic pressure is present prior to the CBC.

**TABLE 32-1.** Indications for Percutaneous Mitral Balloon Valvotomy

| Indication | Class |
|---|---|
| 1. Symptomatic patients (NYHA functional class II, III, or IV), moderate or severe MS and valve morphology favorable for percutaneous balloon valvotomy in the absence of left atrial thrombus or moderate to severe MR | I |
| 2. Asymptomatic patients with moderate or severe MS and valve morphology favorable for percutaneous balloon valvotomy who have pulmonary hypertension (pulmonary artery systolic pressure >50 mm Hg at rest or >60 mm Hg with exercise) in the absence of left atrial thrombus or moderate to severe MR | I |
| 3. Patients with NYHA functional class III to IV symptoms, moderate or severe MS, and a nonpliable calcified valve who are either not candidates for surgery or at high risk for surgery in the absence of left atrial thrombus or moderate to severe MR | IIa |
| 4. Asymptomatic patients, moderate or severe MS, and valve morphology favorable for percutaneous balloon valvotomy who have new onset of atrial fibrillation in the absence of left atrial thrombus or moderate to severe MR | IIb |
| 5. Symptomatic patients (NYHA functional class II, III, or IV) with MV area $\geq 1.5$ cm$^2$ if there is evidence of hemodynamically significant MS based on pulmonary artery systolic pressure >60 mm Hg, pulmonary artery wedge pressure $\geq 25$, or mean MV gradient >15 mm Hg during exercise | IIb |
| 6. Patients in NYHA functional class III to IV with moderate or severe MS and a nonpliable calcified valve as an alternative to surgery | IIb |
| 7. Percutaneous mitral balloon valvotomy is not indicated in patients with mild MS | III |
| 8. Percutaneous mitral balloon valvotomy should not be performed in patients with moderate to severe MR or left atrial thrombus | III |

Data from ACC/AHA 2006 guidelines for the management of patients with valvular heart disease: a report of the American College of Cardiology/American Heart Association Task Force on Practice Guidelines (Writing Committee to revise the 1998 Guidelines for the Management of Patients With Valvular Heart Disease): developed in collaboration with the Society of Cardiovascular Anesthesiologists Endorsed by the Society for Cardiovascular Angiography and Interventions and the Society of Thoracic Surgeons. *J Am Coll Cardiol.* 2006;48:e1-e148.

**TABLE 32-2.** Indications for Surgery for Mitral Stenosis

| Indication | Class |
|---|---|
| 1. Mitral valve surgery (repair if possible) is indicated in patients with symptomatic (NYHA functional class III to IV), moderate to severe MS and valve morphology favorable for repair if (1) percutaneous mitral balloon valvotomy is not available, (2) percutaneous mitral balloon valvotomy is contraindicated because of left atrial thrombus despite anticoagulation or concomitant moderate to severe MR is present, or (3) the valve morphology is not favorable for percutaneous mitral balloon valvotomy in a patient with acceptable operative risk | I |
| 2. Symptomatic patients with moderate to severe MS who also have moderate to severe MR should receive MV replacement, unless valve repair is possible at the time of surgery | I |
| 3. MV replacement is reasonable for patients with severe MS and severe pulmonary hypertension (pulmonary artery systolic pressure >60 to 80 mm Hg) with NYHA functional class I to II symptoms who are not considered candidates for percutaneous mitral balloon valvotomy or surgical MV repair | IIa |
| 4. Asymptomatic patients with moderate or severe MS and valve morphology favorable for repair who have had recurrent episodes of embolic events on adequate anticoagulation | IIb |
| 5. MV repair for MS is not indicated for patients with mild MS | III |
| 6. Closed commissurotomy should not be performed on patients undergoing MV repair; open commissurotomy is the preferred approach | III |

Data from ACC/AHA 2006 guidelines for the management of patients with valvular heart disease: a report of the American College of Cardiology/American Heart Association Task Force on Practice Guidelines (Writing Committee to revise the 1998 Guidelines for the Management of Patients With Valvular Heart Disease): developed in collaboration with the Society of Cardiovascular Anesthesiologists Endorsed by the Society for Cardiovascular Angiography and Interventions and the Society of Thoracic Surgeons. *J Am Coll Cardiol.* 2006; 48:e1-e148.

# SUGGESTED READINGS

Carabello BA. Mitral stenosis. In: Fuster V, Walsh R, Harrington RA, et al, eds. *Hurst's The Heart.* 13th ed. New York, NY: McGraw-Hill; 2011;78:1738-1744.

Bonow RO, Carabello B, Chatterjee K, et al. ACC/AHA guidelines for the management of patients with valvular heart disease: a report of the ACC/AHA taskforce on practice guidelines. *J Am Coll Cardiol.* 2006;48:1-148.

2008 Focused update incorporated into the ACC/AHA 2006 guidelines on the management of patients with valvular heart disease. *Circulation.* 2008;118:e523-e661.

Nishimura RA, Rihal CS, Tajik AJ, et al. Accurate measurement of the transmitral gradient in patients with mitral stenosis: a simultaneous catheterization and Doppler echocardiographic study. *J Am Coll Cardiol.* 1994;2:52-158.

Tuzcu EM, Block PC, Griffin BP, et al. Immediate- and long-term outcome of percutaneous mitral valvotomy in patients 65 years and older. *Circulation.* 1992;85:963-971.

# CHAPTER 33
# MITRAL REGURGITATION

David H. Adams, Blasé A. Carabello, and Javier G. Castillo

## MITRAL REGURGITATION

### ■ DEFINITION, ETIOLOGY, AND PATHOLOGY

Mitral regurgitation (MR) is characterized by an abnormal reversed blood flow from the left ventricle (LV) to the left atrium (LA) due to abnormalities in the mitral apparatus.

Prolapse of the mitral valve leaflets into the left atrium during systole is now the most common cause of primary MR; left ventricular dysfunction is the most common cause of secondary or functional MR. Additional causes include rheumatic carditis, endocarditis, mitral annular calcification, hypertrophic cardiomyopathy, trauma, connective tissue disorders, anorectic agents, and congenital deformities. The competence of the mitral valve depends on the normal structure and function of every part of the mitral apparatus—that is, the leaflets, chordae tendineae, annulus, left atrium, papillary muscles, and LV myocardium surrounding the papillary muscles.

### ■ PATHOPHYSIOLOGY

In MR, the abnormal coaptation of the mitral leaflets creates a *regurgitant orifice* during systole. The systolic pressure gradient between the LV and the LA is the driving force for the regurgitant flow, which results in a *regurgitant volume*. This regurgitant volume represents a percentage of the total ejection of the LV and may be expressed as the *regurgitant fraction*. The regurgitant volume creates a volume overload by entering the LA in systole and the LV in diastole, modifying LV loading and function; it is additive to the systolic output of the right ventricle.

In *acute* MR, the hemodynamic burden is different. The sudden burden of the MR does not allow compensatory dilatation of the LA and LV. Consequently, marked elevations of the LA and pulmonary venous pressures are produced, leading to acute pulmonary edema.

LV dysfunction is a frequent complication of *chronic* MR; its exact mechanism is unknown. The changes in myofiber contractility parallel changes in global LV function and are associated with reduced myofiber content. During diastole, LV relaxation is frequently abnormal, but chamber stiffness is usually reduced. Age and decreased systolic function are associated with increased chamber stiffness.

### ■ CLINICAL MANIFESTATIONS

#### History

Patients with *chronic* MR often are asymptomatic. Even severe MR may be associated with no or minimal symptoms. Fatigue and mild dyspnea on exertion are most common symptoms and are rapidly improved by rest; these progress to orthopnea, paroxysmal nocturnal dyspnea, and peripheral edema.

With severe MR of *acute onset,* symptoms are usually more dramatic—pulmonary edema or congestive heart failure—but may progressively subside with the administration of diuretic and increased LA compliance.

# ■ PHYSICAL FINDINGS

Blood pressure is usually normal. The arterial upstroke is brisk, especially when ejection time is reduced in MR (see also Chapter 1).

On palpation, the cardiac impulse (enlarged LV) is often laterally displaced, diffused, and brief. An apical thrill is characteristic of very severe MR. A left sternal border lift is observed with right ventricular dilatation and may be difficult to distinguish from the LA lift in *later systole* due to the dilated, expansive LA, which is more substernal and lower (see Chapter 1).

The first heart sound is often included in the murmur but may be increased in rheumatic disease. The second heart sound is usually normal but may be paradoxically split if the LV ejection time is markedly shortened. The presence of a third heart sound ($S_3$) is directly related to the volume of the regurgitation. MR is often associated with an early diastolic rumble due to the increased mitral flow in diastole even without mitral stenosis. The $S_3$ and diastolic rumble are low-pitched sounds that may be difficult to detect except in the left lateral decubitus position. An atrial gallop ($S_4$) is heard mainly in MR of recent onset and in ischemic and/or functional MR in sinus rhythm. Midsystolic clicks are markers of mitral valve prolapse and are due to sudden tension of the chordae (discussed later).

The hallmark of MR is the systolic murmur, most often holosystolic, including first and second heart sounds. If an opening snap or $S_3$ is mistakenly interpreted as $S_2$, the murmur may appear midsystolic. The murmur is of a high-pitched and blowing type but may be harsh, especially in mitral valve prolapse syndrome. The maximum intensity is usually at the apex, but it may radiate to the axilla when the anterior leaflet results in greater regurgitation and to the left sternal border when the posterior leaflet results in greater regurgitation. When the posterior leaflet prolapses, the jet is usually superiorly and medially directed, and the murmur radiates toward the base of the heart. When the anterior leaflet prolapses, the murmur may be heard in the back, in the neck, and sometimes on the skull. In those cases where the murmur radiates to the base, it may be difficult to distinguish from the murmur of aortic stenosis or obstructive cardiomyopathy. The murmur decreases with reduction of afterload or LV size and increases with increase of afterload or LV size. Murmur intensity does not increase with postextrasystolic beats because the degree of MR is not increased (see Chapter 1).

Murmurs of shorter duration usually correspond to mild MR; they may be mid- or late systolic in mitral valve prolapse or early systolic in functional MR. The murmur may also be missed, particularly in acute myocardial infarction.

## *Electrocardiogram*

Chronic MR produces LA or LV enlargement, typically manifest by increased amplitude of the P waves and QRS complex. If atrial fibrillation is present, the LA enlargement is associated with coarse fibrillatory waves. RV hypertrophy is uncommon. The electrocardiogram, especially in acute MR, may be entirely normal. When papillary muscle ischemia or infarction is the cause of MR, evidence of inferior or posterior infarction (old or new) may be present.

## *Chest Roentgenogram*

In chronic severe MR, the chest x-ray shows LA and LV enlargement. In rheumatic disease, the valve leaflets may be calcified; with degenerative disease, a calcified mitral annulus is often present. Acute severe MR is usually associated with normal cardiac size and pulmonary edema.

# ■ LABORATORY TESTS

## Echocardiography/Doppler

The echocardiogram is used for defining the etiology of the MR (eg, flail leaflets, severe prolapse, mitral annulus calcification, systolic anterior motion of the anterior leaflet, and endocarditis vegetation) and determining its consequences. The echocardiography/Doppler technique provides an estimate of the severity of the regurgitation by assessing the velocity, width, and length of the regurgitant jet. Color-flow imaging demonstrates the origin and direction of the jet. Accordingly, the jet length, the ratio of the jet area to the left atrial (LA) area, or more simply the size of the jet area have been suggested as good indices of the severity of MR. Small jets, such as those seen in normal subjects, consistently correspond to mild regurgitations.

Color-flow imaging for defining regurgitant lesions has limitations. The extent of a jet is determined by its momentum and thus is determined as much by regurgitant velocity as by regurgitant flow. Also, jets are constrained by the LA and expand more in large atria. The eccentric jets of valvular prolapse depend on the left atrial wall and tend to underestimate regurgitation. In contrast, the central jets of ischemic and functional MR expand markedly in a large atrium and tend to overestimate regurgitation.

Transesophageal echocardiography usually shows larger jets, but does not eliminate these limitations of color-flow imaging. The pulmonary venous velocity profile is useful to assess the degree of regurgitation. Systolic reversal of flow in the pulmonary veins is a strong argument for severe MR. The reliability of several techniques for the quantitative assessment of MR remains to be demonstrated.

## Cardiac Catheterization and Angiography

Cardiac catheterization is utilized to assess hemodynamic status, the severity of MR, LV function, and coronary artery anatomy. A large V wave in the pulmonary capillary wedge pressure tracings suggests MR, but its absence does not exclude MR. The assessment of the degree of regurgitation can be obtained by LV contrast angiography and can be qualitatively graded in three or four grades on the basis of the degree and persistence of opacification of the LA. The hemodynamic response to exercise (eg, cardiac output, pulmonary artery pressure) often helps to determine the need for valve replacement in borderline circumstances.

Exercise testing is often useful for determining the patient's exercise capacity, particularly in those who appear relatively asymptomatic despite severe MR.

# ■ NATURAL HISTORY AND PROGNOSIS

Because of the qualitative and imprecise assessment of the degree of regurgitation, the natural history of MR is poorly defined. Patients with mild rheumatic MR appear to have a good prognosis. The prognosis of patients with echocardiographic mitral valve prolapse and no or mild regurgitation is usually excellent. Some deaths may occur in patients with murmurs of MR, more often when LV function is markedly decreased.

The predictors of poor outcome in patients with MR who are treated medically include severe symptoms (functional classes III to IV), even if the symptoms are transient; pulmonary hypertension; markedly increased LV end-diastolic volume; decreased cardiac output; and reduced LV ejection fraction. A comparison of the outcome of medically and surgically treated patients shows a trend in favor of surgical treatment, especially early surgery, with a definite improvement of outcome with surgery in patients who have decreased systolic LV function.

# ■ MEDICAL TREATMENT

Medical therapy is reserved for symptomatic patients who are being prepared for surgery or are not candidates for surgery. Afterload reduction decreases the amount of regurgitation, not only by reducing the LV systolic pressure but also by decreasing the effective regurgitant orifice area. Diuretic treatment is extremely useful for the control of heart failure and dyspnea. The acute utilization of sodium nitroprusside in unstable patients with severe MR, especially in the context of myocardial infarction, may be lifesaving in patients being prepared for mitral valve surgery.

In patients with AF, rate control is achieved using digoxin and/or β-blockers, diltiazem, and amiodarone. Long-term maintenance of sinus rhythm after cardioversion in patients with severe MR or enlarged LA who are treated medically is usually not possible. Oral anticoagulation should be used in patients with atrial fibrillation (international normalized ratio [INR] 2.0-3.0).

In asymptomatic patients, no specific medical therapy is indicated. For example, chronic afterload reduction is usually not indicated for chronic asymptomatic MR. However, clinical and echocardiographic surveillance for worsening MR, left ventricular dysfunction, and symptoms are important in the asymptomatic patient. Prevention of infective endocarditis with use of prophylactic antibiotics is no longer recommended in patients with MR unless endocarditis has previously occurred. Young patients with rheumatic MR should receive rheumatic fever prophylaxis.

In patients with secondary or functional mitral regurgitation, therapy is directed toward the primary pathophysiologic mechanism, eg, left ventricular dysfunction and/or electromechanical dyssynchrony. For example, the severity of mitral regurgitation generally improves with medical management of systolic heart failure. In addition, cardiac resynchronization therapy is particularly effective at reducing mitral regurgitation when QRS widening (especially a left bundle branch block pattern) complicates systolic heart failure.

# ■ SURGICAL TREATMENT

Patients with severe symptoms due to primary (in contrast to functional) MR should be treated surgically even if their symptoms are markedly improved by medical treatment (**Table 33-1** and Chapter 59). Patients who are functional class I or II but have signs of overt LV dysfunction (LV ejection fraction <60%, end-systolic diameter >45 mm) should be treated surgically, particularly if they are candidates for valve repair or valve replacement with chordal preservation.

In patients with *severe* MR who have no or minimal symptoms and no signs of LV dysfunction, surgery is a reasonable option when it is likely that the mitral valve can be repaired with chordal preservation. This pertains to patients with a low operative risk (1%-2%) and valvular lesions that can be repaired as indicated by echocardiography. Intraoperative transesophageal echocardiography (TEE) should be performed by physicians prior to operation and to monitor the repair procedure and help with decisions warranted by an imperfect result.

Mitral valve reconstruction for MR is usually possible and the surgical procedure of choice. The frequency with which valve repair can be used in patients with MR varies with the experience of the operating team (up to 90% success rate) and the spectrum of underlying valve disease; repair is more often feasible in patients with degenerative valve disease than in those with regurgitation caused by rheumatic valvulitis or endocarditis. LV systolic function and late survival in general are better

**TABLE 33-1.** Recommendations for Mitral Valve Surgery in Non-ischemic Severe Mitral Regurgitation

| Indication | Class |
|---|---|
| 1. Acute symptomatic MR in which repair is likely | I |
| 2. Patients with NYHA functional class II, III, or IV symptoms with normal LV function defined as ejection fraction >0.60 and end-systolic dimension <45 mm | I |
| 3. Symptomatic or asymptomatic patients with mild LV dysfunction, ejection fraction 0.50-0.60, and end-systolic dimension 45-50 mm | I |
| 4. Symptomatic or asymptomatic patients with moderate LV dysfunction, ejection fraction 0.30-0.50, and/or end-systolic dimension 50-55 mm | I |
| 5. Asymptomatic patients with preserved LV function and atrial fibrillation | IIa |
| 6. Asymptomatic patients with preserved LV function and pulmonary hypertension (pulmonary artery systolic pressure >50 mm Hg at rest or >60 mm Hg with exercise) | IIa |
| 7. Asymptomatic patients with ejection fraction 0.50-0.60 and end-systolic dimension <45 mm and asymptomatic patients with ejection fraction >0.60 and end-systolic dimension 45-55 mm | IIa |
| 8. Patients with severe LV dysfunction (ejection fraction <0.30 and/or end-systolic dimension >55 mm) in whom chordal preservation is highly likely | IIa |
| 9. Asymptomatic patients with chronic MR with preserved LV function in whom mitral valve repair is highly likely | IIb |
| 10. Patients with MVP and preserved LV function who have recurrent ventricular arrhythmias despite medical therapy | IIb |
| 11. Asymptomatic patients with preserved LV function in whom significant doubt about the feasibility of repair exists | IIb |

The committee recognizes that there may be variability in the measurement of mitral valve area and that the mean transmitral gradient, pulmonary artery wedge pressure, and pulmonary artery pressure at rest or during exercise should also be taken into consideration.

Data from Bonow RO, Carabello BA, Chatterjee K, et al. ACC/AHA 2006 guidelines for the management of patients with valvular heart disease a report of the American College of Cardiology/American Heart Association Task Force on Practice Guidelines (Writing Committee to revise the 1998 guidelines for the management of patients with valvular heart disease) developed in collaboration with the Society of Cardiovascular Anesthesiologists Endorsed by the Society for Cardiovascular Angiography and Interventions and the Society of Thoracic Surgeons. *J Am Coll Cardiol*. 2006;48 (3):e1-e148. Erratum in: *J Am Coll Cardiol*. 2007;49(9):1014.

with mitral valve repair than with mitral valve replacement because of maintenance of LV function when the chordae are preserved at the time of surgery. In patients whose mitral valves cannot be repaired, mitral valve replacement with chordal preservation is less likely to depress LV function than mitral valve replacement without preservation of the chordae tendineae.

Patients who have *no symptoms* due to *severe* MR and normal LV systolic function who are candidates for mitral valve repair and have severe pulmonary hypertension at rest or with exercise, atrial fibrillation, or recurrent thromboemboli despite anticoagulation therapy are commonly recommended for early surgery if mitral valve repair with preservation of the chordae is the likely procedure.

Percutaneous, nonsurgical methods for mitral valve repair are also in development (**Fig. 33-1**). Technical strategies include (1) "clipping" together of the free edges of the mitral leaflets to produce a two orifice mitral valve and (2) annular size reduction using shortening devices in the coronary sinus. In the recently completed randomized EVEREST II trial, percutaneous repair was inferior to surgical repair to

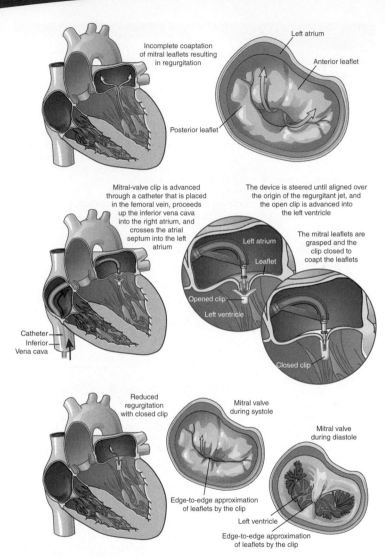

**FIGURE 33-1.** Percutaneous Repair of a Mitral Valve. In patients with mitral regurgitation resulting from incomplete leaflet coaptation, percutaneous mitral-valve repair is performed by means of femoral venous and transseptal access to the left atrium to steer the device toward the origin of the regurgitant jet. A mitral clip is passed through the mitral orifice from the left atrium to the left ventricle and pulled back to grasp the leaflet edges. If reduction of the mitral regurgitation is satisfactory, the device can be locked and then released. A double orifice is created in conjunction with reduction in mitral regurgitation. (Reproduced with permission from Feldman T, et al. Percutaneous Repair or Surgery for Mitral Regurgitation. *NEJM*. 2011; 364:1395.)

decrease the severity of mitral regurgitation but was associated with less morbidity and comparable clinical outcomes.

# MITRAL VALVE PROLAPSE

*Mitral valve prolapse* (MVP) is defined echocardiographically as the systolic billowing of one or both mitral leaflets into the left atrium, with or without mitral regurgitation. The *MVP syndrome* often occurs as a clinical entity with no or only mild mitral regurgitation, and it is frequently associated with unique clinical characteristics when compared with the other causes of mitral regurgitation. Nevertheless, MVP is the most common cause of significant MR and the most frequent substrate for mitral valve endocarditis in the United States. The mitral valve apparatus is a complex structure composed of the mitral annulus, valve leaflets, chordae tendineae, papillary muscles, and supporting left ventricular, left atrial, and aortic walls. Disease processes involving any one or more of these components may result in dysfunction of the valvular apparatus and prolapse of the mitral leaflets toward the left atrium during systole, when LV pressure exceeds left atrial pressure.

In primary MVP (**Table 33-2**), there is interchordal hooding due to leaflet redundancy involving both the rough and the clear zones of the involved leaflets. The basic microscopic feature of primary MVP is marked proliferation of the spongiosa, the delicate myxomatous connective tissue between the atrialis (a thick layer of collagen and elastic tissue forming the atrial aspect of the leaflet) and the fibrosa or ventricularis, which is composed of dense layers of collagen and forms the basic support of the leaflet. Secondary effects of the primary MVP syndrome include fibrosis of the surface of the mitral valve leaflets, thinning and/or elongation of the chordae tendineae, and ventricular friction lesions. Fibrin deposits often form at the mitral valve–left atrial angle. The primary form of MVP may occur in families, where it appears to be inherited as an autosomal dominant trait with varying penetrance. The primary MVP syndrome has also been found with increasing frequency in patients with Marfan's syndrome and in other heritable connective tissue diseases.

Mitral valve leaflet prolapse may also result from postinflammatory changes. Mitral valve prolapse has also been observed in patients with hypertrophic cardiomyopathy, in whom posterior MVP may result from a disproportionally small left ventricular

**TABLE 33-2.** Classification of Mitral Valve Prolapse

Primary mitral valve prolapse
    Familial
    Nonfamilial
    Marfan syndrome
    Other connective tissue diseases
    Cardiomyopathies
    "Flail" mitral valve leaflet(s)
Secondary mitral valve prolapse
    Coronary artery disease
    Rheumatic heart disease
Normal variant
    Inaccurate auscultation
    "Echocardiographic" heart disease

cavity, altered papillary muscle alignment, or a combination of factors. Patients with MVP syndrome must be distinguished from those with normal variations on cardiac auscultation or echocardiograms that are misinterpreted as showing MVP.

# ■ CLINICAL MANIFESTATIONS OF MVP SYNDROME

## Symptoms

The diagnosis of MVP is most commonly made by cardiac auscultation in asymptomatic patients or by echocardiography performed for some other purpose. The patient may be evaluated because of a family history of cardiac disease or occasionally may be referred because of an abnormal resting electrocardiogram. The most common presenting complaint is palpitations, which are usually due to premature ventricular beats. Supraventricular arrhythmias are also frequent; the most common sustained tachycardia is paroxysmal reentry supraventricular tachycardia.

Chest pain is a frequent complaint in patients with the MVP syndrome. It is atypical in most patients without coexistent ischemic heart disease and rarely resembles classic angina pectoris. Dyspnea and fatigue are also frequent symptoms in patients with MVP, including many without severe MR. Objective exercise testing often fails to show an impairment in exercise tolerance, and some patients exhibit distinct episodes of hyperventilation. Neuropsychiatric complaints are not uncommon in patients with MVP: Some have panic attacks and others frank manic-depressive syndromes. Transient cerebral ischemic episodes occur with increased incidence in patients with MVP, and some develop stroke syndromes. Reports of amaurosis fugax, homonymous field loss, and retinal artery occlusion have been described; occasionally the visual loss persists. These signs are likely due to embolization of platelets and fibrin deposits occurring on the atrial side of the mitral valve leaflets. It is important to note that both MVP and panic attacks occur relatively frequently. Accordingly, the occurrence of both syndromes in the same individual would be expected to occur frequently by chance.

## Physical Examination

The presence of thoracic skeletal abnormalities—the most common being scoliosis, pectus excavatum, straightened thoracic spine, and narrowed anteroposterior diameter of the chest—may suggest the diagnosis of the MVP syndrome. The principal cardiac auscultatory feature of this syndrome is the midsystolic click, a high-pitched sound of short duration. The click may vary considerably in intensity and location in systole according to LV loading conditions and contractility. It results from the sudden tension of the mitral valve apparatus as the leaflets prolapse into the left atrium during systole. Multiple systolic clicks may be generated as different portions of the mitral leaflets prolapse at various times during systole. The major feature differentiating the midsystolic click of MVP from that due to other causes is that its timing during systole may be altered by maneuvers that change the hemodynamic conditions.

Dynamic auscultation is often useful for establishing the clinical diagnosis of the MVP syndrome (**Table 33-3**). Changes in the LV end-diastolic volume lead to changes in the timing of the midsystolic click and murmur. When end-diastolic volume is decreased, the critical volume is achieved earlier in systole, and the click-murmur complex occurs shortly after the first heart sound. In general, any maneuver that decreases the end-diastolic LV volume, increases the rate of ventricular contraction, or decreases the resistance to LV ejection of blood causes the MVP to occur early in systole, and the systolic click and murmur to move toward the first heart sound. This occurs when the patient suddenly stands from the supine position, does submaximal hand-grip exercise, or performs the Valsalva maneuver (see Table 33-3).

**TABLE 33-3.** Response of the Murmur of Mitral Valve Prolapse to Interventions

| Intervention | Timing | Intensity |
|---|---|---|
| Standing upright | ← | ↑ |
| Recumbent | → | ↓ or 0 |
| Squatting | → | ↓ or 0 |
| Hand grip | ← | ± |
| Valsalva | ← | ± |
| Amyl nitrite | ± | ↑ |

↑, increase; ↓, decrease; 0, no change; ±, variable; ←, earlier; →, later.

# ■ DIAGNOSTIC STUDIES

## Electrocardiogram

The electrocardiogram (ECG) is usually normal in patients with the MVP syndrome. The most common abnormality in the MVP syndrome is the presence of ST-T-wave depression or T-wave inversion in the inferior leads. MVP is associated with an increased incidence of false-positive exercise ECG results in patients with normal coronary arteries, especially females. Myocardial perfusion imaging with thallium or technetium sestamibi has been useful for differentiating false from true abnormal exercise ECG findings in patients with MVP.

Although arrhythmias may be observed on the resting ECG or during treadmill or bicycle exercise, they are detected more frequently by continuous ambulatory ECG recordings. The reported incidence of documented arrhythmias is higher in patients with MVP; however, most are not life-threatening, and they often do not correlate with the patient's symptoms.

## Echocardiography

As indicated earlier, echocardiography is the most useful noninvasive test for defining MVP. The M-mode echocardiographic definition of MVP includes ≥2-mm posterior displacement of one or both leaflets or holosystolic posterior "hammocking" >3 mm. On 2D echocardiography, systolic displacement of one or both mitral leaflets, particularly when they coapt on the left atrial side of the annular plane in the parasternal long-axis view, indicates a high likelihood of MVP. There is disagreement concerning the reliability of an echocardiographic diagnosis of MVP when these signs are observed only in the apical four-chamber view. The diagnosis of MVP is even more certain when the leaflet thickness is >5 mm during ventricular diastole. Leaflet redundancy is often associated with an elongated mitral annulus and elongated chordae tendineae. On Doppler velocity recordings, the presence or absence of MR is an important consideration, and MVP is more likely when the MR is detected as a high-velocity jet in late systole, midway, or more posterior in the left atrium.

There is no consensus on 2D echocardiographic criteria for MVP. Since echocardiography is a tomographic cross-sectional technique, no single view should be considered diagnostic. The parasternal long-axis view permits visualization of the medial aspect of the anterior mitral leaflet and the middle scallop of the posterior leaflet. If the findings of prolapse are localized to the lateral scallop in the posterior leaflet, they would be best visualized by the apical four-chamber view. All available echocardiographic views should be utilized, with the provision that anterior leaf-let billowing in the four-chamber apical view is not in itself evidence of prolapse; however, a displacement of the posterior leaflet or the coaptation point in any view, including the apical views, suggests the diagnosis of prolapse. The echocardiographic criteria for MVP should include structural changes, such as leaflet thickening, redundancy, annular dilatation, and chordal elongation.

Patients with echocardiographic criteria for the MVP syndrome but without evidence of thickened/redundant leaflets or definite MR are more difficult to classify. If such patients have auscultatory findings typical of MVP, the echocardiogram usually confirms the diagnosis. Two-dimensional/Doppler echocardiography is also useful for defining LA size as well as LV size and function and for the detection and semiquantitation of MR.

## ■ NATURAL HISTORY, PROGNOSIS, AND COMPLICATIONS

In most patient studies, the MVP syndrome is associated with a benign prognosis. The age-adjusted survival rate for both males and females with MVP is similar to that for patients without this common clinical entity. The gradual progression of mitral regurgitation in patients with mitral prolapse, however, may result in progressive dilatation of the LA and LV. LA dilatation often results in atrial fibrillation, and moderate to severe MR eventually results in left ventricular dysfunction and the development of congestive heart failure in certain patients, particularly men. Several long-term prognostic studies suggest that complications occur most commonly in patients with a mitral systolic murmur, thickened redundant mitral valve leaflets, or increased LV or LA size. Sudden death is uncommon but is obviously the most severe complication of mitral valve prolapse. Although sudden death is infrequent, its highest incidence has been reported in the familial form of MVP. Infective endocarditis is a serious complication of MVP but there is no evidence that antibiotic prophylaxis prevents this complication.

In some patients, fibrin emboli are responsible for visual problems consistent with the involvement of the ophthalmic or posterior cerebral circulation. Therefore, it has been recommended that antiplatelet drugs such as aspirin be administered to patients who have MVP syndrome and suspected cerebral emboli. Warfarin therapy is usually reserved for patients with MVP who have atrial fibrillation or poststroke patients with prolapse, particularly when symptoms occur on aspirin therapy. However, neither antiplatelet drugs nor anticoagulants should be prescribed routinely for patients with MVP, since the incidence of embolic phenomena is very low.

## ■ TREATMENT

The majority of patients with the MVP syndrome are asymptomatic. A normal lifestyle and regular exercise are encouraged. Patients with MVP and palpitations associated with sinus tachycardia or mild tachyarrhythmias and those with chest pain, anxiety, or fatigue often respond to therapy with β-blockers. Symptoms of orthostatic hypotension are best treated with volume expansion, preferably by liberalizing fluid and salt intake. In survivors of sudden cardiac death and patients with symptomatic complex arrhythmias, specific antiarrhythmic therapy should be guided by monitoring techniques, including electrophysiologic testing when indicated. Restriction from competitive sports is recommended when moderate LV enlargement, LV dysfunction, uncontrolled tachyarrhythmias, long QT interval, unexplained syncope, prior sudden death, or aortic root enlargement is present, individually or in combination. Asymptomatic patients with MVP and no significant MR can be evaluated clinically every 2 to 3 years. Patients with MVP who have high-risk characteristics, including those with moderate to severe regurgitation, should be followed more frequently, even if no symptoms are present.

## Surgical Considerations

Recommendations for surgery in patients with MVP and MR are the same as for those with other forms of non-ischemic severe MR and include class III to IV symptoms, LV ejection fraction ≤60%, and/or marked increases in LV end-diastolic and end-systolic volumes. Repair is being recommended with increased frequency for functional class II symptoms and suitable anatomy.

# SUGGESTED READINGS

Adams DH, Carabello BA, Castillo JG. Mitral valve regurgitation. In: Fuster V, Walsh R, Harrington RA, et al, eds. *Hurst's The Heart*. 13th ed. New York, NY: McGraw-Hill; 2011:77: 1721-1737.

Bonow RO, Carabello B, Chatterjee K, et al. ACC/AHA guidelines for the management of patients with valvular heart disease. *J Am Coll Cardiol*. 2006; 48:e1-e148. Erratum appears in *J Am Coll Cardiol*. 2007; 49:1014.

Feldman T, Wasserman HS, Herrmann HC, et al. Percutaneous repair or surgery for mitral regurgitation. *N Engl J Med*. 2011; 364:1395.

2008 Focused Update Incorporated into the ACC/AHA 2006 Guidelines on the Management of Patients with Valvular Heart Disease. Circulation 2008;118:e523-e661.

Foster E. Mitral regurgitation due to degenerative mitral valve disease. *N Engl J Med*. 2010;363: 156-165.

Ling LH, Enriquez-Sarano M, Seward JB, et al. Clinical outcome of mitral regurgitation due to flail leaflet. *N Engl J Med*. 1996; 335:1417.

Nishimura R, McGoon MD. Perspectives on mitral valve prolapse. *N Engl J Med*. 1999; 341:48-58.

Nishimura RA, Carabello BA, Faxon DP, et al. ACC/AHA 2008 guideline update on valvular heart disease: focused update on infective endocarditis: a report of the American College of Cardiology/American Heart Association Task Force on Practice Guidelines. *Circulation*. 2008;118(8):887-96.

O'Rourke RA. The syndrome of mitral valve prolapse. In: Albert JA, ed. *Valvular Heart Disease*. New York, NY: Lippincott-Raven; 1999:157-182.

Wilson W, Taubert KA, Gewitz M, et al. Prevention of Endocarditis: Guidelines of the American Heart Association. *Circulation*. 2007;116:1736-1754.

# CHAPTER 34
# TRICUSPID VALVE AND PULMONIC VALVE DISEASE

Pravin M. Shah

Right-sided cardiac valve disease is encountered less frequently when compared to left-sided valve disease and many of the indications for intervention remain uncertain or controversial. Much of what is known about tricuspid and pulmonic valve disease has been derived from the study of adult congenital heart disease and has been extrapolated to other settings. In general, the treatment of right-sided valve disease requires collaboration between the cardiologist, interventional cardiologist, and cardiothoracic surgeon.

# TRICUSPID VALVE DISEASE

## ■ NORMAL ANATOMY

The three leaflets (anterior, posterior, and septal), annulus, and commissures form the valvular apparatus. The chordae tendinae and papillary muscles form the tensor apparatus. The saddle-shaped tricuspid annulus is anchored in part by the fibrous skeleton of the heart. The tricuspid annulus is more prone to dilation when the ventricular cavity enlarges compared to the mitral annulus.

The commissures represent the site along the annulus where the leaflets meet. They always have an underlying papillary muscle and a fanlike array of tendinous cords to anchor and support the leaflets. The papillary muscles can be single or multi-headed and receive tendinous cords from two adjacent leaflets. This dual insertion facilitates closure of the valve during right ventricular systole due to pulling of the leaflets toward each other.

The orifice of the tricuspid valve is triangular in shape and is the largest orifice of the four cardiac valves. This results in lower early and late diastolic inflow velocities into the RV when compared to mitral inflow velocities into the LV. The anterior leaflet is the largest and most mobile of the three leaflets and attaches to the anterior and medial papillary muscles. The posterior leaflet is smaller and appears to be of lesser importance to normal valve function. The septal leaflet attaches directly to the membranous and muscular portions of the ventricular septum leading to its relatively immobile state.

## ■ TRICUSPID VALVE REGURGITATION

### Etiology

Up to 70% to 90% of patients with *structurally normal valves have some degree of tricuspid regurgitation* (TR) in large part due to incomplete coaptation of the leaflets. The vast majority of these patients are asymptomatic and the valve finding is

**TABLE 34-1.** Etiology of Tricuspid Valve Disease

| Primary (Intrinsic) Valve Disease | Secondary (Functional) Valve Disease |
|---|---|
| Infective endocarditis (IV drug use) | Primary RV disease/dilation |
| Rheumatic heart disease (never isolated) | Right ventricular infarction |
| Carcinoid | Dilated cardiomyopathy |
| Myxomatous disease (prolapse) | Elevated right ventricular systolic pressure |
| Endomyocardial fibrosis | Left-sided heart failure |
| Ebstein anomaly | Aortic, mitral, or pulmonic valve |
| Medication use (anorectics and ergot derivatives) | disease |
| Thoracic trauma | Primary pulmonary disease including |
| Iatrogenic (pacemaker lead and repeated | pulmonary arterial HTN of any |
| endomyocardial biopsies) | cause |
| Congenital (non-Ebstein) | Left-to-right shunt |
| Radiation inury | |

considered a normal variant. Pathologic TR can be due to primary (intrinsic) valve disease or more commonly secondary or functional TR (**Table 34-1**). With increasing TR severity, there is an associated worsening prognosis that is independent of ventricular systolic function and pulmonary pressures.

The most common form of primary TR is due to infective endocarditis associated with intravenous drug use. The most common causative organism is *Staphylococcus aureus* followed by coagulase negative staphylococci and beta-hemolytic streptococci. These patients can be extremely difficult to manage due to high recurrence rates associated with medical noncompliance. Another less common condition is valvulopathy related to prescription drug use. The first medications implicated were the anorectics fenfluramine (Pondimin) and dexfenfluramine (Redux). Transthoracic echocardiography (TTE) revealed leaflet retraction and thickening in a subset of patients who subsequently developed murmurs after exposure to the drugs. In a subset of patients who then required valve replacement, histologic evidence displayed a plaque-like process extending across the leaflet surfaces and encasing the chordae tendinae. These findings are similar to the valve changes noted in patients with serotonin-secreting carcinoid tumors and patients taking certain antimigraine drugs (methysergide and ergotamine). In March 2007, the FDA voluntarily withdrew pergolide (Permax), an anti-parkinsonian dopamine agonist with potent serotonin activity, due to similar valulopathic findings suggesting a causal association. Subsequent research has suggested the $5\text{-HT}_{2B}$ receptor to be a key mediator of drug-induced valvular disease.

The most common cause of TR is not intrinsic disease of the valve, but as a consequence of tricuspid annular dilation in the setting of RV dilation and/or pulmonary hypertension. With continued pressure and volume overload of the RV, TR begets TR. Therefore, it is critically important to determine the underlying cause of the dilated annulus since specific therapy aimed at the primary disorder will improve the severity of the TR.

## Diagnosis

The symptoms associated with severe functional TR are those of the associated with RV failure. Dyspnea, fatigue, and exercise intolerance are common due to impaired forward cardiac output. Chest pain and abdominal pain are due to hepatosplenomegaly.

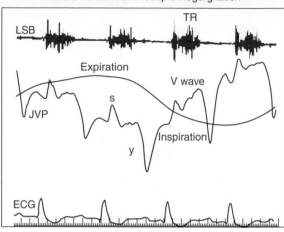

**FIGURE 34-1.** Physical findings of severe tricuspid regurgitation in the setting of right ventricular systolic pressure overload due to pulmonary hypertension. The jugular venous pulse shows a very prominent S (systolic wave) and V wave. With inspiration, there is a significant increase in the height of the S-V wave and the rate of Y descent. There is also a simultaneous increase in the intensity of the pansystolic regurgitant tricuspid murmur. With diuresis, the degree of tricuspid regurgitation and the intensity of the pansystolic regurgitant murmur may decrease or disappear. (Reproduced with permission from Salerni R, et al. Noninvasive graphic evaluation: phonocardiography and echocardiography. In: Frankl WS, Brest AN, eds. *Cardiovascular Clinics: Valvular Heart Disease: Comprehensive Evaluation and Management.* Philadelphia, PA: Davis; 1986;16(2):173-210.)

On physical examination (PE), distended and pulsatile jugular veins with prominent V waves are appreciated (**Fig. 34-1**). Other findings include a precordial impulse of the RV, a holosystolic murmur at either sternal border that increases with inspiration, an accentuated or attenuated P2 (in the setting of pulmonary hypertension [PH]), a pulsatile liver, ascites, peripheral cyanosis, and lower extremity edema. Rivero–Carvallo's sign is an accentuation of the TR murmur with inspiration due to increased venous return to the right side of the heart facilitated by negative intrathoracic pressure. In the absence of PH, even with severe TR, the murmur may be very soft or absent due to the small pressure gradient between the RA and RV.

The electrocardiogram (ECG) frequently shows nonspecific findings compatible with the underlying diagnosis causing the functional TR. Atrial fibrillation is often present, but if sinus rhythm (SR) prevails, right atrial enlargement is often seen with tall and narrow P waves in the inferior leads. In rheumatic disease, there is often biatrial enlargement due to concomitant involvement of the mitral valve. The chest x-ray (CXR) often shows cardiomegaly and obliteration of the retrosternal clear space on the lateral view due to RV enlargement. Prominence of the superior vena cava, distension of the azygous vein, and pleural effusions are often present. The diaphragms may be displaced superiorly due to ascites.

Echocardiography is the reference standard for diagnosis and evaluation of TR. Other cardiac abnormalities that affect tricuspid valve function can be determined as well as determination of RV function and an estimation of the pulmonary pressures using the modified Bernoulli equation. Color flow Doppler is widely used to determine the severity of the regurgitation allowing for visualization of the width of the jet (vena contracta), the spatial orientation of the regurgitant jet area in the receiving chamber (jet area), and flow convergence into the regurgitant orifice (proximal iso-velocity surface area [PISA]). The major criteria for diagnosing severe TR are a vena contracta width greater than 0.7 cm; a PISA radius greater than 0.9 cm; and evidence of systolic flow reversal in the hepatic veins, although this finding is inaccurate in the presence of atrial fibrillation.

In functional TR, dilation of the RA, RV, and tricuspid annulus are by definition present. In addition, there can be findings of paradoxical septal movement reflecting the increased volume within the right ventricle. Specific findings of an apically displaced tricuspid valve and atrialization of the ventricular tissue is seen in Ebstein's anomaly. In patients with endocarditis, vegetations may be seen on the atrial side of the tricuspid valve and/or an associated flail leaflet. Prolapse of the valve may be readily apparent with TTE. Thickened and retracted leaflets are the hallmark of carcinoid valvular disease, which is similar to the findings seen in drug-induced valvular disease due to elevated serotonin levels.

Transesophageal echocardiography (TEE) is rarely needed for TR assessment due to the excellent assessment provided by TTE. Only in those patients with poor acoustic windows should TEE be utilized. Occasionally, in the intraoperative setting, TEE is used to measure the tricuspid annulus diameter and may contribute to surgical decisions regarding TV annuloplasty.

Cardiac catheterization has no role in the diagnosis of TR due to distortion of the TV with placement of catheters into the RV and leading to false assessments with respect to the severity of the TR. However, right heart catheterization is strongly advised in the clinical setting of PH in order to properly document the right ventricular, pulmonary artery, pulmonary capillary wedge pressure, and measurement of cardiac output. These values allow calculation of the transpulmonary gradient and the pulmonary vascular resistance. A systolic PA pressure greater than 55 mm Hg is likely to cause TR with an anatomically normal tricuspid valve, whereas TR occurring with a systolic PA pressure less than 40 mm Hg is likely to reflect a structural abnormality of the valve apparatus.

## Treatment

TR in the absence of right ventricular hypertension is generally well tolerated, as exemplified in patients who have undergone tricuspid valvectomy due to endocarditis where dilation of the RV occurs months or years later. The majority of these patients can be managed with efforts directed to control systemic venous congestion with diuretics, although some patients may go on to develop atrial arrhythmias that will require additional therapy.

Certain patients with severe TR may benefit from surgical intervention, especially if there is concomitant mitral valve disease requiring operative treatment and if there is a class I indication (Level of Evidence: B) according to the most recently published ACC/AHA guidelines (Chapter 59). As a whole, though, the timing of surgical intervention for TR remains controversial, as do the surgical techniques. Differing annuloplasty procedures with and without a supporting ring have been utilized with varying degrees of success. These include plication of the posterior leaflet annulus (bicuspidization), partial purse string reduction in the anterior and posterior leaflet annulus (DeVega annuloplasty), placement of a semirigid ring (Carpentier–Edwards), and placement of a flexible band (Cosgrove annuloplasty system). More recently, there have been clinical evaluations utilizing a three-dimensional annuloplasty system (MC3 ring) in an attempt to preserve atrioventricular dynamics. All of these techniques tend to reduce but do not eliminate TR and every effort should be made to reduce the RV pressure with medications.

Tricuspid valve replacement (TVR) is performed only when annuloplasty is not feasible due to diseased or abnormal valve leaflets and receives a class IIa (Level of Evidence: C) indication for those patients with severe primary TR. When possible, a bioprosthesis is preferred due to high rates of thromboembolic complications in patients with a mechanical prosthesis in the tricuspid position. In patients with conduction system disease, insertion of a permanent epicardial pacing wire at the time of valve surgery can obviate the need for a subsequent transvenous lead across the prosthetic valve.

In contrast to the recommendation for correction of severe symptomatic TR, the guidelines conclude that the weight of evidence is less well established for TV annuloplasty in patients with less than severe TR, who are to undergo MV surgery with a dilated tricuspid annulus in the presence of RV hypertension. Often with correction of the mitral valve disease, the lowering of the left atrial and right ventricular pressures result in significant improvement of the TR; therefore clinical judgment is essential.

Currently, there are no acceptable approved percutaneous techniques available. However, with continued experience and refinement, edge-to-edge valve repair may be an option in the future for those symptomatic patients who are not considered to be optimal surgical candidates.

# TRICUSPID STENOSIS

## ■ ETIOLOGY

Tricuspid stenosis (TS) is a rare clinical entity with RHD accounting for greater than 90% of the cases. In patients with rheumatic mitral valve disease, only 5% to 15% have concurrent TS. There are several conditions that mimic TS by causing obstruction to tricuspid inflow. These include tricuspid atresia, right atrial myxomas (or other tumors), carcinoid syndrome (more likely to cause regurgitation), right atrial thrombus, and bacterial endocarditis.

## ■ DIAGNOSIS

Due to the pressure gradient across the tricuspid valve, the patient with TS notices signs and symptoms related to the elevated RA pressure. The obstruction to forward flow leads to decreased cardiac output and fatigue. Due to the low cardiac output, the lung fields may be clear and the patient may be comfortable while lying supine despite the profound ascites and occasional anasarca. Cardiac findings may be masked by the concomitant mitral stenosis, requiring a high index of suspicion that TS is present.

The cardiac examination may reveal an opening snap at the left lower sternal border. The murmur is usually softer, higher pitched, and shorter in duration than the murmur of MS and increases in intensity with maneuvers which increase tricuspid flow. The presystolic component has a scratchy quality and is the result of atrial contraction when sinus rhythm is present. In the presence of sinus rhythm, jugular venous pulsations reveal a prominent A wave and a diminished rate of Y descent. In atrial fibrillation, it is extremely difficult to diagnose due to the loss of the A wave and the reduction in the intensity of the murmur.

The ECG in sinus rhythm reveals right atrial enlargement and commonly biatrial enlargement due to the concomitant MS. Atrial fibrillation is present in the majority of patients. The CXR is notable for cardiomegaly and enlargement of the right heart border without dilation of the pulmonary artery.

Echocardiographic findings included restricted and thickened leaflets with diastolic doming. There is less calcification and thickening of the tricuspid valves when compared to the mitral valve in patients with combined RHD. A diastolic pressure gradient of 3 to 5 mm Hg is enough to lead to elevated systemic vascular congestion and it rarely exceeds 10 mm Hg. It is extremely important to accurately define the degree of TR as this can impact the decision to proceed with balloon valvotomy.

Right heart catheterization can be performed with simultaneous pressure measurements of the RA and RV. Because a clinically significant obstruction may be present with a minimal gradient (2-4 mm Hg), it is imperative that the transducers be calibrated equisensitive.

## ◼ TREATMENT

Initially, diuretics and sodium restriction may improve the symptoms due to fluid retention. Definitive therapy includes balloon valvotomy; however, reported experience in the literature is limited. Severe TR is a known consequence of this procedure, thus limiting its long-term success when it develops. In patients with severe concomitant MS, TS should not be corrected alone, as this can exacerbate the symptoms of the mitral valve disease due to increased forward cardiac output across the left-sided valve. Therefore, surgical treatment of the TS should be carried out at the same time as the MS.

# PULMONARY VALVE DISEASE

## ◼ NORMAL ANATOMY

The pulmonic valve consists of the annulus, leaflets, and commissures. There are no chordal attachments, thus making the opening and closing a passive process. It lies closest to the chest wall of all cardiac valves with its orifice directed toward the left shoulder.

## ◼ PULMONARY REGURGITATION

### Etiology

The most common etiology of pulmonary regurgitation (PR) is due to dilation of the annulus as a result of pulmonary HTN. Dilation of the pulmonary artery itself may occur in the absence of pulmonary HTN, such as in Marfan syndrome and idiopathic dilatation of the pulmonary artery. PR may also be caused by infective endocarditis or as a late manifestation of previously treated CHD. The two most commonly encountered congenital disorders associated with PR include prior treatment of congenital PS and repair of tetralogy of Fallot (TOF). PR can also develop as a result of primary lesions affecting the valve such as absent or malformed leaflets, which usually occur with other congenital abnormalities.

### Diagnosis

In the setting of severe pulmonary hypertension (PH), the symptoms of the patient are primarily related to the cause of the PH (idiopathic pulmonary arterial hypertension, severe mitral stenosis, Eisenmenger syndrome, etc). *The functional murmur (Graham Steell murmur) is identical to the murmur of aortic regurgitation because the hemodynamics responsible for their production are identical. The differential diagnosis is made by the "company the murmur keeps," and the ancillary findings of both diseases establish the diagnosis.*

The symptoms of organic pulmonary regurgitation may be well tolerated for many years. However, in some patients, the chronic RV overload may cause clinical right ventricular failure. The murmur of organic regurgitation is quite different than the Graham Steell murmur (PR) associated with pulmonary arterial hypertension (PAH).

This organic PR murmur is frequently delayed from the pulmonic closure sound, and then builds up quickly to a crescendo followed by a decrescendo, which ends well before $S_1$ (Chapter 1). Since organic pulmonic regurgitation is usually in the setting of a normal pulmonary artery pressure, the diastolic gradient between the pulmonary artery and right ventricle is very small, resulting in a low-velocity retrograde flow and a lower-pitched murmur. Frequently, there is an associated systolic ejection murmur due to the large stroke volume of the right ventricle.

In the absence of PAH, the ECG may only manifest incomplete right bundle-branch block (RBBB) due to diastolic volume overload. However, when associated with PAH, the ECG traditionally shows RVH. The CXR shows nonspecific signs of prominence of the main pulmonary artery and RV enlargement and the associated findings related to the cause of the PR.

TTE will allow a complete noninvasive evaluation of the morphology and physiology of the PV as well as the size and function of the RV. Abnormal flattening of the interventricular septum may be noted in diastole due to the increased volume in the RV displacing the septum toward the LV cavity. The degree of septal flattening has been shown to correlate with the severity of the PAH. Abnormal Doppler signals in the right ventricular outflow tract (RVOT) with velocity sustained throughout diastole are generally observed in patients with a dilated annulus. In contrast, when the velocity falls during diastole, the PA pressure is usually normal and the PR is due to a primary abnormality of the valve itself.

Due to limitations in echocardiographic imaging of the pulmonic valve due to lung tissue and near-field artifact, Cardiac magnetic resonance imaging (CMR) has become critical to the assessment of PI, particularly when it is associated with congenital heart disease, eg, post-TOF repair. CMR's ability to accurately assess RV volumes, complex cardiac and vascular anatomy, and delineate prior surgical procedures are essential for the surveillance of PI and to plan management strategies.

### Treatment

PR alone is rarely severe enough to require specific treatment. Treatment of the primary condition responsible for the PR will often dramatically improve the degree of PR. However, in the rare CHD patient with severe PR secondary to remote successful repair of TOF and New York Heart Association (NYHA) class II or III symptoms (Chapter 59), surgical consideration may be indicated. In asymptomatic patients, surgical replacement can be considered when there is severe RV dilation and RV dysfunction in order to prevent the development of right heart failure. Under such circumstances, low-risk pulmonary valve replacement (PVR) has been performed with insertion of a homograft or xenograft. Pulmonary percutaneous valve implantation has been performed in the pediatric population and has been used in adults in clinical trials.

# PULMONIC STENOSIS

## ■ ETIOLOGY

Because the pulmonary valve is the least likely valve to be affected by acquired heart disease, virtually all cases of pulmonic stenosis (PS) are congenital. Less common noncongenital causes include the carcinoid syndrome, rheumatic fever, and stenosis of a bioprosthetic valve. Infundibular stenosis is rare as an isolated condition but often accompanies valvular PS due to hypertrophy of the RVOT and typically regresses after correction of the valvular PS. In congenital PS, the valve is either dome shaped due to fusion of the valve leaflets, or thickened and dysplastic resulting in inability of leaflet separation during ventricular systole.

# ■ DIAGNOSIS

Mild and moderate degrees of PS are generally well tolerated. When symptoms from PS develop, they mainly consist of dyspnea on exertion and fatigue due mainly to the limitation of augmentation of right ventricular cardiac output. Severe PS (eg, >60 mm Hg peak gradients) may lead to RV failure and cyanosis in the presence of a concomitant interatrial communication.

The physical examination reveals a basal respirophasic crescendo systolic murmur heard best in the second left interspace. With increasing degrees of obstruction, both the duration of the murmur and the width of the splitting increase. The pulmonic component of the second heart sound may be widely split or difficult to hear. When a respirophasic ejection click is present, it suggests a valvular lesion as opposed to a supravalvular or infravalvular stenosis. A parasternal impulse and a prominent A wave in the JVP are present with significant RV hypertrophy.

The ECG is often normal in mild to moderate PS; however, as the stenosis becomes severe, RA abnormalities, RVH, and RAD are present. In addition RBBB is common, except in Noonan syndrome, where left bundle-branch block may be seen.

Echocardiography is the gold standard to assess the severity of the PS as well as to determine the size and function of the RV. It is a class I recommendation in the ACC/AHA Guidelines (Chapter 59) for the initial evaluation and serial 5- to 10-year follow-up examinations. The guidelines define the severity of the lesion based on the following findings using Doppler techniques:

1. Peak velocity across the PV greater than 4 m/s (peak gradient >60 mm Hg)—severe

2. Peak velocity across the PV greater than 3 m/s and less than 4 m/s (peak gradient 36-60 mm Hg)—moderate

3. Peak velocity across the PV less than 3 m/s (peak gradient <36 mm Hg)—mild

Cardiac catheterization is rarely recommended unless a therapeutic intervention is being considered. Diagnostic cardiac catheterization actually receives a class III indication from the most recent ACC/AHA guidelines as an initial diagnostic strategy (Chapter 59). Cardiac MRI has now become standard in the evaluation of PS when available.

# ■ TREATMENT

The clinical course of children and young adults with PS has been well described. Mild congenital PS is a benign disease that rarely progresses. Those with moderate or severe disease can be improved with either surgery or endovascular techniques. The exception is the presence of Noonan syndrome, which generally requires PVR due to the severely dysplastic valve. Pulmonic valvuloplasty can be performed with low risk to the patient by experienced operators and is associated with excellent long-term outcomes with a low rate of recurrent PS.

# SUGGESTED READINGS

Shah PM. Tricuspid valve, pulmonary valve, and multivalvular disease. In: Fuster V, Walsh R, Harrington RA, et al. *Hurst's The Heart*. 13th ed. New York, NY; 2011; 79: 1745-1756.

ACC/AHA 2008 Guidelines for the Management of Adult Congenital Heart Disease. *Circulation*. 2008;118:xxx-xxx.

Bonow RO, Carabello BA, Chatterjee K, et al. ACC/AHA 2006 practice guidelines for the management of patients with valvular heart disease. *J Am Coll Cardiol*. 2006;48:598-675.

2008 Focused Update Incorporated into the ACC/AHA 2006 Guidelines on the Management of Patients with Valvular Heart Disease. *Circulation.* 2008;118:e523-e661.

Khambadkone S, Coats. L, Taylor A, et al. Percutaneous pulmonary valve implantation in humans. *Circulation.* 2005;112:1189-1197.

McCarthy PM, Bhudia SK, Rajeswaran J, et al. Tricuspid valve repair: durability and risk factors for failure. *J Thorac Cardiovasc Surg.* 2004;127:674-685.

Osterhof T, van Straten A, Vliegen HW, et al. Preoperative thresholds for pulmonary valve replacement in patients with corrected tetralogy of fallot using cardiovascular magnetic resonance. *Circulation.* 2007;116:545-551.

Roth BL. Drugs and valvular heart disease. *N Engl J Med.* 2007;356:6-9.

Sorrell VL, Altbach MI, Kudithpudi V, et al. Cardiac MRI is an important complementary tool to Doppler echocardiography in the management of patients with pulmonary regurgitation. *Echocardiography.* 2007;24:316-328.

Zoghbi WA, Enriquez-Sarano M, Foster E, et al. Recommendations for evaluation of the severity of native valvular regurgitation with two dimensional and Doppler echocardiography. *J Am Soc Echocardiogr.* 2003;16:777-802.

# CHAPTER 35

# PROSTHETIC HEART VALVES: CHOICE OF VALVE AND MANAGEMENT OF THE PATIENT

Joanna Chikwe, Farzan Filsoufi, and Alain Carpentier

A heart valve prosthesis consists of an orifice through which blood flows and an occluding mechanism that closes and opens the orifice. There are two classes of prosthetic heart valves (PHVs): *mechanical prostheses*, with rigid, manufactured occluders; and *biological* or *tissue valves*, with flexible leaflet occluders of animal or human origin. Among the mechanical valves, there are three basic types, depending on whether the occluding mechanism is a reciprocating ball, a tilting disk, or two semicircular hinged leaflets. The biological valves include those whose origin is from the patient, from another human, or from another species.

## PROSTHETIC HEART VALVES

### ■ MECHANICAL VALVES

The first successful PHV, which led to long-term survivors, used a ball-in-cage design and was introduced in 1960. Then came the low-profile disk valves in the early 1970s, followed by bileaflet valves since the early 1980s. Currently, most mechanical valves being implanted are bileaflet valves. Nevertheless, the "current" Starr-Edwards ball valves (models A1200/A1260 and M6120) that were introduced in 1965 have endured until today.

### ■ BIOLOGICAL VALVES

Bioprosthesis (heterograft or xenograft) is a term that was introduced by Carpentier for non-viable valves of biological origin, such as the porcine and bovine pericardial valves. Bioprostheses are mounted on rigid or flexible stents (stented) to which the leaflets and the sewing ring are attached. Nonstented versions are also available (stentless). Pericardial valves are tailored and sewn into a valvular configuration using bovine pericardium as a fabric, resulting in a valve that opens more completely than a porcine valve and thus provides better hemodynamics. Other biological valves are homografts (or allograft) and autografts. A homograft valve is transplanted from another human; the homograft is obtained at autopsy.

# ■ CHOICE OF PROSTHETIC HEART VALVE

The most frequent issue is whether to choose a mechanical or bioprosthetic PHV. The choice is based on balancing the advantages and disadvantages of these two types of PHV (**Tables 35-1** and **35-2**). Mechanical valves are durable but have the problem of thrombogenicity, and thus require lifetime anticoagulation therapy. Biological valves have low thrombogenicity but have the problem of structural valve deterioration (SVD), and thus the risk of reoperation. **Figure 35-1** shows the recommendations based on age (and therefore rate of SVD) and ability to take warfarin anticoagulant therapy. **Figure 35-2** shows the factors to be considered in the choice of PHV for young women with valvular heart disease. **Table 35-3** lists the American College of Cardiologists/American Heart Association (ACC/AHA) recommendations for aortic valve selection. It must be emphasized that all such recommendations cannot apply to each and every patient because there are exceptions, and several factors that must be considered are shown in Table 35-2.

# MANAGEMENT

Patients who have undergone valve replacement are not cured; they still have serious heart disease. They have exchanged native valvular disease for prosthetic valvular disease, and must be followed with great care. **Table 35-4** lists major complications of valve replacement.

Valve prosthesis–patient mismatch (VP–PM) is a unique complication that is commonly underappreciated in clinical practice. No PHV currently used has an effective orifice as large as that of the native valve; consequently, VP–PM occurs. This issue is most relevant in a large patient in whom a prosthesis that is considered "small" in relation to body size was placed for technical reasons. The resulting VP–PM (**Table 35-5**) contributes to incomplete relief of symptoms. Patients with VP–PM have been reported to have worse short-term and long-term outcomes.

---

**TABLE 35-1.** Factors Influencing Operative and Late Mortality After PHV[a]

- Decade of age
- Other valve disease
- Complications of PHV
- Comorbid conditions
- Cardiac
  LV dysfunction, heart failure, NYHA functional class III and IV, CAD, myocardial infarction, CABG, arrhythmias (eg, atrial fibrillation), pulmonary hypertension
- Noncardiac
  Impaired renal function (creatinine clearance), renal dialysis, diabetes, hypertension, dyslipidemia, metabolic syndrome, smoking, liver disease, lung disease (eg, COPD)

CABG, coronary artery bypass graft; CAD, coronary artery disease; COPD, chronic obstructive pulmonary disease; LV, left ventricle; NYHA, New York Heart Association; PHV, prosthetic heart valve.

[a]For operative (30-day mortality) additional factors include emergency surgery > urgent > elective; previous cardiac surgery; perioperative myocardial infarction; and duration of the operation and of aortic cross-clamp time.

Copyright by S. H. Rahimtoola.

**TABLE 35-2.** Deciding Which Prosthetic Heart Valve to Choose

Age of the patient
Comorbid conditions
Expected life span of patient
Long-term known outcomes with prosthetic heart valve
Experience with procedure(s) and prosthetic heart valves by surgical team
Patient's "wishes"
Other extenuating circumstances

Copyright by S. H. Rahimtoola.

All patients with prosthetic valves need appropriate antibiotics for prophylaxis against infective endocarditis (Chapter 37). Patients with rheumatic heart disease continue to need antibiotics as prophylaxis against the recurrence of rheumatic carditis. Adequate antithrombotic therapy is needed for appropriate patients (Chapter 37).

Several syndromes are peculiar to the postoperative period. The postperfusion syndrome usually appears in the third or fourth postoperative week. It is characterized by fever, splenomegaly, and atypical lymphocytes; it is benign and self-limited. The post-pericardiotomy syndrome is characterized by fever and pleuropericarditis. It usually develops in the second or third postoperative week, but can appear as late as 1 year after surgery and sometimes recurs. Although this syndrome is usually self-limited, most patients benefit from taking anti-inflammatory drugs, such as aspirin

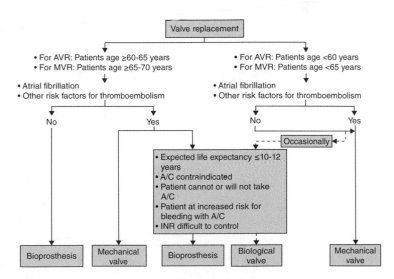

**FIGURE 35-1.** Suggested recommendation for choice of prosthetic heart valves based on age of the patient and the presence of risk factors. (A/C, anticoagulation with warfarin; AVR, aortic valve replacement; INR, international normalized ratio; MVR, mitral valve replacement.) (Rahimtoola SH. Choice of prosthetic heart valve in adult patients. *J Am Coll Cardiol.* 2003;41:893-904.)

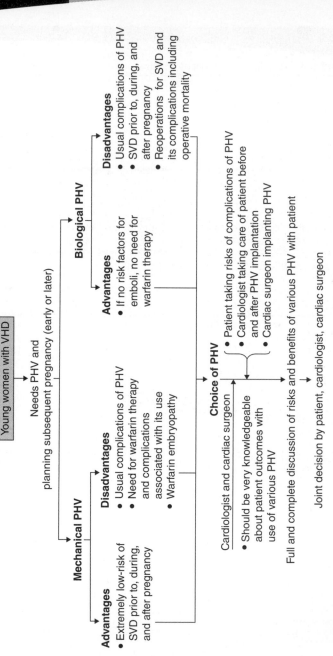

**FIGURE 35-2.** Factors to be considered in the choice of prosthetic heart valve (PHV) for young women with valvular heart disease (VHD). (SVD, structural valve deterioration.) (Hung L, Rahimtoola SH. Prosthetic heart valve and pregnancy. *Circulation.* 2003;107:1240-1246.)

**TABLE 35-3.** Major Criteria for Aortic Valve Selection[a]

**Class I**
1. A mechanical prosthesis is recommended for aortic valve replacement (AVR) in patients with a mechanical valve in the mitral or tricuspid position. (*Level of Evidence: C*)
2. A bioprostheses is recommended for AVR in patients of any age who will not take warfarin or who have major medical contraindications to warfarin therapy. (*Level of Evidence: C*)

**Class IIa**
1. Patient preference is a reasonable consideration in the selection of aortic valve operation and valve prosthesis. A mechanical prosthesis is reasonable for AVR in patients less than 65 years of age who do not have a contraindication for anticoagulation. A bioprosthesis is reasonable for AVR in patients less than 65 years of age who elect to receive this valve for lifestyle considerations after detailed discussions of the risk of anticoagulation versus the likelihood that a second AVR may be necessary in the future. (*Level of Evidence: C*)
2. A bioprosthesis is reasonable for AVR in patients aged 65 years or older without risk factors for thromboembolism. (*Level of Evidence: C*)
3. Aortic valve re-replacement with a homograft is reasonable for patients with active prosthetic valve endocarditis. (*Level of Evidence: C*)

**Class IIb**
1. A bioprosthesis might be considered for AVR in a woman of childbearing age. (*Level of Evidence: C*)

[a]See also Chapter 59.

Data from American College of Cardiology/American Heart Association Task Force on Practice Guidelines; Society of Cardiovascular Anesthesiologists; Society for Cardiovascular Angiography and Interventions; Society of Thoracic Surgeons; Bonow RO, Carabello BA, Kanu C, et al. ACC/AHA 2006 guidelines for the management of patients with valvular heart disease: a report of the American College of Cardiology/American Heart Association Task Force on Practice Guidelines (Writing Committee to revise the 1998 guidelines for the management of patients with valvular heart disease). developed in collaboration with the Society of Cardiovascular Anesthesiologists: endorsed by the Society for Cardiovascular Angiography and Interventions and the Society of Thoracic Surgeons. *Circulation*. 2006;114(5):e84-e231.

**TABLE 35-4.** Major Complications of Valve Replacement

1. Operative mortality
2. Perioperative myocardial infarction
3. Prosthetic endocarditis
4. Prosthetic dehiscence
5. Prosthetic dysfunction
   a. Obstruction: usually thrombotic, occasionally caused by item 3, 4, or 8
   b. Regurgitation
   c. Hemolysis
   d. Structural failure
6. Thromboemboli
7. Hemorrhage with anticoagulant therapy
8. Valve prosthesis–patient mismatch
9. Prosthetic replacement often caused by items 3, 4, or 5; occasionally caused by items 6, 7, or 8
10. Late mortality, including sudden, unexplained death

Reproduced with permission from Rahimtoola SH. Valvular. Heart disease: a perspective. *J Am Coll Cardiol*. 1983;3:199-215.

**TABLE 35-5.** Valve Prosthesis–Patient Mismatch

| Aortic Valve | | |
| --- | --- | --- |
| Severity of Stenosis and of VP–PM after AVR | Valve Area (cm²/m²) | Clinical Status |
| Mild | >0.9 | Asymptomatic |
| Moderate | >0.6-0.9 | Asymptomatic (symptoms with associated conditions) |
| Severe | ≤0.6 | Asymptomatic or symptomatic[a] |
| Mitral Valve | | |
| Severity of Mitral Valve Stenosis and VP–PM after MVR | Valve Area (cm²) | Clinical Status |
| Very mild | >2.0 cm² | Asymptomatic |
| Mild | >1.5-2.0 | Asymptomatic |
| Moderate | 1.1-1.5 | Usually asymptomatic |
| Severe | ≤1.0 cm² | Asymptomatic or symptomatic[b] |

AVR, aortic valve replacement; MVR, mitral valve replacement; VP–PM, valve prosthesis–patient mismatch.

[a]Symptoms: angina, syncope, dyspnea, heart failure, sudden death.

[b]Symptoms associated with left atrial and pulmonary arterial hypertension and low/reduced cardiac output and their consequences.

Reproduced with permission from Rahimtoola SH. Choice of prosthetic heart valve in adult patients. *J Am Coll Cardiol*. 2003;41:893-904.

or indomethacin; a short course of glucocorticoids is also occasionally required. Even though the pericardium is left open at the end of surgery, cardiac tamponade may occur during the first 6 weeks and needs to be relieved. Usually, anticoagulants have been given and the fluid is hemorrhagic. The recommendations for follow-up are shown in **Table 35-6**.

Echocardiography/Doppler is the most useful and practical noninvasive test for assessing valvular function. Fluoroscopy is particularly helpful with mechanical valves since echocardiographic artifacts from the valve can make interpretation difficult.

Pregnancy with PHV poses unique challenges but can be successfully managed through collaboration of the cardiologist and obstetrician (Figures 35-2 and **35-3**).

"Heart failure" after valve replacement may be the result of (1) persistent preoperative left ventricular dysfunction, (2) perioperative myocardial injury, (3) progression of other valve disease, (4) complications of PHV, or (5) associated heart disease such as CAD and systemic arterial hypertension.

Any patient with a PHV who does not improve after the surgery or who later shows deterioration of functional capacity should undergo appropriate testing to determine the cause. For the patient with catastrophic dysfunction, surgery is clearly indicated and urgent.

The management of antithrombotic therapy following valve replacement is discussed in Chapter 37.

**TABLE 35-6.** Suggestions for Follow-Up Strategy of Patient With Prosthetic Heart Valve

History, physical examination, ECG, chest radiograph, echocardiogram/Doppler, complete blood count, serum chemistries, and INR (if indicated) at first postoperative outpatient evaluation.[a]
Radionuclide angiography/CMR to assess LV function if result of echocardiography/Doppler is unsatisfactory.
CMR to assess native and PHV function if results of echocardiography/Doppler are unsatisfactory.
Routine follow-up visits at yearly intervals with earlier reevaluations for change in clinical status.
Routine serial echocardiograms at time of annual follow-up visit at 5 years after bioprosthetic MVR and at 8 years after bioprosthetic AVR even in the absence of change in clinical status.
Other tests, if indicated.

AVR, aortic valve replacement; CMR, cardiovascular magnetic resonance; INR, international normalized ratio; LV, left ventricle; MVR, mitral valve replacement; PHV, prosthetic heart valve.

[a]This evaluation should be performed 4 to 6 weeks after hospital discharge. In some settings, the outpatient echocardiogram may be difficult to obtain; if so, an inpatient echocardiogram may be obtained before hospital discharge. An echocardiogram/Doppler study at 6 to 12 months is essential for proper assessment of severity of valve prosthesis–patient mismatch.

Copyright by S. H. Rahimtoola.

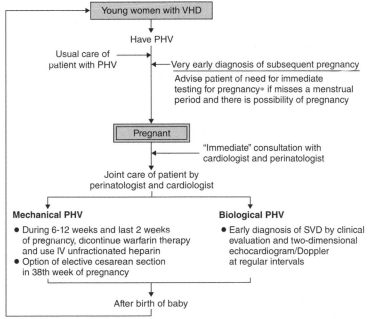

**FIGURE 35-3.** Management of the patient with prosthetic heart valve who becomes pregnant. (PHV, prosthetic heart valve; SVD, structural valve deterioration; VHD, valvular heart disease.) (Hung L, Rahimtoola SH. Prosthetic heart valve and pregnancy. *Circulation*. 2003;107;1240-1246.)

## SUGGESTED READINGS

Chikwe J, Filsoufi F, and Carpentier A. Prosthetic heart valves. In: Fuster V, O'Rourke RA, Walsh R, et al., eds. *Hurst's The Heart*. 13th ed. New York, NY: McGraw-Hill; 2008;80:1757-1773.

Bonow RO, Carabello B, Chatterjee K, et al. ACC/AHA 2006 guidelines for the management of patients with valvular heart disease: a report of the American College of Cardiology/American Heart Association Task Force on Practice Guidelines (writing committee to revise the 1998 Guidelines for the Management of Patients with Valvular Heart Disease). Developed in collaboration with the Society of Cardiovascular Anesthesiologists. Endorsed by the Society for Cardiovascular Angiography and Interventions and the Society of Thoracic Surgeons. *Circulation*. 2006;114:e84-e231. Erratum appears in *Circulation*. 2007;115:e409.

Hung L, Rahimtoola SH. Prosthetic heart valve and pregnancy. *Circulation*. 2003;107;1240-1246.

McAnulty JH, Rahimtoola SH. Antithrombotic therapy for valvular heart disease. In: Fuster V, Alexander RW, O'Rourke RA, et al., eds. *Hurst's The Heart*. 12th ed. New York, NY: McGraw-Hill; 2008:1800-1807.

Rahimtoola SH. Choice of prosthetic heart valve in adult patients. *J Am Coll Cardiol*. 2003;41:893-904.

# CHAPTER 36
# ANTITHROMBOTIC THERAPY FOR VALVULAR HEART DISEASE

## Usman Baber and Valentin Fuster

Although bleeding is a risk with all antithrombotic agents, the frequency and consequences of a stroke outweigh the bleeding risks associated with antithrombotic therapy in most patients with valve disease. This is particularly true in patients with prosthetic heart valves (PHV), but is also true in patients with native valve disease accompanied by comorbid conditions associated with thromboemboli (**Table 36-1**).

Antithrombotic therapy includes antiplatelet agents and anticoagulants. Warfarin, aspirin, unfractionated heparin, and thrombolytic agents are the only antithrombotic agents currently recommended for preventing or treating thromboemboli related to valve disease, although low-molecular-weight heparin is also widely used. The role of other antiplatelet agents, such as clopidogrel, prasugrel, and ticagrelor, and anticoagulants, such as dabigatran and apixaban, remain to be studied in the prevention of thromboemboli associated with valvular heart disease. *There are no randomized trials and few comparative data to guide therapy in preventing thromboemboli in patients with valve disease.*

## NATIVE VALVE DISEASE

Patients with native valve disease require antithrombotic therapy only in the presence of an associated stroke *risk factor*. The two most common associated risk factors are atrial fibrillation and left ventricular (LV) systolic dysfunction.

## ■ RISK OF THROMBOEMBOLI WITH NATIVE VALVE DISEASE

### Atrial Fibrillation

In six large, prospective, randomized trials assessing the value of antithrombotic therapy for primary stroke prevention in patients with nonvalvular, permanent or paroxysmal, atrial fibrillation, the embolic rate (essentially a stroke) was 3% to 8% per year in the placebo arm. Some patients in the studies had valve disease, although patients with severe valvular disease (including all with mitral stenosis or PHV) were excluded. When an individual with native valve disease has associated intermittent or continuous atrial fibrillation, *antithrombotic treatment should be initiated according to the thromboembolic risk as determined by the CHADS2 score (see Chapter 10). In general, most patients will require chronic anticoagulation to minimize thromboembolic risk.*

**TABLE 36-1.** Valve Disease and Antithrombotic Therapy

1. Prevention of thromboemboli should be addressed each time a patient with valve disease is seen.
2. Lifelong antithrombotic therapy is required in patients with atrial fibrillation (paroxysmal or persistent), severe left ventricular dysfunction, or prior thromboembolism.
3. Warfarin therapy is required in all patients with a mechanical prosthesis (see Table 36-2).
4. Antithrombotic therapy should be started early after valve surgery.
5. Warfarin should be avoided in the first trimester of pregnancy.
6. Antithrombotic therapy should be individualized during noncardiac surgery and cardiovascular procedures.

## Left Ventricular Dysfunction

For every decrease in ejection fraction of 5 percentage points, the stroke risk increases by 18% and is almost two-fold when the ejection fraction is <28% when compared to >35%. While antithrombotic therapy is of unproven value, the risk of an embolic event is sufficient that, with or without valve disease, consideration should be given to treatment. Warfarin (INR 2-3) may be considered if the LV ejection fraction (EF) is ≤0.30. There is little evidence that aspirin provides any meaningful benefit.

## Previous Thromboemboli

A thromboembolic event defines patients who are at high risk for having a recurrent event in clinical situations unrelated to native valve disease (eg, in patients with atrial fibrillation or with a PHV). It is unclear whether this is true in patients with native valve disease, but lifelong warfarin therapy should be considered if there are no contraindications to its use.

## ◼ PROSTHETIC HEART VALVES

All patients with mechanical valves require warfarin therapy. Even with the use of warfarin, the risk of thromboemboli in these patients is 1% to 2% per year. The risk of an embolus in patients with biological valves in sinus rhythm is approximately 0.6% to 0.7% per year without antithrombotic therapy.

## ◼ ANTITHROMBOTIC TREATMENT FOR PROSTHETIC VALVES

**Table 36-2** gives an overview of antithrombotic treatment for prosthetic valves.

## Mechanical Valves

All patients with mechanical valves require anticoagulation, usually with warfarin. In patients with an aortic prosthesis without risk factors for emboli, the INR should be between 2.0 and 3.0; in those with risk factors and those with a mitral prosthesis, the INR should be between 2.5 and 3.5. The addition of low-dose aspirin (70-100 mg/d) to warfarin therapy further decreases the risk of thromboembolism and is recommended unless there is a contraindication.

## Biological (Tissue) Valves

Because of an increased risk of thromboemboli during the *first 3 months* after implantation of a biological prosthetic valve, anticoagulation with warfarin is indicated.

**TABLE 36-2.** Antithrombotic Therapy—Prosthetic Heart Valves[a]

| | Mechanical Prosthetic Valves | | | Biological Prosthetic Valves | | |
|---|---|---|---|---|---|---|
| | Warfarin INR 2-3 | Warfarin INR 2.5-3.5 | Aspirin 50-100 mg | Warfarin INR 2-3 | Warfarin INR 2.5-3.5 | Aspirin 50-100 mg |
| First 3 months after valve replacement | | + | ± | | + | ± |
| After first 3 months | | | | | | |
| Aortic valve | + | | ± | | | + |
| Aortic valve + risk factor[b] | + | | + | + | | + |
| Aortic valve + embolus[c] | | + | + | + | | + |
| Mitral valve | | + | ± | | | + |
| Mitral valve + risk factor | | + | + | | + | ± |
| Mitral valve + embolism[c] | | + | + | | + | + |

+, For prevention of thrombosis on prosthetic values; ±, may prevent prosthetic clots; clinical judgment very important for addition of aspirin therapy; INR, international normalized ratio.

[a]Depending on the clinical status of patient, antithrombic therapy must be individualized (see special situations in text).

[b]Risk factors: atrial fibrillation, left ventricle dysfunction, and hypercoagulable state.

[c]Embolus = previous thromboembolism.

Note: In an individual patient, there is a need for clinical judgment ± if aspirin is added to warfarin therapy.

After that time, the tissue valve can be treated in the same way as native valve disease, and warfarin can be discontinued in approximately two-thirds of patients with biological valves. *Associated atrial fibrillation or an LV ejection fraction ≤30% are reasons for lifelong warfarin therapy.*

# SPECIAL CLINICAL SITUATIONS

*In the following situations, there are no randomized studies to provide evidence-based recommendations, so clinical judgment and individualized approaches that weigh the conflicting risks of bleeding and thrombosis are always necessary.*

## ■ SURGERY AND DENTAL CARE

Although antithrombotic therapy must be individualized, some generalizations apply. For procedures in which bleeding is unlikely or would be inconsequential if it occurred, antithrombotic therapy should not be stopped. This can apply to surgery on the skin, dental prophylaxis, or simple treatment for dental caries.

When bleeding is likely or its potential consequences are severe, antithrombotic treatment should be altered. If a patient is on aspirin, it should be discontinued 1 week before the procedure and restarted as soon as it is considered safe by the surgeon or dentist.

For most patients taking warfarin, the drug should be stopped 72 hours before the procedure to achieve an INR ≤1.5. Unless postoperative hemorrhage occurs, warfarin can be restarted within 24 hours after the procedure. Admission to the hospital or a delay in discharge to give heparin is usually unnecessary. Deciding who is at very high risk of thrombosis and thus should require "bridging" with heparin until warfarin can be reinstated may be difficult; clinical judgment is required. Heparin can usually be reserved for patients who have had a prior thromboembolism, patients with demonstrated thrombotic problems when previously off therapy, and patients with two or more risk factors. When used, heparin should be started 24 hours after warfarin is stopped (ie, 48 hours before surgery) and stopped 6 to 12 hours before the procedure. Heparin should be restarted as early, after surgery, as bleeding stability allows and the partial thromboplastin time (aPTT) maintained at a "therapeutic level" until warfarin is restarted and the desired INR can be achieved. Home administration and management of unfractionated heparin (and warfarin) or low-molecular-weight heparins are often used to minimize hospitalization but such practices remain outside the specific guideline recommendations.

## ■ CARDIAC CATHETERIZATION AND ANGIOGRAPHY

Neither antiplatelet therapy nor heparin generally need to be stopped for these procedures. Cardiac catheterization can be performed with a patient taking warfarin, but preferably, the drug should be stopped 72 hours before the procedure and restarted after the procedure on the same day. If a patient is at very high risk of thromboembolism, heparin should be started 48 hours before the procedure and continued until warfarin is restarted and the desired INR is achieved.

## ■ CORONARY ARTERY STENTS

Many patients with valve disease require a stent as treatment for coronary artery disease. A thienopyridine agent, usually clopidogrel, is used for at least 1 month (and up to 12 months or more for drug-eluting stents) to prevent stent thrombosis. Clopidogrel has no proven efficacy in preventing thromboemboli in patients with a PHV, so continuation of warfarin is recommended in patients with mechanical prostheses. If these patients are also on aspirin (along with warfarin), it would seem prudent that it be stopped given the concerns of bleeding, but this is unproved. Patients with tissue valves taking aspirin should continue that drug after stent insertion.

## ■ PREGNANCY

Indications for antithrombotic therapy are not altered by pregnancy but treatment regimens have to be adjusted due to risks to fetal development and concerns for fetal and maternal bleeding. The incidence of warfarin-related embryopathy is 3% to 25% when the drug is taken in the first 3 months (particularly weeks 6 to 12) and it may be dose related. Heparin does not cross the placenta, but like warfarin, can be ineffective or cause maternal bleeding. Given these concerns, it is recommended that the pregnant woman requiring anticoagulation use heparin for the first 3 months and then switch to warfarin. At 1 to 3 weeks before anticipated labor and delivery, warfarin should be discontinued and heparin restarted. The use of low-molecular-weight heparin should be individualized.

## ■ THERAPY AT THE TIME OF A THROMBOEMBOLIC EVENT

### Acute Management

Data and opinions about optimal timing for initiating or continuing anticoagulants in patients in whom an embolus is the presumed cause of a stroke are conflicting. Antithrombotic therapy should be withheld or stopped for 72 hours because of excessive rates of conversion from nonhemorrhagic to hemorrhagic stroke. If a computed tomography (CT) scan at 3 days reveals little or no hemorrhage, heparin should be administered to maintain an aPTT at the lower end of the therapeutic level until warfarin, started at the same time, results in the desired INR. If the CT scan demonstrates significant hemorrhage, antithrombotic therapy should be withheld until the bleed has been treated or has stabilized (7-14 days). Concomitant involvement of neurologist is strongly suggested since therapy must usually be highly individualized.

### Long-Term Management

If the embolic event occurs when a patient is *off* antithrombotic therapy, long-term warfarin therapy is required. If the embolic event occurs while the patient is *on* adequate antithrombotic treatment for PHV, therapy should be altered as follows:

- If on warfarin, with an INR of 2 to 3: increase dose to achieve an INR of 2.5 to 3.5.
- If on warfarin, with an INR of 2.5 to 3.5: add aspirin 50 to 100 mg/d.
- If on warfarin, with an INR of 2.5 to 3.5, plus aspirin 80 to 100 mg/d: aspirin dose may also need to be increased to 325 mg/d.
- If on aspirin 325 mg/d: switch to warfarin to achieve an INR of 2 to 3.

Status of the PHV should always be reviewed in the setting of thromboembolism and PHV replacement should be considered if the valve is the likely source of the thrombus and medical management as outlined above has failed.

## ■ EXCESSIVE ANTICOAGULATION

In most patients with INR above the therapeutic range, excessive anticoagulation can be managed by withholding warfarin. Patients with PHVs with an INR of 5 to 10 who are not bleeding can be managed by withholding warfarin and administering oral vitamin K, often as an inpatient to monitor for bleeding. In emergency situations, the use of fresh-frozen plasma is preferable to high-dose vitamin $K_1$, especially *parenteral vitamin $K_1$*, because use of the latter increases the *risks of overcorrection to a hypercoagulable state and of anaphylaxis.* Human recombinant factor (rFVIIa), dose 15 to 19 µg/kg body weight, has been used to reverse critically prolonged INR and bleeding complications safely and rapidly.

## ■ THERAPY AT THE TIME OF A BLEED

With significant bleeding, antithrombotic therapy should be stopped and, if the patient is at risk, drug effects should be reversed. If possible, the cause of bleeding should be corrected and antithrombotic therapy restarted as soon as possible. If this is not possible, treatment decisions are difficult. In patients with a mechanical prosthesis or multiple risk factors for thromboemboli, acceptance of intermittent bleeding with acute management of bleeding may be necessary. In valve patients who are at lower risk of emboli or in whom the role of antithrombotic treatment is less clear (eg, LV dysfunction), it may be optimal to withhold chronic therapy or, if a patient is on warfarin, to switch to aspirin. With mechanical PHVs, consideration should be given to replacing the mechanical valve with a biologic valve in some patients (eg, in those who have had multiple, large, life- or organ-threatening bleeds).

## ■ THROMBOSIS OF PROSTHETIC HEART VALVES

PHV obstruction is caused by thrombus in approximately 50%, pannus in 10%, and pannus plus thrombus in 40% of cases. Diagnosis can be difficult, even with echocardiography (transthoracic and/or transesophageal). Pannus is tissue in-growth; therefore, thrombolytic therapy is ineffective; if obstruction is severe, valve replacement is indicated. If a patient has a thrombotic obstruction of a right-sided PHV, thrombolytics are the first choice of therapy as they are successful in 80% to 100% of treated patients.

Left-sided PHV thrombosis (aortic and mitral) is more serious and difficult. With use of thrombolytics, studies show a mortality of 2% to 16% depending on New York Heart Association (NYHA) functional status, thromboembolism in 12% to 15%, major bleeding in 5%, and nondisabling bleeding in 14%. Best results were obtained in patients who are in NYHA functional classes I and II and who have a "small" thrombus. Surgical replacement of the thrombosed PHV is associated with a mortality of 10% to 60%.

## ■ INFECTIVE ENDOCARDITIS

If a patient with valve disease develops endocarditis, continued antithrombotic therapy will need to be individualized. If the patient presents with or develops an embolic event involving the central nervous system, therapy should be as described above for acute embolic events and acute anticoagulation withheld.

## SUGGESTED READINGS

Baber U, Fuster V. Antithrombotic therapy for valvular heart disease. In: Fuster V, O'Rourke RA, Walsh R, et al, eds. *Hurst's The Heart.* 13th ed. New York, NY: McGraw-Hill;2011:81: 1774-1780.

Bates SM, Greer IA, Hirsh J, et al. Use of antithrombotic agents during pregnancy. The seventh ACCP conference on antithrombotic and thrombolytic therapy. *Chest.* 2004;126 (suppl):627S-644S.

Bonow RO, Carabello B, Chatterjee K, et al. ACC/AHA 2006 guidelines for the management of patients with valvular heart disease: a report of the American College of Cardiology/American Heart Association Task Force on Practice Guidelines (Writing Committee to Revise the 1998 Guidelines for the Management of Patients with Valvular Heart Disease). Developed in collaboration with the Society of Cardiovascular Anesthesiologists. Endorsed by the Society for Cardiovascular Angiography and Interventions and the Society of Thoracic Surgeons. *Circulation*. 2006;114:e84-e231.

Freudenberger RS, Schumaecker MM, Homma S. What is the appropriate approach to prevention of thromboembolism in heart failure? *Thromb Haemost*. 2010;103:489-495.

Salem DN, Stein PD, Al-Ahmad A, et al. Antithrombotic therapy in valvular heart disease—native and prosthetic. *Chest*. 2004;126 (suppl):457S-482S.

# CHAPTER 37
# INFECTIVE ENDOCARDITIS

Saptarsi M. Haldar and Patrick T. O'Gara

Infective endocarditis (IE) is a disease caused by microbial infection of the endothelial lining of intracardiac structures and is invariably fatal if untreated. Infection most commonly resides on one or more heart valve leaflets, but may involve mural endocardium, chordal structures, myocardium, and pericardium. The presence of an intracardiac or endovascular device provides a nidus for infection, as well as a barrier to eradication. Despite the diagnosis and treatment of IE, the 6-month mortality rates still approach 25%. Changes in both patient demographics and microbial biology have challenged conventional wisdom.

## EPIDEMIOLOGY

In the first half of the 20th century, IE was predominantly a complication of rheumatic heart disease and poor dentition. In developing countries, rheumatic heart disease remains the most frequent predisposing cardiac condition. However, the epidemiologic features in developed countries have changed considerably. With the aging of the population, an increase in the prevalence of degenerative heart valve disease and in the use of implanted heart valve substitutes and intracardiac devices are now common. The numbers of patients with chronic, predisposing medical comorbidities, such as diabetes, HIV infection, and end-stage renal disease, have also increased, as has the commensurate risk of exposure to nosocomial bacteremia, often with antibiotic resistance. These changing demographics are reflected in two observations. First, the median age of patients with IE gradually increased from 30 to 40 years in the pre-antibiotic era, to 47 to 69 years in the first decade of 21st century. Second, the incidence of IE in developed countries has remained unchanged, despite the reduction in rheumatic heart disease over the last half century.

## PATHOGENESIS

The hallmark of IE is persistent endocardial or endovascular infection causing continuous bacteremia. Importantly, IE is a relatively uncommon consequence of transient bacteremia and not all organisms can effectively colonize or invade the endovascular space. It is apparent that complex series of host–pathogen interactions conspire in the development of IE lesions, including the integrity of the vascular endothelium, the host immune system, hemostatic mechanisms, cardiac anatomic characteristics, microbial properties, and the peripheral events that cause the bacteremia. Experimental data suggest that host endothelial damage is the key predisposing insult, supported by the observation that vegetations are most likely to form in areas where blood-flow injury is likely to occur—on the ventricular side of semilunar valves and the atrial side of AV valves.

# MICROBIOLOGY

A wide range of microorganisms can cause IE, but only a few species account for the vast majority of cases. Streptococci and staphylococci are the cause of over 80% of IE cases in which a responsible organism is identified. Streptococcal species were historically the most common group of pathogens, but more recent data identify *Staphylococcus aureus* as the most frequently isolated agent worldwide. Moreover, the rate of antibiotic resistance among causative organisms is increasing.

## ■ NATIVE VALVE ENDOCARDITIS

### *Streptococci*

Viridans group streptococci, or alpha-hemolytic streptococci, are a frequent cause of community-acquired native valve endocarditis (NVE) and are responsible for 30% to 65% of cases of NVE in older children and adults. They are normal residents of the oropharynx and easily gain access to the circulation following dental or gingival trauma. The viridans streptococci comprise several species, of which *S sanguis, S bovis, S mutans,* and *S mitior* are most commonly isolated in cases of IE. *S bovis,* a normal inhabitant of the human gastrointestinal (GI) tract, is noteworthy as IE caused by this organism is strongly suggestive of GI malignancy, polyp formation, or diverticular disease. Colonoscopy should be performed when this organism is detected in the blood.

The *Enterococcus* spp., formerly classified as group D streptococci, are now defined as a distinct genus. The incidence of enterococcal endocarditis appears to be rising, responsible for 5% to 18% of cases of NVE, the vast majority of which are due to *E faecalis* (80%) or *E faecium* (10%). These organisms are normal inhabitants of the GI and genitourinary tracts and may enter the bloodstream after manipulation of the colon, urethra, or bladder (eg, Foley catheterization, colonoscopy).

Group A *Streptococcus* rarely cause IE in the contemporary era. Before 1945, however, *S pneumoniae* caused approximately 10% of IE cases, often resulting in an acute, fulminant illness associated with severe valve damage, perivalvular extension, embolic complications, pericarditis, meningitis, and high mortality (25%-50%).

Group B streptococci (eg, *S agalactiae*) are chiefly responsible for infections in the neonate and parturient, although the organism can also be isolated from diabetic foot ulcers. Risk factors for group B streptococcal bacteremia in adults include obstetric complications, diabetes, carcinoma, liver failure, alcoholism, and injection drug use (IDU).

### *Staphylococci*

*Staphylococcus aureus* causes 80% to 90% of staphylococcal IE and is the most common cause of "acute" IE. Emerging data from the International Consortium on Endocarditis (ICE) suggest that *S aureus* has become the leading cause of IE worldwide. The mucous membranes of the anterior nasopharynx are the most common sites of colonization, and approximately 30% of normal persons carry *S aureus*. High-risk individuals include patients on dialysis, type I diabetics, burn victims, persons with HIV, injection drug users, patients with certain chronic dermatologic conditions, and patients with recent surgical incisions. *S aureus* IE is frequently fulminant when it involves left-sided cardiac valves and often results in major complications such as heart failure, perivalvular extension with conduction disturbances, embolization, and metastatic infection. Not surprisingly, *S aureus* as a causative organism is an independent predictor of poor prognosis in IE and is associated with a 25% to 30% mortality rate. As many as 50% of patients with left-sided native valve IE (NVE) due to *S aureus* will require surgery. Right-sided (tricuspid valve) IE with *S aureus*, by contrast, is most frequently a complication of IDU, is associated with a high incidence of septic pulmonary embolization, but carries only a 2% to 4% case fatality rate.

The coagulase negative staphylococci (CoNS) are constituents of normal human skin flora and are much less likely to infect normal endocardial surfaces. *S epidermidis* is an important causative agent in prosthetic valve and device-related endocarditis. NVE caused by CoNS occurs mainly in patients with preexisting valvular heart disease.

## Gram-Negative Bacilli

IE due to gram-negative bacilli (GNB) is uncommon and tends to occur in IDUs, immunocompromised patients, patients with advanced liver disease, and prosthetic heart valve recipients. The fastidious gram-negative rods of the HACEK (*Haemophilus* species, *Actinobacillus actinomycetemcomitans, Cardiobacterium hominis, Eikenella corrodens,* and *Kingella* species) group reside normally in the oropharynx and are responsible for a very small (~1%) proportion of cases of NVE, usually involving abnormal valve tissue. Because of their growth requirements ($CO_2$), they may take 3 to 4 weeks to grow in culture and have gained notoriety for their implicated role in certain cases of culture-negative IE.

The ricksettial organism, *Coxiella burnetii,* is the causative agent of Q fever and is a relevant cause of IE in areas where cattle, sheep, and goat farming are common. Cases of IE caused by *C burnetii* are well documented in the developed world. As the organism is extremely difficult to culture, the diagnosis is best made serologically using antibody titers. *Bartonella* species, the etiologic agent in cat scratch disease, have been recently described as an important cause of IE among both homeless men and HIV-infected patients. The diagnosis can be confirmed with special culture or polymerase chain reaction (PCR) techniques.

## Fungal IE

Fungal endocarditis is a relatively new syndrome associated with exceedingly high mortality (survival rates <20%). Patients who develop fungal IE often have multiple predisposing conditions that include an immunocompromised state, the use of endovascular devices, and previous reconstructive cardiac surgery. *Candida* and *Aspergillus* species are the most common causes of fungal IE and are associated with large, bulky vegetations that can obstruct valve orifices and embolize to large vessels. Blood cultures are usually positive in cases of *Candida* IE, whereas they are rarely positive with *Aspergillus*. Fungal endocarditis is an indication for surgical replacement of an infected valve. Cure usually requires combination fungicidal (amphotericin) and surgical treatment, followed by long-term suppressive therapy with an oral antifungal agent.

## Culture-Negative IE

Blood cultures are negative in up to 20% of patients with IE diagnosed by strict criteria. Failure to isolate a microorganism may be the result of inadequate culture technique, a highly fastidious organism or a nonbacterial pathogen as the causative agent, or previous administration of antimicrobial therapy prior to blood culture acquisition. The latter is an extremely important consideration as the administration of antibiotics prior to drawing blood cultures can reduce the recovery rate of bacterial pathogens by nearly one-third. There are numerous noninfectious causes of endocarditis that may behave like culture negative IE, including those that are related to neoplasia (nonbacterial thrombotic endocarditis, NBTE), autoimmune diseases (antiphospholipid antibody syndrome, SLE), or the post-cardiac surgical state (thrombi, stitches).

## ■ PROSTHETIC VALVE ENDOCARDITIS

Prosthetic valve endocarditis (PVE) represents approximately 10% to 30% of all IE cases. Although many of the general principles applicable to native valve IE are relevant, there are important considerations specific to PVE (see also Chapter 35). After valve replacement, the incidence of PVE is approximately 1% to 3% at 1 year and 3% to 6% at 5 years. Although the current evidence is not definitive, PVE can be broadly divided into two groups based on the time of onset after valve surgery—early PVE and late PVE. Early PVE is defined as endocarditis that develops within the first 2 months to 1 year after valve surgery. During this period, the vast majority of causative organisms are nosocomially acquired with a predominance of staphylococci, notably coagulase-negative species (*S epidermidis*). In contrast to early PVE, the spectrum of causative organisms in late PVE resembles that of NVE. Complication rates with PVE are high and surgery is often required even in the absence of documented perivalvular extension.

# APPROACH TO THE PATIENT WITH SUSPECTED INFECTIVE ENDOCARDITIS

The history should focus on predisposing factors such as IDU, a prior history of IE, recent exposures, the presence of an intracardiac device or indwelling central venous catheter, congenital or acquired valvular heart disease, and other congenital heart disease. The patient may report fever, fatigue, anorexia, weight loss, night sweats, joint pain, or back pain. Features on clinical examination that raise suspicion for IE include fever, a new heart murmur, signs of heart failure, and vascular and immunologic phenomena. Examples of classic IE-related findings (**Fig. 37-1**) include major arterial emboli with pulse deficits, septic pulmonary emboli (with right-sided IE),

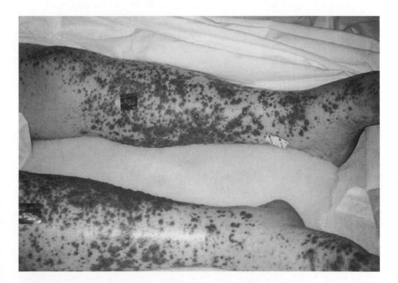

**FIGURE 37-1.** Cutaneous purpura fulminans in a patient with *S abiotrophia* native valve endocarditis of the mitral and aortic valves.

mycotic brain aneurysms with intracranial hemorrhage, mucosal or conjunctival petechiae, splinter hemorrhages of the nailbeds, palpable purpuric skin rashes, Janeway lesions (small, flat, irregular erythematous spots on the palms and soles), Osler nodes (tender, erythematous nodules occurring in the pulp of the fingers), Roth spots (cytoid bodies and associated hemorrhage caused by microinfarction of retinal vessels), and urinary red cell casts suggestive of glomerulonephritis.

The diagnosis of IE rests on the ability to demonstrate endocardial involvement of infection and persistent bacteremia. The proper acquisition of blood cultures prior to initiation of antimicrobial therapy is essential. Echocardiography should be used to assess for the presence of endocardial involvement (vegetations, abscess formation, and new valvular regurgitation). These clinical, microbiologic, and echocardiographic features are the foundation for the Modified Duke Criteria, a set of integrated findings, which has become the standard for diagnosis of IE (**Tables 37-1** and **37-2**).

Once the diagnosis is made and appropriate therapy initiated, patients should be closely monitored for complications and repeat blood cultures should be obtained to ensure sterilization. Persistent fever beyond 1 week of appropriate therapy should raise suspicion for intracardiac extension or satellite abscess formation. In the absence of complications, the first several days of intravenous antibiotics are administered in the hospital and the remaining course provided via a central venous catheter (PICC line) as an outpatient with careful follow-up. Patients should be maintained on telemetry while in hospital; the need for surveillance electrocardiograms (ECGs) during outpatient therapy is dictated by the location of the infection and the predicted likelihood of conduction disturbances. Patients should also be monitored for antimicrobial toxicity, particularly with aminoglycoside use. Routine surveillance echocardiography during therapy is not necessary unless complications develop or cardiac surgery is considered. At the completion of therapy, transthoracic echocardiography (TTE) may be performed to establish a new "post-IE baseline." After successful therapy, patients with IE should be followed longitudinally for progressive valvular and ventricular dysfunction. Patients with successfully treated IE are at high risk for the development of future episodes of IE and should receive antibiotic prophylaxis for procedures, as recommended by current guidelines.

# ◼ DIAGNOSIS OF INFECTIVE ENDOCARDITIS

Ineffective endocarditis is defined as an infection on any structure within the heart, including on normal or damaged endothelial surfaces (eg, myocardium and valvular structures), prosthetic heart valves, and implanted devices (eg, pacemakers, ICDs, ventricular assist devices, and surgical shunts). The diagnosis of IE relies chiefly on the following factors: (1) an initial clinical suspicion, especially in a patient with identifiable risk factors; (2) microbiologic data (blood cultures demonstrating continuous bacteremia or cultures of vegetative lesions removed surgically); and (3) the results of echocardiographic imaging. Diagnosis is straightforward in only a minority of patients who present with a defined predisposing condition and the classic manifestations of fever, evidence of active valvulitis, peripheral emboli, immunologic or vascular phenomena, and bacteremia. In the majority of patients, however, IE has an extremely variable clinical presentation.

# ◼ CLINICAL CRITERIA

The modified Duke criteria (see Tables 37-1 and 37-2) have become the current standard for diagnosis and clinical research and have been validated in numerous subsequent studies. A diagnosis of "definite IE" is established clinically by evidence of two major criteria, one major plus three minor criteria, or five minor criteria. Patients identified with "possible IE" (one major plus one minor criterion or three minor criteria) should be treated for IE until the diagnosis is satisfactorily excluded.

**TABLE 37-1.** Definition of Terms Used in the Proposed Modified Duke Criteria for the Diagnosis of Infective Endocarditis[a]

**Major Criteria**

Blood culture positive for IE

Typical microorganisms consistent with IE from two separate blood cultures:

Viridans streptococci, *Streptococcus bovis*, HACEK group, *Staphylococcus aureus*; or community-acquired enterococci in the absence of a primary focus; or

Microorganisms consistent with IE from persistently positive blood cultures, defined as follows:

At least two positive cultures of blood samples drawn more than 12 h apart; or

All of three or a majority of greater than four separate cultures of blood (with first and last sample drawn at least 1 h apart)

**Single positive blood culture for *Coxiella burnetii* or anti-phase 1 IgG antibody titer greater than 1:800**

Evidence of endocardial involvement

Echocardiogram positive for IE (TEE recommended in patients with prosthetic valves, rated at least "possible IE" by clinical criteria, or complicated IE [paravalvular abscess]; TTE as first test in other patients), defined as follows:

Oscillating intracardiac mass on valve or supporting structures, in the path of regurgitant jets, or on implanted material in the absence of an alternative anatomic explanation; or

Abscess; or

New partial dehiscence of prosthetic valve

New valvular regurgitation (worsening or changing of preexisting murmur not sufficient)

**Minor Criteria**

Predisposition, predisposing heart condition, or injection drug use

Fever, temperature greater than 38°C

Vascular phenomena, major arterial emboli, septic pulmonary infarcts, mycotic aneurysm, intracranial hemorrhage, conjunctival

Hemorrhages, and Janeway lesions

Immunologic phenomena; glomerulonephritis, Osler nodes, Roth spots, and rheumatoid factor

Microbiological evidence: positive blood culture but does not meet a major criterion,[b] or serologic evidence of active infection

With organism consistent with IE

**Echocardiographic minor criteria eliminated**

IE, infective endocarditis; TEE, transesophageal echocardiography; TTE, transthoracic echocardiography.

[a]Modifications are shown in bold type.

[b]Excludes single positive cultures for coagulase-negative staphylococci and organisms that do not cause endocarditis.

Reprinted with permission from Li JS, Sexton DJ, Mick N, et al. Proposed modifications to the Duke criteria for diagnosis of infective endocarditis. *Clin Infect Dis.* 2000;30:8.

The importance of obtaining blood cultures by appropriate methods, prior to the institution of antibiotics, cannot be overemphasized. Three separate sets of blood cultures obtained from different venipuncture sites over 24 hours are recommended.

# ■ ECHOCARDIOGRAPHY IN INFECTIVE ENDOCARDITIS

All patients with suspected IE should undergo prompt echocardiographic assessment. There are several TTE findings suggestive of endocarditis, including vegetations,

**TABLE 37-2.** Definition of Infective Endocarditis According to the Proposed Modified Duke Criteria[a]

Definite infective endocarditis
  Pathologic criteria
    (1) Microorganisms demonstrated by culture or histological examination of a vegetation, a vegetation that has embolized; or Intracardiac abscess specimen; or
    (2) Pathologic lesions; vegetation, or intracardiac abscess confirmed by histological examination showing active endocarditis
  Clinical criteria
    (1) Two major criteria; or
    (2) One major criterion and three minor criteria; or
    (3) Five minor criteria
  Possible infective endocarditis
    (1) **One major criterion and one minor criterion;** or
    (2) **Three minor criteria**
  Rejected
    (1) Firm alternate diagnosis explaining evidence of infective endocarditis; or
    (2) Resolution of infective endocarditis syndrome with antibiotic therapy for less than 4 days; or
    (3) No pathologic evidence of infective endocarditis at surgery or autopsy, with antibiotic therapy for less than 4 days; or
    (4) Does not meet criteria for possible infective endocarditis, as noted above

[a]Modifications are shown in bold type.

Reprinted with permission from Li JS, Sexton DJ, Mick N, et al. Proposed modifications to the Duke criteria for the diagnosis of infective endocarditis. *Clin Infect Dis.* 2000;30:633-638.

evidence of periannular tissue destruction, aneurysms or fistula formation, leaflet perforation, or prosthetic valve dehiscence.

Although there remains some debate regarding the optimal initial approach, the vast majority of patients undergo transthoracic (TTE) imaging first because of its immediate availability. A low threshold to pursue transesophageal (TEE) imaging is appropriate, as dictated by the clinical circumstances, the adequacy of the TTE images, and the potential need for early surgical planning and intervention. The performance characteristics of TTE and TEE are summarized in **Table 37-3**. TEE should be performed expeditiously in patients with high-risk clinical features at presentation (eg, suspected *S aureus* infection of the aortic valve and root), known congenital heart disease, or suboptimal TTE images. For patients undergoing cardiac surgery for IE, intraoperative TEE is routine. TEE should also be considered for patients with catheter-associated *S aureus* bacteremia to predict the indicated duration of antibiotic therapy (ie, 2 weeks versus 4 weeks). In uncomplicated cases of IE, a single echocardiographic

**TABLE 37-3.** Aggregate Performance Characteristics of TTE and TEE in the Diagnosis of IE

|  | Sensitivity (%) | Specificity (%) |
|---|---|---|
| TTE | 60-65 | 98 |
| TEE | 85-95 | 85-98 |

study is usually sufficient. However, with complex IE, serial echocardiographic examinations may help determine prognosis and guide surgical intervention.

# ACUTE COMPLICATIONS

Complication rates with IE have remained relatively unchanged despite advances in diagnosis and antimicrobial therapy. Complications can generally be related to local extension of infection (eg, valve ring abscess, fistulae, conduction block), destruction of or interference with intracardiac structures (eg, leaflet perforation or valvular obstruction), embolization (eg, stroke, septic pulmonary emboli), bacteremia/sepsis (eg, multisystem organ failure), and immune complex disease (eg, glomerulonephritis).

## ■ HEART FAILURE

Heart failure is the most frequent major complication of IE; its development portends an adverse outcome with medical therapy alone and is usually an indication for surgical intervention. Reduced LV systolic function is the most powerful predictor of an adverse outcome following surgery. Heart failure in IE is most often related to acute, severe valvular dysfunction owing either to leaflet destruction or interference with normal coaptation. It may also occur from rupture of infected mitral chordae, obstruction due to bulky vegetations, the development of intracardiac shunts, or prosthetic valve dehiscence. Heart failure may also develop more gradually as a function of continued valve incompetence and worsening ventricular function, following otherwise successful antibiotic treatment. Heart failure is most commonly associated with aortic valve IE, followed by mitral valve, and then tricuspid valve involvement. Inappropriate bradycardia, which can develop if the infection extends into the conduction system leading to atrioventricular block or if the patient receives a β-blocker, can be catastrophic.

## ■ EMBOLIZATION

Embolization is a dreaded complication of IE. Central nervous system (CNS) involvement is most common; stroke comprises up to 65% of embolic events and may be the presenting sign of IE in up to 14% of cases. CNS embolization can present with subtle neurologic abnormalities, as seen with microembolization, or with sudden hemiplegia and obtundation, as seen with a ruptured mycotic aneurysm and intracranial hemorrhage (ICH) or with a large embolic stroke. Up to 90% of CNS emboli lodge in the distribution of the middle cerebral artery, and carry a high mortality rate. Any patient with suspected or definite IE who develops neurologic symptoms should promptly undergo neurologic imaging and be considered to have CNS embolization until proved otherwise.

Emboli may also involve other organ systems including the liver, spleen, kidneys, and lungs. Metastatic sites of infection may appear in the spine or para-spinous space, and may be the cause of prolonged fever or bacteremia despite appropriate antimicrobial therapy. Septic pulmonary emboli are present in the majority of cases of right-sided IE related to IDU.

## ■ MYCOTIC ANEURYSMS

Mycotic aneurysms (MA) represent a small but dangerous subset of embolic complications. They occur most frequently in the intracranial arteries and have a particular predilection for the middle cerebral artery and its branches. The overall mortality rate among IE patients with intracranial MAs is 60%, and approaches 80% if rupture occurs.

Screening patients with definite IE for the presence of intracranial MAs is not currently recommended and neurovascular imaging is reserved for symptomatic patients or for selected patients undergoing surgery for IE.

## ■ PERIANNULAR EXTENSION OF INFECTION

Extension or spread of infection beyond the valve annulus is a very concerning development that usually presages the need for surgical therapy. Findings such as persistent fever and bacteremia despite antibiotic therapy, heart failure, or new conduction block should raise suspicion for this complication. Periannular extension may occur in 10% to 40% of all native valve IE and >50% of prosthetic valve IE and complicates aortic valve IE more commonly than either mitral or tricuspid valve IE.

## ■ RENAL DYSFUNCTION

Renal dysfunction is a common complication of IE and is often multifactorial in nature given the high incidence of preexisting renal disease, immune complex disease, drug-induced nephrotoxicity, and hemodynamic perturbations.

# ANTIMICROBIAL THERAPY

## ■ GENERAL PRINCIPLES

Rapid institution of appropriate parenteral antibiotic therapy is the single most important initial intervention in the treatment of suspected or proven IE. Given the rising rate of antimicrobial resistance among causative organisms, therapy is predicated on the identification of the causative isolate and delineation of its antibiotic sensitivities. An infectious disease specialist should supervise the dose, duration, and method of delivery (IV or IM) of antimicrobial therapy with longitudinal follow-up. Serum antibiotic levels should be monitored where appropriate and renal and hepatic function assayed when indicated. A recent American Heart Association Scientific Statement addresses antimicrobial therapy for IE in detail (**Tables 37-4** to **37-10**).

## ■ CHOICE OF ANTIBIOTICS

The lesions of IE are extremely difficult to eradicate, as the infection exists in a sequestered area of impaired host defense. Thus, IE requires weeks of parenteral antibiotic therapy, preferably with a drug with bactericidal activity against the offending organism. Combination antimicrobial therapy may provide more rapid bactericidal effect and in certain circumstances acts synergistically. All patients should have surveillance blood cultures obtained 2 to 3 days after the initiation of antibiotic therapy to ensure efficacy. Most patients will require long-term venous access via a PICC or Hickman line for a 4- to 6-week course of antibiotics. Patients should remain in an inpatient setting during the initial phase of treatment when complications are most likely, after which selected low-risk patients can be considered for outpatient parenteral antibiotic therapy (OPAT).

## ■ EMPIRIC ANTIBIOTIC THERAPY

Initial empiric antibiotic therapy (ie, before blood culture results are available) should cover *S aureus*, the many species of streptococci that can cause IE, and *E faecalis*. Thus, a combination of a beta-lactamase-resistant penicillin (nafcilllin), or vancomycin for penicillin allergic patients, and gentamicin, is often used.

**TABLE 37-4.** Therapy of Native Valve Endocarditis Caused by Highly Penicillin-Susceptible Viridans-Group Streptococci and *Streptococcus bovis*

| Regimen | Dosage[a] and Route | Duration (wk) | Comments |
|---|---|---|---|
| Aqueous crystalline penicillin G sodium | 12-18 million U per 24 h IV either continuously or in 4-6 equally divided doses | 4 | Preferred in most patients greater than 65 years of age or patients with impairment of 8th cranial nerve function or renal function |
| *Or* | | | |
| Ceftriaxone sodium | 2 g per 24 h IV/IM in 1 dose<br>Pediatric dose[b]: penicillin 200 000 U/kg per 24 h IV in 4-6 equally divided doses; ceftriaxone 100 mg per 24 h IV/IM in 1 dose | 4 | |
| Aqueous crystalline penicillin G sodium | 12-18 million U per 24 h IV either continuously or in 6 equally divided doses | 2 | 2 wk regimen not intended for patients with known cardiac or extracardiac abscess or for those with creatinine clearance of less than 20 mL/min, impaired 8th cranial nerve function, or *Abiotrophia, Granulicatella*, or *Gemella* spp. infection. Gentamicin dosage should be adjusted to achieve peak serum concentration of 3-4 μg/mL and trough serum concentration of less than 1 μg/mL when 3 divided doses are used; nomogram used for single daily dosing |
| *Or* | | | |
| Ceftriaxone sodium | 2 g per 24 h IV/IM in 1 dose | 2 | |

*(Continued)*

**TABLE 37-4.** Therapy of Native Valve Endocarditis Caused by Highly Penicillin-Susceptible Viridans-Group Streptococci and *Streptococcus bovis* (Continued)

| Regimen | Dosage[a] and Route | Duration (wk) | Comments |
|---|---|---|---|
| *Plus* | | | |
| Gentamicin sulfate[c] | 3 mg/kg per 24 h IV/IM in 1 dose<br>Pediatric dose[e]: penicillin 200 000 U/kg per 24 h IV in 4-6 equally divided doses; ceftriaxone 100 mg/kg per 24 h IV/IM in 1 dose; gentamicin 3 mg/kg per 24 h IV/IM in 1 dose or 3 equally divided doses[d] | 2 | |
| Vancomycin hydrochloride[e] | 30 mg/kg per 24 h IV in 2 equally divided doses not to exceed 2 g per 24 h unless concentrations in serum are inappropriately low<br>Pediatric dose: 40 mg/kg per 24 h IV in 2 or 3 equally divided doses | 2 | Vancomycin therapy recommended only for patients unable to tolerate penicillin or ceftriaxone; vancomycin dosage should be adjusted to obtain peak (1 h after infusion completed) serum concentration of 30-45 μg/mL and a trough concentration range of 10-15 μg/mL |

Minimum inhibitory concentration less than or equal to 0.12 μg/mL.

[a]The recommended dosages are for patients with normal renal function.

[b]Pediatric dose should not exceed that of a normal adult.

[c]Other potentially nephrotoxic drugs (eg, nonsteroidal anti-inflammatory drugs) should be used with caution in patients receiving gentamicin therapy.

[d]Data for once-daily dosing of aminoglycosides for children exist, but no data for treatment of infective endocarditis exists.

[e]Vancomycin dosages should be infused during course of at least 1 h to reduce risk of histamine-release "red man" syndrome.

Modified from Baddour LM, Wilson WR, Bayer AS, et al. Infective endocarditis: diagnosis, antimicrobial therapy, and management of complications. A statement for healthcare professionals from the Committee on Rheumatic Fever, Endocarditis, and Kawasaki Disease, Council on Cardiovascular Disease in the Young, and the Councils on Clinical Cardiology, Stroke, and Cardiovascular Surgery and Anesthesia, American Heart Association. *Circulation.* 2005;111:e394-e434.

**TABLE 37-5.** Therapy of Native Valve Endocarditis Caused by Strains of Viridans Group Streptococci and *Streptococcus bovis* Relatively Resistant to Penicillin

| Regimen | Dosage[a] and Route | Duration (wk) | Comments |
|---|---|---|---|
| Aqueous crystalline penicillin G sodium | 24 million U per 24 h IV either continuously or in 4-6 equally divided doses | 4 | Patients with endocarditis caused by penicillin-resistant (MIC greater than 0.5 µg/mL) strains should be treated with regimen recommended for enterococcal endocarditis |
| *Or* | | | |
| Ceftriaxone sodium | 2 g per 24 h IV/IM in 1 dose | 4 | Recommended for enterococcal endocarditis (see Table 37-6) |
| *Plus* | | | |
| Gentamicin sulfate[b] | 3 mg/kg per 24 h IV/IM in 1 dose  Pediatric dose[c]: penicillin 300 000 U per 24 h IV in 4-6 equally divided doses; ceftriaxone 100 mg/kg per 24 IV/IM in 1 dose; gentamicin 3 mg/kg per 24 h IV/IM in 1 dose or 3 equally divided doses | 2 | |
| Vancomycin hydrochloride | 30 mg/kg per 24 h IV in 2 equally divided doses not to exceed 2 g per 24 h, unless serum concentration are inappropriately low  Pediatric dose: 40 mg/kg per 24 h in 2 or 3 equally divided doses | 4 | Vancomycin[d] therapy is recommended only for patients unable to tolerate penicillin or ceftriaxone therapy |

IM, intramuscular; IV, intravenous; MIC, minimum inhibitory concentration.

Minimum inhibitory concentration (MIC) greater than 0.12 µg/mL to less than or equal to 0.5 µg/mL.

[a]Dosages recommended are for patients with normal renal function.

[b]See Table 37-7 for appropriate dosages of gentamicin.

[c]Pediatric dose should not exceed that of a normal adult.

[d]See Table 37-7 for appropriate dosages of vancomycin.

Modified from Baddour LM, Wilson WR, Bayer AS, et al. Infective endocarditis: diagnosis, antimicrobial therapy, and management of complications. A statement for healthcare professionals from the Committee on Rheumatic Fever, Endocarditis, and Kawasaki Disease, Council on Cardiovascular Disease in the Young, and the Councils on Clinical Cardiology, Stroke, and Cardiovascular Surgery and Anesthesia, American Heart Association. *Circulation*. 2005;111:e394-e434.

**TABLE 37-6.** Therapy for Native Valve or Prosthetic Valve Enterococcal Endocarditis Caused by Strains Susceptible to Penicillin, Gentamicin, and Vancomycin

| Regimen | Dosage[a] and Route | Duration (wk) | Comments |
|---|---|---|---|
| Ampicillin sodium | 12 g per 24 h IV in 6 equally divided doses | 4-6 | Native valve: 4-wk therapy recommended for patients with symptoms of illness less than or equal to 3 mo; 6-wk therapy recommended for patients with symptoms greater than 3 mo |
| *Or* Aqueous crystalline penicillin G sodium | 18-30 million U per 24 h IV either continuously or in 6 equally divided doses | 4-6 | Prosthetic valve or other prosthetic cardiac material: minimum of 6-wk therapy recommended |
| *Plus* Gentamicin sulfate[b] | 3 mg/kg per 24 h IV/IM in 3 equally divided doses Pediatric dose[c]: ampicillin 300 mg/kg per 24 h IV in 4-6 equally divided doses; penicillin 300 000 U/kg per 24 h IV in 4-6 equally divided doses; gentamicin 3 mg/kg per 24 h IV/IM in 3 equally divided doses | 4-6 | |
| Vancomycin hydrochloride[d] | 30 mg/kg per 24 h IV in 2 equally divided doses | 6 | Vancomycin therapy is recommended only for patients unable to tolerate penicillin or ampicillin |
| *Plus* Gentamicin sulfate | 3 mg/kg per 24 h IV/IM in 3 equally divided doses Pediatric dose: vancomycin 40 mg/kg per 24 h IV in 2 or 3 equally divided doses; gentamicin 3 mg/kg per 24 h IV/IM in 3 equally divided doses | 6 | 6 wk of vancomycin therapy recommended because of decreased activity against enterococci |

IM, intramuscular; IV, intravenous.

[a]Dosages recommended are for patients with normal renal function.

[b]Dosage of gentamicin should be adjusted to achieve peak serum concentration of 3-4 µg/mL and a trough concentration of less than 1 µg/mL. Patients with a creatinine clearance of less than 50 mL/min should be treated in consultation with an infectious diseases specialist.

[c]Pediatric dose should not exceed that of a normal adult.

[d]See Table 37-7 for appropriate dosing of vancomycin.

Modified from Baddour LM, Wilson WR, Bayer AS, et al. Infective endocarditis: diagnosis, antimicrobial therapy, and management of complications. A statement for healthcare professionals from the Committee on Rheumatic Fever, Endocarditis, and Kawasaki Disease, Council on Cardiovascular Disease in the Young, and the Councils on Clinical Cardiology, Stroke, and Cardiovascular Surgery and Anesthesia, American Heart Association. *Circulation.* 2005;111:e394-e434. See full document for treatment regimens of resistant organisms.

**TABLE 37-7.** Therapy for Endocarditis Caused by Staphylococci in the Absence of Prosthetic Materials

| Regimen | Dosage[a] and Route | Duration | Comments |
|---|---|---|---|
| **Oxacillin-susceptible strains** | | | |
| Nafcillin or oxacillin[b] | 12 g per 24 h IV in 4-6 equally divided doses | 6 wk | For complicated right-sided IE and for left-sided IE; for uncomplicated right-sided IE, 2 wk |
| **With** | | | |
| Optional addition of gentamicin sulfate[c] | 3 mg/kg per 24 h IV/IM in 2 or 3 equally divided doses Pediatric dose[e]: nafcillin or oxacillin 200 mg/kg per 24 h IV in 4-6 equally divided doses; gentamicin 3 mg/kg per 24 h IV/IM in 3 equally divided doses | 3-5 d | Clinical benefit of aminoglycosides has not been established |
| For penicillin-allergic (nonanaphylactoid type) patients: | | | Consider skin testing for oxacillin susceptible staphylococci and questionable history of immediate-type hypersensitivity to penicillin |
| Cefazolin | 6 g per 24 h IV in 3 equally divided doses | 6 wk | Cephalosporins should be avoided in patients with anaphylactoid-type hypersensitivity to beta-lactams; vancomycin should be used in these cases[d] |

*(Continued)*

**TABLE 37-7.** Therapy for Endocarditis Caused by Staphylococci in the Absence of Prosthetic Materials (Continued)

| Regimen | Dosage[a] and Route | Duration | Comments |
|---|---|---|---|
| **With** | | | |
| Optional addition of gentamicin sulfate | 3 mg/kg per 24 h IV/IM in 2 or 3 equally divided doses<br>Pediatric dose: cefazolin 100 mg/kg per 24 h IV in 3 equally divided doses; gentamicin 3 mg/kg per 24 h IV/IM in 3 equally divided doses | 3-5 d | Clinical benefit of aminoglycosides has not been established |
| Oxacillin-resistant strains vancomycin | 30 mg/kg per 24 h IV in 2 equally divided doses<br>Pediatric dose: 40 mg/kg per 24 h IV in 2 or 3 equally divided doses | 6 wk | Adjust vancomycin dosage to achieve 1-h serum concentration of 30-45 μg/mL and trough concentration of 10-15 μg/mL |

IE, infective endocarditis; IM, intramuscular; IV, intravenous.

[a]Dosages recommended are for patients with normal renal function.

[b]Penicillin G 24 million U per 24 h IV in four to six equally divided doses may be used in place of nafcillin or oxacillin if strain is penicillin susceptible (minimum inhibitory concentration less than or equal to 0.1 μg/mL) and dose does not produce beta-lactamase.

[c]Gentamicin should be administered in close temporal proximity to vancomycin, nafcillin, or oxacillin dosing.

[d]Pediatric dose should not exceed that of a normal adult.

Modified from Baddour LM, Wilson WR, Bayer AS, et al. Infective endocarditis: diagnosis, antimicrobial therapy, and management of complications. A statement for healthcare professionals from the Committee on Rheumatic Fever, Endocarditis, and Kawasaki Disease, Council on Cardiovascular Disease in the Young, and the Councils on Clinical Cardiology, Stroke, and Cardiovascular Surgery and Anesthesia, American Heart Association. *Circulation.* 2005;111:e394-e434.

**TABLE 37-8.** Therapy for Prosthetic Valve Endocarditis Caused by Staphylococci

| Regimen | Dosage[a] and Route | Duration (wk) | Comments |
|---|---|---|---|
| **Oxacillin-susceptible strains** | | | |
| Nafcillin or oxacillin | 12 g per 24 h IV in 6 equally divided doses | At least 6 | Penicillin G 24 million U per 24 h IV in 4 to 6 equally divided doses may be used in place of nafcillin or oxacillin if strain is penicillin susceptible (minimum inhibitory concentration less than or equal to 0.1 μg/mL) and does not produce beta-lactamase; vancomycin should be used in patients with immediate-type hypersensitivity reactions to beta-lactam antibiotics (see Table 37-7 for dosing guidelines); cefazolin may be substituted for nafcillin or oxacillin in patients with nonimmediate-type hypersensitivity reactions to penicillins |
| *Plus* | | | |
| Rifampin | 900 mg per 24 h IV/PO in 3 equally divided doses | At least 6 | |
| *Plus* | | | |
| Gentamicin[b] | 3 mg/kg per 24 h IV/IM in 2 or 3 equally divided doses<br>Pediatric dose[c]: nafcillin or oxacillin 200 mg/kg/h IV in 4-6 equally divided doses; rifampin 20 mg/kg per 24 h IV/PO in 3 equally divided doses; gentamicin 3 mg/kg per 24 h IV/IM in 3 equally divided doses | 2 | |

*(Continued)*

**TABLE 37-8.** Therapy for Prosthetic Valve Endocarditis Caused by Staphylococci (Continued)

| Regimen | Dosage[a] and Route | Duration (wk) | Comments |
|---|---|---|---|
| **Oxacillin-resistant strains** | | | |
| Vancomycin | 30 mg/kg per 24 h in 2 equally divided doses | At least 6 | Adjust vancomycin to achieve 1-h serum concentration of 30-45 µg/mL and trough concentration of 10-15 µg/mL |
| *Plus* | | | |
| Rifampin | 900 mg/kg per 24 h IV/PO in 3 equally divided doses | At least 6 | |
| *Plus* | | | |
| Gentamicin[b] | 3 mg/kg per 24 h IV/IM in 2 or 3 equally divided doses | 2 | |
| | Pediatric dose: vancomycin 40 mg/kg per 24 h IV in 2 or 3 equally divided doses; rifampin 20 mg/kg per 24 h IV/PO in 3 equally divided doses (up to adult dose); gentamicin 3 mg/kg per 24 h IV or IM in 3 equally divided doses | | |

IM, intramuscular; IV, intravenous; PO, by mouth.

[a]Dosages recommended are for patients with normal renal function.

[b]Gentamicin should be administered in close proximity to vancomycin, nafcillin, or oxacillin dosing.

[c]Pediatric dose should not exceed that of a normal adult.

Modified from Baddour LM, Wilson WR, Bayer AS, et al. Infective endocarditis: diagnosis, antimicrobial therapy, and management of complications. A statement for healthcare professionals from the Committee on Rheumatic Fever, Endocarditis, and Kawasaki Disease, Council on Cardiovascular Disease in the Young, and the Councils on Clinical Cardiology, Stroke, and Cardiovascular Surgery and Anesthesia, American Heart Association. *Circulation.* 2005;1:e394-e434.

**TABLE 37-9.** Therapy for Both Native and Prosthetic Valve Endocarditis Caused by HACEK[a] Microorganisms

| Regimen | Dosage and Route | Duration (wk) | Comments |
|---|---|---|---|
| Ceftriaxone sodium | 2 g per 24 h IV/IM in 1 dose[b] | 4 | Cefotaxime or another third- or fourth-generation cephalosporin may be substituted |
| Or | | | |
| Ampicillin-sulbactam[c] | 12 g per 24 h IV in 4 equally divided doses | 4 | |
| Or | | | |
| Ciprofloxacin[c,d] | 1000 mg per 24 h PO or 800 mg per 24 h IV in 2 equally divided doses<br>Pediatric dose[e]: ceftriaxone 100 mg/kg per 24 h IV/IM once daily; ampicillin-sulbactam 300 mg/kg per 24 h IV divided into 4 or 6 equally divided doses; ciprofloxacin 20-30 mg/kg per 24 h IV/PO in 2 equally divided doses | 4 | Fluoroquinolone therapy recommended only for patients unable to tolerate cephalosporin and ampicillin therapy; levofloxacin, gatifloxacin, or moxifloxacin may be substituted; fluoroquinolones generally not recommended for patients less than 18 years old. Prosthetic valve: Patients with endocarditis involving prosthetic cardiac valve or other prosthetic cardiac material should be treated for 6 wk |

IM, intramuscular; IV, intravenous; PO, by mouth.

[a]Haemophilus parainfluenzae, Haemophilus aphrophilus, Actinobacillus actinomycetemcomitans, Cardiobacterium hominis, Eikenella corrodens, and Kingella kingae.

[b]Patients should be informed that intramuscular injection of ceftriaxone is painful.

[c]Dosage recommended for patients with normal renal function.

[d]Fluoroquinolones are highly active in vitro against HACEK microorganisms. Published data on use of fluoroquinolone therapy for endocarditis caused by HACED are minimal.

[e]Pediatric dose should not exceed that of a normal adult.

Modified from Baddour LM, Wilson WR, Bayer AS, et al. Infective endocarditis: diagnosis, antimicrobial therapy, and management of complications. A statement for healthcare professionals from the Committee on Rheumatic Fever, Endocarditis, and Kawasaki Disease, Council on Cardiovascular Disease in the Young, and the Councils on Clinical Cardiology, Stroke, and Cardiovascular Surgery and Anesthesia, American Heart Association. *Circulation.* 2005;111:e394-e434.

**TABLE 37-10.** Therapy for Culture-Negative Endocarditis Including Bartonella Endocarditis

| Regimen | Dosage[a] and Route | Duration (wk) | Comments |
|---|---|---|---|
| **Native Valve** | | | |
| Ampicillin-sulbactam | 12 g per 24 h IV in 4 equally divided doses | 4-6 | Patients with culture-negative endocarditis should be treated with consultation with an infectious diseases specialist |
| *Plus* | | | |
| Gentamicin sulfate[b] | 3 mg/kg per 24 h IV/IM in 2 equally divided doses | 4-6 | |
| Vancomycin[c] | 30 mg/kg per 24 h IV in 2 equally divided doses | 4-6 | Vancomycin recommended only for patients unable to tolerate penicillins |
| *Plus* | | | |
| Gentamicin sulfate | 3 mg/kg per 24 h IV/IM in 3 equally divided doses | 4-6 | |
| *Plus* | | | |
| Ciprofloxacin | 1000 mg per 24 h PO or 800 mg per 24 h IV in 2 equally divided doses | 4-6 | |
| | Pediatric dose[d]: ampicillin-sulbactam 300 mg/kg per 24 h IV in 4-6 equally divided doses; gentamicin 3 mg/kg per 24 h IV/IM in 3 equally divided doses; vancomycin 40 mg/kg per 24 h in 2 or 3 equally divided doses; ciprofloxacin 20-30 mg/kg per 24 h IV/PO in 2 equally divided doses | | |

| | | | |
|---|---|---|---|
| **Prosthetic valve (early—less than or equal to 1 year)** | | | |
| Vancomycin | 30 mg/kg per 24 h IV in 2 equally divided doses | 6 | |
| **Plus** | | | |
| Gentamicin sulfate | 3 mg/kg per 24 h IV/IM in 3 equally divided doses | 2 | |
| **Plus** | | | |
| Cefepime | 6 g per 24 h IV in 3 equally divided doses | 6 | |
| **Plus** | | | |
| Rifampin | 900 mg per 24 h PO/IV in 3 equally divided doses | 6 | |
| | Pediatric dose: vancomycin 40 mg/kg per 24 h IV in 2 or 3 equally divided doses; gentamicin 3 mg per kg per 24 h IV/IM in 3 equally divided doses; cefepime 150 mg/kg per 24 h IV in 3 equally divided doses; rifampin 20 mg/kg per 24 h PO/IV in 3 equally divided doses | | |
| **Prosthetic valve (late—greater than 1 year)** | | 6 | Same regimens as listed above for native valve endocarditis |
| **Suspected Bartonella, culture negative** | | | |
| Ceftriaxone sodium | 2 g per 24 h IV/IM in 1 dose | 6 | Patients with Bartonella endocarditis should be treated in consultation with an infectious diseases specialist |
| **Plus** | | | |
| Gentamicin sulfate | 3 mg/kg per 24 h IV/IM in 3 equally divided doses | 2 | |
| **with/without** | | | |
| Doxycycline | 200 mg/kg per 24 h IV/PO in 2 equally divided doses | | |

*(Continued)*

**TABLE 37-10.** Therapy for Culture-Negative Endocarditis Including Bartonella Endocarditis (Continued)

| Regimen | Dosage[a] and Route | Duration (wk) | Comments |
|---|---|---|---|
| Documented *Bartonella* culture postive | | | |
| Doxycycline | 200 mg per 24 h IV or PO in 2 equally divided doses | 6 | If gentamicin cannot be given, then replace with rifampin, 600 mg per 24 h PO/IV in 2 equally divided doses |
| *Plus* | | | |
| Gentamicin sulfate | 3 mg/kg per 24 h IV/IM in 3 equally divided doses<br>Pediatric dose: ceftriaxone 100 mg/kg per 24 h IV/IM once daily; gentamicin 3 mg/kg per 24 h IV/IM in 3 equally divided doses; doxycycline 2-4 mg/kg per 24 h IV/PO in 2 equally divided doses; rifampin 20 mg/kg per 24 h PO/IV in 2 equally divided doses | 2 | |

IM, intramuscular; IV, intravenous; PO, by mouth.

[a]Dosages recommended are for patients with normal renal function.

[b]See Table 37-7 for appropriate dosing of gentamicin.

[c]See Table 37-7 for appropriate dosing of vancomycin.

[d]Pediatric dose should not exceed that of a normal adult.

Modified from Baddour LM, Wilson WR, Bayer AS, et al. Infective endocarditis: diagnosis, antimicrobial therapy, and management of complications. A statement for healthcare professionals from the Committee on Rheumatic Fever, Endocarditis, and Kawasaki Disease, Council on Cardiovascular Disease in the Young, and the Councils on Clinical Cardiology, Stroke, and Cardiovascular Surgery and Anesthesia, American Heart Association. *Circulation.* 2005;111:e394-e434.

# ANTIPLATELET AND ANTITHROMBIN THERAPY

Despite their theoretical benefit, there are no human studies that support the use of either antiplatelet or antithrombin therapy to prevent embolic complications or to hasten antibiotic cure. Moreover, small uncontrolled studies suggest that antithrombin therapy actually increases the risk of intracranial hemorrhage following CNS embolization. For patients who generally require anticoagulation (eg, patients with chronic atrial fibrillation or a mechanical heart valve), warfarin should be immediately discontinued on admission and IV unfractionated heparin cautiously substituted at the time when bleeding risk is deemed acceptably low.

# SURGICAL THERAPY

The decision to undertake cardiac surgery for the treatment of IE can be extremely challenging, and there are no randomized clinical trials to guide practice. Early surgical intervention may be prudent in many situations and early surgical consultation is therefore critical. The most recent ACC/AHA guidelines for surgery in IE are summarized in **Tables 37-11** and **37-12**.

---

**TABLE 37-11.** Indications for Surgery for Native Valve Endocarditis

**Class I**
1. Surgery of the native valve is indicated in patients with acute infective endocarditis who present with valve stenosis or regurgitation resulting in heart failure. *(Level of Evidence: B)*
2. Surgery of the native valve is indicated in patients with acute infective endocarditis who present with AR or MR with hemodynamic evidence of elevated LV end-diastolic or left atrial pressures (eg, premature closure of MV with AR, rapid decelerating MR signal by continuous-wave Doppler (V-wave cutoff sign), or moderate to severe pulmonary hypertension). *(Level of Evidence: B)*
3. Surgery of the native valve is indicated in patients with infective endocarditis caused by fungal or other highly resistant organisms. *(Level of Evidence: B)*
4. Surgery of the native valve is indicated in patients with infective endocarditis complicated by heart block, annular or aortic abscess, or destructive penetrating lesions (eg, sinus of Valsalva to right atrium, right ventricle, or left atrium fistula; mitral leaflet perforation with aortic valve endocarditis; or infection in annulus fibrosa). *(Level of Evidence: B)*

**Class IIa**
Surgery of the native valve is reasonable in patients with infective endocarditis who present with recurrent emboli and persistent vegetations despite appropriate antibiotic therapy. *(Level of Evidence: C)*

**Class IIb**
Surgery of the native valve may be considered in patients with infective endocarditis who present with mobile vegetations in excess of 10 mm with or without emboli. *(Level of Evidence: C)*

---

Data from American College of Cardiology; American Heart Association Task Force on Practice Guidelines (Writing Committee to revise the 1998 guidelines for the management of patients with valvular heart disease); Society of Cardiovascular Anesthesiologists; Bonow RO, Carabello BA, Chatterjee K, et al. ACC/AHA 2006 guidelines for the management of patients with valvular heart disease: a report of the American College of Cardiology/American Heart Association Task Force on Practice Guidelines (Writing Committee to revise the 1998 guidelines for the management of patients with valvular heart disease) developed in collaboration with the Society of Cardiovascular Anesthesiologists endorsed by the Society for Cardiovascular Angiography and Interventions and the Society of Thoracic Surgeons. *J Am Coll Cardiol.* 2006;48(3):e1-e148.

**TABLE 37-12.** Indications for Surgery for Prosthetic Valve Endocarditis

**Class I**

1. Consultation with a cardiac surgeon is indicated for patients with infective endocarditis of a prosthetic valve. *(Level of Evidence: C)*
2. Surgery is indicated for patients with infective endocarditis of a prosthetic valve who present with heart failure. *(Level of Evidence: B)*
3. Surgery is indicated for patients with infective endocarditis of a prosthetic valve who present with dehiscence evidence by cine fluoroscopy or echocardiography. *(Level of Evidence: B)*
4. Surgery is indicated for patients with infective endocarditis of a prosthetic valve who present with evidence of increasing obstruction or worsening regurgitation. *(Level of Evidence: C)*
5. Surgery is indicated for patients with infective endocarditis of a prosthetic valve who present with complications, for example, abscess formation. *(Level of Evidence: C)*

**Class IIa**

Surgery is reasonable for patients with infective endocarditis of a prosthetic valve who present with evidence of persistent bacteremia or recurrent emboli despite appropriate antibiotic treatment. *(Level of Evidence: C)*

Surgery is reasonable for patients with infective endocarditis of a prosthetic valve who present with relapsing infection. *(Level of Evidence: C)*

**Class III**

Routine surgery is not indicated for patients with uncomplicated infective endocarditis of a prosthetic valve caused by first infection with a sensitive organism. *(Level of Evidence: C)*

Data from American College of Cardiology; American Heart Association Task Force on Practice Guidelines (Writing Committee to revise the 1998 guidelines for the management of patients with valvular heart disease); Society of Cardiovascular Anesthesiologists; Bonow RO, Carabello BA, Chatterjee K, et al. ACC/AHA 2006 guidelines for the management of patients with valvular heart disease: a report of the American College of Cardiology/American Heart Association Task Force on Practice Guidelines (Writing Committee to revise the 1998 guidelines for the management of patients with valvular heart disease) developed in collaboration with the Society of Cardiovascular Anesthesiologists endorsed by the Society for Cardiovascular Angiography and Interventions and the Society of Thoracic Surgeons. *J Am Coll Cardiol.* 2006;48(3):e1-e148.

For NVE, the primary indication for surgery in the active phase of infection is the development of heart failure from either valve stenosis or regurgitation. Valve surgery is indicated for the treatment of fungal or other highly resistant organisms, and for treatment of intracardiac abscess, perforation, fistulous tracts, and false aneurysms. Surgery is reasonable for patients with recurrent emboli and persistent vegetations and for patients with persistent bacteremia despite several days (5-7) of appropriate antibiotic therapy in the absence of a metastatic focus of infection. Surgery to prevent embolization can be considered for treatment of large valve repair. Indications for surgery in patients with PVE are similar, although early surgery may be considered for selected patients with PVE despite demonstration of perivalular extension or heart failure.

The timing of surgery following CNS embolization in either native or prosthetic valve endocarditis is problematic due to the risk of hemorrhagic transformation. It is generally advisable to wait at least 5 to 7 days after bland CNS infarction, and as long as 4 weeks after primary CNS hemorrhage (eg, from a ruptured mycotic aneurysm) before undertaking cardiac surgery.

# PROGNOSIS

Patients with IE are an extremely heterogeneous group with varying comorbidities, causative organisms, and complications. Overall mortality can approach 20% to 25%. Accurate prognostic classification may help inform individual treatment decisions. Retrospective studies have identified high-risk features that include advanced age, diabetes mellitus, female gender, heart failure, renal dysfunction, *S aureus*, an embolic event, and vegetation length >1.5 cm. Although the decision to undertake early surgery for the treatment of IE must be made on an individual basis, these data provide a useful means to target aggressive medical and surgical interventions to high-risk patient groups.

# PREVENTION

Antibiotic prophylaxis for IE remains challenging, as there is little evidence from well-designed human trials regarding its efficacy. The prophylaxis guidelines underwent substantial revision in 2007 and now substantially fewer patients are recommended for IE prophylaxis. The changes reflect consensus that IE is much more likely to result from frequent exposure to random bacteremias associated with daily activities than from bacteria caused by a dental, GI tract, or GU tract manipulation. In addition, the population-wide risk of antibiotic-associated adverse events is thought to exceed the benefits from widespread prophylactic antibiotic therapy.

Antibiotic prophylaxis is now only recommended for cardiac conditions associated with the highest risk of adverse outcome (**Table 37-13**). Patients at highest risk should receive prophylaxis when undergoing dental procedures that involve

---

**TABLE 37-13.** Cardiac Conditions Associated With Highest Risk of Adverse Outcome From Endocarditis for Which Prophylaxis in Dental and Respiratory Procedures is Reasonable

Prosthetic cardiac or prosthetic material used for cardiac valve repair
Previous IE
Congenital heart disease (CHD)[a]
    Unrepaired cyanotic CHD, including palliative shunts and conduits
    Completely repaired congenital heart defect with prosthetic material or device, whether placed by surgery or by catheter intervention, during the first 6 months after the procedure[b]
    Repaired CHD with residual defects at the site or adjacent to the site of a prosthetic patch or prosthetic device (which inhibit endothelialization)
Cardiac transplantation recipients who develop cardiac valvulopathy

[a]Except for the conditions listed above, antibiotic prophylaxis is no longer recommended for any other forms of CHD.

[b]Prophylaxis is reasonable because endothelialization of prosthetic material occurs within 6 months after the procedure.

Adapted with permission from Wilson T, Taubert KA, Gewitz M, et al. Prevention of infective endocarditis: guidelines from the American Heart Association. A guideline from the American Heart Association Rheumatic Fever, Endocarditis, and Kawasaki Disease Committee, Council on Cardiovascular Disease in the Young, and the Council on Clinical Cardiology, Council on Cardiovascular Surgery and Anesthesia, and the Quality of Care and Outcomes Research Interdisciplinary Working Group. *Circulation.* 2007;116:1745.

**TABLE 37-14.** Antibiotic Regimens for IE Prophylaxis

| Situation | Agent | Single Dose 30-60 min Before Procedure | |
|---|---|---|---|
| | | Adults | Children |
| Oral | Amoxicillin | 2 g | 50 mg/kg |
| Unable to take oral medication | Ampicillin Or | 2 g IM or IV | 50 mg/kg IM or IV |
| | Cefazolin or Ceftriaxone | 1 g IM or IV | 50 mg/kg IM or IV |
| Allergic to penicillins or Ampicillins–oral | Cephalexin [a,b] Or | 2 g | 50 mg/kg |
| | Clindamycin Or | 600 mg | 20 mg/kg |
| | Azithromycin or Clarithromycin | 500 mg | 15 mg/kg |
| Allergic to penicillins or ampicillin and unable to take oral medication | Cefazolin or Ceftriazone[b] Or | 1 g IM or IV | 50 mg/kg IM or IV |
| | Clindamycin | 600 mg IM or IV | 20 mg/kg IM or IV |

IM, intramuscular; IV, intravenous.

[a]Or other first- or second-generation oral cephalosporin in equivalent adult or pediatric dosage.

[b]Cephalosporins should not be used in an individual with a history of anaphylaxis, angioedema, or urticaria with penicillins or ampicillin.

Adapted with permission from Wilson T, Taubert KA, Gewitz M, et al. Prevention of infective endocarditis: guidelines from the American Heart Association. A guideline from the American Heart Association Rheumatic Fever, Endocarditis, and Kawasaki Disease Committee, Council on Cardiovascular Disease in the Young, and the Council on Clinical Cardiology, Council on Cardiovascular Surgery and Anesthesia, and the Quality of Care and Outcomes Research Interdisciplinary Working Group. *Circulation.* 2007;116:1747.

the manipulation of gingival tissue, periapical region of the teeth, or perforation of the oral mucosa. Prophylaxis is also reasonable for invasive procedures of the respiratory tract that involve incision or biopsy of respiratory mucosa. Importantly, antibiotic prophylaxis is no longer recommended for GU or GI tract procedures. Recommendations for procedure-specific antibiotic prophylaxis regimens are provided in **Table 37-14**.

# SUGGESTED READINGS

Haldar SM, O'Gara PT. Infective endocarditis. In: Fuster V, Walsh R, Harrington RA, et al, eds. *Hurst's The Heart.* 13th ed. New York, NY: McGraw-Hill; 2011: 86: 1940-1969.

Baddour LM, Wilson WR, Bayer AS, et al. Infective endocarditis: diagnosis, antimicrobial therapy, and management of complications. A statement for healthcare professionals from the Committee on Rheumatic Fever, Endocarditis, and Kawasaki Disease, Council on Cardiovascular Disease in the Young, and the Councils on Clinical Cardiology, Stroke, and Cardiovascular Surgery and Anesthesia, American Heart Association. Endorsed by the Infectious Diseases Society of America. *Circulation.* 2005;111:e394-e434.

Bonow RO, Carabello BA, Kanu C, et al. ACC/AHA 2006 guidelines for the management of patients with valvular heart disease: a report of the American College of Cardiology/American Heart Association Task Force on Practice Guidelines (writing committee to revise the

1998 Guidelines for the Management of Patients with Valvular Heart Disease). Developed in collaboration with the Society of Cardiovascular Anesthesiologists. Endorsed by the Society for Cardiovascular Angiography and Interventions and the Society of Thoracic Surgeons. *Circulation.* 2006;114:e84-e231.

Cheitlin MD, Armstrong WF, Aurigemma GP, et al. ACC/AHA/ASE 2003 guideline update for the clinical application of echocardiography: summary article. A report of the American College of Cardiology/American Heart Association Task Force on Practice Guidelines (ACC/AHA/ASE Committee to Update the 1997 Guidelines for the Clinical Application of Echocardiography). *J Am Soc Echocardiogr.* 2003;16:1091-1110.

Lalani T, Cabell CH, Benjamin DK, et al. Analysis of the impact of early surgery on in-hospital mortality of native valve endocarditis *Circulation.* 2010;121:1005-1013.

Levy DM. Centenary of William Osler's 1885 Gulstonian lectures and their place in the history of bacterial endocarditis. *J R Soc Med.* 1985:78:1039-1046.

Li JS, Sexton DJ, Mick N, et al. Proposed modifications to the Duke criteria for the diagnosis of infective endocarditis. *Clin Infect Dis.* 2000;30:633-638.

Mylonakis E, Calderwood SB. Infective endocarditis in adults. *N Engl J Med.* 2001;345:1318-1330.

Netzer RO, Altwegg SC, Zollinger E, et al. Infective endocarditis: determinants of long term outcome. *Heart.* 2002;88:61–66.

Vikram HR, Buenconsejo J, Hasbun R, et al. Impact of valve surgery on 6-month mortality in adults with complicated, left-sided native valve endocarditis: a propensity analysis. *JAMA.* 2003;290:3250-3521.

Wilson, T, Taubert, KA, Gewitz, M, et al. Prevention of infective endocarditis: a guideline from the American Heart Association Rheumatic Fever, Endocarditis, and Kawasaki Disease Committee, Council on Cardiovascular Disease in the Young, and the Council on Clinical Cardiology, Council on Cardiovascular Surgery and Anesthesia, and the Quality of Care and Outcomes Research Interdisciplinary Working Group. *Circulation.* 2007;116:1736-1754.

# CHAPTER 38
# DILATED CARDIOMYOPATHIES

Luisa Mestroni, Edward M. Gilbert, Brian D. Lowes,
and Michael R. Bristow

## BACKGROUND AND HISTORICAL PERSPECTIVE

The primary and secondary dilated cardiomyopathies are the most common causes of chronic heart failure. The clinical syndrome of heart failure is a complex process where the primary pathophysiology is quickly obscured by a variety of superimposed secondary adaptive, maladaptive, and counterregulatory processes. Despite improvements in the treatment of heart failure introduced in the last 10 years, including the general availability of cardiac transplantation and better medical treatment, clinical outcome following the onset of symptoms has not changed substantially. The mortality remains high (median survival of 1.7 years for men and 3.2 years for women), the natural history is progressive, the cost excessive, and disability and morbidity among the highest of any disease or disease syndrome.

## THE CLASSIFICATION OF CARDIOMYOPATHIES

The 1995 World Health Organization/International Society and Federation of Cardiology (WHO/ISFC) classification of cardiomyopathies was recently revised to accommodate several rapidly emerging realities, in particular the identification of new disease entities, advances in diagnosis, and knowledge of etiology of previously unknown types of heart muscle disease.

The classifications of cardiomyopathies are shown in **Table 38-1** (See also Chapters 42 and 43). The WHO/ISFC classification of cardiomyopathy was mainly based on the global anatomic description of chamber dimensions in systole and diastole. Thus, the dilated and restrictive categories had definitions based on left ventricular (LV) dimensions or volume, which also define function via calculated ejection fraction. The novel AHA Scientific Statement emphasizes the genetic determinants of cardiomyopathies. Thus, dilated and restrictive cardiomyopathies are defined as *mixed* cardiomyopathies (predominantly nongenetic); however, hypertrophic cardiomyopathy (HCM), caused by mutations in contractile proteins, and other rare forms of cardiomyopathy including arrhythmogenic right ventricular cardiomyopathy/arrhythmogenic right ventricular dysplasia (ARVC/ARVD) and left ventricular noncompaction (LVNC), which also turned out to be completely genetic in basis, are defined as *genetic* cardiomyopathies. The third category concerns *acquired* cardiomyopathies, such as peripartum- and tachycardia-induced cardiomyopathies. Conversely, genetic cardiomyopathies without unique phenotypes and

**TABLE 38-1.** Classification of the Cardiomyopathies

| Category | Definition |
| --- | --- |
| Genetic | |
| I. Hypertrophic (HCM) | $\uparrow\uparrow$ septal and $\uparrow$ posterior wall thickness, myofibrillar disarray |
| | Mutation in sarcomeric protein, autosomal dominant inheritance |
| II. Arrhythmogenic RV (ARVC/ARVD) | Fibrofatty replacement of RV myocardium |
| III. LV noncompaction | Spongy LV cavity (apex) |
| IV. Glycogen storage diseases | Danon disease, PRKAG2 |
| V. Ion channelopathies | Conduction defects, LQTS, Brugada syndrome, SQTS, CPVT, Asian SUNDS |
| Mixed | |
| I. Dilated (DCM) | $\uparrow$ EDV $\uparrow$ ESV; low EF |
| II. Restrictive (RCM) | $\uparrow$ EDV, $\leftrightarrow$ ESV; $\uparrow$ FP, $\leftrightarrow$ EF |
| Acquired | |
| I. Myocarditis | Inflammatory process |
| II. Stress provoked (*tako-tsubo*) | Reversible LV dysfunction |
| III. Peripartum | Third trimester or 5 months after pregnancy |
| IV. Tachycardia induced | Following prolonged periods of SVT or VT |
| V. Infants of insulin-dependent diabetic mothers | |

ARVC, arrhythmogenic right ventricular cardiomyopathy; ARVD, arrhythmogenic right ventricular dysplasia; CM, cardiomyopathy; CPVT, catecholaminergic polymorphic ventricular tachycardia; EDV, end-diastolic volume; ESV, end-systolic volume; EF, ejection fraction; FP, filling pressure; HCM, hypertrophic cardiomyopathy; LQTS, long QT syndrome; LV, left ventricular; RV, right ventricular; SQTS, short QT syndrome; SVT, supraventricular tachycardia; SUNDS, sudden unexplained death syndrome; VT, ventricular tachycardia.

involvement of a generalized multiorgan disorder, such as the dilated cardiomyopathy of Becker–Duchenne, are defined as *secondary* cardiomyopathies. This distinction is arbitrary and may inevitably cause significant overlap between primary and secondary cardiomyopathies.

# MOLECULAR MECHANISMS IN CARDIOMYOPATHIES

There are three general mechanisms whereby altered gene expression leads to myocardial dysfunction:

1. A single gene defect, as in lamin A/C gene mutations (dilated cardiomyopathy) or beta-myosin heavy chain (hypertrophic cardiomyopathy)
2. Polymorphic variation in modifier genes, such as is present in many components of the renin–angiotensin, adrenergic, and endothelin systems
3. Maladaptive regulated expression of completely normal genes, as in secondary dilated cardiomyopathies (muscular dystrophies).

Multiple gene defects have been identified that can produce a dilated cardiomyopathy in humans, as discussed in more detail in the section on familial forms of dilated cardiomyopathy. These include mutations in genes encoding proteins of the cytoskeleton, such as dystrophin; nuclear envelope, such as lamin A/C; sarcomere, such as cardiac beta-myosin heavy chain (beta-MHC) and alpha-myosin heavy chain (alpha-MHC); ion channels, like SCN5A; desmosome; and signaling pathways, such as transcriptional and $Ca^{2+}$-cycling regulators. The most current and complete compilation of known genetic cardiomyopathies is available through the Online Mendelian Inheritance in Man (www.OMIM.org).

Genes exhibit polymorphic variation; for example, normal variants of genes exist in the population that are of slightly different size or sequence. Some gene polymorphisms are associated with differences in function of the expressed protein gene product, and some differences in function likely account for the *biological variation* routinely encountered in population studies of disease susceptibility or clinical response to treatment.

Examples of modifier genes that may have an impact on the natural history of a dilated cardiomyopathy include the angiotensin-converting enzyme (ACE) *DD* genotype, where individuals are homozygous for the *deletion* variant, which is associated with increased circulating and cardiac tissue ACE activity. The *DD* genotype appears to be a risk factor for early remodeling after MI and for the development of end-stage ischemic and idiopathic dilated cardiomyopathy. Other potentially important polymorphic variants that may influence the natural history of a cardiomyopathy involve the angiotensin $AT_1$ receptor, β-2–adrenergic receptors, the α-2C–adrenergic receptor with or without a β-1–receptor polymorphism, and the endothelin receptor type A.

Polymorphic variations can also influence the response to medications. Patients with the *DD* genotype, who were found to have a worse prognosis, at the same time appeared to respond significantly better to β-blocker therapy compared to the other genotypes (*II* and *ID*). Similarly, a polymorphism within a conserved region of the β-1–adrenergic receptor ([389]arginine) increases the response to isotropic therapy (isoproterenol) and is associated with a reduction of mortality in patients treated with the β-blocker bucindolol.

1. Altered or maladaptive expression of a completely normal *wild-type* gene is most commonly seen in the progression to myocardial failure, which is the natural history of virtually all cardiomyopathies once they are established. Examples in this category include down-regulation of β-1–adrenergic receptors, alpha-MHC, and the *SERCA2* (sarcoplasmic reticulum [SR] $Ca^{2+}$ adenosine triphosphatase [ATPase]) genes and upregulation in the atrial natriuretic peptide (*ANP*), beta-*MHC, ACE,* tumor necrosis factor alpha (*TNF*-alpha), endothelin, and beta-adrenergic receptor kinase (*BARK*) genes. For instance, in patients who respond to treatment by increasing LV ejection fraction, β-blocker therapy may restore some aspects of altered gene expression, increasing the expression of sarcoplasmic-reticulum calcium ATPase and of alpha-MHC, and decreasing beta-MHC.

Tissue preparations and myocytes isolated from failing human hearts exhibit evidence of decreased contractile function. Assuming that loading conditions and ischemia are not adversely affecting cardiac myocyte function, progressive myocardial failure in dilated cardiomyopathies is most likely caused by myocardial cell loss or changes in the gene expression of proteins that regulate or produce muscle contraction. **Figures 38-1** and **38-2** summarize these general points and emphasize the central roles of the renin-angiotensin system (RAS) and adrenergic nervous system (ANS) in promoting cell loss, growth and remodeling, and altered gene expression.

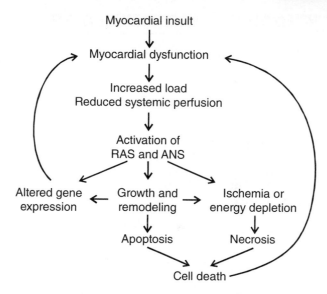

**FIGURE 38-1.** Relationship of neurohormonal activation and production of cardiac myocyte loss due to apoptosis and necrosis and altered gene expression. Cell loss and altered gene expression result in more myocardial dysfunction, and a vicious cycle is established. (RAS, renin-angiotensin system; ANS, autonomic nervous system.)

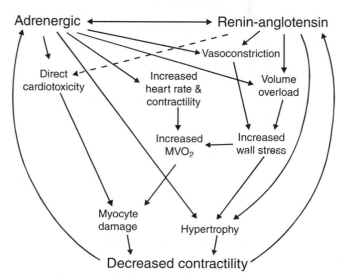

**FIGURE 38-2.** Heart failure compensatory mechanisms activated to support the failing heart. Lighter-colored type areas indicate physiologic mechanisms that stabilize pump function.

# SELECTED DILATED CARDIOMYOPATHIES

## ■ ISCHEMIC CARDIOMYOPATHY

*Ischemic cardiomyopathy* is commonly defined as a dilated cardiomyopathy when there is a history of MI or evidence of clinically significant (ie, ≥70% narrowing of a major epicardial artery) coronary artery disease, in whom the degree of myocardial dysfunction and ventricular dilatation is not explained solely by the extent of previous infarction or the degree of ongoing ischemia (**Table 38-2**). Dilatation of the LV and a decrease in ejection fraction occurs in up to 40% of subjects within 12 to 24 months following an anterior MI and in a smaller percentage of subjects following an inferior MI. The gross pathology of ischemic cardiomyopathy includes transmural or subendocardial scarring. The histopathology of the noninfarcted regions is similar to changes that occur in dilated cardiomyopathy (DCM), as discussed below. Acute ischemia may introduce a state of "stunning" that results in transient reversible myocardial dysfunction. Chronic ischemia may result in a state of "hibernation" in which the myocardial contractile state is depressed in order to match the decreased metabolic requirements in the setting of limited myocardial perfusion. In both settings, timely revascularization is necessary to reverse the contractile abnormality. However, concomitant medical management with ACE inhibitors, beta blockade, aldosterone antagonists and resynchronization (when appropriate) is also paramount.

## ■ HYPERTENSION AND CARDIOMYOPATHY

Hypertension is a major risk factor for heart failure and the phenotypic expression is highly variable. It includes dilated cardiomyopathies with eccentric hypertrophy, systolic dysfunction with and without concentric hypertrophy, and diastolic dysfunction. A *hypertensive dilated cardiomyopathy* is diagnosed when ventricular dilatation and depressed systolic function remain after correction of the hypertension. Importantly, the 2006 AHA Scientific Statement did not include hypertensive myocardial disease in the formal classification of cardiomyopathies.

The cornerstone of management is aggressive control of hypertension with RAS and adrenergic antagonists and additional agents as needed.

## ■ IDIOPATHIC DILATED CARDIOMYOPATHY

DCM is diagnosed by excluding significant coronary artery disease, valvular abnormalities, and other causes. DCM is a relatively common cause of heart failure, with an estimated prevalence rate of 0.04%; incidence rates vary from 0.005% to 0.006%. The incidence of DCM increases with age and males are affected at a higher rate than females. Although the diagnosis is not difficult, problems arise when an apparent DCM presents in someone with a history of hypertension or excessive alcohol intake. Alcohol is likely when the intake has exceeded 80 g/d for males and 40 g/d for females for >5 years; hypertension may be primary when blood pressure has been poorly controlled for years. Histologic features are nonspecific and consist of myocardial cell hypertrophy and varying amounts of increased interstitial fibrosis.

It is important to recognize that DCM may be familial in as many as 35% to 50%. Obtaining a careful family history is essential and screening of first-degree relatives should be considered. The analysis of the phenotype identifies a wide range of clinical and pathologic forms indicating genetic heterogeneity. Most familial patients present with autosomal dominant inheritance and a phenotype characterized by low and age-related penetrance (which is the proportion of carriers who manifest the disease). It is estimated that only 20% of gene carriers younger than the age of 20 display the disease phenotype.

**TABLE 38-2.** Types of Dilated Cardiomyopathies

Ischemic insult (*ischemic cardiomyopathy*)
Valvular disease (mitral regurgitation, aortic stenosis); (*valvular cardiomyopathy*)
Chronic hypertension (*hypertensive cardiomyopathy*)
Tachyarrhythmias (supraventricular, ventricular, atrial flutter)
Familial (autosomal dominant, autosomal recessive, X-linked, matrilinear)
Idiopathic
   Toxins
   Ethanol
   Chemotherapeutic agents (anthracyclines such as doxorubicin and daunorubicin)
   Cobalt
   Antiretroviral agents (zidovudine, didanosine, zalcitabine)
   Phenothiazines
   Carbon monoxide
   Lithium
   Lead
   Cocaine
   Mercury
Metabolic abnormalities
   Nutritional deficiencies (thiamine, selenium, carnitine, protein)
   Endocrinologic disorders (hypothyroidism, acromegaly, thyrotoxicosis, Cushing
   disease, pheochromocytoma, catecholamines, diabetes mellitus)
   Electrolyte disturbances (hypocalcemia, hypophosphatemia)
Infectious
   Viral (coxsackievirus, cytomegalovirus, HIV, adenovirus, HSV)
   Rickettsial
   Bacterial
   Mycobacterial
   Spirochetal
   Fungal
   Parasitic (toxoplasmosis, trichinosis, Chagas disease)
Autoimmune/collagen disorders
   Systemic lupus erythematosus
Juvenile rheumatoid arthritis
   Polyarteritis nodosa
   Kawasaki disease
   Collagen vascular disorders (scleroderma, lupus erythematosus, dermatomyositis)
Infiltrative disorders
   Hemochromatosis
Amyloidosis
   Sarcoidosis
Endomyocardial disorders
   Hypereosinophilic syndrome (Löffler endocarditis)
   Endomyocardial fibrosis
Hypersensitivity myocarditis
Peripartum/postpartum dysfunction
   Arrhythmogenic right ventricular dysplasia or cardiomyopathy
Infantile histiocytoid
Neuromuscular dystrophies
   Becker or Duchenne muscular dystrophy, X-linked cardioskeletal myopathy
Facioscapulohumeral muscular dystrophy
   Erb limb-girdle dystrophy
   Myotonic dystrophy
Friedreich ataxia
   Emery–Dreifuss muscular dystrophy
Inborn errors of metabolism
Mitochondrial cardiomyopathies
Keshan cardiomyopathy

Familial dilated cardiomyopathy can be caused by mutations of a large number of genes (www.OMIM.org) involved in various myocardial functions including the *sarcomere,* the *cytoskeleton/sarcolemma/nuclear envelope, ion channels,* the *desmosome,* and *signaling pathways.* Specific characteristics of the phenotype can help in the identification of the disease gene. The detection of an altered creatine kinase (CK) level can indicate the existence of a subclinical skeletal muscle disease. In these patients an X-linked inheritance suggests mutations in the dystrophin gene (eg, muscular dystrophy). An autosomal dominant transmission and the presence of conduction defects, arrhythmia, and increased CK levels suggest mutations in the lamin A/C gene. In *laminopathies,* the phenotype of the affected relatives can be very variable, from a pure DCM to a mild Emery-Dreifuss–like or limb-girdle–like muscle dystrophy (Erb disease). An autosomal recessive transmission of dilated cardiomyopathy may occur in mutations of sarcoglycan genes, which encode for dystrophin complex–associated proteins. Defects in other structural proteins, such as *desmoplakin,* may result in syndromic DCM (eg, Carvajal syndrome associated with woolly hair and keratoderma).

Other heritable neuromuscular dystrophies associated with cardiomyopathy include Becker, Duchenne, and X-linked cardioskeletal myopathy, myotonic dystrophy (Steinert disease), congenital myotonic dystrophy, familial centronuclear myopathy, Kugelberg–Welander syndrome, Friedreich ataxia, and Barth syndrome. The myocardial involvement, natural history, and prognosis of each of these disorders are variable. Duchenne dystrophy is an X-linked disease of the dystrophic gene with proximal muscle weakness and cardiomyopathy. Patients with myotonic dystrophy present between age 20 and 50 years, and death usually results from respiratory and/or cardiorespiratory failure. The ECG frequently shows a straight posterior myocardial infarction.

Familial investigations require sensitive diagnostic criteria that are able to detect minor cardiac abnormalities in relatives of the proband. These abnormalities include dilatation without systolic dysfunction, subtle abnormalities in contractility, arrhythmia, and other abnormalities. Formal genetic testing may be useful as well, particularly to ascertain risk of developing the phenotype as well as helping to define clinical course in affected relatives. For example, the lamin A/C gene is associated with conduction delays as well as high mortality and morbidity.

Several immune regulatory abnormalities have been identified in DCM. A clinical and pathologic syndrome that is similar to DCM may develop after resolution of viral myocarditis in animal models and biopsy-proven myocarditis in human subjects. This has led to speculation that DCM may develop in some individuals as a result of subclinical viral myocarditis.

The prognosis of primary DCM is generally better than for ischemic cardiomyopathy. Therapy for DCM is no different than for any other form of systolic heart failure and should include RAS and adrenergic antagonists, judicious use of diuretics, and appropriate resynchronization and defibrillator therapy. Approximately 10% of DCM subjects treated with beta-adrenergic blockade will normalize their myocardial function. Among genetic causes of DCM, *laminopathies* (caused by mutations in the lamin A/C gene) have been associated with a rapidly fatal course, making genetic testing an important tool in the clinical management of these patients.

# ■ POSTPARTUM CARDIOMYOPATHY

Post- or peripartum cardiomyopathy is defined as the presentation of systolic dysfunction and clinical heart failure during the last trimester of pregnancy or within 6 months of delivery. Postpartum cardiomyopathy is likely a heterogeneous group of disorders, consisting of the addition of the hemodynamic load of pregnancy to a variety of underlying myocardial processes including hypertensive heart disease, familial or idiopathic dilated cardiomyopathy, and myocarditis. The incidence of peripartum cardiomyopathy varies from 1 in 3000 to 1 in 15 000 pregnancies in the United States. A much higher incidence is observed in Africa (1 in 3000) and Haiti (1 in 350). Predisposing factors include black race, obesity, multiple gestations, preeclampsia, chronic hypertension, and age greater than 30 years.

Endomyocardial biopsy can reveal myocarditis in as many as 50% of these women, but generally the findings are nonspecific. Prolactin may play a role in the disease through pro-inflammatory mechanisms once oxidatively modified during pregnancy. Blockade of prolactin with the dopaminergic agonist, bromocriptine, has been reported in case series of peripartum cardiomyopathy.

Delivery of the baby may be curative in some but the clinical course is highly variable with some achieving complete recovery and others ultimately requiring transplantation. Patients with higher ejection fractions and smaller ventricular diastolic dimensions at the time of diagnosis have a better long-term prognosis. Further pregnancies are generally recommended against but risk of recurrent disease appears to be decreased in those who have complete normalization of cardiac function.

## ■ ALCOHOL CARDIOMYOPATHY

An *alcohol cardiomyopathy* is said to be present when other causes of a dilated cardiomyopathy have been excluded and there is a history of heavy, sustained alcohol intake (eg, 80 g of alcohol per day for males and 40 g for females over years). However, in susceptible individuals it is likely that lower amounts of intake can produce a cardiomyopathy. The histologic features of alcohol cardiomyopathy are nonspecific and do not differ from DCM. Other than history, the only potentially distinguishing feature between DCM and alcohol cardiomyopathy is that the latter may present with a relatively high cardiac output. The pathophysiology of alcohol cardiomyopathy is thought to be related to the toxic effects of alcohol, plus, in some subjects, nutritional components such as thiamine deficiency. Genetic factors may predispose to alcoholic cardiomyopathy, like the ACE *DD* polymorphism.

The treatment of alcohol cardiomyopathy does not differ from that of DCM except for the need for total abstinence from alcohol. However, recovery of myocardial function is unpredictable with abstinence.

## SUGGESTED READINGS

Mestroni L, Gilbert EM, Lowes BD, Bristow MR. Dilated cardiomyopathies. In: Fuster V, Walsh R, Harrigton RA, et al, eds. *Hurst's The Heart.* 13th ed. New York, NY: McGraw-Hill; 2011; 32:821-836.

Bristow MR. β-Adrenergic receptor blockade in chronic heart failure. *Circulation.* 2000;101: 558-569.

Fett JD, Christie LG, Carraway RD, et al. Five-year prospective study of the incidence and prognosis of peripartum cardiomyopathy at a single institution. *Mayo Clin Proc.* 2005;80: 1602-1606.

Hershberger RE, Lindenfeld J, Mestroni L, et al. Genetic evaluation of cardiomyopathy: a heart failure society of America practice guideline. *J Cardiac Fail.* 2009;15:83-97.

Mann DL, Bristow MR. Mechanisms and models in heart failure: the biomedical model and beyond. *Circulation.* 2005;111:2837-2849.

Maron BJ, Towbin JA, Thiene G, et al. Contemporary definitions and classification of the cardiomyopathies. *Circulation.* 2006;113:1807-1816.

McKusick VA. Online Mendelian Inheritance in Man (OMIM). In: McKusick-Nathans Institute for Genetic Medicine, Johns Hopkins University (Baltimore, MD) and National Center for Biotechnology Information, National Library of Medicine (Bethesda, MD); 2000. Available at www.ncbi.nim.nih.gov/Omim/. Accessed September 5, 2012.

Taylor MRG, Fain P, Sinagra G, et al. Natural history of dilated cardiomyopathy due to lamin A/C gene mutations. *J Am Coll Cardiol.* 2003;41:771-780.

# CHAPTER 39
# HYPERTROPHIC CARDIOMYOPATHY

Steve R. Ommen, Rick A. Nishimura, and A. Jamil Tajik

Hypertrophic cardiomyopathy (HCM) was first introduced by Jeare in 1958, when he published the pathologic findings of young patients who had died suddenly. Described as idiopathic hypertrophic subaortic stenosis, muscular subaortic stenosis, and hypertrophic obstructive cardiomyopathy, *HCM* is now the preferred term by the World Health Organization for clinically unexplained left ventricular hypertrophy and small ventricular cavity characteristic of this entity. HCM is perhaps the most common genetic cardiovascular disease caused by a missense mutation in one of at least ten genes encoding proteins of the sarcomere and contractile apparatus. Two-hundred different mutations have now been identified; these lead to myofibrillar disarray and fibrosis. HCM is an autosomal dominant trait with a prevalence of approximately 1 per 500 people, and it is a common cause of sudden death in young people, particularly in trained athletes below 30 years of age. The characteristic features of HCM include an increase in left ventricular (LV) wall thickness without ventricular chamber dilatation and normal or hypercontractile LV function. LV outflow tract obstruction (LVOT) is present in <30% of cases. The most common sites of ventricular involvement include the septum, apex, and midventricle. The pathophysiologic abnormalities in patients with HCM consist of interrelated processes including dynamic LVOT obstruction, diastolic dysfunction, mitral regurgitation (MR), myocardial ischemia, and cardiac arrhythmias.

## PATHOLOGY

Pathologic examination of the heart in HCM often reveals asymmetrical septal hypertrophy (ASH) with a small- or normal-sized LV cavity and left atrial (LA) enlargement. Many variants of HCM exist, including hypertrophy of regions other than the septum, eg, apical, as well as concentric hypertrophy. The mitral valve is usually normal but may be thickened, enlarged, and elongated. Endocardial thickening in the LVOT may be present. There may be anomalous papillary muscle insertion into the anterior mitral leaflet.

Histologic examination reveals myocardial disarray consisting of short runs of hypertrophied, nonparallel myofibers distributed in a disorganized fashion and interrupted by connective tissue, resulting in the characteristic "whirling" pattern. These areas of disorganization and fibrosis are thought to be the source for the ventricular arrhythmias commonly found in HCM.

The intramural coronary arteries may be small secondary to intimal hyperplasia, which results in thickened walls and narrowed lumina. These abnormal intramural coronary arteries may contribute to microvascular angina in the absence of epicardial coronary atherosclerosis.

# CLINICAL MANIFESTATIONS

Dyspnea, angina pectoris, presyncope/syncope, and sudden death are symptoms found in patients with HCM. Although the majority of such patients are asymptomatic, dyspnea is the most common complaint. Dyspnea occurs as a result of a stiff, noncompliant ventricle, resulting in an elevated LV end-diastolic pressure (LVEDP) and abnormal ventricular relaxation. Concomitant dynamic LVOT obstruction and MR may be present. Angina pectoris occurs frequently as well. Also patients commonly experience impaired consciousness (syncope, near-syncope, or dizziness), palpitations, and occasionally orthopnea or paroxysmal nocturnal dyspnea when more advanced stages of heart failure evolve. Syncope is not uncommon, resulting from either a hemodynamic abnormality or a rhythm disturbance. Some 20% of older patients with HCM may experience atrial fibrillation, which can lead to clinical deterioration and increase the risk of systemic embolization.

## ■ PHYSICAL EXAMINATION

The classic physical findings of HCM usually occur only in the presence of an LVOT pressure gradient. Examination of the neck veins reveals a prominent A wave due to a stiff, noncompliant ventricle, elevated pulmonary pressures, or right ventricular outflow obstruction. The carotid pulse is typically bifid with a brisk upstroke, declining in midsystole (secondary to a sudden deceleration of the blood due to midsystolic obstruction) and then having a secondary rise (the subsequent tidal wave), which reflects the classic "spike and dome" configuration. Palpation of the precordium may reveal an apical impulse that is usually sustained and frequently bifid; it may have the classic "triple ripple" (a presystolic and a double systolic movement of the apical impulse). On auscultation, $S_1$ may be normal or loud; $S_2$ may be physiologic or paradoxically split if there is severe LVH, left bundle-branch block, or severe LVOT obstruction. An $S_4$ is usually present. The murmur of HCM is a harsh crescendo-decrescendo systolic murmur heard best along the left lower sternal border and at the apex. The murmur decreases with maneuvers that increase LV volume, such as squatting, leg lifting, or handgrip. Conversely, maneuvers that decrease LV volume—such as standing, the Valsalva maneuver, or amyl nitrite inhalation—tend to increase LVOT obstruction and cause the murmur to increase in intensity. The most useful maneuver is squatting. The murmur may radiate to the base, apex, or axilla but seldom to the neck. Concomitant MR is often present and may be distinguished from the murmur of HCM by location (apical) and character; MR is more holosystolic and does not increase in intensity in the post-premature ventricular contraction (PVC), as does HCM.

# DIAGNOSTIC TESTS

## ■ ELECTROCARDIOGRAM

The 12-lead electrocardiogram (ECG) is very useful in screening for HCM, as a normal ECG virtually eliminates the diagnosis. Common ECG findings include LV hypertrophy (found in 80% of patients), left atrial enlargement, left anterior hemiblock, left bundle-branch block, PVCs, left axis deviation, abnormal Q waves, or poor R-wave progression across the precordium (representing pseudoinfarction). Prominent T-wave inversion across the precordium may be found in patients with the apical variety of HCM. Findings of preexcitation (delta wave) may be present. Atrial fibrillation is not uncommonly found. However, there is no pathognomonic ECG pattern for HCM.

## ■ HOLTER MONITORING

Holter monitoring is frequently utilized to identify patients with high-risk features of sudden cardiac death (SCD). Although the rhythm is typically normal sinus, monitoring may reveal atrial fibrillation, PVCs, and episodes of supraventricular and ventricular arrhythmias.

## ■ CHEST X-RAY

The chest x-ray may be completely normal in the asymptomatic patient. Left atrial enlargement, pulmonary artery engorgement, and edema may be present when LV filling pressures are elevated. The cardiac silhouette is often enlarged, and the left cardiac border may be prominent secondary to LVH. Mitral annular calcification may be seen. The absence of aortic root dilation and aortic valve calcium help to differentiate these patients from those with aortic valve stenosis.

# DIAGNOSTIC EVALUATION

The critical diagnostic issue is to document left ventricular hypertrophy and a diminished ventricular cavity in the absence of a physiologic reason such as hypertension, outflow obstruction (eg, aortic stenosis), and even competitive athletics. Rarely, metabolic disorders may produce the same phenotype, eg, alpha-galactosidase deficiency and Fabry disease.

## ■ ECHOCARDIOGRAPHY

Two-dimensional echocardiography is considered the "gold standard" for diagnosing HCM. Echocardiographic features of HCM include LVH (classically asymmetric) in a nondilated left ventricle with normal systolic function and impaired diastolic function. Although asymmetric septal hypertrophy is the most common morphologic type of HCM, there is considerable variability in the pattern of hypertrophy found in HCM, including involvement of the free wall, the LV apex, and the posterior-basal walls. Concentric hypertrophy may also be present. There is often abnormal anterior displacement of the mitral valve as a result of posterior bulging of the septum. Systolic anterior motion (SAM) of the mitral valve with ventricular septal contact is responsible for dynamic obstruction to LV outflow. Doppler echocardiography can accurately assess the magnitude and dynamic characteristics of the outflow pressure gradient, the severity of dynamic outflow obstruction, and the diastolic filling and relaxation abnormalities. All first-degree family members should undergo echocardiography: every year for the adolescent child aged 12 to 18 and then every 5 years until the sixth to seventh decades of life (**Table 39-1**).

## ■ EXERCISE STRESS TESTING

Exercise stress testing is useful for the objective measurement of exercise tolerance and may help in prognostic evaluation. PVCs, arrhythmias such as atrial fibrillation, ventricular tachycardia, and nonsustained ventricular tachycardia may be provoked during exercise. An abnormal blood pressure response to exercise may occur (**Table 39-2**). Myocardial perfusion imaging with thallium 201 or technetium 99m may demonstrate fixed or reversible perfusion defects suggesting areas of myocardial scar or ischemia even in the absence of atherothrombotic coronary heart disease and is therefore of limited utility.

**TABLE 39-1.** Echocardiographic Features of Obstructive Hypertrophic Cardiomyopathy

Decreased LV systolic dimensions
Asymmetrical septal hypertrophy with a ratio of septum to posterior wall 1.5:1 or greater
Systolic anterior motion of the mitral valve
Delayed closure of the mitral valve
Midsystolic closure of the aortic valve
Left atrial enlargement
Mitral regurgitation
Dagger-shaped late peaking continuous-wave Doppler with resting gradient >30 mm Hg

# ■ MAGNETIC RESONANCE IMAGING

Magnetic resonances imaging (MRI) is the current gold standard for defining the pathologic features associated with hypertrophic cardiomyopathy. MRI is particularly useful in demonstrating hypertrophy when echocardiographic images are visually limited, planning surgical approaches, and quantifying scar burden which may have predictive ability in sudden death.

# ■ HEMODYNAMICS

Cardiac catheterization and angiography should be performed when mechanical intervention is contemplated or there is a concern for epicardial coronary artery disease. When cardiac catheterization is performed, both left and right heart catheterization should be done—in addition to standard coronary angiography—to evaluate for pulmonary hypertension. Left ventriculography should be performed with the RAO projection at 30 degrees and the LAO projection at 60 degrees, with cranial angulation so as to better visualize the septum. Ideally, simultaneous aortic and LV pressures should be measured as the pigtail catheter is pulled back to the LVOT obstruction. Aortic pressure tracings may demonstrate the "spike and dome" configuration (**Fig. 39-1**). The Brockenbrough- Braunwald-Morrow sign may occur

**TABLE 39-2.** Risk Factors for Sudden Cardiac Death in Patients with Hypertrophic Cardiomyopathy

Cardiac arrest (ventricular fibrillation)
Spontaneous sustained ventricular tachycardia
Family history of sudden HCM-related death (2 or more first-degree relatives <40 years of age)
Syncope (2 or more episodes in 1 year)
Nonsustained ventricular tachycardia on Holter ECG monitoring or exercise testing (3 or more consecutive PVCs)
Abnormal blood pressure response with exertion (drop in BP >10 mm Hg or failure to rise >25 mm Hg)
Massive LV hypertrophy (LV thickness >30 mm by echocardiography) LV outflow tract obstruction
Presence of microvascular obstruction detected on MRI or nuclear imaging
High-risk genetic defect within the beta-myosin heavy-chain Arg403Gln, Arg453Cys, and Arg719Trp

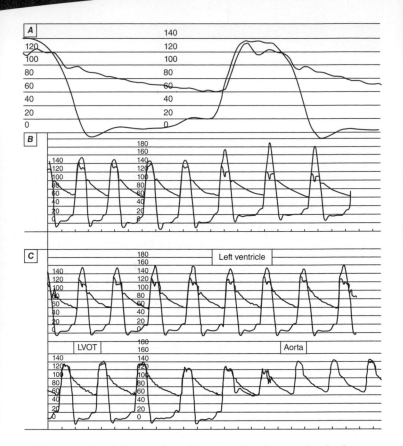

**FIGURE 39-1.** Left ventricular (LV) and LV outflow tract (LVOT) tracings. **A.** Aortic tracing demonstrating spike and dome. **B.** LV and aortic pressure tracing demonstrating increase in peak-to-peak gradient with Valsalva maneuver. **C.** Simultaneous LV and aortic pressure tracings during pull-back from LV to LVOT to aorta.

in the beat following a PVC, which leads to an increase in the LV volume and contractility, resulting in an increase of the LVOT gradient and a decrease in the aortic pulse pressure. Patients who have minimal resting gradients during catheterization should undergo provocation with Valsalva, post-PVC, or exercise. Provocation with dobutamine is generally not recommended, as this can elicit a significant gradient in a hyperdynamic LV without true HCM. A significant gradient can occur without provocation in elderly patients with hypertension and hypovolemia and in the hypovolemic postoperative patient receiving inotropic support (see Fig. 39-1).

# NATURAL HISTORY

The natural history of HCM is variable. Published studies from tertiary referral centers indicate that the annualized mortality from HCM is between 2% and 6%.

However, these centers tend to evaluate a higher proportion of symptomatic and functionally limited patients. Mortality from unselected regional populations is reported at an annual rate of about 1%. The majority of patients are asymptomatic and experience little or no disability, many achieving normal life expectancy. Children between 1 and 15 years of age have an annual mortality of about 6%. Patients with and without LVOT obstruction are equally at risk for sudden death. Premature SCD may occur in the asymptomatic or symptomatic patient. HCM is the most common cause of sudden death in young competitive athletes, frequently occurring during or immediately following physical activity. The primary mechanism of sudden death usually is ventricular tachycardia or fibrillation; however, syncope may result from outflow obstruction as well as brady- and tachyarrhythmias (see Table 39-2). Progressive symptoms of heart failure may occur and can be exacerbated by atrial fibrillation.

Although many patients live their entire lives without functional limitation, some may begin to experience heart failure after having no symptoms for many decades. A small group of patients will have progressive symptoms of heart failure and will eventually develop the "end stage" or "burned out" stage of HCM, when LV systolic function becomes significantly impaired. This occurs as a result of dilation of the LV cavity due to continued wall stress/tension, causing LV wall thinning and eventual loss of the dynamic outflow tract gradient. In addition to heart failure, other complications of HCM include atrial fibrillation, systemic embolization, and infective endocarditis. Pregnancy is usually well tolerated as long as the patient is kept well hydrated (see Table 39-2).

# TREATMENT

All patients with HCM should be evaluated on an annual basis and risk-stratified for the occurrence of SCD. Reevaluation should take place whenever there is a perceived change in clinical status. Patients should be advised against strenuous competitive athletics. The implantable cardioverter/ defibrillator (ICD) can be offered to the high-risk patient to prevent SCD (see Table 39-2). Symptomatic patients can be treated with a β-blocker or a calcium-channel blocker; patients unresponsive to these agents can be treated with disopyramide, which has potent negative inotropic effects. The therapeutic dose of either β-blocker or verapamil should be titrated for symptomatic relief or a resting heart rate of 50 to 60 beats per minute. Alternatives to medical therapy in obstructive HCM include surgical septal myectomy, alcohol ablation, and rarely dual-chamber pacing. Heart failure is notoriously difficult to treat and some patients require heart transplantation (**Fig. 39-2**).

β-blockers work in HCM by decreasing contractility and heart rate, which promotes diastolic filling, ventricular relaxation, and reduction of myocardial oxygen consumption. β-blockers are the preferred drug strategy for patients with chest pain and/or dyspnea. Standard doses are often sufficient to relieve disabling symptoms and decrease the outflow tract gradient. The calcium-channel blockers, diltiazem, and verapamil can also be used to increase LV volume and improve LV isovolumic relaxation. However, verapamil, in particular, has been associated with provoking pulmonary edema and SCD and should be used cautiously.

Dysopyramide is a type IA antiarrhythmic agent with negative inotropic properties. In patients with a resting gradient and severe symptoms, dysopyramide has been shown to reduce the LVOT gradient and myocardial contractility and to improve LV diastolic filling. Doses of 300 to 600 mg/d may be required but may be complicated by significant anticholinergic side effects such as thirst, constipation, urinary retention, and exacerbation of glaucoma.

The use of afterload-reducing agents is usually *contraindicated* in patients with HCM; however, a small percentage of patients develop systolic heart failure during

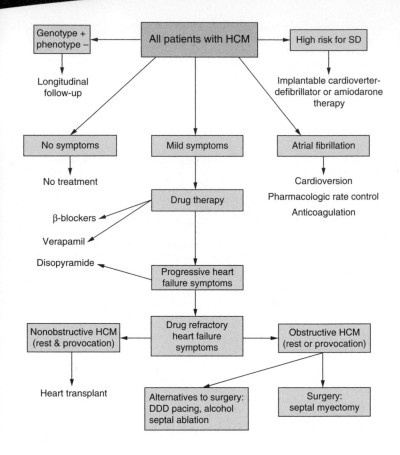

**FIGURE 39-2.** Primary treatment strategies for patients with hypertrophic cardiomyopathy.

the "burnt out" stage of HCM. Appropriate medical therapy can include afterload reduction with agents such as angiotensin-converting enzyme (ACE) inhibitors or angiotension II receptor blockers, digitalis, or even diuretics. Cardiac transplantation is a consideration in this small subgroup of patients.

Despite maximal medical therapy, a small subgroup of patients with HCM will continue to have severe, debilitating symptoms. Patients who have New York Heart Association (NYHA) class III or IV symptoms, are on maximal medical therapy, and have a resting or provocable LVOT gradient ≥30 mm Hg may be candidates for *surgical septal myectomy*. *Alcohol septal ablation* and *dual-chamber pacing* are less invasive alternative methods to septal myectomy.

Surgical septal myectomy has been performed for well over 40 years; The Morrow procedure is considered the gold standard for ameliorating LVOT obstruction and symptoms in both adults and in children. Although septal myectomy is successful in relieving symptoms, the occurrence of SCD is not diminished. Occasionally, amelioration of the LVOT gradient may not correct the MR that can accompany HCM with

LVOT obstruction; concomitant mitral valve repair/replacement should then be performed during septal myectomy. Although the operative risk of septal myectomy is acceptably low, between 1% and 2%, possible complications of septal myectomy include left bundle-branch block, complete heart block, aortic regurgitation, and iatrogenic ventricular septal defects.

An alternative to surgical myectomy is *alcohol septal ablation*. Septal ablation is based on the introduction of alcohol into a septal perforator to create a "controlled" myocardial infarction of the proximal ventricular septum. This procedure was first performed in 1995; it produces akinesis or hypokinesis of the proximal septum, thus reducing LVOT obstruction and decreasing SAM of the mitral valve and MR. Results are comparable to those of septal myectomy. Mortality and morbidity associated with septal ablation in *experienced* centers are similar to those of septal myectomy. Complications include right bundle-branch block, AV block, coronary artery dissection, and large anteroseptal myocardial infarction. Septal ablation creates an arrhythmogenic substrate that can lead to an increased risk of lethal arrhythmias. Long-term follow-up (>10 years) is lacking and considerable controversy exists regarding the optimal primary approach, eg, alcohol septal ablation versus surgical myectomy. Many authorities advocate surgical myectomy as the treatment of choice, particularly in younger patients, and reserve alcohol septal ablation for poor surgical candidates.

Dual-chamber pacing was initially reported to provide a substantial reduction in LVOT gradients and amelioration of symptoms in many patients. However, subsequent studies have not been able to consistently replicate early dramatic benefits. Subjective improvement did not correlate with objective measurements of exercise capacity and oxygen consumption. Dual-chamber pacing is clearly inferior to surgical myectomy and alcohol septal ablation in improving hemodynamics and relieving symptoms.

## SUGGESTED READINGS

Ommen SR, Nishimura RA, Tajik AJ. Hypertrophic cardiomyopathy. In: Fuster V, O'Rourke RA, Walsh RA, et al., eds. *Hurst's The Heart*. 13th ed. New York, NY: McGraw-Hill; 2008; 33: 837-864.

Maron B. Contemporary insights and strategies for risk stratification and prevention of sudden cardiac death in hypertrophic cardiomyopathy. *Circulation.* 2010; 121:445-456.

Maron BJ, McKenna WJ, Danielson GK, et al. ACC/ESC clinical expert consensus document on hypertrophic cardiomyopathy: a report of the American College of Cardiology Task Force on Clinical Expert Consensus Documents and the European Society of Cardiology Committee for Practice Guidelines (Committee to Develop an Expert Consensus Document on Hypertrophic Cardiomyopathy). *J Am Coll Cardiol.* 2003;42:1678-1713.

Maron BJ, Shen WK, Link MS, et al. Efficacy of implantable cardioverter-defibrillators for the prevention of sudden death in patients with hypertrophic cardiomyopathy. *N Engl J Med.* 2000;342:365-373.

Sorajja P, Valeti U, Nishimura RA, et al. Outcome of alcohol septal ablation for obstructive hypertrophic cardiomyopathy. *Circulation.* 2008;118:131-139.

Spirito P, Bellone P, Harris KM, et al. Magnitude of left ventricular hypertrophy predicts the risk of sudden death in hypertrophic cardiomyopathy. *N Engl J Med.* 2000;342:1778-1785.

# CHAPTER 40
# RESTRICTIVE, OBLITERATIVE, AND INFILTRATIVE CARDIOMYOPATHIES

Brian D. Hoit

## RESTRICTIVE CARDIOMYOPATHY

According to a recent consensus document from the American Heart Association, the preferred classification of cardiomyopathies should be either primary (ie, predominantly confined to the heart) or secondary (ie, as part of a generalized systemic disorder). *Restrictive cardiomyopathy* refers to an idiopathic or systemic myocardial disorder characterized by restrictive filling, normal or reduced ventricular volumes, and normal or nearly normal systolic ventricular function (**Table 40-1**). Striking elevation of the jugular venous pulse and prominent X and especially Y descents are characteristic. A reduced stroke volume and tachycardia may be seen in severe cases. The apical impulse is nondisplaced and systolic murmurs of atrioventricular regurgitation and filling sounds marking the abrupt cessation of rapid early diastolic filling are common.

Electrocardiographic abnormalities, such as abnormal voltage, atrial and ventricular arrhythmias, and conduction disturbances are frequent. Atrial enlargement and pericardial effusion may produce an enlarged cardiac silhouette on the chest radiogram, and pleural effusions and signs of pulmonary congestion may also be present. Echocardiography reveals normal or reduced ventricular dimensions, variable systolic function, and increased atrial dimensions. A dominant early diastolic mitral "E" velocity (increased E/A ratio), an increased pulmonary venous atrial systolic "A" reversal velocity and duration, as well as shortened mitral deceleration time are typical features on Doppler.

Several clinical, imaging, and hemodynamic features are helpful in distinguishing restrictive cardiomyopathy from constrictive pericarditis (**Table 40-2**). Although Doppler techniques have assumed an important role in characterizing the nature of transvalvular filling and helping to make this clinically crucial distinction, rigorous studies of the sensitivity and specificity of these Doppler findings are lacking. Thus, the diagnostic certainty is related to the number of "pathognomonic" findings in concert with clinical information and additional imaging studies. Magnetic resonance imaging (MRI) and computed tomography (CT) are useful in that pericardial thickness can be accurately assessed. B-type natriuretic peptide (BNP) levels are markedly elevated in patients with restrictive cardiomyopathy compared to constrictive pericarditis.

Right- and left-sided heart catheterization is performed to document the diagnosis, assess severity, and sometimes establish the etiology by means of endomyocardial biopsy.

**TABLE 40-1.** Classification of the Restrictive Cardiomyopathies

**Myocardial**
1. Noninfiltrative cardiomyopathies
    Idiopathic
    Familial
    Pseudoxanthoma elasticum
    Scleroderma
2. Infiltrative cardiomyopathies
    Amyloidosis
    Sarcoidosis
    Gaucher disease
3. Storage disease
    Hemochromatosis
    Fabry disease
    Glycogen storage diseases

**Endomyocardial**
1. Obliterative
    Endomyocardial fibrosis
    Hypereosinophilic syndrome
2. Nonobliterative
    Carcinoid
    Malignant infiltration
    Iatrogenic (radiation, drugs)

**TABLE 40-2.** Clinical and Hemodynamic Features That Help to Distinguish Restrictive Cardiomyopathy From Constrictive Pericarditis

|  | Restrictive Cardiomyopathy | Constrictive Pericarditis |
|---|---|---|
| History | Systemic disease that involves the myocardium, multiple myeloma, amyloidosis, cardiac transplant | Acute pericarditis, cardiac surgery, radiation therapy, chest trauma, systemic disease involving the pericardium |
| Chest radiogram | Absence of calcification | Helpful when calcification persists |
|  | Massive atrial enlargement | Moderate atrial enlargement |
| Electrocardiogram | Bundle-branch blocks, AV block | Abnormal repolarization |
| CT/MRI | Normal pericardium | Helpful if thickened (>4 mm) pericardium |
| Hemodynamics | Helpful if unequal diastolic pressures | Diastolic equilibration |
|  | Concordant effect of respiration on diastolic pressures | Dip and plateau |
| Biopsy | Fibrosis, hypertrophy, infiltration | Normal |

AV, atrioventricular; CT, computed tomography; MRI, magnetic resonance imaging.

The venous pressure is elevated and the deep decline of the right atrial Y descent is striking. The right ventricular (RV) systolic pressure is often elevated, and the early portion of diastole is characterized by a deep, sharp dip followed by a plateau (square root sign), during which no further increase in right ventricular pressure occurs. These hemodynamic features are similar to those of *constrictive pericarditis* and may create further diagnostic confusion. Although it is not uncommon for the pulmonary wedge and the right atrial pressures to be identical, a higher left than RV filling pressure favors the diagnosis of restrictive cardiomyopathy. The demonstration of respiratory systolic ventricular discordance is the most specific and sensitive hemodynamic finding for constriction; its absence strongly suggests restriction, not constriction, is present.

Treatment of restrictive cardiomyopathy is empiric and directed toward the treatment of diastolic heart failure. Judicious use of diuretics is warranted in view of the steep pressure-volume relation of the ventricles and the need to maintain a relatively high filling pressure. Vasodilators may also jeopardize ventricular filling and should be used cautiously. In appropriate candidates, transplantation is necessary but complicated by the need for biventricular mechanical circulatory support if pharmacologic support is inadequate as a clinical "bridge" to transplantation.

# ■ NONFILTRATIVE RESTRICTIVE CARDIOMYOPATHIES

Idiopathic restrictive cardiomyopathy may involve myocardium, conduction tissue, and skeletal muscle, with resultant restrictive ventricular filling and heart failure, atrioventricular (AV) block, and distal skeletal myopathy, respectively. Although not generally considered familial, several small families with both autosomal dominant and recessive patterns of inheritance have been reported, and missense mutations in human cardiac troponin I (genetic causes of hypertrophic cardiomyopathy) have been reported. In addition, a heterogeneous group of autosomal dominant disorders are characterized by skeletal myopathy and cardiac conduction abnormalities and are causally related to the desmin gene (which may also cause a dilated cardiomyopathy). Myocyte hypertrophy and fibrosis on endomyocardial biopsy are characteristic. Although idiopathic restrictive cardiomyopathy initially may have a protracted course, the prognosis is poor in older patients (particularly males) with increasing signs of systemic and pulmonary venous congestion, atrial fibrillation, and marked left atrial enlargement (>60 mm).

Pseudoxanthoma elasticum is a rare disorder, characterized by fragmentation and calcification of elastic fibers that uncommonly causes restrictive cardiomyopathy. Radiation therapy to the chest (see Chapter 42) may produce restrictive physiology and heart failure but often cannot be separated from concomitant constrictive pericarditis.

# ■ INFILTRATIVE RESTRICTIVE CARDIOMYOPATHIES

## Amyloidosis

Amyloidosis is a systemic disorder characterized by interstitial deposition of amyloid protein fibrils in multiple organs. Cardiac involvement is most common in immunoglobulin amyloidosis (AL type), which is caused by several conditions including primary amyloidosis and plasma cell dyscrasias such as multiple myeloma. Senile amyloidosis, which typically involves the atria, can affect one-quarter of patients older than the age of 80 years and is due to wild type transthyretin. A mutant form of transthyretin is responsible for a familial disorder, which produces peripheral and autonomic neuropathy in addition to cardiac disease. Cardiac deposition of amyloid protein (protein A) may also occur in secondary amyloidosis due to chronic inflammation or autoimmune disease. Cardiac involvement is uncommon in hemo-dialysis-associated (beta-2) amyloidosis.

Amyloid deposits may be interstitial and widespread, resulting in restrictive cardiomyopathy or localized to (1) conduction tissue, resulting in heart block and ventricular arrhythmias (especially in familial amyloidosis); (2) the cardiac valves, resulting in valvular regurgitation; (3) the pericardium, resulting in constriction; (4) the coronary arteries, resulting in ischemia; and (5) the pulmonary vasculature, causing pulmonary hypertension and cor pulmonale. In some cases, the clinical picture is dominated by autonomic neuropathy and nephropathy and cardiac involvement is unrecognized. Cardiac manifestations often progress from being asymptomatic to biventricular failure. The cardiac silhouette on the chest radiogram may be normal or moderately enlarged. Electrocardiographic changes include decreased voltage, pseudoinfarction, and left axis deviation. Arrhythmias and conduction disturbances may dominate the clinical course. The echocardiogram may reveal symmetrical wall thickness involving the right and left ventricles (LV wall thickness is an important prognostic variable), a small or normal LV cavity with variably depressed systolic function, atrial and vena caval dilatation, thickening of the interatrial septum and valves, and a small pericardial effusion. Highly reflective echoes producing a "granular or sparkling appearance" and occurring in a patchy distribution are characteristic echocardiographic findings but are neither sensitive nor specific (**Fig. 40-1**).

The earliest sign of amyloid cardiomyopathy is impaired LV relaxation, manifest by a mitral Doppler E/A ratio <1 and increased isovolumic relaxation and transmitral diastolic deceleration times. The restrictive pattern of LV filling—a transmitral E/A ratio ≥2 without respiratory variation, transmitral diastolic deceleration time

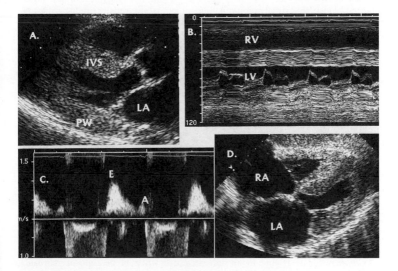

**FIGURE 40-1.** M-mode 2-dimensional and Doppler echocardiograms from a patient with biopsyproven amyloidosis causing hemodynamic restriction. Left ventricular systolic function is mildly impaired, wall thickness is increased, and there is biatrial enlargement. **A.** Parasternal long axis view. **B.** M-mode through the thickened mitral valve. **C.** Doppler of restrictive diastolic mitral inflow and systolic mitral regurgitation. **D.** Subcostal four-chamber view. A, late diastolic transmitral velocity; E, early diastolic transmitral velocity; IVS, interventricular septum; LA, left atrium; LV, left ventricle; PW, left ventricular posterior wall; RA, right atrium; RV, right ventricle.

<150 millisecond, and an isovolumic relaxation time ≤70 millisecond—is a strong predictor of cardiac death. The infiltrative pathology associated with amyloidosis may also be detected using MRI which shows a diffuse subendocardial hyperenhancement.

The variable clinical, diagnostic, and prognostic features reflect the location, nature, and extent of amyloid deposition and the temporal course of the disease. Serum and urine protein electrophoresis or immune fixation electrophoresis is diagnostic in most cases of primary amyloidosis, but monoclonal protein may not be secreted. Endomyocardial biopsy of the right ventricle is definitive, which also allows for hemodynamic assessment. Abdominal fat aspirate can also be attempted but is not commonly definitive.

The treatment of amyloidosis is difficult. Patients are sensitive to digoxin and calcium-channel blockers, and vasodilators and diuretics are poorly tolerated due to the steep LV pressure–volume relation. Angiotensin-converting enzyme inhibitors have been used with varying response rates. Amiodarone and ibutalide are effective drugs for patients with atrial fibrillation. For patients with symptomatic bradycardia or high-grade conduction system disease, a pacemaker should be implanted. Chemotherapy with melphalan, dexamethasone, lenalidomide, and bortezomib have been used to primary AL amyloidosis. Chemotherapy with combined autologous stem cell and cardiac transplantation can be considered in highly selected patients. Combined liver and heart transplantation may be lifesaving in patients with familial amyloidosis.

## Other Infiltrative Cardiomyopathies

Noncaseating granulomas involve the heart in *sarcoidosis* in as many as 50% of patients but are frequently subclinical. The combination of extracardiac manifestations and cardiac abnormalities favors a presumptive diagnosis of sarcoidosis without biopsy. Interstitial granulomatous inflammation initially produces diastolic dysfunction and later may produce systolic abnormalities. Localized thinning and dilatation of the basilar left ventricle are characteristic and the non-vascular distribution distinguishes the changes from the scarring of ischemic heart disease. Restrictive cardiomyopathy is uncommon; more often, sarcoid pulmonary involvement produces pulmonary hypertension and right heart failure. High-grade AV block and ventricular arrhythmias are principal manifestations and may result in syncope and sudden cardiac death. The electrocardiogram (ECG) most commonly demonstrates T-wave and conduction abnormalities and with extensive myocardial involvement, pseudoinfarct patterns may appear. Thallium-201 and gallium-67 have been used to indicate areas of myocardial involvement and are used to predict the response to corticosteroids. MRI may detect sarcoid granulomata or scar and can have characteristic findings. Endomyocardial biopsy is useful but, because of sampling error, may be falsely negative. A strong presumptive diagnosis can be made from clinical criteria that include evidence of myocardial abnormalities and histologic evidence of extra-cardiac sarcoidosis. Treatment with prednisone for symptomatic patients is warranted in highly suspicious or proven cases because the cardiac granuloma may be sensitive. High-grade AV nodal block usually requires a permanent pacemaker, and in patients at high risk for sudden cardiac death, an implantable cardioverter defibrillator is appropriate. Cardiac transplantation is an appropriate consideration for intractable heart failure or arrhythmia.

*Gaucher disease* is due to an inherited deficiency of beta-glucocerebroside, which results in the accumulation of cerebroside in the reticuloendothelial system, brain, and heart. Diffuse interstitial infiltration of the left ventricle occurs, leading to reduced LV compliance and decreased cardiac output, but is often subclinical. Ventricular and valvular thickening and pericardial effusions are seen on echocardiography. Enzyme replacement therapy with alglucerase (the placental derivative) and imiglucerase (the recombinant form) is effective treatment of Gaucher disease but is costly.

# STORAGE DISEASES

Myocardial iron deposition in *hemochromatosis* (genetic or transfusion related) *usually* produces dilated cardiomyopathy, but it may cause restrictive cardiomyopathy; congestive heart failure, arrhythmia, and conduction disturbances are common. The clinical features of hemochromatosis are due to accumulation of iron in the heart, pancreas, skin, liver, anterior pituitary, and gonads. Interstitial fibrosis is variable and unrelated to the extent of iron deposition, which occurs within the myocyte; secondarily, myocardial fibrosis may develop. Findings consistent with either dilated or restrictive cardiomyopathy may be seen. Granular sparkling and atrial enlargement may be observed but are nonspecific signs. CT and MRI may demonstrate subclinical cardiac involvement, and tissue characterization may be possible with MRI. Endomyocardial biopsy is confirmatory. Repeated phlebotomy is recommended for primary hemochromatosis, and the chelating agent desferroxamine is often beneficial in secondary hemochromatosis. Cardiac transplantation (with or without liver transplantation) may be considered in selected cases.

*Fabry disease* is characterized by glycolipid accumulation from a deficiency in alpha-galactosidase in the myocardium as well as the vascular and valvular endothelium and may present as a hypertrophic cardiomyopathy with concomitant vascular disease. Definitive diagnosis may require endomyocardial biopsy with electron microscopic evaluation of the myocardium. Assessment of a serum alpha-galactosidase level can be helpful. Enzyme replacement therapy has proven effective but is limited by cost and the availability of the enzyme.

*Pompe disease* is due to an autosomal recessive deficiency of acid maltase that causes glycogen deposition in the heart and skeletal muscles. The echocardiographic manifestations may be indistinguishable from those of hypertrophic obstructive cardiomyopathy. Adults with *glycogen storage type III disease* (debranching enzyme deficiency) may have marked LVH on echocardiography.

Two new disorders (LAMP-2 and Danon disease) belonging to the subgroup that includes Pompe and Fabry disease have clinical manifestations predominantly limited to the heart. The nonsarcomeric protein mutations in two genes involved in cardiac metabolism (the gama-2–regulatory subunit of the AMP-activated protein kinase and lysosome-associated membrane protein-2) are reported to be responsible for primary cardiac glycogen storage diseases in older children and adults; the clinical presentation resembles hypertrophic cardiomyopathy.

# ENDOMYOCARDIAL DISEASES

Endomyocardial diseases that cause obliterative cardiomyopathy include *endomyocardial fibrosis* (EMF) and *hypereosinophilic (Loeffler)* syndrome. Endomyocardial disease is characterized by endocardial fibrosis of the apex and subvalvular regions of one or both ventricles, resulting in restriction to inflow to the affected ventricle. Although the clinical presentations of the endomyocardial diseases differ, their pathology and therefore the cardiac imaging studies are generally similar. A search for parasitic disease or evidence for eosinophilic malignancies should be considered in Loffler's syndrome. Anthracyclines and methysergide can cause EMF. Echocardiography reveals apical obliteration of the ventricles, apical thrombus, echodensities in the endocardium, and small ventricular and large atrial cavities. Involvement of the posterior mitral and tricuspid valve leaflets results in mitral and tricuspid regurgitation; less commonly, restricted motion may produce stenosis. Sparing of the outflow tracts is characteristic. Typical patterns of restriction, mitral and tricuspid regurgitation, and less often, stenosis are seen on Doppler. Not surprisingly, the location, extent, and severity of involvement determine the clinical picture.

Medical therapy of Loeffler is often ineffective and frustrating. Treatment consists of symptomatic relief, anticoagulants, corticosteroids, hydroxyurea, and interferon alpha; palliative surgery can be considered in the late, fibrotic stage. Surgical excision of fibrotic endocardium and valve replacement may offer symptomatic improvement, but at the expense of high operative mortality. The prognosis of advanced disease is grave (50% 2-year mortality) but is considerably better in those with milder disease.

*Carcinoid syndrome* results from metastatic carcinoid tumors and consists of cutaneous flushing, diarrhea, and bronchoconstriction; involvement of the heart occurs as a late complication of carcinoid syndrome in approximately 50% of patients. Although tricuspid and pulmonic stenosis and regurgitation dominate the clinical picture, restrictive cardiomyopathy may occur.

## SUGGESTED READINGS

Hoit BD. Restrictive, obliterative, and infiltrative cardiomyopathies. In: Fuster V, Walsh R, Harrington RA, et al, eds. *Hurst's The Heart*. 13th ed. New York, NY: McGraw-Hill; 2011; 34: 865-875.

Bhattacharyya S, Davur J, Dreyfus G, et al. Carcinoid heart disease. *Circulation* 2007;116:2860-2865.

Falk R. Cardiac amyloidosis. A treatable disease, often overlooked. *Circulation*. 2011;124: 1079-1085.

Maron BJ, Towbin JA, Thiene G, et al. American Heart Association; Council on Clinical Cardiology, Heart Failure and Transplantation Committee; Quality of Care and Outcomes Research and Functional Genomics and Translational Biology Interdisciplinary Working Groups; Council on Epidemiology and Prevention. Contemporary definitions and classification of the cardiomyopathies: an American Heart Association Scientific Statement from the Council on Clinical Cardiology, Heart Failure and Transplantation Committee; Quality of Care and Outcomes Research and Functional Genomics and Translational Biology Interdisciplinary Working Groups; and Council on Epidemiology and Prevention. *Circulation*. 2006;113:1807-1816.

Patel MR, Cawley PJ, Heitner JF, et al. Detection of myocardial damage in patients with sarcoidosis. *Circulation*. 2009;120:1969-1977.

# CHAPTER 41
# MYOCARDITIS AND SPECIFIC CARDIOMYOPATHIES

Sean P. Pinney and Donna M. Mancini

Myocarditis (**Table 41-1**) encompasses a wide spectrum of diseases that have as their final common pathway left ventricular dysfunction and the syndrome of congestive heart failure (CHF). Cardiomyopathies may be primary or secondary—that is, resulting from specific cardiac or systemic disorders (see Chapters 38 and 42). Although routine endomyocardial biopsy is generally of low yield, in this group of diseases it can be diagnostic (**Table 41-2**).

## MYOCARDITIS

*Myocarditis* means inflammation of the myocardium. Myocardial dysfunction from viral myocarditis can be caused by 2 distinct phases of myocardial cell damage—the first caused by direct viral infection and the second caused by the host's immune response or apoptotic death (**Fig. 41-1**). Multiple infectious etiologies (Table 41-1) have been implicated as the cause of myocarditis, the most common being viral, specifically, the enterovirus coxsackie virus B and more recently parvovirus. The discovery of myocarditis in 1% to 9% of routine postmortem examinations suggests that myocarditis may be a cause of sudden, unexpected death.

The clinical manifestations of myocarditis are variable, ranging from an asymptomatic or self-limited disease to profound cardiogenic shock. Cardiac involvement typically occurs 7 to 10 days following an antecedent viral syndrome or systemic illness, which occurs in 60% of patients. Chest pain can occur in up to 35% of patients and may be associated with pericarditis or result from myocardial ischemia. Syncope and sudden cardiac death can be the initial presentations of myocarditis in some patients, presumably due to complete heart block or ventricular tachycardia.

Physical examination findings in acute myocarditis include fever, tachycardia, and signs of CHF. The first heart sound may be soft and a summation gallop may be present. An apical systolic murmur of mitral regurgitation may be auscultated. A pericardial friction rub may be present. Laboratory findings are generally nondiagnostic and demonstrate leukocytosis, eosinophilia, elevated ESR, and occasionally elevated titers to cardiotropic viruses. A 4-fold rise in IgG or IgM antibody titers documents only the response to a recent viral infection and does not indicate active myocarditis and rarely helpful. An increase in the myocardial band (MB) of creatine phosphokinase (CPK) is observed in approximately 10% of patients, although troponin assays are proving to be more sensitive. The classic clinical triad of preceding viral illness, pericarditis, and associated laboratory abnormalities used to diagnose coxsackie virus B–induced myocarditis is present in fewer than 10% of histologically proven cases. The electrocardiogram (ECG) most frequently shows sinus tachycardia.

**TABLE 41-1.** Causes of Myocarditis

| Disease | Etiologies | Comment |
|---|---|---|
| **Infectious** | | |
| Viral | Viruses | The most common etiology of infectious myocarditis in North America is viral infection by coxsackie- or echoviruses. Most episodes are self-limited and asymptomatic. In patients with symptoms of congestive heart failure (CHF), acute and chronic viral titers are needed along with endomyocardial biopsy to confirm the diagnosis. |
| | Coxsackievirus, echovirus, HIV, Epstein-Barr virus, influenza, cytomegalovirus, adenovirus, hepatitis (A and B), mumps, poliovirus, rabies, respiratory syncytial virus, rubella, vaccinia, varicella zoster, arbovirus | |
| Bacterial | Bacteria | In South America, the most common cause of myocarditis is Chagas disease, caused by the bite of the reduviid bug carrying parasite *Trypanosoma cruzi.* |
| | *Corynebacterium diphtheriae, Streptococcus pyogenes, Staphylococcus aureus, Haemophilus pneumoniae, Salmonella* spp., *Neisseria gonorrhoeae,* leptospirosis, the Lyme disease, syphilis, brucellosis, tuberculosis, actinomycosis, *Chlamydia* spp., *Coxiella burnetii, Mycoplasma pneumoniae, Rickettsia* spp. | |
| Fungal | Fungi | |
| | *Candida* spp, *Aspergillus* spp., histoplasmosis, blastomycosis, cryptococcosis, coccidioidomycosis | |
| Parasitic | Parasites | |
| | Toxoplasmosis, schistosomiasis, trichinosis | |
| Infiltrative | Sarcoid | Myocardial inflammation may be present on biopsy. Routine and special stains are extremely valuable in confirming these diagnoses. |
| | Giant cell | Generally a fulminant disease with a high mortality. May recur after transplant. |

| Hypersensitivity/eosinophilic | *Antibiotics* <br> Sulfonamides, penicillins, cefaclor, chloramphenicol, amphotericin E, tetracycline, streptomycin <br> *Antituberculous drugs* <br> Isoniazid, para-aminosalicylic acid <br> *Anticonvulsants* <br> Phenindione, phenytoin, carbamazepine, phenobarbital <br> *Antidepressants* <br> Amitriptyline, desipramine <br> *Anti-inflammatories* <br> Indomethicin, phenylbutazone, oxyphenylbutazone <br> *Diuretics* <br> Acetazolamide, chlorthalidone, hydrochlorothiazide, spironolactone <br> *Others* <br> Methyldopa, sulforylureas, interleukin-2, interleukin-4, tetanus toxoid | Treatment is discontinuation of the offending agent with or without steroids. Potentially reversible. |
| Toxins | Cocaine, cyclophosphamide, emetine, lithium, methysergide, phenothiazines, interferon alpha, interleukin-2, doxorubicin, cobalt, lead, chloroquine, hydrocarbons, carbon monoxide, anabolic steroids | Potentially reversible for some toxins. |
| Radiation | Past history of lymphoma | |

**TABLE 41-2.** Diseases Diagnosed by Endomyocardial Biopsy

1. Myocarditis
   - Giant-cell arteritis
   - Cytomegalovirus infection
   - Toxoplasmosis
   - Chagas disease
   - Rheumatic fever
   - Lyme disease
2. Infiltrative cardiomyopathy
   - Amyloid
   - Sarcoid
   - Hemochromatosis
   - Carcinoid
   - Hypereosinophilic cardiomyopathy
   - Glycogen storage disease
   - Cardiac tumors
3. Toxins
   - Doxorubicin
   - Chloroquine
   - Radiation injury
4. Genetic conditions
   - Fabry disease
   - Kearns–Sayre syndrome
   - Right ventricular dysplasia

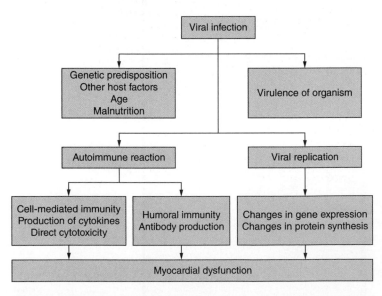

**FIGURE 41-1.** Flow diagram illustrating various factors that contribute to the development of myocardial dysfunction after viral infection.

Diffuse ST- and T-wave changes, prolonged QT intervals, conduction delay, low voltage (from myocardial edema), and even acute pseudoinfarct patterns can also occur. Echocardiography can reveal LV systolic dysfunction in patients with a normal-sized LV cavity. Segmental wall-motion abnormalities and increased wall thickness secondary to inflammation may be present. Ventricular thrombi are seen in 15% of patients. Tissue alterations associated with myocarditis can be identifiable using MRI. Use of transverse relaxation time (T2)-weighted images may visualize tissue edema with active myocarditis, and gadolinium-enhanced MRI has been used to characterize inflammatory changes; *endomyocardial biopsy* can confirm the diagnosis. Because myocarditis can be focal, 4 to 6 samples are obtained to reduce sampling error to <5%. Active myocarditis is defined pathologically as inflammatory infiltrate with myocyte necrosis. As resolution of myocarditis can occur within 4 days of initial biopsy, endomyocardial biopsy should be applied quickly to maximize diagnostic yield. The *Dallas criteria* separate initial biopsies into myocarditis, borderline myocarditis, or no myocarditis. Alternative classification schemes combine histopathologic and clinical criteria, and divide myocarditis into 4 subgroups—fulminant, acute, chronic active, and chronic persistent. These categories provide prognostic information and suggest which patients can or cannot benefit from immunosuppressive therapy.

Approximately 40% of patients with acute myocarditis will completely recover. One-third will be left with mild myocardial dysfunction to significant heart failure. One-quarter will either die or require cardiac transplantation. For patients with histopathologic confirmation of myocarditis, the 1-year survival is approximately 80%, and 5-year survival is in the range of 50% to 60%. Predictors of recovery include the degree of LV dysfunction at presentation, shorter duration of disease, and less intensive drug therapy. Paradoxically, patients with fulminant myocarditis—defined as rapid onset of symptoms, fever, and severe hemodynamic compromise—have a better survival than patients with acute nonfulminant myocarditis.

Treatment of acute myocarditis is supportive. Diuretics, angiotensin-converting enzyme inhibitors, blockers, and aldosterone antagonists should be given in the proper clinical context. Digoxin can increase the expression of inflammatory cytokines and should be used cautiously. When acute myocarditis presents with profound hemodynamic collapse, mechanical circulatory support devices can be used to bridge patients either to cardiac transplantation or to recovery. Anti-inflammatory therapy does not appear to be of benefit although commonly used. The Multicenter Myocarditis Treatment Trial randomized patients with biopsy-proven myocarditis to conventional medical therapy versus steroid/azathioprine or steroid/cyclosporine immunosuppression. Treatment with immunosuppression failed to demonstrate an improvement of ejection fraction, mortality, or attenuate clinical disease. High-dose immunoglobulin (IVIG) is also not effective when compared to placebo. Thus, the routine use of immunosuppressive therapy in myocarditis is not supported. However, myocarditis due to hypersensitivity, sarcoid, and giant cell may be immunoresponsive and should generally be empirically treated with immunosuppressive agents.

# ■ CHAGAS DISEASE

American trypanosomiasis, or Chagas disease, is the most common cause of CHF in rural South and Central America. The disease results from the bite of the reduviid bug, leading to infection with *Trypanosoma cruzi*. Cardiac injury is thought to be immunologically mediated.

In the acute phase, hematogenous spread of the parasite leads to invasion of various organ systems and an intense inflammatory reaction. Patients experience fever, sweating, myalgias, and myocarditis. The case fatality rate is approximately 5%. Survivors enter an asymptomatic latent phase, but 20% to 30% will develop a chronic form of the disease up to 20 years after the initial infection. The chronic stage is a result of gradual tissue destruction. The gastrointestinal tract and heart are the most common sites of involvement, with the primary cause of death being cardiac failure. Fibrosis of myofibrils and the Purkinje fibers leads to cardiomegaly, CHF, heart block, and arrhythmias.

Diagnosis of the acute disease depends on the discovery of trypomastigotes in the blood of the infected individual. Endomyocardial biopsy can show parasites in one-quarter of individuals. Chronic infection can be confirmed by complement-fixation test and positive serologic tests (such as the indirect immunofluorescent antibody, enzyme-linked immunosorbent assays, and hemagglutination tests) together with symptoms and signs compatible with Chagas disease. Echocardiography can demonstrate segmental wall-motion abnormalities—specifically apical aneurysms. ECG findings include complete heart block, atrioventricular (AV) block, or right bundle-branch block with or without fascicular block. Treatment of chronic Chagas disease is symptomatic and includes a pacemaker for complete heart block, an implantable cardioverter-defibrillator for recurrent ventricular arrhythmia, and standard therapy for CHF. Antiparasitic agents, such as nifurtimox and benzimidazole eradicate parasitemia during the acute phase, should be administered for untreated disease, and can be used as prophylaxis in the setting of immunosuppression. The role of immunosuppression therapy for chagasic myocarditis is controversial, and heart transplantation is effective for end-stage refractory cardiac disease.

## ■ LYME CARDITIS

Lyme disease results from infection with the spirochete *Borrelia burgdorferi*, introduced by a tick bite. The initial presenting symptom in patients with the disease who progress to cardiac involvement is frequently complete heart block. LV dysfunction is seen but rare. Endomyocardial biopsy can show active myocarditis; spirochetes are rarely observed. Treatment should include intravenous ceftriaxone and temporary pacing as needed.

## ■ RHEUMATIC CARDITIS

Acute rheumatic fever can occur following group A streptococcal pharyngitis. Clinical diagnosis is made using the *Jones criteria*. The major manifestations are carditis, polyarthritis, chorea, erythema marginatum, subcutaneous nodules, and evidence of preceding streptococcal infection. Minor criteria are nonspecific findings, such as fever, arthralgia, previous rheumatic fever or rheumatic heart disease, elevated erythrocyte sedimentation rate (ESR) or C-reactive protein, and prolonged PR interval. Diagnosis is made by the presence of 2 major criteria or 1 major and 2 minor criteria. Two-thirds of patients present with an antecedent pharyngitis, followed by symptoms of rheumatic fever in 1 to 5 weeks. Heart failure is observed in only 5% to 10% of cases. Severe carditis is usually mild, and valvular lesions predominate. Physical examination is notable for fever and the Carey-Coombs murmur, significant for mitral valvulitis. The mitral valve is involved 3 times as often as the aortic valve. ECG findings include PR prolongation and non-specific ST–T-wave changes. Endomyocardial biopsy demonstrates the pathognomonic Aschoff body, a persistent inflammatory lesion. Laboratory tests suggestive of rheumatic fever include antibodies to antistreptolysin O and anti-DNAse B, an elevated ESR, and elevated CRP. Aspirin and penicillin are the mainstays of therapy, although corticosteroids can provide symptomatic relief. Once rheumatic fever is diagnosed, antibiotic prophylaxis with penicillin is required to prevent recurrent episodes.

# NONINFECTIVE MYOCARDITIS

## ■ HYPERSENSITIVITY

Hypersensitivity myocarditis is thought to be caused by an allergic drug reaction and is characterized by peripheral eosinophilia and infiltration into the myocardium by eosinophils, multinucleated giant cells, and leukocytes. Methyldopa, the penicillins, sulfonamides, tetracycline, and the antituberculous drugs are the pharmaceuticals most commonly associated with this entity. Treatment included stopping the offending agent and corticosteroids therapy.

## ■ GIANT-CELL MYOCARDITIS

Giant-cell myocarditis is an extremely rare but aggressive form of myocarditis, typically progressive and unresponsive to medical therapy. This disease is most prevalent in young adults, and an association with other autoimmune disorders is reported in approximately 20% of cases. Diagnosis is made by endomyocardial biopsy. Widespread or multifocal necrosis with a mixed inflammatory infiltrate including lymphocytes and histiocytes is required for histologic diagnosis. Eosinophils are frequently noted, as are multinucleated giant cells in the absence of granuloma. The clinical course is usually characterized by rapidly progressive heart failure and is frequently associated with refractory ventricular arrhythmia. It is almost uniformly and rapidly fatal. Case reports and the Giant-Cell Myocarditis Registry suggest that treatment with immunosuppressive regimens, but not steroids alone, can extend transplant-free survival by a few months. Mechanical circulatory support may be required as a bridge to transplant, and rare cases of complete recovery have been described. Cardiac transplantation represents the best treatment option despite the possibility of recurrence in the transplanted heart.

# CARDIOMYOPATHY CAUSED BY ENDOCRINE DISORDERS

Thyroid hormone excess or deficiency can lead to reversible cardiomyopathy. Thyroid hormone metabolism is frequently abnormal in patients with heart failure. Changes in cardiac function are mediated by triiodothyronine ($T_3$) regulation of cardiac-specific genes. Hypothyroidism can result in decreased cardiac output, increased peripheral vascular resistance, and impaired exercise performance. Thyroid toxicity can lead to the development of both high- and low-output cardiac failure. A prolonged tachycardia and high-output state caused by thyrotoxicosis is thought eventually to produce LV dilation. A consequent progressive decline in systolic function leads to low-output heart failure.

Pheochromocytoma produces hypertension, swelling, palpitations, and orthostatic hypotension. Although progression to cardiac involvement is unusual, catecholamine-induced myocarditis has been reported. Patients typically die of cardiovascular causes as aggressive disease can lead to heart failure or malignant ventricular arrhythmias. Cardiac abnormalities are reversible with tumor resection.

Acromegalic cardiomyopathy appears to be a specific entity that develops in 10% to 20% of patients with excess growth hormone production. The initial increased cardiac output and decreased total peripheral resistance triggered by increased growth hormone levels over time result in myocyte hypertrophy with fibrosis leading to impaired diastolic function and finally systolic dysfunction. Heart failure in these patients is particularly resistant to conventional therapy presumably due to the higher collagen content in the acromegalic heart. Inflammatory and degenerative damage to the sinoatrial and AV nodes can lead to sudden death. Pituitary surgery and irradiation remain the mainstays of therapy, although the cardiac abnormalities may persist despite a fall in growth hormone levels.

# CARDIOMYOPATHIES ASSOCIATED WITH NUTRITIONAL DEFICIENCIES

Thiamine deficiency may result in wet beriberi, a clinical syndrome characterized by high-output cardiac failure and severe lactic acidosis. Dramatic hemodynamic improvements are seen after bolus infusion of thiamine. Untreated, beriberi can be fatal. Vitamin D deficiency, or rickets, and vitamin D excess are associated with cardiovascular morbidity and mortality.

Cardiomyopathy associated with inadequate dietary intake of selenium is termed *Keshan disease.* Low selenium levels have been documented in patients receiving total parenteral nutrition. Whether the cardiomyopathy results from the actual selenium deficiency or the selenium deficiency increases susceptibility to cardiotropic viruses is unclear. Its incidence is dramatically reduced with supplementation of sodium selenite.

L-Carnitine is essential in the transport of long-chain fatty acids into mitochondria, where they undergo β-oxidation. Normal hearts obtain approximately 60% of total energy production from fatty acid oxidation. Primary carnitine deficiencies result from several genetic disorders and can lead to cardiomyopathy within 3 to 4 years of birth, which responds to carnitine supplementation. Secondary carnitine deficiencies are more common and are associated with liver disease, renal disease, dietary insufficiencies (chronic total parenteral nutrition, malabsorption), diabetes mellitus, and defects in acyl-CoA metabolism.

# TAKO-TSUBO CARDIOMYOPATHY

Also termed *broken heart syndrome* or *stress cardiomyopathy*, Tako-tsubo cardiomyopathy is a reversible cardiomyopathy characterized by apical ballooning observed on left ventriculography. The etiology appears to be related to adrenergic excess and/or sensitivity. Differences in the density of β-adrenergic receptors in the apex and base of the heart can account for the apical ballooning. Other potential mechanisms include coronary vasospasm, microvascular dysfunction, and/or localized myocarditis. The clinical presentation is generally preceded by a stressful emotional, physical, or psychological event. Symptoms include chest pain, dyspnea, and syncope. Cardiac enzymes are usually only modestly elevated. The most common ECG finding is anterior ST elevations and subsequent giant T-wave inversion. Echocardiography reveals mild to severe LV dysfunction with anteroapical akinesis or dyskinesis. MRI shows mid to apical LV dyskinesis without delayed gadolinium hyperenhancement consistent with myocardial viability. Coronary angiography is normal and endomyocardial biopsy is nondiagnostic. Recovery of LV function is usual and occurs over a period of days to weeks.

# NONCOMPACTION CARDIOMYOPATHY

LV noncompaction cardiomyopathy is a genetically heterogenous disorder that may or may not be associated with other congenital abnormalities (see www.OMIM.org). In the absence of coexistent congenital defects, this disorder is called *isolated noncompaction of the left ventricle.* The underlying mechanism is postulated to be caused by intrauterine arrest of myocardial development leading to diffuse prominent deep trabeculations in hypertrophied and hypokinetic segments in the left ventricle.

Ventricular arrhythmias, embolic events, and heart failure, which can occur in two-thirds of patients, are the most common sequelae. Diastolic dysfunction can occur from both abnormal relaxation and restricted filling from the prominent trabeculae. Diagnosis is made by echocardiography or MRI. Anticoagulation to prevent embolization and close monitoring for arrhythmias with early use of implantable defibrillators are key aspects of patient management.

## SUGGESTED READINGS

Pinney SP, Mancini DM. Myocarditis and specific cardiomyopathies. In: Fuster V, Walsh R, Harrington RA, et al, eds. *Hurst's The Heart*. 13th ed. New York, NY: McGraw-Hill; 2011;35: 876-894.

Cooper LT, Baughman KL, Feldman AM, et al. The role of endomyocardial biopsy in the management of cardiovascular disease. *J Am Coll Cardiol*. 2007;50:1914-1931.

Cooper LT, Berry GJ, Shabetai R. Idiopathic giant-cell myocarditis—natural history and treatment. *N Engl J Med*. 1997;336:1860-1866.

Eitel I, Eitel I, von Knobelsdorff-Brenkenhoff F, et al. Clinical characteristics and CMR findings in stress (Takotsubo) cardiomyopathy. *JAMA*. 2011;306:277-286.

Magnani JW, Dec GW. Myocarditis: current trends in diagnosis and treatment. *Circulation*. 2006;113:876-890.

Mason JW, O'Connell JB, Herskowitz A, et al. A clinical trial of immunosuppressive therapy for myocarditis. *N Engl J Med*. 1995;333:269-275.

McCarthy R, Boehmer J, Hruban R, et al. Long-term outcome of fulminant myocarditis as compared with acute (nonfulminant) myocarditis. *N Engl J Med*. 2000;342:690-695.

McNamara DM, Holubkov R, Starling RC, et al. Controlled trial of intravenous immune globulin in recent-onset dilated cardiomyopathy. *Circulation*. 2001;103:2254-2259.

# CHAPTER 42
# THE HEART AND NONCARDIAC DRUGS, ELECTRICITY, POISONS, AND RADIATION

Andrew L. Smith and Wendy M. Book

## NONCARDIAC DRUGS

### ■ CHEMOTHERAPEUTIC AGENTS

Chemotherapeutic agents may cause acute or chronic cardiovascular toxicity (**Tables 42-1** and **42-2**). The increased recognition of these toxicities and the increased survival of cancer patients have led to the development of cardio-oncology. Cardiomyopathy has been classically associated with the anthracy-clines (doxorubicin, daunorubicin, epirubicin, idarubicin, and mitoxantrone). Cyclophosphamide has been associated with reversible systolic dysfunction and occasionally hemorrhagic myocarditis. Interleukin-2 and interferon alpha may cause hypotension and rarely cardiomyopathy. 5-Fluorouracil has been associated with coronary vasospasm. Amsacrine and paclitaxel have been associated with cardiac arrhythmias. Herceptin given in combination with doxorubicin may cause systolic dysfunction. "Targeted chemotherapy" with tyrosine kinase inhibitors (through interruption of growth factor signaling as either monoclonal antibodies or small molecule ligands) has been very effective in many previously untreat-able cancers but may be associated with cardiovascular toxicity (Table 42-2). For example, imatinib (Gleevec) and sunitinib (Sutent) can be associated with hyper-tension and heart failure.

### Anthracyclines

Doxorubicin (Adriamycin) and daunorubicin (Cerubidine) cause dose-related cardiotoxicity through oxidant-mediated free-radical damage. Acute cardiac toxic-ity may occur after the initial doses. The *early or acute cardiotoxicity* manifests as a pericarditis-myocarditis syndrome and is not dose-related. LV dysfunction is rarely seen, but arrhythmias, abnormalities of conduction, decreased QRS voltage, and nonspecific ST-segment and T-wave abnormalities are commonly observed. The prognosis is good, with quick resolution on discontinuation of therapy. Chronic cardiotoxicity occurs within months of therapy. Late cardiac systolic dysfunction occurring years later is also seen. Diffuse left ventricular (LV) dysfunction occurs in up to 7% of patients receiving 450 mg/m$^2$ of doxorubicin. Mediastinal radiation, advanced age, hypertension, and coronary artery disease are risk factors for anthracycline-related

**TABLE 42–1.** Drugs That Can Cause Torsade de Pointes

| |
|---|
| **Drugs commonly involved** |
| Dofetilide |
| Ibutilide |
| Procainamide |
| Quinidine |
| Sotalol |
| Bepridil |
| **Other drugs (<1% incidence)** |
| Amiodarone |
| Arsenic trioxide |
| Cisapride |
| Anti-infective agents: clarithromycin, erythromycin, halofantrine, pentamidine, sparfloxacin |
| Antiemetic agents: domperidone, droperidol |
| Antipsychotic agents: chlorpromazine, haloperidol, mesoridazine, thioridazine, pimozide |
| Methadone |

Adapted with permission from Roden DM. Drug therapy: drug-induced prolongation of the QT interval. *N Engl J Med*. 2004;350:1013-1022.

myocardial toxicity and ventricular dysfunction may present at cumulative doses lower than 450 mg/m$^2$ in this setting.

Toxicity is less with liposomal preparations and prolonged infusions in order to avoid high peak concentrations. Dexrazoxane, an iron-chelating agent, is approved as a preventive strategy in women with breast cancer after cumulative doses of doxorubicin of greater than 300 mg/m$^2$.

Although the diagnosis of anthracycline cardiomyopathy can be made clinically, the definitive diagnosis requires histologic confirmation with endomyocardial biopsy. However, in clinical practice, serial surveillance biopsies are rarely done during anthracycline therapy; instead, ventricular function is followed noninvasively with either echocardiography or MUGA and a decline of 5 percentage points is typically used to define clinically relevant toxicity.

Once cardiomyopathy develops, treatment is similar to that with other forms of systolic dysfunction. The clinical course varies from fulminant heart failure to gradually progressive deterioration. In some patients, systolic dysfunction is reversible. The best management of anthracycline cardiotoxicity is prevention by limiting dosage. Coadministration of β-blockers has also been demonstrated to have cardioprotective effects.

Trastuzumab (Herceptin) is a monoclonal antibody directed against the human epidermal growth receptor 2 (HER-2) receptor protein on breast cancer cells that is associated with an increased risk of heart failure. The incidence of heart failure can range from 7% with monotherapy to 28% when trastuzumab is used in association with anthracyclines and cyclophosphamide. Its use without combined anthracycline therapy carries a much lower risk and is usually reversible.

In contrast to the anthracyclines, cardiotoxicity associated with cyclophosphamide is not dose-related. Pericarditis, systolic dysfunction, arrhythmias, and myocardial can occur. Prior LV dysfunction is a risk factor for development of significant cardiomyopathy with cyclophosphamide. Although mortality is not trivial, survivors exhibit no residual cardiac abnormalities.

**TABLE 42-2.** Kinase Inhibitors in Cancer

| Agent | Class | Target(s) | Malignancies | Cardiovascular Toxicity/(Rate)/Type |
|---|---|---|---|---|
| Imatinib (Gleevec) | TKI | Abl1/2, PDGFRα/β, Kit | CML, Ph+ B-cell ALL, CMMl, HES, GIST | Yes/(low)/HF |
| Dasatinib (Sprycel) | TKI | Abl1/2, PDGFRα/β, Kit, SRC family | CML | Yes/(low to moderate)ᵃ/HF, generalized edema |
| Nilotinib (Tasigna) | TKI | Abl1/2, PDGFRα/β, Kit | CML | Yes/(low)ᵇ/QT prolongation, rare sudden death |
| Sunitinib (Sutent) | TKI | VEGFR1/2/3, Kit, PDGFRα/β, RET, CSF-1R, FLT3 | RGG, GIST | Yes/(moderate)/HF, hypertension |
| Lapatinib (Tykerb) | TKI | EGFR (ERBB1), ERBB2 | HER2⁺ breast cancer | No |
| Sorafenib (Nexavar) | TKI S/TKI | Raf-1/B-Raf, VEGFR2/3, PDGFRα/β, Kit, FLT3 | RCC, melanoma | Yes/(low)/ACS, hypertension, HF |
| Gefitinib (Iressa) | TKI | EGFR (ERBB1) | NSCLC | Noᶜ |
| Erlotinib (Tarceva) | TKI | EGFR (ERBB1) | NSCLC, pancreatic cancer | Noᶜ |
| Temsirolimus (Torisel) | Novel | mTOR (indirect; binds to FKBP12 and complex inhibits mTOR) | RCC | Noᶜ |
| Trastuzumab (Herceptin) | mAb | ERBB2 | HER2⁺ breast cancer | Yes/(moderate)/HF |
| Bevacizumab (Avastin) | mAb | VEGF-A | Colorectal cancer, NSCLC | Yes/(low to moderate)ᵃ/arterial thrombosis, hypertension |
| Cetuximab (Erbitux) | mAb | EGFR (ERBB1) | Colorectal cancer, squamous cell carcinoma of head/neck | Noᶜ |
| Panitumumab (Vectibix) | mAb | EGFR (ERBB1) | Colorectal | Noᶜ |
| Rituximab (Rituxan) | mAb | CD20 | B-cell lymphoma | Unknown |

| Alemtuzumab (Campath) | mAb | CD52 | B-cell CLL | Yes (in patients with mycosis fungoides/Sézary syndrome[15])/HF |
|---|---|---|---|---|
| Lestaurtinib[a] | TKI | JAK2/FLT3 | PCV, IMF | Unknown |
| Pazopanib[a] | TKI | VEGFRs; PDGFRs; Kit | RCC | Unknown |
| Vandetanib[a] | TKI | VEGFR/EGFR | NSCLC | Unknown |
| Cediranib[b] | TKI | VEGFR | NSCLC | Unknown |
| Alvocidib[b] | S/TKI | CDK | CLL | Unknown |
| Enzastaurin[b] | S/TKI | PKCβ | B-cell lymphoma | Unknown |

ACS, acute coronary syndrome; ALL, acute lymphocytic leukemia; CDK, cyclin-dependent kinase; CLL, chronic lymphocytic leukemia; CMML chronic myelomonocytic leukemia; HES, hypereosinophilic syndrome; HF, heart failure; IMF, idiopathic myelofibrosis; mAb, monoclonal antibody; mTOR, mammalian target of rapamycin; NSCLC, non–small-cell lung cancer; PCV, polycythemia vera; PKC, protein kinase C; S/TKI, serine/threonine kinase inhibitor.

Please see text for additional abbreviations. For agents not yet FDA approved, efficacy in malignancies is projected.

[a]NDA expected 2008.

[b]NDA expected 2010.

[c]Effect on left ventricular ejection fraction has not been determined, and therefore these represent best guesses.

Reproduced with permission from Chen MH, Kerkelä R, Force T. Mechanisms of cardiac dysfunction with tyrosine kinase inhibitor cancer therapeutics. *Circulation.* 2008;118:84-95.

# ■ PSYCHOTROPIC AGENTS

## Tricyclic Antidepressants

Tricyclic antidepressants (TAs) have potentially serious cardiovascular effects, including tachycardia, orthostatic hypotension, electrocardiogram (ECG) changes, and depression of LV function. They have electrophysiologic properties similar to those of the type IA antiarrhythmics and are contraindicated in the recovery phase following myocardial infarction. The threshold for the use of TAs should rise as the severity of heart disease increases or when there is QT prolongation.

TA overdose is lethal in approximately 2% of patients, generally related to cardiac complications. Initial clinical status and initial serum drug levels are not predictive of prognosis. QRS prolongation is a sign of toxicity but is an insensitive finding. Gastric lavage, repeat dosing of activated charcoal, and sodium bicarbonate therapy are appropriate treatment strategies. Type I antiarrhythmics should not be used for cardiac rhythm disturbances. Sodium bicarbonate is the initial therapy for ventricular arrhythmias. Hypotension refractory to volume loading and bicarbonate therapy should be treated with vasopressors such as norepinephrine, or vasopressor doses of dopamine.

## Other Psychotropic Agents

The selective serotonin reuptake inhibitors (SSRIs) have rarely been associated with orthostatic hypotension and bradycardia. These drugs may affect the cytochrome P450 system and interfere with other cardiovascular drugs. Case reports of cardiac toxicity are rare. Orthostatic hypotension is common. The major concern with these agents is interaction with tyramine-containing substances, resulting in hypertensive crisis. Lithium may suppress automaticity, particularly of the sinus node. ECG changes may simulate hypokalemia, including T-wave inversion, prominent U waves, and QT prolongation. Overdose with lithium may result in severe bradycardia. Phenothiazine antipsychotic agents, including chlorpromazine and thioridazine, can produce tachycardia, postural hypotension, T-wave changes, QT prolongation, and bundle-branch block. An increased incidence of cardiac complications including myocarditis, pericarditis, and cardiomyopathy is seen with the neuroleptic agent clozapine which is used in the treatment of schizophrenia.

# ■ DRUGS CAUSING TORSADES DE POINTES

Tricyclics, phenothiazine, and other psychotropic agents may prolong the QT interval and induce torsade de pointes. Other toxic causes of torsade de pointes are haloperidol, terfenadine, astemizole, cisapride, pentamidine, probucol, arsenic, organophosphates, and liquid protein diets. Clinicians should consult available databases if torsade de pointes occurs since known and suspected drugs are increasing (see www.qtdrugs.org).

# ■ MISCELLANEOUS DRUGS WITH CARDIOVASCULAR TOXICITY

Valvular heart disease resembling that seen with carcinoid syndrome has been associated with the antimigraine drugs methysergide and ergotamine, the weight loss medications dexfenfluramine and fenfluramine, and possibly pergolide, used to treat Parkinson disease.

Chloroquine and hydroxychloroquine can cause skeletal and rarely heart muscle disease. When cardiac involvement occurs, features of restrictive cardiomyopathy are most common. Acute chloroquine poisoning results in hypotension, tachycardia, and prolongation of the QRS; it is often fatal.

Sumatriptan, in addition to ergotamine and methysergide, is used to treat migraines. It is a selective serotonin type I agonist and may cause *coronary artery vasospasm*. Sumatriptan should not be taken within 24 hours of treatment with ergotamine-like medications because of the risk of prolonged vasoconstriction. Ergotamine, methysergide, and sumatriptan are generally contraindicated in patients with obstructive coronary artery disease because of vasoconstrictor effects and the possibility of precipitating angina.

Illicit use of androgens is a problem in competitive athletes and body builders. Data on human toxicity are limited. Stanozolol and nandrolone have been associated with marked lipid abnormalities and an increase in coronary atherosclerosis. These agents may also cause LV hypertrophy and hypertension. (Complementary and alternative medicines and the heart are discussed in Chapter 60).

## ■ COCAINE AND METHAMPHETAMINES

Cocaine is a common drug of abuse and has broad cardiovascular toxicity. Chest pain is the most common reason for cocaine users to seek medical attention. The evaluation of cocaine-related chest pain is difficult. Approximately 6% of patients presenting to emergency departments with cocaine-related chest pain have myocardial infarction. They are often young men without other risk factors for coronary artery disease except tobacco smoking. The quality or duration of the chest discomfort is often not predictive of infarction. Because young patients often have early repolarization patterns on the ECG, ST-segment elevation in leads $V_1$ to $V_3$ may be confused with acute infarction. Patients may require cardiac monitoring for 6 to 12 hours, until enzymes have excluded infarction. Other cardiovascular effects include premature atherosclerosis, heart failure, ventricular and atrial arrhythmias, sudden death, and aortic dissection.

Patients presenting with anxiety, tachycardia, and/or hypertension may respond well to benzodiazepines. Nitroglycerin may reverse coronary vasoconstriction induced by cocaine. Aspirin may prevent thrombus formation. Patients not responding to these measures may benefit from phentolamine or from calcium-channel blocker therapy with verapamil. β-adrenergic antagonists should generally be avoided due to unopposed α-mediated vasoconstriction. In documented cocaine-related myocardial infarction, thrombolytic therapy is highly effective. However, emergency coronary angiography may be necessary to distinguish patients with acute infarction from those with ST-segment elevation due to early repolarization. Intravenous sodium bicarbonate and magnesium may be beneficial.

The biological effects of methamphetamines are similar to those of cocaine, but vasoconstriction is less. Cardiovascular toxicity is common and includes tachycardia, hypertension, and arrhythmias. Chest pain and myocardial infarction are less common than with cocaine. Chronic use may result in a catecholamine-mediated dilated cardiomyopathy.

# ELECTRICITY

## ■ ENVIRONMENTAL ACCIDENTS

The immediate cardiac effect of injury due to lightning or electric equipment may be asystole or ventricular fibrillation. Cardiac arrest may also result from apnea and hypoxia. Atrial and ventricular arrhythmias, conduction abnormalities, and LV dysfunction may occur. Cardiac abnormalities occur due to direct myocardial injury or central nervous system injury, with intense catecholamine release. Hypertension and tachycardia may be managed with β-blocking agents.

Cardiopulmonary resuscitation should be continued for a prolonged period after apparent death from lightning, since late recovery may occur. In lightning strikes involving multiple victims, attention should first be directed to those who are "apparently dead," since lightning victims with vital signs generally survive without immediate medical attention and those without vital signs may recover after prolonged resuscitation.

## ■ ELECTROCONVULSIVE THERAPY

Electroconvulsive therapy (ECT) may produce cardiac arrhythmias and ECG changes during the first few minutes after the shock. ECT produces brief, intense stimulation of the central nervous system. Cardiovascular complications may result from this stimulation or from the drugs used to modify the response. Patients with coronary artery disease should be pretreated with a β-blocker to blunt tachycardia and hypertension and to reduce the frequency of ventricular ectopic beats. Patients with cardiac pacemakers can safely undergo ECT.

# POISONS

Snake venoms affect the coagulation system, cellular components of the blood, endothelium, nervous system, and heart. Cardiac arrhythmias, severe hypotension, and cardiac arrest may occur. Multiple pulmonary emboli may be seen in patients who survive 12 hours or longer. Scorpion venom may cause hypertension, myocardial infarction, arrhythmias, conduction disturbances, and myocarditis.

Scorpion fish cause envenomation that may result in rhythm disturbances and heart failure. Ingestion of pufferfish may cause severe bradycardia and cardiovascular collapse. Stingray venom contains phosphodiesterases and rarely may cause cardiac rhythm disturbances.

Halogenated hydrocarbons are used in fire extinguishers, solvents, refrigerants, pesticides, and plastics, paints, and glues. They can suppress myocardial contractility and produce arrhythmias and sudden death.

Carbon monoxide poisoning produces myocardial ischemia usually manifest by ST-segment and T-wave changes and atrial and ventricular arrhythmias. Extensive myocardial necrosis and cardiomyopathy can occur.

# RADIATION

Radiation to the mediastinum can affect the pericardium, myocardium, endocardium, valves, and capillaries of the heart. Radiation may cause acute pericarditis, chronic pericarditis, and pericardial constriction. Pericardial involvement is most frequent 4 to 6 months after radiation therapy.

Clinically important myocardial dysfunction related to radiation generally occurs in combination with pericardial disease. Myocardial fibrosis may result in diastolic dysfunction and, less commonly, systolic dysfunction. Radiation-induced valvular heart disease is rare but usually involves the aortic or mitral valves. Premature coronary artery disease may occur after radiation therapy and often involves the coronary ostia.

Radiation may result in fibrosis of the nodal and infranodal pathways. Right bundle-branch block is especially common; complete heart block is rare.

# SUGGESTED READINGS

Smith AL, Book WM. Effect of noncardiac drugs, electricity, poisons, and radiation on the heart. In: Fuster V, Walsh R, Harrington RA, et al, eds. *Hurst's The Heart*. 13th ed. New York, NY: McGraw-Hill; 2011:94:2085-2095.

Adams MJ, Hardenbergh PH, Constine LS, et al. Radiation-associated cardiovascular disease. *Crit Rev Oncol Hematol*. 2003;45:55-75.

Chen MH, Kerkelä R, Force T. Mechanisms of cardiac dysfunction with tyrosine kinase inhibitor cancer therapeutics. *Circulation*. 2008;118:84-95.

De Smet PAGM. Herbal remedies. *N Engl J Med*. 2002;347:2046-2056.

Jain S, Bandi V. Electrical and lightning injuries. *Crit Care Clin*. 1999;15:319-331.

Kloner RA, Rezkalla SH. Cocaine and the heart. *N Engl J Med*. 2003;348:487-488.

Roden DM. Drug therapy: drug-induced prolongation of the QT interval. *N Engl J Med*. 2004;350:1013-1022.

Roth BL. Drugs and valvular heart disease. *N Engl J Med*. 2007;356:6-9.

Witchel HJ, Hancox JC, Nutt DJ. Psychotropic drugs, cardiac arrhythmia, and sudden death. *J Clin Psychopharmacol*. 2003;23:58-77.

# CHAPTER 43
# DISEASES OF THE PERICARDIUM

Brian D. Hoit

The pericardium consists of an inner visceral and an outer parietal layer, between which there is a potential space, the pericardial cavity, which normally contains up to 50 mL of plasma infiltrate. Despite serving many important functions (**Table 43-1**), the pericardium is not essential for life and no adverse consequences follow either congenital absence or surgical removal of the pericardium. Thus, clinicopathologic processes involving the pericardium are understandably few; indeed, pericardial heart disease comprises only pericarditis and its complications (tamponade and constriction) and congenital lesions. Nevertheless, the pericardium is affected by virtually every category of disease (**Table 43-2**).

## ACUTE PERICARDITIS

Acute fibrinous or dry pericarditis is a syndrome characterized by typical chest pain, a pericardial friction rub, and specific electrocardiographic (ECG) changes. It should be emphasized that the quality, severity, and location of pain vary greatly. The ECG may either confirm the clinical suspicion of pericardial disease or first alert the clinician to the presence of pericarditis. Serial tracings may be needed to distinguish the ST-segment elevations caused by acute pericarditis from those caused by acute myocardial infarction (MI) or normal early repolarization. The ST–T-wave changes in acute pericarditis are diffuse and have characteristic evolutionary changes (**Fig. 43-1**).

The chest radiograph is frequently normal, but may reveal an enlarged cardiac silhouette (a moderate or large pericardial effusion) as well as provide evidence of the underlying etiology. When an effusion is present, echocardiography estimates the volume of pericardial fluid, identifies cardiac tamponade, suggests the basis of pericarditis, and documents concomitant acute myocarditis. Nonspecific blood markers of inflammation usually increase in cases of acute pericarditis, and serum cardiac isoenzymes may increase with extensive epicarditis. Many patients presenting with acute, idiopathic pericarditis have increased serum troponin I levels, often within the range considered diagnostic for acute myocardial infarction.

Hospitalization is often warranted for most patients who present with an initial episode of acute pericarditis in order to determine the etiology and to observe for the development of cardiac tamponade. Acute pericarditis usually responds to oral non-steroidal anti-inflammatory drugs (NSAIDs). Prophylaxis against gastrointestinal bleeding with histamine-2 antagonists or proton-pump inhibitors is warranted, particularly in those at high risk or who require longer durations of treatment. Addition of colchicine to NSAID therapy is effective for the acute episode and may prevent recurrences. Indomethacin reduces coronary blood flow and should be avoided. Chest pain is usually alleviated in 1 to 2 days, and the friction rub and ST-segment elevation resolve shortly thereafter. Most mild cases of idiopathic and viral pericarditis are adequately treated in 1 to 4 days. However, the duration of therapy is variable

**TABLE 43-1.** Functions of the Pericardium

Mechanical
  Effects on chambers
    Limits short-term cardiac distention
    Facilitates cardiac chamber coupling and interaction
    Maintains pressure–volume relation of the cardiac chambers and output from them
    Maintains geometry of left ventricle
  Effects on whole heart
    Lubricates, minimizes friction
    Equalizes gravitation, inertial, hydrostatic forces
    Mechanical barrier to infection
Immunologic
Vasomotor
Fibrinolytic
Modulation of myocyte structure, function, and gene expression
Vehicle for drug delivery and gene therapy

and patients should be treated until an effusion, if present, has resolved. The intensity of therapy is dictated by the distress of the patient; narcotics may be required for severe pain. Cases not responsive to NSAIDs and colchicine may necessitate systemic corticosteroids therapy for a week to control pain, with the dosage tapered rapidly thereafter. Corticosteroids should be avoided unless there is a specific indication, such as uremic pericarditis and connective tissue disease, as they enhance viral multiplication and may produce recurrences when the dosage is tapered.

Colchicine decreases recurrence rates and duration of pericardial pain and should be considered early in the course of initial and recurrent pericarditis. Painful recurrences of pericarditis may respond to NSAIDs, but commonly require high-dose corticosteroids. Using the lowest possible dose, alternate-day therapy, combinations with nonsteroidal drugs, or colchicine should minimize the risks of long-term steroids. Intrapericardial administration of triamcinolone has been shown to relieve symptoms in patients with recurrent autoreactive myopericarditis, and azathioprine has also been used to prevent recurrent episodes. Pericardiectomy should be considered only when repeated attempts at medical treatment have clearly failed.

# PERICARDIAL EFFUSION

Accumulation of transudate, exudate, or blood in the pericardial sac is a frequent complication of pericardial disease and should be sought in all patients with acute pericarditis. Chronic effusive pericarditis may be associated with large, asymptomatic effusions. Transudative effusions (hydropericardium) occur in heart failure and other states associated with chronic salt and water retention, and exudative effusions occur in a large number of the infectious and inflammatory types of pericarditis. Although frank hemorrhagic effusions suggest recent intrapericardial bleeding, sanguineous and serosanguineous effusions occur in many infectious and inflammatory disorders. Chylous pericarditis implies injury or obstruction to the thoracic duct, and cholesterol pericarditis is either idiopathic or associated with hypothyroidism, rheumatoid arthritis, or tuberculosis.

*Echocardiography* is the *procedure of choice* for the diagnosis of pericardial effusion. Computed tomography (CT) and magnetic resonance imaging (MRI) may be

**TABLE 43-2.** Causes of Pericardial Heart Disease

Idiopathic
Infectious
    Bacterial
    Viral
    Mycobacterial
    Fungal
    Protozoal
    AIDS-associated
Neoplastic
    Primary
    Secondary (breast, lung, melanoma, lymphoma, leukemia)
Immune/inflammatory
    Connective tissue diseases (rheumatoid arthritis, systemic lupus erythematosus, scleroderma, acute
        rheumatic fever, dermatomyositis, mixed connective tissue disease, Wegener granulomatosis)
    Arteritis (temporal arteritis, polyarteritis nodosa, Takayasu arteritis)
    Acute myocardial infarction (MI) and post-MI (Dressler syndrome)
    Postcardiotomy
    Posttraumatic
Metabolic
    Nephrogenic
    Aortic dissection
    Myxedema
    Amyloidosis
Iatrogenic
    Radiation injury
    Instrument/device trauma (implantable defibrillator, pacemakers, catheters)
    Drugs (hydralazine, procainamide, daunorubicin, isoniazid, anticoagulants, cyclosporine,
        methysergide, phenytoin, dantrolene, mesalazine)
    Cardiac resuscitation
Traumatic
    Blunt trauma
    Penetrating trauma
    Surgical trauma
Congenital
    Pericardial cysts
    Congenital absence of pericardium

useful to identify loculated or atypically loculated pericardial effusions and to characterize the nature of the effusion. Epicardial fat may mimic an effusion, but is slightly echogenic and tends to move in concert with the heart, 2 characteristics that help distinguish it from an effusion, which is generally echolucent and motionless.

The etiology of a pericardial effusion is difficult to determine on historical or clinical grounds. Specific diagnoses are possible using visual, cytologic, and immunologic analysis of the pericardial effusion and pericardioscopic-guided biopsy.

The approach to the management of a moderate-to-large pericardial effusion is shown in **Fig. 43-2**. Drainage of a pericardial effusion is usually unnecessary unless either purulent pericarditis is suspected or cardiac tamponade supervenes, although on occasion pericardiocentesis is needed to establish the etiology of a hemodynamically insignificant effusion. Persistent or progressive effusion, particularly when the cause is uncertain, also warrants pericardiocentesis. In the case of myocardial infarction,

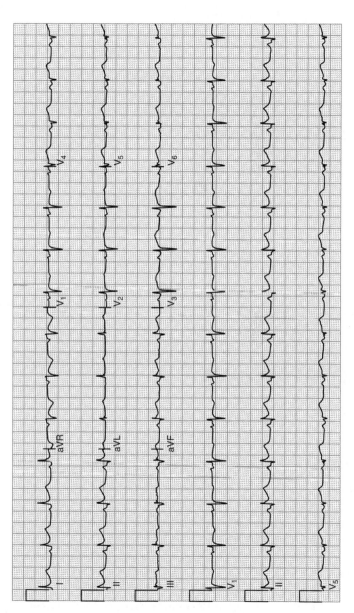

**FIGURE 43-1.** Note diffuse upward concave ST-segment elevations (usually <5 mm) and PR-segment depression (except aVR). Such changes may persist for days followed by return of ST segment to baseline before T wave inverts in contrast to the changes of myocardial infarction (eg, T-wave inversion preceding return of ST segment to baseline).

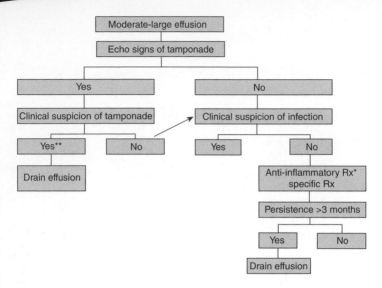

**FIGURE 43-2.** Algorithm for the management of moderate to large pericardial effusions. (*Anti-inflammatory treatment if there are signs of pericarditis. **Right heart catheterization may be required.)

the presence of a circumferential effusion greater than 1 cm is strongly suggestive of myocardial rupture and more extensive cardiac imaging (eg, transesophageal echocardiography or cardiac MRI) is mandatory.

# CARDIAC TAMPONADE

Cardiac tamponade is a hemodynamic condition caused by a pericardial effusion and characterized by equal elevation of atrial, ventricular diastolic, and pericardial pressures; an exaggerated inspiratory decrease in arterial systolic pressure (pulsus paradoxus); and arterial hypotension. Although the absolute intracardiac pressures are elevated, the transmural pressures are practically zero or even negative. The greatly reduced preload is responsible for the fall in cardiac output, and when compensatory mechanisms are exhausted, arterial pressure decreases.

Cardiac tamponade may be acute or chronic and should be viewed hemodynamically as a continuum, ranging from mild (pericardial pressure <10 mm Hg) to severe (pericardial pressure >20 mm Hg). Mild cardiac tamponade is frequently asymptomatic, whereas moderate and especially severe tamponade produces precordial discomfort and dyspnea. Both the severity of cardiac tamponade and the time course of pericardial fluid accumulation dictate symptoms and physical findings. Careful inspection of the jugular venous pulse waveform is essential for the diagnosis; compression of the heart by pericardial fluid results in a characteristic loss of the venous Y descent. An inspiratory decline of systolic arterial pressure exceeding 10 mm Hg defines pulsus paradoxus, a phenomenon with complex and multifactorial origins. However, in the presence of coexisting left ventricular disease, atrial septal defects, or aortic insufficiency, *pulsus paradoxus may not develop*. Low voltage on the ECG and/or electrical alternans should raise the suspicion of cardiac tamponade; unless even a brief delay might prove life threatening, an echocardiogram should be obtained.

During inspiration, greater-than-normal increases in right ventricular dimensions and decreases in left ventricular dimensions occur in many cases of tamponade. These respiratory changes also accompany other conditions associated with pulsus paradoxus, such as chronic obstructive lung disease and pulmonary embolism. Diastolic collapse of the right ventricle and right atrium, which reflects negative transmural pressure, is useful but neither sensitive nor specific as for tamponade. Exaggerated respiratory variation in transvalvular and venous velocities measured by Doppler echocardiography (flow velocity pulsus paradoxus) also helps to diagnose cardiac tamponade. It is important to remember that clinically significant tamponade is a clinical diagnosis and *echocardiographic signs of tamponade* are not by themselves an indication for pericardiocentesis. Although the absence of any cardiac chamber collapse has a high negative predictive value (92%), the positive predictive value is reduced (58%). Although positive and negative predictive values are high (82% and 88%, respectively) for abnormal right-sided venous flows (ie, systolic predominance and expiratory diastolic reversal), they often cannot be evaluated due to imaging limitations.

The pericardial, right atrial, pulmonary capillary wedge, and pulmonary artery diastolic pressures are elevated and equal; the degree of elevation is related to both the severity of tamponade and the patient's intravascular volume status. The right atrial and wedge pressure tracings reveal an attenuated or absent Y descent. Cardiac output is reduced and systemic vascular resistance is elevated.

Removal of small amounts of pericardial fluid (~50 mL) produces considerable symptomatic and hemodynamic improvement because of the steep pericardial pressure–volume relation. Unless there is concomitant cardiac disease or coexisting constriction, removal of all of the pericardial fluid normalizes pericardial, atrial, ventricular diastolic and arterial pressures, and cardiac output. Drainage of the pericardial fluid using a catheter minimizes trauma, allows measurement of pericardial pressure and instillation of drugs into the pericardium, and helps prevent (but does not guarantee) reaccumulation of pericardial fluid. Extended (3 ± 2 days) catheter drainage is associated with lower recurrence rates over a 4-year follow-up. Generally speaking, drainage should continue until the volume of the aspirated volume is less than 25 mL/d.

Although pericardiocentesis may provide effective relief and has relatively simple logistic and personnel requirements, *surgical drainage* offers several advantages. These include complete drainage, access to pericardial tissue for histopathologic and microbiological diagnoses, the ability to drain loculated effusions, and the avoidance of the risk of traumatic injury due to blind placement of a needle into the pericardial sac. The choice between needle pericardiocentesis, ideally performed under echocardiographic guidance, and surgical drainage depends on institutional resources and physician experience, the etiology of the effusion, the need for diagnostic tissue samples, and the patient's prognosis. In either case, pericardial fluid should be sent for smear, culture, and cytology. Repeat pericardiocentesis, sclerotherapy with tetracycline, surgical creation of a pericardial window, or pericardiectomy may treat recurrent effusions. A pericardial window is usually placed in patients with malignant effusions, and pericardiectomy may be required for recurrent effusions in dialysis patients. In critically ill patients, pericardial windows created percutaneously with a balloon catheter have been described.

# CONSTRICTIVE PERICARDITIS

Constrictive pericarditis is a condition in which a thickened, scarred, and often calcified pericardium limits diastolic filling of the ventricles. Although acute pericarditis from most causes may eventuate in constrictive pericarditis, it is an uncommon complication and is dependent on the etiology of the acute pericarditis. Idiopathic or viral idiopathic rarely progresses to constriction; neoplastic, bacterial, and radiation causes are more likely to develop constriction.

Constrictive pericarditis resembles the congestive states of heart failure and chronic liver disease. Patients generally complain of fatigue, dyspnea, weight gain, abdominal discomfort, nausea, and increased abdominal girth. Physical findings include ascites, hepatosplenomegaly, edema, and wasting; often these lead to an erroneous diagnosis of hepatic cirrhosis. The venous pressure is elevated and displays deep Y and often deep X descents, and it fails to decrease with inspiration (Kussmaul sign). Kussmaul sign lacks specificity, as it is seen also in cases of restrictive cardiomyopathy, right ventricular failure and infarction, and tricuspid stenosis. A pericardial knock, similar in timing to the third heart sound, is pathognomonic but occurs infrequently. Pulsus paradoxus may occur with associated pericardial effusion (effusive-constrictive pericarditis).

Low QRS voltage and nonspecific P- and T-wave changes are common; atrial fibrillation is seen in approximately one-third of cases and atrial flutter less often. The cardiac silhouette may be normal or enlarged, and pericardial calcification is present in less than half of the cases. Pericardial thickening and calcification and abnormal ventricular filling produce characteristic but insensitive and nonspecific changes on the M-mode echocardiogram; these reflect abnormal filling of the ventricles. However, a normal study virtually rules out the diagnosis. Because of the close physiologic similarities of constrictive pericarditis and restrictive cardiomyopathy, increased pericardial thickness detected by CT is the most reliable means of distinguishing between the 2 disorders. Accurate definition of pericardial thickness and its distribution are also possible with MRI.

Cardiac catheterization is used to confirm the clinical suspicion of pericardial disease, uncover occult constriction, diagnose effusive-constrictive disease, and identify associated coronary, myocardial, and valvular disease. Endomyocardial biopsy is sometimes necessary to exclude restrictive cardiomyopathy.

Pericardiectomy is the definitive treatment for constrictive pericarditis but is unwarranted either in very early constriction or in severe, advanced disease, when the risk of surgery is excessive (30%-40% mortality) and the benefits are diminished. Involvement of the visceral pericardium and evidence for myocardial fibrosis also increase the surgical risk. Symptomatic relief may take several months following pericardiectomy. Postoperative normalization of cardiac pressures may be incomplete in a significant number of patients.

Evidence of transient (acute) constriction may occur in about 15% of patients with acute effusive pericarditis. Therefore, before proceeding with pericardiectomy, the possibility that pericardial constriction may be reversible and amenable to medical therapy should be considered. Constrictive pericarditis may resolve spontaneously or in response to various combinations of nonsteroidal anti-inflammatory agents, colchicines, steroids, and antibiotics. Diuretics and digoxin are useful in patients who are not candidates for pericardiectomy because of their high surgical risk.

Effusive-constrictive pericarditis is an uncommon entity, which occurs when pericardial fluid accumulates between the thickened layers of pericardium. The hemodynamic picture is consistent with tamponade prior to pericardiocentesis and constrictive pericarditis afterward. Invasive hemodynamic assessment is required for the evaluation of effusive-constrictive pericarditis.

# CONGENITAL PERICARDIAL HEART DISEASE

Congenital absence of the pericardium is an uncommon anomaly, usually involving a portion or the whole of the left parietal pericardium. Its presence is usually suspected from the chest radiogram and echocardiogram. Contrast-enhanced CT and

MRI reliably establish the anatomy of the defect. Pericardial cysts are rare remnants of defective embryologic development and are benign; their importance lies in differentiation from neoplasm.

# SUGGESTED READINGS

Hoit BD. Pericardial disease. In: Fuster V, Walsh R, Harringtron RA, et al. *Hurst's The Heart*. 13th ed. New York, NY: McGraw-Hill; 85;2011:1915-1939.

Hoit BD. Management of effusive and constrictive pericardial heart disease. *Circulation*. 2002;105:2939-2942.

Maisch B, Seferovic PM, Ristic AD, et al. Guidelines on the diagnosis and management of pericardial diseases executive summary; the task force on the diagnosis and management of pericardial diseases of the European Society of Cardiology. *Eur Heart J*. 2004;25:587-610.

Imazio M. Risk of constrictive pericarditis after acute pericarditis. *Circulation*. 2011; 124:1270-1275.

Imazio M, Brucato A, Cemin R, et al. Colchicine for recurrent pericarditis (CORP): a randomized trial. *Ann Intern Med*. 2011;155:409-414.

# CHAPTER 44
# CARDIOVASCULAR DISEASES CAUSED BY GENETIC ABNORMALITIES

Ali J. Marian, Ramon Brugada, and Robert Roberts

Genetic factors play a role in many cardiovascular diseases (CVDs), from familial disorders such as congenital long QT syndrome to complex, nonfamilial phenotypes, such as atherosclerosis. Molecular genetics, in conjunction with cytogenetics, provides the opportunity to decipher the genetic basis and pathogenesis of cardiovascular diseases. In this chapter, several cardiac genetic disorders are reviewed.

## ESSENTIALS OF GENETIC DISORDERS

There are approximately 23 000 genes in the human genome. The gene or genes inherited constitute a person's *genotype*. *Phenotype*, on the other hand, comprises the physical, physiologic, or biochemical features that the individual manifests, which are determined by both genetic makeup and the influence of myriad environmental factors. The percentage of individuals with a genetic mutation who also have one or more features of the genetic disease is referred to as the *penetrance*. Penetrance is an all-or-none phenomenon: any manifestation, however minute, indicates that the gene is penetrant in that individual. *Nonpenetrance* refers to lack of any observable phenotype. This feature is to be distinguished from *expressivity,* which refers to the variable nature of the clinical phenotype, such as severity. Thus, by definition, to have expressivity, the trait must be penetrant.

The most important part of an evaluation for genetic disease is the family history. The individual with the problem who brought the family to medical attention is known as the *proband* or index case. Information should generally be collected on all first-, second-, and third-degree relatives of the proband. A pedigree chart is then generated. Pregnancy and family histories can then be used in conjunction with the findings on physical examination to derive a potential etiologic diagnosis and to plan for further diagnostic studies. Prognosis and recurrence risk are closely tied to an accurate diagnosis and its probable etiology. Genetic counseling should provide information about the diagnosis, possible etiology, and prognosis of a disease. In addition, psychosocial issues, reproductive options, and the availability of prenatal diagnosis should be discussed. Genetic counseling should be nondirective, providing information in a nonjudgmental, unbiased manner. The family should then be able to make decisions based on medical information in the context of their religious, moral, cultural, and social backgrounds and their financial situation. The accelerated pace of progress in gene discovery, molecular medicine, and molecular diagnostics has begun to allow for improved genetic counseling and holds the promise of future genetic therapy. As knowledge about the genetic basis of disease grows, however, so too does the potential for discriminatory health insurance policies to exclude individuals who are at risk for an illness or to charge prohibitively high rates on the basis of predetermined illness.

# CARDIOVASCULAR ABNORMALITIES CAUSED BY CHROMOSOMAL DEFECTS

**Table 44-1** lists chromosomal defects that cause cardiovascular abnormalities. Two commonly encountered syndromes due to chromosomal defects—Down syndrome and Turner syndrome—are reviewed here.

## ■ DOWN SYNDROME

Down syndrome, or trisomy 21, is a major cause of mental retardation and congenital heart disease. The incidence of Down syndrome is approximately 1 in 700 live births. The risk of having a live-born with Down syndrome increases with maternal age. Clinical manifestations include congenital anomalies of the heart and gastrointestinal tract, epicanthal folds, flattened facial profile, small and rounded ears, upslanted palpebral fissures, excess nuchal skin, and brachycephaly. Cardiac abnormalities are present in approximately half of cases, most commonly atrioventricular canal defects and isolated ventricular septal defects (VSDs). Isolated secundum atrial septal defect (ASD) and tetralogy of Fallot are also encountered.

**TABLE 44-1.** Partial List of Chromosomal Abnormalities Associated With Heart Disease

| Chromosome Defect | Syndrome | Cardiac Phenotype |
|---|---|---|
| 45X | Turner syndrome | Coarctation of the aorta, ASD, aortic stenosis |
| Trisomy 5 | | Interrupted aortic arch |
| Trisomy 13 | Patau syndrome | CHD, VSD |
| Trisomy 18 | Edwards syndrome | CHD, VSD |
| Partial trisomy 20q | | Dextrocardia |
| Trisomy 21 | Down syndrome | CHD, ASD, VSD, PDA |
| Trisomy 22 | | VSD |
| Partial tetrasomy 22 | Schmid–Fraccaro syndrome | CHD |
| | | Anomalous pulmonary venous return |
| Deletion 4p | Wolf–Hirschhorn syndrome | CHD |
| Deletion 7q11.23 | Williams syndrome | CHD, supravalvular aortic stenosis, hypertension, MVP |
| Deletion paternal 15q11 | Prader–Willi syndrome | CHD |
| Deletion 17p | Miller–Dieker syndrome | CHD, ASD |
| Deletion 22q11 | CATCH-22, DiGeorge, and velocardiofacial syndromes | CHD |
| Rearrangement 5p15.1–3 | Cri du chat | CHD |
| Recombination chromosome 8 | San Luis Valley syndrome | Tetralogy of Fallot |

ASD, atrial septal defect; CHD, congenital heart disease; MVP, mitral valve prolapse; PDA, patent ductus arteriosus; VSD, ventricular septal defect.

Down syndrome is caused by trisomy 21. It is full trisomy in 95%, chromosomal translocation in 2%, and mosaic in 3%. Most errors in meiosis leading to trisomy 21 are of maternal origin and occur during the first meiosis in two-thirds and during the second meiosis in one-fifth of cases. *DSCR1* (Down syndrome critical region) encodes for calcipressin 1, a calcineurin A inhibitor. It is abundantly expressed in the heart and brain and is a candidate gene for both the cardiac anomalies and the mental retardation.

## ■ TURNER SYNDROME

Turner syndrome is characterized by a constellation of findings that result from partial or complete monosomy of the X chromosome. It is the most common chromosomal abnormality in females, with an incidence of 1 per 2500 to 3000 live-born girls. The phenotype is variable and often mild with short stature, low-set ears, broad chest with widely spaced nipples, peripheral lymphedema, and ovarian dysgenesis; intelligence is normal. Cardiac abnormalities are common, with a prevalence estimated between 23% and 40%. The most common are bicuspid aortic valve in 10% to 20% and coarctation of aorta, present in 10% of adult cases. A variety of other cardiac defects may also occur, usually other left heart abnormalities such as aortic stenosis, dilated ascending aorta, and hypoplastic left heart syndrome (HLHS). Women with Turner syndrome are more susceptible to aortic aneurysms and ischemic heart disease.

Turner syndrome is caused by complete or partial absence of an X chromosome. The most common karyotype is monosomy X (45,X). Approximately 5% to 10% of the cases have duplication of the long arm of one X (46,X,i[Xq]) and the rest have mosaicism.

# GENETIC BASIS OF SPECIFIC CONGENITAL HEART DISEASES

A number of congenital heart diseases occur in isolation and are not part of complex phenotypes as observed in chromosomal abnormalities. Recently, the causal genes for several congenital heart diseases have been identified. Preliminary studies depict a common theme in the pathogenesis of isolated congenital heart defects that implicates deficiency of several transcriptional factors that regulate cardiac gene expression during embryogenesis.

## ■ SUPRAVALVULAR AORTIC STENOSIS

Supravalvular aortic stenosis is an autosomal dominant disease characterized by discrete narrowing of the ascending aorta above the level of the sinusus of Valsalva. It commonly occurs as a phenotype of Williams syndrome (or Williams–Beuren syndrome) in conjunction with mental retardation in some and exceptional talents in others, hypercalcemia, elfin facies, and stenosis of major arteries. The prevalence of supravalvular aortic stenosis is estimated to be 1 in 25 000 live births.

The gene responsible for supravalvular aortic stenosis was initially mapped to chromosome 7q11.23 and subsequently identified as *ELN,* encoding elastin. Almost all cases of isolated supravalvular aortic stenosis are caused by *ELN* mutations. Mutations result in elastin deficiency, which in the vascular system leads to inelasticity of the vessel wall and subsequent fibrosis as a result of an altered stress–strain relation (elastin arteriopathy).

# ■ FAMILIAL ATRIAL SEPTAL DEFECT

ASD is among the most common congenital heart diseases, with an estimated incidence of 1 in 1000 live births. ASD is usually sporadic; however, familial ASD with an autosomal dominant mode of inheritance has also been described. The first gene identified for familial ASD was *NKX2–5 (CSX1)*. The gene is located on 5q35 and encodes NKX2.5, a predominantly cardiac-specific transcription factor that regulates expression of several cardiac genes. The spectrum of clinical phenotypes caused by mutations in NKX2.5 extends beyond secundum ASD to include VSDs, tetralogy of Fallot, subvalvular aortic stenosis, and pulmonary atresia.

A second causal gene for familial ASD with an autosomal dominant mode of inheritance is *GATA4* on chromosome 8p22-23. Mutations diminish DNA-binding affinity and transcriptional activity of GATA4 transcription factor and block its physical interaction with TBX5, another transcription factor involved in the pathogenesis of congenital heart disease.

A third causal gene for familial ASD is *MYH6*, which is located in chromosome 14q12 and encodes myosin heavy chain 6. The MYH6 protein is expressed at high levels in atrial tissues and plays an important role in the formation of the interatrial septum.

# ■ HOLT–ORAM SYNDROME

Holt–Oram syndrome is a rare autosomal dominant inherited disorder characterized by anomalies of the heart and upper extremities, hence the name *hand–heart syndrome*. The most common congenital heart defects are ASD and VSD, followed by conduction system abnormalities and atrial fibrillation. Less common cardiac abnormalities include truncus arteriosus, mitral valve defects, patent ductus arteriosus (PDA), and tetralogy of Fallot. Anomalies of the upper limb vary from mild malformation of the carpal bones to phocomelia.

Mutations in *TBX5* on chromosome 12q24, which codes for transcription factor TBX5, are responsible for the cardiac and skeletal abnormalities in Holt–Oram syndrome. A number of mutations have been described, resulting in reduced expression of TBX5.

# FAMILIAL MYXOMA SYNDROME

Myxomas are the most common cardiac tumors and are generally sporadic. In approximately 10% of cases, however, myxomas are familial with an autosomal dominant mode of inheritance. Familial myxoma commonly occurs as a part of *Carney complex* with the constellation of cardiac myxoma, endocrine disorders, and skin pigmentation. LAMB (*l*entigines, *a*trial myxoma, *m*ucocutaneous myxoma, *b*lue nevi) and NAME (*n*evi, *a*trial myxoma, *m*yxoid neurofibromata, *e*phelides) syndromes are considered variants of Carney complex. The majority of familial cardiac myxomas (Carney complex) are caused by mutations in the *PRKRA1A* gene on chromosome 17q24, which encodes the alpha-regulatory subunit of cyclic adenosine monophosphate (cAMP)–dependent protein kinase.

# ■ GENETIC DISEASES OF CARDIAC MUSCLE

The term *cardiomyopathy* denotes a disorder in which there is a primary defect in the myocardium, affecting cardiac myocyte structure and/or function. Cardiomyopathies are commonly classified into 4 groups according to their phenotypic characteristics: hypertrophic, dilated, restrictive, and arrhythmogenic right ventricular cardiomyopathy (see also Chapter 38). Each of these groups exhibits important genetic influences.

# ■ HYPERTROPHIC CARDIOMYOPATHY

Hypertrophic cardiomyopathy (HCM) is an autosomal dominant disease diagnosed clinically by the presence of unexplained cardiac hypertrophy (see also Chapter 39). The prevalence of HCM is approximately 1 in 500 in young adults and likely higher in the elderly population because of age-dependent penetrance. The pathologic hallmark of HCM is cardiac *myocyte disarray*. Other pathologic features of HCM include myocyte hypertrophy, interstitial fibrosis, thickening of the media of intramural coronary arteries, and often a malpositioned mitral valve with elongated leaflets. Most patients with HCM are asymptomatic or only mildly symptomatic; symptoms are usually related to heart failure or arrhythmia. HCM is the most common cause of sudden cardiac death (SCD) in young, competitive athletes, accounting for almost half of all cases of SCD in athletes younger than 35 years in the United States. However, in the absence of major risk factors for SCD, HCM has a relatively benign course, with an estimated annual mortality of about 1% in the adult population.

HCM is a genetically heterogeneous disease. Approximately two-thirds of patients have a family history of HCM; in the remainder, the disease is sporadic. Both familial and sporadic cases are caused by mutations in sarcomeric proteins. In 1990, an arginine-to-glutamine substitution at codon 403 (R403Q) in the β-myosin heavy chain (MHC) was identified as the first causal mutation. Since then, more than 300 different mutations in over a dozen genes encoding sarcomeric proteins have been identified (**Table 44-2**). Systematic screening of sarcomeric genes suggests that mutations

**TABLE 44-2.** Causal Genes for Hypertrophic Cardiomyopathy (Sarcomeric Genes)

| Gene | Symbol | Locus | Frequency | Predominant Mutations |
|---|---|---|---|---|
| β-Myosin heavy chain | *MYH7* | 14q12 | ~ 30% | Missenses |
| Myosin-binding protein C | *MYBPC3* | 11p11.2 | ~ 30% | Splice-junction and insertion/deletion |
| Cardiac troponin T | *TNNT2* | 1q32 | ~ 5% | Missenses |
| Cardiac troponin I | *TNNI3* | 19p13.2 | ~ 5% | Missense and deletion |
| α-Tropomyosin | *TPM1* | 15q22.1 | ~ 5% | Missenses |
| Essential myosin light chain | *MYL3* | 3p21.3 | <5% | Missenses |
| Regulatory myosin light chain | *MYL2* | 12q23-24.3 | <5% | Missense and 1 truncation |
| Cardiac α-actin | *ACTC* | 15q11 | <5% | Missense mutations |
| Titin | *TTN* | 2q24.1 | <5% | Missense mutations |
| Telethonin (Tcap) | *TCAP* | 17q2 | Rare | Missense mutations |
| α-Myosin heavy chain | *MYH6* | 14q1 | Rare | Missense and rearrangement mutations (association) |
| Cardiac troponin C | *TNNC1* | 3p21.3-3p14.3 | Rare | Missense mutations (association) |
| Cardiac myosin light peptide kinase | *MYLK2* | 20q13.3 | Rare | Point mutations (association) |
| Caveolin 3 | *CAV3* | 3p25 | Rare | Point mutations (association) |
| Phospholamban | *PLN* | 6p22.1 | Rare | Point mutations (association) |
| Myozenin 2 | *MYOZ2* | 4q26-q27 | Rare | Missenses |

in *MYH7* and *MYBPC3,* which encode β-MHC and myosin-binding protein C (MBP-C), respectively, are the most common causes of human HCM, accounting for approximately one-half of all cases. Mutations in *TNNT2* and *TNNI3,* encoding cardiac troponin T and I, respectively, are less common, each accounting for approximately 5% of HCM cases. Overall, the causal genes and mutations for over two-thirds of HCM cases have been identified. The genes accounting for the remainder are yet to be identified or are a result of genes inducing a phenocopy (described later).

A remarkable feature of HCM is the broad spectrum of its phenotypic expression, with respect to both the degree of cardiac hypertrophy and the risk of SCD. This variability is multifactorial. Causal genes and specific mutations are the major determinants of the expressivity of cardiac phenotype. Mutations in *MYH7* are generally associated with early-onset HCM with extensive hypertrophy and a high incidence of SCD, yet there is variability among different *MYH7* mutations. On the other hand, the phenotype in the majority of patients with *MYBPC3* mutations is relatively mild. The age of onset of clinical symptoms tends to be late, the degree of cardiac hypertrophy less severe, and the incidence of SCD low. However, "malignant" mutations have been described that are associated with severe hypertrophy and a high incidence of SCD. The risk of SCD in HCM caused by mutations in *MYH7* and *MYBPC3* is partially reflective of the severity of hypertrophy: mutations associated with mild hypertrophy generally carry a relatively benign prognosis and those with severe hypertrophy indicate a high incidence of SCD. This is in contrast to HCM caused by mutations in *TNNT2,* which is characterized by mild cardiac hypertrophy but extensive myocyte disarray and a high incidence of SCD.

Genes other than the causal genes also affect the phenotype in HCM. They are termed *modifier genes.* Unlike the causal genes, modifier genes are neither necessary nor sufficient to cause HCM. However, they can influence the severity of cardiac hypertrophy and the risk of SCD. *ACE,* encoding angiotensin-I-converting enzyme 1 (ACE-1), was the first gene implicated as a modifier of cardiac phenotype in human HCM. Since then, variants of endothelin-1 (*EDN1*), tumor necrosis factor-α (*TNF-α*), angiotensinogen (*AGT*), angiotensin II receptor 1 (*AGTR1*), and platelet-activating factor acetylhydrolase (*PLA2G7*) have also been associated with the severity of the cardiac hypertrophy. Finally, the environment contributes to the phenotypic expression of HCM. The not-uncommon finding of HCM in young competitive athletes who succumb to SCD suggests that intense physical exertion may worsen the cardiac phenotype. Moreover, the absence of hypertrophy early in life, the fact that hypertrophy often spares the low-pressure right ventricle, despite equal expression of mutant sarcomeric protein in both ventricles, and the attenuation of hypertrophy through pharmacologic intervention (at least in animal models) all serve to support the important contribution of the environment to the development of hypertrophy in HCM.

Unexplained cardiac hypertrophy, which clinically denotes HCM, also occurs in other settings, including metabolic disorders, mitochondrial diseases, and triplet repeat syndromes. Although the gross phenotype is similar, the pathogenesis and prognosis of hypertrophy caused by different classes of mutant proteins differ. Therefore, such conditions are considered *phenocopy* (diseases mimicking HCM). The prevalence of HCM phenocopy is not precisely known. Given the prevalence of each particular HCM phenocopy, it is expected that phenocopy accounts for approximately 5% to 10% of cases with the clinical diagnosis of HCM. The distinction between true HCM and HCM phenocopy is important as there may be specific treatments available for some phenocopies. A prototypic example of HCM phenocopy is Fabry disease, an X-linked lysosomal storage disease. Fabry disease is present in 1% to 3% of cases with the clinical diagnosis of HCM in the adult population. The phenotype results from deficiency of α-galactosidase A (α-Gal A). The deficiency of the enzyme results in deposits of glycosphingolipids in multiple organs, including the heart. Cardiac hypertrophy, which is often indistinguishable from true HCM, is associated with high QRS voltage, conduction defects, and cardiac arrhythmias. Fabry disease is treatable by enzyme replacement.

# ■ DILATED CARDIOMYOPATHY

Dilated cardiomyopathy (DCM) is a primary disease of the myocardium manifested (see also Chapter 38) by dilation of the left (and often right) ventricle and a decline in its contractility. It has a prevalence of 40 cases per 100 000 individuals and an incidence of 5 to 8 cases per 100 000 persons. Patients with DCM are often asymptomatic in the early stages but eventually develop symptoms and signs of heart failure and arrhythmia. A family history of DCM is present in approximately half of all index cases with idiopathic DCM; in the remainder, DCM is considered sporadic. Familial DCM is commonly inherited as an autosomal dominant disease, which clinically manifests during the third and fourth decades of life. Multiple causal genes for autosomal dominant DCM have been identified, including several that encode sarcomeric proteins, which are also implicated in HCM (see the previous section). Thus, despite the contrasting phenotypes of HCM and DCM, mutations in sarcomeric genes can cause either phenotype. Several other of the known causal genes for DCM encode myocyte cytoskeleton proteins (**Table 44-3**). The phenotype of DCM is determined not only by many heterogeneous causal mutations but also by modifier genes and environmental factors. Genetic studies to identify modifier genes for DCM are largely restricted to SNP-association studies (see Chapter 38).

Finally, DCM is often a feature of various genetic multiorgan disorders. Examples include X-linked muscular dystrophies (Duchenne and Becker muscular dystrophies, Emery–Dreifuss syndrome, and Barth syndrome); certain trinucleotide repeat syndromes (myotonic dystrophy, Friedreich ataxia); metabolic disorders (Pompe disease, Refsum disease); and mitochondrial diseases (Kearns–Sayre syndrome, primary L-carnitine deficiency).

# ■ RESTRICTIVE CARDIOMYOPATHY

Restrictive cardiomyopathy (RCM) is a heart-muscle disease characterized by severely enlarged atria as a result of elevated right and left ventricular filling pressures, normal or reduced ventricular volumes, and, usually, preserved global systolic function. The clinical manifestations are those of heart failure, often with predominance of right-sided signs and symptoms. The age of onset of the disease is variable, and the prognosis is relatively poor. RCM can occur because of systemic infiltrative disorders, such as amyloidosis and sarcoidosis, as well as storage diseases, such as Fabry disease. Although such disorders are also genetic in etiology, RCM in such disorders is an indirect consequence, and not a primary myocardial abnormality.

Familial RCM with an autosomal dominant form of inheritance in conjunction with skeletal myopathy and atrioventricular conduction defects has been described. Two causal genes for RCM—*DES* encoding desmin and *TNNI3* encoding cardiac troponin I—have been identified. Desmin is an intermediary filament that is also involved in desminopathies involving skeletal muscles as well as the heart. Mutations in *TNNI3*, which are known to cause HCM and DCM, also cause RCM. RCM also occurs in patients with Noonan syndrome, which is caused by mutations in the protein tyrosine phosphatase, nonreceptor type II. The pathogenesis of RCM remains largely unknown.

# ■ ARRHYTHMOGENIC RIGHT VENTRICULAR CARDIOMYOPATHY

Arrhythmogenic right ventricular cardiomyopathy (ARVC) is an uncommon cardiomyopathy with characteristic pathologic and clinical features. The pathologic phenotype is characterized by gradual replacement of cardiac myocytes by adipocytes and fibrosis. The clinical phenotype comprises ventricular arrhythmias, primarily originating from the right ventricle, SCD and heart failure. ARVC is an

**TABLE 44-3.** Causal Genes for Dilated Cardiomyopathy (DCM)

| Gene | Symbol | Locus | Inheritance | Mutations/ Frequency/Context |
|---|---|---|---|---|
| **Sarcomeric/Cytoskeletal** | | | | |
| Cardiac α-actin | ACTC | 15q11-14 | AD | Missense/uncommon; also causes HCM |
| β-Myosin heavy chain | MYH7 | 14q11-13 | AD | Missense/~5%; also causes HCM |
| Cardiac troponin T | TNNT2 | 1q32 | AD | Missense/uncommon; also causes HCM |
| α-Tropomyosin | TPM1 | 15q22.1 | AD | Missense/rare; also causes HCM |
| Cypher/ZASP: LIM domain binding 3 | LDB3 | 10q22.3-q23.2 | Sporadic and familial | |
| Titin | TTN | 2q24.1 | AD | Missense/uncommon; also causes HCM |
| Telethonin (T-cap) | TCAP | 17q12 | | |
| **Cytoskeletal** | | | | |
| α-Sarcoglycan | SGCA | 17q21 | AD | Limb–girdle muscular dystrophy |
| β-Sarcoglycan | SGCB | 4q12 | AD | |
| δ-Sarcoglycan | SGCD | 5q33-34 | AD AR | |
| Dystrophin | DMD | Xp21 | X-linked | Duchenne and Becker Muscular dystrophy |
| Muscle LIM protein | MLP (CSRP3) | 11q15.1 | AD | Rare, founder effect in families described |
| **Intermediary Filaments** | | | | |
| Desmin | DES | 2q35 | AD | Also causes RCM and desminopathies |
| αB-crystallin | CRYAB | 11q35 | | Desminopathy |
| **Nuclear Proteins** | | | | |
| Lamin A/C | LMNA | 1q21.2 | AD | DCM, conduction defect, muscular dystrophy, lipodystrophy, insulin resistance |
| Emerin | EMD | Xq28 | X-linked | Emery–Dreifuss syndrome |
| Vinculin | VCL | 10q22.1-q23 | Sporadic | Metavincluin isoform |
| **Cell Junction Molecules** | | | | |
| Desmoplakin | DSP | 6p23-25 10q21-23 | AR AD | Also causes ARVC |

(Continued)

**TABLE 44-3.** Causal Genes for Dilated Cardiomyopathy (DCM) (Continued)

| Gene | Symbol | Locus | Inheritance | Mutations/ Frequency/Context |
|---|---|---|---|---|
| **Unknown** | | | | |
| Taffazin (G4.5) | *TAZ* | Xq28 | X-linked | Barth syndrome |
| | | 1q32 | | |
| | | 2q14-22 | | |
| | | 2q31 | | |
| | | 3p22-25 | | |
| | | 6q23-24 | | |
| | | 9q13-22 | | |
| | | 10q21-23 | AD | |
| | | 7p12.1-7q21 | | |

AD, autosomal dominant; AR, autosomal recessive; ARVC, arrhythmogenic right ventricular cardiomyopathy; DCM, dilated cardiomyopathy; HCM, hypertrophic cardiomyopathy; RCM, restrictive cardiomyopathy.

important cause of SCD in apparently healthy individuals. In the US population, it accounts for 3% to 4% of SCD associated with physical activity in young athletes. In some reports, ARVC was found in up to 25% of the cases of nontraumatic SCD.

ARVC is a genetic disease that is estimated to be familial in approximately 30% to 50% of the cases. The most common mode of inheritance is autosomal dominant. Recessive forms in conjunction with keratoderma and woolly hair (Naxos disease) or with predominant involvement of the left ventricle (Carvajal syndrome) also have been described and referred to as *cardiocutaneous syndrome*. The genetic basis of ARVC is partially known. Chromosomal loci have been mapped (**Table 44-4**).

**TABLE 44-4.** Chromosomal Loci and Causal Genes for Arrhythmogenic Right Ventricular Dysplasia

| | Chromosome | Symbol | Protein | Function |
|---|---|---|---|---|
| ARVC1 | 14q24.3 | *TGFβ3* | Transforming growth factor-β-3 | Mitotic and trophic factor |
| ARVC2[a] | 14q42.2-q43 | *RYR2* | Ryanodine receptor 2 | Calcium channel |
| ARVC3 | 1q12-q22 | | | |
| ARVC4 | 2q32.1 | | | |
| ARVD5 | 3p23 | | | |
| ARVD6 | 10p12-p14 | | | |
| ARVD7 | 10q22 | | | |
| ARVC8 | 6p24 | *DSP* | Desmoplakin | Desmosomes |
| ARVC9 | 12p11 | *PKP2* | Plakophilin 2 | Desmosomes |
| | 18q12.1 | *DSG2* | Desmoglein 2 | Desmosomes |
| Naxos disease | 17q21 | *JUP* | Plakoglobin | Desmosomes |

[a]Phenocopy. *RYR2* mutations cause catecholaminergic polymorphic ventricular tachycardia and not true arrhythmogenic right ventricular cardiomyopathy.

Mutations in *PKP2*, which encodes for plakophilin 2, appear to be the most common causes of ARVC, accounting for approximately 20% of the cases. Mutations in *DSG2* and *DSP*, which encode for desmoglein 2 and desmoplakin, respectively, each account for approximately 10% to 15% of the cases of ARVC. The molecular pathogenesis of ARVC is unknown.

# GENETIC DISEASES OF CARDIAC RHYTHM AND CONDUCTION

Cardiac rhythm and conduction abnormalities can occur as the primary phenotypes of genetic disorders that affect ion channels and their regulators (**Table 44-5**). Several of these are reviewed below.

## ■ BRUGADA SYNDROME AND ITS VARIANTS

Brugada syndrome is characterized by syncope or SCD in the setting of a structurally normal heart and a distinctive ECG pattern consisting of *ST-segment elevation in $V_1$ to $V_3$, usually with a right bundle-branch block*. Episodes of syncope and sudden death are caused by fast polymorphic ventricular tachycardia or ventricular fibrillation. Brugada syndrome often manifests in subjects in the third or fourth decades of life, and occasionally in infants as SIDS. Recent studies suggest sudden unexpected death syndrome (SUDS), which is prevalent in Southeast Asia, is a form of Brugada syndrome. Death often occurs at night and more commonly in male subjects (male to female ratio is 10:1). Electrocardiographically, the disease is identical to Brugada syndrome.

In 1998, *SCN5A*, the cardiac sodium channel gene, was identified as the first, and thus far the only, causal gene for Brugada syndrome. More than 60 different mutations in *SCN5A* have been identified that collectively account for approximately 25% of all cases with Brugada syndrome. As in many other genetic disorders, Brugada syndrome also exhibits locus heterogeneity, and a second locus on chromosome 3 has been mapped; however, the causal gene has not yet been identified. Biophysical characterization of mutations in *SCN5A* suggests that mutations decrease the sodium current availability by 2 main mechanisms: decreased expression of the mutant channel or acceleration of inactivation of the channel.

Mutations of *SCN5A* can lead to a large spectrum of phenotypes, including Brugada syndrome, LQT3, isolated progressive cardiac conduction defect, idiopathic ventricular fibrillation, atrial standstill, and SUDS. The phenotypes are all considered allelic variants.

## ■ LONG QT SYNDROME

Long QT syndrome (LQTS) is a disease of ventricular repolarization identified by the prolongation of the QT interval on ECG. Clinical manifestations include syncopal episodes and SCD due to polymorphic ventricular tachycardia (torsade de pointes) and ventricular fibrillation. LQTS is either acquired or congenital. Two patterns of inheritance have been described in the congenital LQT syndrome: (1) autosomal dominant disease, described by Romano and Ward, which is more common; and (2) autosomal recessive disease, described by Jervell and Lange Nielsen, which is associated with deafness.

### Autosomal Dominant LQT Syndrome (Romano–Ward Syndrome)

The first locus for the autosomal dominant disease was mapped to chromosome 11 in 1991. Since then 7 other loci have been mapped (see Table 44-5). Most genes

**TABLE 44-5.** Genetic Disorders Causing Cardiac Arrhythmias in the Absence of Structural Heart Disease (Primary Rhythm Disorders)

|  | Rhythm | Inheritance | Locus | Gene |
|---|---|---|---|---|
| **Supraventricular** |  |  |  |  |
| Atrial fibrillation | AF | AD | 10q22 | — |
|  |  | AD | 11p15 | *KCNQ1* |
|  |  | AD | 21q22 | *KCNE2* |
|  |  | AD | 11q13 | *KCNE3* |
|  |  | AD | 17q23 | *KCNJ2* |
|  |  | AD | 12p13 | *KCNA5* |
|  |  | AD | 1q21 | *GJA5* |
|  |  | AD | 6q14-16 | — |
|  |  | AR | 5p13 | — |
| Atrial standstill | SND, AF | AD | 3p21 | *SCN5A* |
| Sick sinus syndrome | SND | AD | 15q24 | *HCN4* |
|  |  | AR | 3p21 | *SCN5A* |
| Absent sinus rhythm | SND, AF | AD | — | — |
| WPW | AVRT | AD | — | — |
| Familial PJRT | AVRT | AD | — | — |
| **Conduction Disorders** |  |  |  |  |
| PCCD | AVB | AD | 19q13 | — |
|  |  |  | 3p21 | *SCN5A* |
| **Ventricular** |  |  |  |  |
| LQT syndrome (RW) | TdP | AD |  |  |
| LQT1 |  |  | 11p15 | *KCNQ1* |
| LQT2 |  |  | 7q35 | *HERG* |
| LQT3 |  |  | 3p21 | *SCN5A* |
| LQT4 |  |  | 4q25 | *ANKB* |
| LQT5 |  |  | 21q22 | *minK* |
| LQT6 |  |  | 21q22 | *MiRP1* |
| LQT7 |  |  | 17q23 | *KCNJ2* |
| LQT8 |  |  | 12p13 | *CACNA1C* |
| LQT syndrome (JLN) | TdP | AR | 11p15 | *KCNQ1* |
|  |  |  | 21q22 | *minK* |
| SQT syndrome | VF | AD |  |  |
| SQT1 |  |  | 7q35 | *HERG* |
| SQT2 |  |  | 11p15 | *KCNQ1* |
| SQT3 |  |  | 17q23 | *KCNJ2* |
| Catecholaminergic PVT | VT | AD | 1q42 | *RYR2* |
|  |  | AR | 1p13-p11 | *CASQ2* |
| Brugada syndrome | VT/VF | AD | 3p21 | *SCN5A* |

AD, autosomal dominant; AF, atrial fibrillation; AR, autosomal recessive; AVB, atrioventricular block; AVRT, atrioventricular reentrant tachycardia; JLN, Jervell and Lange–Nielsen; LQT, long QT; PCCD, progressive cardiac conduction defect; PJRT, paroxysmal junctional reentrant tachycardia; RW, Romano–Ward; SND, sinus node dysfunction; TdP, torsade de pointes; VF, ventricular fibrillation; VT, ventricular tachycardia; WPW, Wolff–Parkinson–White syndrome.

identified encode proteins that make up potassium channels. *KCNQ1* and *mink* encode for the α- and β-subunits of the slow-activating delayed rectifier potassium channel ($I_{Ks}$) and are mutated in LQT1 and 5, respectively. *HERG* and *MiRP1* encode for the α- and β-subunits of the rapid-activating delayed rectifier potassium channel ($I_{Kr}$) and are mutated in LQT2 and 6, respectively. In addition, *KCNJ2* encodes the inward rectifier potassium channel Kir2.1, defective in LQT7 (also known as *Andersen syndrome*). Mutations in all 5 of these genes cause decreased function in the corresponding potassium channels and consequently a prolongation in the action potential and in the QT interval. On the other hand, 2 forms of LQTS involve channels other than potassium. LQT3 is the result of mutations in *SCN5A*, the gene that encodes the cardiac sodium channel, and the same one implicated in Brugada syndrome (see previous section). However here, a gain-of-function mutation is at play resulting in delayed inactivation of the channel, as opposed to Brugada syndrome, in which inactivation is accelerated. Similarly, in LQT8, also known as *Timothy syndrome*, gain of function mutations in *CACNA1C*, the gene that encodes the subunit of the L-type calcium channel increase the inward calcium current and prolong action potential duration. Finally, 1 form of congenital LQTS is not caused by a mutation in a gene encoding a channel protein at all. LQT4 appears to be caused by a defect in *ANKB*, which encodes for ankyrin-B, a cell membrane anchoring protein.

Several genotype–phenotype correlation studies have been performed to identify the genetic determinants of triggering events, ECG phenotype, and response to therapy. These studies have predominantly focused on the 3 most common forms of LQT syndrome: LQT1, LQT2, and LQT3. In general, individuals with LQT1 exhibit symptoms during physical activity, such as swimming, and have a T wave of long duration on ECG. Individuals with LQT2 usually develop symptoms related to auditory stimuli, and the T wave is small or notched. In contrast, subjects with LQT3 are symptomatic during sleep and the ECG shows a very late T wave with a prolonged ST segment. Mutations also carry prognostic significance, and in all 3 groups (LQT1, 2, and 3), there is a correlation between cardiac events and the QT interval. Although β-blockers are considered the first line of therapy in patients with LQT1, they have not been shown to be beneficial in patients with LQT3, who have a slower heart rate. Preliminary data suggest LQT3 patients might benefit from $Na^{1+}$ channel blockers, such as mexiletine, but long-term evidence is not yet available.

## Autosomal Recessive LQT Syndrome (Jervell and Lange–Nielsen Syndrome)

The autosomal recessive forms of the LQT syndrome, which are also associated with sensorineuronal deafness, have been linked to mutations in the genes encoding $I_{Ks}$ current, namely *KVLQT1* and *mink*. For the LQT phenotype to express, patients must inherit a mutation from both parents. Consequently, it is less common than the Romano–Ward syndrome but is associated with a longer QT interval and a more malignant course. The phenotype could also arise in recessive forms when different mutations in the same gene are inherited from the parents (compound heterozygote).

## ■ SHORT QT SYNDROME

The short QT syndrome is a newly described disease characterized by the presence of the QT interval shortening on ECG and clinically by episodes of syncope, paroxysmal atrial fibrillation, and/or life-threatening cardiac arrhythmias. Short QT syndrome usually affects young individuals with no structural heart disease. It may be present in sporadic cases as well as in families. It was originally described in 2000. In 2003, a link was established between the short QT syndrome and familial sudden death with the first clinical report of 2 families with short QT syndrome and a high incidence of SCD. Three genes, all encoding for potassium channels, have thus far been discovered: *KCNH2, KCNQ1,* and *KCNJ2* (see Table 44-5). Biophysical analyses have demonstrated that mutations in each of these genes that cause short QT syndrome result in channel "gain of function" and consequently shortening of the action potential.

## ■ PROGRESSIVE FAMILIAL HEART BLOCK

Familial heart block is an autosomal dominant disease of the cardiac conduction system characterized by development of bundle-branch block and gradual progression to complete heart block. Two forms have been recognized: in type I, the onset is early and the disease is rapidly progressive; in type II, the onset is later in life and the QRS complex is often narrow and AV nodal block predominates. Clinical features of the disease include syncope, SCD, and Stokes–Adams attacks. A locus has been identified in chromosome 19q13, but the gene has not yet been identified. Mutations in *SCN5A* have been identified in some families with familial heart block. In addition, AV block in conjunction with congenital heart disease such as ASD (NKX2.5 mutations) as well as DCM (lamin A/C mutations) have been described.

## ■ CATECHOLAMINERGIC POLYMORPHIC VENTRICULAR TACHYCARDIA

Catecholaminergic polymorphic ventricular tachycardia (CPVT) is an autosomal-dominant inherited disease with a mortality rate of approximately 30% by the age of 30 years. Phenotypically, it is characterized by runs of bidirectional and polymorphic ventricular tachycardia in response to vigorous exercise in the absence of evidence of structural myocardial disease. CPVT is caused by mutations in ryanodine receptors (*RYR2* on 1q42), calcium-activated calcium channels responsible for the release of this ion from the sarcoplasmic reticulum. A recessive form of familial polymorphic ventricular tachycardia has also been described and mapped to 1p13.3-p11. Mutation screening identified a missense mutation in calsequestrin 2 (*CASQ2*) to be responsible for the disease. CASQ2 is involved in the same pathway as RYR2 to control calcium release from the sarcoplasmic reticulum.

## ■ SICK SINUS SYNDROME

Sick sinus syndrome (SSS) is characterized by the occurrence of sinus bradycardia, sinus arrest, and chronotropic incompetence. Sinus node dysfunction has been linked to loss of function mutations in *HCN4* and, in recessive form, to *SCN5A*. *HCN4* contributes to native f-channels in the sinoatrial node, the natural cardiac pacemaker region. In 2006, a loss of function defect in *HCN4* was also linked to familial sinus bradycardia. *SCN5A* encodes the cardiac sodium channel implicated in Brugada syndrome and LQT3 (see the preceding text).

## ■ FAMILIAL ATRIAL FIBRILLATION

Atria fibrillation (AF) in the absence of known causes of secondary AF may be a familial disorder. The mode of inheritance appears autosomal dominant. The first causal gene for familial AF was identified as the *KCNQ1*, also responsible for LQT1. The mutation for AF is a gain of function mutation, in contrast to the loss of function mutations observed in patients with LQT1. Links between *KCNE2, KCNE3, KCNJ2,* and *KCNA5* and AF have confirmed the role of mutations in channels responsible for potassium currents in the development of AF.

# ■ FAMILIAL WOLFF–PARKINSON–WHITE SYNDROME

Familial Wolff–Parkinson–White (WPW) syndrome is a rare syndrome with autosomal dominant mode of inheritance. It occurs in isolation or in conjunction with other disorders, such as HCM and Pompe disease. It is characterized by palpitations, syncope as a result of supraventricular arrhythmias and evidence of preexcitation on the resting ECG. The phenotype of WPW in conjunction with HCM and conduction defects was found in patients with mutations in *PRKAG2*, which encodes AMP-activated protein kinase.

# GENETIC BASIS OF CARDIAC DISEASE IN CONNECTIVE TISSUE DISORDERS

Several connective tissue disorders have cardiovascular manifestations. Marfan's and Ehlers–Danlos syndromes are reviewed below (see also Chapters 49 and 52).

# ■ MARFAN SYNDROME

Marfan syndrome is a primary disorder of connective tissue with an estimated incidence of 1 per 5000 population. It is characterized by increased height, disproportionately long limbs and digits, increased joint laxity, and lens dislocation or subluxation. Cardiovascular manifestations include progressive dilation of the aortic root, aortic aneurysm and dissection, and aortic and mitral valve prolapse. The age of onset of the clinical manifestations of Marfan syndrome is variable, but cardiac phenotypes commonly occur in the third or fourth decades. Aortic dissection is the leading cause of premature death in patients with Marfan syndrome.

Marfan syndrome is an autosomal dominant disease. The first causal gene to be identified is the *FBN1*, which is located on 15q15.23 and encodes fibrillin. Fibrillin is the major component of extracellular microfibrils in both elastic and nonelastic connective tissues. More than 600 nonrecurring unique mutations in *FBN1* have been described. Mutations are spread throughout most of the gene, and the frequency of each particular mutation is relatively low, thus making screening for mutations tedious. There is significant variability in the phenotypic expression of Marfan syndrome, partly attributable to locus and allelic heterogeneity and partly to the effect of modifier genes and perhaps environmental factors. A phenocopy of Marfan syndrome is congenital contractural arachnodactyly (CCA), characterized by severe kyphoscoliosis, generalized osteopenia, flexion contractures of the fingers, abnormally shaped ears, and, less frequently, mitral regurgitation and congenital heart disease. Recently, point mutations in the *FBN2* gene have been described as causes of contractural arachnodactyly.

The pathogenesis of Marfan syndrome entails decreased expression levels of the fibrillin protein and reduced deposition of fibrillin in vascular adventitia, resulting in weakening of the adventitia and consequent aneurysm formation.

# ■ EHLERS–DANLOS SYNDROME

Ehlers–Danlos syndrome (EDS) is a relatively uncommon group of hereditary connective tissue disorders. There are 6 primary subtypes and several rarer variants; most are the result of defective collagen synthesis. Cardiovascular abnormalities are most common in EDS classic type (formerly EDS I and II) and EDS vascular type (formerly EDS IV). EDS classic type is caused by deficient types V and I collagen and is characterized by hyperextensible skin, joint hypermobility, mitral valve prolapse, and aortic dilation. The disorder is transmitted in an autosomal dominant fashion through genes *COL5A1* on 9q34.2-q34.3, *COL5A2* on 2q31, and *COL1A1* on 17q21.3-22.1. Ehlers–Danlos type IV is considered the most malignant form of the disease because of proneness to spontaneous rupture of the bowel and large arteries (including coronary arteries and the aorta) and a high incidence of pregnancy-related complications. It is caused by mutations in *COL3A1*, which is located on 2q31 and encodes type III procollagen.

## SUGGESTED READINGS

Marian AJ, Brugada R, Roberts R. Cardiovascular diseases caused by genetic abnormalities. In: Fuster V, Walsh R, Harrington RA, et al, eds. *Hurst's The Heart*. 13th ed. New York, NY: McGraw-Hill; 2011;82:1781-1826.

Jain MK, Proweller A, Walsh RA. Principles of molecular cardiology. In: Fuster V, Walsh R, Harrington RA, et al, eds. *Hurst's The Heart*. 13th ed. New York, NY: McGraw-Hill; 2011;6:118-137.

Keren A, Syrris P, McKenna WJ. Hypertrophic cardiomyopathy: the genetic determinants of clinical disease expression. *Nat Clin Pract Cardiovasc Med*. 2008;5:158-168.

# CHAPTER 45
# CONGENITAL HEART DISEASE IN ADULTS

## Jamil A. Aboulhosn and John S. Child

The incidence of moderate and severe forms of congenital heart disease (CHD) is 6 per 1000 live births. Without early medical or surgical treatment, the majority of patients with complex CHD would not survive to adulthood. Surgical and medical advances have dramatically improved prognosis; more than 85% of patients with CHD survive to reach adulthood. Many adults with CHD may never require surgical intervention. The most common defects incidentally encountered in adulthood are

1. Small ventricular septal defect (VSD)
2. Secundum atrial septal defect (ASD)
3. Mild/moderate pulmonary stenosis
4. Bicuspid aortic valve
5. Mitral valve prolapse

Adults with CHD usually present in 1 of 3 ways: (1) with a history of prior surgery (palliative or reparative) during childhood (**Table 45-1**), (2) with a known cardiac lesion without prior intervention, or (3) with an unrecognized defect that is diagnosed in adulthood. With the exception of simple ligation of a small patent ductus arteriosus early in life, there are generally no surgical/interventional cures, and all have certain potential sequelae and complications (**Table 45-2**). Cyanotic adults require special care and consideration (**Table 45-3**). Cyanosis results from shunting of deoxygenated blood to the systemic circulation, eg, because of pulmonary stenosis (as in tetralogy of Fallot) or as a result of suprasystemic pulmonary vascular resistance (Eisenmenger syndrome). In cyanotic congenital heart disease, palliative surgeries are attempts to increase pulmonary blood flow (**Fig. 45-1**). All adults with unrepaired, palliated, or repaired CHD contend with certain medical considerations (**Table 45-4**). As the patient with CHD makes the transition from adolescence to adulthood, it is imperative that the patient understand the nature and implications of his or her heart problem and what interventions have or need to be performed. Appropriate advice and guidance should be available regarding employment, insurance, socialization, contraception, and exercise.

## SELECTED LESIONS

### ■ ATRIAL SEPTAL DEFECT

Seventy-five percent of ASDs are ostium secundum defects; these are among the most common anomalies in adulthood. Twenty percent are ostium primum defects, and 5% are sinus venosus defects.

Associated lesions must be ruled out (cleft mitral valve and inlet VSD in primum defect, anomalous pulmonary venous return in venosus defect) (**Fig. 45-2**).

**TABLE 45-1.** Selected Palliative Surgical Shunts Used for Treatment of Cyanotic Congenital Heart Disease

| Type of Procedure | Description |
|---|---|
| Blalock-Taussig shunt | Subclavian artery to pulmonary artery |
| Potts shunt | Descending aorta to left pulmonary artery |
| Waterston shunt | Ascending aorta to right pulmonary artery |
| Fontan operation | Inferior vena cava (via graft, eg, "tunnel") to pulmonary artery |
| Glenn shunt | Superior vena cava to right pulmonary artery |
| Bidirectional Glenn | End-to-side SVC to pulmonary arteries |

Patients are frequently asymptomatic in early adulthood, presenting because of a murmur or abnormal electrocardiogram (ECG) or chest x-ray (CXR). Auscultation reveals fixed splitting of the second heart sound. Most eventually become symptomatic later in life related to chronic right ventricular (RV) volume overload, pulmonary hypertension, atrial arrhythmias, and rarely paradoxical embolization. Left ventricular (LV) diastolic dysfunction related to age and systemic hypertension may increase left to right shunt with age.

Typical ECG findings in secundum ASD include right axis deviation and incomplete right bundle-branch block (RBBB). Primum ASD presents with left axis deviation.

**TABLE 45-2.** Surgical Considerations in the Care of the Adult With Congenital Heart Disease

| | |
|---|---|
| Type of procedure | May be palliative (eg, systemic-to-pulmonary artery shunt) or reparative. Rarely curative. |
| Procedural sequelae | Certain procedures have known sequelae (eg, transannular patch repair of tetralogy of Fallot with resultant severe pulmonary regurgitation) that over time may lead to heart failure or arrhythmias (RV failure, VT, SVT). |
| Durability of materials used in surgical repair | Valves/conduits have limited durability and may require multiple replacements throughout life. Close follow-up needed. |
| Sternal/thoracic reentry | Reoperation poses a higher risk than first operations. They are more risky when an extracardiac conduit or high-pressure ventricular chamber lies beneath the sternum. |
| Transplantation | Ultimate therapeutic option; however, stringent criteria for transplant listing may exclude some CHD patients (eg, failing Fontan patients with congestive hepatopathy). Higher rate of organ rejection in CHD patients who have had multiple blood transfusions during previous surgeries. Higher risk of perioperative bleeding in patients with previous sternotomies/thoracotomies. |
| Noncardiac surgery | Frequent cause of morbidity and mortality in the adult with congenital heart disease. High-risk patients benefit from special expertise, particularly with cardiac anesthesia. |

RV, right ventricular; SVT, supraventricular tachycardia VT, ventricular tachycardia.

**TABLE 45-3.** Issues in the Care of the Patient With Cyanotic Heart Disease

| | |
|---|---|
| Erythrocytosis | This is a physiologic response to chronic hypoxia. Hyperviscosity symptoms may occur if Hgb ≥20 g/dL (headache, dizziness, fatigue), usually caused by dehydration. Hydration is the preferred initial treatment. Phlebotomy is rarely required. |
| Phlebotomy | Perform only if Hgb is >20 g/dL and there are symptoms of hyperviscosity. Remove 500 mL of whole blood at a time, and always replace with an equal amount of dextrose or saline. |
| Iron deficiency | Common and may be secondary to injudicious phlebotomies. Iron deficient microcytic red blood cells are less deformable, have decreased oxygen carrying capacity and increase blood viscosity, as well as increased risk of stroke. |
| Bleeding | Secondary to coagulation factor deficiency, thrombocytopenia and platelet dysfunction, and increased vascular permeability. Hemoptysis is common in those with severe pulmonary hypertension. Anticoagulants and antiplatelet agents are generally avoided unless definitely required for another indication (eg, indwelling catheters or pacemaker leads in a patient with a right-to-left shunt and risk of thromboembolism). |
| Cardiovascular | Supraventricular arrhythmias in 50%. Ventricular arrhythmias in 15%. Right ventricular dysfunction and right heart failure may occur. Elevated left ventricular filling pressures are common and may be related to abnormal septal motion in those with right ventricular pressure overload. Systemic arterial atherosclerosis is generally absent, but pulmonary arterial atherosclerosis is common. In situ pulmonary artery thrombi are common. |
| Other | Hyperuricemia with occasional gout, renal dysfunction, paradoxical embolization (use filters in all IV lines), cerebral abscesses, hemoptysis, kyphoscoliosis, infective endocarditis (high risk—all patients should be given prophylaxis for bacteremic procedures). Pregnancy ill-advised because of fetal risk and maternal risk (especially if severe pulmonary hypertension is present). |

## Management

Closure should be considered in symptomatic or asymptomatic patients with a shunt of any significance (Qp/Qs ≥1.5, where Qp is pulmonary blood flow and Qs is systemic blood flow) or with RV volume overload. Most have symptomatic improvement. Transcatheter device closure is commonly used for secundum ASD. There is a very low risk of mortality with device or surgical closure. There is a shorter hospital stay and less morbidity with device closure compared to surgery. Surgery is needed in patients with other forms of ASD, large defects, or those with anomalous pulmonary veins. Closure of the ASD in adult life does not prevent atrial arrhythmias.

## ■ VENTRICULAR SEPTAL DEFECT

There are 4 types of VSDs: perimembranous (most common), muscular (most common in infancy and childhood but the majority will spontaneously close), inlet (associated with primum ASD and cleft mitral valve), and outlet (Fig. 45-2).

## Clinical Presentation

The spectrum of isolated VSDs encountered in the adult patient usually consists of the following:

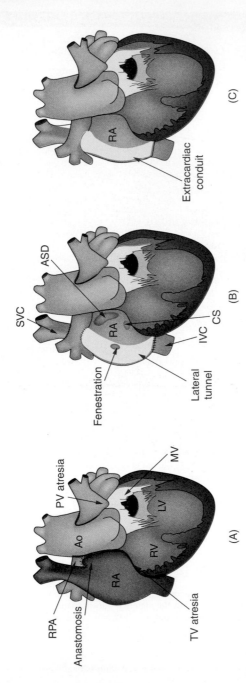

**FIGURE 45-1.** Most commonly used modifications of the Fontan operation. **A.** Right atrial (RA) to pulmonary artery (PA) Fontan connection with the right atrial appendage directly sutured to the RPA in a patient with tricuspid and pulmonary atresia. The right ventricle (RV), left ventricle (LV), mitral valve (MV), right pulmonary artery (RPA), and aorta (Ao) are labeled. **B.** The fenestrated lateral tunnel Fontan in which a synthetic material (eg, Gore-Tex) is used to extend a tunnel along the inside lateral wall of right atrium to the RPA, and the superior vena cava (SVC) is sutured directly to the right pulmonary artery. The fenestration in the wall of the synthetic conduit allows right-to-left shunting and depressurization of the lateral tunnel at the expense of systemic desaturation. **C.** Extracardiac Fontan operation is the current standard. The entire RA is bypassed by a synthetic conduit from the inferior vena cava directly to the RPA. The SVC is sutured directly to the RPA.

**TABLE 45-4.** Medical Considerations in Adults With Congenital Heart Disease

| | |
|---|---|
| Ventricular function | Certain CHD subtypes are at increased risk of progressive ventricular dysfunction (eg, single ventricle physiology systemic RV or RV with pressure and/or volume overload). Benefits of established heart failure regimens in other cardiomyopathic diseases often guide medical treatment of CHD patients with ventricular dysfunction; however, there are limited prospective or randomized data to support the efficacy in CHD. |
| Arrhythmias | Arrhythmias are common and the primary reason most well-repaired and stable adults with CHD seek emergent or urgent medical attention. Underlying hemodynamic problems should always be sought. Atrial arrhythmias are frequently not well tolerated and need to be aggressively treated. VT may be secondary to fibrosis, ventricular dilation, or reentry adjacent to a surgical scar. Sudden cardiac death risk is high in certain subgroups and AICDs may be needed; however, inappropriate shocks are a common problem. |
| Conduction disease | Intrinsic or postoperative sinus node disease and AV node dysfunction common. Pacing may require epicardial lead placement in certain situations. Multisite ventricular pacing is preferable in patients with low ejection fraction, dyssynchrony, or those requiring ventricular pacing secondary to heart block. |
| Endocarditis | Both operated and unoperated patients are at risk. Patients need meticulous dental, skin, and nail care. Antibiotic prophylaxis is important. American Heart Association guidelines from 2007 recommend antibiotic prophylaxis for bacteremic procedures in a small subset of patients (cyanotic CHD, prosthetic valve, recently implanted prosthetic material). |
| Pregnancy | As a rule, stenotic lesions, severe pulmonary hypertension and right-to-left shunts are tolerated poorly, whereas regurgitant lesions and left-to-right shunts do better. Patients need very close follow-up and should deliver in centers with appropriate expertise. Vaginal delivery with epidural anesthesia is usually preferable. Infective endocarditis prophylaxis in certain subsets. Discussion of CHD transmission risk to the fetus, genetic considerations, fetal echocardiography in most patients at 20-22 weeks gestation. |
| Contraception | Estrogen-containing regimens increase thromboembolic risk. Progesterone-based regimens are preferable in patients at increased risk (Fontan patients, right-to-left shunts). |
| Exercise | Exercise testing is a useful tool to assess fitness level, determine hemodynamic response to exercise, rule out exertion-induced tachyarrhythmias, evaluate chronotropic competence, and provide an exercise prescription. As a rule, heavy isometric exercise is contraindicated. |

AICD, automatic implantable cardiac defibrillator; AV, atrioventricular; CHD, congenital heart disease; RV, right ventricle; VT, ventricular tachycardia.

1. Small restrictive defects or defects that have closed partially. The pulmonary vascular resistance is not significantly elevated and the left-to-right shunt magnitude is mild ($Q_p/Q_s \leq 1.5:1$). The intensity of the precordial holosystolic murmur is inversely related to the size of the defect; therefore a loud and harsh holosystolic murmur is commonly present with these small shunts.

2. Large nonrestrictive defects in cyanotic patients who have developed the Eisenmenger complex, with systemic levels of pulmonary vascular resistance and shunt reversal (right-to-left).

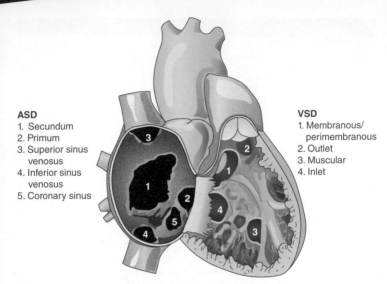

**ASD**
1. Secundum
2. Primum
3. Superior sinus venosus
4. Inferior sinus venosus
5. Coronary sinus

**VSD**
1. Membranous/ perimembranous
2. Outlet
3. Muscular
4. Inlet

**FIGURE 45-2.** Types of atrial septal defects (ASDs) and ventricular septal defects (VSDs) in order of prevalence in adults with CHD.

3. Patients with moderately restrictive defects ($Q_p/Q_s \geq 1.6{:}1$ and $\leq 2{:}1$) who have not undergone closure. These patients often have mild to moderate pulmonary hypertension.

4. Patients who have had their defects closed in childhood. These patients may have VSD patch leaks.

Perimembranous or outlet defects may be associated with aortic regurgitation due to cusp prolapse.

## Management

A small restrictive defect does not require surgical repair unless it is causing hemodynamically significant aortic regurgitation. Patients have a significant risk of endocarditis. Larger defects may be repaired in the absence of severe pulmonary hypertension and severely elevated pulmonary vascular resistance (>10 Wood U/m$^2$), which incurs a high perioperative risk. Transcatheter device occlusion of muscular and perimembranous VSD is feasible, and early trials demonstrate a good safety and efficacy profile. Patients with pulmonary hypertension may derive symptomatic and functional benefits from pulmonary vasodilators—endothelin blockade (bosentan), phosphodiesterase-5 inhibition (sildenafil or tadalafil), and prostacyclin analogues.

## ■ ATRIOVENTRICULAR CANAL DEFECT

*Atrioventricular canal defect* (AVCD) is an umbrella term for endocardial cushion defects representing a spectrum of lesions involving the atrial and ventricular septum, atrioventricular valves, and the LV outflow tract. Defects are classified into "partial" or "complete" forms. The "partial" form may be a primum ASD but no VSD. The "complete" form includes both a primum ASD and an inlet VSD. Deficiency of the inlet ventricular septum plus abnormalities of the atrioventricular valves (overriding, straddling, and/or cleft) commonly occur. Subaortic stenosis is a common association often caused by chordal attachments of the cleft anterior mitral valve to the LV outflow septum; it may also occur de novo following surgical repair. The diagnosis may be missed until adulthood, and patients have a presentation similar to that of secundum ASD, often with coexistent mitral regurgitation.

The typical ECG shows left axis deviation and incomplete RBBB. Primum ASD is the most common cardiac lesion seen in Down syndrome. If a complete and nonrestrictive VSD is not repaired early in childhood, it results in Eisenmenger physiology.

## Management

The complete form requires early surgical repair (age <6 months) to prevent pulmonary hypertension and pulmonary vascular disease. Residual mitral regurgitation is common and frequently must be managed surgically. In the partial form, the need for and timing of repair are dictated by the hemodynamic severity of the dominant lesion. Surgical closure of the defect is usually indicated, with repair of the mitral cleft if necessary.

# ■ TETRALOGY OF FALLOT

Tetralogy of Fallot is the most common cyanotic congenital heart malformation and one of the first complex lesions to be successfully repaired; it occurs in 7% to 10% of children with CHD. The 4 characteristic findings are (1) malaligned VSD, (2) RV outflow and/or pulmonary valve/artery stenosis or atresia, (3) dextroposed overriding aorta, and (4) RV hypertrophy.

Pentalogy of Fallot consists of additional ASD or patent foramen ovale.

## Clinical Presentation

Most patients will have had palliation and/or intracardiac repair during childhood. Rarely, they present in adulthood without prior surgery (pulmonary outflow tract obstruction is mild in those patients with acyanotic or pink tetralogy of Fallot).

The type of surgical intervention predicts long-term complications. If the repair involved a pulmonary valvectomy or the use of a transannular patch, resultant severe pulmonary regurgitation is the rule. This is usually tolerated for 1 to 2 decades but ultimately leads to RV enlargement and dysfunction, tricuspid regurgitation, and supraventricular and ventricular arrhythmias.

Other important issues after repair include recurrent RV outflow tract obstruction, residual VSD, peripheral pulmonary stenosis, and the development of RV outflow tract aneurysm after patch outflow repair. Aortic root dilation is common and aortic valve regurgitation may occur.

There is an increased risk of ventricular arrhythmias and sudden cardiac death, especially in patients with elevated LV filling pressure, known or inducible ventricular tachycardia, prior ventriculotomy incision, severe pulmonary regurgitation, prior palliative shunt, and QRS duration ≥180 milliseconds.

## Management

Timing of pulmonary valve replacement for pulmonary insufficiency is controversial but most experts agree that symptomatic patients, those with ventricular arrhythmias, and those with progressive RV enlargement and/or dysfunction (eg, RV end diastolic volume >160 cc/m$^2$) should undergo valve replacement. Reoperation should be considered for a large residual VSD ($Q_p/Q_s$ ≥1.5:1), significant residual RV outflow tract obstruction, large RV outflow tract aneurysm, or hemodynamically significant aortic regurgitation.

Placement of an implantable cardiac defibrillator is recommended in patients with clinical evidence of sustained or nonsustained ventricular tachycardia and those with inducible sustained ventricular tachycardia.

# ■ ISOLATED PULMONARY STENOSIS

In the adult, this is usually due to a trileaflet pulmonary valve with fused commissures, less commonly due to a dysplastic valve as seen in Noonan syndrome (webbed neck, hypertelorism, low-set ears, small chin, and deformed auricles). Subpulmonary infundibular stenosis is common. Survival to adulthood is common.

## Management

Moderate stenosis is usually well tolerated. Balloon valvuloplasty should be considered if the peak gradient is ≥40 mm Hg. Regression of subpulmonary infundibular stenosis is the norm following valvuloplasty.

# ■ LEFT VENTRICULAR OUTFLOW TRACT OBSTRUCTION

## Clinical Presentation

Obstruction may be valvular (usually bicuspid valve), subvalvular (discrete membrane, more diffuse tunnel, or mitral chordal attachments), or supravalvular (ie, William syndrome). Multilevel obstruction is common. Common associations include parachute mitral valve and aortic coarctation (Shone complex). VSD is also commonly associated. Aortic regurgitation is commonly associated with valvular and subvalvular forms. Medial abnormalities of the ascending aorta commonly result in dilation and may lead to dissection.

## Management

The development of symptoms (angina, dyspnea, or syncope) mandates intervention in aortic valve stenosis. In asymptomatic patients, intervention may be considered if the stenosis is severe. Surgical valvotomy and transcatheter balloon valvuloplasty can relieve obstruction in young patients with mobile and minimally calcified valves with a risk of resultant regurgitation. Valve replacement may be necessary for valves unsuitable for valvotomy, and various prostheses are available (mechanical, bioprostheses, and Ross procedure). For subvalvular obstruction, surgical intervention may consist of membrane excision together with myotomy and myectomy. Multilevel obstruction may require a Konno procedure (aortic annulus enlargement, aortic valve replacement, and ventricular septal myotomy with patch enlargement). Supravalvular stenosis requires surgical excision with end-to-end anastomosis, aortoplasty, or graft placement.

# ■ COARCTATION OF THE AORTA

## Clinical Presentation

In most unrepaired adults, the lesion consists of a discrete narrowing in the descending aorta just distal to the origin of the left subclavian artery. It is often discovered in asymptomatic patients who are found to have upper limb hypertension. A bicuspid valve occurs in up to 50% of patients. An associated aortopathy predisposes the aorta to aneurysm formation and dissection and to development of cerebral aneurysms. Death occurs from complications of hypertension, including stroke, aortic dissection, congestive heart failure, and premature coronary artery disease.

## Management

Assessment of severity includes a combination of measuring upper and lower limb blood pressure, measuring blood pressure response to exercise, and estimating pressure gradients at rest and with exercise using Doppler echocardiography. Cross-sectional imaging modalities (magnetic resonance imaging [MRI] and computed tomography [CT]) are very useful in delineating anatomy and planning interventions.

Intervention may be considered if the peak gradient across the coarctation is ≥20 mm Hg. Surgical repair is well established, with a low complication rate. Techniques include end-to-end anastomosis, patch grafting, and the use of a subclavian flap. Percutaneous balloon angioplasty with stenting for primary and recurrent coarctation is an attractive option in selected patients. Stent implantation is preferable to angioplasty alone.

Patients with successfully treated coarctation often continue to have systemic arterial hypertension despite the absence of significant residual coarctation. Late repair (>14 years of age) is associated with higher rates of hypertension and decreased survival.

## ■ TRANSPOSITION OF THE GREAT ARTERIES

In complete transposition of the great arteries, or d-TGA, the aorta arises from the RV and the pulmonary artery arises from the LV (ventriculoarterial discordance). This causes deoxygenated systemic venous flow to be directed to the aorta and pulmonary venous flow directed to the lungs. Survival to adulthood without intervention is rare. Frequent associations include VSD, LV outflow tract obstruction, and coronary anomalies.

Creation or enlargement of an existing ASD by transcatheter balloon septostomy or surgical septectomy in the infant with d-TGA allows enough left-to-right shunting of oxygenated blood to keep the patient alive.

The early corrective surgical approach consisted of atrial switch, which redirected atrial flow through the creation of a baffle, so that systemic venous blood was diverted to the LV and pulmonary venous flow to the RV (Mustard and Senning operations; **Fig. 45-3**).

Given all of the above intermediate-/long-term complications of the atrial switch operation, since the early 1980s, the surgical approach has consisted of anatomic repair by reconnecting the aorta to the LV and the pulmonary artery to the RV, and coronary artery reimplantation (arterial switch).

## Late Results

Mustard and Senning patients need close follow-up. Long-term survival is >80%; however, over 50% of patients will develop sinus node dysfunction, arrhythmias, baffle-related problems, valve regurgitation, or RV failure.

Long-term results in adults with arterial switch appear promising. Long-term problems include coronary kinking and ischemia, neoaortic valve regurgitation, and neoaortic and neopulmonary artery aneurysms or stenoses.

## ■ CONGENITALLY CORRECTED TRANSPOSITION OF THE GREAT ARTERIES

In this anomaly (L-TGA), the aorta arises from the RV and the pulmonary artery arises from the LV (ventriculoarterial discordance). In addition, the left atrium enters the RV and the right atrium enters the LV (atrioventricular discordance). From a circulatory oxygenation standpoint, these patients are "congenitally corrected." The pulmonary and systemic circulations run in series, not in parallel as with d-TGA. There is ventricular inversion and the respective atrioventricular valves follow the ventricles. The morphologic RV, however, still functions as a systemic ventricle.

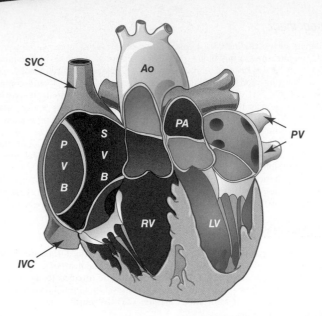

**FIGURE 45-3.** D-Transposition of the great arteries status-post atrial switch procedure (Senning or Mustard) characterized by "baffling" of deoxygenated blood from the superior vena cava (SVC) and inferior vena cava (IVC) via a systemic venous baffle (SVB) to the left ventricle (LV) and thereafter to the pulmonary artery (PA). Oxygenated blood returns to the heart via pulmonary veins (PV) and is "baffled" via a pulmonary venous baffle (PVB) to the right ventricle (RV), which serves as the systemic ventricle and pumps into an anteriorly dextraposed aorta (Ao).

Fewer than 10% of patients are free of associated abnormalities, which include VSD (membranous or muscular) in up to 80%, pulmonic stenosis (valvar or subvalvar) in up to 70%, and tricuspid valve abnormalities (usually Ebstein) in 33%.

Patients are frequently diagnosed in adulthood, when they present with heart block or exercise intolerance secondary to systemic AV valve regurgitation.

## Management

The conduction system is intrinsically abnormal in this condition and progressive heart block is common. Patients frequently require pacing. Significant systemic (tricuspid) AV valve regurgitation requires replacement with a prosthesis before ventricular dysfunction occurs. Since the RV is a systemic ventricle and is frequently abnormal, patients may benefit from heart failure therapies, but no prospective randomized data support this.

## ■ EBSTEIN ANOMALY OF THE TRICUSPID VALVE

### Clinical Presentation

The Ebstein anomaly is characterized by apical displacement of the septal leaflet of the tricuspid valve into the RV cavity. The RV is divided into a proximal "atrialized" portion and a distal "functional" portion. The effective volume of the functional RV is often small. The anterior leaflet is usually excessively long and may have attachments to the RV free wall. The "atrialized" portion of the RV is usually thin because of congenital absence of myocardium. The effective right atrium (+ atrialized RV) is invariably large and becomes more so in the presence of tricuspid regurgitation, which is a very common occurrence. An ASD or patent foramen ovale is present in more than one-third of the cases. Other associated lesions include pulmonary stenosis, VSD, and patent ductus arteriosus. Twenty-five percent of patients have 1 or more accessory pathways with ventricular preexcitation (usually right-sided). Patients often present in adulthood with arrhythmias or exercise intolerance.

## Management

If functionally mild, TR may not require intervention. Progressive RV dysfunction, impaired functional capacity, right-to-left shunting, and/or paradoxical embolization require surgical intervention.

If a large, mobile anterior leaflet is present, the tricuspid valve may be repaired. Otherwise, a biological prosthesis is usually inserted. The ASD will also be closed, and any accessory pathways can be interrupted at the time of surgical repair.

In patients with severe RV dysfunction, a "one-and-a-half" ventricle repair may be useful. This consists of tricuspid valve repair or replacement along with a "Glenn" shunt (superior vena cava attached to right pulmonary artery) in order to offload the dysfunctional RV.

# SUGGESTED READINGS

Aboulhosn J, Child JS. Congenital heart disease in adults. In: Fuster V, Walsh R, Harrington RA, et al, eds. *Hurst's The Heart*. 13th ed New York, NY: McGraw-Hill; 2011;84:1884-1914.

Ammash N, Connolly H, Abel M, et al. Noncardiac surgery in Eisenmenger syndrome. *J Am Coll Cardiol*. 1999;33:222-227.

Brickner ME, Hillis LD, Lange RA. Congenital heart disease in adults. First of two parts. *N Engl J Med*. 2000;342:256-263.

Brickner ME, Hillis LD, Lange RA. Congenital heart disease in adults. Second of two parts. *N Engl J Med*. 2000;342:334-342.

Canadian Cardiovascular Society. Consensus conference on adult congenital heart disease, Montreal, 1996.

Osterhof T, van Straten A, Vliegen HW, et al. Preoperative thresholds for pulmonary valve replacement in patients with corrected tetralogy of Fallot using cardiovascular magnetic resonance. *Circulation*. 2007;116:545-551.

Warnes CA, Williams RG, Bashore TM, et al. 2008 ACC/AHA guidelines on the management of adults with congenital heart disease : a report of the American College of Cardiology/ American Heart Association Task Force on Practice Guidelines (Writing Committee to Develop Guidelines on the Management of Adults With Congenital Heart Disease). Developed in Collaboration With the American Society of Echocardiography, Heart Rhythm Society, International Society for Adult Congenital Heart Disease, Society for Cardiovascular Angiography and Interventions, and Society of Thoracic Surgeons. *J Am Coll Cardiol*. 2008;52(23):e143-e263.

# CHAPTER 46

# PERIOPERATIVE EVALUATION OF PATIENTS WITH KNOWN OR SUSPECTED CARDIOVASCULAR DISEASE WHO UNDERGO NONCARDIAC SURGERY

Debabrata Mukherjee and Kim A. Eagle

Each year 50 000 patients suffer a perioperative myocardial infarction in the United States and more than half of the 40 000 perioperative deaths are caused by cardiac events. Most perioperative cardiac morbidity and mortality is related to myocardial ischemia, congestive heart failure, or arrhythmia. The aims of perioperative evaluation are 2-fold: first, to identify patients at increased risk of an adverse perioperative cardiac event; second, to identify patients with a poor long-term prognosis due to cardiovascular disease who come to medical attention only because another noncardiac problem leads to noncardiac surgery.

## CLINICAL DETERMINANTS OF PERIOPERATIVE CARDIOVASCULAR RISK

The majority of patients at increased risk of adverse perioperative cardiac events can be identified by performing a careful history, physical examination, and review of the resting 12-lead electrocardiogram (ECG). Current recommendations of the American College of Cardiology (ACC) and the American Heart Association (AHA) designate risk factors as belonging to 3 groups: major, intermediate, and minor (**Table 46-1**).

## ■ HISTORY

Risk factors recognized as predictive of increased perioperative risk include advanced age, poor functional capacity, and prior history of coronary artery disease, congestive heart failure, arrhythmia, valvular heart disease, diabetes mellitus, uncontrolled systemic hypertension, renal insufficiency, and stroke. Because most symptoms of

**TABLE 46-1.** Clinical Predictors of Increased Perioperative Cardiovascular Risk

**Major Predictors**
Acute or recent myocardial infarction[a] with evidence of ischemia based on symptoms or noninvasive testing
Unstable or severe[b] angina (Canadian class III or IV)
Decompensated heart failure
High-grade atrioventricular block
Symptomatic ventricular arrhythmias with underlying heart disease
Supraventricular arrthythmias with uncontrolled ventricular rate
Severe valvular heart disease

**Intermediate Predictors**
Mild angina pectoris (1 or 2)
Prior myocardial infarction by history or Q waves on ECG
Compensated or prior heart failure
Diabetes mellitus (particularly insulin-dependent)
Renal insufficiency (creatinine ≥2.0 mg/dL)

**Minor Predictors**
Advanced age
Abnormal ECG (left ventricular hypertrophy, left bundle-branch block, ST-T abnormalities)
Rhythm other than sinus (eg, atrial fibrillation)
Low functional capacity (inability to climb 1 flight of stairs with a bag of groceries)
History of stroke
Uncontrolled systemic hypertension

[a]Recent myocardial infarction is defined as greater than 7 days but less than or equal to 1 month; acute myocardial infarction is within 7 days.
[b]May include stable angina in patients who are usually sedentary.

cardiac disease are either associated exclusively with or exacerbated by increased physical activity, significant noncardiac limitations in physical capacity are associated with inherent problems in the ability to detect symptoms of underlying cardiac disease and thereby to diagnose it. Impaired conditioning, poor cardiac reserve, poor respiratory reserve, or a combination of these disorders results in a poor functional capacity and in a reduced ability to accommodate the cardiovascular stresses that may accompany noncardiac surgery.

# PHYSICAL EXAMINATION

Systemic hypertension, elevated jugular venous pressure, pulmonary rales, the presence of a third heart sound, murmurs suggestive of significant valvular heart disease, and vascular bruits all may identify a patient as having a higher perioperative risk.

## ■ COMORBID DISEASES

Patients with diabetes mellitus, restrictive or obstructive pulmonary disease, renal dysfunction, and anemia all have an increased risk of concomitant cardiac

**TABLE 46-2.** Cardiac Risk Stratification for Different Types of Surgical Procedures

High Risk (reported cardiac risk[a] >5%)
Emergency major operations, particularly in the elderly
Aortic, major vascular, and peripheral vascular surgery
Extensive operations with large volume shifts and/or blood loss

Intermediate Risk (reported cardiac risk <5%)
Intraperitoneal and intrathoracic
Carotid endarterectomy
Head and neck surgery
Orthopedic
Prostate

Low Risk[b] (reported cardiac risk <1%)
Endoscopic procedures
Superficial biopsy
Cataract
Breast surgery

[a]Combined incidence of cardiac death and nonfatal myocardial infarction.

[b]Does not generally require further preoperative cardiac testing.

complications during the perioperative period. Optimization of management and control of noncardiac conditions may therefore reduce the risk of cardiac morbidity in the perioperative period.

## ■ SURGERY-SPECIFIC RISKS

Emergency procedures are associated with a 2- to 5-fold increase in perioperative cardiac risk compared with elective procedures. Other types of noncardiac surgery associated with high perioperative risk include aortic and peripheral vascular surgery and prolonged abdominal, thoracic, or head and neck procedures with large fluid shifts. The ACC/AHA task force report on perioperative cardiac evaluation stratifies noncardiac surgical procedures as high, intermediate, and low cardiac risk (**Table 46-2**). See also Chapter 57.

Perioperative anesthesia technique influences the patient's cardiac physiology and may affect the perioperative cardiac risk. Opioid-based anesthesia generally does not affect cardiovascular function; however, the commonly employed inhalational agents cause afterload reduction and decreased myocardial contractility. Hemodynamic affects are minimal when spinal anesthesia is used for infrainguinal procedures, whereas the higher dermatomal levels of spinal anesthesia required for abdominal procedures may be associated with significant hemodynamic effects, including hypotension and reflex tachycardia.

## CLINICAL ASSESSMENT OF PERIOPERATIVE RISK

A general algorithm for use in determining the need for further cardiac testing prior to surgery is shown in **Fig. 46-1**.

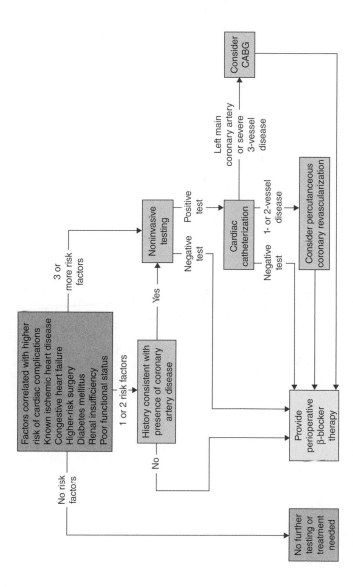

**FIGURE 46-1.** A general algorithm for use in determining the need for further cardiac testing prior to noncardiac surgery.

# ■ PREOPERATIVE TESTING

## Resting Left Ventricular Function

Unless recently defined, preoperative assessment of left ventricular systolic function should be performed among patients with poorly controlled congestive heart failure and should be considered among patients with prior congestive heart failure and among those with dyspnea of unknown cause.

## Functional Testing and Risk of Coronary Artery Disease

Because clinical factors usually serve to identify patients at low or high risk of an adverse cardiac event after noncardiac surgery, preoperative stress testing typically has the greatest utility among patients at intermediate risk. An exercise ECG study allows assessment of functional capacity as well as evaluation for the evidence of coronary artery disease based on ST-segment analysis and hemodynamics. Performance of exercise echocardiographic testing or exercise myocardial perfusion imaging should be considered in the presence of significant resting ECG abnormalities that preclude diagnostic testing for coronary artery disease, such as left bundle-branch block, left ventricular hypertrophy with strain, or digitalis effect.

## Exercise Testing

Preoperative cardiac stress testing is useful in the objective assessment of functional capacity, to identify patients at risk of perioperative myocardial ischemia or cardiac arrhythmias, and to aid in the assessment of long-term as well as perioperative prognosis. In a general population, the mean sensitivity and specificity of exercise ST–T-wave ECG studies for the detection of coronary artery disease are 68% and 77%, respectively. The mortality rate was 5% per year or more among a high-risk subset, comprising 12% of the total population, who were able to achieve an exercise workload of less than Bruce stage I and had an abnormal exercise ECG. In contrast, mortality was less than 1% per year among a low-risk subset comprising 34% of the total population, who were able to achieve at least Bruce stage III with a normal exercise ECG response.

## Nonexercise Stress Testing

Approximately 30% to 50% of patients undergoing noncardiac surgery are unable to achieve an adequate exercise workload for a diagnostic study. In these patients, pharmacologic stress testing for the detection of coronary artery disease can be performed using 1 of 2 general methods. Infusion of the adrenergic agonist dobutamine results in increases in heart rate, myocardial contractility, and, to a lesser degree, blood pressure, resulting in increased myocardial oxygen demand. In the setting of a limited oxygen supply, increased demand causes myocardial ischemia, which is detected as a regional wall-motion abnormality on echocardiographic imaging. Alternatively, pharmacologic "stress" can be achieved using the coronary vasodilators dipyridamole or adenosine.

Although any abnormality on thallium scintigraphy is suggestive of coronary artery disease and is associated with a higher perioperative cardiac risk compared with patients who have normal scans, perioperative cardiac risk associated with a fixed perfusion defect is substantially lower than that associated with perfusion redistribution. In addition, the size of a perfusion defect is directly related to perioperative cardiac risk.

# PREOPERATIVE THERAPY FOR CORONARY ARTERY DISEASE

## ■ CORONARY REVASCULARIZATION

There are no large prospective randomized trials testing the impact of either preoperative coronary artery bypass grafting or percutaneous transluminal coronary angioplasty on perioperative cardiac morbidity and mortality rates. However, several retrospective studies suggest that patients having undergone previous successful surgical coronary revascularization have a low risk of perioperative cardiac events during noncardiac surgery. The risk of death is comparable to that found among patients without clinical indications suggestive of coronary artery disease. The Bypass Angioplasty Revascularization Investigation (BARI) trial investigated 1049 patients undergoing noncardiac surgery and found a low incidence of myocardial infarction or death among patients having undergone either coronary artery bypass surgery or percutaneous angioplasty. The absence of any evident difference between groups suggests that the previous percutaneous coronary angioplasty confers a protection from perioperative cardiac events that is similar to that conferred by surgical revascularization. However, based on the limited data available, indications for percutaneous coronary angioplasty among patients undergoing preoperative evaluation should be considered the same as for the general population.

The optimal timing of noncardiac surgery has not been defined for those patients requiring percutaneous revascularization. Patients who have gone more than 6 months after percutaneous coronary angioplasty with no evidence of recurrent ischemia could be considered to have undergone successful revascularization, presumably with a low perioperative risk. Elective surgery within the first 28 days after the placement of a bare-metal stent has been associated with a high risk of catastrophic events attributed to potential stent thrombosis. The timing for surgery following the placement of a drug-eluting stent also remains unkown. **Figure 46-2** represents a proposed strategy for minimization of stent thrombosis in patients undergoing surgical procedures.

## ■ MEDICAL THERAPY FOR CORONARY ARTERY DISEASE

Although data are lacking to support the empiric use of nitroglycerin or calcium-channel blockers, there is increasing evidence that the empiric use of perioperative β-blockers reduces the risk of an adverse cardiac event in medium- and high-risk patients undergoing vascular surgery. When data from the prospective trials evaluating the use of perioperative β-blockade are combined, 5 to 30 patients would need to be treated to prevent a single perioperative death. However, β-blockers should be started preoperatively and carefully titrated upward to achieve a heart rate in the 60s and without hypotension.

# MANAGEMENT OF SPECIFIC CONDITIONS

Patients with a variety of medical conditions known to increase cardiovascular risk may require noncardiac surgery. Factors that contribute to increased perioperative risk include interruptions in routine medical therapy as well as physical and mental stresses associated with the surgical procedure and convalescent period. It is important to note that the period of maximum cardiac risk appears to occur in the postoperative period. Because cardiovascular risk is not limited to the intraoperative period, appropriate emphasis should be placed on the treatment of specific conditions throughout all phases of the perioperative period.

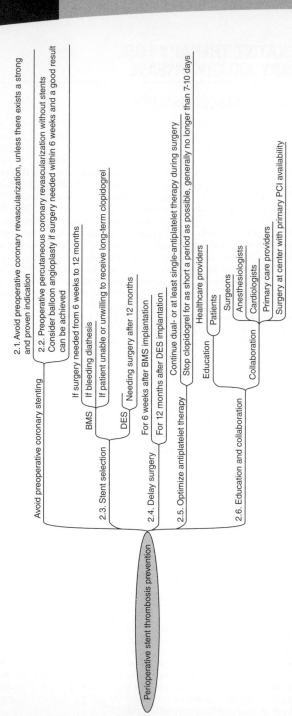

**FIGURE 46-2.** Perioperative strategy for the minimization of potential stent thrombosis. (Reproduced with permission from Brilakis ES, Banerjee S, Berger PB, et al. Perioperative management of patients with coronary stents. *J Am Coll Cardiol.* 2007;49(22):2145-2150.)

# SUGGESTED READINGS

Mukherjee D, Eagle KA. Perioperative evaluation and management of patients with known or suspected cardiovascular disease who undergo noncardiac surgery. In: Fuster V, Walsh R, Harrington RA, et al, eds. *Hurst's The Heart*. 13th ed. New York, NY: McGraw-Hill; 2011;87: 1971-1985.

Reich DL, Mittnacht AJC, Kaplan JA. Anesthesia and the patient with cardiovascular disease. In: Fuster V, Walsh RA, Harrington RA, et al. *Hurst's The Heart*. 13th ed. New York, NY: McGraw-Hill; 2011;88:1986-1994.

Auerbach AD, Goldman L. Beta-blockers and reduction of cardiac events in noncardiac surgery. *JAMA*. 2002;287:1435-1444.

Boden WE, O' Rourke RA, Teo KK, et al. Optimal medical therapy with or without PCI for stable coronary disease. *N Eng J Med*. 2007;356:1503-1516.

Brilakis ES, Banerjee S, Berger PB. Perioperative management of patients with coronary stents. *J Am Coll Cardiol*. 2007;49:2145-2150.

Eagle KA, Rihal CS, Mickel MC, et al. Cardiac risk of noncardiac surgery: influence of coronary artery disease and type of surgery in 3368 operations. CASS Investigators and University of Michigan Heart Care Program. Coronary Artery Surgery Study. *Circulation*. 1997;96: 1882-1887.

Fleisher LA, Beckman JA, Brown KA, et al. ACC/AHA 2007 guidelines on perioperative cardiovascular evaluation and care for noncardiac surgery: a report of the American College of Cardiology/American Heart Association Task Force on Practice Guidelines (Writing Committee to Revise the 2002 Guidelines on Perioperative Cardiovascular Evaluation for Noncardiac Surgery). *J Am Coll Cardiol*. 2007;50:e159-e241.

Kaluza GL, Joseph J, Lee JR, et al. Catastrophic outcomes of noncardiac surgery soon after coronary stenting. *J Am Coll Cardiol*. 2000;35:1288-1294.

Poldermans D, Boersma E. Beta-blocker therapy in noncardiac surgery. *N Eng J Med*. 2005;353:412-414.

# CHAPTER 47
# METABOLIC SYNDROME, OBESITY, AND DIET

Ian Del Conde Pozzi, Scott M. Grundy, and
Sidney C. Smith Jr

The rise in the prevalence of obesity in the United States and worldwide is threatening to undo recent advances in prevention of atherosclerotic cardiovascular disease (ASCVD). Between 1993 and 2008, the proportion of obese adults in the United States increased from 14.5% to 26.7%. It is estimated that approximately 33.8% of US adults aged 20 years and over are obese. Among the complications associated with obesity, cardiovascular events produce the greatest morbidity and mortality. A significant portion of the latter occurs in persons in whom obesity precedes type 2 diabetes. However, diabetes is only one of several conditions that associate strongly with obesity. Others include dyslipidemia, hypertension, systemic inflammation, and a thrombotic tendency. Recently there has been a trend in the cardiovascular field to group all these factors together under the heading of *metabolic syndrome*. In this sense, metabolic syndrome can be taken to represent a multiplex cardiovascular risk factor. This syndrome does not include, but is strongly associated with, other complications of obesity; for example, fatty liver, cholesterol gallstones, obstructive sleep apnea, and polycystic ovarian syndrome. This chapter focuses primarily on metabolic syndrome as a cardiovascular risk factor, with obesity being the primary exogenous factor driving its development.

Metabolic syndrome represents a clustering of cardiovascular risk factors that are amalgamated into a single multiplex risk factor for ASCVD (**Fig. 47-1**). The *metabolic risk factors* that make up the syndrome include atherogenic dyslipidemia, elevated blood pressure, dysglycemia, a prothrombotic state, and a proinflammatory state. Several reports indicate that this clustering of metabolic risk factors cannot be explained by chance alone, hence the use of the term *syndrome*. This suggests that there is a common, underlying etiology of this clustering. Individuals with metabolic syndrome have an approximate doubling of risk for ASCVD and approximately 4-fold higher risk for developing type 2 diabetes compared with those without the syndrome.

## LOW-DENSITY LIPOPROTEIN AND METABOLIC SYNDROME: PARTNERS IN ATHEROGENESIS

The development of atherosclerosis can be considered to occur in 2 stages: injury and response to injury. The primary injurious agents include LDL and other apolipoprotein B (apo B)–containing lipoproteins. The response to injury makes up

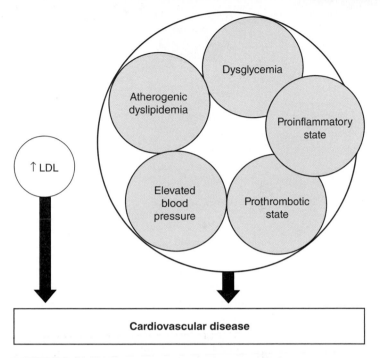

**FIGURE 47-1.** Risk factor partners: elevated low-density lipoprotein (LDL) and metabolic syndrome. The latter is a multiplex risk factor for arteriosclerotic cardiovascular disease and a clustering of atherogenic dyslipidemia, elevated blood pressure, dysglycemia, a prothrombotic state, and a pro-inflammatory state.

a process called inflammation. Metabolic syndrome exacerbates atherogenesis by enhancing the inflammatory response to LDL injury. The key steps in both processes are reviewed briefly.

The first step in the pathogenesis of atherosclerosis is the infiltration of plasma LDL into the arterial intima. The rate of infiltration of LDL depends on 2 factors: (1) the concentration of LDL in the circulation, and (2) the permeability of the arterial wall. A portion of the LDL that infiltrates the vessel wall becomes entrapped into the extracellular matrix. When this occurs, LDL is ripe for modification. When LDL is modified, it acquires the ability to activate various types of cells that play a role in atherogenesis, including endothelial cells, monocyte/macrophages, and smooth muscle cells. All of these changes come under the category of *inflammation* (**Fig. 47-2**). Key changes are endothelial dysfunction, which allows for a more rapid infiltration of LDL into the arterial wall and adherence to circulating monocytes; movement of monocytes into the arterial wall and their activation; proliferation of smooth muscle cells; and enhanced fibrosis. Macrophages are a key player in atherogenesis. They first accumulate lipid and then undergo apoptosis—releasing their excess lipid into lipid pools. Macrophages further produce enzymes, such as metalloproteinases, that degrade the extracellular matrix. These latter 2 changes seemingly create unstable plaques that are prone to rupture and to causation of acute ASCVD events.

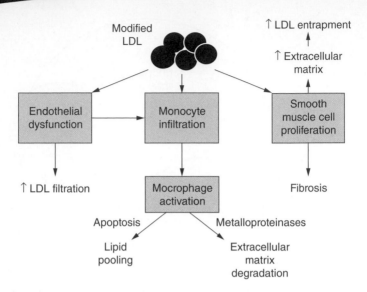

**FIGURE 47-2.** Details of the inflammatory process evoked by modified low-density lipoprotein (LDL). Three cellular systems are affected by modified LDL: endothelial cells, monocytes/macrophages, and smooth muscle cells. Modified LDL causes endothelial dysfunction, allowing increased amounts of LDL to filter into the arterial wall and enhanced attachment of monocytes to the endothelium. It also acts as a chemoattractant to pull monocytes into the arterial wall; at the same time it promotes transformation of monocytes into macrophages and activates them. Activated macrophages ingest modified LDL, become transformed into foam cells, undergo apoptosis to form large lipid pools, and release metalloproteinases to degrade the extracellular matrix. The latter 2 effects lead to destabilization of arteriosclerotic plaques, plaque rupture, and acute cardiovascular events. Finally, modified LDL stimulate smooth muscle cell proliferation for production of collagen fibers, leading to fibrosis of the plaque.

# METABOLIC SYNDROME AND ARTERIAL INFLAMMATION

Each of the components of metabolic syndrome appears to worsen inflammation in plaques. First, in the case of hypertension, an increased hydrostatic pressure in elevated blood pressure can enhance influx of LDL into the arterial wall. Further, hypertension is associated with endothelial dysfunction. Hypertension can be accompanied by increased angiotensin II (A-II), which can induce the expression of vascular adhesion molecule (VCAM)-1 on endothelial cells and cause the release of proinflammatory cytokines (eg, interleukin-6 [IL-6] and monocyte chemotactic protein-1 [MCP-1]). A-II can also increase the expression of proinflammatory cytokines such as IL-6 and MCP-1, and of the leukocyte adhesion molecule VCAM-1, present on endothelial cells. Second, hyperglycemia has been implicated in several ways in the exacerbation of inflammation—formation of inflammatory advanced glycation products, glycation of extracellular matrix enhancing retention of LDL, glycoxidative modification of LDL, and activation of protein kinase C. Third, a key component of atherogenic dyslipidemia is a low high-density lipoprotein (HDL). HDL is believed to be a protective lipoprotein, and if so, most likely exerts its anti-inflammatory effects at multiple levels: It transports excess cholesterol out of macrophages, reducing their atherogenic potential; it prevents conversion of LDL into proinflammatory modified LDL; and it inhibits cytokine-induced expression of cellular adhesion molecules on endothelial cells. Fourth, in metabolic syndrome, there is an increase in circulating cytokines. These cytokines likely act at the level of the arterial wall to enhance the inflammatory response to modified LDL. Finally, a prothrombotic state is characterized by a series of abnormalities that can enhance coagulation, inhibit fibrinolysis, and alter platelet function. Among these factors are increases in plasminogen activator inhibitor-1, fibrinogen, factor VII, factor VIII, factor X, prothrombin fragments F1+2, and von Willebrand factor.

# PATHOGENESIS OF METABOLIC SYNDROME

A simple way to visualize the pathogenesis of metabolic syndrome is illustrated in **Fig. 47-3**. This view identifies an interaction between exogenous and endogenous factors. Obesity is the major exogenous factor, but physical inactivity and excess dietary factors can play a role. Endogenous factors include inherent insulin resistance, dysfunctional adipose tissue, endocrine disorders, and various genetic aberrations. The endogenous factors can be grouped together under the heading of *metabolic susceptibility*. To develop the syndrome, most individuals must be metabolically susceptible. However, even in the presence of susceptibility, the full-blown metabolic syndrome generally will not develop in the absence of exogenous factors (especially obesity).

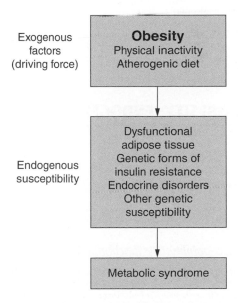

**FIGURE 47-3.** Pathogenic scheme for development of the metabolic syndrome. The syndrome develops as a result of the interaction of exogenous and endogenous factors. The major exogenous factor is obesity, but physical inactivity and atherogenic diet play an important role. Endogenous factors include dysfunctional adipose tissue, genetic forms of insulin resistance, various endocrine disorders, and other genetic susceptibility.

# OBESITY: THE DRIVING FORCE OF METABOLIC SYNDROME

The high prevalence of metabolic syndrome in the United States and worldwide is secondary to a rising prevalence of obesity. Physical inactivity also is associated with a higher prevalence of metabolic syndrome. The mechanisms whereby obesity results in metabolic syndrome are being increasingly understood. Adipose tissue releases several products that appear to worsen metabolic syndrome. The most important is a key fuel source, nonesterified fatty acids (NEFA). During the fasting state, adipose tissue triglyceride undergoes lipolysis and releases NEFA into the circulation. The major enzyme involved in lipolysis is *hormone-sensitive lipase*; the activity of this enzyme is enhanced by catecholamines and suppressed by insulin. If NEFA supply exceeds needs for energy utilization, lipid accumulates in muscle and liver. This accumulation is called *ectopic fat*. When fat accumulates in muscle and the liver, insulin resistance is increased. This change plus other metabolic alterations predisposes to the metabolic syndrome.

Beyond excess fatty acids, other products of adipose tissue are released in abnormal amounts from adipose tissue. One category of products includes the *inflammatory cytokines*, for example, tumor necrosis factor-$\alpha$ (TNF-$\alpha$) and IL-6. Excess cytokine release appears to be secondary to infiltration of adipose tissue with activated macrophages, which can produce these cytokines. The result is a high level of circulating cytokines. These can have several systemic effects: enhancement of insulin resistance in muscle, production of acute-phase reactants (C-reactive protein [CRP] and fibrinogen) by the liver, and exacerbation of inflammation in arteriosclerotic lesions. These cytokines play a key role in the causation of the proinflammatory state of metabolic syndrome.

The adipose tissue likewise can predispose to a prothrombotic state by release of excess amounts of plasminogen activator inhibitor-1, which is released from adipose tissue in response to obesity. Adipose tissue further secretes *leptin*, an appetite suppressant. Leptin levels are high in obesity and seemingly do not suppress the appetite of obese individuals, a condition called *leptin resistance*.

# BEYOND OBESITY: ENDOGENOUS METABOLIC SUSCEPTIBILITY

Only a portion of patients with obesity develop metabolic syndrome. It appears that an individual must be metabolically susceptible to developing the syndrome, and when obesity is acquired, the syndrome becomes manifest. Several factors seemingly contribute to endogenous susceptibility. Among these are dysfunctional adipose tissue, genetic forms of insulin resistance, various endocrine disorders, and other genetic factors. Of particular importance appears to be a dysfunction of adipose tissue.

## Metabolic Susceptibility: Dysfunctional Adipose Tissue

There are at least 4 potential disorders that can contribute to dysfunctional adipose tissue, which in turn will accentuate metabolic syndrome. These include a deficiency of subcutaneous adipose tissue, genetic forms of insulin resistance, dysfunctional adipocytes, and inflammation of adipose tissue (**Fig. 47-4**).

One of the most important of these is a deficiency of subcutaneous adipose tissue. This abnormality is seen in an extreme form in a condition called *lipodystrophy*. Patients with lipodystrophy have little adipose tissue for storage of extra energy; therefore fat is deposited ectopically in the liver and muscle, resulting in the development

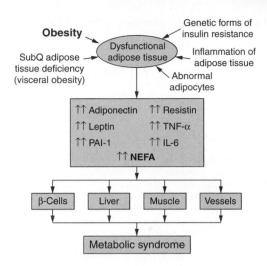

**FIGURE 47-4.** The role of obesity and dysfunctional adipose tissue in causation of the metabolic syndrome. When adipose tissue becomes overloaded with lipid (obesity), it produces abnormal amounts of nonesterified fatty acids (NEFA) and other adipokines. Among the latter are adiponectin, leptin, plasminogen activator inhibitor-1 (PAI-1), resistin, tumor necrosis factor-$\alpha$ (TNF-$\alpha$), interleukin-6 (IL-6), and other inflammatory cytokines. The *protective* adiponectin is produced in subnormal amounts in obese persons. These abnormal products of adipose tissue flood various key tissues—pancreatic $\beta$ cells, liver, muscle, and vessels; their effects in turn give rise to metabolic syndrome or accelerate the development of atherosclerosis at the level of the arterial wall. Additional causes of dysfunctional adipose tissue include a deficiency of subcutaneous adipose tissue, leading to visceral obesity, genetic forms of insulin resistance, abnormal adipocytes, and inflammation of adipose tissue. In the presence of these factors, defects in production of NEFA and adipokines is accentuated, worsening the metabolic syndrome.

of metabolic syndrome. Less severe forms of adipose-tissue deficiency are manifested by an abnormal body fat distribution. Differences in body fat distribution can typically be seen between obese women and men. Women normally have considerable quantities of subcutaneous adipose tissue in the lower body. Only when they are more severely obese does fat begin to accumulate in the upper body. As a result, substantial ectopic fat accumulation is relatively rare. In contrast, men typically have a paucity of lower-body subcutaneous adipose tissue; as a result, they tend to develop upper-body obesity, including considerable amounts of visceral fat as well as ectopic fat. This pattern of fat distribution is called *abdominal obesity*; it is complicated by larger amounts of ectopic fat, which predisposes to metabolic syndrome. There is considerable variation in these trends in both men and women, and some individuals are particularly prone to development of ectopic fat and metabolic syndrome when they become obese.

Dysfunctional forms of adipose tissue further can result from genetic forms of insulin resistance. Insulin is a major regulator of adipose tissue metabolism. When genetic defects occur in insulin signaling in adipocytes, suppression of lipolysis and other products is impaired. In addition, adiponectin release is reduced. All of these will accentuate ectopic fat distribution and metabolic syndrome. Moreover, defective insulin signaling in other tissues such as muscle and liver most likely will accentuate metabolic syndrome. A good example of a genetic form of insulin resistance is found in many persons of South Asian origin. Insulin-resistant South Asians have multiple signs of dysfunctional adipose tissue—elevated NEFA levels, high CRP and leptin levels, and low adiponectin concentrations. These persons are prone to metabolic syndrome and to premature type 2 diabetes and CVD.

Finally, in obese persons, the adipose tissue is invaded with macrophages. The possibility has been raised that activation of these macrophages will result in the production of cytokines that will derange the function of adipocytes. In particular, these cytokines can cause insulin resistance, and the same defects are noted in persons with genetic forms of insulin resistance. Thus *inflammation* of adipose tissue can be yet another factor contributing to dysfunctional adipose tissue and metabolic syndrome.

## Genetic Forms of Insulin Resistance

One hypothesis holds that genetic forms of insulin resistance are the major cause of metabolic syndrome. According to this hypothesis, resistance to the action of insulin is widespread and causes a gross metabolic disturbance in many tissues. This disturbance can account for the multiple metabolic risk factors characteristic of the syndrome. This hypothesis is provocative and has provided a basis for many studies on the causation of metabolic syndrome. The effects of insulin resistance in adipose tissue provide the most direct evidence for the mechanism linking resistance to insulin to metabolic syndrome. Nevertheless, it is certainly possible that widespread metabolic disturbance contributes beyond adipose tissue abnormalities.

## Other Genetic and Metabolic Abnormalities

In view of metabolic differences in men and women, it is likely that endocrine factors play a role in causation of metabolic syndrome. This possibility is heightened by the observation that women with polycystic ovary syndrome are prone to metabolic syndrome. Because patients with hypercorticolism manifest many of the features of the syndrome, abnormalities in cortisol metabolism also have been implicated.

Manifestations of metabolic syndrome vary from individual to individual and also between populations. For example, Asians and Hispanics appear to be particularly susceptible to diabetes, African Americans to hypertension, and Caucasians to dyslipidemia. Certainly all of the features of metabolic syndrome can occur in all of these populations, but prominent features suggest that genetic variation exists and affects manifestations of the syndrome. Research on the genetic basis of ethnic differences has been increasing in the past few years and promises to provide new insights into the causes of variation in expression of the syndrome.

# CLINICAL DIAGNOSIS OF METABOLIC SYNDROME

In 2009 the American Heart Association (AHA), the National Heart, Lung, and Blood Institute (NHLBI), and International Diabetes Federation, along with the World Heart Federation, International Atherosclerosis Society, and the International Association for the Study of Obesity, issued a joint interim statement regarding a common universal definition for the metabolic syndrome. They agreed that the requirement for central obesity as an obligatory component should be dropped, but that waist circumference would continue to be a useful preliminary screening tool. Three of 5 abnormal findings are required for the diagnosis of the metabolic syndrome. With the exception of waist circumference, where national or regional cut points may be used pending further research, a single set of cut points should be used for all other components of the metabolic syndrome (**Table 47-1**). The current recommended waist circumference thresholds for abdominal obesity vary by region and ethnicity (**Table 47-2**).

**TABLE 47-1.** Criteria for Clinical Diagnosis of the Metabolic Syndrome

| Measure | Categorical Cut Points |
|---|---|
| Elevated waist circumference[a] | Population- and country-specific definitions |
| Elevated triglycerides (drug treatment for elevated triglycerides is an alternate indicator[b]) | ≥150 mg/dL (1.7 mmol/L) |
| Reduced HDL-C (drug treatment for reduced HDL-C is an alternate indicator[b]) | <40 mg/dL (1.0 mmol/L) in males; <50 mg/dL (1.3 mmol/L) in females |
| Elevated blood pressure (antihypertensive drug treatment in a patient with a history of hypertension is an alternate indicator) | Systolic ≥130 and/or diastolic ≥85 mm Hg |
| Elevated fasting glucose[c] (drug treatment of elevated glucose is an alternate indicator) | ≥100 mg/dL |

[a]It is recommended that the International Diabetes Foundation (IDF) cut points be used for non-Europeans and either the IDF or American Heart Association/National Heart, Lung, and Blood Institute cut points be used for people of European origin until more data are available.

[b]The most commonly used drugs for elevated triglycerides and reduced HDL-C are fibrates and nicotinic acid. A patient taking one of these drugs can be presumed to have high triglycerides and low HDL-C. High-dose omega-3 fatty acid presumes high triglycerides.

[c]Most patients with type 2 diabetes mellitus will have the metabolic syndrome by the proposed criteria.

HDL-C, high-density lipoprotein cholesterol.

Reproduced with permission from Alberti KGMM, Eckel RH, Grundy SM, et al. Harmonizing the metabolic syndrome. *Circulation.* 2009;120.1640-1645.

# METABOLIC SYNDROME AND RISK FOR ARTERIOSCLEROTIC CARDIOVASCULAR DISEASE

## Long-Term (Lifetime) Risk

In populations at risk, metabolic syndrome is accompanied by an increase in relative risk for ASCVD. In prospective epidemiologic studies, the relative risk for ASCVD events is essentially doubled. It is likely that the 2-fold increase in risk seen in short-term, prospective studies underestimates the long-term impact of the syndrome. The reason is that metabolic risk factors tend to worsen with time. Lipid levels and blood pressure rise with advancing age, and normal glucose levels advance to prediabetes or frank diabetes. Consequently, the earlier metabolic syndrome can be detected and managed, the slower will be the progression.

## Short-Term (10-Year) Risk

At present, more intense clinical intervention is driven by short-term risk for ASCVD. This risk usually is identified as 10-year risk for coronary heart disease (CHD). According to ATP III guidelines, risk can be stratified into 4 categories:

1. *High risk* is a 10-year risk for CHD >20% and includes patients with clinically evident ASCVD, diabetes, or enough other major risk factors to raise the risk to this level.

2. *Moderately high risk* consists of ≥2 major risk factors and a 10-year risk of 10% to 20%.

**TABLE 47-2.** Current Recommended Waist Circumference Thresholds for Abdominal Obesity by Organization

| Population | Organization | Recommended Waist Circumference Threshold for Abdominal Obesity Men | Women |
|---|---|---|---|
| Europid | IDF | ≥94 cm | ≥80 cm |
| Caucasian | WHO | ≥94 cm (increased risk) ≥102 cm (still higher risk) | ≥80 cm (increased risk) ≥88 cm (still higher risk) |
| United States | AHA/NHLBI (ATP III[a] | ≥102 cm | ≥88 cm |
| Canada | Health Canada | ≥102 cm | ≥88 cm |
| European | European Cardiovascular Societies | ≥102 cm | ≥88 cm |
| Asian (including Japanese) | IDF | ≥90 cm | ≥80 cm |
| Asian | WHO | ≥90 cm | ≥80 cm |
| Japanese | Japanese Obesity Society | ≥85 cm | ≥90 cm |
| China | Cooperative Task Force | ≥85 cm | ≥80 cm |
| Middle East, Mediterranean | IDF | ≥94 cm | ≥80 cm |
| Sub-Saharan African | IDF | ≥94 cm | ≥80 cm |
| Ethnic Central and South American | IDF | ≥90 cm | ≥80 cm |

[a]Recent AHA/NHLBI guidelines for metabolic syndrome recognize an increased risk for cardiovascular disease and diabetes at waist-circumference thresholds of ≥94 cm in men and ≥80 cm in women and identify these as optional cut points for individuals or populations with increased insulin resistance.

AHA, American Heart Association; ATP III, National Cholesterol Education Program Adult Treatment Panel III Report; IDF, International Diabetes Foundation; NHLBI, National Heart, Lung, and Blood Institute; WHO, World Health Organization.

Reproduced with permission from Alberti KGMM, Eckel RH, Grundy SM, et al. Harmonizing the metabolic syndrome. *Circulation.* 2009;120:1640-1645.

3. *Moderate risk* exhibits ≥2 risk factors, but a 10-year risk <10%.

4. *Lower-risk* individuals have 0 to 1 risk factor and a 10-year risk <10%.

Most persons with metabolic syndrome can be considered to be at least a moderate risk, but many will have risk >10%.

Framingham risk scoring should be used to estimate 10-year risk in metabolic syndrome patients without established ASCVD or type 2 diabetes mellitus. Because metabolic syndrome is only 1 part of overall risk assessment for ASCVD, it is not an adequate tool to estimate 10-year risk for CHD. These patients must be considered to be at higher lifetime risk for ASCVD, but metabolic syndrome alone is inadequate to guide clinical management for short-term risk reduction.

Although Framingham risk scoring provides a good first-step for estimating risk, other considerations can be brought into play both for confirmation of metabolic syndrome and for estimating 10-year risk in affected patients (**Fig. 47-5**). Besides the simple clinical measures proposed by ATP III, other *emerging risk factors* are commonly present in patients with metabolic syndrome. Identification of abnormalities in these factors can help to confirm the presence of the syndrome. Although these

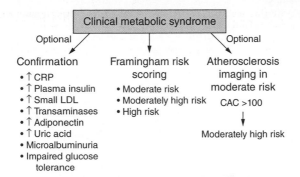

**FIGURE 47-5.** Approaches to cardiovascular risk assessment in patients with clinical evidence of the metabolic syndrome. All such patients should undergo Framingham risk scoring to determine 10-year risk for coronary heart disease (CHD). In addition, as an option, a series of biomarkers can be identified to support and confirm the presence of the metabolic syndrome. Another option is to use atherosclerosis imaging to bolster risk assessment carried out with Framingham scoring. Atherosclerosis imaging in patients with the metabolic syndrome is most appropriate for those found to be at moderate risk (10-year risk for CHD <10%) by Framingham scoring. CAC, coronary artery calcification; CRP, C-reactive protein; LDL, low-density lipoprotein.

emerging risk factors are not required for diagnosis, the presence of several of them will give strong confirmation of the presence of a systemic metabolic disorder. Therefore, their measurement is optional. In addition, confirmation of a higher risk status can be obtained by the finding of significant subclinical atherosclerosis. For example, if a patient with metabolic syndrome found to be at moderate risk by Framingham risk scoring is found to have a higher coronary artery calcification score, this patient might be elevated to a category of moderately high risk if the coronary artery calcification score is >100 Agatston units.

# MANAGEMENT OF UNDERLYING CAUSES

## ■ OVERWEIGHT AND OBESITY

Because obesity is the major driving force behind metabolic syndrome, it is a reasonable primary target of therapy. Clinical guidelines for management of overweight and obesity have been published by the NHLBI and National Institute of Diabetes and Digestive and Kidney Diseases. They distinguish between overweight and obesity by body mass index ranges of 25 to 29.9 kg/m$^2$ and ≥30 kg/m$^2$, respectively. These guideline define abdominal obesity as a waist circumference ≥102 cm (>40 in) in men and ≥88 cm (>35 in) in women. These thresholds were used by ATP III as one of the clinical criteria for metabolic syndrome, but the recent update in diagnostic criteria indicated that some persons can develop metabolic syndrome at lesser waist circumferences. This is particularly the case in certain ethnic groups; for example, the populations of South and Southeast Asia (see Table 47-2).

The initial goal for obesity management is to reduce the body weight by 10% per year; an ultimate goal is to achieve a body mass index <25 kg/m$^2$ over a longer period of time. Obesity guidelines recommend caloric intake and behavioral change as first-line therapies to achieve weight loss. Behavioral change should include increased physical activity as one of its components. A diet that is appropriate for long-term weight reduction should be consistent with current recommendations for a healthy diet in general. Emphasis should be given to reducing consumption of saturated and *trans*-fatty acids and cholesterol, reduced intake of simple sugars, and ample intakes of fruits, vegetables, and whole grains. Some investigators favor a relatively higher intake of unsaturated fatty acids at the expense of carbohydrates. This dietary pattern is similar to that of the *Mediterranean diet*. Behavioral change is the second major requirement for successful weight reduction. Without behavioral change, long-term weight loss will not be possible. It is rarely easy to reverse the lifetime of behavior that resulted in obesity. The earlier in life that obesity (or overweight) can be identified, the more effective will be the intervention. A few behavioral techniques to achieve a long-term weight loss include the following:

- Establishing weight goals (eg, 10% loss of body weight in 1 year)
- Establishing physical activity (eg, exercise 30 minutes daily)
- Learning to avoid situations where overeating is likely to occur
- Identifying circumstances leading to eating binges and avoiding them
- Establishing a regular eating schedule
- Avoiding eating or snacking between meals (eating on schedule)
- Taking smaller portions
- Eating slowly
- Keeping a diet diary (self-monitoring)
- Developing a social support structure
- Learning to manage stressful situations that foster overeating
- Developing a regular schedule for physical activity

Successful weight reduction will reduce all metabolic syndrome risk factors—atherogenic dyslipidemia, blood pressure, plasma glucose, coagulation and fibrinolytic factors, and the proinflammatory state. The Diabetes Prevention Program (DPP) and other studies showed that even moderate weight reduction will delay the conversion of impaired glucose tolerance (IGT)/impaired fasting glucose (IFG) into type 2 diabetes mellitus. Patients with morbid obesity, defined as body mass index >40 kg/m$^2$, or patients with a body mass index >35 kg/m$^2$ with serious obesity-related comorbidities, such as type 2 diabetes mellitus, systemic hypertension, or obstructive sleep apnea, should be considered for bariatric surgery. Surgical intervention in these patients has been shown to be effective in significant improvements in insulin resistance and in decreasing the prevalence of metabolic syndrome. The most clinically relevant impact of surgical weight loss on diabetes mellitus is the ability of the former to reverse the established diabetes mellitus in a large proportion of patients. In a large, long-term, controlled study comparing bariatric surgery and conventional therapy for obesity, established diabetes mellitus was reversed in 21% of the control group, compared to 72% of patients in the surgical group at 2 years of follow-up.

## Physical Inactivity

An extremely high proportion of the United States population is sedentary. There are multiple social trends leading to sedentary life habits. Among these are urbanization, mechanized transportation, reduced manual labor, and a variety of *labor-saving* devices. Physical inactivity is a major contributing cause of metabolic syndrome; moreover, regular physical activity and attaining physical fitness will improve most of metabolic risk factors. Increased physical fitness has been reported to reduce several chronic diseases, including cardiovascular disease.

It is currently recommended that everyone should engage in 30 minutes of moderate-intensity physical activity daily. Even more benefit is achieved by increasing activity to 60 minutes daily. The following are examples of moderate-intensity activity:

- Brisk walking, jogging, swimming, biking, golfing, team sports
- Using simple exercise equipment (eg, treadmills)
- Several short (10 to 15 minutes) bouts of activity (brisk walking)
- Substituting more active leisure activities for sedentary ones (television watching and computer games)

# MANAGEMENT OF METABOLIC RISK FACTORS

Lifestyle therapies are first-line therapies for metabolic syndrome and will improve all of the metabolic risk factors. However, in higher-risk patients, it can be necessary to turn to drug therapies to control the risk factors (**Tables 47-3** and **47-4**). The choice and intensity of drug therapy depends largely on the short-term risk of a patient. Also, the presence of metabolic syndrome itself can influence the particular drugs that are to be chosen.

## Atherogenic Dyslipidemia

This condition is recognized clinically by an increase in serum triglyceride and a reduction in high-density lipoprotein-cholesterol (HDL-C). When triglycerides are elevated, this is usually a sign of an increase in apo B–containing lipoproteins. The primary target of lipid-lowering therapy in all patients is low-density lipoprotein cholesterol (LDL-C), which normally contains most of the apo B (see Table 47-4 for ATP III recommendations for management of elevated LDL-C). In patients with metabolic syndrome who have high triglycerides, a sizable portion of apo B can be in very-low-density lipoprotein (VLDL). For this reason, it is useful to make LDL plus VLDL a secondary target of therapy. An increase in LDL plus VLDL is most readily identified by an elevation of non–HDL-C. The goals for non–HDL-C are 30 mg/dL higher than those for LDL-C. A low level of HDL-C can be considered a tertiary target. After the goals for LDL-C and non–HDL-C have been achieved, consideration can be given to therapies that can raise HDL-C levels.

Clinical trials have been carried out to determine the efficacy of reducing apo B–containing lipoproteins for reducing risk for cardiovascular events. The most effective drugs for reducing apo B–containing lipoproteins are statins. These trials have not specifically targeted patients with metabolic syndrome, but several of them have included subgroups with either metabolic syndrome or type 2 diabetes. Most of the statin trials can be classified as secondary prevention trials, although several have been performed in patients without established ASCVD (primary prevention). The following statin trials have examined outcomes in subgroups with metabolic syndrome or type 2 diabetes: the Air Force Coronary Atherosclerosis Prevention Study (AFCAPS)/Texas Coronary Atherosclerosis Prevention Study (TEXCAPS), WOSCOPS, Scandinavian Simvastatin Survival Study (4S), CARE, LIPID, HPS, Anglo-Scandinavian Cardiac Outcomes Trial (ASCOT), and Treating to New Targets (TNT). In all these virtual trials, patients with either metabolic syndrome or type 2 diabetes benefitted from statin therapy. These trials support the use of drugs that reduce apo B–containing lipoprotein in the treatment of patients with metabolic syndrome. Two clinical trials with statin therapy have specifically targeted type 2 diabetes. In the Collaborative Atorvastatin Diabetes Study (CARDS) trial, statin treatment

**TABLE 47-3.** Therapeutic Goals and Recommendations for Clinical Management of Metabolic Syndrome

| Therapeutic Target and Goals of Therapy | Therapeutic Recommendations |
|---|---|
| **Lifestyle risk factors** | Long-term prevention of CVD and prevention (or treatment) of type 2 diabetes. |
| Abdominal obesity<br>*Goal:*<br>Reduce body weight by 7%-10% during first year of therapy. Continue weight loss thereafter to the extent possible with a goal to ultimately achieve desirable weight (BMI <25 kg/m²) | Consistently encourage weight maintenance/reduction through an appropriate balance of physical activity, caloric intake, and formal behavioral programs when indicated to maintain/achieve a waist circumference of <40 in in men and <35 in in women. Aim initially at a slow reduction of approximately 7%-10% from baseline weight. Even small amounts of weight loss are associated with significant health benefits. |
| Physical inactivity<br>*Goal:* | In patients with established CVD, assess risk with a detailed physical activity history and/or an exercise test to guide prescription. |
| Regular moderate-intensity physical activity. At least 30 min of continuous or intermittent (and preferably ≥60 min) 5 d/wk, but preferably daily | Encourage 30-60 or more min of moderate-intensity aerobic activity such as brisk walking, preferably daily, supplemented by an increase in daily lifestyle activities (eg, pedometer step tracking, walking breaks at work, gardening, household work). Higher exercise times can be achieved by accumulating exercise throughout the day. Encourage resistance training 2 d/wk. Advise medically supervised programs for high-risk patients (eg, recent acute coronary syndrome or revascularization, CHF). |
| Atherogenic diet<br>*Goal:*<br>Reduced intakes of saturated fat, *trans*-fat, and cholesterol | Recommendations: saturated fat <7% of total calories; reduce *trans*-fat; dietary cholesterol <200 mg/dL; total fat 25%-35% of total calories. Most dietary fat should be unsaturated and simple sugars should be limited. |
| **Metabolic risk factors** | Shorter-term prevention of CVD or treatment of type 2 diabetes. |
| Atherogenic dyslipidemia<br>*Goals:* | Elevated LDL-C.<br>Elevated non–HDL-C. |
| Primary target: elevated LDL-C (see Table 47-4 for details) | Follow strategy outlined in Table 47-4 to achieve goal for LDL-C. First option to achieve non–HDL-C goal: intensify LDL-lowering therapy. |
| Secondary target: elevated non–HDL-C | Second option: add fibrate (preferably fenofibrate) or nicotinic acid if non–HDL-C remains relatively high after LDL-lowering drug therapy. |
| High-risk patients[a]: <130 mg/dL (3.4 mmol/L) (optional: <100 mg/dL for very high-risk patients[b]) | Give preference to adding fibrate or nicotinic acid in high-risk patients. |
| Moderately high-risk patients[c]: <160 mg/dL (4.1 mmol/L) Therapeutic option: <130 mg/dL (3.4 mmol/L) | Give preference to avoiding addition of fibrate or nicotinic acid in moderately high-risk or moderate-risk patients.<br>All patients: If TG is ≥500 mg/dL, initiate fibrate or nicotinic acid (before LDL-lowering therapy; treat non–LDL-C to goal after TG-lowering therapy). |
| Moderate-risk patients[d]: <160 mg/dL (4.1 mmol/L) | Reduced HDL-C.<br>Maximize lifestyle therapies: weight reduction and increased physical activity. |
| Lower-risk patients[e]: <190 mg/dL (4.9 mmol/L) | Consider adding fibrate or nicotinic acid after LDL-C–lowering drug therapy as outlined for elevated non–HDL-C. |

(*Continued*)

**TABLE 47-3.** Therapeutic Goals and Recommendations for Clinical Management of Metabolic Syndrome (Continued)

| Therapeutic Target and Goals of Therapy | Therapeutic Recommendations |
|---|---|
| Tertiary target: reduced HDL-C<br>No specific goal: raise HDL-C to extent possible with standard therapies for atherogenic dyslipidemia | |
| Elevated BP<br>*Goals:*<br>Reduce BP to at least achieve a BP of <140/90 mm Hg (or <130/80 mm Hg if diabetes present). Reduce BP further to the extent possible through lifestyle changes | For BP ≥120/80 mm Hg: initiate or maintain lifestyle modification—weight control, increased physical activity, alcohol moderation, sodium reduction, and emphasis on increased consumption of fresh fruits vegetables and low-fat dairy products—in all patients with metabolic syndrome.<br>For BP ≥140/90 mm Hg (or ≥130/80 mm Hg for individuals with chronic kidney disease or diabetes): as tolerated, add BP medication as needed to achieve goal BP. |
| Elevated glucose<br>*Goals:*<br>For IFG, delay progression to type 2 diabetes<br>For diabetes, HbA$_{1c}$<7.0% | For IFG, encourage weight reduction and increased physical activity.<br>For type 2 diabetes, lifestyle therapy, and pharmacotherapy if necessary, should be used to achieve near-normal HbA$_{1c}$ (<7%). Modify other risk factors and behaviors (eg, abdominal obesity, physical inactivity, elevated BP, lipid abnormalities). |
| Prothrombotic state<br>*Goals:*<br>Reduce thrombotic and fibrinolytic risk factors | High-risk patients: initiate and continue low-dose aspirin therapy; in patients with ASCVD, consider clopidogrel if aspirin is contraindicated.<br>Moderately high-risk patients: consider low-dose aspirin prophylaxis |
| Proinflammatory state | Recommendations: no specific therapies beyond lifestyle therapies |

ASCVD, arteriosclerotic cardiovascular disease; BP, blood pressure; BMI, body mass index; CHF, congestive heart failure; CVD, cardiovascular disease; HbA$_{1c}$, glycosylated hemoglobin; HDL-C, high-density lipoprotein-cholesterol; IFG, impaired fasting glucose; LDL-C, low-density lipoprotein-cholesterol; TG, triglyceride; TIA, transient ischemic attack

[a]High-risk patients: those with established arteriosclerotic cardiovascular disease, diabetes, or 10-year risk for coronary heart disease >20%. For cerebrovascular disease, high-risk condition includes TIA or stroke of carotid origin or >50% carotid stenosis.

[b]Very-high-risk patients are those who are likely to have major CVD events in the next few years, and diagnosis depends on clinical assessment. Factors that can confer very high risk include recent acute coronary syndromes, and established CHD plus any of the following: multiple major risk factors (especially diabetes), severe and poorly controlled risk factors (especially continued cigarette smoking), and metabolic syndrome.

[c]Moderately high-risk patients: those with 10-year risk for coronary heart disease 10% to 20%. Factors that favor the therapeutic option of non–HDL-C <100 mg/dL are those that can raise persons to the upper range of moderately high risk: multiple major risk factors, severe and poorly controlled risk factors (especially continued cigarette smoking), metabolic syndrome, and documented advanced subclinical arteriosclerotic disease (eg, coronary calcium or carotid intimal-medial thickness >75th percentile for age and sex).

[d]Moderate-risk patients: those with ≥2 major risk factors and 10-year risk <10%.

[e]Lower-risk patients: those with 0 to 1 major risk factor and 10-year risk <10%.

**TABLE 47-4.** Elevated LDL Cholesterol: Primary Target of Lipid-Lowering Therapy in Persons at Risk for Arteriosclerotic Cardiovascular Disease

| Goals of Therapy | Therapeutic Recommendations |
|---|---|
| High-risk patients[a]: <100 mg/dL (2.6 mmol/L) (for very-high-risk patients[b] in this category, optional goal <70 mg/dL) | High-risk patients: lifestyle therapies[g] plus LDL-C–lowering drug to achieve recommended goal. If baseline LDL-C ≥100 mg/dL, initiate LDL-lowering drug therapy. |
| Moderately high-risk patients[c]: <130 mg/dL (3.4 mmol/L) (for higher-risk patients[d] in this category, optional goal is <100 mg/dL [2.6 mmol/L]) | If on-treatment LDL-C ≥100 mg/dL, intensify LDL-lowering drug therapy (can require LDL-lowering drug combination). If baseline LDL-C <100 mg/dL, initiate LDL-lowering therapy based on clinical judgment (ie, assessment that the patient is at very high risk). |
| Moderate-risk patients[e]: <130 mg/dL (3.4 mmol/L) | Moderately high-risk patients: lifestyle therapies plus LDL-lowering drug if necessary to achieve recommended goal when LDL-C ≥130 mg/dL (3.4 mmol/L) after lifestyle therapies. |
| Low-risk patients[f]: <160 mg/dL (4.9 mmol/L) | If baseline LDL-C is 100-129 mg/dL, LDL-lowering therapy can be introduced if patient's risk is assessed to be in the upper ranges of this risk category. |
| | Moderate-risk patients: lifestyle therapies plus LDL-C–lowering drug if necessary to achieve recommended goal when LDL-C ≥160 mg/dL (4.1 mmol/L) after lifestyle therapies. |
| | Lower-risk patients: lifestyle therapies plus LDL-C–lowering drug if necessary to achieve recommended goal when LDL-C ≥190 mg/dL after lifestyle therapies (for LDL-C 160-189 mg/dL, LDL-lowering drug is optional). |

[a]High-risk patients: those with established arteriosclerotic cardiovascular disease, diabetes, or 10-year risk for coronary heart disease >20%. For cerebrovascular disease, high-risk condition includes TIA or stroke of carotid origin or >50% carotid stenosis.

[b]Very high-risk patients are those who are likely to have major CVD events in the next few years, and diagnosis depends on clinical assessment. Factors that can confer very high risk include recent acute coronary syndromes, and established CHD plus any of the following: multiple major risk factors (especially diabetes), severe and poorly controlled risk factors (especially continued cigarette smoking), and multiple risk factors of the metabolic syndrome.

[c]Moderately high-risk patients: those with 10-year risk for coronary heart disease 10% to 20%.

[d]Factors that can raise persons to the upper range of moderately high risk are multiple major risk factors, severe and poorly controlled risk factors (especially continued cigarette smoking), metabolic syndrome, and documented advanced subclinical arteriosclerotic disease (eg, coronary calcium or carotid intimal-medial thickness >75th percentile for age and sex).

[e]Moderate-risk patients: those with ≥2 major risk factors and 10-year risk <10%.

[f]Lower-risk patients: those with 0 to 1 major risk factor and 10-year risk <10%.

[g]Lifestyle therapies include weight reduction, increased physical activity, and antiatherogenic diet (see Table 47-4 for details).

CHD, coronary heart disease; CVD, cardiovascular disease; LDL-C, low-density lipoprotein cholesterol; TIA, transient ischemic attack.

showed a 37% reduction in major coronary events by reduction of apo B–containing lipoproteins with a statin. In the Atorvastatin Study for Prevention of Coronary Heart Disease Endpoints in Noninsulin-Dependent Diabetes Mellitus (ASPEN) trial, statin therapy showed a trend toward benefit in reduction of ASCVD events, although results for the primary composite ASCVD outcome were not statistically significant.

However, this trial appeared to suffer from inadequate statistical power to allow for a robust testing of the primary hypothesis.

Two other classes of drugs have been used for treatment of atherogenic dyslipidemia. These are nicotinic acid and fibrates. Their primary actions are to reduce triglyceride-rich lipoproteins and to raise HDL. Both lower triglycerides similarly, whereas nicotinic acid raises HDL more than do fibrates. Several clinical trials have been performed with these classes of agents. Again, metabolic syndrome has not been the primary target of therapy. However, subgroup analyses strongly suggest that the greatest reduction in cardiovascular events occurs in patients who have many of the features of metabolic syndrome. The trials (and drugs used) include the Helsinki Heart Study (gemfibrozil), VA-HIT (gemfibrozil), the Stockholm study (clofibrate plus nicotinic acid), BIP (bezafibrate), FIELD (fenofibrate), and the Coronary Drug Project (nicotinic acid). The results of these studies provide a rationale for using either nicotinic acid or a fibrate as *add-on* therapy to statins or other LDL-lowering drugs. One limitation to this combination is the increased risk of muscle toxicity, as high as 1% to 5% in patients taking some fibrates and a statin (eg, lovastatin and atorvastatin) with gemfibrozil. Pravastatin (or perhaps fluvastatin) is the statin of choice in patients treated with gemfibrozil (or other fibric acid derivatives). However, these drugs should be used cautiously and only if the benefit is likely to outweigh the low risk of muscle toxicity. Fenofibrate is the preferred fibrate in patients who require combined therapy with a statin.

For secondary prevention, that is, in patients with established ASCVD, the first goal of therapy is to reduce LDL-C to <100 mg/dL and non–HDL-C to <130 mg/dL. These goals are strongly supported by clinical trial evidence. Recent studies suggest that lowering of LDL-C to well below 100 mg/dL will further reduce risk for future cardiovascular events in patients with established ASCVD. Although the database supporting this lower goal is not as strong as for an LDL-C <100 mg/dL (non–HDL-C <130 mg/dL), the evidence is mounting that "the lower, the better" for apo B–containing lipoproteins in these patients who arc at very high risk for future ASCVD events. For ASCVD patients with either metabolic syndrome or type 2 diabetes, subgroup analysis of clinical trials suggests that further lowering of LDL-C to <70 mg/dL (non–HDL-C to <100 mg/dL) is reasonable.

For primary prevention, the therapeutic goals for lipids depend on the absolute risk of patients. For patients with both the metabolic syndrome and type 2 diabetes, the LDL-C should be reduced to <100 mg/dL (non–HDL-C <130 mg/dL). The same would be true for patients with metabolic syndrome who have a 10-year risk for major coronary events by Framingham scoring of >20%. It is reasonable to reduce LDL-C to <100 mg/dL (non–HDL-C <130 mg/dL) in metabolic syndrome patients whose 10-year risk for CHD is 10% to 20%.

If a decision is made to drive the LDL-C (and non–HDL-C) to the lower ranges, which is considered reasonable for the higher-risk patients with metabolic syndrome, the choice of therapies becomes important. Several alternative approaches are available. For example, it is possible to increase the intensity of statin therapy from standard doses to high doses. The efficacy of this approach has been shown for the TNT trials in patients with metabolic syndrome with or without type 2 diabetes. Besides increasing statin therapy, lower LDL levels can be obtained by combining a standard dose of statins with either ezetimibe or a bile acid sequestrant. To date, the added benefit of such combinations has not been documented through clinical trials. Another alternative is to combine a standard dose of statin with either nicotinic acid or fibrate. Again, however, clinical trials have not been carried out to demonstrate added efficacy.

Finally, the question of whether to specifically target a low HDL level in patients with metabolic syndrome has not been resolved. At present, the only drug that has a substantial HDL-raising potential is nicotinic acid, particularly at high doses where there are side effects. A newer class of drugs that more selectively raise HDL levels is the cholesteryl ester transfer protein (CETP) inhibitors, which includes dalcetrapib and anacetrapib. These agents are currently being studied in large clinical trials to determine whether raising HDL levels translates into improved cardiovascular outcomes.

## Elevated Blood Pressure

Most patients with metabolic syndrome have mild elevation in blood pressure. ATP III defined elevated blood pressure as a component of metabolic syndrome when the blood pressure level is ≥130 mm Hg systolic or ≥85 mm Hg diastolic. The Seventh Report of the Joint National Committee (JNC 7) provides useful guidelines for management of blood pressure. JNC 7 emphasized lifestyle therapy as first-line therapy. When lifestyle changes do not reduce the blood pressure to <140/90 mm Hg, drug therapy must be considered. These guidelines do not identify a priority in choice of drugs. JNC 7 gave priority to diuretics and β-blockers because of proven clinical and cost-effectiveness. However, high doses of these drugs can increase insulin resistance and raise the plasma glucose. Because of the latter, they can convert prediabetes into categorical diabetes. These side effects must be taken into account when diuretics and β-blockers are used in patients with metabolic syndrome and diabetes. Doses of these drugs should be kept as low as possible. Use of aldosterone receptor blockers (eplerenone or spironolactone) is one alternative to thiazides.

Some investigators propose that angiotensin-converting enzyme inhibitors or angiotensin receptor blockers should be first-line therapy in patients with metabolic syndrome. The rationale for this position is based on results of some, but not all, clinical trials. The combination of angiotensin-converting enzyme inhibitors (or angiotensin receptor blockers) plus low-dose thiazide is especially efficacious and appears to be preferable to a high dose of diuretic. Other antihypertensive drugs (calcium channel blockers, $\alpha_1$-blockers, and central $\alpha_2$-blockers) seemingly have no adverse metabolic effect in patients with metabolic syndrome. It is well known that multiple antihypertensive drugs in combination can be required to achieve goals for blood pressure lowering.

In patients with metabolic syndrome, but without type 2 diabetes or chronic renal failure, the goal is to reduce blood pressure to <140/90 mm Hg. When type 2 diabetes or renal failure is present, lowering the pressure to <130/80 mm Hg appears to provide added risk reduction.

## Elevated Plasma Glucose

Approximately one-half of all patients with metabolic syndrome have prediabetes (impaired glucose tolerance and/or impaired fasting glucose). Another one-third with metabolic syndrome have type 2 diabetes. At the same time, approximately three-fourths of persons with prediabetes have metabolic syndrome, and approximately 85% of those with diabetes have the syndrome. Therefore, there is a high prevalence of dysglycemia in patients with metabolic syndrome and vice versa. One of the goals for treatment of prediabetes is to curtail progression to type 2 diabetes. Ample clinical trial evidence shows that progression can be retarded or prevented. The DPP demonstrated that lifestyle change (weight reduction and increased physical activity) will reduce progression of prediabetes to diabetes by approximately 60%. By comparison, the DPP further showed that metformin therapy will reduce conversion by approximately 40%. Although the thiazolidinediones (TZD) (eg, troglitazone, rosiglitazone, and pioglitazone) showed a strong trend toward reduction in conversion of prediabetes to diabetes by as much as 60%, their use has been limited (and stopped definitively in the case of troglitazone) because of increased serious adverse effects (hepatitis in the case of troglitazone, bladder cancer in the case of pioglitazone, and cardiovascular events in the case of rosglitazone).

Patients with type 2 diabetes are at high risk for developing ASCVD. This high risk is largely caused by the coexistence of metabolic syndrome. Therefore, the therapeutic goal for reduction of ASCVD events in patients with type 2 diabetes is to treat all of the risk factors associated with metabolic syndrome. In addition, the LDL-C should be reduced to <100 mg/dL (non–HDL-C to <130 mg/dL); if ASCVD is present simultaneously, further reduction of these lipids to even lower levels is reasonable. The therapeutic options to achieve lower lipid levels were considered previously under the Atherogenic Dyslipidemia section. Blood pressure should be lowered to <130/80 mm Hg, and to <120/80 mm Hg if safe. Every effort should be made to achieve smoking cessation, if the patient with diabetes is a smoker. Finally, the glycosylated hemoglobin (HbA$_{1c}$) levels should be reduced to <7%. Choice of hypoglycemic drugs should be individualized according to available therapies and clinical judgment.

### Prothrombotic State

The only widely used therapy currently available for the routine treatment of a prothrombotic state is aspirin. Other antiplatelet drugs or anticoagulants generally are reserved for special clinical circumstances. Current guidelines indicate that aspirin prophylaxis for the prevention of CHD events is indicated in men when the 10-year risk for CHD is ≥10% as determined by Framingham risk scoring, in high-risk women (>20% 10-year risk for CHD by Framingham Scoring), or when patients have established ASCVD. This recommendation seems appropriate for patients with metabolic syndrome who are known to have increases in prothrombotic factors.

### Proinflammatory State

Metabolic syndrome is characterized by increases in circulating cytokines (eg, TNF-α and IL-6). Secondarily elevations in acute-phase reactants (high sensitivity [hs]–CRP and fibrinogen) can be present. Measurement of hs-CRP is a widely accepted way to identify the presence of a proinflammatory state. The AHA/Center for Disease Control report outlined recommendations for use of hs-CRP as a marker for a proinflammatory state in clinical practice. The hs-CRP can be measured at physician's discretion but is generally most useful in patients whose 10-year risk for CHD is in the range of 10% to 20%. If the hs-CRP level is ≥3 mg/L, therapeutic lifestyle changes should be emphasized. Whether to modify drug therapy based on hs-CRP levels is uncertain.

## CONCLUSION

The cardiovascular specialist and other health care providers must place increased emphasis on the diagnosis and early treatment of patients with metabolic syndrome. Left unchecked, the sharp rise in obesity and its concomitant metabolic risk both in the United States and worldwide will result in a major global increase in cardiovascular events and mortality. A focus on metabolic syndrome will encourage public heath efforts to give more priority to the promotion of weight control and physical activities in their societies. This will require a reconfiguration of health care systems to invest more on preventive medicine.

## SUGGESTED READINGS

Grundy SM, Smith SC Jr. Metabolic syndrome, obesity, and diet. In: Fuster V, Walsh R, Harrington RA, et al, eds. *Hurst's The Heart*. 13th ed. New York, NY: McGraw-Hill; 2011:92:2059-2072.

Eckel RH, Grundy SM, Zimmet PZ. The metabolic syndrome: epidemiology, mechanisms, and therapy. *Lancet*. 2005;365:1415-1428.

Goodman E, Dolan LM, Morrison JA, et al. Factor analysis of clustered cardiovascular risks in adolescence: obesity is the predominant correlate of risk among youth. *Circulation.* 2005;111(15):1970-1977.

Grundy SM, Cleeman JI, Daniels SR, et al. American Heart Association; National Heart, Lung, and Blood Institute. Diagnosis and management of the metabolic syndrome: an American Heart Association/National Heart, Lung, and Blood Institute Scientific Statement. *Circulation.* 2005;112(17):2735-2752.

Novak S, Stapleton LM, Litaker JR, et al. A confirmatory factor analysis evaluation of the coronary heart disease risk factors of metabolic syndrome with emphasis on the insulin resistance factor. *Diabetes Obes Metab.* 2003;5(6):388-396.

Ogden CL, Carroll MD, Curtin LR, et al. Prevalence of overweight and obesity in the United States, 1999-2004. *JAMA.* 2006;295(13):1549-1555.

Smith SC Jr, Allen J, Blair SN, et al. For the AHA/ACC; National Heart, Lung, and Blood Institute. AHA/ACC guidelines for secondary prevention for patients with coronary and other atherosclerotic vascular disease: 2006 update: endorsed by the National Heart, Lung, and Blood Institute. *Circulation.* 2006;113(19):2363-2372.

Tang W, Hong Y, Province MA, et al. Familial clustering for features of the metabolic syndrome: the National Heart, Lung, and Blood Institute (NHLBI) Family Heart Study. *Diabetes Care.* 2006;29(3):631-636.

# CHAPTER 48
# DIABETES AND CARDIOVASCULAR DISEASE

Sameer Bansilal, Michael E. Farkouh, Elliot J. Rayfield,
and Valentin Fuster

## EPIDEMIOLOGY

Globally, diabetes mellitus is a major threat to human health. The number of people with diabetes has increased alarmingly since 1985, and the rate of new cases is escalating. In 1985, an estimated 30 million people worldwide had diabetes; by 2003, it was estimated that approximately 194 million people had diabetes, and this figure is expected to increase to almost 350 million by 2025.

The prevalence of diabetes is higher in developed countries than in developing countries, but the developing world will be hit the hardest by the diabetes epidemic in the future. Increased urbanization, westernization, and economic growth in developing countries have already contributed to a substantial increase in diabetes. Although diabetes is most common among the elderly in many populations, prevalence rates are increasing among young populations in the developing world.

Diabetes mellitus, whether type 1 or type 2, is a very strong risk factor for the development of coronary heart disease (CHD) and stroke (**Table 48-1**). Eighty percent of all deaths among diabetic patients are a result of atherosclerosis, compared with approximately 30% among nondiabetic persons. A large National Institutes of Health (NIH) cohort study revealed that heart disease mortality in the general US population is declining at a much greater rate than it is in diabetic subjects. In fact, diabetic women suffered an increase in heart disease mortality over that period. Among all hospitalizations for diabetic complications, >75% are a consequence of atherosclerosis. An increase in the prevalence of diabetes has been noted, which, in part, can be attributed to the aging of the population and an increase in the rate of obesity and sedentary lifestyle in the United States.

## MANIFESTATIONS OF DIABETES

### ■ DYSGLYCEMIA

The San Antonio Heart Study showed a proportional increase in cardiovascular-related deaths with higher fasting blood glucose levels in type 2 diabetes. Although there are abundant data linking both fasting glucose and impaired glucose tolerance to adverse events, the data demonstrating an improvement in cardiovascular outcomes with an aggressive glucose-lowering treatment strategy have been lacking among patients with type 2 diabetes. Data from the UKPDS study clearly demonstrated a reduction in microvascular complications with intensive glucose control, however, there was not a concomitant significant reduction in macrovascular

**TABLE 48-1.** Clinical Evaluation of Risk Factors for the Development of Cardiovascular Disease in Diabetic Patients

Cigarette smoking
Assess pack-years
Blood pressure
Duration (if known); current and previous medications; assess presence of orthostatic hypertension
Serum lipids and lipoproteins
Dietary habits, alcohol intake, amount of exercise and whether aerobic
Family history of dyslipidemia, eruptive xanthoma, lipemia, retinalis, xanthelasma; thyroid function tests
LDL, HDL, cholesterol, fasting triglycerides
Spot albumin-to-creatinine ratio (in micro- and macroalbuminuria)
Serum creatinine
Do not rely on dipstick protein because negative results may reflect lack of sensitivity of test
Glycemic status
Duration of diabetes; family history of diabetes; vascular, renal, and retinal complications
Laboratory: FPG, hemoglobin $A_{1c}$ every 3 mo; diagnosis: FPG >126 × 2, hemoglobin $A_{1c}$ >6.5%,[3] impaired fasting glucose 110-126 × 2; when in doubt, have patient undergo 2-h oral glucose tolerance test

FPG, fasting blood glucose; HDL, high-density lipoprotein; LDL, low-density lipoprotein.

complications, despite a disproportionate 25% risk of suffering a nonfatal MI or stroke (compared with a 3.4% incidence of developing blindness or a 1% incidence of developing renal failure) during a 10-year period. It is important to remember that UKPDS only studied patients with new-onset diabetes mellitus. Recent data from the Prospective Pioglitazone Clinical Trial in Macrovascular Events (PROACTIVE) study failed to show a significant reduction in the composite macrovascular outcomes with glucose reduction, although the secondary outcome of rate of major adverse cardiac and cerebrovascular events was reduced by a significant 16%.

# ■ DYSLIPIDEMIA

Lipid disorders constitute one of the cornerstones in the cardiovascular management of diabetic patients. Many factors influence the lipid profile in these patients, including glycemic control, whether the diabetes is type 1 or 2, and the presence of diabetic nephropathy. In type 1 diabetes mellitus, the major determinant of the lipid profile is the level of glycemic control. LDL is moderately increased, triglycerides are markedly increased, and HDL is decreased when the level of glycemic control is impaired. For patients with type 2 diabetes, lipid abnormalities are related not only to hyperglycemia but also to the interplay of the insulin-resistant state. Patients with type 2 diabetes may have normal LDL levels but elevated levels of the very-low-density lipoprotein (VLDL) triglycerides moiety and reduced HDL levels. The expected elevation in VLDL triglyceride is usually no more than 100%.

# ■ LDL CHOLESTEROL

Although LDL levels in patients with controlled type 1 or type 2 diabetes may be normal, the atherogenic properties of LDL are increased. There is glycosylation of both apolipoprotein B and the phospholipid component of LDL, which changes LDL clearance and susceptibility to oxidative modifications. The product generated by the combined glycosylation and oxidation of LDL is more atherogenic than is either glycosylated or oxidized LDL alone. Such LDL molecules are taken up more easily by the aortic intimal cells and macrophages, resulting in the formation of foam cells.

Type 2 diabetic patients with insulin resistance have LDL particles that are small and rich with triglycerides but have little cholesterol in them (small, dense LDL). These LDL particles increase the risk of CHD independent of the total LDL level, probably because of their increased susceptibility to oxidative modification.

### Triglycerides and HDL

Diabetic patients have an increase in triglyceride production by the liver, which results in large, triglyceride-rich VLDL particles. Furthermore, the abundance of large triglyceride-rich VLDL is associated with an increase in small, dense, atherogenic LDL particles. Numerous studies show that elevated triglyceride levels are associated with increased risk for CHD in diabetic patients. A low HDL level is a strong risk factor for the development of CHD in the diabetic patient. There is decreased production and increased catabolism of HDL from the hypertriglyceridemia in diabetes. The decreased HDL production is a result of decreased lipoprotein lipase activity.

## ■ HYPERTENSION

The presence of hypertension in diabetic patients significantly increases their risk of micro- and macrovascular complications. It is estimated that 11 million Americans have both diabetes and hypertension. This "deadly duo" increases the cardiovascular event rate 2-fold. Furthermore, hypertension among diabetic patients has been linked with numerous other vascular complications such as nephropathy, retinopathy, the development of cerebrovascular disease, and significant decline in cognitive function in middle-aged diabetic hypertensive patients.

# COMPLICATIONS OF DIABETES

## ■ MICROVASCULAR COMPLICATIONS

### Renal

Nephropathy occurs in 40% of patients with types 1 and 2 diabetes. Risk factors include poor glycemic control, hypertension, and ethnicity (eg, blacks, Mexicans, Pima Indians). **Table 48-2** summarizes the key points for the assessment of renal status in a diabetic patient. The earliest clinical finding of diabetic kidney disease is microalbuminuria, which may occur at a time when renal histology is essentially normal. The Diabetes Control and Complications Trial (DCCT) and the United Kingdom Prospective Diabetes Study (UKPDS) showed that the development and progression of microalbuminuria can be prevented through strict glycemic control.

**TABLE 48-2.** Evaluation of Renal Status

| |
|---|
| **Urine albumin and protein** |
| Yearly screen for microalbumin in types 1 and 2 diabetes; microalbumin-to-creatinine ratio collected in a spot urine, ideally first morning urine specimen (normal <30 mg/g creatinine); must rule out other diseases that cause proteinuria |
| If urine albumin-to-creatinine ratio is >300 mg/g in first morning specimen, macroalbuminuria is present and is usually not reversible with ACE inhibitors; nephrology consult |
| Nephrotic syndrome: urine protein >3 g/d; nephrology consult |
| Other reasons to consult nephrologists are diabetic patients with increasing creatinine from 1.4 to >2.0 mg/dL, elevated creatinine, and symptoms of uremia and microalbuminuria not responding to ACE inhibitor |
| **Urinalysis** |
| Red blood cells, pyuria, and casts require nephrology consult |
| **Blood pressure evaluation** |
| If hypertension is present, exclude secondary causes, including with advancing renal insufficiency |
| Treatment with an ACE inhibitor is preferred first choice even in African Americans (except if precluded by hyperkalemia or other complications) |
| **Blood urea nitrogen, serum creatinine, and glomerular filtration rate** |
| Yearly creatinine clearance should be obtained with 24-h urine collection and serum creatinine; most accurate way to estimate kidney function without using a radioisotope |

ACE, angiotensin-converting enzyme; LDL, low-density lipoprotein; MCP, monocyte chemotactic protein; M-CSF, macrophage colony-stimulating factor; VSMC, vascular smooth muscle cell.

# ■ OPHTHALMOLOGIC COMPLICATIONS

Diabetic retinopathy is the most prevalent microvascular complication, affecting nearly 50% of the diabetic population at a given time and eventually occurring in all diabetic patients. Diabetes remains the leading cause of visual loss in adults. Visual loss from diabetes occurs either as a result of proliferative retinopathy or macular edema.

# ■ MACROVASCULAR MANIFESTATIONS

## Coronary Heart Disease

CHD is strongly associated with type 2 diabetes mellitus and is the leading cause of death regardless of the duration of disease. There is a 2- to 4-fold increase in the relative risk ratio of cardiovascular disease in type 2 diabetes patients compared with the general population. This increase is particularly disproportionate in diabetic women when compared with diabetic men. The protection that premenopausal women have against CHD is not seen if they suffer from diabetes. The degree and duration of hyperglycemia are strong risk factors for the development of microvascular and macrovascular complications. Even impaired glucose tolerance increases cardiovascular risk.

The first detectable sign of a problem in people genetically prone to develop type 2 diabetes is insulin resistance, which can be seen for as long as 15 to 25 years before the onset of diabetes. Several atherogenic factors are associated with insulin resistance, which can start the atherosclerotic process years before clinical hyperglycemia ensues. It is unclear whether the compensatory hyperinsulinemia plays a role in atherosclerosis generation in insulin-resistant patients. A number of prospective studies have shown an association between fasting or postprandial hyperinsulinemia and the future development of CHD.

Hyperglycemia itself plays an important role in enhancing the progression of atherosclerosis in type 2 diabetes. The threshold above which hyperglycemia becomes atherogenic is not known but may be in the range defined as impaired glucose tolerance (ie, fasting plasma glucose level <126 mg/dL with 30-, 60-, or 90-minute plasma glucose concentrations >200 mg/L and a 2-hour plasma glucose level of 140-200 mg/dL during an oral glucose tolerance test). Population-based studies show that the degree of hyperglycemia increases the risk for CHD and cardiovascular events.

### Acute Coronary Syndromes

Diabetic patients represent a high-risk group for developing and surviving acute MI. In particular, patients with type 1 diabetes have a worse outcome than patients with type 2 disease, and diabetic women have almost twice the risk of mortality of diabetic men.

Reperfusion therapy is the cornerstone of the management of acute MI. In a meta-analysis of the major trials comparing thrombolytic therapy to percutaneous coronary intervention (PCI), diabetic patients had significantly higher 30-day mortality when compared with nondiabetic patients (9.4% vs 5.9%, respectively; $p$ <0.001). The advantages of angioplasty over thrombolytic therapy in the diabetic population are comparable to those observed in nondiabetic patients.

### Chronic Coronary Artery Disease

The association between CHD and diabetes is strong and has led to screening strategies in diabetic patients even before they are symptomatic. In addition, diabetic patients often are unaware of myocardial ischemic pain, and thus silent MI and ischemia are markedly increased in this population. There is a heightened concern for the development of sudden cardiac death in those with diabetes.

Therapeutic modalities in diabetic patients with CHD revolve around standard therapy with aspirin, β-blockers, calcium-channel blockers, and nitrates.

### Diabetic Cardiomyopathy

*Diabetic cardiomyopathy* is a term used by clinicians to encompass the multifactorial etiologies of diabetes-related left ventricular failure characterized by both systolic and diastolic function. Diabetes complicated by hypertension represents a particularly high-risk group for the development of congestive heart failure.

### Cerebrovascular Disease

Compared with nondiabetic subjects, the mortality from stroke in diabetic patients is almost 3-fold higher. The small paramedial penetrating arteries are the most common sites of cerebrovascular disease. In addition, diabetes increases the likelihood of severe carotid atherosclerosis. Diabetic patients are likely to suffer increased brain damage with carotid emboli that would result in a transient ischemic attack in a nondiabetic individual.

## MANAGEMENT OF DIABETES AND ITS COMPLICATIONS

The American Diabetes Association (ADA) and American Heart Association (AHA) have published a combined scientific statement to address primary prevention of cardiovascular disease in patients with diabetes.

# ■ THERAPEUTIC LIFESTYLE CHANGES

Steno-2 demonstrated that a comprehensive multifactorial strategy (including lifestyle and pharmacologic interventions) to reduce cardiovascular risk in type 2 diabetic patients with microalbuminuria was highly effective (hazard ratio [HR] = 0.47; 95% confidence interval [CI], 0.24-0.73) when compared with usual care after a mean time of 7.8 years (**Table 48-3**). The number needed to treat to prevent a major cardiovascular event was only 5 patients. The approach included targets of hemoglobin $A_{1c}$ (HbA$_{1c}$) <6.5%, blood pressure <130/80 mm Hg, total cholesterol <175 mg/dL, and triglycerides <150 mg/dL. Patients were prescribed aspirin and an ACE inhibitor or ARB. After 13 years of follow-up, patients randomized to intensive medical management experienced a significant decrease in overall mortality (46%; 95% CI, 32%-89%; $p$ = 0.02), cardiovascular death (57%; 95% CI, 19%-94%; $p$ = 0.01), and combined cardiovascular events (59%; 95% CI, 25%-67%; $p$ <0.001), in addition to experiencing a decrease in the risk of nephropathy and microvascular complications (**Fig. 48-1**). This study validates the multidisciplinary approach to the cardiovascular care of the diabetic patient.

Physical activity is an important component of a comprehensive weight management program. Regular moderate-intensity physical activity enhances long-term weight maintenance. Regular activity also improves insulin sensitivity, glycemic control, and selected risk factors for cardiovascular disease (ie, hypertension and dyslipidemia), and increased aerobic fitness decreases the risk of CHD. Initial physical activity recommendations should be modest, based on the patient's willingness and ability, gradually increasing the duration and frequency to 30 to 45 minutes of moderate aerobic activity 3 to 5 d/wk, when possible. Greater activity levels of at least 1 h/d of moderate (walking) or 30 min/d of vigorous (jogging) activity may be needed to achieve successful long-term weight loss. The American College of Sports Medicine now recommends that resistance training be included in fitness programs for adults with type 2 diabetes. Resistance exercise improves insulin sensitivity to about the same extent as aerobic exercise.

In patients with severe/morbid obesity, surgical options, such as gastric bypass and gastroplasty, may be appropriate and allow significant improvement in glycemic control with reduction or discontinuation of medications. A recent randomized trial of gastric banding compared with conventional therapy showed a greater remission rate of type 2 diabetes through a surgical approach.

# ■ DIABETES EDUCATION

Every patient with diabetes should be provided with diabetes education. Recommendations for glucose testing vary among individuals and depend on the current degree of control and whether the patient is taking a medication that would potentially cause hypoglycemia. For patients to adhere to frequent testing regimens, they must understand what foods, exercise, and circumstances will have an impact on blood glucose levels, as well as how they should modify their behaviors for optimal glycemic control (**Table 48-4** and **Fig. 48-2**).

# ■ DYSGLYCEMIA MANAGEMENT

The medical community has progressively become more and more aggressive about risk factor modification. Multiple trials in cardiovascular prevention have shown that modification of traditional risk factors shows more benefit than glycemic control. Practitioners, however, must realize that because of the importance of glycemic control in preventing microvascular complications, cardiologists have adopted measures to control blood glucose levels.

The AHA and ADA have come to consensus for goals of targets. The HbA$_{1c}$ goal for patients in general is <7%. The American College of Clinical Endocrinology goal

**TABLE 48-3.** Interventions in Diabetes

| Trial | Sample Size | Intervention | Outcome | Follow up | Control Group | Treatment Group | Relative Risk Reduction (%) | p |
|---|---|---|---|---|---|---|---|---|
| | | | REVASCULARIZATION STUDIES | | | | | |
| BARI | 457 | CABG vs PTCA | Survival | 10 y | 57.8% | 45.5% | 21 | 0.025 |
| BARI-Registry | 339 | CABG vs PTCA | Survival | 5 y | 85% | 86% | – | 0.86 |
| EAST | 59 | CABG vs PTCA | Survival | 8 y | 76% | 60% | 21 | 0.23 |
| CABRI | 125 | CABG vs PTCA | Survival | 4 y | 88% | 77% | 12 | NS |
| DUKE | 770 | CABG vs PTCA | Survival | 5 y | 74% | 76% | – | 0.91 |
| ARTS | 208 | CABG vs BMS | Survival | 3 y | 96% | 93% | 3 | 0.39 |
| SOS | 148 | CABG vs BMS | Survival | 5 y | 94.6% | 82.4% | 13 | 0.15 |
| ERACI II | 77 | CABG vs BMS | Survival | 1 y | 95% | 96.4% | – | 0.98 |
| AWESOME | 144 | CABG vs BMS | Survival | 5 y | 66% | 74% | 11 | 0.27 |
| NYS BMS | 17946 | CABG vs BMS | Survival | 3 y | – | – | 31 | Significant |
| NYS DES | 6098 | CABG vs DES | Survival | 18 mo | 91.5% | 93.2% | –3 | 0.75 |
| BARI 2D | 2368 | Revascn vs Medical Rx | CV death, MI, CVA | 5 y | 87.8% | 88.3% | – | 0.97 |
| CARDIA | 600 | CABG vs DES | CV death, MI, CVA | 1 y-TERMINATED | 10.5% | 13% | –25 | 0.39 |
| SYNTAX | 1500 | CABG vs DES | CV death, MI, CVA | 5 y | 12.4% | 17.8% | –43 | <0.001 |
| FREEDOM | 1900 | CABG vs CES | CV death, MI, CVA | 5 y | ONGOING | | | |
| VA-CARDS | 790 | CABG vs DES | CV death, MI | 1 y | UNPUBLISHED-TERMINATED | | | |

(Continued)

**TABLE 48-3.** Interventions in Diabetes (Continued)

| Trial | Sample Size | Intervention | Outcome | Follow-up | Control Group | Treatment Group | Relative Risk Reduction (%) | p |
|---|---|---|---|---|---|---|---|---|
| | | | GLUCOSE CONTROL STUDIES | | | | | |
| UKPDS | 3867 | Intensive glucose lowering | Diabetes related death | 10 y | 11.5% | 10.4% | 10 | 0.34 |
| PROACTIVE | 5238 | Pioglitazone vs placebo | CV death, MI,revascn, vascular intervn/surgery, amputation | 34.5 mo | 21.7% | 19.7% | 10 | 0.095 |
| RECORD | 4447 | Rosiglitazone vs placebo | Hospitaln /CV death | 3.75 y | 9% | 9.7% | -7 | NS |
| ACCORD | 10251 | Intensive Glycemic Control | CV death, MI, CVA | TERMINATED at 4 y | 203 | 257 | -26 | Significant |
| | 4733 | Intensive BP control | CV death, MI, CVA | 5.6 y | 2.09% | 1.87% | 12 | 0.20 |
| | 5518 | Intensive lipid control | CV death, MI, CVA | 5.6 y | 2.4% | 2.2% | 8 | 0.32 |
| | | | HYPERTENSION STUDIES | | | | | |
| HOT | 1501 | BP goals | CV events | 3.8 y | 2.4% | 1.2% | 51 | 0.005 |
| SHEP | 492 | CCB | CV events | 2 y | 57.6% | 22% | 62 | 0.002 |
| HOPE | 3577 | Ramipril vs placebo | CV death, MI, CVA | 4.5y | 19.8% | 15.3% | 25 | 0.004 |
| ADVANCE | 11140 | Perindopril/indapamide | CV death, MI, CVA | 4.3 y | 9.3% | 8.6% | 8 | 0.16 |
| GEMINI | 1235 | Carvedilol vs Metoprolol | Mean change in HbA$_{1c}$ | 35 wk | 0.15% | 0.02% | 87 | 0.004 |
| ONTARGET | 25620 | Telmisartan +ramipril vs ramipril | CV death, MI, CVA, hospn for CHF | 3.5-5.5 y | 16.5 | 16.3 | 1 | NS |
| TRANSCEND | 5776 | Temisartan vs Placebo | | 3.5-5.5 y | 14.4% | 13.5% | 6 | 0.11 |

| | N | Intervention | Endpoints | Duration | | | | |
|---|---|---|---|---|---|---|---|---|
| **LIPID STUDIES** | | | | | | | | |
| CTT | 18686 | Statin | CV death, MI, CVA | 5 y | - | - | 9 | 0.001 |
| VA-HIT | 630 | gemfibrozil vs placebo | CV death, MI, CVA | 5 y | 143 | 97 | 32 | 0.004 |
| FIELD | 9795 | Fenofibrate vs placebo | CHD death, MI | 5 y | 5.2% | 5.9% | 11 | 0.16 |
| AIM-HIGH | 3300 | Niacin+statin vs statin | CV death, MI, CVA, hospitaln for high risk NSTEMI | 3 y | 16.2% | 16.4% | -2 | 0.80 |
| HPS-2 THRIVE | 20000 | Niacin+laropiprant vs placebo | CV death, MI, CVA, revasculn | 4 y | | | ONGOING | |
| **ANTIPLATELET/ANTITHROMBOTIC AGENTS STUDIES** | | | | | | | | |
| APT | 4502 | Clopidogrel | CV death, MI, CVA | 6 mo-2 y | 22.3% | 18.5% | 17 | Significant |
| CREDO | 560 | Clopidogrel vs placebo | CV death, MI, CVA | 1.9 y | - | - | 11.2 | NS |
| CAPRIE | 3866 | Clopidogrel vs placebo | Vasc death, MI,CVA, rehospn | 3 y | 17.7% | 15.6% | 12 | 0.042 |
| CURE | 2840 | Clopidogrel vs placebo | CV death, MI, CVA | 2 y | 16.7 | 14.2 | 15 | NS |
| TRITON- TIMI38 | 3146 | Prasugrel vs Clopidogrel | CV death, MI, CVA | 1 y | 17 | 12.2 | 30 | 0.001 |
| REPLACE-2 | 1624 | bivalirudin vs GP IIa/IIIb | CV death | 1 y | 3.9% | 2.4% | 38 | 0.065 |
| **MULTIFACTORIAL LIFESTYLE INTERVENTION STUDIES** | | | | | | | | |
| STENO-2 | 160 | Multifactorial risk factor intervention | CV death, MI, CVA, CABG,PCI, amputatn, vasc surg | 7.8 y | 44% | 24% | 53 | 0.007 |
| LOOK-AHEAD | 5145 | Sustained wt. loss with diet and exercise | CV death, MI, CVA | 11.5 y | | | ONGOING | |

Modified and updated from Bansilal S, Farkouh ME, Fuster V. Optimal treatment of the diabetic patient witr multivessel disease. *Curr Cardiol Rep.* 2008 Jul;10(4):272-284.

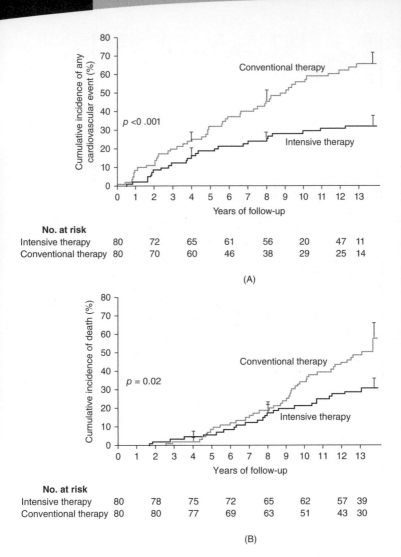

**FIGURE 48-1. A.** Steno-1: incidence of cardiovascular events in diabetics comparing conventional versus intensive therapy. Cumulative events included major cardiovascular events, death due to cardiovascular causes, nonfatal cerebrovascular accident, nonfatal acute myocardial infarction, revascularization, and amputation. **B.** Steno-2: incidence of death due to any cause in diabetics comparing conventional versus intensive treatment. (Reproduced with permission from Gaede P, Lund-Andersen H, Parving HH, et al. Effect of a multifactorial intervention on mortality in type 2 diabetes. *N Engl J Med.* 2008;358(6):580-589.)

is an HbA$_{1c}$ of <6.5%. However, the ideal HbA$_{1c}$ goal for the individual patient is as close to normal (<6%) as possible without significant hypoglycemia. The debate presently is also whether getting to the goal is enough or whether how one gets there is important as well. The Bypass Angioplasty Revascularization Investigation (BARI)

**TABLE 48-4.** Guide to Comprehensive Risk Reduction for Patients With Coronary and Other Vascular Disease Who Have Diabetes

| Risk Intervention | Recommendations |
|---|---|
| **Smoking**<br>Goal: complete cessation | Urge smoking cessation<br>Try NicoDerm patches or Zyban; enroll in smoking cessation program |
| **Blood pressure control**<br><br>Goal: <135/85 mm Hg | Initiate lifestyle modifications such as weight reduction, increased physical activity, alcohol moderation, and sodium restriction in all patients with blood pressure >135/85 mm Hg<br>Add blood pressure medication if blood pressure is not <135/85 mm Hg |
| **Lipid management**<br>Primary goal: LDL ≤100 mg/dL<br>Secondary goals: HDL >35 mg/dL, TG <200 mg/dL | Start AHA Step II Diet in all patients: ≤30% fat, <7% saturated fat, <200 mg/dL cholesterol<br>Assess fasting lipid profile; immediately start cholesterol-lowering drugs when baseline LDL >130 mg/dL<br><br>LDL <100 mg/dL—no drug therapy |

| | LDL 100-129 mg/dL—consider adding drug therapy to diet as follows: | LDL ≥130 mg/dL—add drug therapy as follows: | HDL <35 mg/dL—weight management, physical activity, and smoking cessation |
|---|---|---|---|
| | | Suggested drug therapy | |
| | TG <200 mg/dL<br>Statin or resin | TG 200-400 mg/dL<br>Statin or fibrate | TG >400 mg/dL<br>Consider combined drug therapy (statin + fibrate) |

| Risk Intervention | Recommendations |
|---|---|
| **Glucose control**<br>Goal: nearly normal fasting glucose<br>Goal: HbA$_{1c}$ ≤1% above normal | First-step therapy: lifestyle modifications<br>Second-step therapy: oral hypoglycemic agents (see algorithm in Fig. 48-2)<br>Third-step therapy: insulin therapy (see algorithm)<br>Assess risk, preferably with exercise test, to guide prescription |
| **Physical activity**<br>Goal: minimum 30 min, 3-4 times a week | Encourage minimum of 30-60 min of moderate-intensity activity 3-4 times weekly (eg, walking, jogging, cycling) supplemented by an increase in daily lifestyle activities (eg, walking breaks at work, using stairs, household work)<br>Maximum benefit: 5-6 h/wk<br>Advise medically supervised programs for moderate- to high-risk patients |

*(Continued)*

**TABLE 48-4.** Guide to Comprehensive Risk Reduction for Patients With Coronary and Other Vascular Disease Who Have Diabetes (Continued)

| Risk Intervention | Recommendations |
| --- | --- |
| Weight management | Start intensive dietary therapy and appropriate physical activity, as outlined previously, in patients whose body mass index is ≥25 kg/m$^2$ |
| | Particularly emphasize need for weight loss in patients with hypertension, elevated triglycerides, or elevated glucose levels |
| Antiplatelet agents/anticoagulants | Start aspirin 325 mg/d if not contraindicated |
| | Manage warfarin to INR of 2-3.5 for post-MI patients not able to take aspirin |
| ACE inhibitors in post-MI patients | Start early post-MI in stable high-risk patients (anterior MI, previous MI, Killip class II [S$_3$ gallop, rales, radiographic congestive heart failure]) |
| | Continue indefinitely for all with LV dysfunction (ejection fraction ≤40%) or symptoms of failure |
| | Use as needed to manage blood pressure or symptoms in all other patients |
| β-Blockers | Start in high-risk post-MI patients (arrhythmia, LV dysfunction, inducible ischemia) at 5-28 d; continue for 6 mo minimum; observe usual contraindications; appropriate use of β-blockers not contraindicated in patients with diabetes; use as needed to manage angina, rhythm, or blood pressure in all other patients |
| Estrogen | Observational studies (but not clinical trials) suggest benefit in regard to osteoporosis but not CHD; individualize recommendation consistent with other health risks |

ACE, angiotensin-converting enzyme; AHA, American Heart Association; CHD, coronary heart disease; HbA$_{1c}$, hemoglobin A$_{1c}$; HDL, high-density lipoproteins; INR, international normalized ratio; LDL, low-density lipoprotein; LV, left ventricle; MI, myocardial infarction; TG, triglycerides.

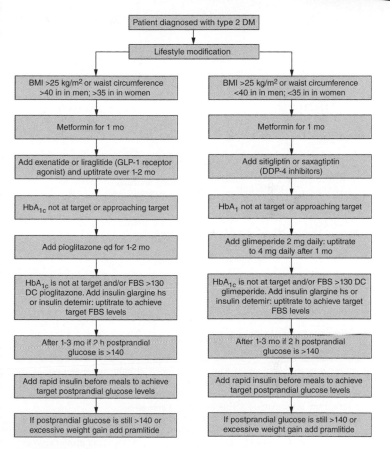

FIGURE 48-2. Algorithm for the management of type 2 diabetes. BMI, body mass index; DM, diabetes mellitus; FBS, fasting blood sugar; HbA$_{1c}$, glycosylated hemoglobin A$_{1c}$; qd, once a day.

2D study provided more data on whether management of insulin resistance with insulin-sensitizing therapies led to better outcomes than insulin-replacing therapies. The study showed that there was no difference in mortality at 5 years whether they used insulin-sensitizing or insulin-replacing therapies.

The guidelines currently recommend treating to target and acknowledge that most type 2 diabetic patients may require more than 1 antidiabetic agent. Most agents have been studied to measure efficacy as monotherapy and across the board

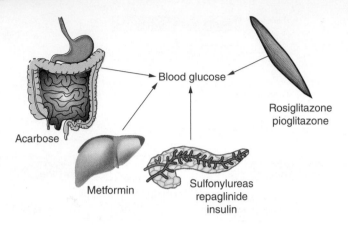

**FIGURE 48-3.** Mechanism of action of hypoglycemic agents.

demonstrate a 40% to 60% reduction in fasting plasma glucose level (**Fig. 48-3**). The following discussion outlines the mechanisms, advantages, and disadvantages of each of these therapies as individual agents.

## Traditional Medications

**Insulin**  Insulin is used in the management of type 1 or type 2 diabetes mellitus as monotherapy or in combination with oral agents. Currently available insulins are synthetic human insulins or analogues of human insulin, which differ in their rate of absorption and duration of action. There are also products that are mixtures of rapid short-acting and intermediate-acting insulins (**Table 48-5**).

There are 4 rapid-acting insulins currently available. Insulin lispro is a rapid-acting insulin analogue in which the amino acids at positions 28 and 29 on the human insulin B chain are reversed. Insulin aspart is a second rapid-acting insulin analogue with a substitution of aspartic acid for proline in position 28 on the B chain. Insulin

**TABLE 48-5.** Insulins

| Type | Name | Onset of Action | Time to Peak Activity | Duration of Action |
|---|---|---|---|---|
| Rapid acting | Aspart | 15 min | 1 h | 3-4 h |
| | Glulisine | 15 min | 30-90 min | 3-5 h |
| | Lispro | 15 min | 1 h | 3-4 h |
| Short acting | Regular | 30-60 min | 2-4 h | 6-8 h |
| Intermediate acting | NPH | 1-3 h | 6-8 h | 12-16 h |
| Long acting | Detemir | 1 h | No peak | About 12 h |
| | Glargine | 1-2 h | No peak | About 24 h |

NPH, neutral protamine Hagedorn.

glulisine is the newest rapid-acting analogue in which the asparagine at position 3 on the B chain is replaced by glutamic acid. These amino acid changes result in a reduced propensity for insulin molecules to form aggregates, providing a more rapid onset and shorter duration of action than RHI. These insulins are used to cover carbohydrates at mealtime to correct for an elevated glucose level and in insulin pumps. The latest rapid-acting insulin is Exubera (a human insulin of rDNA origin), which is inhaled and has an intermediate duration of action (387 minutes) that is faster than lispro and comparable to regular insulin.

Neutral pH protamine Hagedorn (NPH) is an intermediate-acting insulin that is a suspension of RHI with protamine, thus delaying its absorption. NPH can be used at bedtime to normalize fasting glucose and in combination with rapid-acting insulins during the daytime to provide primarily basal coverage.

Insulin glargine is essentially peakless, with a 24-hour duration of action. Insulin detemir is a soluble long-acting human insulin analogue with the elimination of the threonine in position B30 and the addition of a 14-carbon fatty acid chain at position B29. Insulin detemir is absorbed slowly from the injection site and is >98% reversibly bound to albumin in the blood. The basal insulins are used once or twice daily to provide broad coverage.

### Use of Insulin Pumps and Continuous Glucose Monitoring Systems
Insulin pumps are devices with a subcutaneous catheter that deliver continuous subcutaneous insulin infusion. One or more basal rates are preprogrammed by the user, and boluses are taken as needed whenever carbohydrates are ingested. Pumps are generally used in patients with type 1 diabetes but can also be used in patients with type 2 diabetes. Continuous glucose monitoring systems that use a glucose sensor to provide up to 3 days of continuous glucose monitoring in the subcutaneous tissue are available. The record shows glucose patterns and trends that can help in the recognition and prevention of hypoglycemia, hyperglycemia, postprandial glucose excursions, and the effects of exercise.

Multiple other agents are used in the management of diabetes. **Table 48-6** summarizes these agents, and they are described in the following sections.

### Metformin
The mechanism of action of metformin is to decrease hepatic glucose output by inhibiting glucose-6-dehydrogenase activity and stimulating the insulin-induced component of glucose uptake into skeletal muscle and adipocytes.

The starting dose for metformin is 500 mg orally with dinner for 1 week and then 500 mg orally with breakfast and dinner. A sustained-release preparation is available that allows once-daily dosing. Because of its mechanism of action, there is minimal risk for hypoglycemia. This drug should not be used in renal failure or potential hypoxic states, such as congestive heart failure and severe pulmonary disease, because of the risk of lactic acidosis. The risk of lactic acidosis is low and is estimated to be 9 per 100 000 person-years. The most common adverse effects are gastrointestinal—nausea, diarrhea, and abdominal pain—and a metallic taste. It should not be used in patients with impaired renal function (serum creatinine >1.5 mg/dL in men and >1.4 mg/dL in women). Caution should be exercised in prescribing metformin to the elderly. If used in patients older than 80 years, then a normal glomerular filtration rate should be documented. Metformin should be discontinued on the day patients receive an iodinated contrast material for radiographic studies, which can temporarily impair renal function, as well as prior to any surgical procedure. The metformin dose can be resumed 48 hours later if the serum creatinine is in the normal range. Metformin lowers the $HbA_{1c}$ by 1% to 2%.

### Thiazolidinediones
Thiazolidinediones (TZDs) induce peroxisome proliferator-activated receptor (PPAR) γ binding to nuclear receptors in muscle and adipocytes, allowing insulin-stimulated glucose transport.

TZDs lower fasting and postprandial glucose levels, as well as free fatty acid levels. TZDs decrease $HbA_{1c}$ levels by 1% to 1.5%. These agents decrease insulin resistance and possibly preserve β-cell function.

**TABLE 48-6.** Commercially Available (Other Than Insulin) Agents Used to Treat Type 2 Diabetes

| Drug Class | Generic Name | Mechanism of Action | Expected HbA$_{1c}$ Reduction (%) | Daily Dose |
|---|---|---|---|---|
| Biguanide | Metformin | Decreases hepatic glucose output | 1.0-2.0 | 500 mg qd to 1000 mg bid to 850 mg tid |
| Thiazolidinedione | Pioglitazone | PPARα and PPARγ agonist | 1.0-1.5 | 15-45 mg qd |
| | Rosiglitazone | PPARγ agonist | 1.0-1.5 | 2 mg qd or bid, 8 mg qd |
| Sulfonylurea | Glipizide | ↑ β-cell insulin synthesis and release | 1.0-2.0 | 2.5-20 mg qd or bid |
| | Glyburide | ↑ β-cell insulin synthesis and release | | 1.25-10 mg qd or bid |
| | Glimepiride | ↑ β-cell insulin synthesis and release | | 0.5-8 mg qd |
| Meglitinides | Repaglinide | ↑ β-cell insulin synthesis and release | 1.0-2.0 | 0.5-4 mg tid |
| | Nateglinide | ↑ β-cell insulin synthesis and release | 0.5-1.0 | 60-120 mg tid |
| α-Glucosidase inhibitors | Acarbose | α-Glucosidase inhibition (decreased carbohydrate absorption) | 0.5-1.0 | 50-100 mg tid |
| | Miglitol | α-Glucosidase inhibition | 0.5-1.0 | 500-100 mg tid |
| Incretin mimetic | Exenatide | Increasing postprandial insulin, decreasing postprandial glucagon, increasing satiety, and delaying gastric emptying | 0.5-0.9 | 5-10 μg bid |

bid, twice a day; HbA$_{1c}$, hemoglobin A$_{1c}$; PPAR, peroxisome proliferator-activated receptor; tid, three times a day; qd, once a day.

**TZDs and Cardiovascular Outcomes** The TZDs have come under increased scrutiny because of the association with edema and weight gain. When prescribing TZDs, it is essential to balance the risk and benefits. Clearly, patients with congestive heart failure are not candidates for TZD therapy.

**Pioglitazone** The pivotal outcomes trial of pioglitazone, PROACTIVE, did not provide as clear a picture as the surrogate outcomes trials. In this trial, >5000 diabetic patients with established macrovascular complications were randomized to pioglitazone 45 mg/d or placebo. No differences were found in the primary end point, which was a composite of major adverse cardiac event (MACE), leg amputation, peripheral and coronary revascularization, and acute coronary syndrome. However, a key secondary end point of death, MI, and stroke showed a 16% relative risk reduction in favor of pioglitazone (HR = 0.84; 95% CI, 0.72-0.98; $p$ = 0.027). The potential reduction in cardiovascular events associated with pioglitazone is supported by a meta-analysis of 19 trials demonstrating a lower risk for a composite of MACE (HR = 0.82; 95% CI, 0.72-0.94; $p$ = 0.005). A comprehensive meta-analysis did confirm a favorable cardiovascular risk profile for pioglitazone.

**Rosiglitazone** The evidence for a cardioprotective effect of rosiglitazone is not apparent. In fact, the meta-analysis by Nissen and Wolski created a media firestorm by reporting a 43% excess risk for MI and a 60% excess risk for cardiovascular death in type 2 diabetes patients treated with rosiglitazone compared with an active comparator. This meta-analysis was highly criticized for a number of reasons, including pooling trials for which cardiovascular end points were relatively rare and with a great deal of heterogeneity between trials. What was most controversial is that it led to the publishing of an interim analysis of the Rosiglitazone Evaluated for Cardiac Outcome and Regulation of Glycemia in Diabetes (RECORD) trial. Eventually, RECORD was published. The trial randomized >4000 patients in an open-label design. After a mean follow-up of 5.5 years, the addition of rosiglitazone to a combination of metformin and sulfonylurea was found to be noninferior to a combination of metformin and sulfonylurea for the combined end point of cardiovascular hospitalization and cardiovascular death (HR = 0.99; 95% CI, 0.85-1.16). Heart failure causing admission to hospital or death was increased in the rosiglitazone group (HR = 2.10; 95% CI, 1.35-3.27).

**Sulfonylureas** Sulfonylureas are the oldest class of treatment for type 2 diabetes. The mode of action is by stimulating β-cell insulin secretion. The major concern with these agents is hypoglycemia. The second-generation sulfonylureas have a shorter half-life and bind to plasma proteins nonionically, making them less easily displaced from proteins and available for binding to receptors. Commercially available second-generation sulfonylureas are glyburide (1.25-20 mg/d), glipizide (2.5-40 mg/d), and glimepiride (1-8 mg/d). Sulfonylureas decrease the $HbA_{1c}$ by 1% to 2%.

**Meglitinides** Repaglinide is a member of the meglitinide group of insulin secretagogues with a relatively short half-life of 3.7 hours. The drug is taken up to 30 minutes prior to each meal. Repaglinide is particularly useful in the elderly, patients with chronic renal insufficiency, and patients who are erratic eaters. The dose varies between 0.5 and 4 mg before meals. Repaglinide results in a 1% to 2% decrease in $HbA_{1c}$.

Nateglinide has a quicker onset and shorter duration of action than repaglinide. Nateglinide is available as 60- and 120-mg tablets, taken with each meal. It is effective for lowering postprandial glucose levels. Nateglinide results in a 0.5% to 1.0% decrease in $HbA_{1c}$. As with repaglinide, the dose of nateglinide should be omitted if a meal is skipped.

**α-Glucosidase Inhibitors** These agents inhibit α-glucosidases in the brush border of the small intestine, delaying the absorption of complex carbohydrates and they are not systemically absorbed. They are most effective in reducing postprandial blood glucose elevations and can be used as adjunctive therapy with other oral agents. The 2 available agents are acarbose (50-100 mg with meals) and miglitol (50 mg with meals). The adverse effects are flatulence and gastrointestinal discomfort. These medications result in a 0.5% to 1.0% decrease in $HbA_{1c}$ levels and may be useful as an adjunct to other oral hypoglycemic agents with high-carbohydrate meals.

**Amylin** The synthetic human amylin pramlintide is available as an adjunctive treatment for type 1 or 2 diabetic patients who remain uncontrolled with mealtime insulin use. Pramlintide has been shown to decrease glucose fluctuations, improve long-term glycemic control, reduce mealtime insulin requirements, and reduce body

**TABLE 48-7.** Incretins, Incretin Mimetics, and DPP-4 Inhibitors

| Agent | Site of Production | Physiologic Action | Therapeutic Potential |
|---|---|---|---|
| GLP-1 agonist | L cells in ileum and proglucagon derived | Stimulates glucose-dependent insulin secretion and B-cell proliferation and cytoprotection; decreases gastric emptying and postprandial glucagon suppression; increases satiety | Increase insulin secretion in T2DM |
| GIP agonist | K cells in duodenum and proximal jejunum | Stimulates glucose-dependent insulin secretion and B-cell proliferation and cytoprotection; does not inhibit gastric emptying, glucagon secretion, or food intake | Increase insulin secretion in T2DM |
| Exenatide (Byetta) | Synthetic peptide | GLP-1 agonist that potentiates insulin secretion, inhibits glucagon secretion, slows gastric emptying, and promotes satiety; increases growth of pancreatic cells in animals; not known if similar action exists in humans | Increase insulin secretion in T2DM, promote weight loss |
| DDP-4 inhibitors | Synthetic peptides | Delays degradation of GLP-1, extending the action of insulin and suppressing release of glucagon | Increase insulin secretion in T2DM |

DPP-4, dipeptidyl peptidase-4; GIP, glucose-dependent insulinotropic peptide; GLP-1, glucagon-like peptide-1; T2DM, type 2 diabetes mellitus.

weight. Empiric reductions in mealtime insulin doses are recommended at the initiation of pramlintide therapy to decrease the risk of hypoglycemia.

**Incretins** These agents belong to the class of incretin hormones (**Table 48-7**). The first pharmacologic agent available in this class is the glucagon-like peptide-1 (GLP-1) analogue, exenatide. The 2 key incretins are GLP-1 and glucose-dependent insulinotropic peptide (GIP), which are both secreted in the small intestine by the L cells and K cells, respectively.

Exenatide (Byetta) is a synthetic peptide that is a GLP-1 agonist (incretin mimetic). It potentiates insulin secretion and decreases glucagon secretion postprandially. Exenatide delays gastric emptying and promotes satiety, resulting in weight loss. Exenatide is FDA approved as an adjunctive treatment for patients with type 2 diabetes who have not achieved optimal glycemic control on metformin, a sulfonylurea, or both. It can cause nausea, diarrhea, and vomiting, especially when the drug is started, and hypoglycemia when added to a sulfonylurea. A GLP-1 agonist has become clinically available, liraglutide (Victoza). In contrast to exenatide, it is given once daily and can be administered anytime during the day.

**Dipeptidyl Peptidase-4 Inhibitors** The enzyme dipeptidyl peptidase-4 (DPP-4) rapidly degrades GLP-1 and GIP to inactive forms. DPP-4 inhibitors retard peptide degradation of these incretins, allowing therapeutic efficacy. Sitagliptin was the first of this class to be approved by the FDA. The DPP-4 inhibitors are given orally and are weight neutral.

**Cardiovascular Benefits of GLP-1 and DPP-4 Inhibitor Agents**  For the GLP-1 agonists, weight loss may be a key to improved cardiovascular effects. Indirect benefits can arise through reductions in blood pressure and inflammatory markers. In humans with advanced heart failure, those infused with GLP-1 experienced an increase in left ventricular ejection fraction, maximal oxygen consumption, and quality of life when compared with usual care. A number of large cardiovascular outcome trials evaluating DPP-4 inhibitors are in the recruitment phase and should report in the next few years (**Table 48-8**).

# ■ RESULTS OF LARGE CARDIOVASCULAR OUTCOME TRIALS EVALUATING THE ROLE OF GLUCOSE CONTROL

Even after the publication of ACCORD, Action in Diabetes and Vascular Disease: Preterax and Diamicron Modified Release Controlled Evaluation (ADVANCE), and Veterans Affairs Diabetes Trial (VADT), the question of whether glucose management reduces macrovascular events remains unclear (**Table 48-9**).

The UKPDS played a major role in establishing that optimal glycemic targets decreased long-term microvascular complications in type 2 diabetics. Currently, the ADA guidelines target glycemic control at an $HbA_{1c}$ level of <7% without causing significant hypoglycemia.

With the publication of ACCORD, ADVANCE, VADT, Steno-2, and UKPDS (10-year follow-up), there is a greater wealth of evidence, but the question of glycemic control and macrovascular outcomes remains confusing.

The ACCORD trial was a pivotal randomized study sponsored by the National Heart, Lung, and Blood Institute (NHLBI) and including >10 000 individuals with type 2 diabetes and established cardiovascular disease or additional cardiovascular risk factors. In 1 part of the trial, the comparison between tight glycemic control to keep $HbA_{1c}$ levels <6.0% versus conventional control ($HbA_{1c}$ between 7% and 7.9%) and the reduction of combined cardiovascular events (death from cardiovascular causes, nonfatal MI, and cerebrovascular accident) was investigated. ACCORD was stopped prematurely due to a 22% excess in total mortality in the treatment group at 3.5 years. A higher incidence of hypoglycemia, weight gain, and fluid retention was also observed in the intensive treatment group when compared with the conventional treatment group. The investigators suggest that the higher mortality in the aggressively treated group might be associated with the intensity and time to $HbA_{1c}$ level decrease and/or changes in the treatment regimen (ie, changes in drug type and dosage) or the eventual interaction of the different classes of drugs used in high doses and their adverse effects in addition to the combination of all these factors with the clinical characteristics of each patient.

The mechanism for this mortality excess remains unclear, but there was a trend for a 10% reduction in major cardiovascular events overall, with a lower incidence of nonfatal MI (3.6% vs 4.6%; HR, 0.76; 95% CI, 0.62-0.92; $p = 0.004$) with aggressive treatment.

ADVANCE was a randomized, controlled, multicenter study with 11 140 individuals with type 2 diabetes followed for 5 years and randomized into 2 groups: conventional versus intensive glycemic control. In the conventional treatment group, patients could use sulfonylureas other than gliclazide. Compared with the ACCORD cohort, the patients were of similar age but had a lesser duration of diabetes and a lower baseline $HbA_{1c}$. Primary objectives included major macrovascular events (death due to cardiovascular causes, acute MI, and nonfatal cerebrovascular accident) and major microvascular events (development of nephropathy or worsening of nephropathy and retinopathy).

**TABLE 48-8.** CV Safety Trials for New Diabetes Agents

| Study Drug | Name of Study | Sample Size | Population | Outcomes | Will Report |
|---|---|---|---|---|---|
| Canagliflozin | CANVAS | 4331 | DM | CV death+MI+Stroke | 2013 |
| BI 10773 | - | 4000 | DM+ atherosclerotic Ds documented | CV death+MI+Stroke | 2014 |
| Linagliptin | CAROLINA | 6000 | DM+ age/ Atheroscler osclerotic DS/end-organ damage enrichment | CV death+MI+stroke+ hospitalization for angina | 2018 |
| Sitagliptin | TECOS | 14000 | DM+CVD | CV death+MI+stroke+ Hospitalization for angina | 2014 |
| Saxagliptin | SAVOR | 16500 | DM+CVD/ Risk factors enrichment | CV death+MI+stroke | 2015 |
| Alogliptin | EXAMINE | 5400 | DM+ACS | CV death+MI+stroke | 2014 |
| Exenatide | EXSCEL | 9500 | DM | CV death+MI+stroke | 2017 |
| Lixisenatide | ELIXA | 6000 | DM+ACS | CV death+MI+stroke+ hospitalization for angina | 2013 |
| Aleglitazar | ALECARDIO | 6000 | DM+ACS | CV death+MI+stroke | 2015 |
| Liraglutide | LEADER | 8754 | DM+age/ atheros cleroscleroric DS/HF enrichment | CV death+MI+stroke | 2016 |
| Dulaglutide | REWIND | 9622 | DM+age/ atheroscler osclerotic DS/risk factors enrichment | CV death+MI+stroke | 2019 |

A mean follow-up of 5 years indicates that in the group with intensive glycemic control, there was a decrease in $HbA_{1c}$ levels (7.3%-6.5%) and, similar to ACCORD, a significantly lower rate of microvascular events primarily due to a 21% reduction in the occurrence or worsening of nephropathy. Intensive glycemic control had no significant effect on the occurrence of major macrovascular events and death from cardiovascular causes or other causes and did not have an excess in total mortality.

**TABLE 48-9.** Recent Trials Examining the Effect of Glycemic Control on Macrovascular Outcomes

| | UKPDS | ACCORD | ADVANCE | VADT |
|---|---|---|---|---|
| Diabetes duration (y) | Newly diagnosed | 10 (median) | 8 (mean) | 11.5 (mean) |
| Mean age (y) | 53 | 62 | 66 | 60 |
| History of vascular events (%) | Not reported in detail; probably low | 35 | 32 | 40 |
| Duration of intervention (y) | 10 | 3.5 | 5 | 6 |
| Postintervention follow-up | 10 y | None | None | None |
| Primary outcome | Three composite end points | Nonfatal MI, nonfatal stroke, CVD death | Microvascular + macrovascular complications | Nonfatal MI, nonfatal stroke, CVD death, CHF hospitalization, revascularization |
| Medication | Arm A: sulfonylurea/insulin based; arm B: metformin based in obese subjects | All oral drugs and insulin possible | Primarily sulfonylurea based; other oral drugs possible | All oral drugs and insulin possible |
| Achieved HbA$_{1c}$ in active vs control group, median (%) | Arm A: intervention period, 7.0 vs 7.9; follow-up, 7.7 vs 7.7; arm B: intervention period, 7.4 vs 8.0; follow-up, 8.0 vs 8.0 | 6.4 vs 7.5 | 6.5 vs 7.3 (mean) | 6.9 vs 8.4 |
| Hazard ratio for primary outcome ($p$ value or 95% CI) | Arm A: MI 0.85 ($p = 0.014$); arm B: MI 0.67 ($p = .005$) | 0.90 (0.78-1.04) | Macrovascular 0.94 (0.84-0.87 [0.73-1.04] 1.06) | 0.94 (0.84-0.87 [0.73-1.04] 1.06) |
| Hazard ratio for death (95% CI) | Arm A: 0.87 ($p = 0.006$); Arm B: 0.73 ($p = 0.002$) | 1.22 (1.01-1.46) | 0.93 (0.83-1.06) | 1.07 (0.80-1.42) |

ACCORD, Action to Control Cardiovascular Risk in Diabetes; ADVANCE, Action in Diabetes and Vascular Disease: Preterax and Diamicron Modified Release Controlled Evaluation; CHF, congestive heart failure; CI, confidence interval; CVD, cardiovascular disease; HbA$_{1c}$, hemoglobin A$_{1c}$; MI, myocardial infarction; UKPDS, United Kingdom Prospective Diabetes Study; VADT, Veterans Affairs Diabetes Trial.

From Ronnemaa T. Intensive glycemic control and macrovascular disease in type 2 diabetes: a report on the 44th Annual EASD Meeting, Rome, Italy, September 2008. *Rev Diabet Stud.* 2008;5(3):180-183. With permission.

As expected, severe hypoglycemia episodes, although rare, were more frequent in the group receiving intensive treatment (2.7% vs 1.5%; $P <. 001$). However, the study did not show a statistically significant difference in the reduction of macrovascular events.

The VADT trial evaluated type 2 diabetic patients with a longer duration of diabetes and a higher $HbA_{1c}$ than in the ACCORD and ADVANCE trials. After a median follow-up of approximately 6 years, the median $HbA_{1c}$ was reduced from 9.4% to 6.9% in the intensively treated arm. There was a nonsignificant 12% reduction in the primary end point of macrovascular events and no effect of intensive management on overall mortality. The rates of hypoglycemia were high in both arms but greater in the intensive therapy arm (24.1% vs 17.6%).

There are a number of important differences between the ACCORD, ADVANCE, and VADT trials that provide important insight into how to move forward. The use of rosiglitazone was much more frequent in ACCORD patients (92% in the intensive treatment arm). The ACCORD investigators reported that rosiglitazone had no effect on the higher mortality rate found in the intensive control group. The greater frequency of rosiglitazone and insulin administration might explain the greater weight gain observed in the intensive treatment group (average of 3.5 kg). In contrast, the ADVANCE regimen was sulfonylurea based. Because the rate of cardiovascular events in all studies was lower than anticipated, optimal nonglucose medical management has become the cornerstone of therapy.

The UKPDS study, the initial publication of which in 1998 did not show significant effects of tight glycemic control on the incidence of macrovascular complications, recently presented 10-year follow-up data. The trial initially randomized patients to receive conventional or intensive therapy, but after the trial ended, 3277 patients were followed on whatever therapy they were prescribed. In an intent-to-treat analysis based on their initial randomization, the group of patients receiving sulfonylurea or insulin experienced a sustained decrease (at the end of a 10-year follow-up) in the relative risk of any events related to diabetes (9%; $p = 0.04$), microvascular disease (24%; $p = 0.001$), MI (15%; $p = 0.01$), and death due to any cause (13%; $p = 0.007$). In the arm allocated to metformin, there was a significant and sustained decrease in the risk of events related to diabetes (21%; $p = 0.01$), acute MI (33%; $p = 0.005$), and death due to any cause (27%; $p = 0.002$). These results were observed without any difference in $HbA_{1c}$ levels. In addition, postprandial glycemia may also be an important factor in predicting future cardiovascular risk in epidemiologic studies. The Diabetes Epidemiology: Collaborative Analysis of Diagnostic Criteria in Europe (DECODE) study showed that an elevated 2-hour postprandial glucose level was independently associated with an increased mortality (**Fig. 48-4**).

## ■ ESTABLISHING CV SAFETY OF DIABETES MEDICATIONS

Given the recent data from large trials challenging the direct link of glucose lowering with reduction of cardiovascular events and the rosiglitazone debacle, the FDA has mandated establishing CV safety as a prerequisite for the approval of glucose-lowering drugs. This can be done through a meta-analysis of the cumulative data from multiple small phase II and III studies or a single large randomized phase III trial demonstrating noninferiority to placebo and ruling out an excess CV hazard of 1.3. Table 48-8 lists the ongoing CV safety trials for many new diabetes therapies.

## ■ DYSLIPIDEMIA MANAGEMENT

Medical therapy for hyperlipidemia is similar in diabetic and nondiabetic patients, but diabetic patients require special considerations.

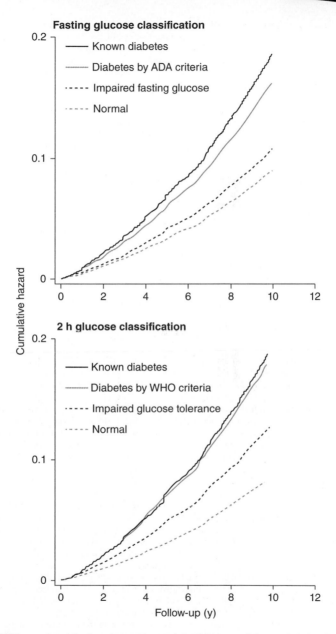

**FIGURE 48-4.** Cumulative hazard curves for American Diabetes Association (ADA) fasting glucose criteria and the World Health Organization (WHO) 2-hour glucose criteria adjusted by age, sex, and study center. (Reprinted from, DECODE Study Group. Glucose tolerance and mortality: comparison of WHO and American Diabetes Association diagnostic criteria. *Lancet.* 1999;354:617-621. Copyright (1999), with permission from Elsevier.)

The hypertriglyceridemia of diabetes can be treated effectively with fibric acid derivatives without an adverse effect on glucose metabolism. Type 2 diabetic patients experience a reduction in the cardiovascular event rate when treated with gemfibrozil. These drugs cause a 5% to 15% decrease in LDL levels in patients with normal triglyceride levels, but in patients with hypertriglyceridemia, LDL levels increase. This elevation is probably caused by the catabolism of the atherogenic LDL particle, resulting in less atherogenic LDL.

The Fenofibrate Intervention and Event Lowering in Diabetes (FIELD) trial studied 9795 patients with diabetes at risk for CHD and showed that fenofibrate was not associated with a difference in the primary composite end point of CHD death or nonfatal MI compared with placebo at 5 years of follow-up. The treatment effect differences, however, may have been attenuated as a consequence of the more frequent use of statins as lipid-lowering therapy in the placebo arm.

Although nicotinic acid lowers both cholesterol and triglyceride levels while increasing HDL levels, it is generally not indicated in diabetes. It has an adverse effect on glycemic control, which results from the induction of insulin resistance. The NIH's multicenter, randomized study called AIM-HIGH (Atherothrombosis Intervention in Metabolic Syndrome with Low HDL/High Triglycerides and Impact on Global Health Outcomes) enrolled 3414 subjects with atherogenic dyslipidemia and established cardiovascular disease to test whether the drug combination of extended-release niacin plus simvastatin is superior to simvastatin alone in delaying time to first major cardiovascular event was stopped early after 3 years of median follow-up for marginal excess in ischemic strokes in the face of neutral benefit. The primary end point—the first event of a composite of CHD death, nonfatal MI, ischemic stroke, hospitalization for ACS or symptom-driven coronary or cerebral revascularization—was similar in the 2 groups, occurring in 282 patients (16.4%) in the niacin group versus 274 patients (16.2%) on placebo.

Bile acid resins can decrease the levels of LDL in diabetic patients, but they can cause a significant increase in triglyceride levels, especially if VLDL levels are already high or if the diabetes is poorly controlled. In patients with high levels of both LDL and VLDL, bile acid resins can be used in low doses in combination with fibric acid derivatives.

Hydroxymethylglutaryl coenzyme A (HMG-CoA) reductase inhibitors—statins—are another group of drugs that are useful in lowering cholesterol levels in type 2 diabetes patients without having an adverse effect on glycemic control. In a study assessing the effectiveness of a cholesterol-lowering drug for secondary prevention of morbidity and mortality in patients with angina or prior MI, simvastatin was found to be more efficacious in diabetic patients than it was in the overall group. The Collaborative Atorvastatin Diabetes Study (CARDS) showed that among 2838 diabetic subjects with at least 1 heart disease risk factor, but without elevated cholesterol levels, randomized to atorvastatin versus placebo and followed up for 3.9 years, statin therapy was associated with a 37% reduction in the primary composite end point of CHD death, fatal MI, hospitalized unstable angina, resuscitated cardiac arrest, coronary revascularization, and stroke. The Heart Protection Study (HPS), with a subgroup of 5963 diabetic patients, showed a 28% reduction in total CHD (nonfatal MI and CHD death), nonfatal and fatal strokes, coronary and noncoronary revascularizations, and major vascular events (total CHD, total stroke, or revascularizations) with simvastatin therapy. Table 48-3 demonstrates the relatively low number needed to treat to prevent a major cardiovascular complication in 3 of the main lipid-lowering trials. These therapies are the cornerstone of diabetic management in the current era.

The NCEP-ATP III reported its executive summary on the treatment of hyperlipidemia. One of the most striking modifications was the raising of patients with diabetes without CHD to the same risk level as someone with CHD. As stated previously, the goal for LDL cholesterol is <100 mg/dL for all those with diabetes regardless of CHD. Patients with a metabolic syndrome were also targeted for aggressive lifestyle modification in this document.

# ■ HYPERTENSION MANAGEMENT

Patients with diabetes should be treated to a systolic blood pressure of 130 mm Hg and a diastolic blood pressure of 80 mm Hg. Patients with a blood pressure ≥140/90 mm Hg should receive drug therapy in addition to lifestyle and behavioral therapy. Multiple drug therapy (2 or more agents at proper doses) is generally required to achieve blood pressure targets. All patients with diabetes and hypertension should be treated with a regimen that includes either an ACE inhibitor or an ARB. If one class is not tolerated, the other should be substituted. If needed to achieve blood pressure targets, a thiazide diuretic should be added as second-line therapy based on the Antihypertensive and Lipid-lowering Treatment to Prevent Heart Attack Trial (ALLHAT) results. The use of calcium-channel blockers is not considered frontline therapy in the current recommendations. They may be used particularly in patients who are intolerant to other first-line therapies.

β-blockers are generally underused in diabetic patients despite convincing evidence dating back to the prethrombolytic era that demonstrated both an early and late survival benefit that was more impressive than that observed in the nondiabetic cohort. The Glycemic Effects in Diabetes Mellitus: Carvedilol-Metoprolol Comparison in Hypertensive (GEMINI) study demonstrated the superiority of carvedilol and metoprolol in achieving a more stabilized glycemic control and reduced insulin resistance in diabetic patients with hypertension who were taking a renin-angiotensin system blocker.

# ■ MANAGEMENT OF NEPHROPATHY

The UKPDS of type 2 diabetics and studies of patients with type 1 diabetes using captopril have shown that control of hypertension slows the progression of nephropathy. The blood pressure should be maintained at <130/85 mm Hg, and angiotensin-converting enzyme (ACE) inhibitors are the preferred antihypertensive agents. The UKPDS, however, showed no difference in blood pressure control with captopril versus atenolol. The benefit of antihypertensive therapy with an ACE inhibitor in type 1 diabetes can be shown early in the course of disease, when microalbuminuria is the only abnormality.

There is insufficient evidence to recommend ACE inhibitors in normotensive patients without microalbuminuria. Nonetheless, physicians should still recommend screening on at least a yearly basis because the risk-to-benefit ratio of diagnosing microalbuminuria justifies treatment with an ACE inhibitor, if not for renal disease alone, then for reducing the incidence of myocardial infarction (MI). Patients on ACE inhibitors should be monitored for potassium because they may develop hyperkalemia in the presence of a type 4 renal tubular acidosis. Sodium restriction is advised because it reduces hypertension. Dietary protein should be adjusted to 0.8 g/kg/d to decrease intraglomerular pressure. More recently, clinical trials evaluating angiotensin receptor blockers (ARBs), including losartan and irbesartan, have demonstrated a significant renal protective effect in the diabetic patient with nephropathy. There were no differences between the ARB and usual care groups with regard to cardiovascular outcomes.

An optimal approach toward diabetic nephropathy combines control of hypertension, preferably with an ACE inhibitor or ARB; glycemic control; sodium restriction; and adjustment of protein intake.

# ■ MANAGEMENT OF DIABETIC CARDIOMYOPATHY

The management of heart failure with preserved left ventricular systolic function usually includes β-blockers and ACE inhibitors, but evidence for this is sparse. Once CHD develops in the diabetic patient, the left ventricular systolic dysfunction that ensues responds to all the same therapies as in the nondiabetic population. The findings of the Heart Outcomes Prevention Evaluation (HOPE) trial suggest that early initiation of ACE inhibition retards the progression to overt congestive heart failure.

# ■ CORONARY REVASCULARIZATION

The management of diabetic patients with CHD entails both pharmacologic and revascularization strategies. Over the past several years, there have been many advances in the medical management of the diabetic patient with CHD. Aspirin, β-blockers, statins, and ACE inhibitors are routinely administered. These agents may provide clinical benefit not only by treating ischemia, but also by stabilizing atherosclerotic plaque and inhibiting endovascular thrombosis, thereby preventing acute coronary events.

## *Options for Revascularization in Diabetic Patients: Coronary Artery Bypass Graft Surgery Versus Balloon Angioplasty*

For the past 2 decades, the question of preferred revascularization strategies—surgery versus PCI, mostly as balloon angioplasty—in patients with obstructive coronary artery disease has led to 13 important randomized clinical trials. There is general consensus that both surgery and percutaneous interventional therapies result in similar death and MI frequency for the overall patient populations evaluated in these studies. The major departure from this observation was highlighted in the BARI trial substudy, wherein there was a clinically meaningful and statistically significant survival benefit favoring coronary artery bypass grafting (CABG) in diabetic patients Specifically, in the BARI randomized trial ($n = 1829$ patients in total), diabetics on oral agent or insulin ($n = 347$) undergoing CABG had a 5-year survival rate of 80.6% compared with 65.5% in the balloon angioplasty arm. In addition, the CABG group had fewer repeat revascularization procedures and less angina. Although this was not a prespecified subgroup analysis according to the BARI protocol, these striking results led to the NIH recommending CABG as the revascularization strategy of choice in diabetics with multivessel coronary artery disease. However, the BARI registry showed no difference in overall long-term survival between CABG and angioplasty patients. In the Northern New England Cardiovascular Disease Study, diabetic patients demonstrated a significant mortality benefit in favor of CABG. [HR was 1.49 ($p = 0.04$) for PCI versus CABG]. Patients with 3-vessel disease had the greatest benefit from CABG.

## *Modern PCI Techniques (Before Drug-Eluting Stents)*

**Bare-Metal Stents** Many of the technical limitations of balloon angioplasty have been overcome by coronary stent implantation during PCI. Stenting is more predictable, giving a more reliable angiographic result in a wide variety of lesion types, and is associated with lower restenosis in many lesion subsets. In the Stent Restenosis Study (STRESS), patients with relatively simple de novo lesions randomized to stent implantation had a 31.6% rate of restenosis compared with 42.1% in the balloon angioplasty group ($p < 0.05$). Similarly, in the Belgium Netherlands Stent (BENESTENT) trial, patients with relatively simple de novo native lesions randomized to stent implantation had a 22% rate of restenosis, compared with 32% in the angioplasty group ($p = 0.02$). What became clear, however, was that diabetic patients were at significantly higher risk for restenosis after either balloon angioplasty or stent implantation compared with nondiabetic patients, as shown in all previous clinical studies on restenosis.

The introduction and generalized application of stenting with bare-metal stents gave promise that by reducing restenosis and preventing repeat revascularizations, diabetic patients may further benefit from a PCI approach, thus achieving parity with CABG as a revascularization strategy. The randomized Arterial Revascularization Trial Study (ARTS) compared the clinical outcomes of aggressive stenting versus CABG surgery in 1205 patients with multivessel coronary disease and demonstrated no important differences in death, MI, or stroke at 1 year. However, there was still a 14% difference, favoring CABG, in 1-year repeat revascularization rates. The diabetes subset from ARTS revealed that multivessel stenting had a poorer 1-year MACE rate compared with CABG (63.4% vs 84.4%; $p$ <0.001); the results were mainly driven by the higher incidence of repeat revascularization after stenting than after CABG (8% repeat of CABG and 14.3% repeat of PCI vs no repeat of CABG and 3.1% repeat of PCI, respectively).

A quantitative analysis of the 1-year clinical outcomes of patients in the ARTS-I, ERACI (Argentine Randomized Trial of Coronary Stents), SOS (Stent or Surgery), and MASS (Medicine, Angioplasty, or Surgery Study)-2 trials showed that PCI with multiple stenting and CABG surgery provided a similar degree of protection against death, MI, and stroke.

## Drug-Eluting Stents

The advent of DESs has revolutionized the field of percutaneous interventions, especially in the diabetic patient. Although DESs have not had a major impact on hard cardiovascular end points such as death and MI, they have been successful in reducing angiographic restenosis and the rates of target-vessel revascularizations. A recent meta-analysis of DES studies showed that for patients with diabetes, the numbers needed to treat to reduce MACEs were 4 patients for SES and 6 patients for PES. **Table 48-10** shows the data for the diabetic patient subsets in the major interventional DES trials with SES and PES.

**SES Versus PES in Diabetic Patients** With the superiority of DESs being established in the diabetic population, the next challenge became the choice of which DES delivers better results—SES or PES. Few studies have compared these major DESs head to head. The ISAR-DIABETES (Intracoronary Stenting and Angiographic Results: Do Diabetic Patients Derive Similar Benefit From Paclitaxel-Eluting and Sirolimus-Eluting Stents?) study enrolled 250 patients with diabetes and coronary disease and randomized patients in a 1:1 ratio to SES and PES. The in-segment late luminal loss was 0.24 mm greater in the PES group compared with the SES group ($p$ = 0.002). Angiographic restenosis was identified in 16.5% of the PES group versus 6.9% of the SES group ($p$ = 0.03). Also the target-lesion revascularization trended toward being higher in the PES group than the SES group (12% vs 6.4%; $p$ = 0.13). However, a meta-analysis of 10 DES trials failed to show a difference in any of the previously mentioned end points in diabetic patients. A recent analysis of a registry of 1320 diabetic patients treated with DESs also concluded that SES and PES are associated with similar rates of revascularization, MACE, and stent thrombosis. The question of which DES is superior for the treatment of diabetic patients remains unclear.

In a subsequent meta-analysis of 13 randomized trials and 16 registries involving >11 000 diabetic patients undergoing PCI, there were no significant differences between SESs and PESs. Overall, the target-vessel revascularization rates with DESs are consistently in the single digits.

## Multivessel Stenting With DESs Versus CABG in Patients With Treated Diabetes

Inadequate data exist for us to be able to evaluate the definitive impact of DES for diabetic patients on long-term outcomes. PCI using DES is being compared

**TABLE 48-10.** Incidence Rate Ratios From Trials of Sirolimus- and Paclitaxel-Eluting Stents and Ratio of Incidence Rate Ratios Comparing Sirolimus With Paclitaxel in Patients With Diabetes

| | IRR (95% Confidence Interval) | | |
| Study | In-Stent Restenosis | TLR | MACE |
|---|---|---|---|
| **Sirolimus trials** | | | |
| SIRIUS (2003) | 0.17 (0.08-0.37) | 0.31 (0.15-0.64) | 0.37 (0.19-0.70) |
| E-SIRIUS (2003) | 0.13 (0.03-0.57) | 0.21 (0.05-0.91) | 0.27 (0.08-0.94) |
| C-SIRIUS (2004) | 0.06 (0.003-1.02) | 1.00 (0.06-15.99) | 1.00 (0.06-15.99) |
| DIABETES (2005) | 0.15 (0.06-0.39) | 0.24 (0.10-0.59) | 0.31 (0.15-0.66) |
| RAVEL (2002) | 0.06 (0.003-0.97) | 0.07 (0.004-1.19) | 0.22 (0.05-0.98) |
| SES-SMART (2004) | NA | NA | NA |
| Combined IRR | 0.15 (0.09-0.25) | 0.27 (0.16-0.45) | 0.33 (0.21-0.51) |
| Heterogeneity[a] | 0.0%; $p = 0.92$ | 0.0%; $p = 0.73$ | 0.0%; $p = 0.89$ |
| **Paclitaxel trials** | | | |
| TAXUS I (2003) | NA | 0 events | 0 events |
| TAXUS II (2003) | NA | 0.16 (0.02-1.25) | NA |
| TAXUS IV (2004) | 0.16 (0.05-0.48) | 0.36 (0.19-0.70) | NA |
| TAXUS VI (2005) | 0.20 (0.05-0.68) | 0.20 (0.04-0.90) | 0.55 (0.21-1.43) |
| Combined IRR | 0.18 (0.08-0.40) | 0.31 (0.18-0.56) | 0.55 (0.21-1.43) |
| Heterogeneity[a] | 0.0%; $p = 0.80$ | 0.0%; $p = 0.62$ | NA |
| RIRR (sirolimus vs paclitaxel) | 0.82 (0.31-2.18); $p = 0.694$ | 0.86 (0.40-1.86); $p = 0.703$ | 0.60 (0.21-1.71); $p = 0.336$ |

[a]$I^2$, test of heterogeneity.

IRR, incidence rate ratio; MACE, major adverse cardiac event; NA, not available; RIRR, ratio of incidence rate ratio; TLR, target-lesion revascularization.

Modified from Stettler C, Allemann S, Egger M, et al. Efficacy of drug eluting stents in patients with and without diabetes mellitus: indirect comparison of controlled trials. *Heart.* 2006;92(5):650-657.

with contemporary CABG in multivessel disease patients with diabetes against the background of aggressive medical therapy in the ongoing NIH/NHLBI-sponsored Future Revascularization Evaluation in Patients With Diabetes Mellitus: Optimal Management of Multivessel Disease (FREEDOM) trial. The Coronary Artery Revascularization in Diabetes (CARDia) and Veterans Affairs Coronary Artery Revascularization in Diabetes (VA-CARDS) trials addressing the question of stenting with DES compared with CABG in diabetic patients were terminated early.

The evaluation of coronary revascularization in diabetic patients was enriched by 2 important recent trials, Synergy Between PCI With Taxus and Cardiac Surgery (SYNTAX) and CARDia. The SYNTAX program consisted of a randomized trial of patients with 3-vessel or left main disease comparing PCI with PESs versus CABG, as well as 2 parallel registries of patients ineligible for PCI or CABG. In the SYNTAX trial, 452 (~28%) of the 1800 patients had diabetes. At 12 months of follow-up, the only difference between PCI and CABG in diabetic patients was the excess of repeat revascularization in the PCI arm (20.3% vs 6.4%; $p$ <0.001). As expected, when compared with nondiabetic patients, the 12-month rate of death, MI, or stroke was higher for the diabetic cohort (10.2% vs 6.8%). Interestingly, when moving across the spectrum of nondiabetes to metabolic syndrome to insulin-treated diabetes, the 12-month major adverse cardiac and cerebrovascular event rate for

CABG was consistent at between 12% and 14%, whereas the major adverse cardiac and cerebrovascular event rates for PCI progressed from 15% in nondiabetes to 30% in insulin-treated diabetes. The SYNTAX investigators intend to follow the patients for up to 5 years.

Another important aspect of the SYNTAX trial was the derivation and evaluation of the SYNTAX scoring system for grading the complexity of coronary artery disease. Simply, the SYNTAX score is the summation of the points assigned for each individual lesion in the coronary tree (divided into 16 segments). The percent stenosis is not included; instead the scoring is assigned according to degree of occlusive versus nonocclusive disease, and the complexity of a given lesion (eg, bifurcation lesion) is factored into the score. Based on angiographic criteria, the investigators demonstrated that patients with higher scores and, thus, more complex disease were more likely to benefit from CABG surgery compared with PCI. This is based on the observation that not all 3-vessel and left main disease is equal. The findings of the SYNTAX trial according to the SYNTAX score are shown in **Fig. 48-5**. Patients with a SYNTAX score >32 appeared to benefit from CABG surgery versus DES PCI.

The CARDia trial evaluated diabetic patients with multivessel disease assigned exclusively to either DES PCI or CABG (**Fig. 48-6**). This 500-patient trial was underpowered to detect important clinical differences in death, MI, or stroke at 12 months. In a noninferiority analysis, the primary event rate was greater in the PCI arm (11.6% vs 10.2%; $p$ = not significant), but this failed to meet statistical significance. PCI was not proven to be noninferior to CABG due to wide 95% CIs. As in SYNTAX, there was an excess in repeat revascularization in the PCI arm. CARDia sets the stage for the FREEDOM trial, which will enroll 1900 subjects with a mean follow-up of 4 years. FREEDOM will report in 2012.

## Comprehensive Meta-Analysis of PCI Versus CABG

A recent meta-analysis by Hlatky et al from the early percutaneous transluminal coronary angioplasty and bare-metal stent era reported results. The diabetes subgroup appeared to fare better with CABG when 5-year findings were pooled.

# ■ SCREENING ASYMPTOMATIC DIABETIC PATIENTS

The recent Detection of Ischemia in Asymptomatic Diabetics (DIAD) trial publication answered an important question in the diabetes and coronary artery disease field—namely, what is the role of routine screening for myocardial ischemia in asymptomatic diabetic patients? For many years, the AHA had advocated for optimal management of coronary risk factors as frontline therapy. Colleagues from the ADA advocated strongly for routine stress testing in these patients. Over 1000 asymptomatic patients were randomized to undergo myocardial perfusion imaging or no screening. After 5 years, there was no difference in the rates of nonfatal MI or cardiac death between the 2 arms (relative risk reduction, 12%; 95% CI, 78%-56%). The DIAD trial demonstrated a very low rate of significant ischemia in the screening arm (~6% with moderate to large perfusion defects) and a very high adherence to a robust medical risk factor modification program. In fact, the excellent medical therapy in DIAD is responsible for a very low 5-year primary event rate. The one question that remains is what is the best therapy for patients with moderate to large perfusion defects if they are to be treated aggressively in an adequately powered trial? If there is no benefit to revascularization in these patients, then there is no rationale to screen for ischemia. Further analysis from BARI 2D may help to address this issue.

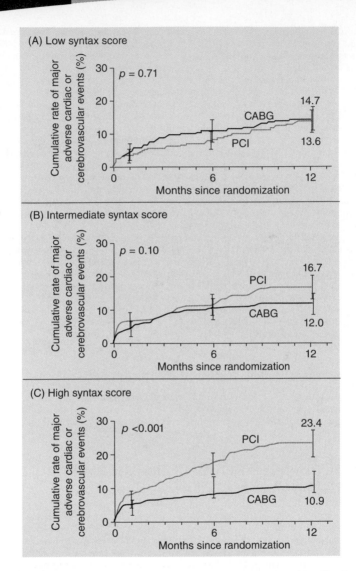

**FIGURE 48-5.** Rates of major adverse cardiac or cerebrovascular events among the study patients, according to treatment group and SYNTAX score category. SYNTAX, Synergy Between PCI With Taxus and Cardiac Surgery. (Reproduced with permission from Serruys PW, Morice MC, Kappetein AP, et al; SYNTAX Investigators. Percutaneous coronary intervention versus coronary-artery bypass grafting for severe coronary artery disease. *N Engl J Med*. 2009;360(10):961-972.)

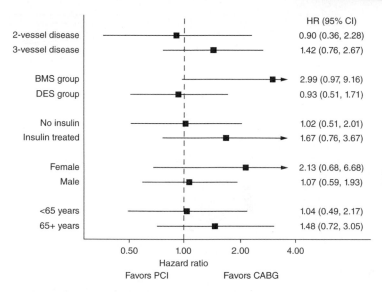

**FIGURE 48-6.** Coronary Artery Revascularization in Diabetes (CARDia) trial: forest plot of death, myocardial infarction, and stroke in key subgroups. BMS, bare-metal stent; CAGB, coronary artery bypass graft; DES, drug-eluting stent; HR, hazard ratio; PCI, percutaneous coronary intervention. (Reproduced with permission from Kapur A, Hall RJ, Malik IS, et al. Randomized comparison of percutaneous coronary intervention with coronary artery bypass grafting in diabetic patients: 1-year results of the CARDia (Coronary Artery Revascularization in Diabetes) trial. *J Am Coll Cardiol*. 2010;55:432-440.)

## ■ CORONARY REVASCULARIZATION COMPARED WITH OPTIMAL MEDICAL THERAPY IN LESS AGGRESSIVE CORONARY ARTERY DISEASE

Approximately one-third of the patients randomized in the Clinical Outcomes Utilizing Revascularization and Aggressive Drug Evaluation (COURAGE) trial were diabetic. The trial demonstrated no difference in the 5-year MACE rate. This required further confirmation. BARI 2D was a multicenter NHLBI-sponsored study to address 2 important questions. First, it addressed the question of whether diabetic patients with relatively mild or no symptoms could be treated with deferred revascularization (optimal medical therapy [OMT] alone) compared with prompt revascularization in addition to OMT. The important feature was that patients were randomized after catheterization with anatomy defined and required at least 1 lesion to be amenable for revascularization. It is critical to emphasize that the decision to undertake PCI or CABG was left to the discretion of the investigators with the caveat that patients with multivessel and more extensive disease were more likely to undergo CABG. Second, BARI 2D addressed that the question of whether treatment with an insulin-sensitizing strategy was superior to a strategy of insulin provision with a target HbA$_{1c}$ of <7.0% in both arms. Patients with left main disease, creatinine >2.0 mg/dL, or HbA$_{1c}$ >13% were excluded.

In the end, 2368 patients were enrolled at 60 international sites, with 1605 in the PCI versus OMT stratum and 763 in the CABG versus OMT stratum (**Fig. 48-7**). As expected, 93% of patients with single-vessel disease were enrolled in the PCI stratum,

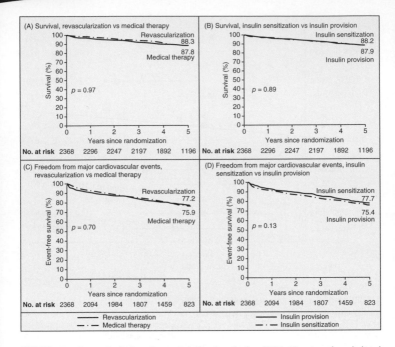

**FIGURE 48-7.** Bypass Angioplasty Revascularization Investigation (BARI) 2D: rates of survival and freedom from major cardiovascular events. (Reproduced with permission from Frye RL, August P, Brooks MM, et al. A randomized trial of therapies for type 2 diabetes and coronary artery disease. *N Engl J Med.* 2009;360(24):2503-2515.)

and conversely, 55% of patients with triple-vessel disease were enrolled in the CABG stratum. The primary outcome measures of the trial demonstrated no difference in 5-year mortality for either the comparison of OMT versus prompt PCI (12.2% vs 11.7%; $p = 0.97$) or the comparison of an insulin-sensitizing versus an insulin-providing strategy (11.8% vs 12.1%; $p = 0.89$). Similarly, the rates of MACE between the 2 principal comparisons did not differ.

BARI 2D was an important contribution because 2 key conclusions can be drawn. First, patients with diabetes who are asymptomatic or have mild symptoms can be first treated with OMT alone. By 5 years, 40% of these patients will require a deferred revascularization procedure. Second, when OMT is applied, the target of HbA$_{1c}$ of 7% can be achieved by an individualized approach. Patient adherence, polypharmacy, weight gain, and edema are all factors that will affect the antidiabetic strategy used. The TZDs were safe in BARI 2D, with a high prescription of rosiglitazone observed.

# FUTURE DIRECTIONS

On the clinical front, there are still many challenges in the prevention and management of diabetic cardiovascular complications. Glycemic control appears to be the mainstay of long-term diabetes management. Thus, development of better therapies and devices (eg, closed-loop pumps, islet and pancreatic transplantations) for achieving and maintaining $HbA_{1c}$ at not only <7%, but in the normal range of <6%, will be a primary goal in the next decade. The emphasis will also be on getting to appropriate targets faster. Clarification of the best glycemic control strategy in preventing CHD is required to validate the hypothesis that an insulin-sensitization strategy may be more cardioprotective than an insulin-providing strategy. The advent of DESs during coronary percutaneous revascularization has led to a reevaluation of the need for coronary bypass surgery in multivessel disease. Finally, the role of gene therapy in the management of diabetic atherosclerotic vascular disease needs to be addressed within the context of all other advances.

## SUGGESTED READINGS

Farkouh ME, Rayfield EJ, Fuster V. Diabetes and cardiovascular disease. In: Fuster V, Walsh R, Harrington RA, et al, eds. *Hurst's The Heart.* 13th ed. New York, NY: McGraw-Hill; 2011; 91:2028-2058.

Action to Control Cardiovascular Risk in Diabetes Study Group. Effects of intensive glucose lowering in type 2 diabetes. *N Engl J Med.* 2008;358:2545-2559.

ADVANCE Collaborative Group. Intensive blood glucose control and vascular outcomes in patients with type 2 diabetes. *N Engl J Med.* 2008;358:2560-2572.

AIM-HIGH Investigators; Boden WE, Probstfield JL, Anderson T, et al. Niacin in patients with low HDL cholesterol levels receiving intensive statin therapy. *N Engl J Med.* 2011;365(24):2255-2267.

American Diabetes Association. Standards of medical care in diabetes—2012. *Diabetes Care.* Jan 2012;35(suppl 1):S11-S63.

Duckworth W, Abraira C, Moritz T, et al. Glucose control and vascular complications in veterans with type 2 diabetes. VADT Investigators. *N Engl J Med.* 2009;360:129-139.

Farkouh ME, Dangas G, Leon MB, et al. Design of the Future REvascularization Evaluation in patients with Diabetes mellitus: Optimal management of Multivessel disease (FREEDOM) Trial. *Am Heart J.* 2008;155(2):215-223.

Frye RL, August P, Brooks MM, et al. A randomized trial of therapies for type 2 diabetes and coronary artery disease. *N Engl J Med.* 2009;360(24):2503-2515.

Hlatky MA, Boothroyd DB, Bravata DM, et al. Coronary artery bypass surgery compared with percutaneous coronary interventions for multivessel disease: a collaborative analysis of individual patient data from ten randomised trials. *Lancet.* 2009;373(9670):1190-1197.

Home PD, Pocock SJ, Beck-Nielsen H, et al. RECORD Study Team. Rosiglitazone evaluated for cardiovascular outcomes in oral agent combination therapy for type 2 diabetes (RECORD): a multicentre, randomised, open-label trial. *Lancet.* 2009;373:2125-2135.

Kapur A, Hall RJ, Malik IS, et al. Randomized comparison of percutaneous coronary intervention with coronary artery bypass grafting in diabetic patients: 1-year results of the CARDia (Coronary Artery Revascularization in Diabetes) Trial. *J Am Coll Cardiol.* 2010;55:432-440.

Serruys PW, Morice MC, Kappetein AP, et al; SYNTAX Investigators. Percutaneous coronary intervention versus coronary-artery bypass grafting for severe coronary artery disease. *N Engl J Med.* 2009;360(10):961-972.

# CHAPTER 49
# RHEUMATOLOGIC DISEASES AND THE CARDIOVASCULAR SYSTEM

Mala S. Kaul, Victor F. Tapson,
E. William St. Clair, and Prashant Vaishnava

Rheumatologic conditions such as systemic lupus erythematosus (SLE), rheumatoid arthritis (RA), and the vasculitides that affect multiple organ systems may also impact the cardiovascular system. These pathologic processes fall in the category of autoimmune diseases, which are initiated by a complex interplay between genetic factors and environmental stimuli. They are presumed to be driven by self-reactive T and B lymphocytes, which, in tandem with a network of endogenous and exogenous signals, activate the immune system, producing tissue inflammation and damage (**Table 49-1**). The effects of autoimmunity on the cardiovascular system may be the result of local or systemic mechanisms. For example, locally aberrant immunity may selectively target the pericardium, myocardium, or conduction system in systemic sclerosis. On the other hand, in patients with SLE or systemic vasculitis, circulating immune complexes may deposit in blood vessels, where they evoke an inflammatory response, which in turn occludes the vessel lumen and causes ischemic manifestations distal to the site of critically limited blood flow. A hypercoagulable state from a condition known as *antiphospholipid antibody syndrome* can lead to thrombotic occlusion, producing myocardial infarction, stroke, or ischemic damage of the visceral organs. Thus diverse pathways of a dysregulated immune system may converge to directly or indirectly damage the heart and vasculature.

This chapter aims to familiarize the cardiovascular specialist with the clinical features of rheumatologic diseases that affect the heart and blood vessels. These diseases derive from chronic inflammation and abnormal tissue repair. This chapter also covers the most common heritable diseases of connective tissue (eg, Marfan syndrome, Ehlers–Danlos pseudoxanthoma elasticum). Unlike autoimmune diseases, these rare disorders mostly result from mutations in specific genes encoding various components of connective tissue that maintain the structural integrity of the vasculature.

# CARDIOVASCULAR MANIFESTATIONS OF SYSTEMIC RHEUMATIC DISEASES

## ■ RHEUMATOID ARTHRITIS

With a worldwide prevalence of 0.5% to 1%, RA ranks as the most common of the systemic autoimmune diseases. RA is a female-predominant disease characterized by a chronic symmetrical polyarthritis with a strong predilection for the small joints

**TABLE 49-1.** Common Clinical and Cardiovascular Manifestations of Systemic Autoimmune Diseases

| Disease | Sex Distribution | Clinical Manifestations | Cardiovascular Manifestations |
|---|---|---|---|
| Rheumatoid arthritis | F>M | Inflammatory polyarthritis, rheumatoid nodules, RF, anti-CCP | Pericarditis, coronary artery disease, cardiomyopathy, congestive heart failure |
| Systemic lupus erythematosus | F>M | Malar rash, arthritis, photosensitivity, serositis, nephritis, +ANA; may have concomitant APS | Pericarditis, Libman-Sacks endocarditis, coronary artery disease, hypertension |
| Inflammatory myopathies | F>M | Proximal muscle weakness, DM with Gottron papules, shawl sign, mechanics hands | Pericarditis, conduction system abnormalities, congestive heart failure, and myocarditis |
| Systemic sclerosis | F>M | Limited form is referred to as CREST. Diffuse form involves proximal skin and visceral organs | Pulmonary hypertension, pericarditis, cardiomyopathy, conduction system disease |
| Seronegative spondyloarthropathy | M>F | Spinal or sacroiliac involvement, enthesitis, absence of rheumatoid factor, and a high incidence of HLA-B27 | Aortitis, conduction system disease |

ANA, antinuclear antibody; APS, antiphospholipid syndrome; CREST, calcinosis, Raynaud syndrome, esophageal dysmotility, sclerodactyly, telangiectasias; anti-CCP, anticyclic citrullinated peptide antibodies; DM, dermatomyositis; RF, rheumatoid factor.

of the hands and feet that often leads to physical impairment and disability. The diagnosis is established on clinical grounds by recognizing the signs and symptoms of joint inflammation. It is supported by the results of laboratory studies and plain radiographs of the hands and feet. Approximately three-quarters of patients with RA test positive for serum rheumatoid factor or anticyclic citrullinated peptide antibodies. Much is known about the pathogenesis of synovial inflammation in RA. Briefly, the synovial tissue is characterized by a chronic inflammatory infiltrate composed chiefly of T cells, B cells, macrophages, fibroblasts, and mast cells. There is increased production of a diverse array of proinflammatory mediators, such as tumor necrosis factor (TNF) α, interleukin (IL) 1, and IL-6, as well as many chemokines that work together to amplify the pathologic response, stimulate proliferation of synovial fibroblasts, upregulate expression of adhesion molecules on blood vessels, and promote angiogenesis.

Although RA is predominately an inflammatory joint disease, it produces systemic effects that can target other organs and tissues. Extra-articular manifestations include fatigue, low-grade fever, Sjögren syndrome, nodules, interstitial lung disease, and vasculitis. In RA, the most common cardiovascular manifestations are pericarditis, valvular disease, cardiomyopathy, coronary vasculitis, ischemic heart disease, and congestive heart failure. While cardiovascular involvement is rarely the presenting manifestation, it may lead to premature death. The pericardium is the most frequently involved cardiac structure in RA.

## Pericarditis

In a necropsy series, evidence of pericarditis can be seen in as many as 54% of cases. Acute, symptomatic pericarditis, however, occurs in fewer than 10% of patients with severe RA. RA patients with acute pericarditis are clinically indistinguishable from those with pericardial disease secondary to nonrheumatic conditions. Symptoms of positional chest pain or a pericardial friction rub may be elicited in up to 55% to 65% of patients. Although in this setting electrocardiograms are often normal, 5% to 10% of patients may manifest abnormalities classically associated with acute pericarditis. Imaging may be useful in confirming the diagnosis of pericarditis. In 1 series, echocardiography revealed a pericardial effusion in 90% of patients with this clinical diagnosis. Aspiration of the pericardial fluid, which is not usually required for diagnosis in the appropriate clinical setting, reveals an elevated white blood cell count, protein, and lactate dehydrogenase; decreased glucose levels; the presence of rheumatoid factor, and a low complement; these features may help to differentiate it from other causes of pericarditis.

In 1 cohort, the occurrence of pericarditis was associated with decreased survival at 10 years. However, it is unlikely that the presence of pericarditis directly contributes to the increased risk of death as the presence of extraarticular disease in general is associated with increased mortality. Constrictive pericarditis, albeit rare, is associated with higher mortality rates than uncomplicated pericarditis. Constrictive pericarditis must be distinguished from restrictive cardiomyopathy, which may result from secondary amyloidosis rarely seen in patients with long-standing RA. Most patients with uncomplicated acute pericarditis will respond to treatment with nonsteroidal anti-inflammatory drugs or corticosteroids. Corticosteroid therapy is generally reserved for patients with moderate to severe pericarditis and usually consists of a short burst of high doses of prednisone (eg, 40-60 mg/d) with subsequent taper over a period of several weeks, depending on the clinical response.

## Valvular Disease

Mitral valve prolapse is frequent. Valvular disease typically presents with nodules and fibrosis of the leaflet, annulus, and subvalvular apparatus. Patients with subcutaneous rheumatoid nodules have a higher rate of mitral valve insufficiency than those without nodules, but unlike patients with rheumatic heart disease, mitral valve disease associated with RA does not lead to valvular stenosis. Patients with severe or symptomatic valvular disease require surgical intervention.

## Cardiomyopathy

RA may cause a cardiomyopathy characterized by focal granulomatous inflammation of the myocardium. The granulomas may involve the conduction system, leading to first-, second-, or third-degree heart block, which usually persists despite immunosuppressive therapy. Rarely, cardiomyopathy may result from secondary amyloidosis, which manifests on echocardiograms as a significant increase in ventricular wall thickness and wall motion abnormalities. Cardiac MRI (cMRI) may be used to differentiate the different causes of cardiomyopathy. In particular, images from cMRI showing delayed enhancement with gadolinium display a characteristic diffuse endocardial hyperenhancement pattern that may suggest cardiac amyloidosis.

## Coronary Vasculitis

Although as many as 20% of patients with RA show histologic evidence of coronary vasculitis by autopsy, the significance of this finding is poorly understood because it rarely occurs as a clinical complication. The diagnosis of coronary vasculitis involving the epicardial vessels may be suggested by the angiographic findings of interspersed areas of smooth-walled stenosis and ectasia as well as focal aneurysms. However, these angiographic features are relatively nonspecific and may be due to atherosclerosis. Recognition of coronary vasculitis is important because it requires treatment with immunosuppressive therapy such as high-dose corticosteroids and possibly other agents.

## Accelerated Coronary Artery Atherosclerosis and Congestive Heart Failure

Overall mortality is increased in patients with RA compared with the general population. It is striking that 40% of deaths in RA are attributable to cardiovascular disease. In a recent study, the prevalence of cardiovascular disease in RA patients was comparable to that of patients with diabetes. Increasing evidence supports a strong link between RA and accelerated atherosclerosis, highlighting it as an important risk factor for cardiovascular disease. Atherosclerosis may be multifocal, and carotid atherosclerosis may predict coronary events in RA.

Systemic inflammation in RA is hypothesized to accelerate atherosclerosis, as well as affect other tissues, such as liver, muscle, and fat, which influence other cardiovascular risk factors (**Fig. 49-1**). Additionally, RA appears to be an independent risk factor

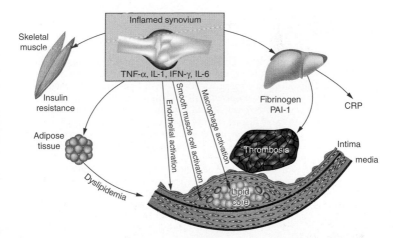

**FIGURE 49-1.** Systemic effects of inflammation in rheumatoid arthritis. The rheumatoid joint expresses high levels of various proinflammatory mediators, including tumor necrosis factor (TNF) α, interleukin (IL) 1, and IL-6, that amplify the inflammatory response. T helper cells secrete interferon-γ (IFN-γ) and IL-17, which in turn activate the cellular constituents of the synovial tissue. These cytokines, which are also found in the vascular endothelium of the atherosclerotic blood vessel, serve to promote coronary artery disease and plaque rupture. Additionally, upregulation of these cytokines influence other cardiovascular risk factors by affecting skeletal muscle, adipose tissue, and the liver, leading to insulin resistance, dyslipidemia, and increased levels of C-reactive protein (CRP), fibrinogen, and plasminogen activator inhibitor-1 (PAI-1), respectively. (Reprinted from Libby P. Role of inflammation in atherosclerosis associated with rheumatoid arthritis. *Am J Med.* 2008;121(10 suppl 1):S21-S31.Copyright © 2008, with permission from Elsevier.)

for multivessel coronary artery disease, and as shown in the Nurses Health Study, women with RA have a 2-fold higher rate of myocardial infarctions compared with controls. Other studies suggest that RA patients are less likely to be symptomatic from ischemic heart disease as non-RA controls and twice as likely to have sudden death and unrecognized myocardial infarction, contributing to a higher incidence of death from coronary atherosclerosis.

Congestive heart failure also contributes to excess cardiovascular mortality in RA. In recent echocardiographic studies, left ventricular systolic dysfunction was 3 times more common in RA patients compared with the general population. Both right and left ventricular diastolic dysfunction has been documented in this disease population despite the lack of clinically evident cardiovascular disease. The mechanisms by which RA patients develop heart failure are unclear. Although in some patients congestive heart failure may develop secondary to ischemic heart disease, most cases of heart failure associated with RA are less likely than other patients with heart failure to have a history of ischemic heart disease, obesity, or hypertension, yet they have significantly increased mortality.

There is currently a lack of evidence-based guidelines for the management and prevention of cardiovascular disease in RA patients. In treating RA, the primary goal is tight control of joint inflammation, which is done using conventional disease modifying antirheumatic agents (eg, methotrexate) as well as biologic therapy (eg, TNF-α inhibitors, tocilizumab, abatacept). TNF-α inhibitors are generally avoided in RA patients with a history of heart failure because of studies showing increased morbidity and mortality in non-RA patients with congestive heart failure who were treated with a TNF-α inhibitor. In general, traditional cardiovascular risk factors should be aggressively managed in patients with RA until further studies have evaluated the relative benefits and risks of this approach.

# ■ SYSTEMIC LUPUS ERYTHEMATOSUS

Systemic lupus erythematosus (SLE) is a systemic autoimmune disease that primarily affects young women, with peak incidence between the ages of 15 and 40 years. In the United States, its prevalence is estimated to be 1 in 2000 individuals and more commonly affects Hispanics and African Americans than Caucasians. Although more than 95% of SLE patients test positive for serum antinuclear antibodies (ANA), not all patients with a positive ANA have SLE. SLE patients are clinically a heterogeneous group, with a wide range of disease severity and spectrum of organ system involvement. Cardiovascular involvement, in particular, occurs commonly in patients with SLE. It is noted in up to 70% of patients by autopsy as well as by abnormalities seen on echocardiography.

The pathogenesis of SLE is likely to be multifactorial with dependence on genetic risk factors. Several lines of evidence support a prominent role for immune complex deposition in disease mechanisms, which may be relevant to the pathogenesis of vasculitis and possibly accelerated atherosclerosis in SLE.

## *Pericarditis*

The most common cardiovascular manifestation of SLE is pericarditis, with up to 42% of patients in one echocardiographic study showing an effusion. Pericardial effusions may be detected at any point in the disease and are usually asymptomatic and small. Acute pericarditis may occur in as many as 20% to 30% of patients with SLE. Rarely, acute pericarditis may be associated with cardiac tamponade; chronic pericarditis may occasionally lead to constriction. Particular attention must be paid to differentiating lupus pericarditis from infectious causes in the setting of concomitant immunosuppressive therapy for SLE. Treatment of lupus pericarditis depends on its severity. Although no therapy is required for asymptomatic, small effusions, symptomatic, acute pericarditis may warrant treatment with nonsteroidal anti-inflammatories or corticosteroids. Acute lupus pericarditis of moderate severity or worse is usually treated with a course of prednisone beginning at 40 to 60 mg daily followed by a subsequent taper in the dose over several weeks according to the clinical response.

## Valvular Disease

The valvular lesions of SLE are noninfectious verrucous vegetations, which can be found on the ventricular surface of the mitral leaflets; this condition is referred to as Libman–Sacks endocarditis (**Fig. 49-2**). Although any of the 4 valves may be affected, valvular abnormalities occur most commonly on the mitral valve, with resultant mitral regurgitation, followed in frequency by the aortic valve. Valvular lesions are not uncommon but usually are asymptomatic. According to one series, more than 50% of patients with SLE had valvular abnormalities by transesophageal echocardiography. The most common abnormality in this study was valvular thickening, followed by vegetations, and then valvular insufficiency. The significance of valve thickening is unknown and may resolve over time or worsen. Complications of valvular vegetations included cerebral and coronary artery thromboembolism, although the absolute risk is very low.

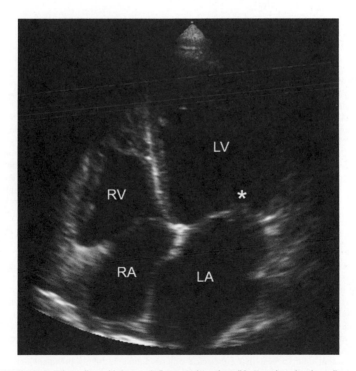

**FIGURE 49-2.** Echocardiographic image of Libman–Sacks endocarditis. Transthoracic echocardiogram (apical 4-chamber view) of a patient with systemic lupus erythematosus and Libman–Sacks endocarditis. Note the thickening and vegetation (*asterisk*) of the mitral valve. LA, left atrium; LV, left ventricle; RA, right atrium; RV, right ventricle.

There is a lack of consensus regarding the use of corticosteroids for treatment of valvular vegetations or other abnormalities. Valve replacement surgery is the usual course of action for the management of patients with clinically symptomatic or hemodynamically significant valve disease.

## Myocardial Disease

Myocardial dysfunction in SLE may result from valvular disease, coronary artery ischemia, or sustained hypertension and in some cases can lead to clinically significant congestive heart failure. Lupus cardiomyopathy, which is defined as a cardiomyopathy in the absence of ischemic disease or hypertension, has been reported in many series but is not well understood from a pathophysiologic perspective. Acute myocarditis should be suspected in any patient with SLE who presents with new-onset arrhythmia, fever, dyspnea, and chest pain. The diagnosis of lupus myocarditis is often based on clinical grounds after evaluation by coronary angiography and other cardiac imaging procedures. Cardiac enzymes are not usually elevated in lupus myocarditis. The role of endomyocardial biopsy is not well established; it is subject to sampling error, and the sensitivity and specificity of the biopsy findings in myocarditis are unknown. Treatment of clinically significant myocarditis typically calls for high doses of prednisone therapy for a prolonged course of 3 to 6 months with or without other immunosuppressive agents.

## Conduction System Disease and Neonatal Lupus

Lupus myocarditis may be complicated by tachyarrhythmias and conduction system disturbances. Additionally, injury to the conduction system, a rare occurrence, may result from small-vessel vasculitis, leading to various forms of heart block. Pericarditis may be associated with atrial fibrillation and flutter, although it is usually transient. Unexplained sinus tachycardia may also occur in SLE patients without obvious cardiac involvement and resolve with steroid therapy.

A conduction system abnormality may occur in infants of mothers with SLE whose serum contains anti-Ro and anti-La antibodies. Some of these mothers may also have been previously diagnosed with primary Sjögren syndrome, whereas others may appear healthy. Fewer than 5% of women with anti-Ro and/or anti-La antibodies will give birth to infants with neonatal lupus syndrome or congenital heart block. Congenital heart block develops from the transmission of maternal anti-Ro and anti-La antibodies to the fetus, causing myocardial inflammation and fibrosis. High-risk mothers with these serologic features should undergo fetal echocardiograms to screen for conduction system abnormalities or evidence of myocardial dysfunction.

## Coronary Artery Disease

Coronary artery disease is prevalent in SLE and has emerged as a significant cause of morbidity and mortality for these patients. Coronary artery disease may result from coronary arteritis or thrombosis but is most often secondary to atherosclerosis. Coronary arteritis, if suspected, may be treated with high doses of corticosteroids, possibly in combination with another potent immunosuppressive agent such as cyclophosphamide. Coronary thrombosis may be associated with the presence of antiphospholipid antibodies (see next section) or embolism from a valvular vegetation, as seen in Libman–Sacks endocarditis.

Recent data suggest that subclinical atherosclerosis is highly prevalent among SLE patients. Women with SLE between the ages of 35 and 44 years are 50 times more likely to have a myocardial infarction than controls. Young women with SLE may have several risk factors for coronary atherosclerosis, such as hypertension, which may be secondary to renal disease and diabetes brought about or worsened by corticosteroid exposure. In epidemiologic studies, SLE has been shown to be an independent risk factor for cardiovascular disease. However, the mechanisms underlying this predisposition are unclear, and their relationship to the systemic inflammatory response in SLE remains an area of investigation. Recently, patients with SLE have been shown to produce proinflammatory forms of high-density lipoprotein that confer an increased risk for atherosclerosis. Because SLE is predominantly a disease of young women, it is important to recognize that this group is at increased risk for coronary artery disease, and prompt evaluation is warranted if they develop any symptoms of cardiac ischemia.

## ▪ ANTIPHOSPHOLIPID SYNDROME

Antiphospholipid syndrome (APS) is a disorder characterized by the clinical triad of recurrent arterial or venous thromboses, pregnancy loss, and thrombocytopenia. Serologically, it is defined by the presence of anticardiolipin antibodies, anti-$\beta_2$ glycoprotein antibodies, or a positive lupus anticoagulant. APS may occur independently, referred to as primary APS, or be associated with SLE or other autoimmune disease, referred to as secondary APS.

Because APS may produce thrombotic occlusion of many different types and sizes of blood vessels, it can produce a variety of cardiovascular manifestations. Valvular disease is the most common APS-related cardiovascular manifestation. It is seen in both primary and secondary APS and is essentially indistinguishable from Libman–Sacks endocarditis. Coronary artery disease and accelerated atherosclerosis have also been associated with APS, although it seems that all types of antiphospholipid antibodies do not equally contribute to atherosclerosis. In a study by Soltész and colleagues, presence of lupus anticoagulant was more frequently associated with venous thrombosis, whereas anticardiolipin antibodies were more often associated with carotid, peripheral, and coronary artery disease.

## ▪ DERMATOMYOSITIS AND POLYMYOSITIS

Dermatomyositis (DM) and polymyositis (PM) are 2 inflammatory muscle diseases with cardiovascular implications. Patients with DM usually present with skin involvement characterized by erythematous scaliness over the knuckles (Gottron papules), elbows, and knees, as well as periorbital swelling and a violaceous rash around the lids, known as a heliotropic rash. They may also display a photo-sensitive rash over the face, chest, and back in a shawl-like distribution. In older patients, DM and PM may evolve as a paraneoplastic syndrome. Although these diseases primarily affect striated muscle, they may also cause cardiovascular complications.

Cardiovascular complications of DM/PM include pericarditis, conduction system abnormalities, congestive heart failure, and myocarditis. Pericardial involvement has been noted most often in patients with overlap syndromes (ie, features of 2 or more connective tissue diseases). Conduction abnormalities, nonspecific ST-T changes, and left ventricular diastolic dysfunction have also been reported in DM/PM. A serious cardiovascular complication is myocardial infarction secondary to coronary vasculitis. Myocarditis may infrequently cause heart failure, although newer imaging modalities, particularly cardiac MRI with gadolinium enhancement, may detect subclinical disease in as many as half the patients with DM/PM and be useful in monitoring response to therapy.

It is important to rule out other forms of myopathy in patients who present with muscle weakness. Patients taking statins may develop a myopathy mimicking inflammatory muscle disease. Statin-related myopathy and inflammatory myopathy may be differentiated by certain aspects of the medical history (eg, statins usually associated with significant myalgia), the results of electromyography, and findings on muscle biopsy, if necessary. For statin-induced myopathy, withdrawal of the offending drug will lead to resolution of the myopathic features. The cornerstone of the treatment for DM/PM is high doses of corticosteroids, usually in doses of 1 mg/kg for several months with a slow taper. Adjunctive therapy often includes methotrexate or azathioprine. Intravenous immunoglobulin may be effective for treating refractory and severe cases.

# ■ SYSTEMIC SCLEROSIS

Systemic sclerosis (or scleroderma) is a rare disorder characterized by microvascular injury and excessive fibrotic changes that can affect multiple organ systems. Most commonly, systemic sclerosis causes hardening of the skin, but can also affect visceral organs, such as lungs, kidneys, and the heart. The diffuse or progressive type of systemic sclerosis results in widespread cutaneous involvement of the distal and proximal extremities as well as the trunk and is usually associated with early and serious visceral involvement. In contrast, limited cutaneous systemic sclerosis, also known as *CREST syndrome*, is characterized by calcinosis cutis, Raynaud phenomenon, esophageal dysmotility, sclerodactyly, and telangiectasias. It may be associated with late involvement of visceral organs, especially increased risk for pulmonary artery hypertension (PAH). Cardiovascular involvement of systemic sclerosis may occur with either the diffuse or limited forms, as well as overlap syndromes in which patients may have features of systemic sclerosis in combination with those of SLE, RA, or polymyositis.

## Pericardial Disease

Pericardial disease in systemic sclerosis is usually benign. On the basis of autopsy results, the incidence of pericardial involvement is approximately 50%, but symptomatic pericarditis only manifests in approximately 16% of patients with diffuse scleroderma and in approximately 30% of patients with limited scleroderma. Pericardial effusions rarely cause symptoms, although they can be detected in approximately 40% of patients by echocardiography. In most cases, the effusion is relatively small and of no clinical consequence. For the treatment of acute pericarditis, nonsteroidal anti-inflammatory therapy is recommended with careful observation of renal function. Corticosteroids are generally considered to be of limited benefit, but they may be lifesaving in the setting of associated myocarditis.

## Myocardial Disease

Although interstitial lung disease (ILD) and PAH are the most common cardiopulmonary conditions that result in increased morbidity and mortality, other cardiac complications may occur in this setting. Localizing to the subendocardial region, areas of "patchy" fibrosis may be the hallmark of the SSc heart and suggest microvascular disease. Left ventricular diastolic dysfunction is a frequent manifestation of systemic sclerosis. Although diastolic dysfunction is common in this disease, it is rarely severe. When severe, diastolic dysfunction may worsen PAH.

## Arrhythmias and Conduction System Disturbances

The most frequent cardiac rhythm disturbance is premature ventricular contractions, often appearing as monomorphic, single ectopic events, or rarely as bigeminy, trigeminy, or pairs. Transient atrial fibrillation, atrial flutter, and paroxysmal supraventricular tachycardia have been reported in 20% to 30% of patients with systemic sclerosis. Nonsustained ventricular tachycardia has been described in 7% to 13%, whereas sudden cardiac death has been reported in 5% to 21% of unselected patients with systemic sclerosis. Conduction disturbances, such as bundle and fascicular blocks, occur in 25% to 75% of patients and appear to be due to fibrosis of the sinoatrial node.

## Pulmonary Arterial Hypertension

PAH is another serious cardiopulmonary complication of systemic sclerosis. Primary pulmonary arteriopathy occurs most commonly in patients with the limited cutaneous form of systemic sclerosis. Although at autopsy 65% to 80% of patients with systemic sclerosis have histopathologic changes consistent with PAH, fewer than 10% develop clinically apparent disease. In systemic sclerosis, the possibility of PAH should always be considered in the setting of dyspnea or right-heart failure. Patients with PAH associated with systemic sclerosis appear to have a worse prognosis than patients with idiopathic PAH, showing an untreated 2-year survival rate as low as 40%. Although there are an increasing number of clinical trials demonstrating the benefit of therapy and likely improvement in prognosis, patients with PAH related to scleroderma still have a less favorable outcome than those with idiopathic PAH.

Randomized clinical trials in patients with PAH have always included patients with idiopathic PAH and PAH associated with systemic sclerosis. These studies have led to approval by the US Food and Drug Administration of 3 prostacyclins (intravenous epoprostenol; intravenous, subcutaneous, and inhaled treprostinil; and inhaled iloprost), 2 oral endothelin receptor antagonists (bosentan and ambrisentan), and 2 oral phosphodiesterase-5 inhibitors (sildenafil and tadalafil). Improvement has been shown using the standard 6-minute walk test, although some studies have shown benefit in pulmonary hemodynamics and quality of life.

Although lung or heart lung transplantation has been performed in patients with ILD or severe PAH due to systemic sclerosis, this approach has been somewhat controversial. Several studies suggest that outcomes of patients with systemic sclerosis undergoing lung transplant were not significantly different from those of patients transplanted for other lung conditions during the same period. Gastrointestinal dysmotility and associated gastroesophageal reflux are substantial concerns, as aspiration has been associated with chronic allograft rejection. Unfortunately, patients with systemic sclerosis and PAH or ILD that might be severe enough for transplant commonly have multiple morbidities that render them less than ideal lung transplant candidates.

## ◼ SERONEGATIVE SPONDYLOARTHROPATHIES

The seronegative spondyloarthropathies are a group of multisystem inflammatory diseases sharing common features, including spinal or sacroiliac involvement, enthesitis (inflammation at the sites where tendons and ligaments insert onto bones), absence of serum rheumatoid factor, and a high incidence of HLA-B27. Among this group of related diseases are ankylosing spondylitis, reactive arthritis (previously referred to as Reiter syndrome), psoriatic arthritis, and inflammatory bowel disease–associated arthritis. In the United States, up to 10% of healthy Caucasians are positive for HLA-B27; the incidence is much lower in African Americans and Asians. HLA-B27 is most strongly associated with ankylosing spondylitis in Caucasians, where this genetic marker occurs in 90% of patients with this disorder. A medical history and examination indicative of inflammatory spinal disease and enthesitis and typical radiographic findings form the basis for diagnosis after excluding other forms of inflammatory arthritis such as RA. In contrast to RA, the spondyloarthropathies occur more commonly in males than females and do not usually involve the small joints of the hands in a symmetrical pattern. Peripheral arthritis tends to involve larger, usually lower extremity joints in an asymmetric distribution.

Among the group of spondyloarthropathies, ankylosing spondylitis and reactive arthritis are most frequently associated with cardiovascular manifestations. The 2 most prevalent cardiovascular manifestations of the spondyloarthropathies are conduction system disease and aortitis, with or without aortic insufficiency. The conduction system disease presents mainly as heart block, which occurs more commonly in males that are HLA-B27 positive; it often requires permanent pacemaker placement. Aortic root involvement is also associated with HLA-B27 in patients with ankylosing spondylitis and reactive arthritis. Aortitis may lead to dilation and stiffening of the aortic root with aortic valvular regurgitation. Aortic valvular regurgitation is usually a late complication of the spondyloarthropathies. It is unknown whether the TNF-α inhibitors will ameliorate cardiovascular manifestations of the spondyloarthropathies. Surgery has been successful for managing severe aortic regurgitation in this setting.

# ■ SYSTEMIC VASCULITIDES

The systemic vasculitides are multisystem diseases whose hallmark is inflammation of blood vessels (**Table 49-2**). Categorization of these diseases is based on the size of vessel involved (small, medium, and large) and the nature of organ system involvement. Vasculitis may be primary or secondary (eg, identifiable trigger such as a drug or infection). Primary vasculitides are presumably due to immune dysregulation in which genetic factors and environmental insults may play roles in their pathogenesis.

## *Giant-Cell (Temporal) Arteritis*

Giant-cell arteritis (GCA), also known as *temporal arteritis*, is the most common vasculitis among patients older than 50 years. It is more common in women than men and seems to be more prevalent in persons of northern European descent than African Americans. The clinical hallmarks of GCA are temporal artery tenderness, headache, jaw claudication, and visual loss. Many patients also manifest constitutional symptoms, such as fatigue and fever, and approximately one-third of cases are associated with polymyalgia rheumatica. Almost all patients with GCA have an elevated sedimentation rate and serum C-reactive protein level. Temporal artery biopsy, the gold standard for diagnosis, shows evidence of chronic granulomatous inflammation involving the entire wall with destruction of elastic laminae. Importantly, the disease may also target the extracranial large artery branches of the aortic arch. Peripheral artery involvement has become increasingly recognized as a complication of GCA and may be the presenting feature of this disease. Signs and symptoms of peripheral large artery involvement include intermittent upper-extremity claudication, decreased or absent peripheral pulses, and bruits over affected vessels.

GCA may also lead to thoracic and abdominal aortic aneurysm. It has been recommended that patients with GCA undergo yearly screening for aortic aneurysm using transthoracic echocardiography and abdominal ultrasonography. Other cardiovascular complications rarely associated with GCA are pericarditis, myocarditis, and coronary arteritis.

Although temporal artery biopsy remains the diagnostic gold standard for GCA, advances in imaging techniques have provided new diagnostic tools for assessing patients with this disease. A noninvasive approach for detecting vasculitis of the temporal arteries is duplex ultrasonography. Ultrasonography of involved temporal arteries demonstrates segmental, concentric hypoechogenic thickening of the arterial wall ("halo sign"). Sonography can also be important in diagnosis, assessment, and follow-up of peripheral artery disease. Computer tomography (CT) angiography and magnetic resonance angiography (MRA) have the added capability of detecting evidence of inflammation in the arterial wall, aneurysms, and luminal

**TABLE 49-2.** Common Clinical and Cardiovascular Manifestations of the Systemic Vasculitides

| Disease | Vessel Size Involved | Clinical Manifestations | Cardiovascular Manifestations |
|---|---|---|---|
| Giant-cell vasculitis | Large | Temporal artery tenderness, headache, jaw claudication, visual loss, most patients >50 years old, highest prevalence in northern Europeans | Aortitis, aortic dissection, limb claudication |
| Takayasu arteritis | Large | Fever, malaise, weight loss, arthralgia, headaches and myalgia; higher prevalence in women in their thirties and Asians | Upper extremity claudication, "pulselessness," chest pain, hypertension from renal artery stenosis |
| Kawasaki disease | Large and medium | Fever, desquamative rash, conjunctivitis, lymphadenopathy; disease of children | Coronary arteritis and aneurysms |
| Wegener granulomatosis | Medium and small | Pansinusitis, nasal blood discharge, oral ulcers, and subglottic stenosis, hemoptysis with pulmonary infiltrates | Pericarditis, cardiomyopathy, and coronary arteritis |
| Churg-Strauss syndrome | Medium and small | Asthma, eosinophilia, and pulmonary infiltrates usually secondary to pulmonary vasculitis | Cardiomyopathy (restrictive or dilated), coronary arteritis |
| Polyarteritis nodosa | Medium | Nodules on the skin, neuropathy in the form of a mononeuritis multiplex, gastrointestinal vasculitis with abdominal pain, hypertension, sparing of the lungs | Congestive heart failure, angina, myocardial infarction, and pericarditis |
| Behçet disease | All sizes | Oral and genital ulcerations | Aortitis |

narrowing (**Fig. 49-3**). Additionally, further information can be ascertained by MRI/MRA about the extent of arterial wall edema using gadolinium enhancement. Because arterial wall edema may correlate with the degree of vessel inflammation, MRI may be more useful than ultrasound for evaluating the extent of vessel inflammation and therefore may be superior for monitoring treatment response.

Corticosteroids are the mainstay of therapy for GCA. High doses of prednisone (0.7-1 mg/kg/d) are employed initially and are then tapered slowly, depending on clinical improvement and the decrease in serum levels of acute phase reactants. Many patients with GCA do not achieve remission with high doses of prednisone and require long-term maintenance with prednisone in low doses. Other immunosuppressive agents, such as methotrexate, may be combined with prednisone, but the evidence supporting their clinical efficacy in this situation remains conflicting. In the absence of any contraindications, low-dose aspirin should be given to all patients with GCA.

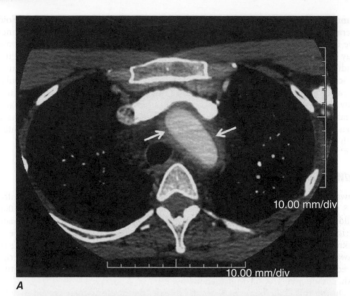

*A*

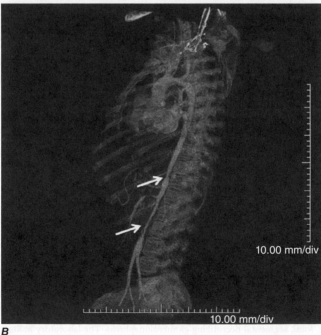

*B*

**FIGURE 49-4.** CT angiogram of Takayasu arteritis. **A.** CT angiogram (axial image) of the aortic arch of a patient with Takayasu arteritis demonstrating marked thickening of the wall of the aortic arch (*arrow*) **B.** Three-dimensional volume rendered image of the abdominal aorta of the same patient demonstrating several areas of narrowing (*arrow*) as a result of vasculitis.

In one study, cardiac involvement, including cardiomyopathy, pericarditis, and coronary arteritis, was described in 6% of 158 patients with WG. Additionally, there have been case reports of aortic regurgitation and high-grade AV block.

Overall, the prognosis for severe WG has improved with the use of corticosteroid therapy combined with daily oral cyclophosphamide. Studies also support the use of methotrexate combined with oral prednisone for treatment of patients with non–life-threatening WG. Surgical replacement of valves and pericardectomy has been performed in this setting for management of severe constrictive pericarditis and valvular dysfunction.

## Churg-Strauss Syndrome

Churg-Strauss syndrome (CSS) is a relatively rare type of systemic vasculitis characterized by a history of asthma, the presence of eosinophilia, and radiographic evidence of pulmonary infiltrates usually secondary to pulmonary vasculitis. Histopathologic lesions usually reveal a small- and medium-sized vessel vasculitis with eosinophilic granulomas, distinguishing it from the medium-sized vessel vasculitis called *polyarteritis nodosa*.

Heart disease is particularly prominent in CSS, with involvement of the cardiovascular system in up to 60% of cases; more importantly, it is the most common cause of death in these patients. The pathophysiology for the development of cardiac disease has not been elucidated, and it is unclear whether manifestations such as cardiomyopathy are a result of small-vessel vasculitis, eosinophilic infiltration of the myocardium leading to fibrosis, or a combination of both processes. Pericardial effusion, myocardial infarction, and myocarditis have also been reported in patients with CSS. Treatment of CSS with corticosteroids is usually very effective in the early stages of disease, although critically ill patients usually require treatment with a second immunosuppressive agent, such as cyclophosphamide.

## Polyarteritis Nodosa

Polyarteritis nodosa (PAN) is another relatively rare vasculitis that predominately affects the medium-sized arteries without granulomas. The evolution of the nosology of the systemic vasculitides has led to some recent confusion between the classification of PAN and microscopic polyangiitis (MPA). Patients with small-vessel involvement such as pulmonary capillaritis or glomerulonephritis are now deemed to have MPA and not classic PAN, and therefore many older studies of PAN have included patients with both classic PAN and MPA. The clinical presentation of PAN varies according to the affected organ system.

Cardiovascular complications of PAN have been reported in approximately 10% of patients in clinical studies and up to 78% in a histologic study. The most common cardiovascular manifestations are congestive heart failure, angina, myocardial infarction, and pericarditis. Various arrhythmias, mainly supraventricular tachycardias, have been associated with PAN, as well as hypertension from renal involvement. Treatment of PAN is similar to that of CSS and the other systemic necrotizing vasculitides. High-dose corticosteroids are the mainstay for initial treatment, with the addition of cytotoxic agents such as cyclophosphamide in severe cases.

# CARDIOVASCULAR MANIFESTATIONS OF CONNECTIVE TISSUE DISEASES

The connective tissue diseases are a group of heritable conditions that can affect skin, joints, and vasculature. The following section reviews the most common connective tissue diseases that affect the cardiovascular system (**Table 49-3**).

**TABLE 49-3.** Cardiovascular Features of Connective Tissue Disease

| Disease | Inheritance | Clinical Features | Cardiovascular Features | Gene |
|---|---|---|---|---|
| Marfan syndrome | AD | Tall stature, arachnodactyly, pectus excavatum, ectopia lentis | Aortic aneurysm/dissection, mitral valve prolapse | *FBN1* |
| Loeys–Dietz syndrome | AD | Hypertelorism, cleft palate/bifid uvula, arachnodactyly, easy bruising, pectus excavatum | Aortic aneurysm with tortuosity (corkscrew strictures), patent ductus arteriosus, bicuspid aortic valves | *TGF-βR* |
| Ehlers–Danlos syndrome | AD or AR | Joint hypermobility, hyperelastic skin, easy bruising (6 types of EDS; type 4 or vascular type is most associated with cardiovascular manifestations) | Aortic aneurysm, mitral valve prolapse | *COL3A1* (for type 4 vascular type) |
| Pseudoxanthoma elasticum | AD or AR | Hyperelastic skin, yellowish papular lesions on neck, axillae, groin, and flexural creases; angioid streaks | Intermittent claudication, coronary artery disease, angina | *ABCC6* |
| Osteogenesis imperfecta | AD | Blue sclerae, hearing loss, easy bruising increased risk of bleeding, and brittle bones (8 types of OI) | Aortic regurgitation, aortic root dilation, aortic dissection, mitral regurgitation | *COL1A1 COL1A2* |

*ABCC*, ATP-binding cassette subfamily C; *COL3A1*, collagen type 3 α-1; *COL1A1, COL1A2*, collagen type 1 α 1 and α 2. *FBN1*, fibrillin-1; *TGF-βR*, transforming growth factor β receptor.

# ■ MARFAN SYNDROME

Marfan syndrome is among the most prevalent of the heritable connective tissue diseases, with an estimated worldwide prevalence of 1 per 3000 to 5000 persons. Although up to one-third of patients have no family history of Marfan syndrome, most cases are inherited as a result of a high penetrance of an autosomal-dominant mutation in the fibrillin (*FBN1*) gene. More than 1000 mutations in the *FBN1* gene have been identified to date. Marfan patients often have a tall stature, long extremities, high-arched palate, joint hypermobility, and ectopia lentis. Additionally, they can have musculoskeletal abnormalities, including a pectus excavatum or carinatum chest deformity or scoliosis. Because some of these features are present in the general population, there has been increased attention given to improving the classification of this disease.

The complications of Marfan syndrome with potential lethality involve the cardiovascular system. Such patients may develop dilation of the proximal ascending aorta, dilation of the proximal pulmonary artery, mitral valve prolapse, and cardiomyopathy. The fibrillin gene encodes proteins essential for the proper formation of microfibrils that uphold the integrity of the extracellular matrix. Patients with Marfan syndrome who have mutations in these genes produce a "weak collagen" in the arterial walls. In the aorta, these changes reduce vessel distensibility and increase wall stiffness. These effects, coupled with the hemodynamic stress in high flow areas, over time, lead to the development of aneurysms, which can produce dissection of the vessel wall and life-threatening complications. Mitral valve prolapse is also commonly associated with Marfan syndrome and occurs in up to one-quarter of patients. It may lead to mitral regurgitation, which, if severe and uncorrected, can result in a dilated cardiomyopathy. Cardiomyopathy in the absence of valvular disease has also been reported in patients with Marfan syndrome and is believed to be secondary to defective cardiac muscle function from fibrillin mutations.

Life expectancy has significantly improved with proper identification and monitoring of patients with Marfan syndrome. The most common causes of death in these patients are rupture of an ascending aortic aneurysm with or without dissection or congestive heart failure from aortic or mitral regurgitation. It is important that Marfan patients be counseled to avoid isometric or strenuous exercise, including contact sports (**Table 49-4**).

**TABLE 49-4.** Task Force 4 Recommendations for Athletes With Marfan Syndrome

| Marfan Syndrome Abnormality | Recommended Sports Participation Level | Class of Recommendation |
|---|---|---|
| No aortic root dilation, moderate to severe mitral regurgitation, or family history of dissection of sudden death[a] | Low and moderate static/low dynamic competitive sports<br>No sports with potential for bodily collision | IA and IIA[b] |
| Aortic root dilation >40 mm, prior surgical aortic root construction, chronic aortic dissection, moderate to severe mitral regurgitation, family history of dissection or sudden death | Low-intensity competitive sports<br>No sports with potential for bodily collision | IA[b] |

[a]These patients should have echocardiographic measurement of aortic root dimension repeated every 6 months.

[b]IA: Evidence obtained from meta-analysis of randomized controlled trials. IIA: Evidence obtained from at least 1 well-designed controlled study without randomization.

Data from Maron BJ, Ackerman MJ, Nishimura RA, et al. Task Force 4: HCM and other cardiomyopathies, mitral valve prolapse, myocarditis, and Marfan syndrome. *J Am Coll Cardiol.* 2005;45(8):1340-1345.

It is currently recommended that all Marfan patients receive the maximum-tolerated dose of a β-blocker. The beneficial effects of β-blockade are reduction in heart rate and in the rate of pressure increase in the aorta that lead to less cumulative stress on the aorta. The use of angiotensin-2-receptor blockers (ARBs) may also slow the rate of progressive aortic dilation.

Patients with Marfan syndrome should undergo annual echocardiograms to evaluate the status of the aortic root and heart valves. Recommendations vary with respect to the optimal time for prophylactic surgical intervention. Generally, however, in an asymptomatic patient, repair of the dilated aorta is recommended when the diameter reaches 45 mm, there has been rapid progression in dilation, or if there is family history of dissection or rupture. After surgical intervention, yearly MRI or CT scan is recommended to monitor the graft.

Finally, female Marfan patients of childbearing age should be counseled regarding the relatively high risk of transmission of their disease to their offspring. Further, if a woman already has aortic root dilation greater than 40-45 mm, pregnancy should be avoided due to the high risk of complications when systemic blood pressure is increased during delivery. If the aortic root is less than 40 mm, then the patient may be allowed to become pregnant. However, the woman must be carefully monitored during pregnancy using transesophageal echocardiography and treated with a β-blocker.

# ■ LOEYS–DIETZ SYNDROME

Loeys–Dietz types I and II are among the more recently recognized of the heritable connective tissue diseases; their associated mutations reside in the genes encoding the transforming growth factor β receptors 1 and 2. Although these patients were previously categorized as having either Marfan syndrome or Ehlers–Danlos syndrome of the vascular type, more sophisticated molecular analysis has led to disease reclassification. Similar to patients with Marfan syndrome, these patients may have aortic aneurysms and musculoskeletal abnormalities such as scoliosis or pectus excavatum. However, patients with type I Loeys–Dietz also display the clinical triad of hypertelorism, either bifid uvula or cleft palate, or both, and generalized vascular aneurysms. The type II patients are characterized by cutaneous manifestations such as velvety translucent skin, easy bruising, and widened atrophic scars that are also seen in patients with Ehlers–Danlos vascular type. Loeys et al. studied 52 affected families and found that patients with Loeys–Dietz type I had shorter lives and underwent cardiovascular surgery earlier than type II patients. There was rapid formation of arterial aneurysms and a high incidence of pregnancy-related complications in both types. Distinguishing patients with Loeys–Dietz syndrome and transforming growth factor β-receptor mutations from patients with Marfan syndrome and Ehlers–Danlos syndrome is important for guiding medical therapy, making decisions about the optimal timing of prophylactic surgery, and management of pregnancy.

# ■ EHLERS–DANLOS SYNDROME

Ehlers–Danlos syndrome comprises a group of disorders that are characterized by hyperextensibility of skin, easy bruising, and joint hypermobility. There are 6 clinical types of Ehlers–Danlos syndrome; the vascular type, or type IV, is associated with mutations of the COL3A1 gene. Its prevalence is estimated to be 1 case per 100 000 to 250 000 people and it primarily affects the cardiovascular system. Ehlers–Danlos of the vascular type, which can mimic Loeys–Dietz syndrome, leads to diffuse vascular aneurysms that have a tendency for spontaneous rupture.

# ■ PSEUDOXANTHOMA ELASTICUM

Pseudoxanthoma elasticum is a rare disorder with an estimated prevalence of between 1 in 25 000 and 100 000 persons that can be transmitted either as an autosomal dominant or recessive trait. It is characterized by progressive accumulation of mineral precipitants within elastic fibers of the skin, eyes, gastrointestinal tract, and blood vessels. Clinically, patients display yellow macules or papules on their skin that have a cobblestone appearance at areas where there is flexion, such as the axillae, groin, and popliteal spaces. They also develop angioid streaks on the retina that represent breaks in Bruch membrane behind the eye. Mutations in the gene *ABCC6* (R1141X) have been implicated in the development of this disease, as well as in the increased risk for developing coronary artery disease in this setting. The vascular manifestations of the disease are secondary to degeneration of the elastic lamina of blood vessels and subsequent calcifications. They include easy bleeding and symptoms of claudication and angina, which are secondary to arterial narrowing.

Echocardiography of affected patients may reveal calcification of the atrial and ventricular endocardium, valves, and calcified thrombi, which can result in mitral valve prolapse, mitral valve stenosis, or restrictive cardiomyopathy. Surgery has been used to remove these calcium deposits, but otherwise, management involves properly identifying these patients, avoiding antiplatelet agents due to their increased risk of bleeding, and managing their cholesterol levels given the increased risk of cardiovascular disease.

# SUGGESTED READINGS

Kaul MS, Tapson VF, Clair EW St. Rheumatologic diseases and the cardiovascular system. In: Fuster V, Walsh R, Harrington RA, et al, eds. *Hurst's The Heart*. 13th ed. New York, NY: McGraw-Hill; 2011:89:1995-2010.

Canadas V, Vilacosta I, Bruna I, Fuster V. Marfan syndrome. Part 1: pathophysiology and diagnosis. *Nat Rev Cardiol*. 2010;7(5):256-265.

Canadas V, Vilacosta I, Bruna I, Fuster V. Marfan syndrome. Part 2: treatment and management of patients. *Nat Rev Cardiol*. 2010;7(5):266-276.

Doria A, Iaccarino L, Sarzi-Puttini P, et al. Cardiac involvement in systemic lupus erythematosus. *Lupus*. 2005;14:683-686.

Giles JT, Post W, Blumenthal RS, et al. Therapy insight: managing cardiovascular risk in patients with rheumatoid arthritis. *Nat Clin Pract Rheumatol*. 2006;2(6):320-329.

Graf J, Scherzer R, Grunfeld C, et al. Levels of C-reactive protein associated with high and very high cardiovascular risk are prevalent in patients with rheumatoid arthritis. *PLoS One*. 2009;4(7):e6242.

Kaloudi O, Matucci Cerinic M. Systemic sclerosis: the heart puzzle. *Rheumatologist*. 2009;3:13-15.

Keane MG, Pyeritz RE. Medical management of Marfan syndrome. *Circulation*. 2008;117(21): 2802-2813.

Liao SL, Elmariah S, van der Zee S, Sealove BA, Fuster V. Does medical therapy for thoracic aortic aneurysms really work? Are beta-blockers truly indicated? *Cardiol Clin*. 2010;28(2):261-269.

Libby P. Role of inflammation in atherosclerosis associated with rheumatoid arthritis. *Am J Med*. 2008;121(10 suppl 1):S21-S31.

Loeys BL, Chen J, Neptune ER, et al. A syndrome of altered cardiovascular, craniofacial, neurocognitive and skeletal development caused by mutations in TGFBR1 or TGFBR2. *Nat Genet*. 2005;37(3):275-281.

Pagnoux C, Guillevin L. Cardiac involvement in small and medium-sized vessel vasculitides. *Lupus*. 2005;14(9):718-722.

Pepin M, Schwarze U, Superti-Furga A, et al. Clinical and genetic features of Ehlers-Danlos syndrome type IV, the vascular type. *N Engl J Med*. 2000;342(10):673-680.

Roldan CA, Shively BK, Crawford MH. An echocardiographic study of valvular heart disease associated with systemic lupus erythematosus. *N Engl J Med*. 1996;335(19):1424-1430.

Roman MJ, Shanker BA, Davis A, et al. Prevalence and correlates of accelerated atherosclerosis in systemic lupus erythematosus. *N Engl J Med*. 2003;349(25):2399-2406.

Roman MJ, Moeller E, Davis A, et al. Preclinical carotid atherosclerosis in patients with rheumatoid arthritis. *Ann Intern Med.* 2006;144(4):249-256.

Sarzi-Puttini P, Atzeni F, Gerli R, et al. Cardiac involvement in systemic rheumatic diseases: an update. *Autoimmun Rev.* 2010;9:849-852.

Schoenfeld Y, Gerli R, Doria A, et al. Accelerated atherosclerosis in autoimmune rheumatic diseases. *Circulation.* 2005;112:3337-3347.

Shores J, Berger KR, Murphy EA, et al. Progression of aortic dilatation and the benefit of long-term beta-adrenergic blockade in Marfan's syndrome. *N Engl J Med.* 1994;330(19):1335-1341.

Solomon DH, Karlson EW, Rimm EB, et al. Cardiovascular morbidity and mortality in women diagnosed with rheumatoid arthritis. *Circulation.* 2003;107(9):1303-1307.

Williams MH, Das SC, Handler CE, et al. Systemic sclerosis associated pulmonary hypertension: improved survival in the current era. *Heart.* 2006;92(7):926-932.

# CHAPTER 50
# WOMEN AND CORONARY ARTERY DISEASE

Judith Z. Goldfinger, Pamela Charney, and Marc A. Miller

Cardiovascular (CV) mortality trends have finally begun to decrease among women in the United States similar to the pattern noted in men since the 1980s (**Fig. 50-1**). The importance of coronary artery disease (CAD) and its prevention in women is receiving increased attention from physicians and the public. An expert panel recently updated effectiveness-based guidelines for the prevention of CAD in women, and sex differences are increasingly being explored. Still, in a survey of primary care physicians, gynecologists, and cardiologists, fewer than 20% were aware that more women than men die annually of CAD. Similarly, in a telephone survey of more than 1000 American women in 2005, only 55% identified heart attack and heart disease as the major cause of mortality for women; this was an improvement from 30% of women surveyed in 1997 (**Fig. 50-2**). In contrast, 61% of the women reported heart disease as the leading cause of mortality in men. Interestingly, the most frequent reason women had not discussed heart health with their physicians was that their providers did not bring up this issue.

## PREVENTION: SEX-SPECIFIC ISSUES

### ■ TOBACCO

Tobacco exposure is the single most important coronary artery risk factor for women and men. In epidemiologic studies, greater tobacco exposure in amount and duration is related to higher CAD events in a dose-related fashion. Median smoking prevalence in 2007 was 21.3% for men and 18.4% for women. Among women, more Native American women smoke (26.8%) than white (20%) or black women (17.3%), with lower rates among Hispanic (11.1%) and Asian women (6.1%). Cigarette smoking has been associated with an earlier age of first myocardial infarction (MI) (see also Chapter 50) and menopause. Because middle-aged women experience less symptomatic CAD than middle-aged men, the increased risk of MI and sudden death related to tobacco use is greater for women than men.

Over the past several decades, American women's personal use of cigarettes has not decreased as dramatically as it has among men (**Fig. 50-3**). The prevalence of cigarette use among women reflects both higher initiation rates and lower initial and long-term cessation rates. However, successful tobacco cessation for women, as for men, dramatically decreases the risk of further coronary events.

Women contemplating smoking cessation are often concerned about weight gain, a common consequence of efforts to stop smoking. Weight gain tends to be higher among women, blacks, and smokers who inhale more than 25 cigarettes per day. Women smokers report that they are unwilling to experience even a minimal weight increase as a result of smoking cessation.

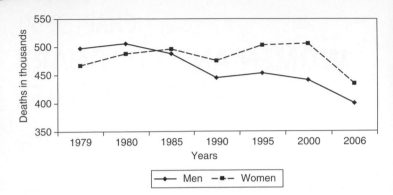

**FIGURE 50-1.** Graph comparing rates of coronary artery disease and mortality for women and men, 1979 to 2006. (From Lloyd-Jones D, Adams RJ, Brown TM, et al. American Heart Association Statistics Committee and Stroke Statistics Subcommittee. Heart disease and stroke statistics–2010 update: a report from the American Heart Association. *Circulation.* 2010 Feb 23;121(7):e46-e215.)

Multiple pharmacologic therapies are available to aid in smoking cessation. Nicotine replacement products roughly double the rate of successful tobacco cessation; all forms (transdermal patch, gum, spray, or lozenge) have similar efficacy at 6 months of follow-up. Bupropion improves tobacco cessation rates in both white and black smokers, and can help minimize weight gain while it is used, although weight gain occurs when it is stopped. Bupropion is contraindicated in patients with

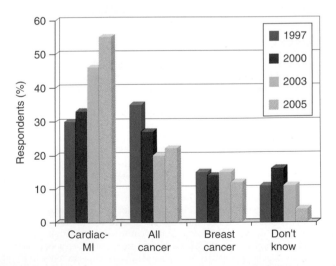

**FIGURE 50-2.** Trends in American women's perception of the leading cause of death in women. MI, myocardial infarction. (Reproduced with permission from Mosca L, Mochari H, Christian A, et al. National Study of Women's Awareness, Preventive Action, and Barriers to Cardiovascular Health. *Circulation.* 2006;113:525-534.)

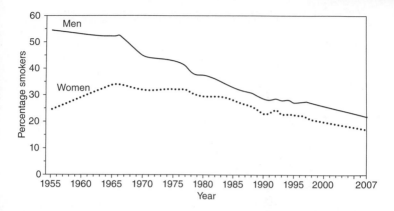

**FIGURE 50-3.** Prevalence of smoking among men and women age 18 years and younger in the United States. Before 1992, current smokers were defined as persons who reported having smoked more than 100 cigarettes and who currently smoked. Since 1992, current smokers have been defined as persons who reported having smoked more than 100 cigarettes during their lifetime and who reported now smoking every day or some days. (Reproduced with permission from Centers for Disease Control and Prevention. State-specific prevalence and trends in adult cigarette smoking–United States, 1998–2007. *MMWR Morb Mortal Wkly Rep.* 2009;58(9):221-226.)

a history of seizures, head trauma, heavy alcohol consumption, anorexia, bulimia, or recent use of monoamine oxidase inhibitors. Physicians can have a powerful effect on smoking cessation. While strong evidence supports avoiding tobacco exposure is important for women, additional research about sex and racial differences is needed.

## ■ DIABETES

Diabetes increases CAD mortality. In the past decade, coronary heart disease (CHD) mortality rates have increased by 23% in diabetic women, but they have decreased by 27% in nondiabetic women. In men with diabetes, mortality rates have declined by 13%, compared to a decrease of 36% in nondiabetic men. A prospective 25-year follow-up from Scotland revealed the highest mortality rates among those with both diabetes and known CHD (**Fig. 50-4**). The higher CAD risk for diabetic women has been noted in multiple population studies. It has been postulated that sex differences in endothelial function, especially endothelial-dependent vasodilation, may play a pathophysiologic role. Diabetic women have CAD rates similar to those of diabetic men, so the usual "female advantage" of later onset of CAD is lost.

The lifetime risk of developing CV disease (CVD) is related to the presence or absence of both diabetes and obesity. In the Framingham Heart Study, over 30 years, CVD occurred in 78% of women with diabetes compared with 38% women without diabetes. In nondiabetic women, CVD occurred in 46.7% of obese women and 34.3% of normal weight women. Most importantly, the risk of CVD over 30 years among obese women with diabetes was 78.8% but was only 54.8% in normal-weight diabetic women.

Compared to diabetic men, diabetic women have higher in-hospital mortality after MI and an increased incidence of congestive heart failure (CHF). In a review of data from the National Registry of Myocardial Infarction (NRMI) II, women's

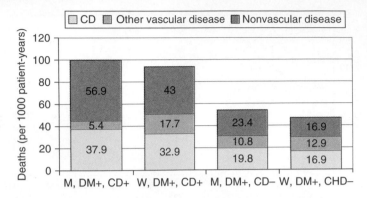

**FIGURE 50-4.** Mortality in diabetic patients followed prospectively for 25 years. Mortality (deaths per 1000 patient-years) from coronary heart disease (CD), other vascular disease, and nonvascular causes in men (M) and women (W) with and without diabetes (DM+ and DM–, respectively) and known coronary heart disease (CD+ and CD–respectively). (Data from Whiteley L, Padmanabhan S, Hole D, et al. Should diabetes be considered a coronary heart disease equivalent? Results from 25 years of follow-up in the Renfrew and Paisley Survey. *Diabetes Care.* 2005;28:1588-1593.)

increased mortality post-MI was associated with hypertension and hyperlipidemia, not glycemic control. It is unclear whether these observations reflect sex differences in risk factors, natural history, or how less aggressive CAD prevention in diabetic women plays a role. In telephone interviews of diabetic patients with CVD in 2001, aspirin use was reported by 54.7% of women and 82.7% of men (risk ratio [RR], 0.81; 95% CI, 0.70-0.90).

For diabetic women, the dose-response hazards of tobacco use have been documented in the Nurses' Health Study with 20 years of follow-up. The relative risk for a CAD event was 2.68 for current diabetic smokers of more than 15 cigarettes daily, 1.66 for current diabetic smokers of fewer than 15 cigarettes daily, and 1.21 for past diabetic smokers, all compared with women who had never smoked (*p* <0.001). Diabetic women who had not smoked for 10 years had a similar risk to nonsmoking diabetic women.

Among participants in the Framingham Heart Study from 1997 to 2005, diabetics at age 50 years had greater increases in body mass index (BMI) and cholesterol compared with nondiabetics at age 60 years and similar decreases in systolic blood pressure and tobacco use. Blood pressure control was achieved only in about 15% of diabetics and 36% of nondiabetics despite the higher CV risk among diabetics. Increased control of other CV risk factors is essential to decrease the overall CV risk associated with diabetes.

Women at risk for developing diabetes include obese women and those who have been diagnosed with gestational diabetes. Greater weight is associated with greater insulin resistance and decreased glucose tolerance. Even a moderate increase in physical activity and avoiding weight gain decreases the risk of developing diabetes.

Women with insulin resistance, characterized by elevated levels of circulating insulin, often have associated glucose intolerance, higher levels of free fatty acids, central obesity, and hypertension and are also at greater risk of developing diabetes. The *metabolic syndrome*, defined in the Third Report of the National Cholesterol Education Program Expert Panel on Detection, Evaluation, and Treatment of High Blood Cholesterol to include obesity, glucose intolerance, hypertension, and lipid abnormalities, occurs in women and men at greater rates with increasing age.

The metabolic syndrome is increasingly diagnosed at an early age; tobacco exposure from 12 to 19 years of age dramatically increases the risk for the metabolic syndrome. Polycystic ovarian syndrome (PCOS), with increased androgens, lower high-density lipoprotein (HDL) levels, and higher triglyceride levels and higher rates of CAD, may affect up to 10% to 20% of women of childbearing age. Women with PCOS, compared with age-, race-, and socioeconomic-matched controls, more often had diabetes, hypertension, and hyperlipidemia and had a higher prevalence of coronary artery calcification. Pharmacologic and lifestyle interventions, including regular exercise and aggressive management of tobacco use, lipoprotein abnormalities, and hypertension may improve prognosis and insulin resistance.

## ■ HYPERTENSION

The prevalence of hypertension increases with advancing age; because life expectancy is greater for women than men, there are more elderly women with hypertension. Although women are more likely to have hypertension than men, there are substantial racial and ethnic variations in hypertension prevalence: black, non-Hispanic women (43.4%) and men (40.4%) have higher rates than white, non-Hispanic women (28.4%) and men (27.5%) or Mexican American women (27.8%) and men (26.7%). Sex differences in autonomic nervous system function may explain difficulties in blood pressure modulation in some premenopausal women when they are exposed to stress or vasoactive drugs.

Both systolic and diastolic blood pressures predicted coronary events in population, cohort, and treatment studies. Framingham data revealed that with a systolic blood pressure above 180 mm Hg, the annual incidence of CHD (angina, coronary insufficiency, MI, or death from these diagnoses) in women older than 65 years was above 30%, but for men older than 65 years, it was approximately 50%. In other epidemiologic studies, higher diastolic blood pressure also predicted greater rates of clinical CAD. Through Framingham data analysis, predictors of new-onset isolated systolic hypertension included female sex, increasing age, and increased BMI during follow-up but not initial BMI. Lowering blood pressure decreases the incidence of first MI and sudden death, although this effect is less dramatic than the decrease in stroke occurrence with blood pressure control.

Sex-specific information about pharmacologic therapy of hypertension with angiotensin-converting enzyme (ACE) inhibitors and thiazide diuretics continues to evolve. ACE inhibitors should be used cautiously in women of reproductive age because teratogenic effects have been documented in the first trimester of pregnancy. Infants with only first-trimester ACE inhibitor exposure had an increased risk of CV and central nervous system malformations (RR, 2.71; CI, 1.72-4.27). Cough, a common side effect of first-generation ACE inhibitors but not the angiotensin receptor blockers (ARBs), occurs more frequently in women than in men. Thiazide diuretics are a preferred first choice in the treatment of hypertension in women as well as men, because of positive effects on bone health.

## ■ LIPIDS

There are sex differences in lipoprotein profiles and the impact of lipids on CV risk. Many experts consider HDL more predictive for women than any other lipoprotein component, with the strongest correlation between low HDL levels and CAD events. Low-density lipoprotein (LDL) levels increase with increasing age and are especially predictive of events in men. Triglyceride levels may be especially important in women. In fact, enlarged waist (>88 cm) combined with elevated triglycerides (≥1.45 mmol/L) best prospectively identified postmenopausal women at CV risk followed over 8 years.

Although secondary prevention with pharmacologic treatment of hyperlipidemia decreases CAD events in women as well as men, these agents are underprescribed for women after MI, and target treatment levels are often not reached. Primary prevention trials for hyperlipidemia in women with HMG-CoA reductase inhibitors (which simultaneously decrease LDL and increase HDL) have not demonstrated a reduction in mortality, perhaps due to low event rates. With the latest cholesterol treatment guidelines, diabetic women are candidates for primary prevention with aggressive treatment of lipid abnormalities. There is still controversy about the cost-to-benefit ratio for aggressive treatment in women at low risk for vascular disease.

# ■ OBESITY

The prevalence of obesity in the United States has increased over the past 40 years. Substantial ethnic and racial differences in obesity as measured by BMI exist (**Fig. 50-5**). Racial differences in BMI, as well as glycosylated hemoglobin, start in childhood, with black and Mexican American girls having less favorable profiles than white girls.

Obesity is linked to multiple cardiac risk factors (including insulin resistance, diabetes, hypertension, and hyperlipidemia) and is independently associated with coronary artery event rates. The pattern of weight distribution is also predictive of coronary events, with more events among women with the "apple" shape, who have a greater abdominal girth, than among those with the "pear" shape, who have more weight on the hips and buttocks. A greater waist circumference increases health risk regardless of BMI.

Increased physical activity or weight loss is associated with a decreased risk of CAD events. Behavioral interventions to decrease weight have been most successful when there is a physical activity component. In the Nurses' Health Study, both

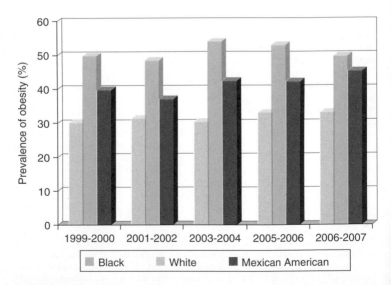

**FIGURE 50-5.** Prevalence of obesity (body mass index ≥30) in the National Health and Nutrition Examination Survey (NHANES) in women age 20 years and older by race and age. (Data from Flegal KM, Carroll MD, Ogden CL, et al. Prevalence and trends in obesity among US adults, 1999–2008. *JAMA.* 2010;303:235-241.)

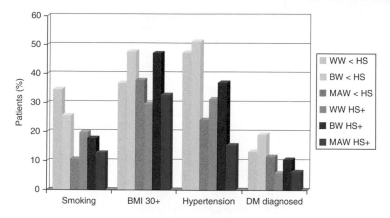

**FIGURE 50-6.** Selected cardiovascular risk factors for women by self-reported race and high school completion (fewer years of formal schooling or at least high school graduation). Smoking and diabetes data from the Behavioral Risk Factor Surveillance System and Obesity (body mass index [BMI] ≥30) or hypertension defined by blood pressure above 140/90 mm Hg, self-reported current use of antihypertensive medication, or having been given a hypertension diagnosis by a health professional at least twice from the National Health and Nutrition Survey, 1999 to 2002. BW, black women; DM, diabetes mellitus; HS, high school; MAW, Mexican-American women; WW, white women. (Data from Mensah G, Mokdad A, Ford E, et al. State of disparities in cardiovascular health in the United States. *Circulation.* 2005;111:1233-1241.)

BMI above 25 and physical activity were important predictors of CHD in 20-year follow-up (**Fig. 50-6**). Although new pharmacologic treatments for obesity have been developed, many have been documented to be hazardous.

## ■ PHYSICAL ACTIVITY AND EXERCISE

Women's physiologic response to exercise includes a lower work capacity and oxygen uptake than men. This occurs because women's cardiac output is predominantly increased by increasing heart rate. Men, in comparison, accomplish an increase in cardiac output predominantly by increasing stroke volume. In observing women health professionals over an average of 5 years, women who walked at least 1 hour each week had half the CHD rate as women who did not walk regularly. Women and men benefit from referral to cardiac rehabilitation programs after MI, but fewer women are referred and participate in cardiac rehabilitation.

## ■ MENOPAUSE AND HORMONAL THERAPY

The importance of the menstrual cycle and menopause as risk factors for CAD in women is still being defined. Women with early menopause after gynecologic surgery are thought to be at higher risk for CAD and osteoporosis, but a 1999 analysis from the Nurses' Health Study found only women smokers with a younger age of menopause have a greater risk of CAD.

Although population surveys suggested hormonal therapy after menopause decreased the risk of CAD, women using hormones tended to be healthier and wealthier: they reported less tobacco exposure, greater levels of exercise, and readier access to medical care. The Women's Health Initiative (WHI), a prospective randomized clinical trial of women 50 to 79 years of age, revealed that the combination of estrogen and progestin after menopause increases CAD risk. Estrogen alone does not decrease CAD risk in women without a uterus, and is contraindicated in women with a uterus because of the increased risk of endometrial cancer. In contrast, the observational Nurses' Health Study noted that women beginning hormonal therapy soon after menopause had lower CHD risk (RR, 0.72; 95% CI, 0.56-0.92 for estrogen and progesterone and RR, 0.6; 95% CI, 0.54-0.80 for estrogen alone) than women beginning treatment 10 years after menopause.

National guidelines reflect these results and emphasize modalities for the prevention of heart disease in women that do *not* include hormonal therapy. Hormonal therapy use is currently limited to control severe vasomotor symptoms.

## ■ PSYCHOSOCIAL RISK FACTORS

Both socioeconomic and psychological factors affect the prevalence and outcome of CAD (see Chapter 96). Coronary disease morbidity and mortality are greater among those of lower socioeconomic status (SES). Markers for SES include years of formal education, owning a car, income, sex, parental status, race, and ethnicity.

The prevalence of common CV risk factors were analyzed in white, black, and Mexican Americans comparing individuals with self-reported completion of high school education or fewer years of formal education. As in other population studies, white women had the highest prevalence of smoking, especially those with less education. Obesity, hypertension, and self-reported diabetes were especially prevalent in black women, and obesity levels did not vary by years of education. For all groups, rates of hypertension and self-reported diabetes were more common in those who had not completed high school (see Fig. 50-6). Similarly, in the Coronary Artery Risk Development in Young Adults Study, education level was inversely associated with baseline smoking, BMI, and systolic blood pressure. Positive computed tomography coronary artery calcium levels was also inversely related to education in both sexes and in both blacks and whites.

Exploration of individual women's attitudes has provided additional insights into the incidence of CAD. WHI participants underwent initial psychological evaluations and were then divided into quartiles based on how optimistic versus pessimistic they were. The most optimistic women were characterized by higher education, income, employment rates, and likelihood of attending religious services at least weekly. Optimism did not correlate with race. After eight years of follow up, optimists had lower age-adjusted rates of CHD and all-cause mortality compared with pessimists. These outcomes were independent of other CHD risk factors. Women characterized as cynical and hostile were less educated, had lower incomes, were more likely to use tobacco, and were more sedentary with higher rates of diabetes and depression. Not surprisingly, the optimists were less cynical. The most cynical quartile experienced higher rates of CHD and all-cause mortality.

Depression is diagnosed twice as often in women as in men and affects CAD outcomes. Depressive symptoms were common in the women in the observational arm of the WHI study, which excluded participants with major depression, with significant racial and ethnic variation. Hispanic and American Indian Alaskan Native women had the highest rates of depression, and Asian and Pacific Islander American women had the lowest rates. There were even larger differences by educational level, with 30% prevalence among women with less than an eighth-grade education compared with 13% for women with a college degree. History of CAD symptoms and diagnoses increased the risk of depression to a greater degree than a history of cancer. For women without CAD, history followed for over 4 years, depressive symptoms adjusted for age, and race was independently associated with a 58% higher CVD mortality rate (RR, 1.58; 95% CI, 1.19-2.10). In multivariate analysis, even including pharmacologic treatment of depression, the increased risk persisted.

Depressive symptoms screened for at hospitalization in the Prospective Registry Evaluation Outcomes After Myocardial Infarction: Events and Recovery (PREMIER) study were common (40% of women and 22% of men ≤60 years compared with 21% of women and 15% of men >60 years). In this cohort, the depressed young women had more comorbidity and less favorable health and SES. Only 18% of those who were depressed were discharged with antidepressant medications. Pharmacologic treatment for depression after MI decreases the rate of both recurrent MI and death.

Acute and reversible cardiomyopathy has been documented after profound emotional stress. An acute and reversible severe cardiomyopathy predominantly noted in women was first described in Japan as *takotsubo*. Takotsubo is a stress cardiomyopathy characterized by acute onset of symptoms, usually substernal chest pain or dyspnea, most often associated with ST-segment elevation or T wave inversion, with profound systolic dysfunction and the absence of significant luminal narrowing at angiography. Patients are usually postmenopausal and experience severe emotional or physical distress prior to the onset of cardiac symptoms. Severe left ventricular systolic dysfunction comes in four classic morphologies: ballooning of the apex, both ventricles, midventricle, or the bases. This ballooning usually resolves in anywhere from 5 days to 2 months. Takotsubo cardiomyopathy may be under-diagnosed, with reports varying between less than 2.3% up and 6% to 12% of women presenting with anterior MI. Mortality is low, and patients generally do well with supportive treatment.

## ■ RACE, WOMEN, AND CORONARY ARTERY DISEASE

Racial differences in mortality, risk factors, and physiology have also begun to be considered (see Chapter 104). Black women's CAD mortality rates are related to traditional CAD risk factors as well as racial and socioeconomic issues. Combined analysis of data from the 1986 National Mortality Feedback Survey, the 1985 National Health Interview Survey, and the US Bureau of the Census revealed that black women younger than 55 years had more than twice the rate of CAD mortality (sudden and nonsudden) as young white Americans. CAD death rates for young black women in this study exceeded rates for young men and white women. Importantly, family income, educational level, and occupational status accounted for more of this observed difference than traditional coronary risk factors.

With the application of careful methodology, Mexican American women have CHD mortality rates higher or equal to those of non-Hispanic white American women. This observation is consistent with the higher rates of obesity, hypertension, and diabetes among Mexican American women than among white women, even if tobacco use is less frequent. Fewer data are available on Asian Indian immigrants and those living in India, but preliminary publications report high CAD rates at a young age in both men and women.

## ■ SIGNIFICANT COMORBIDITIES: LUPUS, RHEUMATOID ARTHRITIS, AND MIGRAINE HEADACHES

Increasing attention has been paid to the relationship between medical illness associated with inflammation and the development of CAD. A case-control evaluation using population-based data from the United Kingdom–based General Practice Research Database compared 8688 patients with MI with matched control subjects. A higher risk of MI was seen in patients with systemic lupus erythematosus (SLE) and rheumatoid arthritis (RA).

The increased risk for CAD in patients with SLE is not fully explained by traditional risk factors. Even when 122 SLE patients without clinical CAD were initially assessed, 37.7% had myocardial perfusion defects; with a median of 8.7 years follow-up, there was one MI, and 14 individuals had new-onset angina. Myocardial defects were predictive with an HR of 13.0 (95% CI, 2.8-60.1; $p = 0.001$). Of interest, Framingham risk scores were "low risk."

RA has also been associated with increased CV mortality and morbidity. CAD may occur a decade earlier than expected. Higher rates of CV morbidity and mortality are

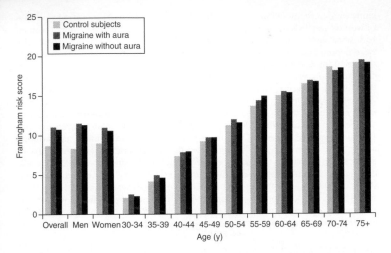

**FIGURE 50-7.** Mean Framingham risk scores as a function of migraine headache status and patient characteristics. (Reproduced with permission from Bigal ME, Kurth T, Santanello N, et al. Migraine and cardiovascular disease: a population-base study. *Neurology.* 2010;74:628-635.)

likely due to inflammation, as demonstrated by elevations in inflammatory markers like tumor necrosis factor-$\alpha$ (TNF–$\alpha$) and interleukin-6 (IL-6) and in CT-obtained coronary calcium scores, as compared with age- and sex-matched control subjects. Both methotrexate and anti-TNF therapies, which decrease the inflammatory process in RA, are associated with lower rates of CAD.

Migraine headaches, especially those with aura, are an evolving risk factor for CAD. Because migraines occur in 18% of American women compared with 6% of men, the CV implications may especially impact the care of women. The Women's Health Study, developed to assess low-dose aspirin for primary prevention, found that women with migraines with aura had more major CVD events, including angina, MI, coronary revascularization, and death from CAD over 10 years of follow-up. Most recently, the American Migraine Perception and Prevention study followed 120 000 US households for 5 years, with more than 9000 individuals surveyed and compared with 10 000 control subjects. Individuals with migraines were more often women (80.3% vs 53%; $p$ <0.0001) and older, and migraine headaches were significantly associated with MI risk. This was reflected in comparison of Framingham scores by migraine type (**Fig. 50-7**). Migraine sufferers were also more likely to have other cardiac risk factors, like diabetes, hypertension, or hyperlipidemia.

# DIAGNOSIS OF CORONARY ARTERY DISEASE IN WOMEN

The risk of CAD increases with older age. Evaluation of CAD and stroke risk in adults aged 35 to 54 years has revealed some important trends comparing 1988 to 1994 with 1999 to 2004. Although the rates of CAD rates are higher for men than women in both time periods, over time, rates are decreasing in men and increasing in women. Except for increasing rates of diabetes among all individuals, cardiac risk factor reduction has occurred more in men than women.

Furthermore, the stroke risk among adults of age 45 to 54 years is twice as high for women as for men.

Because CAD is often diagnosed clinically by a careful history, preconceived biases can affect the perception of CAD risk. Primary care physicians more often rated intermediate-risk women as low risk compared with men with the same risk factors. When physicians viewed a video of different actors (black and white women and men) accompanied by the same written information, the black woman was least likely to be referred for cardiac catheterization. Adequate assessment of CAD risk and severity is required for appropriate evaluation and management to occur.

When CAD is considered as a diagnosis, noninvasive stress testing aids in the assessment of disease presence and severity in individuals with intermediate risk for CAD. More extensive discussion can be found in Chapters 15 and 20, but potential sex differences in noninvasive testing are discussed briefly here. Exercise stress testing has lower sensitivity and specificity in women, in part related to lower ECG voltage. In multiple populations, women have been noted to have more frequent ST–T-wave abnormalities, and so sex-specific criteria have been proposed to compensate for the generally smaller ST-segment changes seen in women. After exercise stress testing, the maximal exercise capacity and heart rate recovery in women are important prognostically. Among asymptomatic women with low-risk Framingham scores, those with lower exercise capacity and slower heart rate recovery are at increased risk for CV death. In women, nuclear stress perfusion testing with thallium can be hindered by attenuation from breast tissue, so technetium may be preferred. Stress echocardiography is highly dependent on operator expertise and may be technically difficult in obese patients.

Patterns of referral for cardiac catheterization may vary by sex, with some appropriate differences. Because cardiac catheterization is less likely to reveal CAD in women, many clinicians initially evaluate women at intermediate risk with stress imaging. For example, anginal symptoms are less predictive of abnormal coronary anatomy in women than men (**Fig. 50-8**). Direct referral to cardiac catheterization

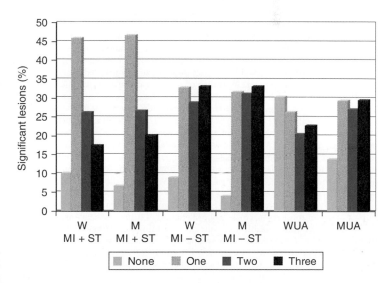

**FIGURE 50-8.** Comparison of chest pain clinical presentation scenarios and risk of having coronary artery disease on testing. M, men; MI, myocardial infarction; UA, unstable angina; W, women. (Data from Snow V, Barry P, Fihn SD, et al. Evaluation of primary care patients with chronic stable angina: guidelines from the American College of Physicians. *Ann Intern Med.* 2004;141:57-64.)

should occur in patients with a high suspicion of significant CAD that might benefit from intervention. In a registry of patients in Alberta, Canada, undergoing cardiac catheterization from 1995 to 2000, women comprised only 29.9% of the cohort. Women were older, had more comorbid conditions, and had a higher 1-year mortality (5.6% vs 4.6%; $p$ <0.001) that occurred early after percutaneous transluminal coronary angioplasty or catheterization.

Exploration of the specific type of coronary lesions identified by sex with early multidetector computed tomographic angiography (MDCTA) studies reveals possible important sex differences. In 416 consecutive symptomatic patients (36% female) without prior known CAD referred for similar reasons, women had higher rates of diabetes and family history of CAD. As might be expected, more women than men had no CAD (23% vs 6%; $p$ <0.0001); women also had less luminal narrowing of 70% or greater (12% vs 25%; $p$ <0.0001). Further use of this methodology may provide important insights into sex differences in the pathophysiology and natural history.

# MANAGEMENT OF CORONARY ARTERY DISEASE IN WOMEN

## ■ ASYMPTOMATIC WOMEN

Some individuals are truly asymptomatic, while others may have atypical symptoms that were not diagnosed as possible CAD. In several population studies, more than 25% of MIs were not clinically recognized, and a history of angina was lacking. After 34 years of Framingham follow-up, 34% of women and 26% of men had MIs unidentified by their physicians. Of these patients, 33% of women and 24% of men had a history of angina compared with 45% of women and 53% of men with recognized MI. Mortality for women is similar after an unrecognized or recognized MI.

For truly asymptomatic women, national guidelines for prevention are developing. Counseling for asymptomatic women about CAD should include a review of the common risk factors and symptoms of CAD as well as encouragement for implementing a healthy lifestyle. The only randomized, controlled trial of aspirin for primary prevention of CVD in women of age 45 years or older was the Women's Health Study, which included more than 39 000 women professionals who received 100 mg of aspirin on alternating days or placebo with 10 years of follow-up. There was a significant decrease in ischemic strokes, but no significant decrease in CV risk or MI. In subgroup analysis, aspirin at 100 mg every other day decreased MI, ischemic stroke, and major CV events in women over age 65. In a recent meta-analysis of international primary prevention data including aspirin doses from 100 mg on alternating days to 500 mg daily, the proportional improvement was similar in women and men, and the smaller number of women may explain the better outcomes for ischemic stroke ( **Fig. 50-9**).

Prospective cohort studies have been used to develop models to predict the impact of one or more risk factors on the likelihood of future coronary artery events. From data in National Health and Nutrition Examination Survey (NHANES) III, more than 90% of CAD events occur among those with at least one of the following risk factors: smoking, blood pressure, low LDL and HDL level, and glucose intolerance. When multiple individual risk factors are present, the cumulative risk of CAD is greater than the sum of its parts.

Clustered risk factors were an important predictor in the Framingham Offspring Study (patients aged 30-74 years at enrollment), in which 17% of all participants had 3 of the 6 risk factors (lowest-quintile HDL cholesterol, highest-quintile cholesterol, BMI, systolic blood pressure, triglycerides, and glucose). With 16 years of follow-up

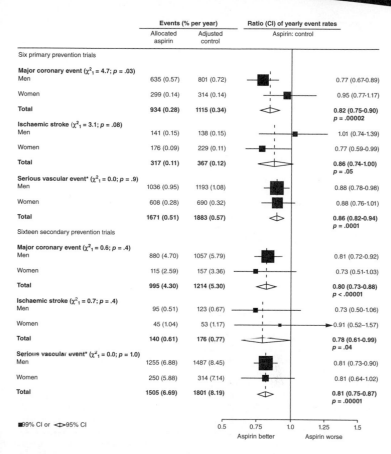

**FIGURE 50-9.** Selected outcomes in primary and secondary prevention trials of aspirin by sex. CI, confidence interval. (Reproduced with permission from Antithrombotic Trialists Collaboration. Aspirin in the primary and secondary prevention of vascular disease: collaborative meta-analysis of individual participant data from randomized trials. *Lancet.* 2009;373:1849-1860.)

for coronary artery events (MI or sudden death), there were 79 first coronary artery events among the 1818 women who were initially free of symptomatic CAD compared with 229 events among the 1759 men. However, CAD events were associated with 3 or more risk factors for 48% of the CAD events in women and 20% of the CAD events in men.

The 2007 guidelines for cardiovascular disease prevention in women created a new algorithm for risk stratification in women: "at high risk" includes documented CVD, diabetes, end-stage or chronic kidney disease, or 10-year predicted risk for CHD >20% based on the Framingham risk score; "at risk" due to the presence of 1 or more major cardiac risk factors, metabolic syndrome, evidence of subclinical vascular disease, or poor exercise tolerance on treadmill testing; and "at optimal risk" with a Framingham risk score <10%, no major cardiac risk factors, and adherence to a healthy lifestyle. The 2011 guidelines also included this algorithm.

# ■ ANGINA

As described from Framingham data, the first presentation of symptomatic CAD is typically angina in women and MI in men. The prevalence of angina is similar in women and men, but women have less angiographic documented CAD. Although less severe obstruction decreases the need for surgery and stents, the prognosis and treatment require additional physician efforts. As the spectrum of CAD in women is further explored, alternative pathophysiologic models have been proposed (**Fig. 50-10**).

The clinical diagnosis of angina can be challenging. Women generally visit physicians more often than men and report more symptoms, including chest pain. Women compared with men with angina more frequently report angina with emotional or mental stress. Too often, older women ascribe their decreased ability to complete housework or walk to getting old.

The prognosis after the clinical diagnosis of angina is evolving. Daly et al reported on the evaluation and medical care of 3779 men and women diagnosed with stable angina between March and December 2002 who were seen by cardiologists throughout study centers in Europe for the first time or for the first consultation in at least 1 year. Women were less likely to receive antiplatelet or statin medications, referral for exercise stress testing (0.81; 95% CI, 0.69-0.95), or coronary angiography (0.59; 95% CI, 0.48-0.73). Similar to other studies, anginal symptoms in women are less predictive of abnormal coronary anatomy than in men (see Fig. 50-9). Coronary angiography was completed in 34% of women and 47% of men; even after adjustment for multiple clinical factors, women were 40% to 50% less likely to undergo angiography. Results of the completed angiography revealed coronary disease among 63% of women compared with 87% of men. Women had less revascularization and yet more death and nonfatal MI during 1 year of follow-up than men (2.09; 95% CI, 1.13-3.85). Major clinical events after 1 year occurred at higher rates among those with CAD on angiography than those with only a clinical diagnosis of angina. Therefore, women with angina, even without substantial coronary obstruction, should receive aggressive CV risk factor management.

Natural history data can help guide the care of women without obstructive CAD. The degree of coronary artery obstruction predicted outcomes at 5 years, specifically hospital admissions for heart failure and stroke. The CV event rate increased with more documented obstruction and the increased prevalence of CV risk factors (see Fig. 50-1 at cardiac catheterization). A subset of women without obstructive disease underwent magnetic resonance spectroscopy with handgrip exercising. Outcomes over the next 3 years correlated with whether there was an ischemic response (43% if abnormal and 13% if normal). Although one prospective study of focused stress reduction in women decreased mortality, more research is needed.

The relationship between the menstrual cycle and vascular spasm has received some attention. The menstrual cycle can be divided into menstrual, follicular (from menses to ovulation, high estrogen levels), and luteal (ovulation to menses, low estrogen and high progesterone levels) phases using historical timing, basal body temperature, bleeding patterns, and laboratory results. In a study of premenopausal women with a history of vasospastic angina and normal cardiac catheterization, all cardiac medication was held for a full menstrual cycle, with assessment of morning estrogen and progesterone levels, ST-Holter monitoring, and flow-mediated dilation measurement of the brachial artery. The average number of ischemic episodes was greatest in the luteal phase, inversely correlated with flow-mediated vasodilation of the brachial artery. Other studies have also raised speculation about the importance of documenting when in the menstrual cycle a stress test is completed. More research is required to determine the clinical significance of these findings.

Secondary prevention should be initiated with the diagnosis of angina, including control of risk factors and appropriate pharmacologic therapies (aspirin and lipid-lowering agents but usually not hormone replacement therapy).

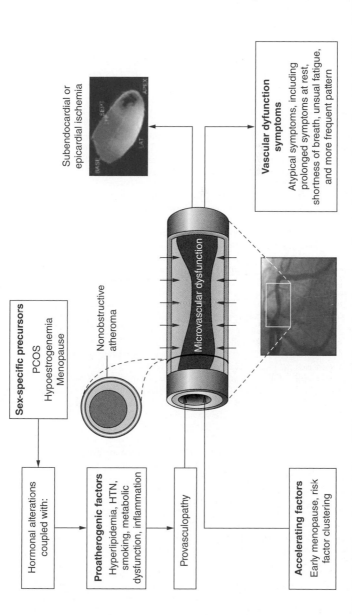

**FIGURE 50-10.** Model of microvascular angina in women. HTN, hypertension; PCOS, polycystic ovarian syndrome. (Reproduced with permission from Shaw LJ, Bugiardini R, Merz NB. Women and ischemic heart disease: evolving knowledge *J Am Coll of Cardiol.* 2009;54:1561-1575.)

# ACUTE CORONARY ISCHEMIA, INCLUDING ACUTE MYOCARDIAL INFARCTION

There are substantial sex differences in the presentation and natural history of acute coronary ischemia, including both unstable angina and MI. Anatomic lesions may be less common in women, because of differences in vascular tone and microvascular or endothelial dysfunction. Women with acute ischemia may present with upper abdominal symptoms like nausea, neck or jaw pain, or shortness of breath, rather than crushing chest pain. Atypical symptoms are more common in older patients and those with diabetes.

Sex differences in the spectrum of acute coronary ischemic events, natural history, and 5-year prognosis were explored in Alberta, Canada, from 1993 through 2000. More women than men were diagnosed with unstable angina (32.3% compared with 24.1%; $p$ <0.001), and women had lower rates of inpatient angiography within 6 months. Whereas crude mortality rates for women and men with unstable angina were similar, women over age 65 had a survival advantage in multivariate analysis (HR, 0.81; 95% CI, 0.72-0.92).

Sex differences with MI and during follow-up have been increasingly considered. After MI, women were nearly as likely to have cardiac catheterization, angioplasty, or stenting but still underwent CABG less often (adjusted prevalence ratio [PR], 0.78; 95% CI, 0.77-0.79). This is consistent with women having lower rates of multivessel obstructive disease. Through the 1990s in the Worcester, Massachusetts metropolitan area, there has been increased use of catheterization and percutaneous coronary interventions (PCIs) after MI with greater increases for women than men.

Data from the Thrombogenic Factors and Recurrent Coronary Events (THROMBO) trial on patients who had survived at least 2 months after MI and that included 26% women showed that the women were older and had higher rates of hypertension, diabetes, and pulmonary congestion than men. Similar rates of ST-elevation MI were noted in women and men, but in 3.5 years of follow-up, women had a higher rate of cardiac events (30% women, 22% men; $p$ = 0.02). After a week, persistent anterior ST elevations in women and persistent lateral ST depression in men increased the rate of recurrent cardiac events.

The interaction of sex and age was explored with data available from the NRMI II. As in other data sets, women with MI are often older and have more comorbid conditions than men. Analysis of the interaction of sex and age revealed that the 30-day mortality after MI was approximately twice as great for women aged 30 to 50 years compared with men of the same age and progressively decreased with increasing age until reaching unity at age 75 years (**Fig. 50-11** ).

Clinical trial data are more complex. Of note, women are generally underrepresented in clinical trials. Sex differences in mortality after acute coronary syndrome admissions were analyzed from data from 11 independent clinical trials completed at Duke Clinical Research Institute. Women were older and had more comorbidities, including hypertension, diabetes, hyperlipidemia, and heart failure. More men were smokers or had prior MI. Before adjustments for comorbidities, women had a higher mortality with ST-elevation MI and lower mortality compared with men for non–ST-elevation MI and unstable angina. After adjustment for comorbidities, differences were only significant for women with ST-elevation MI despite women having less occlusive disease.

There has been less study of sex differences in health status and morbidity 30 days after MI. In a retrospective analysis of PREMIER (Prospective Registry Evaluating Myocardial Infarction) enrollment from 2003 to 2004, 32% of participants were women. The women were older and more often had hypertension, diabetes, chronic obstructive pulmonary disease (COPD), non–ST-elevation MI, and unstable angina than men. Women were as likely to have catheterization but less often had revascularization. On phone interviews at about 30 days, more than 25% of both women

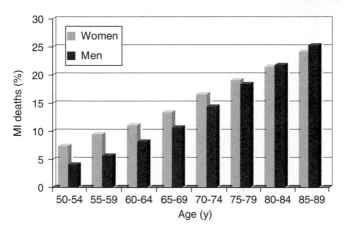

**FIGURE 50-11.** Mortality after myocardial infarction: sex differences by age. (From Vaccarino V, Parsons L, Every NR, et al. Sex-based differences in early mortality after myocardial infarction. *N Engl J Med.* 1999;341:217-225.)

and men experienced angina, but women reported poorer quality of life and physical functioning.

Acute MI in pregnancy was reviewed among a 2000 to 2002 Nationwide Inpatient Survey; the rate was 6.2 per 100 000 deliveries in the United States (3-4 times higher than nonpregnant women in the same age range). Most MIs occurred during an admission for pregnancy (73%), but 27% occurred during a postpartum admission. The most substantial risk factor was increasing age older than 20 years. In multivariate analysis, the most prominent risk factors were thrombophilia, hypertension, age 35 years and older compared with age younger than 20 years, smoking, bleeding requiring blood transfusion, diabetes, and black race. Of women with pregnancy-related MI, 45% had cardiac catheterization and 45% had subsequent intervention (angioplasty, stent placement, or surgery). Coronary artery dissection as a complication may occur. The mortality rate for MI during pregnancy was 5.1%.

Although medical therapy that provides survival advantage after MI has been well defined, women have historically received these treatments less and do not reach blood pressure and lipid goals as often as men. In long-term follow-up after MI, women tend to have more angina and CHF despite better systolic left ventricular function.

Aggressive management of associated risk factors after MI may especially benefit women. In the Third National Health and Nutrition Survey, a focus on secondary prevention revealed women, blacks, and those of ages 46 to 65 years were more likely to have more than 2 poorly controlled major risk factors. Cardiac rehabilitation is equally effective for women, but participation continues to be lower for women than men after MI (age-adjusted OR, 1.8; 95% CI, 1.5-2.1).

## ■ INTERVENTIONS FOR CORONARY ARTERY DISEASE

Understanding of sex differences in the prevalence and complications of PCIs and CABG surgery is evolving. At least 33% of PCIs are performed in women. The development of smaller coronary artery catheters only partially decreased the sex difference in complications. Women are more likely to experience short-term vascular complication rates, including problems at the access site, retroperitoneal bleeding, and higher transfusion requirements, which may be due to older age at time of procedure, more medical comorbidities, and longer duration of symptoms compared with men. In the American College of Cardiology National Cardiovascular Registry from 2004 to 2006, there were no sex differences in the use of drug-eluting stents. Women were less often discharged with aspirin or statins and yet had lower subacute stent thrombosis (0.43 vs 0.57%; $p = 0.0003$).

CABG surgery is more commonly performed in men than women. In a population-based study in Ontario, Canada, from 1991 to 2002, only 22% of those who underwent CABG were women. Although the internal mammary artery (IMA) is associated with the best short- and long-term results, women have lower rates of IMA use. Reasons for avoiding IMA grafts might include smaller size, higher rates of diabetes in women undergoing CABG, and the decreased use of IMA grafting in the setting of osteoporosis. After hospital discharge, women had a lower mortality rate but more readmissions (without analysis of reason for readmission).

CABG complications was explored among 9218 Michigan Medicare beneficiaries who had CABG from 1997 to 1998; 37.6% were women. During the CABG hospitalization, the infection rate was 16.1% for women compared with 9.8% for men ($p <0.001$). The most common sites of infection were respiratory followed by urinary tract, gastrointestinal, and skin. Infections requested mortality for both women and men during the hospitalization and at 30 and 100 days after CABG. Of interest, 96% of the sex difference at 100-day mortality was related to infection. In a study of off-pump CABG, women had more wound infections and longer hospitalizations. Among patients at least 75 years old at the time of CABG in the Society of Thoracic Surgeons' voluntary database, women were more likely to have emergency surgery and had higher operative mortality, more pulmonary and vascular complications, and longer hospitalizations.

# ■ CONGESTIVE HEART FAILURE

CHF prevalence has continued to increase as life expectancy has increased. The cause has been shifting from low systolic ejection fraction (EF) from CAD to preserved systolic function from hypertension, especially in those older than 70 years. Mortality and morbidity, including hospitalization rates, are substantial regardless of EF. Mortality rates among those younger than 65 years at diagnosis are lower for women than men (70% compared with 80%).

Women with CHF tend to have preserved systolic function and are generally older, with higher rates of hypertension, and less CAD. In the Alberta Provincial Project for Outcome Assessment in Coronary Heart Disease (APPROACH) cohort, among the 80% of enrollees with a documented EF, women more often had preserved EF (women were 46.2% of those with preserved EF compared with 30.6% of those with low EF). Women with CHF were also older and had higher rates of hypertension. Morality over 6.5 years was greater among patients with low EF (<50%) than those with preserved systolic function regardless of sex (women with low EF HR, 1.5; 95% CI, 1.1-2.0; men with low EF HR, 1.6; 95% CI, 1.2-2.1).

Although the use of implantable cardioverter-defibrillators (ICDs) has increased among patients with low EF, the lower rate of participation of women in clinical trials has limited sex-specific analysis. Completion of a pooled analysis of the 5 prospective, randomized clinical trials that published mortality data by sex was complicated by substantial design heterogeneity. None of these trials revealed a statistically significant mortality benefit for women (pooled analysis HR, 1.01; 95% CI, 0.76-1.33; $p = 0.95$).

As in other areas, pharmacologic treatment for CHF has included limited assessment for sex-specific differences. Significant sex outcome differences were noted in a post-hoc analysis of the randomized clinical trial of the Digitalis Investigation

Group, in which 6800 participants with stable CHF and an EF of 45% or below were randomized to digoxin or a placebo. Mortality overall was higher in women randomized to digoxin than to placebo (33.1% vs 28.9%) compared with men where the difference was not significant. Multivariate analysis for women receiving digoxin revealed an adjusted all-cause mortality HR of 1.23 (95% CI, 1.02-1.47).

## ■ SUDDEN DEATH

Sudden death occurs more often in American men than women (1.3-1.4:1). Rates have not changed for American women but are decreasing for American men. Whereas out-of-hospital cardiac arrest in men is associated with ventricular tachycardia and fibrillation, women have higher rates of asystole and pulseless electrical activity. In an evaluation of 2568 sudden death cases in Oregon from 2002 to 2007, women were 36% of the sample and were less likely to have evidence of previously recognized CAD or severe left ventricular dysfunction (EF ≤35%). In the Nurses' Health Study, high levels of phobic anxiety in women were associated with an increased risk of fatal CAD, including sudden death, even after controlling for comorbidities. Also, the prognosis of silent MI requires further exploration; sudden death is one possible sequela, as documented in an autopsy study where 2 of the 51 women with sudden death had a documented prior MI, but 35% of the sample had evidence of a prior MI. The acute thrombus associated with plaque erosion (often noted in early atherosclerosis) occurred more often in younger women smokers without obesity, high cholesterol, or elevated glycohemoglobin. In comparison, plaque rupture was more often found in older women.

## ARRHYTHMIAS

Women generally have a higher heart rate than men and respond to increasing cardiac demand by increasing heart rate rather than increasing stroke volume. Women in their seventh decade with a heart rate above 77 bpm had substantially higher CV (>77 bpm; ROR, 13.99, 95% CI, 1.93-101.16) and all-cause mortality rates (>77 bpm; ROR, 3.71; 95% CI, 1.41-9.80) than women with slower pulses with 6 years of follow-up after controlling for potential confounders such as prior CVD, smoking, hypertension, activity level, and anemia. When women exposed to β-blockers were excluded, the results were more dramatic. This association was not statistically significant in men within the same cohort.

Sex differences in the incidence and management of arrhythmias have been noted. There is a female predominance of atrioventricular node reentrant tachycardia and orthodromic supraventricular tachycardia, but men are more likely to have atrial and ventricular fibrillation, sudden death from ventricular tachycardia and fibrillation, and atrioventricular reentry associated with Wolff-Parkinson-White syndrome. In a prospective study of initially healthy women followed for more than 12 years, the incidence of atrial fibrillation was greater with higher systolic and diastolic blood pressure even with blood pressures less than 140/90 mm Hg. Although the use of radiofrequency catheter ablation for the treatment of supraventricular reentrant tachycardias has been increasing, there are limited data on sex differences.

Implantable ICDs are used in men more often than in women. In a meta-analysis of ICD for primary prevention, there was only a 12% reduction in death from any cause for women compared with a 24% mortality reduction in men. In consecutive patients receiving ICDs in Ottawa, fewer women received ICDs for primary (male:female ratio, 8.5:1; *p* <0.01) and secondary prevention (male:female ratio, 4.5:1; *p* <0.01). The women had more CHF and diabetes but less ischemic heart disease. The discharge rate was similar regardless of sex. Complications of ICD insertion are more common in women. A recent meta-analysis raises questions about ICD benefit among women with advanced heart failure.

Overall, women have a higher risk of dying of atrial fibrillation compared with age- and sex-matched control subjects (OR for men, 1.5; for women, 1.9). In a randomized controlled trial comparing rate and rhythm control in patients with atrial fibrillation despite prior electrical cardioversion, the primary end points (composite of death from CVD, heart failure, thromboembolism complications, bleeding, the need for pacemaker implantation, or severe adverse effects of antiarrhythmic agents) had important sex differences. For women, rhythm control had substantially worse outcomes with an absolute difference of 21.5 (95% CI, 30.8-2.1). Therefore, it may be beneficial to focus on rate rather than rhythm control for women in persistent atrial fibrillation. Women are also less likely to be anticoagulated for atrial fibrillation than men. Anticoagulation may be especially important for women; a recent prospective study of patients with atrial fibrillation found that for those not taking warfarin sodium (Coumadin), women had higher embolism rates than men (3.5% compared with 1.8%; RR, 1.6; 95% CI, 1.3-1.9) after multivariable analysis. Interestingly, in this study, women on warfarin sodium (Coumadin) developed less intracranial bleeding than men. Women are also less likely to receive pacemakers.

Drug-induced torsade de pointes occurs more commonly in women than men. Risk factors may include the greater prevalence of congenital prolonged QT syndrome and higher rates of adverse drug reactions. A prospective study on the impact of the menstrual cycle on the development of torsade de pointes revealed the greatest increase in QT interval was seen in women during menses and in their ovulatory phase, compared with men and with women during the luteal phase of menstruation. QT intervals also vary by race and ethnicity; for example, Asian women have a QTc that is 10 milliseconds longer than other ethnic groups.

# SUMMARY

Significant differences in individual patient factors that affect diagnosis and management are emerging. Further exploration of these differences will improve care for individual patients. Identification of CAD in women can be improved by assessing possible angina symptoms and screening high-risk women. Women with clinical symptoms or documented CAD, even without documented lesions at catheterization, should receive aggressive secondary prevention. All physicians and patients must focus on primary and secondary prevention for both women and men.

# SUGGESTED READINGS

Charney P. Women and coronary artery disease. In: Fuster V, Walsh R, Harrington RA, et al. *Hurst's the Heart*. 13th ed. New York, NY: McGraw-Hill; 2011;103:2226-2240.

Berger JS, Elliot L, Gallup D, et al. Sex differences in mortality following acute coronary syndromes. *JAMA*. 2009;302(8):874-882.

Charney P, ed. *Coronary Artery Disease in Women: Prevention, Diagnosis and Management*. Philadelphia, PA: American College of Physicians; 1999.

Eitel I, von Knobelsdorff-Brenkenhoff F, Bernhardt P, et al. Clinical characteristics and cardiovascular magnetic resonance findings in stress (takotsubo) cardiomyopathy. *JAMA*. 2011 Jul 20;306(3):277-286.

Ghanbari H, Dalloul G, Hasan R, et al. Effectiveness of implantable cardioverter-defibrillators for the primary prevention of sudden cardiac death in women with advanced heart failure: a meta-analysis of randomized controlled trials. *Arch Intern Med*. 2009;169:1500-1506.

Guru V, Fremes SE, Austin PC, et al. Gender differences in outcomes after hospital discharge from coronary artery bypass grafting. *Circulation*. 2006;113:507-513.

Mosca L, Benjamin EJ, Kathy B, et al. Effectiveness-based guidelines for the prevention of cardio-vascular disease in women: 2011 Update. *Circulation.* 2011;123:1243-1262.

Mosca L, Linfante A, Benjamin E, et al. National Study of Physician Awareness and Adherence to Cardiovascular Disease Prevention Guidelines. *Circulation.* 2005;111:499-510.

Ridker PM, Cook NR, Lee IM, et al. A randomized trial of low-dose aspirin in the primary prevention of cardiovascular disease in women. *N Engl J Med.* 2005;352:1293-1304.

Schulman KA, Berlin JA, Harless W, et al. The effect of race and sex on physician's recommendations for cardiac catheterization. *N Engl J Med.* 1999;340:618-626.

# CHAPTER 51
# HEART DISEASE AND PREGNANCY

Jennifer Conroy, John H. McAnulty, Craig S. Broberg, and James Metcalfe

## HEART DISEASE ISSUES UNIQUE TO PREGNANCY

Heart disease is the second most common cause of maternal death in Western countries (suicide is first). Maternal health is a major determinant of fetal health. Fetal safety is an important consideration and generally informs the selection of diagnostics and therapies in the management of heart disease in pregnant women. Ultimately, however, maternal health is the highest priority. Sometimes the risk for the mother is sufficient to recommend avoidance or interruption of pregnancy (**Table 51-1**). For those who continue with pregnancy, diagnostic studies, drugs, or surgery may increase fetal loss, result in teratogenicity, or alter fetal growth. Additionally, uterine blood flow may already be compromised in a woman with heart disease, further increasing the possibility of inadequate uterine perfusion. Specific issues for newborns include potentially jeopardized early infant nourishment in the setting of severe maternal illness, transmission of cardiac medication to the infant via breast milk, and finally the potential loss of the mother due to heart disease.

The combination of heart disease with pregnancy exceeds the expertise of most care providers and, in fact, exceeds the capabilities of any single care provider. Care is best given by an experienced team that includes counselors, primary care providers, obstetricians, cardiologists, anesthesiologists, and pediatricians. Any woman with heart disease contemplating pregnancy should be educated by experienced care providers before conception.

## CLINICAL CONSIDERATIONS

### ■ CONTRACEPTION

All of the advantages and disadvantages of each method of birth control apply to women with heart disease. Any method can be considered for most women with heart disease, but potential fluid retention with depoprogesterone should guide its use. Although thromboemboli are of concern in many forms of heart disease, use of drugs with estrogen is safe in the nonsmoker if the estradiol content is less than 35 μg per tablet. Women at higher risk (WHO Class 3) should consider alternate forms of contraception besides combined hormonal contraceptives. Women with highest risk cardiac disease (WHO Class 4) should consider progesterone-only forms of contraception and intrauterine devices.

# ■ PRECONCEPTION

Antenatal care should include a discussion of the vulnerability issues explored above. The patient should be told which medications to avoid during pregnancy. Angiotensin-converting enzyme (ACE) inhibitors, and angiotensin II receptor blockers (ARBs) should be stopped. Consideration should be given to discontinuing warfarin. (see discussion of drugs below). Any needed diagnostic tests or interventions should be performed before risk to the fetus becomes a factor.

# ■ FIRST TRIMESTER

Once pregnancy is confirmed, medications should be re-assessed, again avoiding medications with teratogenic effects. Aspirin should be considered in cyanotic patients. If not already done, referral to an appropriate center of expertise with heart disease and pregnancy should begin. Parents should be educated on warning symptoms, need for scheduled imaging, optimal site for delivery, and type of delivery.

# ■ SECOND AND THIRD TRIMESTERS

The expected hemodynamic changes associated with pregnancy reach their peak near the 20th week. Women should be advised of the likely sensation of dyspnea. An obstetrician should monitor fetal growth and determine the need for fetal echocardiography.

If a pregnancy is at the 24th week or beyond and the mother develops a life-threatening situation such as uncontrollable pulmonary edema or a situation requiring emergency surgery, a cesarean section delivery should be considered.

# ■ LABOR AND DELIVERY

Labor and delivery place great demands on the cardiovascular system. Vaginal delivery is optimal in most patients with heart disease. However, if the second stage of labor is excessively painful or prolonged, the obstetricians should plan on assisted delivery (with forceps or vacuum suction) to shorten the second stage and should consider an assisted delivery depending on the severity of the mother's heart disease. Induced labor or cesarean section should be reserved for obstetrical indications or worsening cardiovascular function. Exceptions to this include patients with extremely high-risk heart disease, including Eisenmenger syndrome and Marfan syndrome with aortic root dilatation, in whom an appropriately planned early delivery can be performed when the fetus is adequately mature. Oxytocin should be avoided because of potential hypotension.

In most cases, lumbar epidural anesthesia using low-dose techniques for cardiostability with a pudendal nerve block to minimize pain is effective and least likely to result in hemodynamic compromise and should be favored over general anesthesia. Antibiotic prophylaxis against bacterial endocarditis at the time of labor and delivery is practiced by most experienced centers. If it is used, new guidelines suggest it should be limited to women with previous endocarditis, a prosthetic valve, complex cyanotic heart disease, or a cardiac transplant.

# ■ POSTPARTUM

Successful delivery does not mean the mother is out of danger; a large proportion of maternal deaths occur more than 1 week after delivery. Hemodynamic and electrocardiographic (ECG) monitoring should be continued for 48 to 72 hours in those with severe abnormalities (eg, pulmonary hypertension, cyanotic lesions, severe obstructive lesions, or a severe cardiomyopathy). Important changes in clotting factors normally prevent excessive uterine bleeding but may disrupt the fragile balance of factors in cyanotic patients. Warfarin can be reinstated carefully after delivery when necessary.

**TABLE 51-1.** Cardiovascular Abnormalities Placing a Mother and Infant at Extremely High Risk

| |
|---|
| **Advise avoidance or interruption of pregnancy** |
|    Pulmonary hypertension |
|    Dilated cardiomyopathy with congestive failure |
|    Marfan syndrome with dilated aortic root |
|    Cyanotic congenital heart disease |
| **Pregnancy counseling and close clinical follow-up required** |
|    Prosthetic valve |
|    Coarctation of the aorta |
|    Marfan syndrome |
|    Dilated cardiomyopathy in asymptomatic women |
|    Obstructive lesions |

Modified from McAnulty JH, Morton M J, Ueland K. The heart and pregnancy. *Curr Probl Cardiol.* 1988;13:589-665. Reproduced with permission from the publisher and authors.

# CARDIOVASCULAR ADJUSTMENTS DURING A NORMAL PREGNANCY

Maternal adaptation to pregnancy includes remarkable cardiovascular changes. These explain in part why some cardiac abnormalities are poorly tolerated during pregnancy (Table 51-1).

Resting cardiac output (CO) increases by more than 40% during pregnancy, reaching its highest levels by the 20th week (**Fig. 51-1**). Its early increase is caused

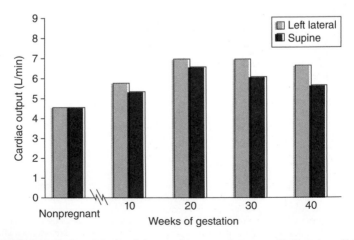

**FIGURE 51-1.** Cardiac output values during normal pregnancy when measured in the supine and left lateral positions. The values are derived from measurements made in many studies.

mainly by an increase in stroke volume, with heart rate increasing gradually throughout pregnancy (**Fig. 51-2**). The ejection fraction does not change. In the third trimester, CO is significantly affected by body position (Fig. 51-1) because the enlarged uterus reduces venous return from the lower extremities. In general, this results in few or no symptoms, but in some women, maintenance of the supine position may result in symptomatic hypotension. Symptoms of this *supine hypotensive syndrome of pregnancy* can be corrected by having the woman turn onto her side.

Blood pressure decreases slightly in early pregnancy. Systemic vascular resistance decreases until the 20th week and then gradually increases through the remainder of pregnancy (Fig. 51-2). The mother's oxygen consumption (which includes that of her fetus) increases by 20% within the first 20 weeks of pregnancy and increases steadily to a level that is approximately 30% above the nonpregnant level at the time of delivery. This increase is caused by both the metabolic needs of the fetus and the increased metabolic needs of the mother. These changes are better tolerated in patients with volume overload lesions (valvular regurgitation or shunts) than in patients with fixed output (obstructive valves, coarctation, or pulmonary hypertension).

Pregnancy results in a redistribution of blood flow (**Fig. 51-3**). In nonpregnant women, uterine blood flow is approximately 100 mL/min (2% of the CO); it increases to approximately 1200 mL/min at term, a value approaching the mother's blood flow to her own kidneys. During pregnancy, uterine blood vessels are maximally dilated. Excitement, heat, anxiety, exercise, and a decrease in venous return all decrease uterine blood flow. Vasoconstriction caused by endogenous catecholamines, vasoconstrictive drugs, maternal mechanical pulmonary ventilation, and some anesthetics, as well as that associated with preeclampsia and eclampsia, may decrease perfusion of the uterus.

At the beginning of labor, CO measured in the supine position increases to more than 7 L/min and to more than 9 L/min with each uterine contraction. Administration of epidural anesthesia reduces this CO to approximately 8 L/min, and the use of general anesthesia reduces it still further. After delivery, the CO briefly approaches 10 L/min (7-8 L/min with cesarean section); it then decreases rapidly to near-normal, nonpregnant values within a few weeks after delivery. A slight elevation in CO may persist for as long as 1 year. The increase in maternal CO in women with twins or triplets is only slightly greater than that in women with single pregnancies.

## ■ HEMODYNAMIC CHANGES WITH EXERCISE

Pregnancy changes the hemodynamic response to exercise. For any given level of exercise in the sitting position, the CO is greater than in nonpregnant women, and maximum CO is reached at lower exercise levels. During pregnancy, expected effects of conditioning or training on stroke volume are not seen, possibly because of uterine compression of the inferior vena cava or the increased venous capacitance. Exercise during pregnancy is not clearly any more dangerous or beneficial to a woman with heart disease than when she is not pregnant. While there is an insufficient amount of data to suggest that healthy pregnant women should avoid recreational exercise, an argument can be made for advising women with heart disease to keep the exercise level below that which causes symptoms.

## ■ MECHANISMS FOR HEMODYNAMIC CHANGES

The mechanisms involving this adaptation to pregnancy are not totally understood. They can in part be caused by volume change. Total body water increases steadily throughout pregnancy by 6 to 8 L (most is extracellular). Sodium retention results in an excess accumulation of 500 to 900 mEq by the time of delivery. As early as

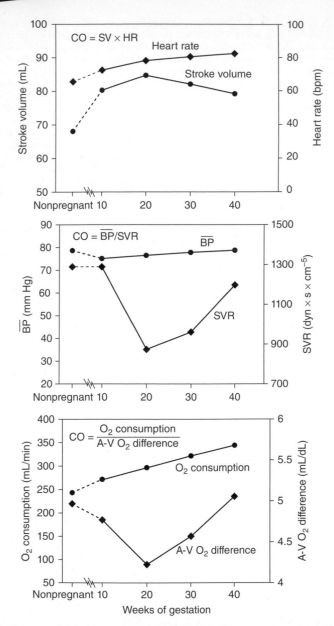

**FIGURE 51-2.** The cardiac output (CO) can be determined from other parameters in at least 3 ways: CO = Heart rate (HR) × Stroke volume (SV); CO = Mean arterial pressure (blood pressure) − Right atrial (RA) pressure/Systemic vascular resistance (SVR); CO = Oxygen ($O_2$) consumption/arteriovenous (AV) $O_2$ difference. The expected values for these parameters measured in the supine position during pregnancy are based on information acquired from many studies.

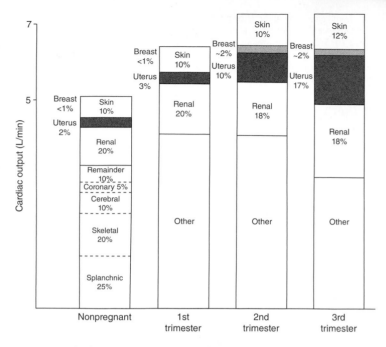

**FIGURE 51-3.** The changes in cardiac output and its distribution at rest in nonpregnant women. Data used in this graph are fragmentary, especially early in pregnancy. They presumably vary significantly with position, exertion, and other activity.

6 weeks after conception, plasma volume increases, approaching its maximum of 1.5 to 2 times normal by the second trimester, where it stays throughout the pregnancy. The red blood cell mass also increases but not to the same degree. Thus, the hematocrit decreases, although rarely to less than 30%.

Vascular alterations also contribute to the hemodynamic changes of pregnancy. Arterial compliance is increased. Venous capacitance increases as well, although there is an increase in venous vascular tone. These changes are advantageous in maintaining the hemodynamics of a normal pregnancy. There can be disadvantages as well; vascular accidents, when they occur in women, frequently do so during pregnancy. Additionally, the venous changes can explain, in part, the increase in thromboemboli during pregnancy. The ultimate cause of these recognized changes is uncertain. Complex interactions of the renin-angiotensin-aldosterone system, prostaglandins, nitric oxide, and atrial and brain natriuretic factors contribute to the fluid and sodium changes.

# DIAGNOSIS OF HEART DISEASE

## ■ CLINICAL EVALUATION

In a normal pregnancy, symptoms (dyspnea, fatigue) and signs (a third heart sound [$S_3$], pedal edema) mimic those of heart disease, making diagnosis difficult. Symptoms that should alert a caregiver to the possibility of heart disease include limiting dyspnea or orthopnea, hemoptysis, syncope with exertion, or chest pain clearly related to effort. On examination, cyanosis or clubbing, a loud systolic murmur (grade 3 or louder) or any diastolic murmur suggests heart disease. Venous hums or internal mammary flow sounds (the mammary souffle), which have diastolic components, are findings during a normal pregnancy.

## ◼ DIAGNOSTIC STUDIES

Echocardiography is safe and is so diagnostically useful that overuse, expense, and potential misinterpretations are the only significant concerns. Chamber dimensions and velocity measurements need to be interpreted considering the hemodynamic changes outlined above.

Electrocardiography is safe, although pregnancy makes interpretation of ST-T wave variations even more difficult than usual. Inferior ST-segment depression is common enough to possibly be the result of a normal pregnancy. There is a leftward shift of the QRS axis during pregnancy, but true axis deviation (−30 degrees) implies heart disease.

Cardiac magnetic resonance imaging (MRI) is also generally safe during pregnancy, although administration of gadolinium is contraindicated.

All radiation procedures, including computed tomography (CT), nuclear scans, and catheterization, should be avoided unless absolutely necessary. If a study is required, it should be delayed to as late in pregnancy as possible, the radiation dose should be kept to a minimum, and shielding of the fetus should be optimized.

# CARDIOVASCULAR DRUGS AND PREGNANCY

Nearly all cardiac drugs cross the placenta and are secreted in breast milk. Because information about the use of any drug is incomplete, it is best to avoid drug use, but if required for maternal safety, drugs should not be withheld. Although limited because of incomplete data, a US Food and Drug Administration (FDA) classification of drugs as they relate to fetal safety provides broad guidance for drug use during pregnancy (**Table 51-2**).

## ◼ DIURETICS

Diuretics can and should be used for treatment of congestive heart failure that is uncontrolled by sodium restriction and for the treatment of hypertension. Furosemide, which is often used, is FDA class C. Diuretics should not be used for prophylaxis against toxemia or for treatment of pedal edema.

## ◼ INOTROPIC AGENTS

The indications for the use of digoxin (FDA class C) are not changed by pregnancy. The same dose of digoxin in general will yield lower maternal serum levels during pregnancy than in the nonpregnant state. Fetal serum levels approximate those in the mother.

When intravenous (IV) inotropic or vasopressor agents are required, the standard agents (dopamine, dobutamine, and norepinephrine; FDA class B and C) can be used, but the fetus is jeopardized because all such agents increase resistance to uterine blood flow and can stimulate uterine contractions. In animal models, ephedrine is an appropriate initial vasopressor drug as it does not adversely affect uterine blood flow.

**TABLE 51-2.** Fetal Drug Risk

| FDA Pregnancy Category | |
|---|---|
| A | Human and animal studies have not shown fetal risk. |
| | *Use for maternal safety and symptoms appropriate.[a]* |
| B | No adequate human studies. Animal studies have not shown fetal risk. |
| | *Use for maternal safety or severe symptoms appropriate.* |
| C | No adequate studies in humans. Teratogenicity has been shown in animal studies. |
| | *Use for maternal safety may be justified.* |
| D | Demonstrated fetal risk in human (and animal) studies. |
| | *Maternal safety would seem to be the only justification for use during pregnancy.* |
| X | Demonstrated fetal risk in human and animal studies of sufficient severity to recommend that drug not be used during pregnancy. |
| | *Only extreme maternal safety issues justify use.* |

[a]Italicized recommendations are those of authors.

Data from *Federal Register.* Vol 73, No. 104. May 29, 2008.

There is little information about the clinical efficacy or safety of the phosphodiesterase inhibitors (amrinone, milrinone) in pregnancy. Milrinone is FDA class C.

# ■ ADRENERGIC RECEPTOR-BLOCKING AGENTS

The use of β-blockers for the usual cardiac clinical indications is reasonable. Metoprolol (FDA class C) is favored over atenolol (FDA class D). If these agents are used during pregnancy, it is appropriate to monitor fetal and newborn infant heart rate, blood sugar, and respiratory status.

Experience with the α-blocking agents phenoxybenzamine and phentolamine (FDA class C) is sparse. Clonidine, prazosin, and labetalol, with their mixed α- and β-blocking effects, have been used for the treatment of hypertension during pregnancy without clear detrimental effects.

# ■ CALCIUM CHANNEL BLOCKING DRUGS

The dihydropyridine agents are effective antihypertensive and afterload-reducing agents that have been used without any adverse effect on fetuses or newborn infants. If a nondihydropyridine agent is required, verapamil (FDA class C) is favored over diltiazem (FDA class C). The calcium channel blockers cause relaxation of the uterus; nifedipine has been used for this purpose.

# ■ ANTIARRHYTHMIC AGENTS

When atrioventricular (AV) node blockade is required during pregnancy, β-blockers, calcium blockers, adenosine, or digoxin can be used. It is preferable to avoid the standard antiarrhythmic drugs unless essential for management of recurrent arrhythmias or for maternal safety. If IV drug therapy is required, lidocaine (FDA class B) or procainamide (FDA class C) provide reasonable first-line therapy; there is limited reported experience with IV amiodarone or ibutilide (FDA class C).

If oral antiarrhythmic therapy is necessary, flecainide (FDA class C) and sotalol (FDA class B) are often given to the mother to treat the fetus. Quinidine has also been used frequently. Information about procainamide, disopyramide, mexiletine, and dofetilide (FDA class C) is sparse. Amiodarone (FDA class D) should be avoided unless its use is essential for maternal or fetal safety. Dronedarone is FDA class X and should not be used in pregnancy.

# ■ VASODILATOR AGENTS

For a true hypertensive crisis or emergency afterload and preload reduction, nitroprusside (FDA class C) is the vasodilator drug of choice. A concern that its metabolite, cyanide, can be detected in the fetus has not been a demonstrated significant problem in humans. Concern about toxicity is a reason to replace it with alternative drugs such as parenteral hydralazine, nitroglycerin, or labetalol (FDA class C) when the most acute situation is made more stable.

Chronic afterload reduction to treat hypertension, aortic or mitral regurgitation, or ventricular dysfunction during pregnancy has been achieved with the calcium blocking drugs, hydralazine, and methyldopa. Adverse fetal effects have not been reported.

ACE inhibitors (FDA class C in the first trimester and class D in the remaining trimesters) increase the risk of major congenital abnormality and are *contraindicated in pregnancy*. A series of case reports of similar problems with the ARBs suggest that their use should be avoided.

# ■ PULMONARY VASCULAR DILATOR DRUGS

Prostaglandins (epoprostenol and iloprost), phosphodiesterase type 5 inhibitors (sildenafil), and nitric oxide (FDA classes B and C) have been used successfully as vasodilators to treat pulmonary hypertension with no reported adverse maternal or fetal effects. The endothelin receptor blocker bosentan (FDA class X) should not be used.

# ■ ANTITHROMBOTIC AGENTS

Warfarin is FDA class X and has been historically contraindicated during the first 3 months (particularly weeks 6-12) of pregnancy because of the incidence of malformations that comprise the *warfarin embryopathy syndrome* (facial abnormalities, optic atrophy, digital abnormalities, epithelial changes, and mental impairment). Most recent data suggest this risk may be dose related. Studies suggest doses greater than 5 mg/d increase the occurrence of warfarin embryopathy.

Heparin does not cross the placenta; fetal risk is minimal, although maternal bleeding can occur. If heparin is used, sufficient dosing is essential to prevent thromboemboli. Self-administered subcutaneous high-dose unfractionated heparin (UFH; 200-300 U/kg subcutaneously every 12 hours) or low molecular weight heparin (LMWH; eg, enoxaparin 1 mg/kg subcutaneously every 12 hours) are reasonable options. If used, a factor Xa level should be assessed initially, titrating the drug to achieve trough levels (11 hours after dose) of more than 0.6 U/mL. Although peak levels (1-2 hours after a dose) relate to bleeding risk, the emphasis should be on avoiding insufficient trough levels (particularly when using this therapy in women with prosthetic heart valves; see later). The activated partial thromboplastin time is less reliable for managing heparin use during pregnancy. When anticoagulation is required, traditional recommendations have been UFH and, more recently, LMWH for the first trimester, switching to warfarin for the next 5 months with a return to heparin therapy before and through labor and delivery.

Antiplatelet agents cross the placenta and increase the chance of maternal bleeding. Aspirin has been associated with an increased incidence of abortion and fetal growth retardation. Its inhibition of prostaglandin synthesis may result in closure of the ductus arteriosus during fetal life. Still, it has frequently been used and even recommended by some as prophylaxis against preeclampsia. These trade-offs are difficult to evaluate; we suggest aspirin should be used when needed for maternal safety. Data on the effects of the thienopyridines (clopidogrel and prasugrel), ticagrelor, and the IIb/IIIa glycoprotein platelet receptor inhibitors during pregnancy are anecdotal and minimal. There is also no information on the safety of the direct thrombin inhibitors during pregnancy in women.

# MANAGEMENT OF CARDIOVASCULAR SYNDROMES

## ◼ LOW CARDIAC OUTPUT SYNDROME

Although potentially treatable causes such as tamponade, severe valvular stenosis, or cardiomyopathy should be considered, low CO is most often caused by intravascular volume depletion. This is particularly dangerous in those with lesions that limit blood flow, such as pulmonary hypertension, aortic or pulmonic valve stenosis, hypertrophic cardiomyopathy (HCM), or mitral stenosis. Measures to prevent or treat a decrease in central blood volume are outlined in **Table 51-3.**

## ◼ CONGESTIVE HEART FAILURE

The management of congestive heart failure during pregnancy should not differ greatly from that at other times *except* that the ACE inhibitors and ARBs should not

---

**TABLE 51-3.** Measures to Protect Against a Decrease in Central Blood Volume

| |
|---|
| **Acute** |
| Position |
|     45-60 degree left lateral |
|     10 degree Trendelenburg |
| Volume administration: Glucose-free saline |
| Drugs: Ephedrine if unresponsive to fluid replacement |
| Anesthetics (if required) |
|     Regional: Serial small boluses |
|     General: Emphasis on benzodiazepines and narcotics, low-dose inhalation agents |
| **Chronic** |
| Full leg stockings |
| Avoid vasodilatation drugs |

be used. Congestive heart failure is one situation in which maintaining a woman in the supine position can be beneficial by causing preload reduction with obstruction of return of blood from the inferior vena cava to the heart.

Diastolic ventricular dysfunction is rarely described in pregnancy. Cautious titration of diuretics seems appropriate for symptomatic women with pulmonary rales and an elevated central venous pressure.

## ■ THROMBOEMBOLIC COMPLICATIONS

The risk of venous thromboemboli increases 5-fold during and immediately after pregnancy, prophylactic antithrombotic therapy (using the drugs and schedule described earlier) is indicated in those at high risk for a thromboembolic complication, including women with thromboemboli during a previous pregnancy, antithrombin III deficiency, protein C deficiency, protein S deficiency, and the anticardiolipin antibody syndrome. Prothrombin gene mutations and factor V mutation resulting in the resistance to activated protein C (found in 3%-5% of the population) may eventually be shown to be a reason for prophylaxis as well.

If a thrombus or embolus is identified, strategies for anticoagulation include the use of intravenous heparin, subcutaneous low molecular weight heparin, or subcutaneous unfractionated heparin. Close monitoring is essential for successful therapy. If a thromboembolus is life threatening (eg, a massive pulmonary embolus or a thrombosed prosthetic valve), thrombolytic therapy may be used.

## ■ HYPERTENSION

Hypertension can be present before pregnancy (in 1%-5%) and persist throughout pregnancy, or it can develop with pregnancy. When associated with proteinuria, pedal edema, central nervous system (CNS) irritability, elevation of liver enzymes, and coagulation disturbances, the hypertension syndrome is called *preeclampsia*. If convulsions occur, the diagnosis is *eclampsia*. Preeclampsia increases maternal risk and may cause fetal growth retardation. Maternal and fetal morbidity and mortality increase still further with eclampsia.

Keeping the systolic blood pressure below 160 mm Hg and the diastolic blood pressure below 100 mm Hg provides a margin of safety against severe hypertensive episodes. Unless the patient has previously demonstrated salt-sensitive hypertension, sodium restriction is inadvisable. Concern about hypovolemia is a reason to bypass a thiazide diuretic as first-line therapy. A dihydropyridine calcium blocker (eg, sustained-release nifedipine) seems to be the optimal alternative. Large experience with $\alpha$ methyldopa shows it is effective without adverse effects on the fetus. $\beta_1$-Selective blockers and labetalol have been proven to be effective. ACE inhibitors and ARBs *should not be used*. Direct renin inhibitors should be similarly avoided.

## ■ PULMONARY HYPERTENSION

In the setting of pulmonary hypertension, maternal mortality ranges from 30% to 70%. If severe pulmonary hypertension is recognized early in the pregnancy, interruption of the pregnancy is advised. If the pulmonary hypertension is recognized late in pregnancy, close follow-up is required. Pulmonary vasodilators can be used when pressures are high and a woman is symptomatic (see drug descriptions earlier). At the time of labor and delivery, a central venous line allows adequate fluid administration, and a radial artery catheter makes determinations of blood pressure and oxygen saturation easier. These lines should be used for 48 to 72 hours after delivery.

# ◼ ARRHYTHMIAS

The rules for treatment should be the same as in nonpregnant patients with the possible exception that a rhythm causing hemodynamic instability should be treated somewhat more rapidly because of concern about diversion of blood flow away from the uterus.

*Atrial* or *ventricular premature beats* and *sinus tachycardia* are common and beyond identifying and correcting any reversible causes do not require specific treatment.

*Paroxysmal supraventricular tachycardia* is the most common sustained abnormal rhythm occurring with pregnancy. Initial treatment with vagal maneuvers is appropriate. If urgent treatment is required, IV adenosine, verapamil, or cardioversion can be used. If recurrent episodes necessitate a daily drug, verapamil or a β-blocker is often effective.

*Atrial fibrillation* and *flutter* should be treated as in nonpregnant women. If these rhythms occur in a woman with mitral stenosis, severe LV dysfunction, or a previous thromboembolic event, antithrombotic therapy is indicated. If necessary for refractory arrhythmias, radiofrequency catheter ablation can be performed, optimally later in pregnancy and with radiation shielding.

Emergency management of rapid ventricular tachycardia or ventricular fibrillation should be as recommended for nonpregnant women. If possible, during acute management, the women should be rolled to her left side to enhance blood return from the lower extremities. Pregnancies have been successful in women with implanted cardioverter/defibrillators; treatment shocks have no demonstrated adverse effects on the fetus.

*Repolarization abnormalities* that predispose young adults to ventricular fibrillation are not well characterized during pregnancy. Most is known about the prolonged QT-interval syndrome. If this is recognized (usually from transient arrhythmia symptoms) and it is an acquired form, the presumed cause (usually a drug) should be eliminated. If the syndrome is congenital, β-blocker therapy during pregnancy is recommended although unproven. Implantable defibrillators have been used with recurrent ventricular arrhythmias, but their value remains unproven in this syndrome even when it is unrelated to pregnancy. In patients with a congenital syndrome, transmission with autosomal dominance can affect the fetus. Arrhythmogenic RV dysplasia and Brugada syndrome are even less well characterized with little information related to pregnancy.

*Bradyarrhythmias* can occur during pregnancy and treatment is generally not required unless the patient has clear hemodynamic compromise. Reversible causes should be sought. Complete heart block, which in this age group is most likely to be congenital in origin, is consistent with a successful pregnancy. If required, a permanent pacemaker can be inserted.

# ◼ LOSS-OF-CONSCIOUSNESS SPELLS

If a seizure disorder cannot be excluded as a cause, appropriate evaluation with electroencephalography is indicated. If a seizure is unlikely or excluded, the syndrome of syncope should include a consideration of the usual causes, most of which are caused by an imbalance of vascular volume and tone or by cardiac arrhythmias.

# ◼ MYOCARDIAL INFARCTION

Acute myocardial infarction should prompt consideration of immediate reperfusion. If stent placement is indicated, maximal radiation shielding of the uterus is required. If early in pregnancy, a bare metal stent may be preferable to a drug-eluting stent given the lack of evidence about the safe use of clopidogrel, prasugrel, or ticagrelor during pregnancy and limited clinical experience with drug eluting stents in pregnancy. Thrombolytic agents can be used though should be reserved for emergency situations when there is limited access to PCI.

## ◼ ENDOCARDITIS

The clinical presentation of endocarditis is the same during pregnancy as at other times. Infection with *Streptococcus* spp. is the most common cause. IV drug abusers are more likely to have staphylococcal infections, and women with genitourinary tract infections are more likely to have gram-negative infections, most commonly caused by *Escherichia coli*. If endocarditis does occur, it should be treated aggressively with medical therapy, and the usual indications for surgery are appropriate during pregnancy. If open-heart surgery is required late in pregnancy, simultaneous cesarean section should be considered. Antibiotic prophylaxis against endocarditis is discussed above (under Labor and Delivery).

## ◼ AORTIC DISSECTION

Aortic dissection is an increasing cause of maternal mortality. It generally occurs in conjunction with Marfan syndrome, a bicuspid aortic valve, or coarctation. If suspected, evaluation with ultrasonography, MRI, or CT is appropriate. If found, measures to protect the mother are essential. If major surgery is considered necessary and the pregnancy exceeds 24 weeks, delivery should be considered.

# SPECIFIC FORMS OF HEART DISEASE

## ◼ VALVULAR HEART DISEASE

Worldwide, rheumatic fever is the predominant cause of valve disease encountered during pregnancy. In affluent countries congenital and ischemic heart disease predominate. Management of valve disease through pregnancy is largely the same regardless of the cause. An exception is that those with rheumatic fever as the cause should be advised of antibiotic prophylaxis against a recurrence, even during pregnancy.

### *Mitral Stenosis*

In pregnancy, mitral stenosis is typically the most poorly tolerated valve lesion. The increased CO, tachycardia, and fluid retention of pregnancy can double the resting pressure gradient across a stenotic mitral valve. Symptoms generally become apparent by the 20th week and can be aggravated still further at the time of labor and delivery. Maternal death is rare when careful attention is paid to the management of congestive heart failure.

In a woman with symptomatic mitral stenosis, balloon valvuloplasty or valve surgery should be performed before conception. If mitral stenosis is first recognized during pregnancy and symptoms develop, standard medical therapy is appropriate, including careful fluid management. If this does not control symptoms, balloon valvuloplasty can be performed (with appropriate radiation shielding of the fetus). Mitral valve surgical commissurotomy or valve replacement has been performed, but fetal loss exceeds 30%. Atrial fibrillation is of particular concern during pregnancy. Immediate treatment of a rapid ventricular response should include IV verapamil or cardioversion.

## Mitral Regurgitation

In general, mitral regurgitation is well tolerated during pregnancy. If it is severe, symptomatic, or associated with LV dysfunction, valve repair before pregnancy is recommended. One cause of mitral regurgitation is *mitral valve prolapse.* Pregnancy can alter examination findings, but rare associated arrhythmias, endocarditis, cerebral emboli, and hemodynamically significant regurgitation are no more likely to occur during pregnancy than at other times.

## Aortic Stenosis

Pregnancy in the presence of aortic valve stenosis can be successful, but if stenosis is severe, maternal deaths have occurred and congestive heart failure is common. Aortic valve stenosis is most often caused by a bicuspid aortic valve, which is associated with an increased risk of aortic dissection. Even if tolerated during pregnancy, aortic valve stenosis may affect subsequent maternal functional capabilities and survival.

If severe aortic valve stenosis is recognized before pregnancy, balloon valvuloplasty or a surgical commissurotomy is recommended prior to conception. If pregnancy does occur in the presence of severe aortic stenosis, measures to avoid hypovolemia are particularly important. If congestive heart failure develops, it can be treated as previously described. If severe symptoms persist, a balloon valvuloplasty or aortic valve surgery can be performed during pregnancy, the latter being associated with increased fetal loss.

## Aortic Regurgitation

Aortic regurgitation is a reason to consider Marfan syndrome as a cause (see later); otherwise, it is generally well tolerated during pregnancy. If it is severe, symptomatic, or associated with LV dysfunction, valve surgery should be considered before pregnancy. If congestive heart failure occurs with pregnancy, treatment should include afterload reduction. *ACE inhibitors and ARBs should be avoided.* If endocarditis occurs and the infection is not rapidly controlled, mortality with medical therapy is high, and surgical therapy is indicated. If this occurs late in pregnancy, consideration of associated cesarean section is appropriate.

## Pulmonic Valve Disease

Many women with pulmonic valve disease will have had previous valve commissurotomy or balloon valvuloplasty for valve stenosis or as part of the correction of tetralogy of Fallot. The residual stenosis and invariable regurgitation are potential concerns but in general do not adversely affect the outcome of pregnancy. The occasional patient with significant pulmonic valve stenosis who has not been treated appears to tolerate pregnancy well. Intravascular volume depletion should be avoided. If severe symptoms (recurrent syncope, uncontrolled dyspnea, and chest pain) occur, balloon valvuloplasty can be performed.

## Tricuspid Valve Disease

Significant tricuspid valve disease is also uncommon during pregnancy, although still encountered in patients with Ebstein anomaly (see later). This regurgitation usually requires no specific therapy during pregnancy. Tricuspid stenosis is rare. If it is encountered, avoidance of intravascular volume depletion seems to be important.

## *Prosthetic Heart Valve Disease*

One or more of the major associated complications of prosthetic heart valve disease—thromboemboli, bleeding (from anticoagulation), endocarditis, valve dysfunction, reoperation, or death—affects patients at a rate greater than 5% per year throughout their lives. Pregnancy increases the risk of each of these complications, and the prosthetic valve and its treatment can adversely affect the fetus. All of these are reasons that a prosthetic valve is a relative contraindication to pregnancy. Selection of the appropriate prosthesis for a young woman should include consideration of future pregnancies.

**Mechanical Valves** Durability is the strong advantage of these valves. The disadvantage is the need for anticoagulation. While there is no consensus amongst various professional societies on a single optimal strategy for anticoagulation during pregnancy, there is no question that the choice must be informed by patient preferences and weighing of risks and benefits. The American College of Cardiology/American Heart Association (ACC/AHA) guidelines recommend heparin during weeks 6 and 12 of the first trimester, then warfarin until the 35th week, and then a return to heparin through labor and delivery. Full-dose subcutaneous heparin should be dose adjusted to maintain a "high therapeutic level" by following factor Xa levels. LMWH is an appealing alternative. Complications have occurred because of insufficient dosing, a reason to be certain that trough transfer Xa levels are above 0.6 U/mL, even if resulting in relatively high levels at other times. Low dose aspirin is recommended additionally in the second and third trimesters. Guidelines from the European Society of Cardiology, balancing the lower risk of embryopathy with warfarin doses <5 mg and the higher incidence of valve thrombosis when heparin or LMWH was used, recommend that warfarin be continued throughout the pregnancy. If the warfarin dose exceeds 5 mg, substitution with dose-adjusted heparin or LMWH between weeks 6 and 12 is reasonable. Low dose aspirin is not recommended. Finally, the American College of Chest Physicians recommend that warfarin throughout pregnancy is reasonable for select high risk patients (history of thromboembolism, atrial fibrillation, left ventricular dysfunction, prosthesis in mitral position, or first generation prosthesis) assuming the warfarin dose is <5 mg. Low dose aspirin is additionally recommended in these high risk patients. Irrespective of the strategy for anticoagulation, close follow-up and careful monitoring of levels is essential. Patients should be counseled on all of the risks and benefits associated with the use of different anticoagulants.

**Bioprosthetic (Tissue) Valves** The advantage of these valves is that anticoagulation is usually not required. The trade-off, however, of using these valves to avoid anticoagulation is decreased durability. Homografts are preferable to heterografts in this regard, with 10-year failure rates as low as 18% with the former and as high as 72% with the latter.

## ■ CONGENITAL HEART DISEASE

Congenital heart disease is now the most common heart disease encountered in women of childbearing age in the United States. In many, it has been altered by surgery. Overall, maternal complications during pregnancy occur in more than 10% with congenital heart disease.

Each abnormality is unique, but some issues apply to all. First, some abnormalities significantly increase the risk of maternal morbidity and mortality during pregnancy. In addition to the specific abnormalities presented in Table 51-1, maternal risk can be estimated from clinical variables. A point-score system for variables predicting adverse maternal events was developed from an observational study and validated in prospective studies of pregnant women ( **Table 51-4**). The majority of adverse maternal cardiovascular events were congestive heart failure and arrhythmias.

**TABLE 51-4.** Predictors of Adverse Maternal Cardiovascular Events During Pregnancy

NYHA Functional class III or IV or cyanosis

Previous cardiovascular event

Left heart obstruction

Ejection fraction ≤0.40

| Predictive value of adverse maternal events if each of the above is given 1 point | |
|---|---|
| No. of points | Adverse maternal CV events (%)[a] |
| 0 | 4-12 |
| 1 | 27-30 |
| >1 | 62-100 |

CV, cardiovascular; NYHA, New York Heart Association.

[a]Lower rates data from Siu SC, Sermer M, Coleman JM, et al. Prospective multicenter study of pregnancy outcomes in women with heart disease. *Circulation.* 2001;104(5):515-521; and higher rates data from Khairy P, Ouyang DW, Fernandes SM, et al. Pregnancy outcomes in women with congenital heart disease. *Circulation.* 2006;113(4):517-524.

Maternal mortality was less than 1%, but it is important to note that relatively few women with the abnormalities listed in Fig. 51-1 were included.

Second, there is an increased risk of fetal death. This increases with the severity of the maternal lesions.

Third, the presence of a congenital cardiac abnormality in either parent or in a sibling increases the risk of cardiac and other congenital abnormalities in the fetus.

## Left-to-Right Shunts

Although left-to-right shunting increases the chances of pulmonary hypertension, RV failure, arrhythmias, and emboli, it is not certain that these complications are accentuated by a pregnancy. The degree of shunting is generally not affected by pregnancy because the resistances of the systemic and pulmonary vascular circuits fall to a similar degree. The RV volume overload associated with the shunts is generally well tolerated during pregnancy.

*Atrial septal defects* are the most common cause of left-to-right shunts and can occasionally be first diagnosed at the time of pregnancy. Pregnancy is generally well tolerated as long as pulmonary vascular resistance is normal (<3.0 Wood units). Transcutaneous closure with an occluder device should make pregnancy even safer, but there is rarely a need to offer this if the woman is already pregnant.

*Ventricular septal defects* are the most common congenital abnormality in children. *Patent ductus arteriosus* is also common. In adults, these lesions will most likely have either closed spontaneously; been closed surgically; or be small, restrictive lesions without hemodynamic effect (although a loud murmur will be audible). A large, unclosed defect will most likely have resulted in Eisenmenger physiology, which is highly dangerous for pregnancy, as discussed above. Otherwise, these lesions are generally well tolerated in pregnancy, with a small risk of arrhythmia or congestive heart failure.

## Right-to-Left Shunt (Cyanotic Heart Disease)

Right-to-left shunting may occur through septal defects when pulmonary vascular resistance exceeds systemic vascular resistance (Eisenmenger physiology) or when there is an obstruction to RV outflow and pulmonary vascular resistance is normal (most often tetralogy of Fallot or pulmonary atresia). All are forms of *cyanotic* heart disease. The presence of cyanosis, especially when sufficient to result in elevated hemoglobin levels, is associated with high fetal loss, prematurity, and reduced infant birth weights. When pulmonary hypertension is not present, maternal mortality is significantly less, but women are at increased risk of heart failure (~15%) thromboemboli, arrhythmias, and endocarditis (4.5%). Providers should consider aspirin as antiplatelet therapy and early delivery if fetal maturity allows.

Eisenmenger syndrome is a contraindication to pregnancy and it is advisable to offer interruption of pregnancy early on if conception occurs. A woman who opts to continue should be put on bedrest, heparin, and oxygen for at least the third trimester and should be monitored closely in the postpartum period without premature hospital discharge. Pulmonary vasodilator drugs can be considered (see above).

*Tetralogy of Fallot* is the most common form of right-to-left shunting resulting from obstruction to pulmonary flow when pulmonary vascular resistance is normal. If it is uncorrected, successful pregnancy can be achieved, but maternal mortality is high, and fetal loss can exceed 50%. After surgical correction of the defect, maternal mortality does not clearly exceed that of a woman without heart disease.

Women with pulmonary atresia that has been corrected by a Fontan procedure in childhood will, similar to those who have had surgery for tetralogy of Fallot, no longer be cyanotic. The most common issues will be pulmonic valve regurgitation, RV pulmonary artery conduit stenosis (in pulmonary atresia), or ventricular tachycardia.

## Obstructive Lesions

Two recommendations apply in women with obstructive cardiac lesions. First, volume depletion should be avoided because it may result in a significant decrease in CO whether the obstruction is on the left or right side of the heart. Second, surgical or catheter treatment for a left- or right-sided obstructive lesion is recommended before pregnancy. During pregnancy, these procedures should be reserved for patients with severe congestive failure or fetal distress.

Congenital bicuspid aortic stenosis is likely the most common obstructive lesion encountered in pregnancy and its management is described above. Two other LV obstructive disease processes warrant further discussion: coarctation of the aorta and hypertrophic obstructive cardiomyopathy (HOCM).

## Coarctation of the Aorta

Hypertension, ascending aortic aneurysm, aortic dissection or rupture, stenosis or restenosis at the coarctation site, and the presence of intracranial aneurysms are all factors which may impact the outcome of pregnancies in women with corrected or uncorrected coarctation. Surgical correction before pregnancy reduces the risk of aortic dissection or rupture. A similar effect of catheter dilatation and stenting on subsequent pregnancies would seem likely, but information is limited. If pregnancy occurs in a woman with a coarctation, blood pressure control with β-blockers is mandatory, although it may result in reduced placental circulation and needs to be monitored closely. It is not clear whether mechanical treatment decreases the rate of rupture of associated intracranial aneurysms.

## Hypertrophic Obstructive Cardiomyopathy

Dynamic outflow obstruction may worsen in pregnant women with HOCM. The decrease in peripheral vascular resistance and peripheral pooling of blood during pregnancy may cause hypotension and the intermittent high catecholamine state of pregnancy may increase LV outflow tract obstruction. It is not clear that pregnancy increases the approximately 1% to 3% chance per year of sudden death, but deaths with pregnancy can exceed 1%. It is important to avoid hypovolemia. β-Blocker therapy is recommended at the time of labor and delivery.

## Complex Congenital Lesions

Maternal and fetal morbidity and mortality are high, particularly when complex abnormalities result in maternal cyanosis or marked functional limitation. Still, surgery has made pregnancy a consideration.

**Transposition of the Great Vessels** Women with dextro (D)-transposition of the great arteries (some with single ventricles) can become pregnant. The little available information indicates very poor maternal and fetal outcomes. Partial or complete surgical correction of the lesion before pregnancy improves the outcome for the mother as well as the fetus. If L-transposition (congenitally *corrected* transposition) is not complicated by cyanosis, ventricular dysfunction, or heart block, pregnancy should be well tolerated.

**Ebstein Anomaly** This condition encompasses a spectrum that can be mild and unrecognized during pregnancy or severe and can be associated with abnormalities in addition to that of the tricuspid valve. Increasing problems of RV dysfunction, obstruction to right-sided heart flow, and right-to-left shunting resulting in cyanosis may occur. Maternal morbidity and mortality are low if the patient does not have severe disease. Significant right-to-left shunting is a reason to avoid pregnancy.

**Single Ventricle/Fontan** Often patients with a single functional ventricle will have been palliated in childhood with some variant of the Fontan procedure, during which venous blood flows passively to the pulmonary capillary bed. As adults these patients are at risk of venous thromboembolism, atrial arrhythmia, and low-output heart failure, and complications related to chronic elevation of central venous pressure, including hepatic congestion and protein-losing enteropathy. Because cardiac output remains relatively fixed because of limitations of pulmonary blood flow, cardiovascular complications, usually heart failure symptoms or arrhythmia, occur in 10% to 20% of pregnant patients. There is a high risk of fetal loss (~30%-50%) and prematurity (38%).

**Marfan Syndrome** Women with Marfan syndrome require specialized attention. The risk of death from aortic rupture or dissection during pregnancy is high (3%) in women with Marfan syndrome and exceeds 10% if the aortic root is greater than 40 mm by echocardiography. For that reason regular monitoring of the aortic root diameter is required. Activity should be restricted and hypertension should be prevented. Although unproven, prophylactic use of β-blockers during pregnancy seems reasonable. Caesarean delivery is recommended to avoid the hemodynamic stresses of labor.

## ■ MYOCARDIAL DISEASE

### Dilated Cardiomyopathy

In women who have had or have a dilated cardiomyopathy, whether congenital or because of a recognized cause, the risks to the mother and child are sufficient to recommend avoidance of pregnancy. This recommendation comes from the observation of outcomes of women with an isolated dilated cardiomyopathy as well as from those with LV dysfunction associated with other cardiovascular abnormalities. It also comes from the observations of those who develop *peripartum cardiomyopathy* in the last month of pregnancy or within 5 months of delivery. Mortality in a group of these young women was 9% in one series, most within 2 years of delivery. In women with dilated cardiomyopathy during pregnancy, standard treatment for heart failure, thromboemboli, and arrhythmias is appropriate. If ventricular function does not return to normal after pregnancy, subsequent pregnancies have been associated with maternal mortality rates of 19% to 50% and an increased need for cardiac transplantation. Even in those whose LV function returns to normal, deaths have been reported with subsequent pregnancies.

### Hypertrophic Cardiomyopathy

Obstructive, *nonconcentric* HCM has been discussed. Concentric HCM may be the result of aortic stenosis or hypertension. If the cause is unexplained, there is little information about its significance during pregnancy.

## ◼ ISCHEMIC HEART DISEASE

Chest discomfort is common during a normal pregnancy and for the most part is caused by abdominal distension or gastroesophageal reflux. Coronary artery disease (CAD) is an uncommon but possible (and increasing) cause. Previously, CAD during pregnancy has been most commonly attributed to infrequent phenomena, such as dissection of the coronary artery, spasm, emboli, vasculitis, or anomalous origin of a left coronary artery. An observed increase in maternal deaths from myocardial ischemia is more likely to be attributable to an increase in atherosclerotic risk factors in conjunction with an increase in pregnancies at older ages. An ECG and exercise stress test can help with the diagnosis. If essential, MRI of the proximal coronary arteries (gadolinium should be avoided) is safe and worthwhile. Thallium imaging or angiography can be performed if absolutely necessary. When it is suspected or demonstrated, CAD should be treated with standard medical therapy; angioplasty or bypass surgery can be performed at an experienced center (see Myocardial Infarction on page 637.).

# PREGNANCY AFTER CARDIAC TRANSPLANTATION

Many cardiac transplant recipients are women of childbearing age. Successful pregnancies after transplantation have been reported, but the potential hazards to the mother and fetus—which include maternal heart failure, immunosuppressive therapy, maternal infections, and serial diagnostic studies—have already been recognized as causing problems in fetuses and newborns. A shortened maternal life span must also be considered when a patient is counseled about the advisability of pregnancy.

## SUGGESTED READINGS

McAnulty JH, Broberg CS, Metcalfe J. Heart disease and pregnancy. In: Fuster V, Walsh R, Harrington RA, et al. *Hurst's The Heart.* 13th ed. New York, NY: McGraw-Hill; 2011; 97: 2146-2158.

Avila WS, Rossi EG, Ramires JA, et al. Pregnancy in patients with heart disease: experience with 1,000 cases. *Clin Cardiol.* 2003;26:135-142.

Bates SM, Greer IA, Pabinger I, Sofaer S, Hirsh J. Venous thromboembolism, thrombophilia, antithrombotic therapy, and pregnancy: American College of Chest Physicians Evidence-Based Clinical Practice. *Chest.* 2008;133:844S-886S.

Bonow RO, Carabello BA, Chatterjee K, et al. 2008 focused update incorporated into the ACC/AHA 2006 guidelines for the management of patients with valvular heart disease: a report of the American College of Cardiology/American Heart Association Task Force on Practice Guidelines (Writing Committee to revise the 1998 guidelines for the management of patients with valvular heart disease). Endorsed by the Society of Cardiovascular Anesthesiologists, Society for Cardiovascular Angiography and Interventions, and Society of Thoracic Surgeons. *J Am Coll Cardiol.* 2008;52, e1-e142.

Capeless EL, Clapp JF. Cardiovascular changes in early phase of pregnancy. *Am J Obstet Gynecol.* 1989;161:1449-1453.

Elkayam U, Bitar F. Valvular heart disease and pregnancy: part II: prosthetic valves. *J Am Coll Cardiol.* 2005;46: 403-410.

Hameed A, Karaalp IS, Tummala PP, et al. The effect of valvular heart disease on maternal and fetal outcome of pregnancy. *J Am Coll Cardiol.* 2001;37(3):893-899.

Khairy P, Ouyang DW, Fernandes SM, et al. Pregnancy outcomes in women with congenital heart disease. *Circulation.* 2006;113(4):517-524.

Kron J, Conti JB. Arrhythmias in the pregnant patient: current concepts in evaluation and management. *J Interv Card Electrophysiol.* 2007;19(2):95-107

Regitz-Zagrosek V, Blomstrom LC, Borghi C, et al. ESC Guidelines on the management of cardiovascular diseases during pregnancy: the Task Force on the Management of Cardiovascular Diseases during Pregnancy of the European Society of Cardiology (ESC). *Eur Heart J.* 2011;32:3147-3197.

Safgfasg Elkayam U. Clinical characteristics of peripartum cardiomyopathy in the United States: diagnosis, prognosis, and management. *J Am Coll Cardiol.* 2011;58(7):659-670.

Siu SC, Sermer M, Coleman JM, et al. Prospective multicenter study of pregnancy outcomes in women with heart disease. *Circulation.* 2001;104(5):515-521.

Siu SC, Colman JM, Sorensen S, et al. Adverse neonatal and cardiac outcomes are more common in pregnant women with cardiac disease. *Circulation.* 2002;105(18):2179-2184.

Stergiopoulos K, Shiang E, Bench T. Pregnancy in patients with pre-existing cardiomyopathies. *J Am Coll Cardiol.* 2011; 58(4): 337-350

Uebing A, Steer PJ, Yentis SM, et al. Pregnancy and congenital heart disease. *BMJ.* 2006;332(7538):401-406.

# CHAPTER 52
# AORTIC VALVE DISEASE

Sammy Elmariah, Rosario V. Freeman,
Marc A. Miller, and Catherine M. Otto

## EPIDEMIOLOGY

The prevalence of significant aortic valvular heart disease (moderate severity or worse) increases with age, present in only 0.7% of those age 18 to 44 years but increasing to 13.3% of adults 75 years and older. Compared with other types of clinically significant valve disease seen on echocardiography, native aortic valve stenosis is the most common (34%) in the Euro Heart Survey, followed by previous valve surgery (28%), mitral regurgitation (25%), and multivalve disease (20%).

### ■ CAUSES OF AORTIC VALVE DISEASE

Aortic stenosis typically is due to disease of the valve leaflets. Aortic regurgitation may be due to leaflet or aortic root disease (**Tables 52-1** and **52-2**). The primary causes of aortic leaflet disease are a congenitally abnormal (often bicuspid) valve, calcific valve disease, or rheumatic valve disease. Abnormalities of the aorta that result in valve dysfunction include genetic connective tissue disorders, such as Marfan syndrome, or other causes of aortic root dilation, such as systemic inflammatory disorders, including systemic lupus erythematosus or rheumatoid arthritis. Rarely, the use of some pharmacologic agents, such as serotonin inhibitors, results in leaflet thickening and valve regurgitation.

### ■ CALCIFIC AORTIC VALVE DISEASE

Calcific aortic valve disease (CAVD) is abnormal calcification of the valve leaflets, characterized by involvement of the leaflet bases, relative sparing of the leaflet edges, and absence of commissural fusion. CAVD spans the range from mild focal areas of valve thickening without impairment of leaflet motion, called aortic sclerosis, to significant obstruction of LV outflow, called calcific aortic stenosis (**Fig. 52-1**). CAVD may be present on an anatomically normal trileaflet aortic valve or on a congenitally bicuspid valve. Once severe calcification is present, it may be difficult to identify the number of leaflets with certainty on clinical imaging.

### Prevalence

Aortic valve sclerosis was present in 26% of adults older than 65 years and 48% of those older than 85 years of age in the US population-based Cardiovascular Health Study (CHS), which included 5621 adults. Similarly, in the Finnish Helsinki Aging Study, 21% of adults aged 55 to 71 years had aortic sclerosis on echocardiography. Aortic sclerosis may progress over time to stenosis. Severe calcific aortic stenosis occurs in approximately 2% to 4% of adults older than 65 years, with increasing prevalence with age. Of the approximately 50 000 aortic valve replacements performed

**TABLE 52-1.** Causes of Aortic Stenosis

**Common**
Bicuspid aortic valve
Calcific aortic valve disease
Rheumatic valve disease

**Uncommon**
Congenital aortic stenosis
Homozygous type II hyperlipoproteinemia
Metabolic infiltrative disorders (eg, Fabry disease)
Systemic lupus erythematosus
Ochronosis with alkaptonuria

**Nonvalvular left ventricular outflow obstruction**
Subaortic membrane
Hypertrophic cardiomyopathy
Supravalvular aortic stenosis (eg, Williams syndrome)

**TABLE 52-2.** Causes of Aortic Regurgitation

**Leaflet abnormalities**
Chronic regurgitation
    Bicuspid aortic valve
    Calcific valve disease
    Rheumatic valve disease
    Myxomatous valve disease
    Rheumatoid arthritis
    Nonbacterial thrombotic endocarditis
    Systemic lupus erythematosus
    Pharmacologic agents
Acute regurgitation
    Endocarditis
    Iatrogenic leaflet damage
    Ruptured leaflet fenestration
    Blunt chest trauma

**Abnormalities of the aorta**
Chronic regurgitation
    Marfan syndrome
    Bicuspid aortic valve disease
    Hypertensive aortic dilation
    Familial aortic aneurysm
    Cardiovascular syphilis
    Ankylosing spondylitis
    Other systemic inflammatory disorders
Acute regurgitation
    Aortic dissection

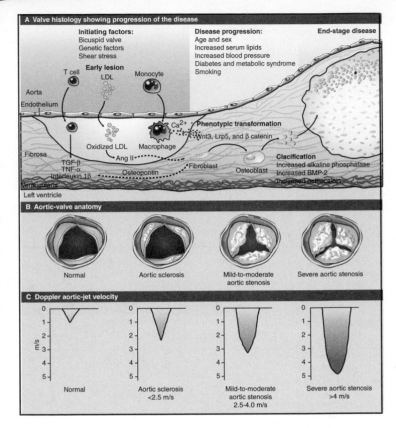

**FIGURE 52-1.** ( **A**) In the early lesion of calcific aortic valve disease there is subendothelial accumulation of oxidized low-density lipoprotein (LDL), production of angiotensin II, and inflammation with T lymphocytes and macrophages. With disease progression, there is production of proteins that mediate tissue calcification, such as osteopontin, osteocalcin, and bone morphogenic protein 2, and leaflet fibroblasts undergo phenotypic transformation to osteoblasts. Inflammatory signaling pathways, including tumor necrosis factor (TNF) α, tumor growth factor (TGF) β, the complement system, C-reactive protein, and interleukin-1β are activated. Microscopic extracellular calcification, seen in the early lesion, progresses to areas of frank bone formation in end-stage disease. Macroscopically, there is progressive leaflet thickening and calcification ( **B**) which leads to outflow obstruction and a corresponding increase in the Doppler aortic-jet velocity ( **C**). (Reproduced with permission from Otto CM. *N Engl J Med.* 2008;359(13):1395-1398. Copyright © 2008 Massachusetts Medical Society. All rights reserved.)

annually in the United States, the vast majority are for aortic stenosis. On the basis of pathologic examination of surgically removed valves, approximately 50% of calcified valves removed at surgery are congenitally bicuspid and approximately 50% are due to calcification of a trileaflet valve.

## Pathophysiology

At the tissue level, the early lesion of CAVD is characterized by focal subendothelial lesions on the aortic side of the leaflet, with extension of the disease process into the adjacent fibrosa. These early lesions resemble atherosclerosis and contain extracellular lipid, including oxidized low-density lipoprotein (LDL), an inflammatory cell infiltrate with macrophages and T lymphocytes, and microscopic tissue calcification. There is evidence of angiotensin-converting enzyme production by a subset of macrophages, along with proteins associated with tissue calcification. Studies of surgically excised valves and animal models of CAVD suggest that disease progression involves phenotypic transformation of valvular interstitial cells, with subsequent osteogenesis resulting in cartilage and bone formation in end-stage disease (Fig. 52-1).

## Genetics and Clinical Risk Factors

Development of CAVD is associated with several anatomic, genetic, and clinical factors. The strongest predictor of CAVD development is a congenitally bicuspid valve. However, genetic factors may be important, even in those with an anatomically trileaflet valve. A study from France showed geographic clustering of aortic stenosis cases where families with multiple affected members over several generations were identified. Additionally, case control studies looking at specific candidate genes have shown genetic polymorphisms associated with CAVD, including variants of the vitamin D receptor, estrogen receptor, apolipoprotein E4, and interleukin 10 alleles.

Clinical factors associated with CAVD have been examined in several large population-based studies. Clinical factors associated with CAVD have included older age, male gender, elevated serum lipoprotein(a) and LDL levels, hypertension, smoking status, diabetes and metabolic syndrome, renal dysfunction, and abnormalities in calcium and phosphate metabolism, and shorter stature. The strength of these associations with CAVD is comparable to that seen with atherosclerotic disease. Other supporting data for an association of CAVD with atherosclerotic risk factors is the presence of accelerated CAVD in the aortic sinuses and root seen early in life in patients with homozygous type II hyperlipoproteinemia. It remains unclear whether clinical risk factors associated with CAVD presence also predict disease progression.

## Clinical Outcomes

Early CAVD (aortic sclerosis) progresses to severe valve obstruction (aortic stenosis) in some, but not all, individuals. Progression from sclerosis to stenosis over a 5-year interval was observed in approximately 9% of the Cardiovascular Health Study (CHS) population (all were older than 65 years). In a study of more than 2000 patients with aortic sclerosis, the average time progression from aortic sclerosis diagnosis to severe aortic stenosis was 8 years, with 10% developing mild stenosis, 3% developing moderate stenosis, and 3% developing severe stenosis.

Even in the absence of significant outflow obstruction, the presence of aortic sclerosis has been associated with adverse clinical outcomes, and this risk persists even in those who do not progress to aortic stenosis. In the CHS study, in which all participants had no known coronary artery disease, the relative risk of cardiovascular death over 5 years was 1.52 (95% CI, 1.12-2.05) compared with those with a normal aortic valve, even after correction for associated baseline clinical factors. In the LIFE hypertension study, the risk associated with aortic sclerosis was additive to the risk of underlying coronary artery disease for an adverse cardiovascular event ( **Fig. 52-2**). The mechanism of the increased risk associated with aortic sclerosis is unclear, but it is likely that aortic sclerosis is a marker of increased risk of atherosclerotic disease, reflecting a susceptible genetic background, an unidentified clinical risk factor, or a generalized inflammatory process.

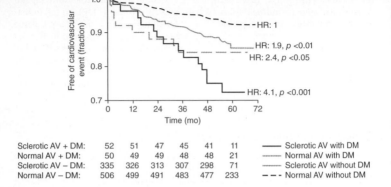

**FIGURE 52-2.** Kaplan-Meier plot showing lower freedom from cardiovascular events in patients with aortic sclerosis compared with those with normal aortic valves (AV). Freedom from cardiovascular events was lower in those with preexisting diabetes mellitus (DM) and was worst in those with both aortic sclerosis and DM. The number of patients at risk are at the bottom of the figure. Hazard ratios (HR) were calculated using Cox regression analysis. (Reproduced with permission from Olsen MH et al. *Am J Cardiol.* 2005;95(1):132-136.)

# ■ BICUSPID AORTIC VALVE DISEASE

## Prevalence and Genetics

A congenitally bicuspid aortic valve (BAV) is common, present in 1% to 2% of all people; 70% to 80% of cases are in men. In some cases, small family studies suggest an autosomal-dominant inheritance pattern. Recently, in a large family with 11 cases of congenital heart disease in 5 generations, a specific defect in the *NOTCH1* gene was identified in association with a BAV and calcific aortic stenosis.

## Pathophysiology

The BAV phenotype may be described based on leaflet morphology. The most common phenotype, occurring in 80% of patients, is congenital fusion of the right and left coronary cusps, resulting in valve opening in a right-left orientation with larger right-sided leaflet. Congenital fusion of the right and noncoronary cusps occurs in the remaining 20% of cases, resulting in an anterior-posterior opening with a larger anterior leaflet.

The abnormal mechanical stress and altered shear stress of a BAV are associated with progressive valve calcification, although genetic factors, such as the *NOTCH1* gene, and a more aggressive inflammatory process may predispose these patients to abnormal tissue calcification. At the tissue level, calcific stenosis of a BAV appears similar to calcific stenosis of a trileaflet valve, and the term CAVD encompasses both bicuspid and trileaflet valve anatomy.

A BAV may be incompetent due to inadequate leaflet coaptation. In addition, in a subset of cases, the BAV phenotype is associated with an aortopathy. Compared with matched patients with a trileaflet aortic valve, patients with BAV have larger ascending aortic dimensions, a faster rate of aortic dilation, and altered aortic elasticity. The pattern of aortic dilation and risk of dissection are not related to valve hemodynamics (eg, severity of stenosis or regurgitation), but preliminary studies suggest a relationship with the specific valve morphology.

## Clinical Outcomes

Overall, long-term survival of adults with BAV does not differ from the general population; however, valve-related clinical events are common. Valve function is normal in the vast majority of patients until the sixth or seventh decade of life, when calcific changes result in severe stenosis, on average a decade earlier than stenosis of a trileaflet valve. Although aortic stenosis is the most common sequelae of a BAV, approximately 15% to 20% of BAVs have inadequate diastolic closure leading to aortic regurgitation. Clinical presentation for significant BAV regurgitation is usually in young adulthood (20-40 years of age) and typically requires valve replacement. Indications for valve replacement are most often due to symptom onset or for prevention of heart failure based on progressive ventricular dilation or early systolic dysfunction. Compared with patients with a normal aortic valve, the risk of aortic dissection is significant. Overall, approximately 7% of aortic dissections occur in people <40 years of age. In this subgroup, 50% have Marfan syndrome, 34% have hypertensive heart disease, 19% have a familial aneurysm, 12% have had prior aortic valve replacement, and 9% have a native BAV. In a consecutive series of 642 adults with a BAV (mean age 35 ± 16 years, 68% men) followed for approximately 9 years, clinical outcomes occurred in 25%. These outcomes included aortic valve replacement (with or without concurrent aortic root surgery) in 22%, heart failure in 2%, aortic complications in 2%, and cardiac death in 3%. Predictors of adverse clinical outcomes were age more than 30 years and greater than mild aortic stenosis or regurgitation.

## ■ RHEUMATIC AORTIC VALVE DISEASE

### Prevalence

Worldwide, rheumatic fever is the most common cause of valvular heart disease, with an estimated prevalence of 15.6 million persons. The geographic prevalence of deaths due to rheumatic valve disease per 100 000 population varies from as high as 6 to 7 in Southeast Asia and the Western Pacific; a mid-range of 4 to 5 in Africa, Europe, and the Eastern Mediterranean; to a low of 1.8 in the Americas. Rheumatic disease primarily affects the mitral valve, with secondary aortic valve involvement seen in approximately one-third of patients, typically resulting in combined aortic stenosis and regurgitation.

### Pathophysiology

Rheumatic valve disease occurs as a consequence of rheumatic fever. In Europe and North America, there is an interval of approximately 15 years between acute rheumatic fever and clinically evident valve disease. A shorter interval between the acute illness and valve dysfunction is seen in areas with a higher prevalence of recurrent rheumatic fever. The anatomic hallmark of rheumatic valve disease is fusion of valve commissures. The mitral valve is uniformly affected with commissural thickening and fusion leading to mitral stenosis. When there is chordal involvement, with thickening and shortening of the subvalvular apparatus, mitral leaflet coaptation is adversely affected and there is concomitant mitral regurgitation. A similar disease process affects the aortic valve with thickening of leaflet edges and commissural fusion, resulting in a central triangular systolic valve orifice and valve stenosis. With increased leaflet stiffness and deformity, aortic regurgitation may also occur. At the tissue level, rheumatic valve leaflets show thickening and fibrosis, with typical rheumatic features including Aschoff bodies, leukocyte infiltration, and prominent neovascularization. Ultimately, superimposed calcification and fibrosis, similar to CAVD, are seen.

## Clinical Outcomes

Mitral valve involvement is usually predominant and often defines the clinical course and management. Compared with CAVD, rheumatic aortic stenosis generally progresses more slowly, although natural history studies are limited and the disease course may be accelerated with recurrent episodes of rheumatic fever, emphasizing the importance of secondary prevention in patients with rheumatic valve disease. In addition, CAVD may become superimposed on the rheumatic valve with disease progression related to calcific disease rather than to the rheumatic process per se.

## ■ AORTIC VALVE STENOSIS

### Valve Opening and Flow Dynamics

The cross-sectional area of the normal aortic valve in systole is only slightly less than the size of the adjacent LV outflow tract so that blood is ejected from the LV at a low velocity (approximately 1 m/s) as a smooth column of blood with parallel streamlines across the flow area. For any transaortic volume flow, aortic velocity and the pressure gradient increase with worsening LV outflow obstruction. The magnitude of increase in jet velocity varies with the volume flow rate. Therefore, in those with severe stenosis, but only a low stroke volume, such as in those with LV systolic dysfunction, there may only be a moderate increase in aortic velocity.

The normal adult aortic valve area is between 3.0 and 4.0 cm². A normal cardiac output can be maintained without a significant increase in aortic velocity until valve area is reduced to approximately 25% to 30% of normal. With decreases in valve area below 1 cm², very small changes in orifice area lead to marked changes in transvalvular pressure gradient and hemodynamic load. LV systolic pressure increases in proportion to the severity of valve obstruction, with the potential energy in the difference (or gradient) between LV and aortic pressure converted into kinetic energy as blood is ejected at high velocity across the valve.

The normal aortic valve area depends on body size, with an increase in valve area from birth to adulthood corresponding to the increase in lean body mass. In adults, valve area can be indexed for body size, typically using body-surface area, although it is not clear that indexing is necessary, nor that body surface area is the best method of indexing. A simple clinical approach is to consider the ratio of the velocity in the LV outflow tract (the patient's normal valve size) to the aortic velocity. A normal ratio is close to 1.0; a ratio of 0.25 indicates a valve area 25% of expected for that patient. The standard clinical hemodynamic parameters of aortic stenosis severity are as follows:

- Transaortic velocity
- Mean transaortic pressure gradient
- Aortic valve area

Definitions for mild, moderate, and severe aortic stenosis are shown in **Table 52-3**. This table provides only a guideline for clinical practice; in an individual patient, not all parameters will fit in the same category, and between patients, there is considerable variability in the degree of valve stenosis resulting in clinical symptoms. Other measures of aortic valve hemodynamics have been proposed and may be useful in some situations, but are not routinely recommended. These measures include LV stroke work loss, recovered pressure gradient, energy loss index, and valvuloarterial impedance.

### Coronary Blood Flow

Approximately 50% of adults with severe aortic stenosis have concurrent coronary artery disease. Even in the absence of associated atherosclerotic coronary disease,

**TABLE 52-3.** Hemodynamic Severity of Aortic Valve Stenosis

| | Aortic sclerosis | Mild | Moderate | Severe |
|---|---|---|---|---|
| Aortic jet velocity (m/s) | ≤2.5 m/s | 2.6-2.9 | 3.0-4.0 | >4.0 |
| Mean gradient (mm Hg) | – | <20(<30[a]) | 20-40[b] (30-50[a]) | >40[b](>50[a]) |
| AVA (cm²) | – | >1.5 | 1.0-1.5 | <1.0 |
| Indexed AVA (cm²/m²) | | >0.85 | 0.60-0.85 | <0.6 |
| Velocity ratio | | >0.50 | 0.25-0.50 | <0.25 |

[a]Indicates the European Society of Cardiology (ESC) mean gradient classification.

[b]Indicates the American College of Cardiology (ACC) classification.

Modified from Baumgartner H, Hung J, Bermejo J, et al. Echocardiographic assessment of valve stenosis: EAE/ASE recommendations for clinical practice. *J Am Soc Echocardiogr*. 2009;22(1):1-23.

there is limited coronary flow reserve because the increase in coronary vessel size often fails to match the increase in LV mass. Additionally, the adequacy of myocardial oxygen delivery is limited by decreased capillary density and increased diastolic wall stress. Mismatch in myocardial oxygen supply and demand is initially evident in the subendothelium and is likely the pathophysiologic basis of angina in the absence of epicardial coronary stenosis.

## LV Response to Pressure Overload

Aortic stenosis imposes an increased pressure load on the LV, resulting in *compensatory* LV hypertrophy. *LV hypertrophy* is defined as an increase in LV mass when compared with normal standards based on body size and sex and may be due to an increase in wall thickness with a normal chamber size (concentric hypertrophy) or an increase in LV size with relatively normal wall thickness (eccentric hypertrophy). When aortic stenosis is present, a compensatory increase in LV wall thickness serves to maintain normal wall stress ($\sigma$) because wall stress is proportional to LV pressure ($P$) and radius ($r$) and inversely related to wall thickness ($Th$):

$$\sigma = (p \times r)/2Th$$

Thus the typical response of the left ventricle as aortic stenosis severity gradually progresses is symmetrically increased LV wall thickness, with no change in chamber size. The presence and severity of LV hypertrophy varies from patient to patient. Concurrent hypertension may result in excessive LV hypertrophy due to the additional hemodynamic afterload of increased systemic vascular resistance. Although somewhat related to the severity of valve obstruction, not all patients develop hypertrophy. An increase in LV mass is seen in 81% of women but only 54% of men with severe aortic stenosis. In women, the increase in LV mass is due to a marked increase in wall thickness with a small chamber size and normal or hyperdynamic systolic function, with evidence of diastolic dysfunction. In contrast, men more often have only a mild increase in wall thickness with an increase in chamber size.

In most patients with aortic stenosis, LV ejection fraction and wall stress remain normal due to LV compensatory mechanisms to increase wall thickness. However, the increase in afterload may eventually exceed the compensatory LV response, resulting in *afterload mismatch* and impaired LV systolic function. The concept of afterload mismatch is preservation of myocardial contractile function, but impaired systolic function due to high afterload. In this scenario, LV systolic function should improve if afterload is relieved with replacement of the stenotic valve. Clinical experience supports this concept, with LV ejection fraction usually improving after valve replacement for severe aortic stenosis (average improvement ~10 ejection fraction units).

## Low-Flow Low-Gradient Aortic Stenosis

A small subset of patients with aortic stenosis develop impaired myocardial contractility that does not improve after valve replacement. Most of these patients have decreased systolic function due to coronary artery disease or a concurrent cardiomyopathy. A few have long-standing, untreated severe aortic stenosis, resulting in irreversible myocardial dysfunction. This is a complication that can be prevented by valve replacement at symptom onset or at onset of LV dysfunction, as recommended in current guidelines.

Although aortic valve area varies less than aortic velocity (or pressure gradient), with changes in transaortic volume flow rate, the degree of valve leaflet opening can vary in some situations. At the extreme, there is no aortic leaflet motion when there is no transaortic flow, even with normal valve leaflets. In patients with aortic stenosis and concurrent LV systolic dysfunction, full aortic leaflet opening may be reduced due to a low stroke volume, rather than to severe valve obstruction. In this scenario, the calculated valve area reflects the actual leaflet opening, not the maximal leaflet opening possible if cardiac output were normal. Thus it can be difficult to identify severe stenosis resulting in LV dysfunction (true stenosis) from primary myocardial dysfunction with only moderate aortic stenosis (pseudostenosis). Distinguishing these patients can be achieved with evaluation of valve hemodynamics during low-dose pharmacologic augmentation of cardiac output with either dobutamine (via increased contractility) or nitroprusside (via vasodilation). With these modalities, the change in aortic velocity and valve area is assessed as the transaortic volume flow rate increases. Severe stenosis is present if aortic velocity increases to at least 4.0 m/s or if aortic valve area remains 1.0 cm$^2$ or smaller in the setting of increased stroke volume or ejection fraction by at least 20%. These patients benefit from valve replacement. In contrast, stenosis is only moderate if aortic velocity remains less than 4.0 m/s and valve area increases to greater than 1.0 cm$^2$ with an increase in stroke volume. For these patients, valve replacement is less likely to be beneficial. The failure of ejection fraction and transaortic flow rate to increase at all with dobutamine is called *lack of contractile reserve* and connotes poor prognosis with either medical or surgical therapy.

Low-output aortic stenosis also may be seen in patients with a normal ejection fraction but small transaortic stroke volume. These patients have normal LV systolic function both visually and on measurement of ejection fraction but have a small LV chamber size due to myocardial hypertrophy, often in conjunction with diastolic dysfunction that further limits ventricular filling. Although aortic velocity and pressure gradient are relatively low in these patients, calculated aortic valve area is small and correctly reflects the severity of valve obstruction. Concurrent systemic hypertension can also hinder interpretation of aortic valve hemodynamics because increased systemic vascular resistance may reduce forward stroke volume, resulting in underestimation of the severity of valve disease. Ideally, valve stenosis severity should be remeasured after normalization of blood pressure in these patients.

## ■ DIAGNOSIS

Most patients initially diagnosed with aortic stenosis are asymptomatic; patients are identified when a murmur is noted on physical examination. Increased flow velocity and turbulent flow across the narrowed valve results in a systolic crescendo-decrescendo (ejection) murmur heard loudest over the proximal ascending aorta in the right parasternal third or fourth intercostal space (aortic region). The murmur usually radiates to the carotids and can be distinguished from a carotid bruit by a similar tonal quality and timing relative to the primary murmur. In older patients, the murmur may radiate to the apex instead of the carotids, termed the *Gallavardin phenomenon* (**Table 52-4**). A systolic murmur is sensitive, but not specific for diagnosis of aortic stenosis. A very loud ejection murmur, grade 4/6 or higher, particularly with an associated parasternal thrill, suggests severe stenosis. However, murmur severity alone does not correlate well with disease severity because most patients with significant stenosis have only a grade 2/6 or 3/6 murmur. Moreover, many patients with a systolic murmur actually have a benign murmur due to aortic valve sclerosis or mitral regurgitation.

With progressive stenosis severity, the aortic component of the second heart sound ($S_2$) becomes muffled or absent because the thickened leaflets no longer generate a valve closure sound. As such, a single $S_2$ is consistent with severe stenosis; normal physiologic splitting of $S_2$ reliably excludes severe valve obstruction. An $S_4$ is common with diastolic dysfunction and increased atrial contribution to LV filling. An $S_3$ gallop is present only late in the disease and indicates severely elevated filling pressures. In young adults with congenital stenosis, a systolic ejection click may be present due to sudden tensing as the fused leaflets reach their limit of excursion in early to mid systole. This finding is rarely appreciated in older adults (Table 52-4). A delayed and diminished (*parvus et tardus*) carotid upstroke is a key physical finding

**TABLE 52-4.** Common Clinical Findings in Aortic Stenosis

| Clinical history |
| --- |
| Exertional dyspnea |
| Decreased exercise tolerance |
| Angina |
| Heart failure |
| Exertional dizziness/syncope |

| Physical examination |
| --- |
| Systolic ejection murmur (right parasternal third or fourth intercostal space) |
| Parasternal thrill |
| Radiation of murmur to carotid artery |
| Radiation of murmur to the apex (Gallavardin phenomenon) |
| Delayed and diminished (parvus and tardus) carotid upstroke |
| Single $S_2$ |
| $S_4$ gallop |

| Echocardiography |
| --- |
| Aortic leaflet calcification |
| Stenosis severity |
|     Aortic peak velocity |
|     Mean transaortic gradient |
|     Aortic valve area |
| Normal left ventricular (LV) chamber size with normal systolic function |
| Concentric LV hypertrophy |
| Evidence of LV diastolic dysfunction |
| Pulmonary hypertension |

in aortic stenosis and correlates with stenosis severity and increased likelihood of symptom onset. Concurrent hypertension may mask this finding because increased arterial stiffness will result in an apparently normal carotid impulse despite valve obstruction.

Initial echocardiography is appropriate when aortic stenosis is suspected by history (cardiopulmonary symptoms) or physical examination (newly diagnosed grade 2/6 or louder systolic murmur). Echocardiographic visualization of leaflet anatomy allows identification of valve disease etiology, and stenosis severity is evaluated using Doppler data. By echocardiography, LV chamber size usually appears normal, with concentric hypertrophy and preserved systolic function. There is often evidence of diastolic dysfunction, with left atrial enlargement and diminished septal myocardial tissue velocity. Other associated abnormalities may include aortic dilation, coexisting mitral valve disease, and pulmonary hypertension.

In rare cases where echocardiography findings are discrepant from patient symptoms or clinical examination, cardiac catheterization may be used for direct measurement of transaortic pressure gradients. However, current guidelines discourage crossing the aortic valve with catheters unless necessary, given the potential risk of cerebral embolization. ECG findings are not sensitive for aortic stenosis diagnosis and are related to associated findings, such as LV hypertrophy with increased QRS voltage, ST-T wave changes (strain pattern), and left atrial enlargement. Chest CT and cardiac MRI are not recommended for initial diagnostic evaluation, although these modalities may provide further visualization of aortic root anatomy and dimensions in patients with a BAV.

# ■ CLINICAL COURSE

In mild to moderate aortic stenosis, prospective studies of hemodynamic progression document a mean yearly rate of increase in aortic jet velocity of 0.3 m/s per year, a mean increase in transaortic pressure gradient of 4 to 7 mm Hg per year, and a mean decrease in valve area of 0.1 cm$^2$ per year. Although mean rates of hemodynamic progression are comparable across studies, there is marked individual variation, with some patients showing an increase in mean systolic gradients as high as 15 to 20 mm Hg per year. Clinical factors associated with a more rapid progression are not fully defined but include the baseline severity of stenosis, the degree of leaflet calcification, and etiology of valve disease.

## Symptoms Due to Aortic Stenosis

The classic symptoms of aortic stenosis are angina, syncope, and heart failure. Typically, patients with stenosis remain asymptomatic for many years, despite a gradual progressive obstruction to LV outflow and increased intracavitary LV pressure. Symptom onset occurs at the point when cardiac output cannot be increased adequately across the narrowed valve to meet metabolic demands. Thus initial symptoms nearly always occur with exertion. There is wide individual variability in the severity of outflow obstruction that produces symptoms. Over a third of patients who are symptomatic do not yet have critical aortic stenosis. A hemodynamic evaluation of stenosis severity, usually by echocardiography, is important to ensure that valve obstruction is the cause of symptoms, as stenosis that is only mild or moderate is unlikely to be the culprit.

In the absence of preceding symptoms, primary syncope attributable to aortic stenosis is uncommon. Potential contributors to exertional syncope include an exaggerated LV baroreceptor response to exercise with associated peripheral vasodilation and an inability to augment cardiac output across the fixed outflow obstruction. Arrhythmic contributors to syncope are less likely, but may include exercise-induced transient bradycardia and atrial fibrillation. Primary ventricular arrhythmias in aortic stenosis are rare.

Symptoms of heart failure are usually due to diastolic dysfunction. Increased afterload leads to concentric LV hypertrophy as a mechanism to maintain normal wall stress. As stenosis severity and hypertrophy progresses, there is a decrease in LV compliance and increase in LV end-diastolic pressure. In these patients, atrial fibrillation, with loss of the atrial contractile contribution to diastolic filling, can lead to severe clinical deterioration. Clinical progression to systolic dysfunction, particularly in the absence of symptoms, is rare. Contributing causes for decreased systolic function may include ischemic heart disease or mitral regurgitation.

Pulmonary hypertension in aortic stenosis is common. In a study of 388 symptomatic patients with aortic stenosis who underwent cardiac catheterization, approximately 50% had mild to moderate pulmonary hypertension and approximately 15% had severe pulmonary hypertension. Believed to be due to diastolic dysfunction and elevated LV end-diastolic pressure, recognition of pulmonary hypertension is important because it is associated with a more severe clinical picture and poorer long-term prognosis, even in those who have undergone aortic valve replacement.

Another clinical finding seen in patients with aortic stenosis is an increased bleeding tendency; this is thought to be due to acquired platelet dysfunction resulting from mechanical disruption of von Willebrand multimers, with turbulent blood flow through the narrowed valve and triggered platelet clearance. Commonly manifesting as chronic gastrointestinal or mucosal bleeding, this abnormality can be seen in the majority of patients with severe aortic stenosis, and the magnitude of abnormality is directly related to stenosis severity.

## Clinical Outcomes

Natural history studies of aortic stenosis document low mortality rates in patients who remain symptom free. Symptom presence is the strongest predictor of adverse outcomes with moderate to severe aortic stenosis, despite individual variation in the hemodynamic severity of valve obstruction at symptom onset. If left untreated, symptomatic patients with severe stenosis have a dismal prognosis. In a study following symptomatic patients who refused surgery, average survival was only 2 years, with a 5-year survival less than 20%. Thus current clinical guideline recommendations predicate timing of valve replacement on symptom onset. Valve replacement in symptomatic patients is nearly always followed by improvement in symptoms and survival.

All patients with aortic stenosis have some hemodynamic progression of stenosis over time; symptom onset eventually occurs once stenosis is severe, typically the seventh or eighth decade of life with stenosis of a trileaflet valve and the sixth or seventh decade of life with stenosis of a BAV. Patients who progress to severe stenosis may initially be asymptomatic, but most develop symptoms within a few years of diagnosis. Thus, monitoring for symptom onset is critical once stenosis of any severity is diagnosed.

The strongest predictor of disease progression and symptom onset is the severity of aortic stenosis at initial presentation. In a prospective study of 123 adult patients with asymptomatic aortic stenosis, fewer than 26% remained symptom free after 5 years; the rate of symptom onset was 8% per year when aortic jet velocity was less than 3 m/s per year and 17% per year in those with an aortic velocity between 3 and 4 m/s per year. Other predictors of symptom onset include older age, the rate of change in jet velocity over time, the extent of valvular calcification, concurrent coronary artery disease, and functional status. Higher-risk asymptomatic patients includes those with ejection fraction <50%, an annual increase in aortic jet velocity of ≥0.3 m/s per year, moderate to severe leaflet calcification, and marked LV hypertrophy.

Low-gradient low-output aortic stenosis, defined as a valve area less than 1.0 cm$^2$ with a mean transaortic pressure gradient <30 mm Hg, occurs in patients with LV systolic dysfunction, which results in a low transaortic volume flow rate. Compared with those with normal LV systolic function, perioperative mortality is significant, usually with some degree of persistent, postoperative heart failure. Importantly, however, systolic dysfunction is not a contraindication for valve replacement. Surgery is still recommended because the clinical course is nearly always improved compared with that seen with conservative management, with improvements in both survival and ventricular performance. Evidence for contractile reserve on dobutamine stress echocardiography in this patient population is predictive of significantly improved clinical outcomes after valve replacement.

Less commonly, low-gradient aortic stenosis is seen in patients with normal LV function. Overall clinical outcomes are worse compared with those with higher transaortic gradients. In a study of 512 patients with severe aortic stenosis and a normal LV ejection fraction, patients with low flow aortic stenosis ($n = 181$) had a significantly lower 3-year survival compared with patients with a normal flow rate ($n = 331$) (76% vs 86%; $p = 0.006$).

## Periodic Evaluation

In asymptomatic patients with aortic stenosis, a conservative approach with close clinical follow-up and serial echocardiography is reasonable. Current clinical guidelines for management of valvular heart disease recommend intervals for echocardiographic monitoring that vary with stenosis severity: yearly for severe stenosis, every 1 to 2 years for moderate stenosis, and every 3 to 5 years for mild stenosis. In addition, at least annual clinical visits with the patient's care providers for symptom monitoring is recommended (**Table 52-5**).

**TABLE 52-5.** Serial Evaluation in Asymptomatic Patients

| | Clinical Follow-Up | Echocardiography |
|---|---|---|
| **Aortic stenosis** | | |
| Mild | At least yearly | Every 3-5 y |
| Moderate | At least yearly | Every 1-2 y |
| Severe | At least yearly | Yearly |
| **Aortic regurgitation** | | |
| Mild | At least yearly | Every 2-3 y |
| Moderate | At least yearly | Every 1-2 y |
| Severe (normal LV size) | At least yearly | At least yearly |
| Severe (increased LV size) | At least yearly | Every 6-12 mo |
| **Bicuspid AV, screen as above for stenosis or regurgitation or additionally** | | |
| If ascending aorta >4.0 cm | At least yearly | Yearly (additional modalities: CT or MRI) |

AV, aortic valve; CT, computed tomographic imaging; MRI, magnetic resonance imaging.

Data from Bonow RO, Carabello BA, Chatterjee K, et al. ACC/AHA 2006 guidelines for the management of patients with valvular heart disease: a report of the American College of Cardiology/American Heart Association Task Force on Practice Guidelines (Writing committee to revise the 1998 guidelines for the management of patients with valvular heart disease) developed in collaboration with the Society of Cardiovascular Anesthesiologists endorsed by the Society for Cardiovascular Angiography and Interventions and the Society of Thoracic Surgeons. *J Am Coll Cardiol.* 2006;48(13):e1-e148.

If symptom determination is equivocal, stress testing can be a helpful adjunct. During stress testing, an increase in the mean transaortic pressure gradient ≥18 mm Hg or an abnormal exercise test (ischemic ECG changes or blunted blood pressure response) has been shown to be predictive of cardiac events. Stress testing can be performed safely when monitored by an experienced physician, but should be ended promptly if the patient develops symptoms or has a blunted blood pressure response (<20 mm Hg increase with exercise). Because symptom onset may be insidious or may be masked by other comorbidities that cause similar symptoms, brain natriuretic peptide (BNP) has also been investigated as a more objective marker to discriminate early symptoms of heart failure and to identify patients earlier who might benefit from surgery. Serum BNP has been associated with stenosis severity and predict the short-term development of symptoms.

## ■ MEDICAL THERAPY TO PREVENT PROGRESSION

Based on the overlap in clinical risk factors between CAVD and atherosclerosis and the similarities in the disease processes at the tissue level, it was hypothesized that lipid lowering might prevent progressive valve obstruction in adults with CAVD. Although initial data with statin therapy from retrospective observational studies was promising, prospective randomized trials have not convincingly shown a significant benefit of statin therapy to slow disease progression in the valve leaflets. The SALTIRE trial prospectively enrolled 155 adults with calcific aortic stenosis (aortic jet velocity >2.5 m/s) randomly assigned to atorvastatin 80 mg/d or placebo. At a median follow-up of 25 months, there was no difference in the rate of increase in aortic jet velocity or of progression of aortic valve calcification. Similarly, the SEAS trial prospectively enrolled 1873 adults with mild to moderate aortic stenosis (mean aortic jet velocity of 3.1 m/s) randomly assigned to simvastatin plus ezetimibe or placebo. At a median follow-up of 52 months, there was no difference in increase in aortic jet velocity or cardiovascular outcomes. In the most recent prospective trial, the ASTRONOMER trial, there was again no significant difference in aortic stenosis progression in patients treated with a HMG Co-A reductase inhibitor (rosuvastatin) compared to placebo over a median follow-up of 3.5 years. ASTRONOMER was a randomized, double-blind, placebo-controlled trial of asymptomatic patients with mild to moderate AS and no clinical indication for lipid lowering. The findings of the SEAS, SALTAIRE, and now, ASTRONOMER all suggest that treatment with an HMG Co-A reductase inhibitor is not associated with a reduction in aortic stenosis progression and should not be used as primary prevention or a primary treatment strategy for aortic stenosis.

It has also been suggested that angiotensin converting enzyme (ACE) inhibitors might have a potential benefit on LV remodeling and LV hypertrophic changes seen in aortic stenosis. However, in a large retrospective cohort study examining use of ACE inhibitors in patients with aortic stenosis, 134 of 211 subjects receiving ACE inhibitors had no significant difference on the rate of CAVD progression.

Nitrogen-containing bisphosphonates inhibit the cholesterol biosynthesis pathway resulting in several anti-atherosclerotic pleiotropic effects. In addition, their inhibition of bone resorption may indirectly reduce calcification of cardiovascular tissues. Together, these properties suggest a role for bisphosphonates in slowing the progression of calcific valve disease. In fact, several small, retrospective studies have demonstrated that bisphosphonate therapy is associated with slowed progression of AS. Additionally, an analysis from the Multi-Ethnic Study of Atherosclerosis (MESA) suggests that bisphosphonates may be beneficially related to valve and vascular calcification in older subjects. Prospective studies are needed to determine whether these agents are of clinical value in managing patients with aortic stenosis.

# ■ TIMING OF SURGERY FOR AORTIC STENOSIS

## Symptomatic Severe Aortic Stenosis

Given the grim prognosis if valve obstruction is not relieved, surgical valve replacement should be considered in all symptomatic patients, regardless of age or comorbidities (Fig. 52-3 and Table 52-6). Importantly, early symptom identification may be missed, particularly in the elderly, where a decline in exercise tolerance may be attributed to "old age." Older age is not a contraindication for valve replacement, as symptomatic patients who undergo valve replacement have nearly normalized age-corrected postoperative survival.

Patients should be carefully educated on the symptoms of aortic stenosis and instructed to promptly relay onset to providers. In patients with equivocal or unclear symptom status, exercise testing or serum BNP levels may be an adjunct to identify patients who are nearing symptom onset. If exercise testing is performed, patients with reduced exercise tolerance or a blunted blood pressure rise (<20 mm Hg) should be considered for valve replacement because these findings indicate probable symptoms. In patients who initially present with acute, decompensated heart failure due to severe aortic stenosis, cautious administration of nitroprusside has been shown to transiently improve hemodynamic status and myocardial performance as a bridge to surgery.

Approximately 30% of patients with symptomatic aortic stenosis are denied surgery due to comorbid conditions. Historically, these patients have had limited therapeutic options. Percutaneous balloon valvuloplasty has been used in this setting for palliation as the procedure results in a modest reduction in outflow gradient and symptoms. However, residual obstruction from leaflet thickening and annular

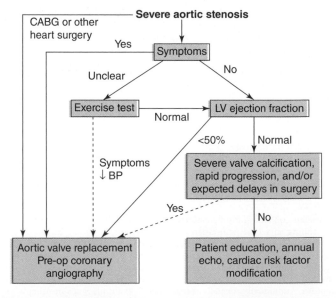

**FIGURE 52-3.** Suggested algorithm for clinical management of adults with severe aortic stenosis. BP, blood pressure; CABG, coronary artery bypass grafting; LV, left ventricular. [Modified from Bonow RO et al. *Circulation.* 2008;118(15):e523-e661.]

**TABLE 52-6.** Measures of Aortic Regurgitation Severity

| Parameter | Mild (%) | Moderate (%) | Severe (%) |
|---|---|---|---|
| Jet width/LVOT | <25 | 25-65 | >65 |
| Vena contracta (cm) | <0.3 | 0.3-0.6 | >0.6 |
| Pressure half-time (ms) | >500 | 200-500 | <200 |
| Regurgitant volume (mL/beat) | <30 | 30-60 | >60 |
| Regurgitant fraction (%) | <30 | 30-50 | >50 |
| Regurgitant orifice area (cm²) | <0.10 | 0.1-0.3 | >0.30 |

LVOT, left ventricular outflow tract.

Data from Zoghbi WA, Enriquez-Sarano M, Foster E, et al. Recommendations for evaluation of the severity of native valvular regurgitation with two-dimensional and Doppler echocardiography. *J Am Soc Echocardiogr.* 2003;16:777-802.

calcification often remains, and symptoms typically recur within 6 to 12 months. In addition, survival benefit has not been demonstrated after valvuloplasty. Consequently, practice guidelines consider aortic valvuloplasty acceptable for palliation or as a bridge to surgery in hemodynamically unstable patients. Percutaneous balloon valvuloplasty may also be useful in rheumatic heart disease, in patients with severe aortic stenosis in need of major, noncardiac surgery, and in rare situations, as a diagnostic technique to definitively determine whether patient symptoms are indeed secondary to severe AS prior to subjecting them to more high-risk procedures such as aortic valve replacement.

More recently, transcatheter aortic valve replacement (TAVR) has emerged as a viable option for high-risk patients with symptomatic severe aortic stenosis. Currently, 2 TAVR technologies have been extensively studied and are gaining acceptance: the Edwards SAPIEN (Edwards LifeSciences, Irving, CA, USA) and the Medtronic CoreValve (Medtronic Inc, Minneapolis, MN, USA) transcatheter heart valve system. The SAPIEN valve is composed of bovine pericardial leaflets mounted within a balloon-expandable stent; whereas, the CoreValve contains porcine pericardial leaflets within a self-expanding stent. The PARTNER trial, utilizing the SAPIEN valve, recently demonstrated a dramatic reduction in the rate of death from any cause at 1-year follow-up in inoperable patients (hazard ratio 0.55; 95% CI, 0.40-0.74). In high-risk operable patients (predicted operative risk ≥15%), transcatheter and surgical aortic valve replacement resulted in similar 1-year survival. The CoreValve US Pivotal Trial is currently ongoing, but data from its international use has been equally promising.

## Asymptomatic Severe Aortic Stenosis

Prophylactic valve replacement in asymptomatic patients with severe aortic stenosis is not recommended because outcomes are excellent in the absence of symptoms. Given that the overall risk of sudden cardiac death is less than 1% in asymptomatic patients, the perioperative morbidity and mortality risk incurred would outweigh benefit. Potential complications of a prosthetic valve include endocarditis, prosthesis dysfunction, and morbidity associated with anticoagulation, all of which combined occur at a rate of approximately 3% per year. Moreover, aortic valve replacement may not necessarily abolish the risk of sudden death. In addition, the hemodynamic severity of aortic stenosis at symptom onset is variable. The lack of an absolute "cutoff" to predict symptom onset precludes prophylactic valve replacement for hemodynamic indices alone, as the patient may remain asymptomatic for some time, potentially negating the need for surgery altogether.

However, individual consideration of prophylactic valve replacement is made in certain patient groups, including those with moderate to severe stenosis undergoing other cardiac surgery and those with severe aortic stenosis with mitigating circumstances, such as women contemplating pregnancy, patients who plan activities that involve severe exertion, and those who live in areas remote from medical care, which might delay prompt intervention at symptom onset. Additionally, in patients who are asymptomatic and with a low expected operative mortality, earlier surgery might be considered if stenosis is extremely severe and there is a high likelihood of rapid disease progression (Table 52-6).

## Low-Output Low-Gradient Aortic Stenosis

Determining the potential benefit and timing of surgery in patients who present with both LV systolic dysfunction and aortic stenosis is problematic because valve replacement in this population is associated with significant postoperative morbidity and mortality. Nonetheless, surgery should be strongly considered in any patient with low-output severe stenosis because valve replacement is associated with better survival and clinical outcome than conservative treatment alone. In a report of 52 patients with ejection fraction ≤35% and transvalvular mean gradient less than 30 mm Hg, perioperative mortality was 21%, and overall survival at 5 years was 39%. Importantly, among those who were able to survive the perioperative time period, significant postoperative improvements in functional status and ejection fraction were seen. Postoperative outcome is most improved for patients with low-output stenosis where contractile reserve is demonstrated during preoperative dobutamine testing (>20% increase in stroke volume or >10 mm Hg increase in mean transaortic pressure gradient). Although clinical improvement in low-output aortic stenosis patients is greatest where contractile reserve is established, even those without contractile reserve demonstrate some improvement in postoperative ejection fraction and functional class. Therefore, given the very high mortality rate in these patients without surgery, consideration of a surgical approach in all patients with low-output stenosis should be made.

## ■ AORTIC VALVE REGURGITATION

### Regurgitant Orifice and Flow Dynamics

Incomplete closure of the aortic valve in diastole results in retrograde flow from the aorta back into the LV in diastole. The volume of retrograde blood flow is determined by the diastolic pressure difference between the aorta and LV, the size of the regurgitant orifice, the duration of diastole, and the relative compliance of the aorta and LV. Both a greater pressure difference between the chambers and a larger orifice area are associated with a greater degree of regurgitation. However, the interaction of physiologic variables affecting regurgitant severity can be complex. For example, with exercise, the rate of backflow per heartbeat increases due to the increase in systemic blood pressure, but the duration of diastole decreases due to tachycardia, so that regurgitant volume is unchanged.

Aortic regurgitant severity is described in terms of the amount of backflow of blood across the aortic valve in diastole. The volume leaking across the valve on each beat is multiplied by heart rate to yield *regurgitant volume,* measured in liters per minutes. *Regurgitant fraction* is the ratio of regurgitant volume to the total volume of blood ejected by the ventricle, expressed as a percentage. The actual size of the regurgitant orifice, or *regurgitant orifice area* (ROA), is likely the most robust measure of disease severity. This is calculated based on the continuity principle.

Regurgitant orifice area is calculated by dividing the regurgitant volume on a single beat (mL or cm$^3$) by the velocity time integral of flow (VTI$_{RJ}$) in the regurgitant jet through the narrowed orifice (cm):

$$ROA\ (cm^2) = RV(cm^3)/VTI_{RJ}\ (cm)$$

Regurgitant volume can be measured by Doppler echocardiography as the difference between the total stroke volume ejected by the ventricle forward across the aortic valve (in systole) and the forward stroke volume delivered to the systemic vasculature measured by the antegrade flow rate across the pulmonic or mitral valve. Total stroke volume can be measured by echocardiography, cardiac MRI, or LV angiography as the difference between end-diastolic and end-systolic volume. Regurgitant volume also can be measured by cardiac MRI based on systolic and diastolic Q-flow in the proximal ascending aorta.

Aortic pulse pressure is increased in patients with aortic regurgitation because increased antegrade stroke volume results in high systolic aortic pressure, whereas backflow of blood across the valve in diastole results in a low diastolic pressure. The distance that retrograde diastolic flow in the aorta extends downstream correlates with regurgitant severity; moderate regurgitation is associated with holodiastolic flow reversal in the proximal descending aorta, whereas severe regurgitation results in holodiastolic flow reversal in the abdominal aorta. With chronic regurgitation, LV diastolic pressures are usually normal because a more compliant LV allows a large LV volume at a low diastolic pressure (a shallow slope of the diastole pressure–volume relationship). This physiology is reflected in the velocity of the aortic regurgitant flow, with the velocity and timing reflecting the instantaneous aortic to LV pressure difference. In addition, in chronic regurgitation, aortic regurgitation is high velocity, reflecting a large pressure difference, with a flat slope from early to late diastole, reflecting normal LV diastolic pressures and only a slight decrease in diastolic aortic pressure.

## Coronary Blood Flow

Coronary blood flow is altered by aortic regurgitation by 2 factors. First, decreased diastolic aortic pressure results in a lower pressure difference between the aorta and coronary vasculature and a decreased diastolic perfusion pressure. Second, although increased LV mass and wall stress lead to a compensatory increase in coronary artery size, this increase is often inadequate to meet the higher LV oxygen demands.

## LV Response to Volume Overload

With chronic aortic regurgitation, the LV dilates, initially with increased compliance, to maintain normal forward stroke volume and normal aortic diastolic pressure (**Fig. 52-4**). LV volume reflects total stroke volume, which increases in direct proportion to the severity of aortic regurgitation. In addition to the LV volume overload imposed by the regurgitant lesion, there is also progressive increases in LV pressure as the larger stroke volume is ejected against peripheral systemic vascular resistance. Despite increased end-systolic pressure, wall stress is maintained by a compensatory increase in wall thickness. Combined volume and pressure overload results in a marked increase in LV mass (much greater than with any other valve lesion) and a substantial increase in LV size. The shape of the LV is affected, becoming more spherical, with apical rounding to accommodate the volume load.

Generally, LV systolic function remains normal for many years with chronic aortic regurgitation, even as the ventricle dilates. Clinical evaluation for diastolic function is problematic as the LV accommodates both normal LV inflow across the mitral valve and the diastolic flow across the incompetent aortic valve. Chronic volume and pressure overload do eventually result in LV systolic dysfunction.

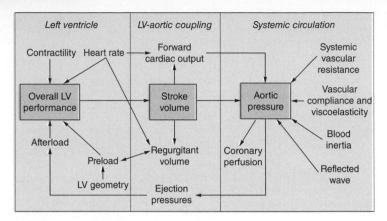

**FIGURE 52-4.** Pathophysiology of chronic aortic regurgitation. Left ventricular (LV) stroke volume includes forward cardiac output and regurgitant volume. Although increased stroke volume increases systemic systolic ejection pressure and aortic pressure, increased regurgitant volume lowers systemic diastolic pressures and, as a result, coronary perfusion. Compensatory mechanisms of the LV to maintain cardiac output despite increased regurgitant volume include dilation and remodeling of the LV. When compensatory mechanisms fail, there is adverse effect on LV contractility. The volume of regurgitant flow is determined by the diastolic pressure difference between the aorta and LV, the size of the regurgitant orifice, the duration of diastole, and the relative compliance of the aorta and LV. [Modified with permission from Borow KM and Marcus RH. *J Am Coll Cardiol.* 1991;17(4):898-900.]

Initially, systolic performance is impaired due to afterload mismatch so that LV size and systolic function return to normal if valve replacement is promptly performed. However, in more advanced cases, patients develop irreversible LV dysfunction that does not improve or only partially improves after valve replacement. Optimal timing of valve replacement in these patients is challenging because clinical measures of ventricular performance vary with changes in preload and afterload, both of which are altered in chronic aortic regurgitation.

Both prospective natural history studies and retrospective surgical series have shown that the strongest predictors of postoperative ejection fraction in patients with chronic regurgitation are the preoperative ejection fraction and end-systolic dimension. Ejection fraction is dependent on preload and afterload so is not an ideal measure, whereas end-systolic dimension is relatively independent of preload and only mildly affected by afterload. These parameters are now used in clinical practice to guide timing of valve replacement in adults with chronic asymptomatic aortic regurgitation.

## ■ DIAGNOSIS

In chronic, compensated aortic regurgitation, the LV dilates to accommodate the progressive increase in regurgitant volume yet still maintain a normal cardiac output. In this phase of the disease, which can last for decades, patients are usually asymptomatic. The diagnosis is made when a diastolic murmur is heard on physical examination, an enlarged heart is noted on chest radiography, or as an incidental finding on echocardiography.

Physical examination findings consistent with chronic aortic regurgitation include a holodiastolic decrescendo murmur heard best at the left sternal border at end expiration with the patient leaning forward. The murmur may be difficult to discern and is often not heard by less experienced observers. Murmur intensity is not necessarily predictive of regurgitant severity. A mid-diastolic rumble at the cardiac apex (*Austin-Flint murmur*) may be heard with severe aortic regurgitation. The mechanism of this murmur is attributed to partial closure of the anterior mitral valve leaflet with turbulent transmitral flow or vibrations caused by the regurgitant jet hitting the LV free wall. Given the increased overall stroke volume, a functional systolic "flow" murmur may also be present, but is usually soft unless stenosis is also present. LV enlargement, if present, is evidenced by a diffuse and laterally displaced LV apical impulse as well as an $S_3$ gallop **(Table 52-7 )**.

The pulse pressure is widened with prominent (bounding) peripheral pulses due to the rapid decrease in aortic pressure in diastole as blood flows retrograde across the aortic valve. The widened pulse pressure accounts for the peripheral vascular physical findings of aortic regurgitation, including bounding carotid pulses (Corrigan pulse), head bobbing (Du Musset sign), and systolic pulsations in the fingernail beds on gentle pressure (Quincke pulses). Diastolic retrograde flow in the distal aorta (Duroziez sign) may be appreciated during slight compression of the femoral artery with a stethoscope (Table 52-7).

Echocardiography is diagnostic for the cause and severity of aortic regurgitation. Anatomy and morphology of the aortic valve and aortic root are generally well seen with transthoracic imaging. However, transesophageal echocardiography may be needed to more closely evaluate valve anatomy, paravalvular abscess, or aortic dissection. If aortic dilation or dissection is suspected, other imaging options for the aorta are CT or MRI, which may better delineate the location and extent of the aortic dilation and the presence of an intimal flap. Doppler echocardiography allows for quantitative evaluation of regurgitation severity as described above (Table 52-6). Other elements of the echocardiographic examination include quantitative measurements of LV chamber size and systolic function, specifically end-diastolic and end-systolic minor axis dimensions and ventricular volumes derived from 2-dimensional or 3-dimensional approaches, along with calculation of LV ejection fraction. Cardiac MRI also allows measurement of LV chamber size and volumes, ejection fraction, and aortic dimensions, but is not typically the initial diagnostic study of choice.

**TABLE 52-7.** Findings in Acute and Chronic Severe Aortic Regurgitation

|  | Acute | Chronic |
| --- | --- | --- |
| Cardiogenic shock | Present | Absent |
| Diastolic LV pressure | Increased | Normal |
| Diastolic LV volume | Normal | Increased |
| Pulse pressure | Normal | Increased |
| Diastolic murmur | Soft, early, harsh | Holodiastolic, decrescendo |
| Mid-diastolic rumble (Austin-Flint murmur) | May be present | May be present |
| $S_1$ | Soft | Normal |
| $S_2$ | Loud $P_2$ | Normal |
| $S_3$ | Present | Absent |
| LV size | Normal | Increased |

LV, left ventricular.

Adapted with permission from Stout KK, Verrier ED. Acute valvular regurgitation. *Circulation.* 2009;119(25):3232-3241.

Aortic regurgitation severity and regurgitant volume can be measured with cardiac MRI based on systolic and diastolic Q-flow in the proximal ascending aorta.

There are no specific ECG abnormalities associated with aortic regurgitation, although evidence for LV hypertrophy is often seen. Chest radiography may show an enlarged LV, a dilated aorta, or evidence of heart failure, but these findings are not specific for aortic regurgitation. Exercise stress testing may be useful when the history is equivocal and symptom status is uncertain, and some centers advocate evaluation of ejection fraction with stress to detect early LV systolic dysfunction.

# ■ CLINICAL COURSE

In patients with only mild aortic regurgitation, regurgitant volume is well tolerated and there is no detectable long-term effect on LV chamber size or systolic function. Most patients with mild regurgitation do not have progressive disease and do not develop symptoms or require intervention. The strongest factor predicting disease progression in patients with mild regurgitation is the underlying etiology of aortic valve disease. For example, mild regurgitation due to hypertension or aortic sclerosis is benign and rarely progresses to pathologic disease. In contrast, aortic regurgitation due to a BAV or in a patient with Marfan syndrome will likely be progressive, eventually requiring surgical intervention on either the aortic valve, the aortic root, or both.

For severe aortic regurgitation, the primary determinants of survival after valve replacement are regurgitant severity, preoperative cardiopulmonary symptoms, and preoperative LV size and function. The significance of clinical symptoms was demonstrated in a follow-up study of 246 patients with more than moderate aortic regurgitation. Those with preoperative functional New York Heart Association (NYHA) class III or IV heart failure symptoms had an annual mortality of 25%, while mildly symptomatic patients (NYHA class II symptoms) had an annual mortality of only 6%. Outcome is poor in symptomatic patients with conservative management alone; annual mortality rates without surgery are more than 10% in those with angina and increase to more than 20% in those with overt heart failure. Therefore, clinical guidelines recommend surgery in any symptomatic patient.

Most patients with severe regurgitation develop symptoms prompting valve replacement before there is evidence of LV systolic dysfunction. The latency period during which asymptomatic patients with significant aortic regurgitation maintain preserved systolic function can be prolonged. In asymptomatic patients with preserved systolic function, disease progression is generally slow, with an average rate of progression to symptoms or LV dysfunction of approximately 4% per year. Sudden cardiac death is rare, occurring at a rate of less than 1% per year. If valve replacement is delayed to the point at which effects of chronic volume overload have resulted in an irreversible decline in LV contractility, long-term clinical outcome is worse, with less recovery of LV postoperative ejection fraction and a higher likelihood of persistent heart failure. Importantly, up to 25% of asymptomatic patients remain asymptomatic despite development of overt LV dysfunction. Therefore, once aortic regurgitation is diagnosed, serial echocardiography with internal clinical evaluation is critical to monitor LV size and systolic function.

The severity of aortic regurgitation is associated with clinical outcome. A recent study of 251 asymptomatic adult patients (mean age 60 years) with aortic regurgitation and ejection fraction ≥50% demonstrated the value of quantitative measures of regurgitant severity in predicting cardiac events (death, heart failure, and new atrial fibrillation). These measures were predictive of prognosis, with a 10-year survival of 69% ± 9% in those with severe regurgitation compared with 92% ± 4% in those with mild regurgitation ($p = 0.05$).

Identifying asymptomatic patients with severe regurgitation at the clinical point just before symptom onset or early evidence of LV dysfunction is challenging. Some centers advocate for measures of LV function during stress testing to aid in timing of valve replacement. In a study of 104 asymptomatic or minimally symptomatic patients with aortic regurgitation and normal LV function prospectively followed for a mean of 7.3 years, the strongest predictor of future decreased LV function, symptom onset, need for surgery, or sudden death was the exercise-induced change in LV ejection fraction. However, several patient series have demonstrated that the most robust predictors of symptom onset or LV dysfunction in chronic regurgitation are preoperative LV size and ejection fraction. Therefore, current consensus guidelines rely on resting measures of LV size and function to determine timing of surgical intervention for asymptomatic patients.

### Periodic Evaluation

Timing of periodic imaging in adults with chronic aortic regurgitation is based on the cause of valve disease, the severity of regurgitation, LV size, and LV systolic function. The presence of an anatomic valve abnormality (such as BAV) or aortic root dilation mandates more frequent evaluation. With mild aortic regurgitation of any cause and a normal LV, a repeat study in 2 to 3 years is reasonable. When moderate regurgitation is present with a normal LV, repeat evaluation in 1 to 2 years is appropriate (Table 52-5). However, annual echocardiography is recommended when severe regurgitation is present, with even more frequent evaluation when there is associated LV dilation. The frequency of evaluation should be modified (earlier) based on intercurrent clinical events or in the setting of a superimposed hemodynamic burden, such as pregnancy or noncardiac surgery. Conversely, the interval between evaluations may be extended if serial studies show only mild to moderate disease with no change on serial studies.

## MEDICAL THERAPY TO PREVENT PROGRESSION

The physiology of aortic regurgitation suggests that afterload reduction might reduce regurgitant severity by decreasing the diastolic pressure gradient across the aortic valve while simultaneously reducing the force (LV wall stress) required to eject the stroke volume into the aorta in systole. Several studies have investigated the utility of vasodilator pharmacologic agents, such as nifedipine or ACE inhibitors, in chronic asymptomatic severe aortic regurgitation to prevent progression. Variable effects have been observed in small clinical trials, with some studies showing slowing of the rate of LV dilation and others showing no effect. In a prospective randomized trial of nifedipine versus digoxin, there was a lower rate of progressive LV dilation requiring valve replacement in the vasodilator group. However, a more recent randomized prospective study showed no benefit for nifedipine or enalapril compared with placebo in terms of reducing regurgitant volume, preventing LV dilation or dysfunction, or delaying valve surgery. Therefore, current guidelines provide only a weak recommendation for use of afterload reduction therapy in asymptomatic severe aortic regurgitation with LV dilation but normal systolic function. The choice of which agent to prescribe is not clear, but given the demonstrable benefit of ACE inhibitors in other causes of LV dysfunction, these agents are often the first line of choice, particularly in patients who are also hypertensive. β-Blockers should be avoided due to bradycardia, which would lengthen time in diastole and increase the regurgitant volume load on the heart.

In symptomatic patients with severe aortic regurgitation, surgery is the primary therapeutic intervention. Pharmacologic afterload reduction may be helpful in patients who are not surgical candidates or for stabilizing patients with acute decompensation in the preoperative period. Regardless of the initial response to therapy, however, these agents do not supplant valve replacement if surgical criteria are otherwise met.

In adults with aortic enlargement in association with aortic valve disease, optimal blood pressure control is strongly recommended. Data on the effects of pharmacologic therapy on the rate of aortic dilation are limited. Current recommendations as provided in treatment guidelines are largely based on expert clinical experience. If aortic dilation is due to a systemic connective tissue disorder, such as Marfan syndrome, and there is less than moderate aortic regurgitation, β-blockade is recommended and ACE inhibitor therapy may be considered. When aortic dilation is associated with BAV disease, it is reasonable to treat if surgery is not yet indicated for valve dysfunction or if aortic diameter has not yet met surgical indications.

## ■ TIMING OF SURGERY FOR AORTIC REGURGITATION

Timing of surgery for chronic aortic regurgitation is predicated on the presence of symptoms attributable to regurgitation or evidence of adverse hemodynamic consequences, such as LV enlargement or systolic dysfunction. Valve replacement is indicated in all symptomatic patients, regardless of baseline LV systolic function. In patients with equivocal or unclear symptom status, exercise testing or serum BNP levels may be a valuable adjunct ( **Fig. 52-5** and Table 52-6).

In asymptomatic patients, the risks of valve surgery and a prosthetic valve must be balanced against the potential benefit of preventing long-term LV dysfunction. The strongest predictors of postoperative outcome and LV function include preoperative

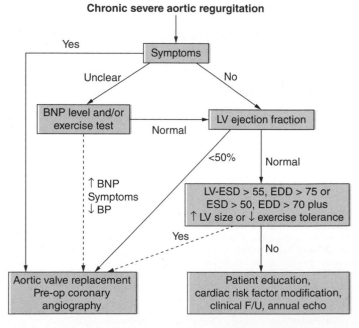

**FIGURE 52-5.** Suggested algorithm for management of adult's with severe chronic aortic regurgitation. BNP, brain natriuretic peptide; BP, blood pressure; EDD, end-diastolic diameter; ESD, end-systolic diameter; F/U, follow-up; LV, left ventricular. (Modified from Bonow RO et al. *Circulation.* 2008;118(15):e523-e661.)

functional class, end-systolic LV dimension, and resting ejection fraction. Therefore, in asymptomatic patients with severe regurgitation, valve surgery is appropriate when there is evidence of early systolic dysfunction manifested as reduced ejection fraction or excessive LV dilation (Table 52-6).

Current guidelines recommend intervention when severe regurgitation is present and LV ejection fraction falls below 50%, end-systolic dimension exceeds 55 mm, or end-diastolic dimension is more than 75 mm, or in those undergoing other cardiac surgery (Table 52-6). The European Society of Cardiology guidelines are more aggressive, recommending intervention when the end-systolic dimension exceeds 50 mm, or end-diastolic dimension is more than 70 mm. Importantly, when contemplating LV measurements and surgical indication, consideration of body size should be made, as patients with smaller stature, particularly women, are less likely to reach these criteria. In these cases, evidence of a progressive change in LV size and ejection fraction by serial clinical imaging studies should prompt consideration of earlier intervention.

If preoperative systolic function is already reduced at the time of surgery, perioperative mortality increases significantly, but there is still a demonstrable mortality benefit if patients proceed to surgery. Additionally, valve replacement in this population has been associated with a postoperative improvement in LV systolic function (absolute increase in LV ejection fraction by ~5%), decreased progression to heart failure, and prolonged survival. With relief of the chronic pressure and volume overload of aortic regurgitation, LV dilation and function typically normalize after valve replacement. These beneficial effects are greatest if the duration of systolic dysfunction is short (less than approximately 1 year). Postoperatively, most of the normalization of LV size occurs within the first 2 weeks of surgery.

## ■ OTHER CONSIDERATIONS

### Acute Aortic Regurgitation

The physiology of acute aortic regurgitation differs from that of chronic aortic regurgitation. Unlike the gradual process of ventricular adaptation to an increasing volume load, in acute regurgitation, the nondilated left ventricle is suddenly exposed to acute volume overload; the left ventricle is typically small, with markedly elevated diastolic pressure. In the extreme case, aortic and LV end-diastolic pressure are equalized. Forward cardiac output is reduced, even when systolic function appears normal, because the total stroke volume can increase only slightly with a nondilated ventricle, and much of the blood ejected in systole returns to the LV immediately in diastole and thus does not reach the systemic vasculature.

Elements of the clinical presentation characteristic of chronic regurgitation, such as a widened pulse pressure, are less prominent in acute regurgitation due to a decrease in mean arterial pressure (hypotension) and inadequate time for compensatory changes in LV chamber size and function to augment forward stroke volume. Physical examination in acute aortic regurgitation is consistent with cardiogenic shock and pulmonary edema. The murmur of acute regurgitation, lower pitched and earlier in diastole compared with that of chronic regurgitation, may be difficult to discern if the patient is tachycardic and hypotensive or may be mistaken for a systolic murmur. This error can be avoided by using the carotid pulse for timing, revealing the diastolic timing of this atypical murmur. Peripheral signs of regurgitation are usually absent unless the patient has acute regurgitation superimposed on chronic regurgitation. However, other clinical findings associated with the underlying cause of acute regurgitation often support the diagnosis. Examples include inequality of upper-extremity blood pressures for aortic dissection or systemic signs of endocarditis.

Acute aortic regurgitation is a surgical emergency. Without surgery, cardiovascular mortality is high, most commonly due to cardiogenic shock, pulmonary edema, and ventricular arrhythmias. If there is delay to surgery, hemodynamic stabilization may be attempted with inotropic agents and peripheral vasodilators to enhance forward flow. However, these measures do not supplant valve surgery. Additionally, in patients with hemodynamic instability, support with an intra-aortic balloon pump is contraindicated because diastolic inflation of the balloon will worsen regurgitation. In patients with acute regurgitation due to dissection, aortic root replacement in addition to valve surgery is also indicated. In those with endocarditis, aggressive medical therapy is indicated, but surgery should not be delayed if patients remain hemodynamically unstable despite medical therapy. Antibiotic therapy alone is typically inadequate to completely clear the infection, particularly if there is a paravalvular abscess.

## Mixed Aortic Regurgitation and Stenosis

Most patients with aortic valve disease have predominant stenosis or regurgitation so that timing of surgical intervention is based on the criteria for the primary hemodynamic abnormality. In the subset of patients with balanced moderate stenosis and moderate regurgitation, clinical decision making should be individualized. Even when the degree of independent stenosis or independent regurgitation would be unlikely to cause symptoms or LV dysfunction alone, when both are present, the combination may become hemodynamically significant. Aortic valve disease is likely the cause of symptom onset with mixed stenosis and regurgitation if no other cause for symptoms is identified. If LV dilation or systolic dysfunction is present, the same principle applies; valve disease is the likely cause of the LV abnormality unless an alternate plausible explanation is evident.

## ■ RISK OF VALVE SURGERY

Once symptoms are present, the risk of aortic valve surgery is lower than the risk without surgery regardless of patient age. However, operative mortality does increase with age and, more dramatically, with comorbid conditions such as pulmonary disease, renal dysfunction, hepatic disease, and hematologic abnormalities. Overall operative mortality rates for valve replacement are as low as 1%, increasing to 9% in higher-risk patients. Risk is higher with emergency valve procedures, hemodynamically unstable patients, repeat surgical procedures, LV dysfunction, and coexisting coronary disease. Surgical risk can be estimated using one of several tools. The Ambler score is a valve surgery–specific score published by the Society for CT Surgery in Great Britain and Ireland, based on outcomes in more than 32 000 patients undergoing valve surgery. The score was developed using data from 16 679 patients and then validated in a subsequent cohort of 16 160 patients and is a point-based score with a lookup table for estimated operative mortality. The EuroSCORE and the Society of Thoracic Surgery score are based on large numbers of patients and can be calculated with an online interactive web site based on multiple patient and clinical characteristics. None of these scores is ideal; the EuroSCORE is not specific for valve disease, but also includes risk estimation for other types of cardiac surgery, and likely overestimates risk for aortic valve surgery. An updated EuroSCORE II has been developed and is currently available online; however, predictive accuracy for valve surgery remains to be determined. The Society of Thoracic Surgery score, in contrast, appears to be more reliable but may underestimate risk. In addition, other factors such as nutritional status, clinical fragility, aortic root calcification, and cognitive status are not fully accounted in these models. For most adults, the risk of valve surgery for aortic valve disease is acceptable. In very high-risk patients, decision making is individualized, and alternate management strategies such as transcatheter valve implantation (for aortic stenosis) or palliative medical therapy may be considered.

# ■ OUTCOMES AFTER VALVE REPLACEMENT

Long-term survival after aortic valve replacement is 80% at 3 years, with an age-corrected survival postoperatively that is nearly normalized. Postoperative morbidity is primarily dependent on that associated with placement of a prosthetic valve, including thromboembolism, bleeding complications from anticoagulation, prosthetic valve dysfunction, and endocarditis (occurrence ~3% per year). If LV dilation or systolic dysfunction persists postoperatively, standard approaches for medical therapy of LV systolic dysfunction are appropriate.

After valve replacement for aortic stenosis, LV systolic function generally remains preserved. However, diastolic dysfunction may persist after relief of the outflow obstruction. In the early postoperative period, diastolic dysfunction may manifest as a very narrow "pre-load window" with low cardiac outputs when filling pressures are low; in these patients, with even a slight increase in filling pressures, pulmonary congestion ensues.

For aortic regurgitation, the prognostic benefit of following recommended guidelines on timing of valve replacement was demonstrated prospectively in 170 patients where one-third underwent recommended early surgery and nearly two-thirds underwent "too late" surgery as defined by symptoms, an LV ejection fraction <45%, or an end-systolic dimension >55 mm. At a mean follow-up of 10 years, cardiac mortality was significantly higher in the patients who underwent "too late" surgery (28% vs 9%), primarily due to heart failure or sudden cardiac death. In a study of 125 patients who underwent valve replacement for chronic regurgitation and who were followed a mean duration of 13.3 years, postoperative mortality rate was approximately 2.5% per year and predictors of survival were younger age, lower preoperative NYHA class, smaller LV size, and a postoperative reduction in LV end-diastolic dimension of >20%.

# SUGGESTED READINGS

Freeman RV, Otto CM. Aortic valve disease. In: Fuster V, Walsh RA, Harrington RA, et al, eds. *Hurst's The Heart.* 13th ed. New York, NY: McGraw-Hill; 2011;76:1692-1720.

Bonow RO, Carabello BA, Chatterjee K, et al. ACC/AHA 2006 guidelines for the management of patients with valvular heart disease: a report of the American College of Cardiology/American Heart Association Task Force on Practice Guidelines (Writing Committee to Revise the 1998 guidelines for the management of patients with valvular heart disease) developed in collaboration with the Society of Cardiovascular Anesthesiologists endorsed by the Society for Cardiovascular Angiography and Interventions and the Society of Thoracic Surgeons. *Circulation.* 2008;118(15):e523-e661.

Evangelista A, Tornos P, Sambola A, et al. Long-term vasodilator therapy in patients with severe aortic regurgitation. *N Engl J Med.* 2005;353(13):1342-1349.

Garg V, Muth AN, Ransom JF, et al. Mutations in NOTCH1 cause aortic valve disease. *Nature.* 2005;437(7056):270-274.

Leon MB, Smith CR, Mack M, et al. Transcatheter aortic-valve implantation for aortic stenosis in patients who cannot undergo surgery. *N Engl J Med.* 2010;363:1597-1607.

Nkomo VT, Gardin JM, Skelton TN, et al. Burden of valvular heart diseases: a population-based study. *Lancet.* 2006;368:1005-1011.

Otto CM, Lind BK, Kitzman DW, et al. Association of aortic-valve sclerosis with cardiovascular mortality and morbidity in the elderly. *N Engl J Med.* 1999;341:142-147.

Rossebø AB, Pedersen TR, Boman K, et al. Intensive lipid lowering with simvastatin and ezetimibe in aortic stenosis. *N Engl J Med.* 2008;359(13):1343-1356.

Tzemos N, Therrien J, Yip J, et al. Outcomes in adults with bicuspid aortic valves. *JAMA.* 2008;300(11):1317-1325.

Zoghbi WA, Enriquez-Sarano M, Foster E, et al. Recommendations for evaluation of the severity of native valvular regurgitation with two-dimensional and Doppler echocardiography. *J Am Soc Echocardiogr.* 2003;16:777-802.

# CHAPTER 53
# CEREBROVASCULAR DISEASE AND NEUROLOGIC MANIFESTATIONS OF HEART DISEASE

Torsten Vahl, Megan C. Leary, and Louis R. Caplan

## BRAIN AND CEREBROVASCULAR COMPLICATIONS OF HEART DISEASE

Stroke is a common and devastating disease, the third leading cause of death and the leading cause of disability in the United States. Cardiogenic stroke can occur due to (1) embolism, (2) pump function failure and hypoperfusion of the brain, and (3) drugs given to treat cardiac disease have neurologic adverse effects.

## ■ DIRECT CARDIOGENIC BRAIN EMBOLISM

### Etiology

Cardiogenic cerebral embolism is responsible for approximately 20% of ischemic strokes. However, because many patients have coexisting cardiac and extracranial vascular disease, criteria for the diagnosis of cardiac embolism remain controversial even today. As more advanced diagnostic techniques have been developed, more causative cardiac abnormalities and their association with stroke have been recognized. Cardiac sources of brain emboli can be divided into 3 groups and are listed in **Table 53-1**.

The risk of embolism varies within individual cardiac abnormalities depending on many factors. For example, in patients with AF, associated congestive heart failure, hypertension, patient age, diabetes mellitus, duration, chronic versus intermittent fibrillation, and atrial size all influence embolic risk.

**Atrial Fibrillation** Persistent and paroxysmal atrial fibrillation (AF) is a potent predictor of first and recurrent stroke, with >75 000 attributed cases annually. In patients with brain emboli caused by a cardiac source, there is a history of nonvalvular AF in roughly one-half of all cases, of left ventricular thrombus in almost one-third, and of valvular heart disease in one-fourth. Stroke prevention in patients with AF and other heart diseases will be discussed later on in this chapter.

**Intracavitary Thrombus** Intracavitary thrombus caused by acute MI occurs in an estimated one-third of patients within the first 2 weeks after anterior MI and in an even greater proportion of patients with large left ventricular apex infarcts. Stroke is less common among uncomplicated MI patients but can occur in up to 12% of patients with acute MI complicated by a left ventricular thrombus. The rate of stroke

**TABLE 53-1.** Cardiac Sources of Brain Emboli

1. **Cardiac wall and chamber abnormalities**
   Cardiomyopathies
   Hypokinetic and akinetic ventricular segments after myocardial infarction
   Atrial septal aneurysms
   Ventricular aneurysms
   Cardiac tumors
   Septal defects
   Patent foramen ovale

2. **Valve disorders**
   Rheumatic mitral and aortic valve disease
   Prosthetic valves
   Bacterial endocarditis
   Fibrous and fibrinous endocardial lesions
   Mitral valve prolapse
   Mitral annulus calcification

3. **Arrhythmias**
   Atrial fibrillation
   Sick sinus syndrome

is higher in patients with anterior rather than inferior infarcts and may reach up to 20% in those with large anteroseptal MI. The incidence of embolism is highest during the period of active thrombus formation in the first 1 to 3 months, with substantial risk remaining even beyond the acute phase in patients with persistent myocardial dysfunction, congestive heart failure, or AF.

**Congestive Heart Failure** Congestive heart failure affects >4 million Americans and increases stroke risk by a factor of 2 to 3, accounting for an estimated 10% of ischemic strokes. In patients with non-ischemic dilated cardiomyopathy, the rate of stroke is similar to that of cardiomyopathy caused by ischemic heart disease. An estimated 72 000 initial strokes annually are associated with left ventricular systolic dysfunction, and the 5-year recurrent stroke rate in patients with cardiac failure has been reported as high as 45%.

## Valvular Heart Disease

**Rheumatic Mitral Valve Disease** Recurrent embolism occurs in 30% to 60% of patients with rheumatic mitral valve disease and a history of a previous embolic event. Between 60% and 65% of these recurrences develop the first year, many within the first 6 months. Mitral valvuloplasty does not appear to eliminate the risk of embolism.

**Mitral Valve Prolapse** Mitral valve prolapse (MVP) is the most common form of valve disease in adults and is generally benign. MVP as a source of embolic stroke continues to be controversial. Several small clinical series have reported cerebral embolism in MVP patients who lacked other possible embolic sources. Patients with MVP also may have other disorders such as AF, syncope, and migraine. The rate of recurrent stroke in patients with MVP as the only known cause is very low.

**Mitral Annulus Calcification** Mitral annulus calcification (MAC) is an important, often unrecognized cause of embolism. Several series show a convincing relation between MAC and brain emboli and stroke. Bacterial endocarditis can also develop on the MAC. Anticoagulation does not prevent calcific emboli. The decision to use antiplatelet agents versus anticoagulants should include consideration of other potential comorbid factors such as AF, which can occur 12 times more often in patients with MAC than it would in those without MAC.

**Aortic Valve Disease** Aortic valve disease, in isolation, is not often associated with systemic embolism. Although there are isolated case reports of patients who had strokes from spontaneous aortic valve calcific emboli, few trials of selected patients with stroke and aortic valve disease exist at present. One prospective analysis of 815 patients with calcification of the aortic valve (with or without stenosis) did not show any association between either of the 2 aortic valvular lesions and stroke. Current treatment recommendations in these cases are based on larger antiplatelet trials of stroke and transient ischemic attack (TIA) patients.

*Fibrous and fibrinous lesions of the heart valves and endocardium* are associated with certain medical conditions. Similar valve lesions occur in patients with systemic lupus erythematosus (Libman–Sacks endocarditis), antiphospholipid antibody syndrome, and cancer and other debilitating diseases (nonbacterial thrombotic endocarditis). Mobile fibrous strands are also often found during echocardiography. Fibrin-platelet aggregates may attach to these fibrous and fibrinous lesions.

**Infective Endocarditis** Embolic complications are common in patients who have *infective endocarditis*. Mycotic aneurysms can cause fatal subarachnoid bleeding. Bleeding can also result from vascular necrosis as a result of an infected embolus. Embolization usually stops when infection is controlled. Warfarin does not prevent embolization and is contraindicated unless there are other important lesions such as prosthetic valves or pulmonary embolism. In children and young adults with congenital heart defects, especially those with right-to-left shunts and polycythemia, brain abscess is an important complication.

**Noncardiac Emboli** Emboli often arise from sources other than the heart, such as the aorta, proximal arteries (*intra-arterial* or so-called *local embolism*), leg veins (*paradoxical emboli*), fat in the liver or bones (*fat embolism*), and materials introduced by the patient or physician (drug particles or air). The types of embolic material vary (**Table 53-2**). *Atheromatous plaques in the aortic arch and ascending aorta* are an important source of embolism to the brain. Ulcerated atheromatous plaques are often found at necropsy in patients with ischemic strokes, especially in those in whom the stroke etiology was not determined during life. Transesophageal echocardiography (TEE) often shows these atheromas, but technical factors limit visualization of the entire arch. Large (>4 mm), protruding mobile aortic atheromas are especially likely to cause embolic strokes and are associated with a high rate of recurrent strokes. Use of oral anticoagulants rather than antiplatelet agents is recommended in these patients.

## ■ ONSET, CLINICAL COURSE, AND DIAGNOSTIC APPROACHES TO BRAIN EMBOLI

Warning signs of stroke can include sudden hemiparesis, hemisensory loss, confusion, trouble in speaking or understanding, visual loss, diplopia, ataxia, vertigo, or sudden severe headache with no known cause. Most embolic events occur during activities of daily living, but some embolic strokes have their onset during rest or sleep. Sudden coughing, sneezing, or arising at night to urinate can precipitate embolism. Although the deficit is most often maximal at outset, 11% of embolic stroke patients in the Harvard Stroke Registry had a stuttering or stepwise course, whereas 10% had fluctuations or progressive deficits. Later progression, if it occurs,

**TABLE 53-2.** Embolic Materials

| Cardiac | Intra-arterial |
|---|---|
| 1. Red fibrin-dependent thrombi | 1. Red fibrin-dependent thrombi |
| 2. White platelet-fibrin nidi | 2. White platelet-fibrin nidi |
| 3. Material from marantic endocarditis | 3. Combined fibrin-platelet and fibrin-dependent clots |
| 4. Bacteria from vegetations | 4. Cholesterol crystals |
| 5. Calcium from valves and mitral annulus calcification | 5. Atheromatous plaque debris |
| 6. Myxoma cells and debris | 6. Calcium from vascular calcifications |
| | 7. Air |
| | 8. Mucin from tumors |
| | 9. Talc or microcrystalline cellulose from injected drugs |

is usually within the first 48 hours. Progression is usually caused by distal passage of emboli. *Nonsudden* embolism is explained by an embolus moving from its initial location, as demonstrated by angiography, to a more distal branch. Early angiography has a very high rate of showing intracranial emboli, but angiography after 48 hours shows a much lower rate of blockage. More recently, transcranial Doppler (TCD) sonography has shown a high incidence of middle cerebral artery (MCA) blockage acutely in patients with sudden-onset hemispheric strokes; but later, recanalization of the MCA and normalization of the intracranial blood velocities occur. As in all large infarcts, brain edema and swelling may develop during the 24 to 72 hours after stroke with headache, decreased alertness, and worsening of neurologic signs. The edema is often cytotoxic (inside cells) and usually does not respond to corticosteroid treatment.

Emboli usually cause occlusion of distal branches and produce surface infarcts that are roughly triangular, with the apex of the triangle pointing inward. CT and MRI findings can suggest the presence of embolism by the location and shape of the lesion, presence of superficial wedge-shaped infarcts in multiple different vascular territories, and hemorrhagic infarction, as well as visualization of thrombi within arteries. MRI, particularly with the use of MR diffusion-weighted and MR gradient recall echo (GRE) imaging, is more sensitive for detection of acute brain infarcts than is CT and is also superior in detecting hemorrhagic infarction by imaging hemosiderin. Hemorrhagic infarction has long been considered characteristic of embolism, especially when the artery leading to the infarct is patent. The mechanism of hemorrhagic infarction is reperfusion of ischemic zones after iatrogenic opening of an occluded artery (eg, endarterectomy, fibrinolytic treatment) or after restoration of the circulation after a period of systemic hypoperfusion. Hemorrhage occurs into proximal reperfused regions of brain infarcts. At times, it is also possible to image the acute embolus on CT and also via MRI with T2-weighted gradient echo imaging.

In unselected series of stroke patients, transthoracic echocardiography (TTE) has been variably useful in detecting sources. TTE is useful in patients with known cardiac disease to clarify potential embolic sources and heart function, in young patients without stroke risk factors, and in stroke patients who do not have lacunar infarction or ultrasound evidence of intrinsic atherostenosis of a major extracranial and intracranial artery. TEE provides much better visualization of the aorta, atria, cardiac valves, and septal regions. The use of an echo-enhancing agent such as agitated saline helps detect intracardiac shunts.

Cerebral embolic signals are now detected by monitoring with TCD. Embolic particles passing under TCD probes produce transient, short-duration, high-intensity signals referred to as *HITS* (high-intensity transient signals).

# ■ PREVENTION AND TREATMENT

## Rheumatic Mitral Stenosis and Atrial Fibrillation

**Warfarin** Early studies showed that warfarin was effective in preventing brain embolism in patients with both rheumatic mitral stenosis and AF. Previously, the intensity of anticoagulation was higher than that currently used, and brain hemorrhages and other bleeding complications were common. Trials have now shown that lower dose warfarin (international normalized ratio [INR] 2.0-3.0) is also effective in preventing brain emboli in patients with nonrheumatic AF. The CHADS$_2$ score is used for the risk assessment of embolic events to guide anticoagulant therapy. Warfarin is more effective than aspirin in preventing strokes in patients with AF who do not have valvular disease. A meta-analysis of 5 randomized controlled trials (AFASAK, SPAF, BAATAF, CAFA, SPINAF) demonstrated that AF patients taking Warfarin have a 68% reduction in their stroke risk compared with Placebo. The available data suggests that the optimal intensity of oral anticoagulation for stroke prevention in patients with AF appears to be a target INR of 2.0 to 3.0. However, the narrow therapeutic margin of warfarin, in addition to associated food and drug interactions, requires frequent INR testing and dosage adjustments. These liabilities likely contribute to underuse of warfarin and alternative therapies are needed.

Although many trials have demonstrated the superiority of adjusted-dose warfarin over antiplatelet therapy for stroke prevention, participants in those trials tended to be younger (typically 70 years old) than the AF patients commonly encountered in clinical practice (typically late 70s with a substantial fraction of octogenarians). The Birmingham Atrial Fibrillation Treatment in the Aged (BAFTA) trial addressed this issue, randomizing 973 AF patients with age ≥75 years to adjusted-dose warfarin versus aspirin 75 mg/d. The stroke rate was 5% on aspirin and nearly halved by warfarin. Surprisingly, major hemorrhage rates were similar in both groups. It is of note that 40% of patients had received warfarin previously, potentially biasing toward lower bleeding rates. The investigators concluded that "these data lend support to the use of anticoagulation for all people aged over 75 years who have AF, unless there are contraindications or the patient decides that the size of the benefit is not worth the inconvenience of treatment."

**Antiplatelet Agents** The Atrial Fibrillation Clopidogrel Trial with Irbesartan for Prevention of Vascular Events (ACTIVE) evaluated the safety and efficacy of the combination of aspirin plus clopidogrel in AF patients who were unsuitable candidates for vitamin K antagonist therapy. In those patients, the addition of clopidogrel to aspirin did reduce the risk of major vascular events, especially stroke, but also increased the risk of major hemorrhage.

**Direct Thrombin Inhibitors** Dabigatran is an oral direct thrombin inhibitor that has also been compared with warfarin in a noninferiority trial (RE-LY). In this trial, 18 113 patients with AF were assigned to dabigatran 110 mg twice a day, dabigatran 150 mg twice a day, or adjusted-dose warfarin. Dabigatran was found, at the 110-mg dose, to have similar rates of stroke and systemic embolism as well as lower rates of major hemorrhage. The 150-mg dose had lower rates of stroke and embolism but similar rates of major hemorrhage. However, the rate of MI was higher in both dabigatran groups.

Other agents, particularly factor Xa inhibitors are being tested as well in patients with AF. For example, the ROCKET AF (Rivaroxaban Once Daily Oral Direct Factor Xa Inhibition Compared with Vitamin K Antagonism for Prevention of Stroke and

Embolism Trial in Atrial Fibrillation) study was a prospective, randomized, double-blind, multicenter, event-driven, noninferiority study comparing the efficacy and safety of rivaroxaban, an oral, once-daily, direct factor Xa inhibitor with adjusted-dose warfarin in patients with nonvalvular AF. In the intention-to-treat analysis, the primary end point of stroke or systemic embolism occurred 2.1% per year in the rivaroxaban group and 2.4% per year in the warfarin group. Thus, rivaroxaban was noninferior to warfarin with respect to stroke prevention and there was no difference in major or nonmajor bleeding between the 2 groups. However, fatal and intracranial bleeding was significantly reduced in patients treated with rivaroxaban.

Apixaban, also a factor Xa inhibitor, was compared with warfarin in the ARISTOTLE trial. Patients treated with apixaban 5 mg twice daily had a significant reduction in the primary end point of ischemic or hemorrhagic stroke or systemic embolism. In addition, apixaban treatment lowered the rates of death from any cause significantly from 3.94% to 3.52% compared with warfarin.

The timing of the initiation of warfarin anticoagulation after embolic stroke remains controversial. Embolic brain infarcts often become hemorrhagic and serious brain hemorrhage has occurred after anticoagulation. Large infarcts, hypertension, large bolus doses of heparin, and excessive anticoagulation have been associated with hemorrhage. Because most hemorrhagic transformations occur within 48 hours, the recommendations of the Cerebral Embolism Task Force were to avoid early anticoagulation in patients with large infarcts or hemorrhagic transformation on repeat CT. Studies of patients with cerebral and cerebellar hemorrhagic infarction show that, in the vast majority, the cause is embolic, hemorrhagic infarction occurs equally with and without anticoagulation, and the development of hemorrhagic infarction is rarely accompanied by clinical worsening. Patients with hemorrhagic transformation who were continued on anticoagulants did not worsen. The risk of re-embolism must be balanced against the small but definite risk of important bleeding. However, if the patient has a large brain infarct, heparin should be delayed, and bolus heparin infusions should be avoided. If the risk for re-embolism is high, immediate heparinization is advisable; whereas if the risk seems low, it is prudent to delay anticoagulants for at least 48 hours. One study showed that patients with AF with embolic strokes who were treated with well-controlled heparin anticoagulation soon after stroke onset fared better than did patients treated later.

# PARADOXICAL EMBOLISM

Although once considered rare, emboli entering the systemic circulation through right-to-left shunting of blood are now often recognized with the advent of newer diagnostic technologies. By far the most common potential intracardiac shunt is a residual patent foramen ovale (PFO). The high frequency of PFOs in the normal adult population has made it difficult to be certain in an individual stroke patient with a PFO whether paradoxical embolism through the PFO was the cause of the stroke or whether the PFO was merely an incidental finding. Autopsy series have shown that approximately 30% of adults have a probe PFO at necropsy. Echocardiographic studies have shown that PFOs are more common in patients with an undetermined cause of stroke than in those in whom another etiology has been defined. Lechat and coworkers, using TTE with contrast injection during Valsalva maneuver, demonstrated right-to-left shunting through a PFO in 56% of patients with cryptogenic stroke, in comparison to 10% of the patients in the control group.

Review of series of patients with paradoxical embolism through a PFO and the authors' experience allow the derivation of 5 criteria that, when 4 or more are met, establish the presence of paradoxical embolism with a high degree of certainty:

1. A situation that promotes thrombosis of leg or pelvic veins (eg, long sitting in one position, such as prolonged airplane flight, or recent surgery)

2. Increased coagulability (eg, the use of oral contraceptives, presence of factor V Leiden, dehydration)

3. The sudden onset of stroke during sexual intercourse, straining at stool, or other activity that includes a Valsalva maneuver or that promotes right-to-left shunting of blood

4. Pulmonary embolism within a short time before or after the neurologic ischemic event

5. The absence of other putative causes of stroke after thorough evaluation

Current treatment options for future stroke prevention in patients with PFO and ischemic stroke include medical therapy, open or minimally invasive cardiac surgical closure, and transcatheter closure. Before any treatment option is selected, it is important to confirm that the stroke is indeed cryptogenic. The treating physician should exclude all other possible contributing causes to the stroke, including a coexisting hypercoagulable state and deep venous thrombosis (with or without May–Thurner syndrome). Once this has been done, with regard to medical therapies, antiplatelet therapy is reasonable for future stroke prevention in cryptogenic stroke patients with a first ischemic stroke/TIA plus an isolated PFO. In patients with a cryptogenic stroke and an atrial septal aneurysm, evidence is insufficient to determine whether warfarin or aspirin is superior in preventing recurrent stroke or death, but minor bleeding is more frequent with warfarin. Warfarin is considered to be an appropriate treatment option in the subgroup of PFO/ischemic stroke patients with concomitant hypercoagulable state or venous thrombosis.

A benefit of transcatheter closure over medical therapy for future stroke prevention is currently not supported by any prospective randomized clinical trials. A recent review of 10 nonrandomized unblended transcatheter closure studies for secondary stroke prevention reported a reduction of recurrent neurologic events in transcatheter closure patients compared with medically treated patients. However, a recent prospective randomized clinical trial, CLOSURE I, failed to demonstrate a clinical benefit. Small, separate trials have also suggested that, in highly symptomatic migraineurs with a history of PFO and stroke, transcatheter closure can also result in improvement of migraine severity in a high percentage of patients. At the time of this publication, transcatheter closure is not FDA approved for use after a first ischemic stroke in PFO patients; however, in PFO patients who fail medical therapy and have a second ischemic cerebral event, it is a treatment option to consider.

With regard to surgical closure of symptomatic PFO, there is no clear evidence at present that it is superior to medical or endovascular therapy for secondary stroke prevention. More recently, widespread use of intraoperative TEE during cardiac surgery has resulted in frequent discoveries of incidental asymptomatic PFOs. Recent data supports that patients with an incidentally repaired PFO had 2.47 times greater odds of having a postoperative stroke compared with those with unrepaired PFO (there was no difference in long-term survival). These findings of increased short-term postoperative stroke risk should discourage the routine closure of incidentally detected PFO for now. Further studies to assess whether any subgroup of PFO patients may benefit from closure will be important in the future.

# BRAIN HYPOPERFUSION (CARDIAC PUMP FAILURE)

After cardiopulmonary resuscitation (CPR), the heart often recovers in individuals whose brain has been irreversibly damaged by ischemic-anoxic damage. Cardiologists must become very familiar with the pathology, signs, and prognosis of brain dysfunction after periods of circulatory failure.

Different brain regions have selective vulnerability to hypoxic-ischemic damage. Regions that are most remote and at the edges of major vascular supply are more liable to sustain hypoperfusion injury. These zones are usually referred to as *border zones* or *watersheds*. The cerebral cortex and hippocampus are particularly vulnerable to injury. In the cerebral cortex, the border zone regions are between the anterior cerebral artery (ACA) and MCA and between the MCA and posterior cerebral artery (PCA). The basal ganglia and thalamus are most involved if hypoxia is severe but some circulation is preserved. This situation applies most to hanging, strangulation, drowning, and carbon monoxide exposure. Cerebellar neurons may also be selectively injured.

When circulatory arrest is complete and abrupt, brainstem nuclei are especially vulnerable to necrosis in young humans and experimental animals. When hypoxia and ischemia are especially severe, the spinal cord may also be damaged. When cortical damage is severe and protracted, cytotoxic edema causes massive brain swelling, with cessation of blood flow and brain death.

## ■ CLINICAL FINDINGS

Very severe hypoxic-ischemic damage can lead to mortal injury to the cortex and brainstem, irreversible coma, and brain death. When initially examined, such patients have no brainstem reflexes and no response to stimuli except perhaps a decerebration response. These findings do not improve and respiratory control is absent or lost.

When cerebral cortical damage is very severe but brainstem reflexes are preserved, there is no meaningful response to the environment. Automatic facial movements such as blinking, tongue protrusion, and yawning usually persist. The eyes may rest slightly up and move from side to side. When this state does not improve, it is referred to as the *persistent vegetative state* or *wakefulness without awareness*. Laminar cortical necrosis can cause seizures (multifocal myoclonic twitches or jerks of the facial and limb muscles), which are difficult to control with anticonvulsants.

With severe hypoperfusion ACA-MCA border zone injury, there is weakness of the arms and proximal lower extremities with preservation of face, leg, and foot movement (the "man in a barrel" syndrome). With MCA-PCA ischemia, the symptoms and signs are predominantly visual. Patients describe difficulty in seeing and inability to integrate the features of large objects or scenes despite retained capacity to see small objects in some parts of their visual fields. Reading is impossible. There are features of Balint syndrome. Apathy, inertia, and amnesia are also common. Patients cannot make new memories and have patchy, retrograde amnesia for events during and before hospitalization. This Korsakoff-type syndrome is caused by hippocampal damage and may not be fully reversible. Amnesia may be accompanied by visual abnormalities, apathy, and confusion, or may be isolated.

## ■ PROGNOSIS

Shortly after resuscitation or arrest, patients with less severe cerebral injuries show some reactivity to the environment. Eye opening and restless limb movements develop. The eyes may fixate on objects. Noise, a flashlight, or a gentle pinch may arouse patients to react to stimuli. Soon patients awaken fully and may begin to speak. Cognitive and behavioral abnormalities may be detected after the patient awakens, depending on the degree of injury.

Prognostic signs and variables have been extensively studied. The initial neurologic findings and their course are helpful in predicting outcome. Among patients who have meaningful responses to pain at 1 hour, almost all survivors have preserved intellectual function. Patients who do not respond to pain by 24 hours typically either die or remain in a vegetative state. Being comatose predicts a poor prognosis. *Thus, 2 simple observations—the presence or absence of coma and the response to pain—predict neurologic outcome very early.* Recurrent myoclonus is also a poor prognostic sign.

## ■ DIAGNOSTIC TESTING

Neuroimaging and other tests have proved to be relatively unhelpful in contrast to the neurologic examination. CT is used to exclude other causes of coma such as brain hemorrhage. Electroencephalography is helpful in studying cortical activity in unresponsive patients. TCD may be helpful in the evaluation of brain death.

## ■ TREATMENT

Other than maintaining adequate circulation and oxygenation, treatment has not helped to improve outcome. Increased blood sugar correlates with poor outcome. A multifaceted approach to therapy has been most successful.

# NEUROLOGIC EFFECTS OF CARDIAC DRUGS AND CARDIAC ENCEPHALOPATHY

Drugs given to patients with cardiac disease often have neurologic adverse effects. Digitalis can cause visual hallucinations, yellow vision, and general confusion. Digitalis levels need not be excessively elevated; the symptoms disappear with drug cessation. Quinidine can cause delirium, seizures, coma, vertigo, tinnitus, and visual blurring. Similar toxicity has been seen with lithium. Patients may become acutely comatose while being treated with intravenous lidocaine. This effect has been associated with the accidental administration of very large doses; more common CNS effects of less extreme toxicity include sedation, irritability, and twitching. The latter may progress to seizures accompanied by respiratory depression. Amiodarone can cause ataxia, weakness, tremors, paresthesias, visual symptoms, a Parkinsonian-like syndrome, and occasionally delirium.

Patients with congestive heart failure often develop an encephalopathy characterized by decreased alertness, sleepiness, decrease in all intellectual functions, asterixis, and variability of alertness and cognitive functions from hour to hour. These patients may not have pulmonary, liver, or renal failure or electrolyte abnormalities. This cardiac encephalopathy is probably multifactoral.

# NEUROLOGIC AND CEREBROVASCULAR COMPLICATIONS OF ENDOVASCULAR CARDIAC PROCEDURES AND CARDIAC SURGERY

Patients with heart disease are diagnosed, treated, and at times even cured with a variety of cardiac procedures. Although the implicit goal with any cardiac intervention (diagnostic or therapeutic) is to improve a patient's quality of life, these procedures often carry risk as well as the possibility of benefit.

# ENDOVASCULAR CARDIAC DIAGNOSTIC AND THERAPEUTIC PROCEDURES

## ■ CARDIAC CATHETERIZATION

Stroke and TIA are known complications of heart catheterization, occurring in up to 10 of 1000 patients. Neurologic complications of cardiac catheterization are not limited to elderly patients but can also occur in children. In the absence of atherosclerosis, the suspected catheterization-related stroke mechanisms included intracranial hemorrhage caused by intraprocedure anticoagulation as well as cerebral embolism from local clot. Other potential mechanisms for cerebrovascular events during cardiac angiography may include catheter tip thromboembolism, atherosclerotic plaque or cholesterol embolism, air emboli, arterial vasospasm, and/or hypotension.

# ■ ELECTROPHYSIOLOGIC PROCEDURES AND ELECTRICAL CARDIOVERSION

Thromboembolic stroke can be a complication of cardiac electrophysiologic procedures, including radiofrequency catheter ablation of arrhythmia. Multicenter data are limited; however, the stroke risk appears to be <2%. Additionally, electrical cardioversion may be used in the treatment of AF and atrial flutter. Stroke caused by direct current cardioversion has been estimated to occur in 1.3% of cardioverted patients. Anticoagulation before and after cardioversion lowers the risk of embolism.

# ■ PERCUTANEOUS CLOSURE OF THE LEFT ATRIAL APPENDAGE

In patients with nonvalvular AF, embolic stroke is thought to be associated with left atrial appendage (LAA) thrombi. One multicenter, randomized, noninferiority trial found that percutaneous closure of the LAA was noninferior to warfarin treatment. In the future, closure of the LAA might provide an alternative to chronic warfarin for stroke prevention in patients with nonvalvular AF. A second study investigated percutaneous closure of the LAA in patients who were not warfarin candidates. At the 5-year follow-up, the annualized stroke/TIA rate was 3.8% per year, which was lower than predicted.

# ■ PERCUTANEOUS VALVULOPLASTY AND TRANSCATHETER VALVE REPLACEMENT

Surgical treatment, specifically valve replacement, is still the definitive treatment of choice for most patients with aortic stenosis. Aortic valvuloplasty provides only transient and modest benefit for aortic stenosis, with a significant risk of stroke and vascular injury. However, it can stabilize patients who require additional attention prior to undergoing surgery. Additionally, percutaneous approaches to valve implantation are now available for selected patients. Technical and device issues are still being refined, and some percutaneous treatments are showing promise in ongoing clinical trials. Percutaneous balloon aortic and mitral valvuloplasties have been complicated by stroke. Sudden coma has also been reported after percutaneous balloon mitral valvuloplasty. In the Partner trial (cohort B) Transcatheter aortic valve implantation (TAVI) led to a reduction in mortality compared with standard therapy in patients with severe aortic stenosis who were not candidates for surgical valve replacement. However, when compared to surgical aortic valve replacement, the stroke rates in high-risk patients with severe aortic stenosis undergoing TAVI were twice as high at 1 year (Partner trial, cohort A).

# ■ INTRA-AORTIC BALLOON PUMP

Intra-aortic balloon pumps (IABPs) are used in patients with severe left ventricular failure or cardiogenic shock. The IABP is inserted into the patient's midthoracic aorta to maintain adequate perfusion. Spinal cord infarcts can occur in patients with IABPs caused by local thromboembolism, aortic dissection, aortic atherosclerotic plaque rupture, or local hypoperfusion.

# CARDIOVASCULAR SURGERY

Coronary artery bypass graft (CABG) surgery is the most common major cardiovascular operation performed. The frequency of abnormalities of intellectual function and behavior after cardiac surgery is high. Preoperative diagnoses of diabetes, history of prior stroke, older age, female sex, smoking, hypertension, left main coronary disease, mild renal impairment (defined as serum creatinine 1.47-2.25 mg/dL), and high-sensitivity preoperative C-reactive protein (defined as high-sensitivity C-reactive protein concentration ≥3.3 mg/L) have all been identified to increase perioperative stroke risk. Additionally, preoperative stroke and TIA are also risk factors for in-hospital mortality. The cerebrovascular risk depends on the particular procedure performed. Estimations of stroke risk for isolated CABG range from 0.8% to 3.8%. A particular patient's risk of perioperative stroke may be estimated using the Society of Thoracic Surgeons 2008 cardiac surgery risk models, which include outcomes for stroke, as well as deep sternal wound infection, reoperation, prolonged ventilation, and renal failure, among other morbidities. Several variables were forced into each model to ensure face validity (eg, the permanent stroke model includes AF as a variable).

The majority of studies presented in the current literature suggest that there is a decrease in postoperative stroke rates in patients undergoing off-pump CABG compared with patients undergoing the traditional on-pump operation, but conflicts in the literature do exist. One potential explanation for the discrepancy is that the temporal pattern of stroke after CABG was not distinguished in all studies. Perhaps the difference in the early stroke etiology between off- and on-pump CABG could be explained by the difference in clamp use between these CABG procedures.

Another reason for the discrepancies in the data may be that many of the above studies also did not differentiate between clampless and partial clamp off-pump techniques. Aortic no-touch technique decreased the incidence of stroke (0.2% vs 2.2%) in one study, whereas partial aortic clamping increased this risk 28-fold.

## ■ ATHEROTHROMBOTIC, HEMODYNAMICALLY MEDIATED BRAIN INFARCTS

An estimated 12% of patients requiring CABG also have significant carotid artery disease. One major concern regarding cardiac surgery patients has been whether the hemodynamic stress of heart surgery leads to underperfusion of areas supplied by already stenotic or occluded arteries, resulting in brain infarcts. This concern underlies neck auscultation for bruits, ultrasound carotid artery testing, and cerebral angiography prior to CABG. However, hemodynamically induced infarction related to preexisting atherosclerotic occlusive cervicocranial arterial disease is a rare complication of heart surgery. Asymptomatic patients with carotid bruits have a very low rate of stroke after elective surgery. However, the risk of perioperative stroke does increase with increasing severity of carotid stenosis. Uncertainty exists about whether carotid endarterectomy (CEA) performed simultaneously or prior to CABG improves perioperative stroke risk. Stroke rates vary greatly in those undergoing combined CEA-CABG as opposed to staged procedures. Carotid artery stenting (CAS) has been recently introduced as an alternative revascularization modality in high-risk patients. Although some studies suggest that endovascular CAS for both symptomatic and asymptomatic carotid artery disease prior to CABG is safe and without an increased risk of stroke, conflicts again arise in the literature. Whether CAS should be performed prior to CABG is still a point of debate at this time.

# ■ BRAIN EMBOLISM

One point against a hemodynamic or hypoperfusion cause of many strokes is their timing. It appears that strokes may occur more frequently *after* recovery from the anesthetic. If the mechanism of stroke were hemodynamic, the major circulatory stress would be intraoperative and patients would at least awaken from anesthesia with the deficit. In 2 studies in which the authors record the timing of coronary artery bypass surgery-related strokes, only 16% and 17% of patients had deficits noted immediately postoperatively. The distribution of infarcts and their multiplicity on neuroimaging scans were most consistent with embolism. In cardiac surgery patients, the preponderance of evidence suggests that macroemboli (>200 μm in diameter) and microemboli are responsible for most neurologic complications. Macroemboli (associated with atherosclerotic plaque disruption or rupture) are believed to precipitate focal deficits, whereas particulate microemboli (white blood cell and platelet aggregates, fat, or air) may be implicated in more subtle diffuse cognitive dysfunction.

Given that atherosclerosis of the ascending aorta is a risk for perioperative stroke, it was postulated that avoiding direct manipulation of this area may improve neurologic outcome postoperatively. Epiaortic ultrasound scanning is thought to be superior to both manual palpation of the ascending aorta and TEE in detecting atherosclerosis, particularly noncalcified plaque. It has led to modifications in surgical management in patients undergoing CABG, such as modification of cannulation, clamping, or anastomotic technique, and temperature management. One study suggested that the application of aortic clamping or cardiopulmonary bypass was not a risk when the ascending aorta was evaluated using epiaortic ultrasound. Thromboembolic infarction often occurs in the days following surgery when cessation of anticoagulation is necessary. Postoperative activation of coagulation factors in cardiac surgery patients can promote hypercoagulability. Disseminated intravascular coagulation, acquired antithrombin III deficiency, and acquired protein C deficiencies are not uncommon. Activation of the coagulation-fibrinolytic system can persist for 2 months after cardiopulmonary bypass surgery. In some patients, hypercoagulability related to surgery can precipitate occlusive thrombosis in atherostenotic arteries, and the newly formed thrombus can lead to intra-arterial embolism. Cardiac, aortic, and intra-arterial embolism accounts for the vast majority of cardiac surgery-related focal neurologic deficits.

# ■ POSTOPERATIVE ENCEPHALOPATHY: MICROEMBOLI AND OTHER CAUSES

Gilman described a diffuse CNS disorder following open heart surgery (characterized by altered levels of consciousness and activity and confusion) that is now referred to as *encephalopathy*. Clinical and imaging studies usually do not show important focal neurologic signs or large focal infarcts. The incidence of encephalopathy varies. In one series, 57 (3.4%) of 1669 CABG patients had postoperative mental state changes including delirium and encephalopathy. In the Cleveland Clinic prospective series, 11.6% of patients were encephalopathic on the fourth postoperative day. Additionally, the incidence of encephalopathy also varies depending on the cardiac procedure itself. Compared with conventional on-pump CABG, off-pump CABG has been shown to reduce postoperative neuropsychological dysfunction in elderly patients with severe systemic atherosclerosis.

Encephalopathy has multiple causes. A necropsy study of patients who died after cardiopulmonary bypass or angiography has awakened interest in this subject. Focal, small capillary and arteriolar dilatations (SCADs) were commonly found in the brain. Approximately one-half of the SCADs show birefringent crystalline material within the dilated capillaries. SCADs could, at least in part, explain the decreased cerebral blood flow found during cardiopulmonary bypass. SCADs are iatrogenically generated microemboli, but as yet, their origin is unknown. Their morphology is most consistent with air or fat.

Other causes of encephalopathy are common. Diffuse hypoxic-ischemic insults from hypotension and hypoperfusion do occur. Postoperative cognitive dysfunction at 1 week after surgery has been associated with increasing age and shorter duration of hospital stay. Cognitive dysfunction at 3 months after CABG has also been associated with increasing age and with diabetes mellitus. Lastly, drugs are a common cause of encephalopathy in the postoperative period. Particularly important are haloperidol, narcotics, and sedatives. Morphine is sometimes used heavily intraoperatively, and can result in opiate withdrawal with restlessness and hyperactivity. Agitation and restlessness are often early signs of organic encephalopathy and may lead to the administration of haloperidol, barbiturates, phenothiazines, or benzodiazepines for calming and sedation. When these drugs wear off and the patient begins to awaken, agitation may occur, and more sedatives may be given. Haloperidol causes rigidity, restlessness, agitation, hallucinations, and confusion. In experimental animals, haloperidol delays recovery from strokes by months, and its use is not advised. Phenothiazines and sedatives are also problematic; *in general, use of sedatives and narcotics should be minimized, and they should be tapered as soon as possible.*

## ■ POSTOPERATIVE INTRACRANIAL HEMORRHAGE

Intracerebral or subarachnoid hemorrhages have occasionally been reported after cardiac surgery, most commonly in children who had repair of congenital heart disease or in cardiac transplantation patients. The postulated mechanism involves an abrupt increase in brain blood flow with rupture of small intracranial arteries unprepared for the new load. Usually, there is a prolonged period when cardiac output is low, and this output is suddenly increased by the surgery. Abrupt increases in brain blood flow or pressure in other situations have also been associated with intracerebral hemorrhage.

## ■ STROKE MIMICS: POSTOPERATIVE PERIPHERAL NERVE COMPLICATIONS

Brachial plexus and peripheral nerve lesions frequently develop after cardiac surgery and can be confused with CNS complications. In one series, new peripheral nervous system deficits occurred in 13% of patients. The most common deficit is a unilateral brachial plexopathy characterized by shoulder pain and usually weakness and numbness of one hand. It is probably caused by either sternal retraction or positioning of the arm during surgery, with traction on the lower trunk of the brachial plexus. Ulnar, peroneal, and saphenous nerve injuries are also common and are also related to positioning. Diaphragmatic and vocal cord paralyses are likely related to local effects of the cardiac surgery on the recurrent laryngeal and phrenic nerves. Postoperative Horner syndrome may be caused by manipulation of the sympathetic chain, but carotid dissection (particularly in surgical patients undergoing aortic dissection repair) should be excluded.

# CARDIAC EFFECTS OF BRAIN LESIONS

## ■ CARDIAC LESIONS

The 2 most common lesions found in the hearts of patients dying with acute CNS lesions are patchy regions of myocardial necrosis and subendocardial hemorrhage.

The abnormalities range from eosinophilic staining of cells with preserved striations to transformation of myocardial cells into dense eosinophilic contraction bands. These changes have been referred to as *myocytolysis.* One study found a high incidence of myocardial abnormalities in patients dying of brain lesions that increase intracranial pressure rapidly. Stress-related release of catecholamines and possibly corticosteroids may be responsible, in part, for the cardiac lesions found in patients with CNS lesions. Adrenoreceptor polymorphisms can explain increased catecholamine sensitivity and thus increased risk of cardiac injury in patients with subarachnoid hemorrhage and acute ischemic stroke.

# ELECTROCARDIOGRAPHIC AND ENZYME CHANGES

In stroke patients, especially those with subarachnoid hemorrhage (SAH), ECGs may show a prolonged QT interval; giant, wide, roller coaster-inverted T waves; and U waves. These changes are often called *cerebral T waves.* Patients with stroke undergoing continuous ECG monitoring have a high incidence of T wave and ST-segment changes, various arrhythmias, and cardiac enzyme abnormalities. ECG changes may include a prolonged QT interval, depressed ST segments, flat or inverted T waves, and U waves. Less often, tall, peaked T waves and elevated ST segments are noted. Myocardial enzyme release and echocardiographic regional wall motion abnormalities are associated with impaired left ventricular performance after SAH. In severely affected patients, reduction of cardiac output may elevate the risk of vasospasm-induced cerebral ischemia. Cardiac and skeletal muscle enzymes, including the MB isoenzyme of creatine kinase (MB-CK), are often abnormal in stroke patients. During days 4 to 7 after stroke, there is usually a slow increase and later decrease in serum MB-CK levels, a pattern quite different from that found in acute MI; the temporal pattern of cardiac isoenzyme release is more compatible with smoldering low-grade necrosis, such as patchy, focal myocytolysis. The ST-segment and T-wave abnormalities and cardiac arrhythmias correlate significantly with increased levels of MB-CK in stroke patients.

# ARRHYTHMIAS

Various cardiac arrhythmias have been found in stroke patients, most frequently sinus bradycardia and tachycardia and premature ventricular contractions. Some arrhythmias are manifestations of primary cardiac problems, but others are undoubtedly secondary to the brain lesions. The incidence of sinus tachycardia and bradycardia is maximal on the first day after intracerebral hemorrhage. Ventricular bigeminy, atrioventricular dissociation and block, ventricular tachycardia, AF, and bundle-branch blocks are found less often. Arrhythmias are more common in patients who have primary brainstem lesions or brainstem compression.

# ECHOCARDIOGRAPHIC CHANGES

Takotsubo cardiomyopathy is also known as *broken heart syndrome,* as well as *transient left ventricular apical ballooning.* The name *takotsubo* cardiomyopathy was coined because the shape of the end-systolic left ventriculogram resembles an octopus catcher used in Japan. It has been found after severe emotional stress, especially in postmenopausal women, and has been identified in both SAH and ischemic stroke patients. In ischemic stroke patients, it occurs soon after stroke onset, is commonly asymptomatic, and is associated with insular damage.

Echocardiography shows a hyperkinetic basal region and an akinetic apical half of the ventricle, traditionally in the setting of minimal cardiac enzyme release and normal coronary arteries on angiography.

Stimulation of the limbic system, including the insula, can result in marked sympathetic activation. With this unifying pathophysiology of excessive sympathetic discharge, the broken heart syndrome may represent a variant of the regional wall motion abnormality phenomenon associated with SAH. Prognosis is generally very good, with full recovery in most patients; however, there may be increased morbidity in patients with SAH. Thus, it may be reasonable to consider TTE in SAH patients with ECG abnormalities.

## NEUROGENIC PULMONARY EDEMA

Acute pulmonary edema may complicate strokes, especially SAH, subdural hemorrhage, primary spinal cord hemorrhage, and posterior circulation ischemia and/or hemorrhage. Pulmonary edema has been found in 70% of patients with fatal SAH and correlates with the development of increased intracranial pressure. The pulmonary edema can develop despite normal cardiac function. The most relevant imaging method is the chest x-ray, where diffuse hyperintensive infiltrates in both lungs are apparent.

## SUDDEN DEATH

Sudden death associated with stressful situations, including so-called *voodoo death*, must involve CNS mechanisms. However, the role that the CNS plays in precipitating sudden cardiac death is still uncertain. In particular, establishing a cause-effect relationship in the setting of a stroke has been complicated because these patients usually have risk factors for coronary disease as well. However, it is notable that patients with lateral medullary and lateral pontine infarcts die unexpectedly and also have a high incidence of autonomic dysregulation (eg, labile blood pressure, tachycardia).

ECG alterations predictive of sudden death, such as QT prolongation, late ventricular potentials, premature ventricular beats, nonsustained ventricular tachycardia, and the R on T phenomenon, have been described in patients with SAH, intracerebral hemorrhage, and ischemic stroke. Additionally, a higher incidence of ventricular arrhythmias, particularly ventricular fibrillation (the presumed mechanism of sudden death), has been noted in acute stroke patients. Ventricular fibrillation can be reliably elicited by stimulation of cardiac sympathetic nerves in both the normal and the ischemic heart. Postmortem analysis of patients who died suddenly and without any evidence of coronary disease often shows myocytolysis and myofibrillar degeneration (which is observed also in experimental models of hearts subjected to sympathetic overstimulation). Sudden vagotonic stimulation can cause bradycardia and cardiac standstill; however, the effects of vagal stimulation on the development of ventricular arrhythmias are uncertain.

## COEXISTENT VASCULAR DISEASES AFFECTING BOTH HEART AND BRAIN

### ■ ATHEROSCLEROSIS

The most common and important vascular disease that affects both the brain and the heart is atherosclerosis. The most frequent cause of death in stroke patients is coronary artery disease, and extra- and intracranial arterial atherosclerosis is common in patients with coronary artery disease.

## Pathology and Predominant Sites of Disease

In white men, the predominant atherosclerotic lesions involve the origins of the internal carotid artery (ICA) and the vertebral artery (VA) origins in the neck. Fatty streaks and flat plaques first affect the posterior wall of the common carotid artery (CCA). Atherosclerotic plaques at this site do not differ from plaques in the aorta or coronary arteries. At first, plaques expand gradually and encroach on the lumen of the ICA and sometimes the CCA. Atheromatous plaques often develop concurrently at the VA origin or spread from the parent subclavian artery to involve the VA origin. When plaques reach a critical size, they affect turbulence, flow, and motion of the arteries, causing complications to develop within the plaques. Cracking, ulcerations, and mural thrombi develop, and the overlying endothelium is damaged with the development of occlusive thrombi. Fresh thrombi loosely adherent to vascular walls rapidly propagate and embolize. Because the ICA has no nuchal branches, the clot often propagates cranially. In the initial 2 to 3 weeks after the development of an occlusive thrombus, the clot gradually organizes and is much less likely to propagate or embolize. The reduction in cranial blood flow caused by severe stenosis or occlusion of the ICA or VA stimulates development of collateral circulation that usually becomes adequate.

There are important race and sex differences in the distribution of cerebral atherosclerosis. White men usually develop lesions of the ICA and VA origins. Patients with ICA-origin disease have a high frequency of hypercholesterolemia, coronary artery disease, and peripheral vascular occlusive disease. Blacks and individuals of Chinese, Japanese, and Thai ancestry have a much higher incidence of intracranial occlusive disease and a rather low frequency of extracranial disease. Intracranial disease is more prevalent in women and diabetics. Interestingly, patients with intracranial occlusive disease do not have a high incidence of coronary or peripheral vascular occlusive disease.

## Mechanisms of Ischemia

Ischemia in patients with atherosclerotic occlusive lesions is caused by 2 different mechanisms: hypoperfusion and embolism. Hypoperfusion develops only when a critical reduction in luminal diameter causes reduced distal perfusion. When flow is reduced slowly, the brain vasculature has a remarkable capacity to develop collateral circulation. Patients with severe ICA-origin occlusive disease can remain asymptomatic despite marked decrease in blood flow. Even when vascular occlusion is abrupt—as in tying neck arteries to treat brain aneurysms—surprisingly few patients develop persistent brain ischemia. In most patients, within a few days or at most 2 weeks following an arterial occlusion, collateral circulation stabilizes.

Intra-arterial embolism from atherosclerotic lesions is probably a much more frequent and important cause of brain infarction than hypoperfusion. However, decreased perfusion probably limits clearance (washout) of emboli. In patients with anterior circulation infarcts, angiography shows a very high frequency of intra-arterial intracranial emboli distal to an ICA thrombosis. These emboli most often involve the MCA and its branches. If angiography is repeated or performed later than 48 hours after stroke, MCA occlusion is usually not present. Intra-arterial emboli often fragment and move distally. Intra-arterial embolism is also common in the posterior circulation, where the most common donor sites are the VA origin and intracranial VA.

## Clinical Findings

Many patients with atherosclerotic occlusive disease are asymptomatic. The most frequent symptoms of hypoperfusion or embolism are headache, TIAs, and focal neurologic signs from brain infarction. Headaches are caused by vascular distension or brain swelling secondary to infarction. Unaccustomed headaches often precede strokes. TIAs are caused by hypoperfusion or intra-arterial emboli. Frequent, very brief stereotyped TIAs precipitated by postural changes, also known as *limb-shaking TIA*, can suggest a hemodynamic mechanism. In contrast, emboli cause longer, less frequent attacks. In many patients with clinical TIAs (spells <24 hours in duration with no lasting symptoms or signs), neuroimaging tests show brain infarcts.

Neurologic symptoms and signs depend on the region of brain that is ischemic. Table 53-2 outlines the most frequent clinical patterns resulting from occlusions of the major extracranial and intracranial arteries.

## Diagnostic Testing

In most patients, the nature and severity of the brain and vascular lesions causing the stroke can be defined. CT and MRI should localize brain lesions, distinguish between infarcts and hemorrhages, and determine the location, extent, and size of the processes. CT or MRI is usually the first test in patients with suspected stroke because the information allows clinicians to exclude nonvascular disease such as tumor or abscess, differentiate hemorrhage from ischemia, identify the vascular territory involved, and define the extent of brain damaged.

The vascular territory involved should be inferred by the nature of the neurologic symptoms and signs and the location of brain lesions on CT or MRI. Echocardiography, especially TEE, has dramatically improved the ability to detect potential cardiac sources of emboli. Ultrasound techniques can be used to screen for obstructive lesions in the major extracranial and intracranial arteries in both anterior (carotid) and posterior (vertebrobasilar) circulation arteries. TCD ultrasound is used to analyze the presence of intracranial arterial stenoses and provide information about the intracranial effects of extracranial occlusive lesions. The technique takes advantage of the soft spots in the temporal bones and natural foramina (the orbit and foramen magnum) that provide windows for ultrasound recording. Magnetic resonance angiography (MRA) provides an additional method of imaging both the extracranial and intracranial arteries for areas of stenosis and occlusion. CT angiography (CTA), using a spiral (helical) CT machine and dye injected intravenously, can also image the major large craniocervical arteries. Standard catheter angiography is warranted when ultrasound and CTA or MRA have not sufficiently defined the vascular lesion and treatment is clinically feasible.

## Treatment

For rational treatment, know the following: (1) location, nature, and severity of the occlusive lesion, (2) location, extent, and reversibility of the brain lesion, and (3) blood constituents and coagulability. Treatment should *not* be guided solely by the temporal pattern of the symptoms, such as TIA, progressing stroke, or so-called *completed stroke*. These time courses do not predict the cause and mechanism of ischemia, identify whether an infarct is present, or identify patients who will have further or recurrent ischemia.

Physicians should first decide whether or not any specific therapy is indicated. Very severe neurologic deficits, serious intercurrent illnesses (eg, dementia, cancer), and psychosocioeconomic considerations may make patients unsuitable for specific treatments. If treatment is feasible, 2 questions should be considered next: What brain tissue is at risk for further ischemia? What is the benefit-to-risk ratio of specific treatments? To determine the tissue at risk, clinicians consider the cause and the deficit. For example, a man with a slight hemiplegia caused by a small lacunar infarct in the anterior limb of the internal capsule may have infarcted the entire tissue supplied by an occluded small artery. In that case, treatment consists of controlling hypertension, the cause of the microvasculopathy. If, however, that same patient has a small cortical infarct in the precentral gyrus caused by ICA disease, the rest of the ICA territory is at risk for further ischemia, and aggressive treatment is warranted. Newer MRI techniques, such as diffusion-weighted and perfusion MRI, along with MRA, can show, even very soon after symptoms begin, brain tissue that is already infarcted and brain tissue that is underperfused but not yet infarcted.

The Asymptomatic Carotid Artery Study (ACAS) suggested that CEA is slightly better than medical therapy in asymptomatic patients with severe carotid stenosis when the operation is executed by surgeons who have records of very low surgical morbidity and mortality. To be effective, the operative mortality and morbidity of CEA must be ≤2% to 4%.

With regard to medical therapy, for minor and moderate degrees of stenosis in extra- and intracranial arteries, agents that alter platelet aggregation and adhesion are recommended. The most likely mechanism of ischemia in these patients is *white clot*, or platelet fibrin emboli. Aspirin, ticlopidine, clopidogrel, and Aggrenox (a tablet containing aspirin 25 mg and modified-release dipyridamole 200 mg given 2 times a day) have all proven effective in randomized trials in preventing a recurrent stroke after an initial noncardioembolic stroke. There is debate about which individual or antiplatelet therapy should be selected. The results of the Management of Atherothrombosis with Clopidogrel in High-Risk Patients with TIA or Stroke (MATCH) trial assessed patients with a prior stroke or TIA ($n$ = 7599) who were assigned to either clopidogrel 75 mg daily or combination therapy (clopidogrel 75 mg daily plus aspirin 75 mg daily). Primary outcomes observed included ischemic stroke, MI, vascular death, and rehospitalization caused by ischemic event. There was no significant benefit observed in the combination group compared with clopidogrel alone; the risk of major hemorrhage was also increased in the combination therapy group. Thus, although clopidogrel plus aspirin is recommended over aspirin alone for acute coronary syndromes, the MATCH results do not suggest a similar benefit for stroke and TIA patients. Clopidogrel is as effective as ticlopidine and has fewer serious hematologic complications.

The Prevention Regimen for Effectively Avoiding Second Strokes (PROFESS) trial compared the efficacy and safety of aspirin plus extended-release dipyridamole with the efficacy and safety of clopidogrel among patients who had experienced a recent noncardioembolic ischemic stroke. Treatment with the combination therapy was associated with a reduction of 25 ischemic strokes compared with clopidogrel but with an increase of 38 hemorrhagic strokes and 4 strokes of unknown etiology. Despite the increase in bleeds, when stroke recurrence and major hemorrhage were combined into one end point reflecting a benefit-risk relationship, no statistical difference between the 2 groups was noted. So which drug should a physician choose while we are waiting for guideline committees to review the data and make a formal recommendation? There is a range of reasonable conclusions, and the decision should depend on factors such as adverse effects (eg, headache with the combination drug), medical history (eg, angina or stenting, which may warrant clopidogrel), and cost. All factors being equal, our personal preference is clopidogrel.

For patients with severe stenosis of large intracranial arteries, we previously recommended warfarin if there were no contraindications. The randomized, double-blind, multicenter Warfarin-Aspirin Recurrent Stroke Study (WARSS) compared the efficacy of aspirin with warfarin (INR 1.4-2.8) for the prevention of secondary ischemic stroke caused by noncardioembolic sources ($n$ = 2206). Various subgroups, including large-artery atherosclerotic lesions, were evaluated. No significant differences between aspirin and warfarin for secondary stroke prevention or death were found. However, patients treated with warfarin in whom the INRs were in the target range had significantly fewer strokes than patients treated with aspirin. Given the cost of monitoring warfarin and the potential increase in bleeding risk with warfarin use, the authors recommended that antiplatelets be chosen over anticoagulants for stroke prevention in patients with prior noncardioembolic strokes.

The state of the intracranial arteries can be monitored using TCD and/or MRA or CTA. For patients with complete occlusions and with stump emboli-induced ischemic strokes, we still recommend heparin and then warfarin for 2 to 3 months. Heparin should be used without a bolus, and target INR with warfarin should be 2.0 to 3.0.

Thrombolytic drugs, especially recombinant tissue-type plasminogen activator (rt-PA) and streptokinase, have been given intravenously and intra-arterially in patients with acute brain ischemia. In a study in which the arterial lesions were undefined, intravenous therapy with rt-PA given within 90 minutes and 3 hours of ischemia onset, in the aggregate, provided a statistically significant benefit. Additionally, in a more recent study, intravenous t-PA was found to be of overall benefit even when given 3 to 4.5 hours after ischemic stroke symptom onset. Unfortunately, in these and other studies, approximately 6% to 12% of patients treated with thrombolytic agents developed important intracranial bleeding. Uncontrolled studies show that patients with distal intracranial arterial embolic occlusions do well with intravenous thrombolytic therapy. Patients with ICA occlusions in the neck and intracranially rarely reperfuse after intravenous thrombolytic therapy, especially if collateral circulation is poor. Intra-arterially administered prourokinase thrombolysis has also been proven to be very effective in opening blocked intracranial arteries within the anterior circulation. The dose, timing, mode of delivery, and target group for therapy remain unsettled. The authors believe vascular imaging should precede administration of thrombolytic agents. Brain and vascular imaging can guide physicians as to who should receive thrombolytics and by what route.

Because all patients with atherosclerosis are at risk of developing more lesions, control of risk factors is very important and should be begun in the hospital. Risk factors include smoking, hyperlipidemia, obesity, inactivity, and hypertension. Blood pressure should not be excessively lowered during the acute ischemic period because this may decrease flow in collateral arteries. Blood pressure control can be instituted 3 to 4 weeks after the stroke. Rehabilitation must also begin early.

# MANAGEMENT OF COEXISTING CORONARY AND CEREBROVASCULAR DISEASE

In patients considered for cardiac surgery who have symptoms of brain ischemia, it is important to define the extent of cerebrovascular disease preoperatively by non-invasive means (ultrasound and/or MRA), as well as to define cardiac and coronary artery anatomy and function. In some patients with excessive surgical risks, anticoagulation may represent an alternative treatment. Clearly, optimal medical therapy should be instituted preoperatively and continued after surgery.

## ■ SYSTEMIC ARTERIAL HYPERTENSION

High blood pressure, both acute and chronic, damages deep, penetrating small intracranial arteries; accelerates the development of atherosclerosis in the extracranial and large intracranial arteries; and results in ischemic syndromes of lacunar infarction, diffuse ischemic changes in white matter and basal gray matter structures (Binswanger disease), and intracerebral hemorrhage. Hypertension is also frequent in patients with aneurysmal SAH and may contribute to enlargement and rupture of aneurysms.

The 2 major patterns of brain ischemia in patients with hypertension are *discrete lacunar infarcts* and a more *diffuse, patchy, white and gray matter degeneration with gliosis*. Both are caused by sclerotic changes in deep intracerebral arteries and arterioles. The term *lacune* (hole) refers to a small, deep infarct caused by lipohyalinosis of the penetrating artery feeding the ischemic brain tissue. Amyloid angiopathy can also cause small, deep infarcts in normotensive and hypertensive patients. Single lacunes cause discrete clinical syndromes. The most common syndromes are pure motor hemiparesis, pure sensory stroke, ataxic hemiparesis, and the dysarthria–clumsy hand syndrome.

Since the advent of CT and MRI, it has become widely appreciated that hypertensive patients with lacunes often have more diffuse changes in the white matter of the brain, referred to as *leukoariosis*. The clinical picture consists of acute strokes; subacute progression of neurologic signs; dementia; slow shuffling gait disorder; and parkinsonian, pyramidal, and pseudobulbar signs. The clinical signs and gross pathology are identical to those partially described by Otto Binswanger in 1894 and 1895 and by his students Alzheimer and Nissl. The deep arteries are thickened and hyalinized and show lipohyalinosis and sometimes amyloid angiopathy in regions of white matter atrophy and gliosis. Invariably, lacunar infarcts are also found. The diagnosis is made based on the clinical findings, the CT and MRI abnormalities, and the absence of cortical infarcts, larger artery occlusive disease, or cardioembolic sources.

## Hypertensive Intracerebral Hemorrhage

Intracerebral hemorrhage (ICH) accounts for approximately 10% of all strokes. Head trauma, vascular malformations, bleeding diatheses, drugs (especially anticoagulants, amphetamines, and cocaine), amyloid angiopathy, and intracranial aneurysms account for some cases. Traditionally, spontaneous ICH has usually been equated with hypertensive hemorrhage. Many patients, however, have no history of hypertension or associated changes of hypertensive vasculopathy at necropsy. Acute elevations of blood pressure and/or blood flow to the brain (**Table 53-3**) can cause ICH by the sudden increase in blood pressure, causing vessel breakage.

Hypertensive ICH issues from the deep penetrating arteries, so the locations parallel the distribution of these arteries. Hypertensive hematomas develop in the same sites as lacunes; the most frequent locations are the putamen/internal capsule (30%-40%), caudate nucleus (8%), lobar white matter (20%), thalamus (15%), pons (10%), and cerebellum (10%). In fatal hematomas, microaneurysms and lipohyalinosis are prevalent in penetrating arteries, but the hematomas obscure findings in the middle of the lesions. Arterioles or capillaries rupture in the center of the lesion, suddenly increasing local tissue pressure and leading to pressure on adjacent capillaries, which then rupture. As the hematoma gradually grows on its periphery, local tissue pressure and finally intracranial pressure increase until the hematoma is contained. Alternatively, the pressure is decompressed by the lesion, emptying into the ventricular system or into the subarachnoid space on the brain surface.

**Clinical Findings** Patients with ICH most often have a gradual evolution of neurologic signs. The first neurologic signs are related to the bleeding site (eg, left putaminal hematoma patients might first notice right arm weakness or numbness). As the hematoma grows, focal signs worsen. When and if the hematoma increases in size to increase intracranial pressure, headache, vomiting, and decreased levels of alertness develop. In the presence of small, restricted hemorrhages, headache is absent, and the patient remains alert. Headache is absent or not is a very prominent symptom in more than half of patients with ICH. Loss of consciousness is a bad prognostic sign when present.

**Diagnosis** Noncontrast CT, MR-GRE, and MR susceptibility imaging accurately show the location, size, and shape of acute ICHs. Routine MRI (without MR susceptibility or GRE sequences) in the patient with an acute hematoma is more difficult

**TABLE 53-3.** Causes of Acute Changes in Blood Pressure or Blood Flow That Can Result in Intracerebral Hemorrhage

Drugs, especially cocaine and amphetamines
Recent onset of arterial hypertension
Pheochromocytoma
Cold hemorrhages (exposure to freezing ambient temperatures)
Dental chair hemorrhages
Intracranial operations on the fifth cranial nerve
Stereotactic treatment of the fifth cranial nerve for trigeminal neuralgia
Carotid endarterectomy (reflex hypertension and reperfusion)
Cardiac transplantation, especially in children
Surgical repair of congenital heart disease in children
Migraine

to interpret. MRI is superior to CT in imaging arteriovenous malformations and cavernous angiomas. Lumbar puncture is seldom warranted. Atypical location, absence of hypertension, and abnormal vascular echoes on MRI are indications for angiography.

## Prognosis and Treatment

Coma, increased intracranial pressure, and large hematoma size (>3 cm in 1 dimension on CT) all indicate a poor prognosis. Ordinarily, severe systemic hypertension is reduced but not excessively. Patients with ICH can die from increased intracranial pressure. To perfuse the brain and maintain an arteriovenous pressure gradient, the systemic arterial pressure must increase. Overzealous reduction of systemic blood pressure can cause clinical deterioration. The patient's state of alertness and neurologic signs should be carefully monitored, together with the blood pressure.

Recent hematomas in the cerebral lobes, cerebellum, and right putamen are sometimes drained surgically without leaving a major deficit, at times using stereotactic equipment with CT guidance. The indications for drainage are increased intracranial pressure and the presence of lesions that require removal (eg, tumor, arteriovenous malformations, aneurysm). When hematomas resolve, they leave a cavity disconnecting but not destroying the overlying cortex.

Small hematomas usually resolve well without specific therapy except blood pressure control, whereas massive hematomas usually kill or maim patients before they can be treated. Medium-sized hematomas (2-4 cm) that increase intracranial pressure and cause worsening signs or decreased consciousness while patients are under observation are indications for drainage if the hematoma is favorably located.

## ◼ SUBARACHNOID HEMORRHAGE

SAH is not directly caused by hypertension in most cases, although an abrupt increase in blood pressure (eg, caused by cocaine or amphetamines) can sometimes lead to SAH, as can a bleeding diathesis, trauma, and amyloid angiopathy. The most frequent lesions causing SAH are abnormal vessels such as aneurysms and vascular malformations on or near the surface of the brain. SAH describes bleeding directly into the subarachnoid space with rapid dissemination into the cerebrospinal fluid (CSF) pathways. Usually blood is suddenly released under systemic arterial pressure, causing an abrupt increase in intracranial pressure and producing headache, vomiting, and interruption of conscious behavior and memory, at least temporarily. In some patients, the jet and spread of blood cause neckache, backache, or sciatica instead of headache. Patients are usually agitated and restless or sleepy and have a stiff neck.

The most frequent cause of SAH is leakage from a berry aneurysm. Often there has been a past history of a *warning leak or sentinel hemorrhage,* presenting as a sudden-onset headache unusual for the patient that lasts for days and prevents normal activities. Aneurysms are usually located at bifurcations of major intracranial arteries. CT can often suggest the site of rupture if blood is pooled locally near a typical site. Large aneurysms are occasionally visible on contrast-enhanced CT or MRI. CTA and MRA are useful tests for screening for aneurysms. Lumbar puncture is very important in the diagnosis of SAH. The absence of blood in the CSF effectively excludes the diagnosis of SAH if the fluid is examined within 24 hours of the onset of the headache, but bleeds that are very small in volume or older than 72 hours can be missed. The CSF pressure, presence of xanthochromia, and quantification of the hemoglobin and bilirubin content of the CSF by spectrophotometry can help establish and date the bleeding and document increased intracranial pressure.

The 2 most important neurologic complications of aneurysmal SAH are rebleeding and brain ischemia caused by vasoconstriction (so-called vasospasm). Once an aneurysm has ruptured, either a tiny cap of platelets and fibrin seals the point of rupture or continued bleeding leads to death. Lysis of the fibrin cap initiates rebleeding. Surgical clipping of the aneurysmal sac or obliteration of the aneurysm by endovascular use of balloons or other devices should be attempted before rebleeding occurs.

Vasoconstriction of arteries is thought to be caused by blood or blood products that bathe the adventitia of arteries. In the presence of a large accumulation of blood, there is a much higher incidence of arterial vasoconstriction and resultant brain ischemia and infarction. Delayed ischemia can also develop after surgery, as manipulation of vessels can precipitate vasoconstriction. The clinical findings in patients with vasoconstriction are often those of diffuse brain swelling, such as headache, decreased alertness, and confusion. When vasoconstriction is focal, the clinical findings are those of focal ischemia, such as hemiparesis, aphasia, hemianopia, and so on. Vasoconstriction usually has its onset 3 to 5 days after hemorrhage. The peak time for constriction is on days 5 to 9; vasoconstriction usually improves after the second week unless rebleeding occurs.

Vasoconstriction is detected by angiography in 30% to 70% of patients with SAH, depending on the timing of the study. TCD is effective in monitoring for the presence of vasoconstriction. Single-photon emission CT (SPECT) can also show regions of poor perfusion and delayed ischemia.

Many treatments have been tried to prevent or treat vasoconstriction after SAH, including removal of blood by lumbar puncture and at the time of early surgery, pharmacologic agents such as calcium channel blockers to minimize vasospasm, and hypervolemia to prevent ischemia by maintaining perfusion. At present, the most popular approaches are early surgery, nimodipine (a calcium channel blocker), and hypervolemic therapy, especially after aneurysmal clipping. Hypovolemia is common after SAH, as is hyponatremia. Hypervolemia does not reverse the vasoconstriction but helps maintain brain perfusion.

# ■ ARTERIAL DISSECTION

Aortic dissections involving the innominate or common carotid arteries are a well-known cause of stroke and TIA. Less well known are the syndromes produced by dissections of the extracranial and intracranial cervicocephalic arteries, which are especially likely to occur in young, active individuals without risk factors for atherosclerosis or stroke but after trauma or chiropractic or other neck manipulations. They are also associated with fibromuscular dysplasia, $\alpha_1$-antitrypsin deficiency, Marfan syndrome, pseudoxanthoma elasticum, and migraine.

Dissections start with a tear in the media and spread longitudinally, often disrupting adventitial fibers or even rupturing through the adventitia to produce an extravascular hematoma and a false aneurysm, or pseudoaneurysm, within muscle and connective tissue. Intracranially, such a rupture can produce SAH. Other dissections cause arterial obstruction and secondary thrombosis of the narrowed vascular lumen. Most cerebrovascular dissections occur in the extracranial vessels, particularly the pharyngeal portion of the ICA and the nuchal VAs.

Extracranial dissections produce sharp pain and throbbing headache; brain and retinal ischemic episodes, which may occur in rapid-fire attacks (*carotid allegro*); and pressure on adjacent structures, especially cranial nerves X through XII, which exit at the skull base. Strokes, usually from embolization of clots, are common but may have a benign course. Intracranial dissections have a poorer prognosis, often with vascular rupture and SAH. The diagnosis is confirmed by angiography, CT, or MRI. Ultrasound studies can be helpful in suggesting the diagnosis of dissection in the neck.

There is debate regarding the appropriate treatment for cervicocephalic arterial dissection. We would recommend that treatment consist of the use of heparin acutely, followed by warfarin. In patients in whom the dissected artery is initially occluded and remains occluded, warfarin can be stopped after 6 to 12 weeks, and an antiplatelet agent should then be initiated. The authors continue warfarin in other patients until severe luminal narrowing is no longer present, monitoring the dissected arteries with serial noninvasive techniques (ultrasound, CTA, or MRA) every few months. Intracranial dissections with SAH have been treated surgically.

## SUGGESTED READINGS

Leary MC, Caplan LR. Cerebrovascular disease and neurologic manifestations of heart disease. In: Fuster V, Walsh R, Harrington RA, et al, eds. *Hurst's The Heart*. 13th ed. New York, NY: McGraw-Hill;2011:107:2290-2314.

ACTIVE Investigators, Connolly SJ, Pogue J, Hart RG, et al. Effect of clopidogrel added to aspirin in patients with atrial fibrillation. *N Engl J Med*. 2009;360:2066-2078.

Amarenco P, Duyckaerts C, Tzourio C, et al. The prevalence of ulcerated plaques in the aortic arch in patients with stroke. *N Engl J Med*. 1992;326:221-225.

Baker RA, Hallsworth LJ, Knight JL. Stroke after coronary artery bypass grafting. *Ann Thorac Surg*. 2005;80:1746-1750.

Cho KH, Kim JS, Kwon SU, et al. Significance of susceptibility vessel sign on T2-weighted gradient echo imaging for identification of stroke subtypes. *Stroke*. 2005;36:2379-2383.

Connolly SJ, Ezekowitz MD, Yusuf S, et al. Dabigatran versus warfarin in patients with atrial fibrillation. *N Engl J Med*. 2009;361:1139-1151.

Ezekowitz MD, Bridgers SL, James KE, et al. Randomized trials of warfarin for atrial fibrillation. *N Engl J Med*. 1992;327:1451-1453.

Guzman LA, Costa MA, Angiolillo DJ, et al. A systematic review of outcomes in patients with staged carotid artery stenting and coronary artery bypass graft surgery. *Stroke*. 2008;39:362-365.

Kittner SJ, Sharkness CM, Sloan M, et al. Infarcts with a cardiac source of embolism in the NINDS Stroke Data Bank: neurologic examination. *Neurology*. 1992;42:299-302.

Messé SR, Silverman IE, Kizer JR, et al. Quality Standards Subcommittee of the American Academy of Neurology. Practice parameter: recurrent stroke with patent foramen ovale and atrial septal aneurysm: report of the Quality Standards Subcommittee of the American Academy of Neurology. *Neurology*. 2004;62:1042-1050.

# CHAPTER 54
# THE NONSURGICAL APPROACH TO CAROTID DISEASE

Jason Chinitz, Amar Krishnaswamy, Jay Yadav, and Samir R. Kapadia

Carotid artery stenoses, both symptomatic and asymptomatic, increase the risk for ischemic cerebrovascular events. The long-standing gold standard for invasive treatment of these lesions has been surgical carotid endarterectomy (CEA). CEA reduces the risk of stroke for both severe asymptomatic carotid stenosis and moderate or severe symptomatic stenosis when compared with medical management alone.

Surgery, however, is not without limitations. The risk of stroke associated with CEA ranges from 2.9% to 10.7% in major trials. Additionally, the coronary artery disease (CAD) that frequently accompanies carotid atherosclerosis increases the risk of perioperative myocardial infarction (MI), complicating even further the management of these patients. Moreover, several groups of patients have a prohibitively high surgical risk for CEA due to comorbid conditions such as severe coronary atherosclerotic disease, severe left ventricular dysfunction, severe aortic stenosis, a history of head or neck radiation, previous ipsilateral CEA, or contralateral carotid occlusion.

Because of these factors, along with the inherent invasiveness and recovery time associated with surgery, nonsurgical alternatives are an important tool in the management of carotid artery stenosis.

## CAROTID ANATOMY

In most individuals, the right common carotid artery (CCA) originates from the innominate (brachiocephalic) artery, which is typically the first branch of aortic arch, and the left CCA arises as the second branch of the arch. There are, however, many anatomic variants. Up to one-fourth of patients have a common origin of the left common carotid and innominate arteries, and in one-fifth of patients, the left CCA arises directly from the innominate artery. Although historically referred to as *bovine arch* configurations, these 3 variants do not actually resemble the arch of cattle.

**Figure 54-1** demonstrates the commonly used anatomic classification of the origins of the great vessels. Aortic arch classification is based on the relationship of the innominate artery to the top of the arch. In the type I arch, all 3 great vessels originate from the same horizontal plane (Fig. 54-1A); the origin of the innominate artery lies between the horizontal planes of the inner and outer curvature of the aortic arch in the type II arch (Fig. 54-1B); and in the type III arch, the innominate artery arises inferior to the horizontal plane of the inner curvature of the aortic arch (Fig. 54-1C).

The CCA bifurcates into the internal carotid artery (ICA) and the external carotid artery at the level of the C4 to C5 intervertebral space. The ICA continues superiorly

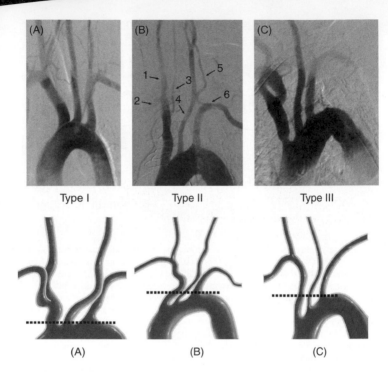

**FIGURE 54-1.** Aortic arch classification. **A.** Type I arch. **B.** Type II arch. **C.** Type III arch. The arch type is dependent on the relationship of the innominate artery to the outer and inner curvatures of the aortic arch. 1. Right common carotid artery; 2. Right subclavian artery; 3. Right vertebral artery; 4. Left common carotid artery; 5. Left vertebral artery; 6. Left subclavian artery. (Reprinted from Krishnaswamy A, Klein JP, Kapadia SR. Clinical cerebrovascular anatomy. *Catheter Cardiovasc Interv.* 2010;75:530-539.)

and gives rise to its first major branch, the ophthalmic artery, in the subarachnoid space. It then bifurcates into the anterior and middle cerebral arteries. The ICA is divided into the prepetrous, petrous, cavernous, and supraclinoid segments (**Fig. 54-2**).

The carotid sinus is located in the ICA just distal to the bifurcation of the CCA and measures approximately 7 mm in diameter in most adults. The sinus contains mechanoreceptors, which are responsible for the carotid sinus reflex.

The external carotid artery has an extensive collateral network; therefore, unilateral stenosis is rarely symptomatic. Severe stenosis or obstruction, however, may cause jaw claudication in patients with concomitant contralateral occlusion.

# CAROTID ATHEROSCLEROTIC DISEASE

## ■ EPIDEMIOLOGY

Stroke is the third leading cause of death in the United States. Approximately 800 000 people experience either an initial or recurrent stoke each year. An estimated 50 000 more women than men suffer a stroke annually, and the risk for a first-ever stroke

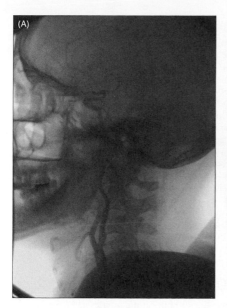 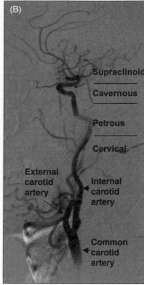

**FIGURE 54-2.** Segments of the internal carotid artery. (Reprinted from Krishnaswamy A, Klein JP, Kapadia SR. Clinical cerebrovascular anatomy. *Catheter Cardiovasc Interv.* 2010;75:530-539.)

is almost 2 times greater for blacks. Ischemic strokes, which are closely related to vascular stenosis, account for 87% of all strokes. Overall, the estimated prevalence of carotid stenosis is 0.5% at 50 years of age and 10% at 80 years of age. In addition to the acute clinical consequences, there are significant long-term effects related to stroke. Stroke is the number 1 cause of long-term disability, with 20% of victims needing institutional care 3 months after the event. Furthermore, nearly a quarter of all stroke patients will die within 1 year following the event, and this number is even higher for those who are above age 65.

## ■ RISK FACTORS

There are several risk factors for the development of carotid atherosclerosis and its associated clinical sequelae. Stroke rates increase in a stepwise fashion with age. Tobacco use imparts a significant risk of stroke that is correlated to usage. Heavy smokers have twice the relative risk (RR) of stroke compared with light smokers, and the risk of stroke is significantly reduced within 2 years of smoking cessation, with a return to baseline at 5 years. Race has also been shown to impart risk. Blacks have twice the age-adjusted risk for stroke compared with non-Hispanic whites, and both male and female blacks are more likely to die secondary to strokes when compared with non-Hispanic whites. Hypertension, diabetes, the metabolic syndrome, male sex, and hypercholesterolemia are additional risk factors that have been shown to impart an elevated risk of carotid disease. Similar to recent work in the coronary realm, inflammation has been shown to be associated with an increased risk of both carotid atherosclerosis and carotid plaque instability.

# ■ NATURAL HISTORY

Once carotid atheromatous lesions have formed, the severity of stenosis and associated symptoms are predictive of the risk of stroke. In asymptomatic carotid stenosis of ≥60%, the annual risk of stroke is approximately 2.1%. The addition of symptoms such as transient ischemic attack (TIA) significantly increases the risk of stroke in patients with even moderate stenosis, and this risk increases in a stepwise fashion with the severity of stenosis. The risk of stroke following a TIA was 40% in the Framingham Study, and two-thirds of these strokes occurred within the first 6 months. There is also a direct correlation between the severity of stenosis and the risk of death. The adjusted RR of death is 1.32 for stenoses <45%, 2.22 for stenoses of 45% to 74%, and 3.24 for stenoses of 75% to 99%. Progressive carotid stenoses are more likely to be associated with adverse events.

Recent guidelines support carotid revascularization in symptomatic patients with carotid stenosis >70% by noninvasive imaging, or >50% as documented by angiography, when the anticipated rate of perioperative stroke or mortality is less than 6%. In asymptomatic patients, the guidelines suggest that CEA is reasonable (class IIa recommendation) when carotid stenosis is >70% and the risk of perioperative stroke, MI, and death is low; carotid stenting is supported only in highly selected asymptomatic pateints.

# ■ CLINICAL PRESENTATION

Carotid bruits can be auscultated over one or both carotid arteries and have a harsh blowing quality associated with them. Evidence of a carotid bruit on physical examination is the most common finding leading to the diagnosis of asymptomatic carotid stenosis. The severity of the bruit, however, has not been shown to be consistently associated with the degree of stenosis, having sensitivity in some series of <30%. Although carotid bruits are poor predictors of the severity of atherosclerosis, they are associated with an increased risk of stroke, MI, and death.

A TIA is the most common presentation of symptomatic carotid stenosis. By definition, a TIA lasts for <24 hours and typically resolves within 30 minutes. Symptoms from a TIA are related to the distribution affected by the area of ischemia. Carotid-related symptoms include aphasia and dysarthria. Visual disturbances, such as ipsilateral amaurosis fugax or contralateral homonymous hemianopia, may also be present. Sensory and motor deficits are typically contralateral. Importantly, TIAs caused by vertebrobasilar insufficiency must be differentiated from those secondary to carotid origin, which can be done with careful history analysis and physical examination. Symptoms related to vertebrobasilar insufficiency include transient cranial nerve findings, diplopia, vertigo, and dysarthria. Motor deficits are ipsilateral, and visual losses are frequently bilateral.

# DIAGNOSIS

## ■ NONINVASIVE TECHNIQUES

### Ultrasonography

**Stenosis Severity** The standard noninvasive method for the evaluation of carotid artery stenosis is duplex ultrasonography. Several studies have encouraged diagnosis of the severity of carotid artery stenosis based on ultrasound alone, without the need for angiography. Results concerning the diagnostic accuracy of carotid ultrasound in the centers participating in the NASCET study, however, cast some doubt on the validity of ultrasound by showing that the sensitivity and specificity of carotid ultrasound were 68% and 67%, respectively. This poor correlation has been attributed to many factors, including variations in patient selection, imaging device performance, and the imaging protocols used.

Ultrasound evaluation fared better in the Asymptomatic Carotid Atherosclerosis Study (ACAS). In this study, centers had to show evidence of Doppler measurements and carotid arteriography correlation; a standard protocol was adopted, which played a part in the specificity of carotid ultrasound being measured above 95%. Corroborating these results, Jahromi and colleagues reported a sensitivity of 98% and a specificity of 88% for diagnosing an angiographic stenosis of >50% using ultrasound. Recent data suggest that carotid ultrasound also has a high accuracy for carotid restenosis after endarterectomy. Nonetheless, despite the overall high sensitivity and specificity for carotid ultrasound, accuracy varies widely according to laboratory. Therefore, properly trained sonographers and a routine quality assurance program are critical to the sensitivity and specificity of results obtained from sonography.

Various criteria have been proposed to diagnose severe carotid stenosis with a high level of accuracy. Different cutoff points for peak systolic and diastolic velocities from the ICA and the ratio of peak systolic velocity from the ICA and CCA have been correlated with severe stenosis. Typically, a >80% stenosis correlates with a systolic velocity >300 to 400 cm/s, a diastolic velocity >100 to 135 cm/s, and an ICA/CCA systolic velocity ratio of >4 to 6. Contralateral occlusion, severe left ventricular (LV) dysfunction, aortic stenosis, and common carotid stenosis are some of the variables that make these measurements less reliable and should be factored in when interpreting carotid ultrasound information.

Recently, 3-dimensional (3D) ultrasound imaging has emerged as an alternative option for volumetric imaging of carotid plaque. While 2-dimensional (2D) ultrasound permits only limited views, 3D imaging provides more information regarding plaque size, composition, and morphology, and thus may aid in the identification of vulnerable carotid plaque. Studies have shown good reproducibility of 3D ultrasound evaluation of plaque volume, morphologic features such as plaque surface irregularity or ulceration, and plaque echodensity. However, the clinical applications of 3D ultrasound are still being determined, and further study is needed to demonstrate superiority of this approach over traditional 2D imaging, as well as its cost-effectiveness.

**Carotid Intima-Medial Thickness** Carotid intima-medial thickness (CIMT) is a measure of the thickness of the intima and media and provides a measure of subclinical atherosclerosis. As such, it has been associated with an increased risk of MI, stroke, and cardiovascular death. Furthermore, it is increasingly being used as a trial end point and even as a surrogate marker for clinical events in large studies. The use of CIMT in routine clinical practice, however, is still being established. Recent data suggests that 3D volume measurements of carotid plaque is more sensitive than CIMT for the evaluation of carotid plaque progression. At this time, it is recommended for patients without established atherosclerotic disease and an intermediate probability of cardiovascular events, in whom the use of preventive therapies is unclear and further risk assessment would be beneficial.

## Magnetic Resonance Angiography

Magnetic resonance angiography (MRA) can be performed using 2 different techniques: time-of-flight (TOF) and contrast-enhanced imaging. TOF imaging is useful in patients with contraindications to the use of gadolinium-based contrast agents. The relative inaccuracy of this method is in large part due to the lengthy time of acquisition (10-15 min), which increases the susceptibility to artifacts and flow disturbances. Some investigators have reported sensitivities as high as 90% but specificities as low as 64%. The advent of 3-dimensional contrast-enhanced MRA provided advancement in the noninvasive examination of the aortic arch and carotid arteries. Advantages of gadolinium-enhanced (GE) MRA for carotid angiography include the ability to image plaque ulcerations, which are often not seen on TOF imaging; lack of flow-related artifacts, which can degrade tortuous vessels by in-plane saturation; short imaging times with excellent signal-to-noise ratio; and the ability to image from the aortic arch to circle of Willis in approximately 30 seconds. The GE MRA technique is limited by interference from contrast in the jugular vein, which may impair visualization of the carotid artery and thereby decrease the sensitivity for measuring stenoses when a long scan time is used. Conversely, using the shorter scan time decreases the spatial resolution.

Multiple investigators have demonstrated sensitivities of 88% to 97% and specificities of 89% to 96% for GE MRA. A recently published meta-analysis comparing GE MRA and TOF found better sensitivity (94.6% vs 91.2%) and specificity (91.9% vs 88.3%) for GE MRA in diagnosing severe (>70%) carotid stenosis. The accuracy of both techniques was relatively poor in diagnosing moderate (50%-69%) stenosis (sensitivities of 65.9% and 37.9% for GE MRA and TOF MRA, respectively), a finding that has been demonstrated by other investigators.

Ultimately, magnetic resonance imaging (MRI) has established itself as a useful noninvasive imaging tool in the evaluation of carotid stenosis. Improved sensitivity and specificity may be provided by concomitant MRA and Doppler ultrasound examination, possibly reducing the need for invasive angiography. Future improvements in MRA technology are also likely to improve its diagnostic capabilities and accuracy.

## Computed Tomography Angiography

In one of the first studies evaluating multislice CT angiography (CTA) for carotid imaging, Sameshima and colleagues examined 128 carotid bifurcations, comparing CTA to Doppler ultrasound and MRA, using conventional angiography as the standard. MRA tended to overestimate stenosis, whereas CTA strongly correlated with conventional angiography ($r = 0.987$, $p < 0.0001$).

A more recently published meta-analysis, however, reported a lower accuracy for CTA. In 684 arteries in 362 patients, CTA demonstrated a sensitivity of 77% and specificity of 95% in diagnosing severe carotid stenosis, a finding that is more consistent with other investigators using strict methodologic criteria. Calcium blooming artifact is the major limiting factor decreasing the ability of CT scan to measure accurate stenosis severity in calcified lesions. Sensitivity (67%) and specificity (79%) in diagnosing moderate stenosis, similar to both MRA and Doppler ultrasound, were much lower. With the advent of more advanced multislice CT scanners and easy availability of CTA than MRA, this technique is quickly becoming popular as a noninvasive diagnostic modality.

## ■ INVASIVE TECHNIQUES

### Angiography

The gold standard for assessing the severity of carotid stenosis severity remains the angiogram. In most situations, digital subtraction angiography is applied when imaging the cervicocerebral circulation. By "subtracting" the bones and soft tissues, the arteries are more clearly visualized. There are several factors that make angiography unique and attractive in its detection of atherosclerotic plaque. It provides high-resolution images of the stenosis and plaque surface and is able to distinguish easily between a high-grade stenosis and occlusion. It allows the simultaneous study of the origin of the neck vessels and intracranial circulation. This is important for the detection of tandem stenoses, which pose diagnostic problems for Doppler ultrasound. The ability to assess collateral circulation as well as the speed of blood flow is quite useful in clinical decision making, particularly in predicting the safety of temporary carotid occlusion associated with either CEA or carotid artery stenting. Additionally, angiography provides information regarding the atherosclerotic lesion and surrounding reference vessel. The risk of transient and permanent neurologic complications with invasive digital subtraction angiography is estimated at 1.3% to 1.8% and 0.5% to 0.6%, respectively.

# MEDICAL MANAGEMENT

Therapies with antiplatelet agents, anticoagulant agents, lipid-lowering agents, and antihypertensive agents have all been studied for reducing the risk of stroke.

## ◼ ANTIPLATELET AGENTS

### Aspirin

The long-standing foundation of antiplatelet therapy in the management of atherosclerotic disease has been aspirin. Aspirin exerts its antiplatelet effect by acetylating platelet cyclooxygenase, thereby irreversibly inhibiting the formation of platelet-dependent thromboxane $A_2$, a potent effector of platelet activation, vasoconstriction, and smooth muscle proliferation. Multiple investigators have demonstrated the efficacy of aspirin in the prevention of stroke. The Antithrombotic Trialists' Collaboration documented, in their meta-analysis of >200 000 patients from 287 randomized trials, the powerful effect of antiplatelet agents (primarily aspirin) in the primary and secondary prevention of both fatal and nonfatal strokes. Specifically, they noted a 25% reduction in nonfatal stroke and a 30% reduction in fatal or nonfatal ischemic stroke. They also found that low doses of daily aspirin (75-150 mg) were just as effective as higher doses (up to 1500 mg). The authors also comment that daily doses of <75 mg may be as effective as higher doses based on their meta-analysis, but they caution that this has been less widely studied and thus remains uncertain. It should be noted that the use of aspirin in low-risk women was called into question by the Women's Health Study, which noted an increased risk of hemorrhagic stroke. In women with documented carotid disease, however, the benefits are likely to outweigh this risk. Therefore, aspirin is recommended for the primary prevention of cardiovascular events in men >45 years old and women >55 years old for whom the benefits are likely to outweigh the risks. All patients with documented carotid disease, stroke, or TIA should receive aspirin, in the absence of a contraindication, to reduce the risk of stroke and other cardiovascular events.

### Thienopyridines

Clopidogrel and ticlopidine are thienopyridines that irreversibly bind the $P2Y_{12}$ subunit of the adenosine diphosphate (ADP) receptor. This blocks ADP-mediated activation of the glycoprotein IIb/IIIa receptor complex, thereby inhibiting fibrinogen activity and platelet aggregation, as well as the action of other platelet agonists such as thrombin and thromboxane $A_2$. The Ticlopidine Aspirin Stroke Study compared the use of ticlopidine and aspirin in patients with a history of TIA, reversible ischemic neurologic deficit, or minor stroke. Ticlopidine significantly reduced the risk of fatal and nonfatal stroke by 24% ($p = 0.011$) compared with aspirin. This effect was even greater during the first year, with a 48% reduction in the risk of stroke. However, due to the complications associated with its use, such as neutropenia and thrombotic thrombocytopenic purpura, the use of ticlopidine has been supplanted by clopidogrel.

The Clopidogrel versus Aspirin in Patients at Risk of Ischemic Events (CAPRIE) trial was a randomized, double-blind trial that compared clopidogrel versus aspirin in patients with a history of recent MI, ischemic stroke, or peripheral vascular disease. Clopidogrel demonstrated an 8.7% RR reduction for the primary outcome of stroke, MI, or vascular death ($p = 0.04$). In the subgroup of patients with a history of a previous stroke, there was a trend toward reducing the risk of adverse events with an RR reduction of 7.3% in favor of clopidogrel ($p = 0.26$).

The role of dual antiplatelet therapy (aspirin plus clopidogrel) in patients at risk for stroke has been studied by multiple investigators. The Management of Atherothrombosis with Clopidogrel in High-Risk Patients with Recent Transient Ischaemic Attack or Ischaemic Stroke (MATCH) trial evaluated dual antiplatelet therapy in 7599 patients with recent stroke or TIA. All patients received clopidogrel 75 mg daily and were randomized to aspirin (75 mg daily) or placebo. After a follow-up of 18 months, the primary end point, a composite of ischemic stroke, MI, vascular death, or rehospitalization for acute ischemia was insignificantly lower for the dual therapy group (15.7% vs 16.7%; $p$ = not significant), although life-threatening bleeding was higher (2.6%) than in the clopidogrel-only group (1.3%; $p < 0.0001$).

The Clopidogrel for High Atherothrombotic Risk and Ischemic Stabilization, Management and Avoidance (CHARISMA) investigators evaluated dual antiplatelet therapy in patients with either clinically overt vascular disease (cardiovascular, cerebrovascular, or peripheral vascular disease) or multiple risk factors. In this study, 15 603 patients were randomized to clopidogrel (75 mg daily) plus aspirin (75-162 mg daily) or to aspirin alone. After a median follow-up of 28 months, the primary end point, which was a composite of cardiovascular death, stroke, or MI, did not differ between the aspirin plus clopidogrel group (6.8%) and the aspirin-only group (7.3%; $p = 0.22$). The subgroup of patients enrolled with prior stroke similarly did not benefit. As seen in MATCH, the risk of bleeding was significantly increased with dual antiplatelet therapy.

Taken together, studies of clopidogrel in the prevention of stroke have established its efficacy when used as monotherapy as an alternative to aspirin. However, the increased risk of bleeding with dual antiplatelet therapy (aspirin plus clopidogrel) and a lack of consistent benefit in clinical outcomes have resulted in a class III (not recommended) designation for use of the combination in stroke or TIA.

## Dipyridamole

Dipyridamole (DP) is an inhibitor of adenosine deaminase and phosphodiesterase, resulting in the accumulation of adenosine, adenine nucleotides, and cyclic adenosine monophosphate (cAMP), which in turn inhibit platelet aggregation and cause vasodilation. The first major trial of extended-release DP (ER-DP) in the secondary prevention of stroke, the European Stroke Prevention Study 2 (ESPS-2), randomized 6602 patients with previous stroke or TIA to aspirin, ER-DP, aspirin plus ER-DP, or neither. Compared with placebo, the risk of stroke was decreased by 18% with aspirin ($p = 0.013$); by 16% with DP alone ($p = 0.039$); and by 37% with combination therapy ($p < 0.001$). The European/Australasian Stroke Prevention in Reversible Ischaemia Trial (ESPRIT) study group randomized 2739 patients with recent (<6 months) TIA or minor stroke to aspirin with or without ($n = 1376$) DP and found a less robust effect from the addition of DP. The primary outcome (composite of death from all vascular causes, nonfatal stroke, nonfatal MI, or major bleeding complication) occurred in 13% of patients on combination therapy and 16% of patients on aspirin alone (hazard ratio [HR] = 0.80; 95% confidence interval [CI], 0.66-0.98) over a period of 3.5 years, or a 1% absolute risk reduction annually (95% CI, 0.1-1.8).

A meta-analysis by De Schryver and colleagues studied the safety and efficacy of ER-DP in 29 trials enrolling a total of 23 019 patients. They found that the addition of ER-DP to aspirin had no significant effect on the rate of vascular death (RR = 0.99; 95% CI, 0.87-1.12) but, in patients with prior ischemic stroke, it did provide a reduction in overall vascular events (RR = 0.88; 95% CI, 0.81-0.95). A study by the Prevention Regimen for Effectively Avoiding Second Strokes (PRoFESS) study group compared aspirin/ER-DP versus clopidogrel in a group of patients with ischemic stroke. The rate of recurrent stroke was not significantly different (HR = 1.01; 95% CI, 0.92-1.11). Although the rate of major bleeding was higher with the aspirin/ER-DP combination (HR = 1.15; 95% CI, 1.00-1.32), the net risk of recurrent stroke or major bleeding was not significantly different (HR = 1.03; 95% CI, 0.95-1.11)

The use of an aspirin/ER-DP combination is recommended by the American Heart Association/American Stroke Association as an alternative first-line treatment for patients with a history of stroke or TIA.

## Cilostazol

Through the inhibition of phosphodiesterase III, cilostazol decreases the degradation of cAMP, resulting in impaired platelet activation and aggregation. There is also the suggestion that cilostazol decreases smooth muscle proliferation, delays the formation of atherosclerosis, and promotes vasodilation. The Cilostazol Stroke Prevention Study randomized 1062 patients with ischemic stroke (<6 months prior to study) to cilostazol or placebo. The active treatment arm experienced a 41.7% reduction in recurrent stroke compared with placebo ($p = 0.015$). Although this was a significant reduction, the comparison to placebo makes the results less applicable to clinical practice.

More recently, the Cilostazol for Prevention of Secondary Stroke (CSPS 2) trial randomized 2757 patients with recent (<26 weeks) ischemic stroke to show non-inferiority of cilostazol vs aspirin. The primary endpoint of recurrent stroke of any kind was reduced with cilostazol (HR = 0.743; 95% CI, 0.564-0.981; $p = 0.0357$), as were hemorrhagic events (HR = 0.458; 95% CI, 0.296-0.711; $p = 0.0004$); however, side effects such as headache, diarrhea, palpitation, dizziness, and tachycardia were more frequent with cilostazol.

Ultimately, these trials raise the possibility that cilostazol is at least as effective as aspirin and possibly safer. However, larger trials will be necessary before definitively establishing a role for cilostazol in the secondary prevention of stroke.

## ■ ANTICOAGULANTS

Although there is evidence that warfarin reduces the risk of stroke in specific subsets of patients, such as those with atrial fibrillation, there is no convincing evidence that it is superior to aspirin in patients with a history of ischemic stroke from a noncardioembolic source. The Stroke Prevention in Reversible Ischemia Trial (SPIRIT) evaluated the use of warfarin (with a target international normalized ratio [INR] of 3.0-4.5) compared with aspirin for the prevention of adverse events in patients with a history of noncardioembolic TIA or stroke. Warfarin was associated with twice the risk of vascular death, stroke, MI, or major bleeding complications compared with aspirin (12.4% vs 5.4%; $p <0.05$). This poor outcome was mainly attributable to excess bleeding complications, including 27 intracranial bleeds associated with warfarin.

The Warfarin Aspirin Recurrent Stroke Study (WARSS) compared warfarin (with a lower target INR of 1.4-2.8) with aspirin in 2206 patients with a history of ischemic, noncardioembolic stroke. The rates of complications, including major hemorrhage, were not statistically different between the 2 treatment groups with the more conservative dosing of warfarin, and there was no difference between aspirin and warfarin for the prevention of recurrent ischemic stroke or death (17% vs 16%; $p = 0.25$).

The Warfarin-Aspirin Symptomatic Intracranial Disease (WASID) trial randomized symptomatic patients (TIA or stroke within 90 days) with a 50% to 99% major intracranial artery stenosis to warfarin (INR 2-3) or aspirin (1300 mg/d). During a mean follow-up of 1.8 years, 4.3% of aspirin patients died compared with 9.7%

of warfarin patients ($p = 0.02$), resulting in early termination of the trial. Warfarin patients had a higher incidence of major hemorrhage (8.3% vs 3.2%; $p = 0.01$) and MI or sudden death (7.3% vs 2.9%; $p = 0.02$).

Taken together, these clinical trials fail to demonstrate a significant benefit for warfarin over aspirin in decreasing the incidence of recurrent stroke in patients with noncardioembolic stroke. Furthermore, the risk of complications such as major bleeding is significantly higher with anticoagulation. Therefore, the use of warfarin to prevent stroke is reserved for patients with a cardioembolic source (eg, mechanical heart valve, atrial fibrillation). Patients with recurrent stroke while on antiplatelet therapy may be another group that benefits from anticoagulation, but this has not been extensively studied.

# ■ ANTIHYPERLIPIDEMICS

The treatment of hyperlipidemia confers a cardiovascular and mortality benefit. Statins are potent inhibitors of 3-hydroxy-3-methylglutaryl–coenzyme A reductase. They have been shown to decrease levels of low-density lipoprotein (LDL) and C-reactive protein, a potent marker of inflammation; upregulate nitric oxide synthase; decrease expression of endothelin-1 mRNA; improve platelet function; and decrease the production of detrimental free radicals. These effects (and likely others still to be discovered) contribute to improved endothelial function and may decrease the progression of atherosclerosis. There are a number of investigators who have demonstrated the beneficial effect of statin therapy on carotid disease.

Multiple trials have shown the benefit of statin therapy to reduce carotid artery plaque, as well as to alter atheroma composition potentially making them less vulnerable. These changes are associated with substantial clinical benefit. Several large meta-analyses have demonstrated a role for statins in the primary prevention of stroke. Bucher and coworkers analyzed the results from >100 000 patients treated with statins, fibrates, resins, or dietary intervention. Only statins were associated with a reduction in the risk of stroke ($p < 0.05$). The Cholesterol Treatment Trialists' (CTT) Collaborators evaluated >90 000 patients from 14 randomized trials of statins, finding a 17% risk reduction of stroke (95% CI, 22%-12%). This risk reduction is robust, occurring in patients with and without CAD. Briel and colleagues demonstrated this by evaluating outcomes for >200 000 patients from 65 trials. They found risk ratio of 0.75 (95% CI, 0.65-0.87) for patients with CAD compared with 0.77 (95% CI, 0.62-0.95) for patients without CAD.

The Stroke Prevention by Aggressive Reduction in Cholesterol Levels (SPARCL) Investigators provided the first major randomized trial of intensive statin use after recent stroke or TIA (1-6 months prior to entry) in patients without a documented history of CAD. They randomly assigned 4731 patients to atorvastatin 80 mg daily versus placebo with a mean follow-up of 4.9 years. LDL levels were significantly reduced with statin therapy (72.9 vs 128.5 mg/dL; $p < 0.001$). The treatment group experienced a 2.2% absolute risk reduction at 5 years (adjusted HR = 0.84; 95% CI, 0.71-0.99; $p = 0.03$) in the primary end point of fatal or nonfatal stroke. Subgroup analysis suggested that the group with carotid stenosis may have had an even greater degree of benefit (HR = 0.67; 95% CI, 0.47-0.94; $p = 0.02$) and experienced a 56% reduction (HR = 0.44; 95% CI, 0.24-0.79; $p = 0.006$) in the need for later carotid revascularization.

In summary, statins have demonstrated an abrogation of plaque progression and stabilization in plaque morphology. These effects (and likely others to be discovered) have translated into significant clinical benefits in the primary and secondary prevention of stroke. Currently, patients with high-risk features such as diabetes, as well as those with documented atherosclerotic disease, are prescribed statin therapy with a goal LDL of <100 mg/dL and consideration of a goal LDL of <70 mg/dL.

## ■ ANTIHYPERTENSIVES

Approximately 50 000 000 Americans have hypertension, a well-established risk factor for a first or recurrent ischemic stroke. A number of trials and meta-analyses have demonstrated a consistent decrease in the risk of stroke or stroke recurrence with antihypertensive treatment. The Heart Outcomes Prevention Evaluation (HOPE) study demonstrated a 24% risk reduction (95% CI, 5%-40%) in the combined end point of stroke, MI, and death for ramipril (vs placebo) in 1013 patients with a history of stroke or TIA. However, in the Perindopril Protection Against Recurrent Stroke Study (PROGRESS) study, the use of angiotensin-converting enzyme inhibitors was associated with a decreased risk of stroke only when combined with the diuretic indapamide (RR reduction vs placebo 28%; 95% CI, 17%-38%; $p < 0.0001$) but not when used alone.

Evidence for the use of angiotensin receptor blockers was provided by the Losartan Intervention for Endpoint Reduction in Hypertension (LIFE) trial, in which the drug reduced the rate of stroke by 25% versus atenolol in patients with a history of hypertension. However, in the PRoFESS trial, Yusuf and colleagues were unable to demonstrate a significant decrease in recurrent stroke for patients using telmisartan (vs placebo) on top of baseline antihypertensive therapy.

Similarly, data exist for the efficacy of calcium channel blockers and diuretics for the reduction of stroke risk. As implied earlier, however, there is substantial controversy in the use of specific antihypertensive agents for the primary or secondary prevention of stroke. Therefore, current recommendations stress only the need for treatment of hypertension to abrogate the risk of stroke.

# HISTORY OF INVASIVE CAROTID TREATMENTS

## ■ CAROTID ENDARTERECTOMY

Historically, carotid artery stenosis has been treated invasively with CEA. It was first reported in 1954, and its use increased steadily until the mid-1980s, when questions arose concerning its effectiveness and safety. Subsequent studies, however—including NASCET, the European Carotid Surgery Trialists' (ECST) collaboration, and the Veterans Affairs Cooperative trial—have all demonstrated a decrease in the risk of stroke for patients with severe, symptomatic carotid stenosis treated with CEA compared with medical management. The ACAS study showed that asymptomatic patients with >60% stenosis treated with CEA had a decreased risk of stroke at 5 years compared with those managed medically.

Although in experienced hands CEA has been proven safe and effective for many patients with carotid stenosis, CEA has limitations because patients treated outside clinical trials may be at higher risk of complications than trial patients. For example, patients operated on by trial hospitals in ACAS and NASCET had a perioperative mortality of 1.4%, despite a mortality of 0.1% in ACAS and 0.6% in NASCET. In patients at high operative risk, the rate of stroke associated with CEA approaches 8% with an equally high rate of perioperative myocardial infarction. As a result, percutaneous treatment has proved to be a promising alternative for many patients with high operative risk.

## ■ CAROTID ANGIOPLASTY

The first reports of percutaneous transluminal angioplasty (PTA) of the carotid artery in humans were made by both Mullan et al. and Kerber et al. in 1980. This was followed by widespread controversy associated with the investigation of carotid PTA. In the 1996 review by Kachel, the results of >500 carotid angioplasties were presented,

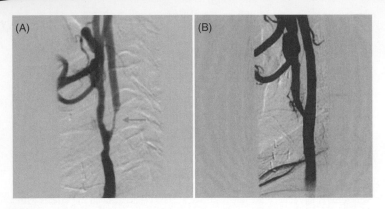

**FIGURE 54-3.** Internal carotid stenosis before **(A)** and after **(B)** stenting.

demonstrating a very low event rate comparable to that of CEA. Concerns such as vascular recoil, distal embolization, and dissection, however, have made stand-alone carotid artery angioplasty a historical procedure that has largely been supplanted by carotid artery stenting with the use of emboli protection devices (EPDs) (**Fig. 54**-3).

# CAROTID ARTERY STENTING

## ■ EARLY EXPERIENCE

Carotid artery stenting (CAS) successfully addressed many of the shortcomings of balloon angioplasty, including vessel recoil and dissection, but introduced its own unique challenges. Because of the superficial nature of the carotid arteries and their vulnerability to external forces, balloon-expandable stents have proved to be poor choices for CAS. Although the stents are easy to place, deformation caused by external compression has been demonstrated. Self-expanding Elgiloy stents (Wallstent) and nitinol stents (Precise, Memotherm, Acculink, Endostent), which continue to exert outward forces, have proven to be better suited for carotid arteries. Most carotid stenting is now performed using nitinol stents because of their better conformability and radial force.

The first reports of stent implantation for the treatment of carotid artery disease were published by Marks et al. Since that time, several large-scale observational series with and without EPDs have been published documenting experience with this method. These are summarized in **Table 54**-1. Most patients included in these reports were at high surgical risk for CEA.

In 2003, Wholey and Al-Mubarek published a global review of carotid stenting. In 11 243 patients, 12 254 carotid artery stents were placed worldwide, with a technical success rate of 98.9%. The risk of stroke at 30 days was 3.3% (2.1% minor and 1.2% major), and the mortality rate was 0.64%. Restenosis was 2.6% and 2.4% at 1 and 2 years, respectively.

## ■ EMBOLI PROTECTION DEVICES

Advancements in the stent platform and the use of EPDs have significantly improved the safety and efficacy of percutaneous carotid intervention and heralded its acceptance

**TABLE 54-1.** Early Carotid Artery Stenting Registries

| Study | Lesions | Success (%) | 30-Day Outcomes Stroke (%) | MI (%) | Death (%) | Restenosis (%) | Follow-up |
|---|---|---|---|---|---|---|---|
| Diethrich et al. | 117 | 99.1 | 8.3 | 0 | 0.9 | 1.7 | 7.6 mo |
| Yadav et al. | 126 | 100 | 6.3 | — | 0.8 | 4.9 | 6 mo |
| Wholey and Al-Mubarek | 12254 | 98.9 | 3.3 | — | 0.64 | 2.6 | 3 y |
| Global Experience[a] | 192 | 99.0 | 2.9 | 0 | 0 | 2.0 | 19 mo |
| Shawl et al. | 100 | 100 | 1.0 | — | 0 | 1.0 | 12 mo |
| Gupta et al. | 88 | 97.7 | 1.2 | 2.3 | 0 | 0 | 30 d |
| Reimers et al.[b] | 604 | 98.0 | 5.8 | — | 1.5 | 3.0 | 36 mo |
| Roubin et al. | 13,481 | 99.2 | 3.4 | — | 0.66 | 2.6 | |
| Total | | | | | | | |

MI, myocardial infarction.

[a]Four thousand two hundred twenty-one patients were treated with emboli protection devices.

[b]Emboli protection (3 filters).

as a treatment in appropriately selected patients. Numerous studies have demonstrated the occurrence of microemboli as detected by transcranial Doppler during CAS and CEA. There are data suggesting a correlation between the number of emboli and neurologic events after CEA. Accordingly, numerous mechanical devices have been developed to prevent the distal embolization of debris during CAS. There are 2 major approaches to emboli prevention devices: filters and occlusion; occlusion can be further subdivided into distal and proximal.

The PercuSurge GuardWire (Medtronic, Santa Rosa, CA) is the prototypical distal occlusive balloon emboli prevention device. A low-pressure balloon is located at the distal tip of a hollow wire. This balloon is inflated after the lesion is crossed and traps any debris released during the percutaneous procedure in the ICA, which is then aspirated prior to deflation of the balloon. The advantages of this system include a low crossing profile and superior wire flexibility. Disadvantages include the occlusive nature of this device, which is not well tolerated in patients without good collateral flow, as well as potential damage to the distal ICA by the device. Additionally, after inflation of the balloon, angiography to localize balloon or stent placement is difficult.

Proximal occlusion balloon systems create retrograde flow in the ICA, which prevents emboli from traveling to the cerebral circulation. Like the GuardWire device, this requires occlusive balloon inflation and can cause vessel damage. Good collateral circulation is also critical. The devices tend to be large and are more difficult to place. Examples of these devices include the Parodi and Mo.Ma devices. The advantage of this approach is that emboli prevention is achieved without crossing the lesion, which is particularly helpful when there is a large clot burden.

The AngioGuard Emboli Capture Guidewire (Cordis, Miami, FL) (**Fig. 54-4**) was the first distal filtration wire system designed to conform to the artery and trap microemboli while maintaining distal flow through a filter umbrella with multiple

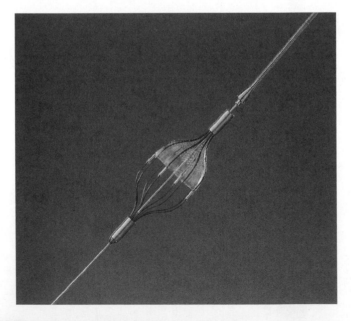

**FIGURE 54-4.** The AngioGuard Emboli Capture Guidewire System.

perfusion pores. The major advantage of filters is the preservation of flow during the intervention and the ability to visualize the vessel with contrast material throughout the procedure. Disadvantages of filters include a larger crossing profile, which may necessitate predilatation prior to placement of the filter distal to the lesion.

Most currently available data are from case series using these devices to perform carotid stenting. The results are very encouraging regarding the efficacy of the devices in reducing procedural stroke compared with retrospective cohorts where these devices were unavailable. Similarly, several single-arm clinical trials evaluating carotid stenting with EPDs have been presented or are ongoing (**Table 54-2**). Many of these trials evaluated patients considered high risk for CEA but nevertheless demonstrated favorable results compared with historical controls.

Kastrup and colleagues systematically reviewed the literature, analyzing outcomes for 896 procedures performed with emboli protection compared with 2537 procedures performed without emboli protection. Patients treated with emboli protection had a 30-day stroke or death incidence of 1.8% compared with 5.5% for patients treated without emboli protection. Likewise, the Endarterectomy versus Angioplasty in Patients with Symptomatic Severe Carotid Stenosis (EVA-3S) trial, a randomized trial comparing CEA to stenting in symptomatic patients, reported outcomes for 80 patients randomized to stenting according to use of an EPD. EVA-3S found a stunning incidence of stroke of 26.7% for patients treated without emboli protection compared with an incidence of 8.6% for patients treated with emboli protection.

Based on robust experience in large trials, emboli prevention devices have become the standard of care for carotid stenting procedure in clinical practice. At this time, there are no studies comparing the safety and efficacy of different emboli prevention devices, and devices are often selected based on operator preference and experience.

# ■ BRIEF REVIEW OF THE CURRENT PROCEDURE

Carotid stenting typically requires an overnight stay, but ambulatory stenting also appears to be safe. The procedure is commonly performed using a 6- to 8-Fr femoral or radial sheath. Heparin is used to achieve an activated clotting time of 250 to 300 seconds. Bivalirudin has been used for carotid stenting, although little data exist comparing bivalirudin with heparin. A guiding catheter or sheath is advanced to the CCA, and the lesion is crossed with an EPD. The EPD is deployed in the ICA, and the lesion is predilated with a small balloon. The lesion is then stented with a self-expanding stent, and the stent is postdilated to the appropriate diameter. The EPD is captured and removed at the end of the procedure. Monitoring of intracardiac filling pressure is helpful in patients with severe LV dysfunction or severe aortic stenosis or in patients who are hemodynamically unstable. Adjunctive treatment with glycoprotein IIb/IIIa inhibitors has been studied in small studies and may be beneficial but has been largely supplanted by emboli prevention devices. Aspirin is continued for life and clopidogrel for at least 1 month after the procedure.

# ■ COMPLICATIONS AND THEIR MANAGEMENT

There are several important issues, some unique to CAS and some similar to those seen in percutaneous coronary intervention, of which the physician must be mindful to avert an adverse and potentially catastrophic outcome. The major periprocedural complications of CAS are stroke, MI, and death. The Stenting and Angioplasty with Protection in Patients at High Risk for Endarterectomy (SAPPHIRE) trial documented a 30-day risk of 5.8% in high-risk patients for these end points. Importantly, the Carotid Revascularization with ev3 Arterial Technology Evolution (CREATE)-Pivotal trial found that independent predictors of death or stroke at 30 days included baseline renal insufficiency, symptomatic carotid stenosis, and duration of filter deployment. The lead-in phase for the Carotid Revascularization Endarterectomy

**TABLE 54-2.** Nonrandomized Clinical Trials of Protected Carotid Artery Stenting

| Study | Patients (No.) | Device | Type of Device | High Risk | 30-Day Death, Myocardial Infarction, or Stroke (%) |
|---|---|---|---|---|---|
| ARCHER-2 | 278 | Accunet OTW | Filter | Yes | 8.6 |
| ARCHER-3 | 145 | Accunet RW | Filter | Yes | 8.3 |
| BEACH | 747 | FilterWire EX/EZ | Filter | Yes | 5.8 |
| CABANA | 1100 | FilterWire EX/EZ | Filter | Yes | Ongoing |
| CABERNET | 454 | FilterWire EX/EZ | Filter | Yes | 3.8 |
| CAPTURE | 1603 (2500 planned) | Accunet | Filter | Yes | 5.1 |
| CAPTURE-2 | ~10 000 | Accunet | Filter | Yes | Ongoing |
| CaRESS | 143 CAS, 254 CEA | GuardWire Plus | Balloon | No | 2 (CAS) vs 3 (CEA) |
| CASES-PMS | 1279 (1493 planned) | AngioGuard | Filter | Yes | 4.8 |
| CREATE-Pivotal | 419 | Spider | Filter | Yes | 6.8 |
| CREATE II | 160 | SpideRX | Filter | Yes | 5.6 |
| EXACT | 1500 | Emboshield | Filter | Yes | 4.6 |
| EPIC | 237 | FiberNet | Filter | Yes | 3.0 |
| MAVErIC I | 99 | GuardWire | Balloon | Yes | 5.1 |
| MAVErIC II | 399 | GuardWire | Balloon | Yes | 5.3 |
| MAVErIC III | 413 | GuardWire | Balloon | Yes | Ongoing |
| MO.MA | 157 | Mo.Ma | Proximal Occlusion | No | 5.7 |
| PRIAMUS | 416 | Mo.Ma | Proximal Occlusion | No | 4.6 |
| RULE-Carotid | 60 | Rubicon | Filter | No | 5.0 |
| SAPPHIRE Worldwide | 10 000 | AngioGuard | Filter | Yes | Ongoing |
| SECURITY | 305 | Emboshield | Filter | Yes | 6.9 |
| SHELTER | 400 | GuardWire | Balloon | Yes | Ongoing |
| VIVA | >500 | Emboshield | Filter | Yes | Ongoing |
| Total (Completed) | 6918 | | | | 4.9 |

CAS, carotid artery stenting; CEA, carotid endarterectomy.

versus Stent Trial (CREST) demonstrated a substantially increased risk of stroke for patients ≥80 years old (12.1%) compared with patients <80 years old (3.2%). Other associated adverse events are intracranial hemorrhage, bradycardia, hypotension, seizures, contrast nephrotoxicities, and access site complications.

Although most ischemic complications occur during the procedure, they can also occur several hours later. Careful neurologic examination is essential to identify these complications. Routine use of cerebral angiography before and after stenting can help identify occluded intracranial vessels. Intra-arterial thrombolytic therapy has been used to treat this complication but with very limited success, reflecting the fact that embolic materials are commonly plaque fragments and not thrombus. Furthermore, the risk of intracranial hemorrhage with this approach is substantial. Mechanical dislodgement of the embolic debris with soft wires may be the best approach to minimize the size of cerebral infraction.

The carotid sinus reflex is most often responsible for the bradycardia and hypotension associated with carotid sinus manipulation. In anticipation of this effect, antihypertensives medications are typically held in the morning of the procedure and, depending on the response to stenting, may also be held until the following morning. Adequate volume expansion is the cornerstone of effective treatment. Atropine is helpful in cases of severe bradycardia. Vasopressors may be required for severe and persistent hypotension. The carotid sinus reflex is typically transient, but it may continue to be a concern for up to 24 hours after the procedure.

On the other side of the spectrum, brisk return of blood flow distal to a chronically ischemic cerebral hemisphere with disordered cerebral autoregulation can lead to problems. Hyperperfusion syndrome is a potentially deadly complication from CAS or CEA. Severe hypertension, critical carotid stenosis, and contralateral carotid occlusion appear to be predisposing factors. Strict monitoring of blood pressure with appropriate treatment is crucial to preventing this. All patients undergoing CAS should be instructed on the importance of medication compliance as well as home blood pressure monitoring. They should be instructed to keep their systolic blood pressure <140 mm Hg. Furthermore, patients must be instructed to monitor for headaches localized to one side associated with nausea, vomiting, and photophobia. Treatment of hyperperfusion syndrome includes strict blood pressure control with the lowering of systolic blood pressure to approximately 100 mm Hg.

# COMPARISONS OF CAS AND CEA

## ■ TRIALS

Although CAS is a less invasive method of treating carotid artery stenosis compared with CEA, extensive evidence of the safety and feasibility of CEA has made it difficult to establish CAS as a viable alternative. Therefore, the initial studies of CAS have involved patients deemed high risk for CEA due to anatomic (eg, high cervical ICA disease, previous neck radiation or surgery) or physiologic (eg, unstable CAD, severe aortic stenosis, significantly depressed ejection fraction, severe pulmonary disease, contralateral ICA occlusion) factors.

The SAPPHIRE trial was published in October 2004 and is a seminal study in carotid intervention as the first randomized controlled trial comparing emboli-protected CAS to CEA. The 334 patients enrolled were either asymptomatic with ≥80% stenosis by ultrasound or symptomatic with ≥50% stenosis. All patients enrolled had a comorbid condition that increased the risk of CEA. The entry inclusion criteria included previous CEA, congestive heart failure, severe CAD, previous radical neck surgery or radiation therapy, and chronic obstructive pulmonary disease. Patients who, in the opinion of a vascular surgeon, could not have surgery were enrolled in a stent registry (409 patients). Patients considered at too high a

**TABLE 54-3.** One- and Three-Year Outcomes from the SAPPHIRE Trial

| | 1-Year Outcomes | | | 3-Year Outcomes | | |
|---|---|---|---|---|---|---|
| Major Event | STENT ($n = 167$) | CEA ($n = 167$) | $p$ | STENT ($n = 167$) | CEA ($n = 167$) | $p$ |
| Death | 7.4% | 13.5% | 0.08 | 18.6% | 21.0% | 0.68 |
| Major ipsilateral stroke | 0.6% | 3.3% | 0.09 | 2.0% | 9.0% | 0.99 |
| Myocardial infarction | 3.0% | 7.5% | 0.07 | 5.4% | 8.4% | 0.39 |
| Cranial nerve palsy | 0 | 4.9% | 0.004 | Not reported | Not reported | NA |
| Target-vessel revascularization | 0.6% | 4.3% | 0.04 | 2.4% | 5.4% | 0.26 |
| Prespecified combined end point[a] | 12.2% | 20.1% | 0.05 | 24.6% | 26.9% | 0.71 |

CEA, carotid endarterectomy; NA, not applicable; SAPPHIRE, Stenting and Angioplasty With Protection in Patients at High Risk for Endarterectomy.

[a]Death, stroke, or myocardial infarction at 30 days plus ipsilateral stroke or death from neurologic causes within 31 days to 1 year or 3 years.

risk for percutaneous management were likewise enrolled in a surgical registry (17 patients). The primary end point of major adverse cardiovascular events (MACE) included death, stroke, or MI within 30 days of the procedure plus death from neurologic causes or ipsilateral stroke up to 1 year. The results are shown in **Table 54-3**. The MACE rate was lower in the percutaneous treatment group compared with the CEA group (12.2% vs 20.1%; $p = 0.05$). In the registry data, the 30-day MACE rate was 7.8% for stenting (32 of 409 patients) and 14.3% (1 of 7 patients) for CEA. There were no significant differences between the 2 groups with regard to either major bleeding (8.3% vs 10.6%; $p = 0.56$) or TIA (3.85% vs 2.0%; $p = 0.5$), but CAS did have an advantage over CEA with regard to cranial nerve injury (0% vs 5.3%; $p < 0.01$). Restenosis rates were not presented. This trial clearly demonstrated a reduction in risk of MACE at 1 year for high-risk patients treated with protected CAS compared with conventional CEA.

Long-term follow-up of patients enrolled in SAPPHIRE was presented by Gurm and colleagues in 2008 (**Fig. 54-5**). Data were available on 260 patients (77.8%) to investigate the prespecified major secondary end point of MACE at 3 years (death, stroke, or MI within 30 days of the procedure or death or ipsilateral stroke between 31 and 1080 days). The end point occurred in 24.6% of the protected CAS group and 26.9% of the CEA group. There was no significant difference in the need for repeat revascularization between CAS and CEA (2.4% vs 5.4%; $p = 0.26$). Therefore, the authors concluded that, at the 3-year follow-up in this group of patients, there was no significant difference in outcome between protected CAS and CEA.

More recent trials randomizing patients to CEA or CAS include the Stent-Supported Percutaneous Angioplasty of the Carotid Artery versus Endarterectomy (SPACE) trial and the EVA-3S trial. The SPACE trial randomized 1200 patients with carotid stenosis of at least 70% by carotid duplex and history of TIA or stroke within 180 days to CEA or CAS. The use of EPDs was not mandated, and they were

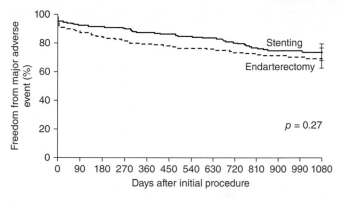

**FIGURE 54-5.** Stenting and Angioplasty With Protection in Patients at High Risk for Endarterectomy (SAPPHIRE) trial long-term results. (Reprinted from Gurm HS, Yadav JS, Fayad P, et al. Long-term results of carotid stenting versus endarterectomy in high-risk patients. *N Engl J Med*. 2008;358(15):1572-1579.)

used in only 27% of cases. Furthermore, patients in SPACE were clearly lower risk than patients in SAPPHIRE. Specifically, exclusion criteria in SPACE included contralateral carotid occlusion, carotid stenosis after endarterectomy, and history of neck radiation, all of which were inclusion criteria for SAPPHIRE. SPACE failed to show noninferiority of CAS for the primary endpoint of ipsilateral stroke or death from any cause within 30 days. Broad application of the results of SPACE is questionable given the high incidence of stroke or death compared with other trials and registries, and the infrequent use of EPDs in the CAS arm. The authors did perform a subgroup analysis and noted no difference in death or stroke for patients treated with embolic protection (7.3%) compared with patients treated without protection (6.7%).

The EVA-3S trial randomized 520 patients with carotid stenosis of at least 60% and a history of TIA or stroke within 120 days to CEA or CAS. Similar to patients in SPACE, patients in EVA-3S were not high risk. The primary end point was the incidence of stroke or death at 30 days. EVA-3S planned to enroll 827 patients but was stopped prematurely because of a significantly higher event rate in the CAS arm. Thirty-day stroke or death occurred in 3.9% of endarterectomy patients compared with 9.6% of stenting patients ($p = 0.01$), driven by a highly significant difference in nonfatal stroke (2.7% vs 8.8%; $p = 0.004$). By 6 months, any stroke or death occurred in 6.1% of endarterectomy patients compared with 11.7% of stenting patients ($p = 0.02$).

The EVA-3S trial also demonstrated important differences in carotid stenting between patients treated with and without cerebral protection. Patients treated with embolic protection had a 30-day incidence of death or stroke of 7.9% compared with 25% for patients not treated with embolic protection ($p = 0.03$). Nonetheless, the RR of stroke or death for stenting over endarterectomy did not differ significantly for the trial before routine embolic protection (RR = 2.0; 95% CI, 0.8-5.0) or after (RR = 3.4; 95% CI, 1.1-10.0, $p = 0.50$). This trial may also have limited general applicability given the high event rate seen in the CAS arm relative to prior studies (30-day incidence of death, MI, or stroke in EVA-3S was 9.6% vs 2.1% in SAPPHIRE), despite including lower risk patients.

The Carotid Revascularization Using Endarterectomy or Stenting Systems (CaRESS) trial was conducted by a consortium of vascular surgeons and reported 4-year outcomes from their prospective, nonrandomized comparative cohort study of patients undergoing protected CAS or CEA. The 397 patients had varying degrees of surgical risk (only 46% were considered high risk), >75% of patients had stenosis >90%, and more than two-thirds were asymptomatic. The primary outcome measures were not significantly different between CAS and CEA, with trends that favored CAS (incidence of any stroke: 8.6% vs 9.6%, $p = 0.444$; death/nonfatal stroke: 21.8% vs 26.5%, $p = 0.361$; and composite of death, nonfatal stroke, and MI: 21.7% vs 27.0%, $p = 0.273$). In the subgroup of patients with symptomatic stenosis, the rate of death, stroke, or MI was significantly lower with CAS than CEA (12.4% vs 33.5%; $p = 0.019$). A similar benefit of CAS was seen in patients <80 years old (13.8% vs 25.3%; $p = 0.030$). Although the limitations of a nonrandomized study and subgroup analysis are valid, CaRESS provides important data regarding the safety and efficacy of protected CAS in a group of patients who are largely not high risk.

The Carotid Revascularization Endarterectomy versus Stenting Trial (CREST) was a multicenter prospective study of 2502 symptomatic and asymptomatic patients (all considered good candidates for surgery) randomized to protected CAS or CEA. CREST found no significant difference in the primary endpoint of death, myocardial infarction or stroke between CAS and CEA (7.2% vs 6.8%, $p = 0.51$) up to 4 years following intervention. In the periprocedural period, stroke was more common with CAS (4.1% vs 2.3%, $p = 0.012$), and myocardial infarction was more common with CEA (2.3% vs 1.1%, $p = 0.032$), though the overall incidence of primary endpoint in the periprocedural period was similar for CAS and CEA. In addition, outcomes were slightly better after CAS for patients <70 years old, and better for CEA in older patients.

It is clear that the safety and efficacy of CAS has improved substantially since its inception due to the use of EPDs, operator proficiency, and better patient selection. The data provided by clinical trials thus far have led the American Heart Association/American Stroke Association to offer a Class I recommendation for CAS as an alternative to CEA in patients with symptomatic stenosis >70% as documented by noninvasive imaging, or >50% by angiography, when the anticipated rate of periprocedural stroke or mortality is less than 6%. Furthermore, the guidelines state that it is reasonable to choose CAS over CEA when revascularization is indicated in patients with neck anatomy unfavorable for surgery (Class IIa). In a similar vein, reimbursement for CAS by the Centers for Medicare and Medicaid Services (CMS) is provided for patients with high surgical risk and symptomatic stenosis of >70%. Furthermore, they provide reimbursement for patients at high risk with symptomatic stenosis between 50% and 69% or asymptomatic stenosis >80% to be enrolled in clinical trials or postapproval studies of CAS. Several trials are currently ongoing to examine the safety and efficacy of CAS in other patient groups and are discussed later.

# ■ SPECIAL SUBGROUPS

There are several patient subgroups that have posed special challenges for the vascular surgeon contemplating a surgical approach to treatment of carotid artery stenosis. Existing data support the use of CAS as a safe and efficacious alternative to CEA in these patients.

## Concomitant Carotid Stenosis and CAD

In patients undergoing coronary artery bypass grafting (CABG), up to 22% have been noted to have asymptomatic carotid stenosis >50%. In these patients, the stroke rate after CABG may be as high as 11%. The management options for carotid stenosis in this setting are controversial but traditionally include either staged or simultaneous

CEA and cardiac surgery. However, both of these strategies carry a high risk of postoperative stroke, MI, and death, even in trials of highly selected patients with low or moderate levels of risk. As a result, there has been a great interest in CAS as an alternative and potentially safer treatment for this group of patients. It should be noted, however, that there is currently no consensus regarding the management of patients with asymptomatic carotid stenosis prior to open-heart surgery (OHS).

Ziada and colleagues evaluated the outcomes of 64 patients with severe carotid and coronary stenoses treated with CAS followed by CABG and compared them to 112 concurrent patients who underwent combined CEA and CABG. There was a significantly higher prevalence of unstable angina, poor LV function, critical aortic valve stenosis, history of TIA or stroke, and history of previous OHS in the CAS group. Although there was no difference in mortality, the CAS patients had a significantly lower incidence of strokes (2% vs 9%; $p = 0.05$) and strokes and MI (6% vs 19%; $p = 0.02$).

Naylor and colleagues conducted a meta-analysis of 11 trials enrolling 760 patients in studies of staged or simultaneous CAS and CABG, the majority of whom (87%) had asymptomatic carotid stenosis. At a follow-up of 30 days after CABG, the rates of ipsilateral stroke, MI, and death were 3.3%, 1.8%, and 5.5%, respectively. Taken together, studies of CAS in patients prior to CABG suggest that this strategy is safe and may significantly abrogate the risks of stroke, MI, and death seen in studies of staged or simultaneous CEA and CABG.

A significant logistical consideration with the use of CAS perisurgically is that of antiplatelet therapy. Although the use of aspirin and clopidogrel is recommended after CAS for a period of at least 2 to 4 weeks, dual antiplatelet therapy does increase the risk of bleeding-related outcomes in patients undergoing OHS. If CABG can be postponed for this period of time, clopidogrel can then be safely held and restarted thereafter. If the need for OHS is more pressing, other strategies that have been suggested include transfer directly after CAS to OHS using aspirin and unfractionated heparin or the use of a heparin and glycoprotein IIb/IIIa inhibitor as a bridge during OHS. Balloon angioplasty without stenting eliminates the need for dual antiplatelet therapy and is also a useful strategy in patients requiring urgent bypass surgery. An interesting strategy still in its infancy is simultaneous CAS and CABG. Versaci and colleagues recently provided encouraging results of their prospective trial of 101 high-risk patients undergoing hybrid CAS/CABG with a 4% risk of the combined end point (stroke, MI, or death).

## Radiation Therapy and Radical Neck Surgery

Radiation therapy is often used as a treatment modality in patients with head and neck cancers. Unfortunately, the incidence of significant carotid stenosis (>50%) is reportedly as high as 19.8% at 5 years and 77.5% at 10 years after therapy. In these patients, tissue dissection is complicated by the extensive fibrosis of the arterial wall and normal tissue planes, and the difficult locations of the lesions, caused by extensive involvement of long segments of the carotid artery above and below the carotid bifurcation, make open access difficult. Carotid stenting has been reported as safe and effective in the treatment of this problem. Retrospective studies suggest that the rate of procedural complications and cardiovascular events with CAS in this group of patients is not significantly different compared with conventional atherosclerotic disease, nor is the rate of post-CAS restenosis. Additionally, the risks of cranial nerve damage and impaired wound healing in this patient group are essentially negated by the use of CAS.

In patients with tracheostomy, cervical spine disease, or other radical neck surgery, access to the ICA, proper patient positioning, and disruption of the normal anatomy may all be affected, prohibiting CEA and favoring CAS. Therefore, carotid stenting can be considered the treatment of choice for carotid stenosis requiring revascularization after cervical radiation or radical neck surgery.

## Recurrent Stenosis After Endarterectomy

Approximately 6% of patients require reoperation for recurrent stenosis after CEA. In retrospective studies, repeat CEA carries a significantly higher risk of stroke and death than first-time CEA (up to 10%), as well as a much higher incidence of cranial nerve injury (approaching 25%). Furthermore, the lesion may also be in an anatomically unfavorable location for surgery. Therefore, there has been significant interest in a percutaneous solution to post-CEA restenosis. A multicenter registry of 14 US centers with 338 patients undergoing CAS of 358 arteries for restenosis after CEA revealed an overall 30-day stroke and death rate of 3.7%. During the follow-up period, there was 1 fatal stroke (0.3%) and 1 nonfatal stroke (0.3%), and there was a 96% rate of freedom from all strokes at 3 years. These results suggest that CAS is an effective treatment alternative for restenosis following CEA and may be safer than repeat surgery.

# FUTURE APPLICATIONS AND TRIALS

The applicability of protected CAS to patients without high surgical risk for CEA, as well as the effect of contemporary optimal medical therapy (OMT) on the incremental benefit from carotid revascularization, has not yet been clearly defined by randomized controlled trials. There are, however, a few ongoing studies aimed at filling this void in the published literature. The International Carotid Stenting Study (ICSS), also known as CAVATAS-2, is a prospective, multicenter trial randomizing non–high-risk patients with symptomatic stenosis to protected CAS or CEA. Similarly, The Transatlantic Asymptomatic Carotid Intervention Trial (TACIT) is expected to enroll 2400 patients with severe asymptomatic stenosis to OMT, OMT plus protected CAS, or OMT plus CEA. Updated information on these trials is available online at www.strokecenter.org and www.clinicaltrials.gov.

# CONCLUSION

Carotid artery atherosclerosis is an important cause of stroke and presents a major public health concern. The management of carotid disease includes antiplatelet therapy, treatment of hyperlipidemia and hypertension, and revascularization in symptomatic patients with moderate or severe stenosis and asymptomatic patients with severe stenosis. Historically, CEA has been the revascularization method of choice, but in recent years, CAS with embolic protection has been established as safe and effective in patients with high surgical risk. Future trials will establish whether the percutaneous treatment of carotid disease can be safely accomplished in patients with low or moderate surgical risk.

# SUGGESTED READINGS

Krishnasawamy A, Yadav J, Kapadia SR. The nonsurgical approach to carotid disease. In: Fuster V, Walsh RA, Harrington RG, eds. *Hurst's The Heart.* 13th ed. New York, NY: McGraw-Hill; 2011:108:2315-2330.

Bates ER, Babb JD, Casey DE, et al. ACCF/SCAI/SVMB/SIR/ASITN 2007 clinical expert consensus document on carotid stenting: a report of the American College of Cardiology Foundation Task Force on Clinical Expert Consensus Documents (ACCF/SCAI/SVMB/SIR/ASITN Clinical Expert Consensus Document Committee on Carotid Stenting). *J Am Coll Cardiol.* 2007;49:126-170.

Brott TG, Halperin JL, Abbara S, et al. 2011 SA/ACCF/AHA/AANN/AANS/ACR/ASNR/CNS/ SAIP/SCAI/SIR/SNIS/SVM/SVS guideline on the management of patients with extracranial carotid and vertebral artery disease. A report of the American College of Cardiology Foundation/American Heart Association Task Force on Practice Guidelines, and the American Stroke Association, American Association of Neuroscience Nurses, American Association of Neurological Surgeons, American College of Radiology, American Society of Neuroradiology, Congress of Neurological Surgeons, Society of Atherosclerosis Imaging and Prevention, Society for Cardiovascular Angiography and Interventions, Society of Interventional Radiology, Society of NeuroInterventional Surgery, Society for Vascular Medicine, and Society for Vascular Surgery. *Circulation* 2011;124:e54-e130.

Gurm HS, Yadav JS, Fayad P, et al. Long-term results of carotid stenting versus endarterectomy in high-risk patients. *N Engl J Med* 2008;358:1572-1579.

Mantese VA, Timaran CH, Chiu D, Begg RJ, Brott TG. The Carotid Revascularization Endarterectomy versus Stenting Trial (CREST): stenting versus carotid endarterectomy for carotid disease. *Stroke* 2010;41:S31-S34.

Mas JL, Chatellier G, Beyssen B. Carotid angioplasty and stenting with and without cerebral protection: clinical alert from the Endarterectomy Versus Angioplasty in Patients With Symptomatic Severe Carotid Stenosis (EVA-3S) trial. *Stroke* 2004;35:18-20.

Sacco RL, Adams R, Albers G, et al. Guidelines for prevention of stroke in patients with ischemic stroke or transient ischemic attack: a statement for healthcare professionals from the American Heart Association/American Stroke Association Council on Stroke: co-sponsored by the Council on Cardiovascular Radiology and Intervention: the American Academy of Neurology affirms the value of this guideline. *Stroke* 2006;37:577-617.

Safian RD, Bacharach JM, Ansel GM, Criado FJ. Carotid stenting with a new system for distal embolic protection and stenting in high-risk patients: the carotid revascularization with ev3 arterial technology evolution (CREATE) feasibility trial. *Catheter Cardiovasc Interv* 2004;63:1-6.

Yadav JS, Wholey MH, Kuntz RE, et al. Protected carotid-artery stenting versus endarterectomy in high-risk patients. *N Engl J Med* 2004;351:1493-1501.

Zarins CK, White RA, Diethrich EB, Shackelton RJ, Siami FS. Carotid revascularization using endarterectomy or stenting systems (CaRESS): 4-year outcomes. *J Endovasc Ther* 2009;16:397-409.

# CHAPTER 55
# DIAGNOSIS AND MANAGEMENT OF DISEASES OF THE PERIPHERAL ARTERIES AND VEINS

Usman Baber, Paul W. Wennberg, and Thom W. Rooke

Peripheral vascular diseases are a diverse collection of disorders that affect all organ systems. Although peripheral arterial disease (PAD) is the disease most commonly encountered by the cardiologist, disease of the lymphatics and veins is equally common (globally more so). For the cardiologist or internist with an interest in vascular disorders, a systematic and comprehensive approach is required. This chapter covers commonly encountered areas of vascular disease, including lymphedema, venous disease, and PAD. Accompanying chapters on aortic and cerebrovascular disease address those areas in more detail.

## ARTERIAL DISEASE

### ■ LOWER EXTREMITY OCCLUSIVE DISEASE

#### Prevalence and Natural History

PAD caused by atherosclerosis is the most common cause of lower extremity ischemic syndromes in Western societies. It is estimated that 10 million people have symptomatic PAD and another 20 to 30 million have asymptomatic disease. Ten percent of individuals over age 60 are affected and its prevalence continues to increase with age. Death directly due to PAD is rare as morbidity and mortality are more often due to concomitant coronary or cerebrovascular disease. Risk factors for PAD are the same as those for coronary artery disease (CAD), with tobacco use and diabetes having an even greater effect. Although the cardiovascular mortality and morbidity of patients with PAD is sobering, the rate of progression of limb symptoms and need for limb revascularization or amputation are low. Need for revascularization due to tissue loss (ulcer) or rest pain is 5% per year. Amputation rates are even lower, at approximately 1% per year.

### ■ CLINICAL PRESENTATION

**Claudication** Literally meaning *limping* (Latin), claudication is a stereotypical, reproducible distress in single or multiple muscle groups of the lower extremity

**TABLE 55-1.** Differential Diagnosis of Claudication

Atherosclerosis obliterans
Arteritis (Takayasu, giant cell)
Embolic disease/acute arterial occlusion
Degenerative joint disease (hip, back, knee)
Spinal stenosis
Myopathy
Thromboangiitis obliterans
Popliteal entrapment
Venous claudication/varicosities
Baker cyst
Deconditioning
Aortic dissection
Aortic coarctation
Retroperitoneal fibrosis

brought on by sustained exercise and relieved by rest. The differential diagnosis of claudication is broad; an abbreviated list is given in **Table 55-1**. With this in mind, information regarding risk for atherosclerosis, current medical problems, prior lower extremity and back trauma, and all vascular and orthopedic procedures should be obtained. The description of claudication symptoms is unique to each patient. Symptom specifics, including onset, progression, and aggravating or alleviating factors, should be rigorously clarified. Commonly, several types of discomfort caused by several etiologies are present. Symptoms are usually described as cramping, but numbness, weakness, giving way, aching, and dull pain are all common adjectives. The distress changes in character and/or location as the flow-limiting lesion(s) progress. When workload is increased by rapid pace, a burden, or walking uphill or over rough terrain, the distance or time to onset will shorten. When the distance to onset or severity abruptly changes, thrombosis in situ or an embolic event should be considered. In general, symptoms occur distal to the level of stenosis or occlusion. Relief with rest is independent of position and is timely, usually complete within 5 minutes. When specific positions are required for relief, musculoskeletal or neurologic disorders should be suspected. Standardized treadmill testing using ABIs at rest and after completion of an exercise protocol confirms the diagnosis, determines the severity, and documents claudication distance for future follow-up.

**Critical Limb Ischemia** Critical limb ischemia may be defined as tissue loss or rest pain in a limb, usually at the distal portion and rarely in the entire limb. Small, localized areas of ischemic pain or ulceration are often caused by minor trauma to an area with poor perfusion rather than progression of disease. It is important to inquire about new shoes, recent nail care, pets, and other potential sources of trauma. Rest pain is present when supine and is often relieved by dependency, such as hanging the limb off the bed or, paradoxically, by walking. Pain may progress to become constant, interrupting sleep, suppressing appetite, inducing weight loss and delirium, and requiring large doses of analgesics for pain relief. Patients may take to sleeping in a chair to get better rest and often will present with edema as a result.

**Pseudoclaudication** Pseudoclaudication is typically of neurogenic origin. The patient with neurogenic claudication describes exercise-induced distress with a dysesthetic quality that clears slowly or requires a specific posture for relief, usually with the hips flexed. Clumsiness may develop as walking continues. Symptoms also occur with prolonged standing or when supine. Compression of the distal spinal cord by hypertrophic bone, disk protrusion, or tumor may be the cause. A history of back injury is common. Arterial and pseudoclaudication often coexist. In this situation, the dominant lesion can be clarified by observing and timing symptoms with standing still and comparing with symptoms during exercise, as well as by measuring the arterial indices before and after exercise.

## Arterial Examination

**Sight** A red or purplish color of the forefoot during dependency (dependent rubor) is common with severe ischemia. Rubor caused by ischemia will change to pallor with elevation, versus cellulitis that may remain rubrous with elevation. Timing the onset of pallor and time to venous refilling can be performed in the examination room. Loss of normal hair growth is also a marker of ischemia.

**Palpation** The aorta, radial, ulnar, subclavian, carotid, temporal, occipital, femoral, popliteal, posterior tibial, and dorsalis pedis arteries are accessible by palpation. Pulses are graded on a scale (**Table 55-2**). If a pulse is not palpable, Doppler examination should be performed to establish whether flow is absent or below the level of detection by palpation. Surface temperature is reduced when perfusion is compromised. Temperature differences are best felt with the dorsum of the fingers; comparison to the contralateral limb or proximal ipsilateral limb should be made.

**Auscultation** Blood pressure should be taken in both arms and should be similar but rarely identical, even when done simultaneously. Respiratory variation, positioning of the arm, and atrial fibrillation are just a few reasons the pressures vary. If a large difference is noted between arms (>14 mm Hg), blood pressures should be rechecked. If still discrepant, simultaneous pressures are done to confirm the finding. The femoral, iliac, aortic, carotid, and subclavian arteries should be auscultated routinely. Simultaneous palpation of a radial artery during auscultation will improve detection of subtle bruits (especially abdominal bruits when bowel sounds are vigorous) and allows accurate timing of bruits. An epigastric bruit that varies

**TABLE 55-2.** Pulse Grading Scale[a]

| Mayo Grade | Physical Findings | ACC/AHA Grade |
|---|---|---|
| 0 | Absent | 0 |
| 1 | Severely reduced—palpable with great difficulty; unable to accurately count pulse | 1 |
| 2 | Moderately reduced—palpable with some difficulty; able to count pulse | 1 |
| 3 | Mildly reduced—easily palpable | 1 |
| 4 | Normal pulse—easily palpable | 2 |
| 5 | Enlarged—widened, possibly aneurysmal | 3 |

ACC/AHA, American College of Cardiology/American Heart Association.

[a]Pulse grading scale. Presence of edema and other physical barriers at time of examination must be taken into account when grading.

with respiration is most often due to compression of the celiac artery by the arcuate ligament of the liver.

## Imaging Studies

**Conventional Angiography**   Conventional angiography is the standard by which all other imaging techniques are judged. It provides reproducible information with very high resolution not yet matched by other modalities. Drawbacks include risk of distal embolization and arterial damage at the puncture site. Iodinated contrast is used with small but real risk of anaphylactoid reaction and contrast nephropathy.

**CT Angiography**   CT angiography (CTA) provides detailed anatomic information without need of arterial access. Iodinated contrast is still required. Three-dimensional (3D) reconstructions can include or exclude bony structures and other organs in the final images and also have the advantage of being 3D, allowing the image to be rotated on an axis. A strong argument may be made for using CTA as an initial imaging modality when percutaneous intervention is unlikely.

**Magnetic Resonance Angiography**   Magnetic resonance angiography (MRA) provides information similar to CTA without the need for iodinated contrast. For those at risk of contrast nephropathy or anaphylactoid reaction, it is a safe and accurate alternative to CTA and conventional angiography. However, those with a low creatinine clearance are at risk of nephrogenic fibrosing dermopathy, also known as *nephrogenic systemic fibrosis*.

**Duplex Ultrasound**   Duplex ultrasound provides safe and reliable data of not only arterial anatomy but also of the hemodynamic effects of stenosis when Doppler flow analysis is incorporated. Contrast is not required, and no ionizing radiation is used. Ultrasound is portable and captures images in real time, allowing both bedside and intraoperative monitoring of therapy.

## Hemodynamic/Functional Studies

**Segmental Pressures**   Segmental pressures and exercise testing provide a simple, reproducible, inexpensive, and accurate method of determining whether or not arterial stenosis is present, the severity of the stenosis, and the approximate location of the stenosis. Pneumatic cuffs are placed around the thigh, calf, ankle, upper or lower arm, or digits. A CWD probe is positioned over the artery at a site distal to the cuff, and the systolic pressure at which arterial flow ceases and resumes is recorded. Each segmental pressure is divided by a reference arterial pressure (the highest brachial artery pressure most commonly) to create an index. The most commonly reported segmental pressure is the ABI. A normal ABI should be ≥1.0, but >0.90 is considered normal in most laboratories. Severe disease is present when the ABI is <0.50 (**Table 55-3**).

The biggest disadvantage of segmental pressure measurement is that it is unreliable in patients with noncompressible or poorly compressible vessels, seen most commonly in diabetes. The stiff vessels are caused by calcium deposition in the media of the arteries (Mönckeberg calcification). Many groups use the great toe index in these patients. The toe-brachial pressure index is considered normal when >0.70. The great toe is most often used, with the second toe as an alternative. Even when the large vessels of the limb are noncompressible, the digital vessels in the toes and fingers often remain noncalcified and can be used to estimate pressure with an appropriate-sized cuff. Pulse volume recording, laser Doppler fluximetry (LDF), and transcutaneous oximetry can be effective in these patients (see following sections).

**Lower Extremity Arterial Exercise Testing**   Lower extremity arterial exercise testing is performed by walking on a treadmill at a standardized protocol. Protocols may be

**TABLE 55-3.** ABI Criteria[a]

|  | Rest | Postexercise | Symptoms | Time (min) |
|---|---|---|---|---|
| Normal | >0.90[b,c] | >0.90 | None | 5 |
| Minimal | >0.90 | <0.90 | None | 5 |
| Mild | >0.80 | >0.50 | Present late | 5 |
| Moderate | <0.80 | <0.50 | Present, limiting | <5 |
| Severe | <0.50 | <0.15 | Early, limiting | <3 |

ABI, ankle-brachial index.

[a]ABI is the systolic blood pressure at the ankle measured in the supine position/systolic blood pressure of the higher arm. Postexercise values are after 5 minutes at a 10% grade at 2 miles per hour (the authors' laboratory protocol; other protocols may be used). Speed may be varied if patient is unable to maintain this speed.

[b]An ABI >1.30 is considered noncompressible, and an alternative means of investigation should be considered.

[c]Some laboratories use 0.95 as the lower limit of normal.

*fixed* (eg, 2 miles per hour at a 10% incline for a maximum of 5 minutes) or graded, increasing speed and/or incline at set intervals, similar to those used in cardiac exercise studies. Select parts of the lower extremity study (ie, ABIs or CWD at the common femoral level) are performed before and after exercise. With exercise, the systolic blood pressure increases as peripheral resistance decreases, resulting in a larger pressure gradient and the resultant lower ABI and abnormal Doppler signals. Therefore, a decrease in ABI or a change in Doppler signal may be detected after exercise (Table 55-3). Even if the resting values are normal, a decreased ABI following exercise predicts an increase in mortality.

**Pulse Volume Recording** Pulse volume recording assesses the magnitude of the arterial impulse entering a limb or segment of a limb. A pneumatic pressure cuff connected to a pressure transducer is placed around the limb and filled with air to a low pressure (typically 40-60 mm Hg). During systole, pulsatile inflow of the arterial system causes distension of the limb. This technique has the advantage of remaining accurate in the setting of poorly compressible vessels.

**Transcutaneous Oxygen** Transcutaneous oxygen pressure measurement ($TCPO_2$) assesses the microcirculation by quantifying the amount of oxygen that diffuses out of the skin. $TCPO_2$ can be used to monitor the effect of therapy such as bypass graft or stenting, sympathectomy, or spinal cord stimulation. It may also predict whether the cutaneous perfusion is adequate for healing at a given amputation site.

## Treatment

The recent American College of Cardiology/American Heart Association (ACC/AHA) practice guidelines on lower extremity PAD summarize the medical and interventional treatment options and level of evidence available (**Table 55-4**).

*Walking programs* should be initiated in all patients with claudication. The effectiveness of a supervised walking program has been well demonstrated, and supervised programs have proven to be more effective than nonsupervised programs. Exercise for 30 minutes 4 to 5 days per week improves functional ability and exercise capacity, and increases total and absolute walking distance from 50% to 300%. Walking should be to near maximal tolerated pain, then rest for relief and repeated.

**TABLE 55-4.** Treatment of PAD ACC/AHA Indications[a]

| Intervention | Class I | Class IIA | Class IIB |
|---|---|---|---|
| Smoking cessation | Yes | | |
| Walking program | Supervised | | Unsupervised |
| Lipid treatment | Statin to LDL <100 | Statin to LDL <70 | Fibric acid derivative High TG/low HDL |
| Antihypertensive treatment | SBP <130; DBP <80 β-Blockade | ACEI (symptomatic) | ACEI (asymptomatic) |
| Diabetes | Proper foot care | HbA$_{1c}$ <7% | |
| Homocysteinemia | | | Folic acid |
| Antiplatelet therapy | Aspirin Clopidogrel | | |
| Pharmacologics | Cilostazol | | Pentoxifylline |
| Supplements | | | L-arginine p-L-carnitine Ginkgo biloba |

ACC, American College of Cardiology; ACEI, angiotensin-converting enzyme inhibitor; AHA, American Heart Association; DBP, diastolic blood pressure; HbA$_{1c}$, hemoglobin A$_{1c}$; HDL, high-density lipoprotein; LDL, low-density lipoprotein; PAD, peripheral arterial disease; SBP, systolic blood pressure; TG, triglyceride.

[a]Summary of AHA/ACC level of evidence guidelines for therapies in claudication.

**Medical Therapy** Smoking cessation is a must for treatment of PAD. Cilostazol is effective in increasing walking distance when used in conjunction with a walking program. Although effective, cilostazol should always be used as part of a comprehensive program, including exercise and risk factor reduction. Antiplatelet agents have long been considered first-line agent for patients with PAD. In the Clopidogrel versus Aspirin in Patients at Risk of Ischemic Events (CAPRIE) trial, clopidogrel monotherapy was superior to aspirin in reducing cardiovascular mortality in PAD patients. Similarly, the addition of clopidogrel to aspirin was more effective than aspirin alone in reducing risk for myocardial infarction among PAD patients enrolled in the Clopidogrel for High Atherothrombotic Risk and Ischemic Stabilization, Management and Avoidance (CHARISMA) trial. Lipid lowering in PAD has been shown to decrease progression of claudication symptoms. Hypertension control should be optimized, recognizing that pressure reduction in the setting of severe stenosis rarely worsens symptoms.

**Revascularization** The indication for revascularization is based on a number of factors, including comorbidities, functional status, and severity of symptoms. Surgical and endovascular treatment strategies are addressed in adjacent chapters. In general, proximal (iliac) stenosis and short-segment occlusion are best treated using an endovascular approach, with long lesions and occlusions best treated surgically. Revascularization should be considered for patients with rest pain, tissue loss, or lifestyle-limiting symptoms refractory to medical therapy.

## Acute Arterial Occlusion

**Presentation** Acute arterial ischemia is a particularly ominous sign, with a 20-day mortality rate of 25%. It presents suddenly as a painful, cold (polar), pale, pulseless limb that progresses to paresthesia and paralysis. Limb viability is at risk if flow is not restored quickly. Severe ischemia is suggested by pallor at rest, profound coolness, tender or hard muscles, and loss of motor and/or sensory functions. The etiology of acute arterial occlusions may be trauma, dissection, thrombosis in situ, or embolism from a proximal source.

**Treatment** Immediate measures are needed to protect the limb and restore blood flow. Heparinization should be started to prevent clot propagation and to stabilize the embolic source(s). Angiography may be required to plan repair when there is preexisting occlusive or aneurysmal disease or when the etiology is unclear. Ideally, all occlusions should be considered for reestablishment of flow, but urgency is governed by the degree of ischemia. If the affected limb is not viable, amputation should be performed as quickly as possible to avoid further complications. When indicated, thrombolysis of acute occlusion can be effective, although the risks of bleeding and stroke must be considered.

## Thromboangiitis Obliterans

Thromboangiitis obliterans (TAO), or Buerger disease, is an inflammatory vasculopathy affecting small- and medium-sized arteries and veins caused by an inflammatory, highly cellular intraluminal thrombus. TAO was thought to be only associated with tobacco use, but cannabis, either on its own or because of contamination with tobacco, causes a similar entity, and its use should also be addressed. Historically, TAO was seen in males in the second through fifth decades. Currently, the incidence in women has risen, reflecting the changed demographics of tobacco use. Clinically, TAO differs from atherosclerosis in that involvement of the upper extremity is common and usually present. The initial involvement is in digital, pedal, and hand vessels frequently with ulceration of 1 or more digits. Rare manifestations include coronary, cerebral, and mesenteric artery lesions. Improvement is possible only after all exposure to tobacco ceases, but the improvement remains variable.

## Giant Cell and Takayasu Arteritis

Takayasu arteritis (TA) and giant cell (temporal) arteritis (GCA) are similar in pathologic process but affect different age groups. TA affects those younger than 40 years, and GCA usually affects those older than 50 years. TA generally involves arteries below the neck, and GCA generally involves arteries above the diaphragm, but involvement of the aorta, subclavian, axillary, renal, iliac, femoral, and superficial femoral arteries has been described in both. Disease is usually bilateral and presents with rapidly progressive symptoms in the setting of a nonspecific systemic illness. Limb-threatening ischemia is rare but does occur when diagnosed late. Both GCA and TA have characteristic clinical and laboratory findings, including an elevated sedimentation rate (>90%, but not in all patients) and typical angiographic features of smooth tapered narrowing of large- and medium-sized arteries. These diseases are unique among arteriopathies in that the acutely stenotic lesions improve rapidly with steroid therapy. Alternative immunosuppressive agents are often used, but corticosteroids remain the mainstay of treatment.

## Fibromuscular Dysplasia

Fibromuscular dysplasia most commonly affects women in the middle years and has been described in almost all arteries. The renal artery is most commonly involved, affecting 4% to 5% of the general population, and is bilateral in approximately 10% of cases. Treatment with angioplasty has generally good outcomes, with stent use reserved for complications such as angioplasty-associated dissection. Surgical repair is reserved for refractory cases or when distal renal disease is present.

## Raynaud Phenomenon

Raynaud phenomenon is diagnosed by history, with the examination and laboratory findings playing a secondary role. The syndrome is classically defined as discoloration episodes of white ischemia, then blue stasis, and then red hyperemia during the recovery phase. In practice, most patients do not describe all 3 phases. Fingers are involved more often than toes. Allen and Brown defined primary Raynaud phenomenon as episodes of bilateral color changes induced by cold or emotion without evidence of ischemia or other disease for 2 years. This represents most cases and, in some sense, can be considered simply an exaggerated response of a normal reflex. The pathophysiology of the exaggerated vasoconstriction is complex but appears to involve both local and systemic pathways. Most patients with primary Raynaud phenomenon require no therapy and quickly learn to keep not only hands but the whole body warm.

Secondary Raynaud phenomenon is caused by another etiology and is present in approximately 10% of patients at initial evaluation. For those without a secondary cause at presentation, one is identified at a rate of 2% per year over a 10-year interval. Causes of secondary Raynaud phenomenon are diverse (**Table 55-5**).

**TABLE 55-5.** Secondary Causes of Raynaud Phenomenon

Collagen vascular disease
   Scleroderma
   Mixed connective tissue disease
   Rheumatoid arthritis
   Myositis
   Sjögren syndrome
   Necrotizing vasculitis
Hematologic disorders
Neurogenic
   Thoracic outlet irritation
   Carpal tunnel syndrome
   Neuropathy
Myxedema
Acromegaly
Pulmonary hypertension
Medications
   β-Blockers
   Ergotamine
   Methysergide
   Vinblastine, bleomycin
   Estrogens
   Imipramine
Microcirculatory diseases
Buerger disease
Hypothenar hammer syndrome
Environmental
   Cold injury
   Vibration syndrome
   Vinyl chloride disease

Treatment of secondary Raynaud is directed at the underlying cause when feasible. Calcium-channel blockers and α-blockers, either as monotherapy or in combination, can blunt the episodes in many patients but may have little impact on ischemic complications. ACEI, angiotensin II receptor inhibition, and endothelin receptor inhibition are promising in the setting of scleroderma.

# ■ VENOUS DISEASE

Venous disease is common with multiple clinical presentations and causes.

## Varicose Veins

Primary varicosities tend to be familial and without other causative events. They often first appear during pregnancy. Prolonged dependency at the place of work may increase the risk of developing varicose veins. Secondary varicosities may be caused by several etiologies, including extrinsic venous compression, prior DVT, congenital lesions, arteriovenous fistulas, right heart disease, or perforator vein incompetence. History, examination, and laboratory evaluation of the deep venous system allow differentiation of primary from secondary varicosities. Symptoms and progression can be improved by graduated compression hose. Ablation of the vein should be considered if complications or discomfort interfere with occupation or lifestyle. Sclerotherapy is effective for small varicosities and larger *spider veins.*

## Superficial Thrombophlebitis

Superficial thrombophlebitis (STP) presents as a tender, erythematous, indurated lesion following the course of a superficial vein that, on palpation, feels like a cord. STP often occurs in varicose veins or at sites of indwelling catheters or recent intravenous injections. Cellulitis is common, and when present, antibiotics should be used. STP is usually self-limited, and recovery may be accelerated by rest, elevation, warm compresses, and anti-inflammatory agents. There is a moderate incidence of concurrent DVT in STP. Evaluation for underlying thrombophilia testing for a clotting abnormality should be considered in the setting of recurrent STP or in those with a strong family history of thrombosis.

## Deep Vein Thrombosis

The morbidity and mortality of DVT are high. Risk factors for DVT and pulmonary embolism have been well defined in several studies (**Table 55-6**). The signs and symptoms of DVT are nonspecific and unreliable. Objective testing to confirm and define the extent of DVT should be obtained whenever the diagnosis is entertained.

Treatment with heparin acutely and warfarin chronically is highly effective in preventing clot propagation and pulmonary embolism. Low-molecular-weight heparins (adjusted for weight) have proven effective in treating DVT and can be used for outpatient management in uncomplicated cases. Heparin-induced thrombocytopenia is common; platelets should be monitored routinely while on heparin. Heparin-induced thrombocytopenia is confirmed by detecting platelet factor 4 antibodies. When present, a direct thrombin inhibitor or danaparoid is used in place of heparin until the warfarin effect is therapeutic.

The duration of treatment with warfarin for optimal risk-to-benefit ratio following DVT is not known. Recent literature suggests treatment for a minimum of 6 months in patients with spontaneous DVT and 3 months for a precipitated DVT, but this decision must be individualized for each case.

**TABLE 55-6.** Risk Factors for Deep Vein Thrombosis

| Transient Cause | Fixed Cause |
| --- | --- |
| Recent surgery | Prior superficial vein thrombosis |
| Hospitalization | Prior deep venous thrombosis |
| Trauma | Residence in health care facility |
| Malignancy | Immobility |
| Hormonal therapy | Age |

## Venous Ulceration

The formation of venous ulceration following DVT is unfortunately common with substantial clinical and economic implications. Ulcers occur at the medial perimalleolar region most often because this area has the highest venous pressure when upright. The excess venous pressure results in a decreased perfusion pressure and chronically hypoxic skin prone to injury. Once ulceration has occurred, successful management requires reduction of the edema by compression and conservative debridement of necrotic tissue and fibrinous eschar. After skin integrity is restored, control of venous hypertension with elastic support hose is required indefinitely.

## Phlegmasia Cerulea Dolens

Phlegmasia cerulea dolens is a rare complication of DVT characterized by acute, massive edema, severe pain, and cyanosis in the setting of extensive iliofemoral thrombosis. One-third of patients die because of pulmonary embolism, and half develop distal gangrene caused by thrombus-induced compartment syndrome. Phlegmasia cerulea dolens is seen most commonly with advanced malignancy or severe infections but can occur following surgery, fractures, and other common precipitants of thrombosis. Treatment includes placement of a caval filter, heparinization, and clot removal by thrombectomy (surgical or endovascular) and possibly thrombolysis.

## ■ LYMPHEDEMA

Globally, lymphedema is the most common vascular disease, affecting 90 to 120 million people. Defined as an abnormal accumulation of lymphatic fluid in the dermal and subcutaneous tissues, lymphedema may be primary or secondary in etiology. Primary lymphedema may be congenital (present at birth) or, more commonly, present in the early teen years (lymphedema praecox) and is more common in females presenting around menarche. Lymphedema tarda presents in later years and is a diagnosis of exclusion because a secondary cause is much more likely in this age group. Trauma, recurrent infection, obstruction, infiltration, and radiation all cause lymphatic vessel damage. Upper extremity lymphedema may occur after axillary node dissection. Recurrent cellulitis is common in patients with lymphedema and may be an initiating, exacerbating, or complicating event.

## Diagnosis and Testing

History and physical examination make the diagnosis in the majority of cases. Unlike edema and lipedema, lymphedema involves the toes and often affects them first. The skin is thickened and takes on an orange peel consistency (*peau d'orange*) A diffuse, flat, warty consistency may affect the skin over time. Dependent edema spares the toes unless secondary lymphedema is present. Lipedema is caused by excess fatty deposits in the leg and may be difficult to differentiate from lymphedema if the foot is not examined. However, with lipedema, the toes are spared and there is often a ridge or fold overhanging the ankle.

## Treatment

Treatment for lymphedema is volume reduction of the limb. Reduction in limb size by elevation, mechanical pumping, or manual massage is effective. Wrapping of the limb, distal to proximal, is required whenever the patient is up. After leg volume is decreased, an elastic compression garment (40-50 mm Hg in strength), should be worn daily and replaced 2-4 and times per year as needed. Early and aggressive treatment of cellulitis and fungal infections of the toes helps to prevent cellulitis.

# SUGGESTED READINGS

Wennberg PW, Rooke TW. Diagnosis and management of diseases of the peripheral arteries and veins. In: Fuster V, Walsh RA, Harrington RG, eds. *Hurst's The Heart*. 13th ed. New York, NY: McGraw-Hill; 2011:109:2331-2346.

Allison MA, Hiatt WR, Hirsch AT, et al. A high ankle-brachial index is associated with increased cardiovascular disease morbidity and lower quality of life. *J Am Coll Cardiol*. 2008;51:1292-1298.

Berger JS, Krantz MJ, Kittelson JM, et al. Aspirin for the prevention of cardiovascular events in patients with peripheral artery disease: a meta-analysis of randomized trials. *JAMA*. 2009;301:1909-1919.

CAPRIE Steering Committee. A randomized, blinded, trial of clopidogrel versus aspiring in patients at risk of ischaemic events (CAPRIE). *Lancet*. 1996;348:1329-1339.

Feringa HH, van Waning VH, Bax JJ, et al. Cardioprotective medication is associated with improved survival in patients with peripheral arterial disease. *J Am Coll Cardiol*. 2006;47:1182-1187.

Giri J, McDermott MM, Greenland P, et al. Statin use and functional decline in patients with and without peripheral arterial disease. *J Am Coll Cardiol*. 2006;47:998-1004.

McDermott MM, Liu K, Greenland P, et al. Functional decline in peripheral arterial disease: associations with the ankle brachial index and leg symptoms. *JAMA*. 2004;292:453-461.

Olin JW. Hypertension and peripheral arterial disease. *Vasc Med*. 2005;10:241-246.

Strandness DE Jr, Dalman RL, Panian S, et al. Effect of cilostazol in patients with intermittent claudication: a randomized, double-blind, placebo-controlled study. *Vasc Endovascular Surg*. 2002;36:83-91.

# CHAPTER 56
# SURGICAL TREATMENT OF CAROTID AND PERIPHERAL VASCULAR DISEASE

Joseph M. Sweeny, Jayer Chung, and Thomas F. Dodson

The discipline of vascular surgery has witnessed a rapid proliferation and remarkable progress in technique, technology, and clinical research. In the past 2 decades, endovascular therapy has become a fundamental part of the vascular specialist's practice, and clinical data supporting its use continues to provide evidence helping to formulate standards of care aimed at improving clinical outcomes in patients with peripheral vascular disease.

## CAROTID REVASCULARIZATION

Stroke remains the third leading cause of death in the United States accounting for 1 of every 18 deaths. The incidence is increasing, with 795 000 new cases per year reported in the United States. Substantial morbidity results from stroke, as approximately 31% of all stroke patients require outpatient rehabilitation and >18% of stroke survivors are unable to return to work. Overall, the national 2009 direct and indirect estimate of the cost of stroke was $68.9 billion, most of which results from a loss of earnings due to the disability of stroke.

Approximately 15% to 20% of strokes originate from carotid atherosclerotic plaques, emboli, or thombi, and several preoperative imaging modalities are available to evaluate the carotid circulation. Arteriography remains the gold standard of preoperative imaging for carotid artery disease but is being used less frequently with increased availability of various noninvasive modalities. Presently, vascular surgeons rely on duplex ultrasound alone or in conjunction with computed tomography angiography (CTA) and magnetic resonance angiography (MRA). Unfortunately, noninvasive studies fail to elucidate all carotid stenoses accurately; therefore, carotid angiography is preferred when there is

- Uncertainty about the accuracy or reliability of the vascular ultrasound results
- Uncertainty about the possibility of complete occlusion of the carotid artery in a patient with ongoing localizing symptoms
- Concern about proximal or intrathoracic disease
- A patient with technically difficult studies caused by variant arterial anatomy
- A patient with symptoms and an indeterminate noninvasive study

Carotid endarterectomy (CEA) remains the most frequently performed procedure to prevent stroke, with approximately 93 000 operations performed in 2009. CEA is performed through a vertical incision along the anterior border of the sternocleidomastoid muscle. An endarterectomy is carried out along a dissection plane in the media of the artery, with the key to the procedure being the attainment of a smooth tapering end point into the internal carotid artery. A dacron or bovine pericardial patch is used in the majority of patients because the overall incidence of recurrent carotid stenosis has been shown to be one-third less frequent when compared with primary repair. It is important to note that autogenous patches are prone to pseudoaneurysm formation, which is avoided with the use of synthetic patches.

Multiple randomized, controlled studies support CEA over medical therapy in both asymptomatic and symptomatic patients. These trials also highlight several subgroups that deserve special attention. Women derive less of a benefit from CEA among asymptomatic patients. Interestingly, women with 50% to 69% symptomatic stenoses also did not show a clear benefit from CEA. CEA also provides a greater benefit in patients with hemispheric strokes or transient ischemic attacks compared with patients with retinal ischemic events. Patients with contralateral carotid occlusion derive less of a benefit from CEA, particularly patients who are asymptomatic at presentation. Furthermore, data regarding technical outcomes in the surgical arms of these studies are derived from centers of excellence; therefore, replication of these outcomes requires referral to vascular surgeons with similar success rates. Patients deriving the greatest benefit from CEA are those who are able to survive for at least 2 years. Therefore, risks of surgery against the potential benefits must be assessed. With these facts in mind, a decision-making process regarding carotid revascularization is outlined in **Table 56-1**.

Data over the past decade regarding carotid artery stenting (CAS) reflect changes in technology. The current registry and randomized, controlled data all use a cerebral protection device to prevent periprocedural emboli from escaping into the cerebral circulation and require practitioners to demonstrate proficiency with the most recent techniques and equipment. None of these trials shows superiority of CAS, with several showing superiority of CEA (**Table 56-2**). These trials have been widely criticized, with detractors citing flaws in patient enrollment, study design, lack of long-term follow-up, and definition of end points. More recently, the Carotid

**TABLE 56-1.** Treatment Plan for Patients With Carotid Disease

| Category of Patient | Treatment |
|---|---|
| **Patients with symptomatic carotid stenosis** | |
| >80% stenosis of internal carotid artery | CEA/CAS indicated |
| 50%-79% stenosis of carotid artery but with vascular laboratory data suggesting closer to 79% | CEA/CAS probably indicated; assess risk factors |
| 50%-79% stenosis of carotid artery but with vascular laboratory data suggesting closer to 50% | CEA/CAS may be indicated; assess risk factors |
| <50% stenosis of carotid artery | Trial of medical therapy |
| **Patients with asymptomatic carotid stenosis** | |
| >80% stenosis of carotid artery | CEA/CAS indicated |
| 50%-79% stenosis of carotid artery but with vascular laboratory data suggesting closer to 79% | CEA/CAS may be indicated; assess risk factors |
| 50%-79% stenosis of carotid artery but with vascular laboratory data suggesting closer to 50% | Revascularization not indicated |
| <50% stenosis of carotid artery | Revascularization not indicated |

CAS, carotid artery stent; CEA, carotid endarterectomy.

**TABLE 56-2.** Results of Randomized Controlled Studies, Nonrandomized Prospective Studies, and Registry Data Studying Carotid Artery Stenting

| | Study and Year | No. of Patients | 30-Day Stroke/Death Rate | |
| --- | --- | --- | --- | --- |
| | | | CAS | CEA |
| Randomized | CREST, 2010 | 2502 | 4.1% | 2.3% |
| | SAPPHIRE, 2004 | 334 | 4.8% | 5.4% |
| | SPACE, 2006 | 1200 | 7.7% | 6.5% |
| | EVA-3S, 2006 | 527 | 9.6% | 3.9% |
| Prospective series | ARCHeR, 2006 | 581 | 6.9% | NA |
| Registry | CREATE, 2006 | 419 | 5.2% | NA |
| | CAPTURE, 2007 | 3500 | 5.7% | NA |

ARCHeR, ACCULINK/ACCUNET for Revascularization of Carotids in High-Risk Patients; CAPTURE, Carotid RX ACCULINK/ACCUNET Post-Approval Trial to Uncover Unanticipated or Rare Events; CAS, carotid artery stenting; CEA, carotid endarterectomy; CREATE, Carotid Revascularization With ev3 Arterial Technology Evolution; CREST, Carotid Revascularization Endarterectomy Versus Stenting Trial; EVA-3S, Endarterectomy Versus Angioplasty in Patients With Severe Symptomatic Carotid Stenosis; NA, not applicable; SAPPHIRE, Stenting and Angioplasty With Protection in Patients at High Risk for Endarterectomy; SPACE, Stents in Patients With Diabetes Mellitus or Metabolic Syndrome.

Revascularization Endarterectomy versus Stenting Trial (CREST) results were published in July 2010. While there was a higher risk of stroke with stenting and a higher risk of myocardial infarction with carotid endarterectomy, "the risk of the composite primary outcome of stroke, myocardial infarction, or death did not differ significantly" among symptomatic and asymptomatic patients with carotid stenosis undergoing either carotid artery stenting or endarterectomy. Interestingly, an interaction between age and treatment efficacy was detected in this trial with a crossover at an age of 70 years. Patients ≥70 years old experienced higher rates of stroke, myocardial infarction, or death compared to patients ≤70 years old—a finding thought to be secondary to greater vascular tortuosity and calcification in elder patients. Future studies will be required as newer modalities, and techniques arise to improve the safety of CAS. Presently, carotid stenting is considered for a select minority of patients who meet criteria for carotid revascularization and who are at a high risk for surgical CEA. In light of these recent trials, the following criteria are a guideline for patient selection for CAS:

- Lesion at C2 or higher, or below the clavicle
- Prior radical neck dissection or neck irradiation
- Contralateral carotid occlusion
- Recurrent carotid stenosis
- Contralateral laryngeal nerve palsy
- Presence of a tracheostomy
- Age ≤70 years
- Class III/IV heart failure or angina pectoris
- Left main or 2-vessel or greater coronary artery disease
- Open-heart surgery within 6 weeks

- Myocardial infarction within 30 days
- Left ventricular ejection fraction ≤30%
- Severe chronic lung or renal disease (dialysis dependent)

For all patients, clopidogrel therapy is recommended before carotid stent placement and for at least 30 days postoperatively.

# UPPER AND LOWER EXTREMITY REVASCULARIZATION

## ■ UPPER EXTREMITY REVASCULARIZATION

Symptomatic ischemia afflicts far fewer patients in the upper extremities than in the lower extremities. In the upper extremities, effort fatigue is a frequent complaint resulting in the need for revascularization, as symptoms of upper arm fatigue are often more functionally disabling than claudication in the lower extremities. Other symptoms of upper extremity ischemia requiring revascularization include vertebrobasilar steal, rest pain, and gangrene. Important physical findings include the pulse examination of both upper extremities and ulceration or gangrene of the digits. Findings on physical examination are often subtle due to rich collateral networks surrounding the shoulder and elbow. Therefore, arteriography is required in most cases to confirm the diagnosis and to appropriately plan operative interventions. Other noninvasive tests, such as segmental blood pressure measurements, ultrasound, and computed tomography, are instrumental in the diagnostic workup of upper extremity ischemia.

Revascularization depends on the location of the culprit lesion and the patients' medical comorbidities. Lesions of the supra-aortic trunks are more commonly associated with atherosclerosis and are most frequently approached via extrathoracic approaches, such as carotid-subclavian artery bypass and transpositions. Transpositions are preferred over bypass given better long-term patency rates. Intrathoracic reconstructions are generally avoided, especially with cardiopulmonary disease or a history of prior sternotomy, because the morbidity is markedly less for transpositions or bypasses; however, if there is disease in the innominate artery or occlusive disease in multiple major vessels, transthoracic reconstructions based on the ascending aorta may be preferable. In all reconstructions, care must be taken to preserve the left internal mammary artery, because of its potential importance in coronary revascularization. For lesions distal to the subclavian artery, bypass, with vein or prosthetic graft, is the predominant modality of revascularization.

More recently, endovascular therapy has been successfully applied to treat many of these lesions. Its long-term durability and efficacy have yet to be fully elucidated, though early results, particularly for lesions of the supra-aortic trunk, are encouraging. In patients who are at high risk for a traditional vascular procedure, endoluminal angioplasty and/or stenting appears favorable. The role of endovascular therapy as the primary treatment modality is still debatable, although it is gaining popularity among peripheral vascular specialists.

## ■ AORTOILIAC AND LOWER EXTREMITY REVASCULARIZATION

Approximately 15% to 20% of the population older than 70 years has objective evidence or symptoms of peripheral arterial disease (PAD). PAD encompasses 2 classic syndromes: intermittent claudication and chronic critical limb ischemia. Both result from reduced blood flow to the lower extremities; however, critical limb ischemia, as the name implies, defines the patient population at greatest risk of limb loss.

Claudication occurs because of an increased demand for blood flow by the muscles that the atherosclerotic vasculature cannot supply. Nonoperative management under close physician supervision is generally appropriate, as only 1 of 4 patients symptomatically worsens over time. Conservative management consists of risk factor modification. Cigarette smoking, diabetes, hypertension, hyperlipidemia, hyperhomocysteinemia, elevated C-reactive protein, and hypercoagulability are modifiable factors or markers that influence the progression of atherosclerosis in PAD. Guidelines for therapy are summarized in the recommendations of the Trans-Atlantic Inter-Society Consensus (TASC) II Working Group.

After control of risk factors, a formal, supervised exercise program is necessary in the treatment of claudication. Exercise training should be performed at least 3 times per week for a minimum of 12 weeks. Patients who stop smoking and participate in a regular exercise program have nearly a 70% likelihood of improving their walking distance. In the absence of congestive heart failure, cilostazol (100 mg orally twice daily) is indicated as an effective therapy to improve symptoms and increase walking distance in patients with intermittent claudication. Antiplatelet therapy (aspirin) is indicated to reduce risk of myocardial infarction, stroke, or vascular death in patients with claudication. Other medications (naftidrofuryl) can be considered according to TASC II Guidelines.

Revascularization, whether endovascular or surgical, is reserved for patients suffering serious impairment of activities important to the patients who have failed conservative management for claudication. Absence of another disease that would limit exercise even if the claudication was improved should be documented. Generally speaking, initial revascularization strategies frequently rely on endovascular techniques, with open surgical intervention reserved for individuals whose arterial anatomy is unfavorable for endovascular procedures. In patients with combined inflow and outflow disease, inflow problems are corrected first. An improvement in inflow may diminish symptoms and, if distal revascularization is needed, reduce the likelihood of distal graft thrombosis from low flow. Focal stenoses or occlusions are often treated with angioplasty alone, with approximately 70% 5-year patency; however, 5-year patency is improved to approximately 80% with the addition of iliac stenting. If open surgical procedures are required, aortofemoral bypass grafts are preferred to aortoiliac bypass grafts because the external iliac artery is often severely diseased. Extra-anatomic bypasses are usually avoided in claudicants; however, the most commonly used extra-anatomic bypass is the femoral-to-femoral bypass, with an anticipated 71% patency at 5 years. There are multiple options to improve outflow in claudicants. The superficial femoral artery and proximal popliteal artery are the most common sites of stenosis or occlusion in patients with intermittent claudication. The most commonly performed operative bypass for the treatment of claudication is the femoral-popliteal artery bypass. Nearly every study that has compared vein with prosthetic conduit for arterial reconstruction of the lower extremity has demonstrated the superiority of vein over prosthetic conduits. Bypass with a prosthetic graft should rarely be necessary for the treatment of mild intermittent claudication because of the increased risk of amputation associated with failure of such grafts. Angioplasty and stenting are now accepted procedures for stenoses and occlusions of the superficial femoral artery, with decreased early morbidity relative to bypass surgery. Technical advances such as hydrophilic wires, improved catheter and balloon design coupled with subintimal angioplasty have improved results of endovascular therapy for chronic total occlusions; however, occlusions >10 cm in length are least suitable to endovascular therapies.

Chronic critical limb ischemia is a process that, if left untreated, may result in amputation. Prompt recognition of the signs of limb-threatening ischemia and the prompt initiation of therapy are necessary. These patients often present with rest pain, nonhealing ulcers, and/or gangrene. Because of the limb-threatening nature of the ischemia, interventions that are often considered to be invasive or risky among claudicants are strongly considered in the critical limb ischemia population. Chronic critical limb ischemia patients are also some of the least healthy patients in vascular surgery, with almost 20% requiring a major amputation or dying within 1 year of lower extremity bypass. Therefore, the decision as to how and when to intervene must be balanced delicately with the patient's comorbid, ambulatory, and social living status.

Patients who have significant necrosis of the weight-bearing portions of the foot, an uncorrectable flexion contracture, paresis of the extremity, refractory ischemic rest pain, sepsis, or a very limited life expectancy caused by comorbid conditions are evaluated for primary amputation. If the patient is ambulatory and has a reasonable operative risk (dependent on cardiac, pulmonary, and renal factors), a revascularization procedure is offered. Arteriography remains the definitive method to delineate the exact level of arterial occlusion and to define the vascular anatomy prior to selecting an intervention. For individuals with combined inflow and outflow disease with critical ischemia, inflow lesions should be addressed first. If symptoms persist, an outflow procedure is warranted. Also, if infection, ischemic ulcers, or gangrenous ulcers are present, an outflow procedure that bypasses all major stenoses and occlusions should be considered. Although the greater saphenous vein is preferred as a conduit for bypass (**Fig. 56-1**), there are a number of alternatives. Besides prosthetic bypasses, arm and lesser saphenous vein grafts, composite sequential bypass using a vein sewn to a prosthetic graft, use of an anastomotic vein patch, and cryopreserved vein allografts are all options when adequate greater saphenous veins are unavailable.

Endovascular therapies are more frequently being used primarily or as an adjunct to lessen the morbidity of a lower extremity bypass to treat critical limb ischemia. Early results with endovascular therapies suggest that they yield equivalent amputation-free survival rates, although larger studies with longer follow-up are required. In contradistinction to claudicants, critical limb ischemia patients with infrapopliteal disease can be treated with endovascular techniques, although there are presently no data to dictate which patients are most suitable for endovascular or open revascularization. For all patients undergoing stent placement, lifelong clopidogrel or aspirin is recommended.

# UPPER AND LOWER EXTREMITY VENOUS THROMBOSIS

## ■ UPPER EXTREMITY VENOUS THROMBOSIS

Recent reports indicate that upper extremity DVT may occur more frequently than previously thought, especially among patients with prior central venous catheter placement, hypercoagulable states, and a history of prior lower extremity DVTs. Moreover, approximately one-third of patients with upper extremity DVT also have a high probability of having a pulmonary embolus by perfusion lung scanning or angiogram. Recurrent thromboembolism is rare, but postphlebitic syndrome occurs in up to one-fourth of patients at 2 years, especially in patients with residual thrombosis. In general, there are 2 classes of upper extremity DVT: primary and secondary.

Patients with primary upper extremity DVTs often present acutely with thrombosis of the subclavian-axillary vein, resulting in swelling of the arm (100%), venous engorgement (82%), pain (73%), and cyanosis (55%). Frequently referred to as *Paget-von Schrötter syndrome*, acute effort thrombosis of the subclavian vein is generally seen in healthy young people after repetitive motion or exercise involving the affected extremity. As many as 10% of patients may develop a pulmonary embolus, and only <10% spontaneously recanalize. The amount of swelling and discomfort is

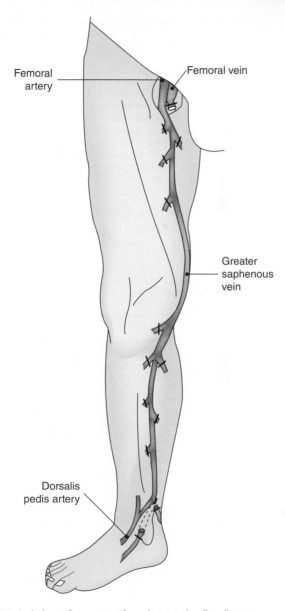

**FIGURE 56-1.** In situ bypass from common femoral artery to dorsalis pedis artery.

related directly to the amount of arm use (venous claudication) because the symptoms are a result of obstruction and not reflux. Therapy involves catheter-directed thrombolysis, followed by surgical decompression of the thoracic outlet. Catheter-directed thrombolysis should ideally be instituted within 2 weeks of the onset of symptoms; otherwise, chronic fibrosis of the vein ensues, resulting in an increased incidence of postphlebitic syndrome. Chronic fibrotic lesions of the vein may be amenable to stenting after successful thoracic outlet decompression, although the long-term outcomes are not known.

Secondary venous thrombosis is caused mainly by indwelling venous catheters, which increase the odds of an upper extremity DVT by 7-fold. The onset of signs and symptoms is more gradual and often subtle. Because of milder symptoms, limited longevity, and reduced activity, most patients are treated conservatively with device removal, anticoagulation therapy, avoidance of excessive use of the affected arm, arm elevation to combat swelling, and the use of an elastic support.

Patients with upper extremity DVT who have contraindications to or unsuccessful use of anticoagulation have been a significant source of concern. Superior vena cava filters are often the only safe option in this group and are placed in an inverted position in the superior vena cava compared with its configuration in the inferior vena cava.

## ■ LOWER EXTREMITY VENOUS THROMBOSIS

In a population of 100 000, an estimated 70 to 113 cases of DVT are diagnosed annually. Thirty-day mortality for DVT and pulmonary embolism is approximately 6% and 15%, respectively. The risk of DVT increases with age with a dramatic increase in risk after age 60, Caucasian ethnicity, past history of DVT, general anesthesia, operations, pregnancy, malignancy, hypercoagulable states, and trauma. Long-term sequelae of DVT comprise the postthrombotic syndrome, a clinical entity of chronic venous insufficiency, and manifest as edema, hyperpigmentation, and ulceration. Postphlebitic syndrome can occur in up to two-thirds of patients, with ulceration occurring in 5% despite adequate anticoagulation.

Present treatment recommendations from the American College of Chest Physicians (ACCP) include acute anticoagulation with heparin, low-molecular-weight heparin, or fondaparinux, in conjunction with warfarin therapy to maintain a goal international normalized ratio (INR) of 2.0 to 3.0 for 6 months. Catheter-directed thrombolytic therapy is often recommended for patients without contraindication to thrombolytics with acute (≤14 days in duration) confirmed iliofemoral or femoropopliteal DVTs, because thrombolysis is more effective at reducing clot burden and deep venous valve function. Ultimately, with preservation of venous valve function, it is thought that postphlebitic sequelae can be avoided. A recent registry study of 473 patients treated with catheter-directed thrombolysis for acute DVT showed that complete lysis can be achieved in approximately one-third of patients, especially if there is no prior history of DVT. One-year patency was 60%, with the initial degree of thrombolysis being most predictive of 1-year patency. The risks of intracranial hemorrhage are low, being reported as <1% in most series. Age >75 years, hypertension, history of prior stroke, female sex, black race, excessive anticoagulation, and low weight are all independent predictors of intracranial hemorrhage. Compression stockings, with pressures of 30 to 40 mm Hg, are necessary adjuncts to help prevent postphlebitic syndrome.

ACCP guidelines recommend placement of IVC filters for patients with a contraindication to anticoagulation and a DVT. Anticoagulation is recommended in conjunction with the IVC filter if the prior contraindication to anticoagulation resolves as the patient convalesces.

## SUMMARY

The management of peripheral vascular disease continues to evolve, reflecting technologic innovations and clinical trials investigating treatment modalities. While surgery continues to be the gold standard in all arterial segments with which endovascular therapy must be compared, endovascular therapies now provide alternative or adjunctive options for patients who may not be optimal candidates for surgery. Prospective randomized controlled trials and long-term natural history studies will clarify the efficacy, role, and durability of both open and endovascular procedures in the future to further optimize patient care.

## SUGGESTED READINGS

Chung J, Dodson T. Surgical treatment of carotid and peripheral vascular disease. In: Fuster V, Walsh R, Harrington RA, et al, eds. *Hurst's The Heart.* 13th ed. New York, NY: McGraw-Hill; 2011:110:2347-2354.

Adam DJ, Beard JD, Cleveland T, et al. Bypass versus angioplasty in severe ischemia of the leg (BASIL): multicentre, randomized controlled trial. *Lancet.* 2005;366:1925-1934.

Brott TG, Halperin JL, Abbara S, et al, ASA/ACCF/AHA/AANN/AANS/ACR/ASNR/CNS/SAIP/SCAI/SIR/SNIS/SVM/SVS guideline on the management of patients with extracranial carotid and vertebral artery disease. *Circulation.*2011;124:e54-e130.

Brott TG, Hobson RW, II, Howard G, et al. Stenting versus endarterectomy for treatment of carotid-artery stenosis. *N Engl J Med.* 2010;363(1):11-23.

Dosluoglu HH, Lall P, Cherr GS, et al. Superior limb salvage with endovascular therapy in octogenarians with critical limb ischemia. *J Vasc Surg.* 2009;50:305-315.

Executive Committee for the Asymptomatic Carotid Atherosclerosis Study. Endarterectomy for asymptomatic carotid artery stenosis. *JAMA.* 1995;10:1421-1428.

Kearon C, Kahn SR, Agnelli G, et al. Antithrombotic therapy for venous thromboembolic disease: American College of Chest Physicians Evidence-Based Clinical Practice Guidelines (8th edition). *Chest.* 2008;133:454S-545S.

Norgren L, Hiatt WR, Dormandy JA, et al. Inter-Society Consensus for the Management of Peripheral Arterial Disease (TASC II). *Eur J Vasc Endovasc Surg.* 2007;33(suppl 1):S1-S75.

Regensteiner J, Ware JE Jr, McCarthy WJ, et al. Effect of cilostazol on treadmill walking, community-based walking ability, and health-related quality of life in patients with intermittent claudication due to peripheral arterial disease: meta-analysis of six randomized controlled trials. *J Am Geriatr Soc.* 2002;50:1939-1946.

Roger, Veronique L, Go Alan S, et al. Heart disease and stroke statistics—2012 update: a report from the American Heart Association Statistic Committee and Stroke Statistics Subcommittee. *Circulation.* 2011[published online December 15, 2011].

# CHAPTER 57
# THERAPEUTIC DECISION MAKING BASED UPON CLINICAL TRIALS AND CLINICAL PRACTICE GUIDELINES

Sameer Bansilal, Ira S. Nash,
Michael E. Farkouh, and Valentin Fuster

Evidence-based medicine is the conscientious, explicit, and judicious use of current best evidence in making decisions about the care of individual patients. The practice of evidence-based medicine means integrating individual clinical expertise with the best available external clinical evidence from systematic research. The development of clinical practice guidelines has paralleled the growth and importance of the focus on medical quality. A discussion of the context in which practice guidelines have achieved their current prominence is followed by a presentation of their development, implementation, and maintenance. Finally, their quality and impact on medical practice are assessed.

## EVIDENCE-BASED MEDICINE: A BUILDING BLOCK FOR CLINICAL PRACTICE GUIDELINES

Evidence-based medicine gives the highest priority to the well-powered randomized controlled trial (RCT). The RCT is the most rigorous form of prospective scientific human experimentation to evaluate a therapeutic intervention (clinical trial) and has become the gold standard design. The RCT begins with an early stage involving evaluation for safety and treating several doses (phase 1), followed by dose-finding studies and those utilizing surrogate markers of effectiveness (phase 2), and finally by outcomes trials for safety and effectiveness (phase 3) It is now common to have phase 4 trials postapproval that afford the opportunity to expand the indications for a given therapy or to further explore safety concerns when events are rare but potentially fatal. The evidence can be best summarized by defining the patient population, the intervention, and the outcomes of interest.

## ■ STUDY PATIENTS

### Inclusion/Exclusion Criteria

The role of bias is a critical feature of what distinguishes clinical trials from clinical practice. The most important form of bias is selection bias whereby subjects enrolled in a trial differ systematically from those individuals in the general population. In EBM, this can lead to a trade-off between internal validity (findings can be applied to the types of patients enrolled in the trial) and external validity (generalizability to a wider population). By restricting the trial cohort to particular age or medical condition criteria, trial results can be skewed against those that are underrepresented. Purists will argue that trial conclusions should be restricted to those that would have met the eligibility criteria. This especially becomes problematic with the systematic exclusion of women and the elderly from many trials and consequent withholding of potentially efficacious therapies from deserving patients.

Simultaneously, data dredging to arrive at conclusions regarding differential effects related to ethnicity, region, or nonprospectively defined postrandomization subgroups leads to erroneous conclusions, which may be refuted when studied prospectively. Secondary analyses of clinical trials should be interpreted as hypothesis generating only.

## Consent Bias

When considering the external validity of a trial, the first issue to address is consent bias. This is a measure of how different a study participant who has provided informed consent is from an eligible patient who has not provided informed consent.

# ■ STUDY DESIGN

The design and conduct of a clinical trial are important factors in assessing the influence of bias. While a double-blind trial is the preferred version, there are advances that can increase the reliability of open-label trials. The prospective, open, blinded end point (PROBE) design mandates an independent clinical events adjudication committee (CEC). The blinding of the adjudicators reduces bias and should be considered in all clinical trials.

Noninferiority trials have taken center stage with the emergence of newer therapies, which offer benefits as regards safety, convenience, or cost, while maintaining efficacy. The noninferiority comparison sets targets for the upper limit of the 95% confidence interval to fall within, based on a difference between the 2 arms that is predetermined. The Consolidated Standards of Reporting Trials (CONSORT) and the FDA have developed standards for nonsuperiority designs, including noninferiority trials to improve the planning, conduct, and quality of reporting.

Another emerging issue is related to adaptive trials, wherein, based on blinded review of aggregate data, the trial may be modulated in multiple ways such as adjusting sample size, terminating 1 subgroup, differential recruitment of subjects, or altering the statistical analysis plan. High degree of transparency needs to be maintained for proper evaluation of the trial by the scientific community in such situations. Similar rules apply as regards stopping of trials for safety of efficacy.

## Observational Versus RCTs Versus Meta-analyses of RCTs

There is a large body of literature evaluating the relative virtues of observational studies compared to RCTs. The argument for the validity of well-conducted observational studies is strong since they can include a wider range of patients and end points and are, therefore, more reflective of the "real world." While they are great tools to assess the role of physician's judgment in patient and therapy selection, they face the challenge of being unable to adjust for baseline risk.

RCTs provide the highest level of evidence and should remain the gold standard for evaluating therapies. The real concern with the field is that with increasingly complex trial designs, active comparator trials, and the tendency to limit follow-up of patients to shorter durations, the gap between the robustness of RCTs and observational studies may be closing. The only solution is to make it easier to perform RCTs and include a wider range of patients.

# STUDY THERAPY

## Cointervention

The importance of cointervention cannot be exaggerated. The background therapy administered to all arms of a randomized trial directly impacts the event rate and therefore the feasibility of the study. In clinical practice, patients often receive different background therapy than in a trial due to less adherence to guidelines and other factors, including cost of these therapies.

In the last decade, clinical trials have begun recruiting in developing countries with less advanced health care systems. This has resulted in faster recruitment at a lower cost since recruitment rates are higher and subsequently trial duration is reduced considerably. The downside of these global trials is that cointerventions such as background medical therapy or interventions with devices are less prevalent because of inaccessibility and economics. This also often involves less access to proven therapies that reduce the baseline risk profile.

# STUDY OUTCOMES

One of the most important aspects of clinical trials is selection of the primary outcome measures. This often shapes how influential the trial is in changing practice down the road. Inappropriate dilution of outcomes with softer, ill-defined components or the choice of a time point for assessment for outcomes which may be clinically less meaningful are common pitfalls for "positive" trials failing to change practice.

## Translating Measures of Benefit/Harm and Statistical Significance Into Practice

One of the most misinterpreted parts of clinical trials is the measure of clinical benefit. Commonly, the findings of RCTs are expressed as relative risk or relative risk reduction (RRR). Relative risk reduction usually remains durable across the spectrum of baseline risk but is misleading when event rates are low. The number needed to treat (NNT), which is clinically more useful, is the inverse of the absolute risk reduction times 100 and has been found to influence clinical decision making to a greater extent than RRR. The NNT or in some cases the number needed to harm (NNH) should be evaluated keeping in mind the time frame to achieve that benefit or accrue that harm.

Clinical trials often fall short of adequately estimating safety concerns that are rare, since they are often significantly underpowered to detect such risks. A means of linking phase 3 clinical trials with phase 4 postmarketing surveillance would be a step in the right direction. The FDA has made great strides in identifying the challenges of late pharmacovigilance. The FDA Amendments Act provides a framework to create such surveillance. The recent controversy of the safety of antidiabetic medications will likely be addressed through this mechanism.

# STUDY REPORTING

## Registration, Publication Bias, Inadequate Reporting

In the past, there has been great concern that only a fraction of trials that are completed actually are eventually published. This has led to a serious form of bias termed *publication bias*.

Recently, the ICMJE has instituted a strategy that only trials that have been preregistered will be published in their member journals. Registration on ClinicalTrials.gov has been widely accepted as the gold standard and is now a requirement for any serious investigation. These repositories are now including a wide spectrum of clinical trials including phase 1 trials.

The reporting of trial results has often been of poor quality and prone to misinterpretation. In response to these observations, the CONSORT group established a 22-item checklist that standardizes trial reporting.

### Limitation of Extending RCT Findings to Individual Patients

The importance of generalizing findings from clinical trials is realized 1 patient at a time. For clinicians doing their best to practice evidence-based medicine, the real question is does this finding apply to the individual patient in front of me? Because of the emerging evidence that shows wide individual variations in the response to given therapies, conventional sub group analyses of RCTs are often inadequate to detect these variations.

### Meta-analysis: Strengths and Limitations

There has been a trend toward pooling of data at either published level or patient level to summarize treatment effects in cardiovascular medicine. The advantages of meta-analysis are that it provides robust information on the direction of effect and helps to understand these effects in important sub groups. There, however, have been many instances where the quality of meta-analysis is poor and unlikely to provide any important contribution.

Clinical trials by their very nature do not capture the patient's role in decision making, and therefore will always be limited in the capacity to change actual clinical practice. This is where clinical judgment, by encompassing clinician experience, will always involve more than the evidence itself.

### Summary

The application of findings from clinical trials to our daily practice is challenging and must always be put into the context of the uniqueness of each patient. The more inclusive the eligibility criteria and the more rigorous the trial design, the more likely that these findings are valid and generalizable to real-world patients.

# CLINICAL PRACTICE GUIDELINES

## ■ DEFINITION

In 1992, the Agency for Healthcare Research and Quality (AHRQ) and the Institute of Medicine defined practice guidelines as "systematically developed statements in which scientific evidence and clinical judgment can be systematically combined to produce clinically valid, operational recommendations for appropriate care that can and will be used to persuade clinicians, patients, and others to change their practices in ways that lead to better health outcomes and lower health care costs."

## ■ AIDS TO CLINICAL PRACTICE

As the perceived need to improve the quality of care has grown, so too has the range of tools available to practitioners. Medical review criteria are "systematically developed statements that can be used to assess the appropriateness of specific health care decisions, services, and outcomes." These are also referred to as performance measures, quality measures, or performance indicators, and are generally derived from clinical practice guidelines and allowed for their application in assessing and improving care. For example, the ACC/AHA guidelines for acute myocardial infarction (AMI) recommend the use of angiotensin-converting enzyme (ACE) inhibitors for AMI patients with a reduced ejection fraction or clinical heart failure. One performance indicator developed by CMS and The Joint Commission for the assessment of the quality of care, and publicly reported for US hospitals, is the percentage of myocardial infarction patients with left ventricular systolic dysfunction and without contraindications to ACE inhibition who actually receive the medication during their hospitalization.

Another quality improvement tool closely related to practice guidelines is a critical pathway. A critical pathway can also be referred to as a critical path, a clinical pathway, a clinical plan, a care map, or a care plan. These are usually locally developed and highly detailed accounts of how the process of care should unfold for a focused episode of care. They typically deal with the direction and coordination of inpatient services for a particular diagnosis or procedure. Developing an explicit statement of this type forces group of providers to examine their practices and achieve local consensus about how care should be delivered. The final products serve as real-time references to those caring for patients.

## ■ GUIDELINE DEVELOPMENT

The utility of a practice guideline depends critically on the process by which it was created. Task Force 1 of the 28th Bethesda Conference of the ACC detailed 8 phases of successful clinical practice guideline development (**Table 57-1**). The AHA and the ACC have collaborated, often in association with international or subspecialty societies, to produce a series of well-respected clinical practice guidelines for cardiovascular care. They have produced a manual for guideline developers which follows these recommendations. International efforts to facilitate guideline development also recommend an explicit work plan that includes defining the precise scope of the endeavor, systematically gathering and evaluating evidence from the medical literature, and synthesizing clear recommendations.

### Limitations of Guideline Process

There are a number of important limitations to the current system for developing guidelines: (1) Governance: the governing body sanctioning the guideline may not include authorities from a wide range of disciplines; (2) unanimity: most often votes on a particular recommendation are divided yet unanimity is projected by the guideline; and, (3) a lack of independent review.

Sniderman and Furberg suggest the following reforms: (1) The required membership should be broad and clearly defined; (2) membership of the committee should be changed from one edition to another; (3) reports should not be issued unanimously if the vote was divided; (4) post a preliminary version on the web and solicit responses; and, (5) all financial relationships with industry should be disclosed. One of the most challenging aspects of weighing evidence to translate into practice comes from the fact that unequivocal data from well-performed trials are often lacking.

While some have advocated for methodologists to write guidelines, it is clear that the users, namely the clinicians, may feel otherwise.

### Level of Evidence

Perhaps no other step in guideline development is as critical as systematically evaluating the strength of the evidence on which recommendations are based.

**TABLE 57-1.** Phases of Guideline Development and Associated Tasks Identified by the 28th Bethesda Conference

**Phase 1. Administrative oversight**
Task 1. Identify specific goals
Task 2. Prioritize possible guideline topics
Task 3. Review the literature to define task, costs, and time line

**Phase 2. Select expert panel**
Task 1. Members must bring expertise, diversity, enthusiasm, and commitment
Task 2. Convene panel electronically (video conference, e-mail) to begin plans
Task 3. Confirm outline, map patient-care algorithm

**Phase 3. Literature search and evidence review**
Task 1. Computerized literature search
Task 2. Match literature to guideline outline, rate evidence
Task 3. Create evidence tables for each topic
Task 4. Base wording of recommendations on strength of relevant evidence

**Phase 4. Consensus process**
Task 1. Converge on recommendations by an explicit process

**Phase 5. Computerize guideline documents in format for clinical use**
Task 1. Link recommendations with related evidence
Task 2. Create preformatted documents to capture data and facilitate care
Task 3. Create database to store information regarding guideline compliance

**Phase 6. Test and revise guideline**
Task 1. Expert panel tests computerized guideline in actual patient care
Task 2. Final revision of guidelines based on testing

**Phase 7. Disseminate guideline**
Task 1. Publish printed version, disseminate computerized version
Task 2. Encourage local customization

**Phase 8. Revise and refine guideline**
Task 1. Maintain ongoing literature review
Task 2. Refine management strategies based on patient outcomes associated with guideline use

Data were derived with permission from Jones RH, Ritchie JL, Fleming BB, et al. Task Force 1: clinical practice guideline development, dissemination and computerization. *J Am Coll Cardiol.* 1997;29:1133-1141.

The most reliable research results come from RCTs. In descending order of reliability (ascending vulnerability to bias), the remaining sources of data are observational studies, case reports, and expert opinion.

The international GRADE (grades of recommendations, assessment, development, and evaluation) working group also recommended that evidence should be weighed on the basis of consistency and directness. Consistency refers to finding a similar direction and magnitude of treatment effects across different studies. Directness refers to the extent to which the studied population, treatments, and outcomes are similar to those to which the guideline applies. Finally, any scheme used to grade evidence to form the basis of clinical practice guidelines should also consider the ease with which it can be applied consistently by guideline developers and the ultimate transparency and utility of the scheme to the guideline users. The evidence grading schemes used in this book are adopted from the ACC and AHA. The 2006 Methodology Manual for ACC/AHA Guideline Writing Committees stipulates that evidence should be characterized as "level" A, B, or C. Level A is defined as "data derived from multiple RCTs or meta-analyses"; level B as "data derived from a single randomized trial, or nonrandomized studies"; level C as "consensus opinion of experts, case studies, or standard of care."

## Classification of Recommendations

The formulation of treatment recommendations rests on making an informed judgment about whether the benefits of a particular intervention outweigh the associated risks, burden, and cost. When this balance is substantially tipped in one direction or the other, and the evidence to support that conclusion is clear, then a strong recommendation about the intervention can be made.

The apparent favorable comparison of benefits over risks also depends critically on how individuals value particular outcomes. As a result, recommendations inevitably involve making judgments about values held by others, which is subjective and often a challenging exercise. Well-designed clinical trials usually involve highly specified patient populations, defined by extensive inclusion and exclusion criteria, although practice guidelines, by their nature, are intended to be broadly applicable. There is no simple formula to reconcile the nature of the evidence and the need for recommendations.

The classification of recommendations of the ACC and AHA is used throughout this book and is summarized in **Table 57-2**.

There is no consistent correlation between level of evidence and class of recommendation. If several large RCTs provide conflicting conclusions, then the quality of the available evidence can be high but the recommendation necessarily weak. However, if there is such universal agreement that a particular element of care is so essential that no RCT is ever likely to be done (eg, the necessity of examining a patient), then a strong recommendation can be appropriate in the absence of rigorous evidence.

## ■ GUIDELINE IMPLEMENTATION

Clinical practice guidelines are tools for improving patient care. Much of that potential can be realized only by changing physician behavior because physicians are responsible for directing care. Even a well-crafted guideline will not benefit patients unless and until it actually changes the way physicians act under particular circumstances. The prevalence of substantial deficiencies in the quality of care despite the ubiquity of clinical practice guidelines suggests strongly that their successful implementation must go beyond making the guidelines themselves accessible through publication in the medical literature or by electronic means. Cabana et al presented a useful taxonomy for the barriers to guideline adoption

**TABLE 57-2.** American College of Cardiology/American Heart Association Classification of Guideline Recommendations

**Class I:** Conditions for which there is evidence and/or general agreement that a given procedure or treatment is useful and effective

**Class II:** Conditions for which there is conflicting evidence and/or a divergence of opinion about the usefulness/efficacy of a procedure or treatment

**Class IIa:** Weight of evidence/opinion is in favor of usefulness/efficacy

**Class IIb:** Usefulness or efficacy is less well established by evidence/opinion

**Class III:** Conditions for which there is evidence and/or general agreement that the procedure/treatment is not useful/effective and in some cases can be harmful

Data from Guyatt G, Gutterman D, Baumann MH, et al. Grading strength of recommendations and quality of evidence in clinical guidelines: report from an American College of Chest Physicians Task Force. *Chest.* 2006;129:174-181.

and implementation. They grouped barriers into those related to physician's knowledge (lack of awareness or lack of familiarity), attitudes (lack of agreement, lack of self-efficacy, lack of outcome expectancy, or the inertia of previous practice), and behavior (external barriers).

Just as the barriers to guideline implementation are diverse, there is no single proven strategy for successful guideline adoption. For guideline developers, close attention to the principles of rigorous data synthesis and the straightforward presentation of well-documented recommendations is essential. Explicit discussion of potential conflicts with other guidelines and the reasons for different recommendations should be included. Guideline writers should include clear statements regarding the limitations of their own guidelines with respect to the patients or conditions to which they apply and consider the practicality of their recommendations.

The AHA program, called "Get With the Guidelines," is intended to promote the use of a small number of key treatments for patients hospitalized with coronary heart disease, acute coronary syndromes, heart failure, and atrial fibrillation. These treatments include, for example, the timely use of aspirin, the assessment and treatment of blood lipid disorders, and the discharge prescription of an ACE inhibitor in patients with left ventricular systolic dysfunction. Hospitals must register as program participants. They then gain access to a web-based data collection instrument for monitoring guideline adherence, which also allows for comparisons of local performance against regional and national data. The "Get With the Guidelines" program also provides a "tool kit" of educational material (including presentation slides), guideline implementation aids (such as standardized admission order sets), and extensive program support. More information is available on the AHA web site.

The ACC-sponsored Guidelines Applied in Practice (GAP) program is a rapid-cycle quality improvement initiative that is also intended to boost adherence with major elements of the ACC/AHA guidelines. The GAP program has separate modules for AMI and congestive heart failure. The myocardial infarction tool kit consists of (1) AMI standard admission orders, (2) a clinical pathway, (3) a pocket guide to care, (4) a patient information form, (5) a patient discharge checklist, (6) chart stickers to alert providers, and, (7) hospital performance charts.

## ▪ GUIDELINE MAINTENANCE

If a particular practice guideline is to remain a useful tool for improving the quality of care, it must maintain its scientific currency and its relevance to clinical practice. Guidelines should keep abreast of changes in the risk and benefit of current practice and interventions, outcomes that are considered important and the value placed on them and importantly changes in available resources. A systematic reassessment of existing guidelines by recognized experts, supplemented by limited searches of the medical literature and operating with prospectively defined criteria for obsolescence, may be the only practical way to ensure timely updates.

Electronic publication and partial, rather than complete, revisions have been used effectively by the AHA and ACC to reduce the revision cycle time for their guidelines that need to be updated.

## ▪ GUIDELINE QUALITY

Several observers have suggested lists of attributes that good practice guidelines should have. The Institute of Medicine report lists 8 important qualities (**Table 57-3**). Validity implies that the guidelines, if adopted, will actually lead to the anticipated improvements in health outcomes and/or cost of care. Reliability or reproducibility is achieved if another group of guideline developers would create equivalent guidelines, if they relied on the same evidence, and if the guidelines are "interpreted and applied consistently by practitioners." Good guidelines should also have clear clinical

**TABLE 57-3.** Desirable Attributes of Clinical Practice Guidelines Identified by the Institute of Medicine

Validity
Reliability
Clinical applicability
Flexibility
Clarity
Multidisciplinary development
Scheduled review
Documentation

Data from Field MJ, Lohr KN, eds. *Guidelines for Clinical Practice: From Development to Use.* Washington, DC: National Academy Press; 1992:4.

applicability, so that they pertain to a broad, well-defined, and explicitly stated population. Guidelines must also allow some flexibility of medical practice and acknowledge the appropriate role of clinical judgment and possible exceptions to broad dictates. Clarity of recommendations is another important attribute and should be promoted through the use of precise definitions of terms, unambiguous recommendations, and a variety of presentation techniques. Ideally, guidelines should be developed through a multidisciplinary process, which elicits the input of a broad range of stakeholders in the field. Finally, the Institute report suggests that good guidelines should be well documented, so that users will know the procedures followed in developing guidelines. It should also include the involved participants, the used evidence, the accepted assumptions and rationales, and the employed analytic methods.

More recently, an international effort, the AGREE (Appraisal of Guidelines, Research and Evaluation) project, has led to the development and validation of a new tool to evaluate guideline quality. The evaluation instrument allows reviewers to use standard criteria to judge guidelines in 6 "domains:" scope and purpose, stakeholder involvement, rigor of development, clarity and presentation, applicability, and editorial independence. Each domain is scored independently on the basis of answers to explicit questions. This tool is rapidly becoming the new international standard for the assessment of guideline quality, and is now available through the AGREE web site in 14 languages. Using the AGREE instrument as part of a systematic review of CHF management guidelines, only 5 of 16 guidelines were of good quality. This suggests that we need to set stronger standards in guideline development. The GRADE working group have developed a systematic approach judging the quality of evidence that supports guideline recommendations.

# ■ GUIDELINE EFFECTIVENESS

With legitimate questions raised over the quality of guidelines and the challenges associated with their development, implementation, and maintenance, what is the evidence that the cardiovascular clinical practice guidelines have actually improved the quality of care? Failure to demonstrate improvements in cardiovascular care through the use of guidelines can represent deficiencies in the applicability or practicality of practice guidelines, the operational failure of implementing them locally, or some combination of both. In addition, it is challenging to perform randomized trials of guideline use. Fortunately, there are data to suggest that guidelines can improve care.

Grimshaw and Russell compiled the most rigorous assessment of the success of practice guidelines, in a variety of medical conditions, in improving the quality of care. They reviewed 59 published reports evaluating the impact of practice guidelines and found that in nearly all cases the implementation of a practice guideline had improved the measured process of care. Of the 11 studies they reviewed that reported a clinical outcome in addition to the process of care, 9 reported significant improvement.

The success of the guideline implementation programs sponsored by the AHA and ACC, detailed earlier in this chapter, also support the usefulness of practice guidelines in improving the quality of cardiovascular care. Greater success in implementing practice guidelines depends in part on the refinement of the guidelines themselves, the more extensive use of clinical information systems to present critical data and guideline recommendations to clinicians at the point of care, and greater sensitivity to the systematic barriers to their adoption.

## ■ FINDING PRACTICE GUIDELINES

Keeping track of the guidelines themselves has become challenging for clinicians and policy makers. Fortunately, there are several ways to find relevant guidelines.

Most clinical practice guidelines are published in peer-reviewed medical journals. Often, the journals are the official publication of the same parent organization that produced the guideline. As a consequence, a computer search of the MEDLINE database of peer-reviewed journals can produce a list of many of the sought guidelines. Each of these organizations also maintains its own web site where practice guidelines are available. The ACC/AHA guidelines and their associated updates are all available at their respective web sites: www.acc.org and www.americanheart.org.

The electronic compendium of guidelines maintained by the National Guideline Clearinghouse is very useful. This searchable web site allows the user to specify the subject and/or sponsor of guidelines. The interface is user-friendly, and the list generated by the search contains links to the specified guideline. So, for example, if one specifies cardiovascular disease, more than 850 listed guidelines are presented, along with suggested search terms (heart disease, vascular disease, etc) and the number of guidelines fitting those search criteria. The links allow a user to go directly from the list to a brief summary of the guideline prepared by the National Guideline Clearinghouse as well as to the full text of a particular guideline, often at the web site of the sponsoring organization.

## ■ CONCLUSION

Assessing and improving the quality of care is a vital component of responsible medical practice. It has taken on increased prominence in recent years because of the widespread evidence of unexplained practice variation, the underuse of effective therapies, and the increasing pressure for accountability at all levels of health care delivery. Clinical practice guidelines have emerged as an important tool to improve the quality of medical care, and cardiovascular medicine has become a particularly fertile ground for their development. A large number of high-quality clinical practice guidelines are now available that address critical issues in cardiovascular medicine. When they are based on dependable, rigorous evidence, written in clear language, and implemented with sensitivity to the myriad local issues that can thwart their success, clinical practice guidelines can help improve patient care.

## SUGGESTED READINGS

Nash IS, Farkouh ME, Fuster V. Therapeutic decision making based upon clinical trials and clinical practice guidelines. In: Fuster V, Walsh R, Harrington RA, et al. *Hurst's The Heart*. 13th ed. New York, NY: McGraw-Hill; 2011;13:228-238.

American Heart Association. Available at: http://www.americanheart.org/presenter. jhtml?identifier=1165.

Antman EM, Anbe DT, Armstrong PW, et al. ACC/AHA guidelines for the management of patients with ST-elevation myocardial infarction: executive summary: a report of the ACC/AHA Task Force on Practice Guidelines (Committee to Revise the 1999 Guidelines on the Management of Patients With Acute Myocardial Infarction). *J Am Coll Cardiol.* 2004;44:671-719.

De Angelis C, Drazen JM, Frizelle FA, et al. Clinical trial registration: a statement from the international committee of medical journal editors. *N Engl J Med.* 2004;351(12):1250-1251.

Eagle KA, Koelling TM, Montoye CK. Primer: implementation of guideline-based programs for coronary care. *Nat Clin Pract Cardiovasc Med.* 2006;3:163-171.

GRADE Working Group. Grading quality of evidence and strength of recommendations. *BMJ.* 2004;328:1490-1497.

Guyatt G, Gutterman D, Baumann MH, et al. Grading strength of recommendations and quality of evidence in clinical guidelines: report from an American College of Chest Physicians Task Force. *Chest.* 2006;129:174-181.

Hay MC, Weisner TS, Subramanian S, et al. Harnessing experience: exploring the gap between evidence-based medicine and clinical practice. *J Eval Clin Pract.* 2008;14(5):707-713.

Kent DM, Hayward RA. Limitations of applying summary results of clinical trials to individual patients: the need for risk stratification. *JAMA.* 2007;298(10):1209-1212.

Methodology Manual for ACC/AHA Guidelines Writing Committees. Available at: http://www.acc.org/clinical/manual/manual_index.htm.

Piaggio G, Elbourne DR, Altman DG, et al; CONSORT Group. Reporting of noninferiority and equivalence randomized trials: an extension of the CONSORT statement. *JAMA.* 2006;295(10):1152-1160.

Psaty BM, Vandenbroucke JP. Opportunities for enhancing the FDA guidance on pharmacovigilance. *JAMA.* 2008;300(8):952-954.

The AGREE Collaboration. Development and validation of an international appraisal instrument for assessing the quality of clinical practice guidelines: the AGREE project. *Qual Saf Health Care.* 2003;12:18-23.

US Department of Health and Human Services. Hospital quality initiatives overview. Available at: http://www.cms.hhs.gov/HospitalQualityInits/.

# CHAPTER 58
# ADVERSE CARDIOVASCULAR DRUG INTERACTIONS AND COMPLICATIONS

Alan D. Enriquez, Ileana L. Piña,
Gerard Oghlakian, and Marc A. Miller

Cardiovascular-targeted pharmacotherapy continues to rapidly evolve as newer agents are sought to fill in gaps in care or to lower adverse reactions of existing therapies. With newer agents, however, benefits are accompanied by new potential reactions. This chapter covers important aspects of adverse drug reactions and reviews pharmacokinetics and pharmacodynamics of commonly used drugs with an emphasis on mechanisms. Specific cardiac disease states are presented, with focused discussion on newer pharmacologic agents that can present challenges to the clinicians faced with the plethora of choices.

Adverse drug reactions (ADRs) are the fourth leading cause of death in patients hospitalized in the United States. ADRs are responsible for approximately 1 of every 16 hospital admissions and occur in as many as 20% of hospitalized patients. The financial burden of ADRs in the United States is staggering, ranging from $30 billion to more than $130 billion annually.

The World Health Organization defines an ADR as "a response to a drug that is noxious and unintended and occurs at doses normally used in man for the prophylaxis, diagnosis and therapy of disease, or for modification of physiological function." ADRs are commonly classified as either type A (augmented) or type B (bizarre) reactions. Type A reactions are predictable based on the pharmacologic characteristics of the agent(s). In contrast, type B reactions are idiosyncratic and unpredictable, and this simple classification system remains in use throughout the literature. Most of the ADRs discussed in this chapter are type A reactions because they are fairly common, predictable, and often preventable.

Patients with heart disease represent a population who are at particularly high risk for ADRs. Certain cardiovascular disease states such as heart failure can influence drug metabolism and elimination by altering end-organ perfusion. Patients with heart disease are often elderly and at increased risk for ADRs due to age-related alterations in renal and hepatic function, the presence of multiple medical comorbidities, and a high prevalence of polypharmacy. ADR risk has been shown to increase exponentially with the number of medications prescribed, and the average nursing home resident takes 7 medications, most for treatment of cardiovascular disease. A patient taking 7 medications has the potential for $6 + 5 + 4 + 3 + 2 + 1 = 21$ possible drug-drug interactions. Lastly, patients with heart disease often require periodic hospitalization and are at highest risk for ADRs after discharge when faced with old medications at home in addition to newly prescribed ones. Thus, medication reconciliation at discharge is critical in patient care. This chapter provides an overview of the adverse reactions associated with the use of cardiovascular drugs. It is organized by disease state rather than by drug class to highlight the clinical relevance of each interaction.

# CLINICAL PHARMACOLOGY

Drug interactions can be classified as being either *pharmacokinetic* or *pharmacodynamic*. Pharmacokinetic interactions alter the delivery of a drug to its site of action, while pharmacodynamic interactions alter the effect of a drug at its site of action. Clinically relevant interactions between drugs can be pharmacokinetic, pharmacodynamic, or both. For example, patients who are taking both amiodarone and digoxin are at increased risk for symptomatic bradycardia. Amiodarone inhibits the clearance of digoxin, resulting in greater delivery to cardiac tissue, a pharmacokinetic interaction. Amiodarone also blocks the AV node, augmenting the effect of digoxin on AV nodal conduction, a pharmacodynamic interaction.

## ■ PHARMACOKINETIC INTERACTIONS

The effective delivery of a drug to its biological target depends on its absorption, distribution, metabolism, and elimination. Pharmacokinetic interactions may occur at any of these steps, leading to either amplification or diminution of the drug's primary effect or its side effects.

### Absorption

Absorption determines drug *bioavailability,* defined as the degree to which a drug becomes available at its site of biologic action. Most orally administered drugs are absorbed by the small intestine, and agents that influence gastrointestinal metabolism, motility, or pH have the potential to interact with numerous drugs. Drugs that increase GI motility (metoclopramide) tend to reduce the bioavailability of other drugs, whereas those that decrease motility (anticholinergic drugs) may increase drug bioavailability by allowing for a longer period of absorption. Drugs may also bind to one another in the GI tract and reduce bioavailability; for example, this can occur when digoxin is concomitantly administered with antacids. The bioavailability of other agents may also be altered by food ingestion.

### Distribution

Once absorbed, many drugs bind to high-affinity sites on plasma proteins such as albumin and establish some degree of equilibrium between free and protein-bound states. The volume of distribution (Vd) is a theoretical measure that reflects how well a drug is removed from the plasma and distributed in tissue. It is related to the serum concentration of a drug by the formula $Vd = D/C$, where $D$ is the drug dose and $C$ is the serum concentration. The pharmacologic effect of a drug is proportional to the concentration of the drug in the free state. Alterations in protein binding can influence the delivery of a drug to its site of action by influencing the proportion of free drug in the plasma. However, the clinical relevance of changes in drug distribution is frequently offset by reciprocal changes in drug elimination.

Drug distribution may also be influenced by the behavior of membrane transport proteins located in cells that comprise the blood-tissue interface of various organs. P-glycoprotein (P-gp) is an ATP-dependent efflux membrane transporter. P-gp has also been isolated from healthy human tissue, including the small intestine, liver, and blood-brain barrier. Several drugs appear to depend on P-gp for intracellular transport, most notably digoxin. Cardiac drugs known to interact with digoxin, such as verapamil and amiodarone, have also been shown to inhibit the activity of P-gp and increase serum digoxin levels.

## Metabolism

Most drugs undergo at least some degree of hepatic metabolism. The liver receives absorbed drugs from the small intestine via the portal vein and converts these relatively hydrophobic agents into water-soluble compounds that are more readily eliminated from the body. Hepatic metabolism consists of 2 phases, biotransformation and conjugation (**Fig. 58-1**). During biotransformation (phase I), drugs are rendered more hydrophilic by oxidation, reduction, or hydrolysis. Phase I is typically followed by conjugation (phase II), during which drugs receive a molecular attachment that can facilitate drug transport within the body. Most drug-drug or drug-nutrient interactions involve the induction or inhibition of phase I metabolic enzymes, and the majority of these interactions involve cytochrome P450 (CYP) isozymes.

CYP is an iron-dependent oxidative enzyme found predominantly within the sarcoplasmic reticulum of hepatocytes. Although more than 30 CYP isozymes have been identified, 6 of them are responsible for more than 90% of human oxidative drug metabolism, and 1, CYP3A4, is involved in the oxidation of half of *all* drugs. CYP inhibition or induction causes the serum concentrations of substrate drugs to increase or decrease, respectively. Many drugs are metabolized by more than 1 CYP isozyme, and CYP induction also increases with hepatic blood flow and decreases with age. **Table 58-1** lists common interactions with the P450 system.

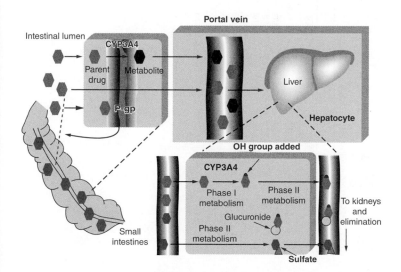

**FIGURE 58-1.** Drug metabolism. Parent drugs enter the portal circulation using protein transport system such as P-glycoprotein (P-gp). Phase 1 metabolism facilitates systemic drug distribution and involves hydrolysis, reduction, or oxidation by enzymes such as cytochrome P450 (CYP) 3A4. Phase 2 metabolism facilitates drug elimination and involves sulfonation and glucuronidation. (Reproduced with permission from Hansten PD: Understanding drug-drug interactins, Science & Medicine 1998;Jan/Feb;5(1):16-25.)

**TABLE 58-1.** Common CYP450 Isozyme Substrates, Inhibitors, and Inducers

| | | | | CYP Isozyme | | | |
|---|---|---|---|---|---|---|---|
| Function | CYP1A2 | CYP2C19 | CYP2C9 | CYP2D6 | CYP2E1 | CYP3A4 | |
| Substrate | Caffeine | Amitriptyline | Amitriptyline | Amitriptyline | Acetaminophen | Aliskiren | |
| | Clozapine | Citalopram | Celecoxib | Clomipramine | Chlorzoxazone | Alprazolam | |
| | Cyclobenzaprine | Clomipramine | Diclofenac | Codeine | Dapsone | Astemizole | |
| | Fluvoxamine | Cyclophosphamide | Flurbiprofen | Desipramine | Enflurane | Buspirone | |
| | Imipramine | Diazepam | Ibuprofen | Dextromethorphan | Ethanol | CCB | |
| | Mexiletine | Imipramine | Losartan | Imipramine | Halothane | Carbamazepine | |
| | Olanzapine | Lansoprazole | Naproxen | Metoprolol | Isoflurane | Cisapride | |
| | Pimozide | Nelfinavir | Phenytoin | Nortriptyline | Isoniazid | Cyclosporine | |
| | Propranolol | Omeprazole | Piroxicam | Oxycodone | | Doxorubicin | |
| | Tacrine | Phenytoin | SMX | Paroxetine | | Erythromycin | |
| | Theophylline | | Tolbutamide | Propafenone | | Etoposide | |
| | Warfarin | | Warfarin | Risperidone | | Fentanyl | |
| | | | | Thioridazine | | HIV PI | |
| | | | | Timolol | | Iphosphamide | |
| | | | | Tramadol | | Lovastatin | |
| | | | | Venlafaxine | | Midazolam | |
| | | | | | | Pimozide | |
| | | | | | | Quinidine | |
| | | | | | | Quinine | |
| | | | | | | Simvastatin | |
| | | | | | | Tacrolimus | |
| | | | | | | Terfenadine | |
| | | | | | | Triazolam | |

| | | | | | | |
|---|---|---|---|---|---|---|
| **Inhibitor** | Cimetidine<br>Ciprofloxacin<br>Citalopram<br>Diltiazem<br>Enoxacin<br>Erythromycin<br>Fluvoxamine<br>Mexiletine<br>Ofloxacin<br>Tacrine<br>Ticlopidine | Cimetidine<br>Felbamate<br>Fluoxetine<br>Fluvoxamine<br>Ketconazole<br>Lansoprazole<br>Omeprazole<br>Paroxetine<br>Ticlopidine | Amiodarone<br>Fluconazole<br>Fluoxetine<br>Fluvastatin<br>Isoniazid<br>Metronidazole<br>Paroxetine<br>Phenylbutazone<br>SMX/TMP<br>Sulfaphenazole<br>Ticlopidine | Amiodarone<br>Chlorpheniramine<br>Fluoxetine<br>Haloperidol<br>Indinavir<br>Paroxetine<br>Propafenone<br>Quinidine<br>Ritonavir<br>Sertraline<br>Thioridazine<br>Ticlopidine | Disulfiram<br>Water cress | Amiodarone<br>Cimetidine<br>Conivaptan<br>Cyclosporine<br>Danazol<br>Diltiazem<br>Fluconazole<br>Grapefruit juice<br>HIV PI<br>Itraconazole<br>Ketoconazole<br>Macrolides<br>Miconazole<br>Nefazodone<br>Omeprazole<br>Quinidine<br>Ritonavir<br>Verapamil |
| **Inducer** | Carbamazepine<br>Tobacco | Carbamazepine<br>Norethindrone | Phenobarbital<br>Rifampin<br>Secobarbital | Ethanol<br>Isoniazid | Tobacco | Carbamazepine<br>Rifabutin<br>Rifampin<br>Ritonavir |

CCB, calcium-channel blockers; HIV PI, HIV protease inhibitors; SMX, sulfamethoxazole; TMP, trimethoprim.

## Elimination

Most drugs are eliminated by the kidneys, either through glomerular filtration, active tubular secretion, or passive tubular reabsorption. Substances that interfere with the function of the kidneys at any of these levels may precipitate a pharmacokinetic drug interaction. The induction or inhibition of P-gp, mentioned previously, may also influence drug elimination.

## ■ PHARMACODYNAMIC INTERACTIONS

Pharmacodynamic interactions occur commonly in the treatment of cardiovascular disease because many cardiac drugs have overlapping physiologic effects. For example, the management of New York Heart Association (NYHA) class III heart failure may include treatment with a β-blocker, angiotensin-converting enzyme inhibitor, and loop diuretic. Each of these drugs can reduce blood pressure, and the development of symptomatic hypotension in such a patient would be considered a pharmacodynamic interaction. Although the clinician should endeavor to avoid antagonistic interactions such as drug-induced hypotension, some pharmacodynamic interactions are therapeutically synergistic. For example, the diuretic metolazone can enhance sodium delivery to the loop of Henle and increase the diuretic effectiveness of loop-acting drugs, such as furosemide.

## ■ OTHER CONTRIBUTORS TO ADVERSE DRUG REACTIONS

### Genetic Factors

Human genetic diversity influences the pharmacokinetics and pharmacodynamics of cardiovascular drugs. The frequency of genetic polymorphisms involving CYP 450 isozymes varies by ethnic group (**Fig. 58-2**), although the clinical relevance of these polymorphisms is not uniform. For example, one-third of Caucasians carry at least 1 variant allele for the gene encoding CYP2C9, which is involved in the

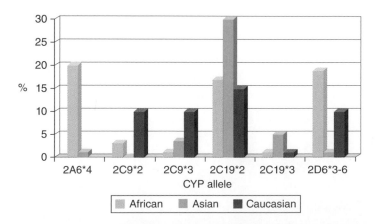

**FIGURE 58-2.** Prevalence of inactive cytochrome P450 (CYP) alleles within various ethnic groups. (Data from Bjornsson TD, Wagner JA, Donahue SR, et al. A review and assessment of potential sources of ethnic differences in drug responsiveness. *J Clin Pharmacol.* 2003;43:943-967.)

metabolism of warfarin. The presence of this polymorphism increases the anticoagulant effect of warfarin, and affected individuals require lower doses and more frequent monitoring. However, although patients with deactivating polymorphisms involving CYP2D6 experience up to a 5-fold increase in serum metoprolol levels compared with unaffected individuals, adverse events and poor tolerability generally do not occur. Polymorphisms involving the expression of α- and β-adrenergic receptor subunits appear to influence responsiveness to antihypertensive drug therapy. Understanding how to incorporate knowledge of an individual's genotype into prescribing pharmacotherapy remains a work in progress.

## Diet

Dietary behavior may influence the pharmacokinetics and pharmacodynamics of certain cardiac drugs. Grapefruit juice is a popular beverage and potent CYP3A4 inhibitor that significantly increases serum levels of commonly used drugs such as simvastatin and felodipine. The anticoagulant effects of warfarin may be substantially reduced in patients who consume vitamin K–rich foods such as lettuce, spinach, avocado, asparagus, and canola oil. Herbal remedies have become enormously popular in recent years, and patients seldom report the use of herbal products.

*Hypericum perforatum* (St. John's wort), a popular herbal remedy for treating depression, decreases plasma levels of digoxin, possibly due to P-gp transport induction. *H. perforatum* also reduces cyclosporine levels and has been implicated as a contributor to acute rejection of a transplanted heart. Black licorice (*Glycyrrhiza glabra*) can raise blood pressure and pharmacodynamically competes with aldosterone antagonists for binding at the mineralocorticoid receptor.

## Age

The elderly are particularly vulnerable to drug-drug interactions. Drug pharmacokinetics may change with advancing age for several reasons. Percent body fat tends to increase with age and may increase the volume of distribution of fat-soluble drugs. Conversely, cachexia can increase serum levels of drugs with a large volume of distribution such as digoxin. Although hepatic metabolism is relatively unaffected by age in the absence of overt liver disease, alterations in hepatic blood flow may reduce the first-pass metabolism of highly extracted drugs. Hepatic metabolism is particularly pertinent in patients with heart failure, especially among patients with right heart failure and peripheral congestion. Glomerular filtration and renal tubular secretion decreases with increasing age and may influence drug clearance. Drug pharmacodynamics are also influenced by age. β-Adrenergic receptor sensitivity decreases with age and may reduce the efficacy of β-blocker therapy. However, aging often accompanies other comorbidities, and age should not a priori change medication target doses, although uptitration should be done with caution. Finally, age-related changes in baroreceptor reflex sensitivity may increase the risk of orthostatic hypotension in elderly patients taking antihypertensive medications.

## Smoking

Cigarette smoking may influence the metabolism of cardiovascular drugs by increasing phase I hepatic enzyme activities. Heavy smoking has been shown to increase the activity of CYP2D6 4-fold when compared with nonsmokers. Increased CYP1A2 activity has also been observed in male smokers, and clinicians should be mindful of the effects of smoking cessation on cardiovascular drugs that are metabolized by CYP1A2.

# HEART FAILURE AND TRANSPLANT

## ■ HEART FAILURE

Heart failure is the most common reason for hospitalization among Medicare recipients, and the number of patients treated for heart failure is expected to increase as the US population ages. Clinical trials of new agents for the treatment of heart failure historically use the previously proven drug as background therapy upon which to test the newest agent. Therefore, heart failure is the classic "add-on-therapy" syndrome, putting patients at risk for the adverse complications of multidrug therapy. In addition, the majority of patients with heart failure have comorbid conditions that are likely to require their own pharmacotherapies. Furthermore, the impaired cardiac output that is characteristic of heart failure may affect drug absorption by slowing gastrointestinal transit time and drug elimination via concomitant renal dysfunction. Therefore, heart failure patients should be considered at high risk for ADRs.

### Thiazolidinediones in Heart Failure

Heart failure is common among patients with advanced diabetes, and diabetes has been identified as one of the risk factors for stage A heart failure. Among the advances of diabetes treatment has been the emergence of the thiazolidinediones (TZDs). These agents improve insulin sensitivity in adipose, muscle, and liver. However, these agents have limited use in patients with heart failure. They can cause fluid retention, worsening edema, and precipitate CHF exacerbations. Rosiglitazone has been associated with an increased incidence of myocardial infarction, and the FDA restricted its use in 2010. Pioglitazone, however, does not appear to have the same cardiovascular risk profile as rosiglitazone. In addition, pioglitazone may have other beneficial cardiovascular effects such as suppressing in-stent neointimal proliferation, possibly due to improvements in endothelial dysfunction. Therefore, these agents should be avoided or used with considerable caution in patients with advanced heart failure. If a TZD is necessary, pioglitazone should be used.

### Aldosterone Antagonists

Aldosterone antagonists, spironolactone and eplerenone, are mainstays in the treatment of chronic heart failure. The efficacy of spironolactone was established in the landmark Randomized Aldactone Evaluation Study (RALES) trial, which showed that the addition of sprinolactone to standard therapy dramatically improved survival in severe heart failure patients. Eplerenone is also an aldosterone antagonist, but it is significantly more selective than spironolactone for the mineralocorticoid receptor over progesterone, androgen, and glucocorticoid receptors. This selectivity leads to a lower incidence of gynecomastia, breast pain, and impotence. Eplerenone, in addition to standard therapy, was shown to significantly reduce mortality in patients post–acute myocardial infarction complicated by left ventricular dysfunction in the EPHESUS trial as well as in patients with mild systolic heart failure (NYHA class II symptoms) in the EMPHASIS-HF trial.

The primary adverse reaction with spironolactone and eplerenone is hyperkalemia, and there is significant potential for pharmacodynamic interactions since heart failure patients are also treated with either ACE inhibitors, ARBs, or, in some cases, both. After the publication of RALES in 1999, the rate of hospitalization for hyperkalemia rose from 2.4 per 1000 patients in 1994 to 11.0 per 1000 patients in 2001, and the associated mortality rose from 0.3 per 1000 to 2.0 per 1000 patients. With the recent publication of EMPHASIS-HF and the indication for aldosterone antagonists in all patients with symptomatic heart failure, usage of these agents is likely to increase further. Thus, the addition of spironolactone or eplerenone must be performed with great caution, and careful monitoring of potassium and renal function is mandatory. In addition, it is important to note that eplerenone is metabolized by CYP3A4, and caution should be exercised with other inhibitors or inducers of CYP3A4.

## β-Adrenergic Receptor Blockers (β-Blockers)

Once thought to be contraindicated in patients with left ventricular systolic dysfunction, certain β-blockers have since been shown to dramatically reduce morbidity and mortality in patients with heart failure. In spite of these significant trials, the administration and dosing of β-blockers requires careful attention to avoid giving "the right drug at the wrong time." β-blockers are negative inotropic agents, and their first effect is to reduce ventricular contractility. However, their biologic effects (reverse remodeling) are time-dependent. Therefore, heart failure patients should be carefully examined to ensure euvolemia before initiating β-blocker therapy. If administered to a volume overloaded patient, β-blockers may contribute to volume excess and precipitate heart failure decompensation, as a mild increase in intravascular volume is common when β-blockers are started or when doses are increased. This volume increase is usually transient and can often be controlled with additional diuretics. β-blockers should be started at very low doses, especially in those with advanced heart failure, and titrated up every 2 to 3 weeks as tolerated. If a patient is admitted with a heart failure exacerbation on maintenance β-blocker therapy, β-blockers may be continued with intensification of diuretic therapy, provided that there is no hemodynamic instability. Appropriate timing and dosing will allow most heart failure patients to initiate and continue these lifesaving drugs.

## Angiotensin-Converting Enzyme Inhibitors

These powerful drugs have been proven to increase survival and decrease hospitalizations in patients with NYHA class II to IV heart failure. Despite these benefits, clinicians continue to both underuse and underdose these agents. Some of the concerns arise from inappropriate timing of administration. As with β-blockers, accurate volume assessment is critical when administering angiotensin-converting enzyme inhibitors (ACEIs) for heart failure. Patients with clinical hypovolemia, frequently due to overly aggressive diuresis, may experience acute renal failure when ACEIs are initiated or increased. However, these changes are usually transient, and avoiding the impulse to aggressively diurese will usually allow successful introduction and uptitration of these important agents. A similar rationale should be applied to ARB administration in heart failure.

## Isosorbide Dinitrate/Hydralazine

The fixed-dose vasodilator combination of isosorbide dinitrate and hydralazine is indicated for treatment of heart failure in African Americans. The African-American Heart Failure Trial (A-HeFT) showed that addition of this drug to optimized background heart failure therapy in symptomatic African American patients was associated with a decrease in mortality of 43%, while also decreasing hospitalization and improving quality of life. Use of isosorbide dinitrate/hydralazine is contraindicated with concurrent use of phosphodiesterase-5 inhibitors. The hydralazine component can, in rare cases, cause a drug-induced lupus-like syndrome. Isosorbide/hydralazine can also cause reflex tachycardia and result in increased myocardial oxygen demand if not used concomitantly with a β-blocker. Whether other forms of nitrates such as the mononitrates can be substituted is a matter of controversy because these alternatives have not been studied in a large clinical trial. Currently, hydralazine dosed separately with a nitrate is frequently administered in lieu of the fixed-dose drug.

## Aspirin

More than 50% of patients with heart failure have coronary artery disease and are likely to be prescribed aspirin for primary or secondary prevention. Post hoc analysis of completed randomized trials had suggested that the benefit of ACE inhibitors in heart failure patients may be attenuated by the concomitant use of aspirin. Indirect evidence of the possible negative effect of aspirin comes from the WATCH trial that compared aspirin, clopidogrel, or warfarin in patients with chronic heart failure. Retrospective analysis revealed that there were significantly more hospitalizations for heart failure in the aspirin group compared to warfarin. However, the totality of evidence in a systematic review of 6 major trials shows no significant differences in cardiovascular outcomes with ACE inhibitor therapy in the presence or absence of aspirin. While it is not recommended to routinely use aspirin in patients with a non-ischemic cardiomyopathy, there is insufficient evidence to withhold aspirin in heart failure patients with significant atherosclerotic disease given its clear benefit.

## Vasopressin Antagonists

Conivaptan and tolvaptan are vasopressin receptor antagonists, a class of drugs that inhibit vasopressin V2 receptors in the basolateral membrane of the collecting duct cells of the kidneys (tolvaptan) or both the V2 and V1 receptors (conivaptan). V1 receptors found in the myocardium and blood vessels are thought to be responsible for peripheral and coronary vasoconstriction. In the kidneys, these drugs lead to a net aquaretic effect (**Fig. 58-3**). The net water loss achieved by this class of medications

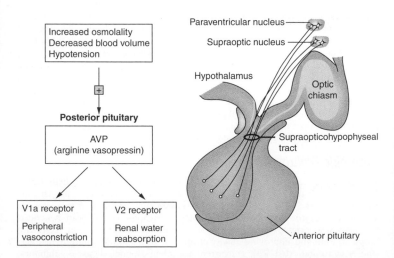

**FIGURE 58-3.** Vasopressin release by the posterior pituitary is stimulated by increased osmolality, hypotension, and hypovolemia. The main 2 effects of vasopressin include vasoconstriction via V1a receptors and water retention via V2 receptors in the kidneys. (Adapted with permission from Oghlakian and Klapholz.)

has been associated with a rise in plasma sodium levels. Conivaptan is approved for the treatment of euvolemic or hypervolemic hyponatremia in hospitalized patients. Conivaptan is available only in intravenous form and is a strong inhibitor of CYP3A4. Therefore, it can increase the levels of many cardiac medications, including digoxin, eplerenone, and everolimus.

Recently, the US Food and Drug Administration (FDA) approved tolvaptan for the treatment of patients with clinically significant hyponatremia in patients with heart failure, cirrhosis, and the syndrome of inappropriate antidiuretic hormone (SIADH). In contrast to conivaptan, tolvaptan is a selective antagonist and administered orally. In the EVEREST trial, which tested tolvaptan against placebo in a group of heart failure patients admitted with volume overload, tolvaptan decreased body weight more than placebo but failed to impact the primary end point of all-cause mortality, cardiovascular mortality, or heart failure hospitalization. Tolvaptan is metabolized in the liver via the CYP3A4 system, and its use is contraindicated in patients on strong inhibitors of CYP3A4. Tolvaptan can also lead to an increase in potassium, which should be closely monitored.

## Doxazosin

α-blockers have been used for many years to treat hypertension. Prazosin was initially developed for hypertension, but its presumed effect of afterload reduction made it an attractive drug for the treatment of heart failure. However, reports of tachyphylaxis and fluid accumulation made the drug difficult to use in heart failure patients, and the drug was no better than placebo in reducing mortality in heart failure patients in the VHeFT trial. More recently, the α-blocker doxazosin was tested in the ALLHAT trial and stopped early due to onset of heart failure. Doxazosin is now being used frequently for symptomatic treatment of prostatic hypertrophy and urinary hesitancy. In patients with advanced heart failure, these agents must be used very cautiously because of the potential for fluid accumulation.

## ■ CARDIAC TRANSPLANT

Cardiac transplant recipients are at unique danger of drug-drug interactions as a result of general unfamiliarity with immunosuppressive drugs by most nontransplant clinicians and the narrow therapeutic window of these agents. Interactions may be inevitable because of the complexities of the medication regimens, and very careful thought is warranted by clinicians caring for this group of patients. It would be challenging, if not impossible, to list each and every ADR for this population. This section selects the most common and potentially dangerous ADRs involving transplant patients. Consultation with a specialist in the care of the cardiac transplant patient may be indicated, especially if medication changes are numerous and/or complex.

## Cyclosporine and Tacrolimus

Cyclosporine (CSA) and tacrolimus (TAC) belong to the family of calcineurin inhibitors that undergo metabolism via hepatic and intestinal CYP3A4. Oral CSA and TAC have incomplete, irregular absorption that varies from patient to patient. **Table 58-2** depicts a variety of interactions with commonly used agents after transplant. It is important to remember that after transplant, hypertension and hyperlipidemia are common due to treatment with calcineurin inhibitors. Therefore, patients will often require ≥1 antihypertensive medications in addition to lipid-lowering therapy. Careful monitoring of CSA and tacrolimus levels is critical to avoid rejection or alternatively excessive levels and side effects.

**TABLE 58-2.** Pharmacokinetic Interactions With Cyclosporine and Tacrolimus

| Drug Class | Examples | Effect | Onset | Management |
|---|---|---|---|---|
| Antihypertensives | Amlodipine Diltiazem Felodipine Nifedipine Verapamil | Increased TAC/CSA effect | Delayed | Monitor TAC/CSA levels 3 times per week. Reduce TAC/CSA dose by 20%-50% with diltiazem or verapamil. |
| Lipid-lowering agents | Atorvastatin Fluvastatin Lovastatin | Increased statin effect with risk for myopathy or rhabdomyolysis | Delayed | Use lowest possible statin dose Consider fluvastatin or pravastatin |
| | Pravastatin Rosuvastatin Simvastatin Ezetimibe | Increased ezetimibe effect Decreased TAC/CSA effect | | Use lowest possible ezetimibe dose Monitor TAC/CSA 2-3 times weekly for first week then weekly for 1 mo |
| | Gemfibrozil Fenofibrate | | | |
| Antiplatelet agents | Clopidogrel Ticlopidine | Decreased clopidogrel metabolite | Delayed | Monitor CSA/TAC levels closely for several months. Monitor for abnormal clotting |
| Azole antifungals | Clotrimazole | Increased TAC/CSA effect | Delayed | Monitor CSA/TAC levels 2-3 times for first week |
| | Fluconazole | Increased TAC/CSA effect | Delayed | Monitor CSA/TAC levels 2-3 times for first week |
| | Itraconazole | Increased TAC/CSA effect Nephrotoxicity | Rapid | Monitor CSA/TAC levels 2-3 times for first week; reduce initial dose of CSA/TAC by 50% |
| | Ketoconazole | Increased TAC/CSA effect Nephrotoxicity and hepatotoxicity | Rapid | Monitor CSA/TAC levels 2-3 times for first week; reduce initial dose of CSA/TAC by 50% Monitor renal and hepatic functions closely |

CSA, cyclosporine; TAC, tacrolimus.

Data from Page RL, Miller GG, Lindenfeld J. Drug therapy in the heart transplant recipient: part IV: drug-drug interactions. *Circulation.* 2005;111:230-239.

**Antihypertensive Agents** Diltiazem is a commonly used antihypertensive in this population due to a positive effect on transplant arteriopathy in a small, randomized study. Diltiazem inhibits both CYP3A4 and P-gp and raises CSA levels 1.5- to 6-fold, requiring a reduction in CSA dosing by 20% to 75%. A similar reduction is necessary for TAC. Dihydropyridine calcium-channel blockers also inhibit the CYP3A4 system and may potentially interact with CSA and TAC.

**Lipid-Lowering Agents** Atorvastatin, simvastatin, and lovastatin are all substrates for CYP3A4 that may interact pharmacokinetically with CSA and TAC, resulting in myopathy or even rhabdomyolysis. Fluvastatin is metabolized primarily by CYP2C9 and pravastatin through other pathways that do not fully involve the CYP enzyme system. Rosuvastatin exhibits minimal metabolism via the CYP enzyme system. With the exception of fluvastatin, all the statins have been associated with rhabdomyolysis when used concomitantly with CSA. When starting statins, the lowest effective dose should be used with careful monitoring for myopathy. If rhabdomyolysis occurs, therapy should be discontinued. Pravastatin appears to have the least accumulation in the presence of CSA.

**Antibiotics** Antibiotics are frequently prescribed for patients after cardiac transplant, particularly during the first posttransplant year, when there is a delicate balance between rejection and overimmunosuppression. Depending on the structure and metabolism of antibiotics, both CSA and TAC are likely to be affected, because many antibiotics are also metabolized by the CYP450 system. For example, clarithromycin is a potent CYP3A inhibitor. The coadministration of TAC and clarithromycin may increase serum TAC levels 4- to 5-fold (**Fig. 58-4**). Another example is the use of fluoroquinolones such as ciprofloxacin or levofloxacin, which are also metabolized by the P450 system. A small study showed that levofloxacin, an agent with limited hepatic metabolism, significantly increased the mean area under the blood concentration-time curve (AUC) of CSA and TAC by approximately 25%.

**Other Drug-Drug Interactions** See Table 58-2 for a complete list.

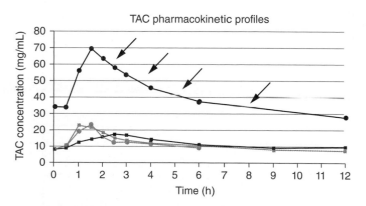

**FIGURE 58-4.** Significant interaction between tacrolimus (TAC) and clarithromycin (CLA). Pharmacokinetic profiles are shown for various TAC doses before CLA (8 mg/d and 6 mg/d), with CLA (4 mg/d, *filled circle*), and 2 months after CLA (4 mg/d, *filled square*). Note the marked increase in serum TAC levels in the presence of CLA despite lower TAC dosing (*arrows*). (Reproduced with permission from Kunicki PK, Sobieszcza ska-Malek M. Pharmacokinetic interaction between tacrolimus and clarithromycin in a heart transplant patient. *Ther Drug Monit.* 2005;29(1):107–108.)

## Sirolimus and Everolimus

The target of rapamycin (TOR) inhibitors are more commonly used in heart transplant recipients. Sirolimus (SIR) was first introduced in the market, and now everolimus (EVER) has been approved for use in cardiac transplant patients. Both of these agents are macrolide immunosuppressants. SIR is extensively metabolized by CYP3A4, and drug interactions are likely. Both of these agents exacerbate hyperlipidemia, and statin use requires the same precautions as with the CYP3A inhibitors. In one study, diltiazem increased SIR levels in healthy subjects, likely due to inhibition of CYP3A4. Thus far, by observation from efficacy data, everolimus levels have not been affected by potential CYP3A4 inhibitors.

**Other Agents**  In current posttransplant practice, it is common to use combinations of agents with the CYP3A inhibitor drugs. The administration time of CSA with SIR may affect SIR pharmacokinetics. When CSA and SIR are administered together, SIR levels increase, possibly due to inhibition of first-pass metabolism. Therefore, SIR should be administered 4 hours after CSA dosing.

**Antifungal Agents**  The azole-derived antifungal agents should be used carefully in combination with SIR or EVER. See **Table 58-3**.

## Mycophenolate Mofetil

Mycophenolate mofetil (MMF) is an antiproliferative drug that is well absorbed after oral administration and is converted to its active metabolite, mycophenolic acid (MPA). MPA is metabolized by glucuronyl transferase and excreted in the urine and bile. When cyclosporine and MMF are given in combination, it may result in lower plasma MMF levels secondary to cyclosporine-induced alterations in biliary clearance. The effects of concurrent tacrolimus administration on MPA exposure are less clear.

**Lipid-Lowering Agents**  Cholestyramine may decrease MMF active compound levels. This decrease is probably due to binding of the recirculating conjugated active compound by cholestyramine, preventing enterohepatic circulation of MMF and loss of the secondary peak. Package labeling recommends that MMF and cholestyramine not be coadministered.

**Other Agents**  The absorption of MMF may be impaired by antacids or iron preparations because of possible chelation complex formation. Therefore, it is advisable to stagger any antacids or iron supplements 2 to 4 hours with MMF administration.

**TABLE 58-3.** Pharmacokinetic Interactions With Sirolimus and Everolimus

| Drug | Effect | Onset | Management |
|------|--------|-------|------------|
| Diltiazem | Increased SIR effect | Delayed | Monitor SIR levels 3 times per week in first week |
| Fluconazole | Increased SIR/EVER effect | Delayed | Monitor SIR/EVER levels for 1-2 wk |
| Itraconazole | Increased SIR/EVER effect | Delayed | Monitor SIR/EVER levels for 1-2 wk |
| Ketoconazole | Increased SIR/EVER effect | Delayed | Avoid combination |
| Voriconazole | Increased SIR/EVER effect | Delayed | Avoid combination |
| Cyclosporine | Increased SIR/EVER effect | Rapid | Administer SIR 4 h after cyclosporine |

EVER, everolimus; SIR, sirolimus.

Data from Page RL, Miller GG, Lindenfeld J. Drug therapy in the heart transplant recipient: part IV: drug-drug interactions. *Circulation*. 2005;111:230-239.

## Azathioprine

Azathioprine is not as widely used today as it was in the 1990s as an antiproliferative agent. The reader is referred to several in-depth discussions of the pharmacokinetics of azathioprine and its potential ADRs.

# CORONARY ARTERY DISEASE

Major technologic and pharmacologic advances over the past 2 decades have substantially improved outcomes in patients with acute and chronic coronary artery disease. The widespread utilization of fibrinolytic, antiplatelet, and catheter-based therapies has dramatically improved the morbidity and mortality of coronary disease. This changing clinical landscape increases the potential for adverse drug interactions.

## ■ FIBRINOLYTIC THERAPY

Although urgent catheter-based coronary revascularization has been shown to be superior to fibrinolytic therapy in patients presenting with ST-segment elevation myocardial infarction (STEMI), lack of timely proximity to interventional cardiology services often precludes this treatment option. Fibrinolysis thus remains an essential component to STEMI management for many patients. All fibrinolytic drugs work by either directly or indirectly promoting the conversion of plasminogen to plasmin, a nonspecific serum protease that lyses fibrin clot and degrades certain clotting factors. The risk for potentially fatal bleeding complications with the use of any fibrinolytic agent is self-evident, and full knowledge of the absolute and relative contraindications of fibrinolytic drugs is mandatory before their use.

The risk for significant pharmacokinetic interactions involving fibrinolytic drugs is low. Fibrinolytics are not dependent on cytochrome P450 metabolism and are not significantly affected by inhibitors and inducers of this enzyme. Agents such as alteplase and saruplase are highly cleared by the liver and thus are theoretically susceptible to reduced hepatic blood flow, which might occur in patients receiving β-blockers, nitrates, or those with cardiogenic shock. There are a few potential pharmacodynamic interactions to consider when using fibrinolytic drugs. Concomitant use of heparin does increase the potential for serious bleeding; however, in general this increased risk does not offset the additive benefit of these drugs with respect to maintaining vessel patency and reducing recurrent ischemic events. The activated partial thromboplastin time (aPTT) should be frequently monitored when heparin is used in conjunction with a fibrinolytic agent and should be maintained between 1.5 and 2.0 times the upper limit of normal. Aspirin does not appear to increase the risk of bleeding when given with fibrinolytic therapy and, in fact, improves mortality. Data from clinical trials suggest that glycoprotein (Gp) IIb/IIIa inhibitors may result in an unacceptably high risk for bleeding when given with full-dose fibrinolytic therapy, and protocols using half-dose fibrinolytics have been uniformly disappointing in failing to improve clinical outcomes.

## ■ ORAL ANTIPLATELET THERAPY

Aggressive platelet inhibition has revolutionized the management of coronary artery disease. Indeed, the broad success of intracoronary stenting is due in part to the development of potent antiplatelet agents that prevent catastrophic early and late stent thrombosis and improve long-term clinical outcomes.

## Aspirin

Aspirin plays a cornerstone role in the secondary prevention of coronary artery disease, and its use is essential along with an adenosine diphosphate (ADP) blocker to reduce the risk of intracoronary stent thrombosis. Like other inhibitors of cyclooxygenase-1, aspirin reduces prostaglandin production, which may attenuate the effects of many antihypertensive drugs. However, this phenomenon is more likely to occur at higher (>100 mg) aspirin doses. Aspirin hypersensitivity, though rare, may result in life-threatening bronchospasm and anaphylaxis. Patients with true aspirin hypersensitivity who have a strong indication for the drug may undergo rapid desensitization within a few hours, preferably under the consultative care of an allergist. Aspirin use in conjunction with anticoagulants can increase the likelihood for significant bleeding complications.

## Ticagrelor

Ticagrelor is a new platelet aggregation inhibitor that was associated with a reduction in the composite of death from vascular causes, myocardial infarction, or stroke when compared with clopidogrel in patients with acute coronary syndromes. There was no difference in the overall rate of major bleeding, but the ticagrelor group did have a higher rate of non–coronary artery bypass grafting-related bleeding. Ticagrelor blocks ADP receptors of subtype P2Y12, but the inhibition is reversible. Unlike the ADP blockers, clopidogrel and prasugrel, ticagrelor is not a prodrug and does not require hepatic activation. It does have some adverse effects, including an increased incidence of bradycardia and dyspnea compared with clopidogrel. Ticagrelor was approved by the FDA in July 2011 for use in acute coronary syndromes.

## Thienopyridines

The thienopyridines (ticlopidine and clopidogrel) inhibit platelet function by binding to platelet surface ADP receptors. Both ticlopidine and clopidogrel, alone or in combination with aspirin, have been shown to reduce the likelihood of recurrent myocardial ischemia or infarction in at-risk populations, and thienopyridine therapy is essential after intracoronary stenting.

**Ticlopidine** Ticlopidine is a potent inhibitor of CYP2D6 and CYP2C19 and thus carries a risk for pharmacokinetic interactions with drugs metabolized by these enzymes. Its use has been associated with adverse hematologic events, including aplastic anemia and thrombotic thrombocytopenic purpura. Since the development of clopidogrel, the use of ticlopidine has been limited largely to patients who are clopidogrel intolerant.

**Clopidogrel** Clopidogrel is associated with fewer adverse reactions than ticlopidine and is administered once daily. Hematologic abnormalities associated with clopidogrel use are rare and rashes are uncommon. Clopidogrel is activated by CYP3A4, and its antiplatelet effects may be attenuated by concurrent use of CYP3A4 inducers such as amiodarone. Pharmacodynamically, clopidogrel use is associated with an increased risk for significant bleeding when given with anticoagulants or other antiplatelet agents, including aspirin. In patients with acute coronary syndromes, the combination of aspirin and clopidogrel has been shown to significantly reduce recurrent adverse cardiac events to a greater degree than it promotes major bleeding. Thus, in this population, *dual* antiplatelet therapy is preferred. In patients with stroke, however, aspirin and clopidogrel may reduce the risk for recurrent events when given *individually*, but, in combination, these drugs do not incrementally reduce event rates enough to justify the increased bleeding risk.

## Clopidogrel and PPI

Some proton pump inhibitors (PPIs) may inhibit the metabolism of clopidogrel to its active metabolite through inhibition of CYP2C19. With this mechanism as a background, some retrospective studies have suggested an increase in cardiovascular events in patients treated with proton pump inhibitors and clopidogrel. Although there does appear to be both a pharmacokinetic and pharmacodynamic interaction when combining these drugs, other observational data have been less compelling regarding a true effect on clinical outcomes. On November 17, 2009, The FDA issued a Health Care Provider alert making clinicians aware of these potential interactions and urging caution in prescribing the drugs concomitantly (http://www.fda.gov). However, since that time, the COGENT trial, which randomized patients taking plavix to omeprazole or placebo, has showed that there was no meaningful cardiovascular interaction between clopidogrel and omeprazole. The ACC/AHA concluded that while a meaningful clinical interaction between PPIs and clopidogrel cannot be excluded, the available data do not suggest a consistent effect on CV outcomes. Thus, clinicians may use PPIs with clopidogrel but need to balance the risks and benefits from cardiovascular and gastrointestinal perspectives.

## Prasugrel

Prasugrel is a new member of the thienopyridine class of ADP receptor inhibitors that inhibits platelet aggregation by irreversibly binding to the P2Y12 receptor. In patients with acute coronary syndromes in the TRITON-TIMI 38 trial, prasugrel (60-mg loading dose followed by 10-mg daily dose) reduced the combined rate of death from cardiovascular causes, nonfatal myocardial infarction, and nonfatal stroke compared with clopidogrel. The difference was primarily driven by the reduction of nonfatal myocardial infarctions. This improvement in outcomes was associated with an increased rate of serious bleeding events and fatal bleeding with prasugrel, though overall mortality did not differ between the groups. In July 2009, the FDA approved prasugrel while issuing a black box warning about its increased bleeding risk and urging caution in certain patient groups. Prasugrel is contraindicated in patients with prior history of TIA or stroke and generally is not recommended in patients older than 75 years. Additional risk factors for bleeding with prasugrel include weight less than 60 kg and its use with other medications that increase the risk of bleeding. Dose reduction to 5-mg daily dose should be considered in patients less than 60 kg, although the data supporting this reduced dosing recommendation are largely based on pharmacokinetic and pharmacodynamic considerations.

## Dipyridamole

Dipyridamole is a potent vasodilator with antiplatelet activity that is often used as the vasodilator in pharmacologic myocardial perfusion imaging studies. It also has a role as an adjunctive antiplatelet agent in certain patients with cerebrovascular disease. However, its role as an effective agent added to other antiplatelet agents in patients with coronary artery disease has not been established. The vasodilatory effects of dipyridamole are antagonized by xanthine derivatives, and adverse reactions to dipyridamole such as bronchospasm, bradycardia, and flushing can be treated with theophylline or aminophylline.

## ■ ANTITHROMBIN THERAPY

Therapeutic anticoagulation with heparinoids and direct thrombin inhibitors has dramatically improved outcomes in patients with coronary artery disease, particularly acute coronary syndromes. The risk for potentially serious bleeding with antithrombin therapy is obvious; however, with appropriate monitoring, the benefit these drugs provide to patients with unstable coronary syndromes far outweighs their collective risk.

# ■ UNFRACTIONATED HEPARIN

Heparin potentiates the effect of antithrombin III, which leads to inactivation of thrombin. Heparin also inactivates several clotting factors and prevents the conversion of fibrinogen to fibrin. Heparin has a half-life of approximately 90 minutes and is metabolized by the liver and reticuloendothelial system. Pharmacokinetic drug interactions involving heparin are rare, and most pharmacodynamic interactions with heparin involve the concurrent use of drugs with antiplatelet or anticoagulant properties. Life-threatening bleeding complications involving heparin can be treated with its antidote, protamine sulfate. Early, abrupt cessation of heparin therapy in patients treated for acute coronary syndromes has been associated with rebound ischemia. Monitoring these individuals for at least 24 hours after heparin cessation is advisable.

One potentially dangerous adverse event associated with heparin use is heparin-induced thrombocytopenia (HIT). Mild thrombocytopenia may occur in as many as 20% of patients beginning heparin therapy and typically resolves within a few days. HIT occurs in 1% to 5% of heparin-exposed patients and is associated with significant thrombocytopenia (<100 000/μL) that typically occurs several days after exposure to any amount of heparin. HIT is caused by autoantibodies directed against the complex of heparin and platelet factor 4 (PF4). These antibodies may trigger platelet activation and produce a prothrombotic state that places affected patients at risk for venous and arterial thrombosis. HIT management includes discontinuation of heparin and anticoagulation with direct thrombin inhibitors and warfarin. A prior history of HIT is considered a contraindication to subsequent heparin therapy.

## *Low-Molecular-Weight Heparin*

Low-molecular-weight heparin (LMWH) is produced by chemical or enzymatic depolymerization of the unfractionated heparin molecule. This process produces small (4000-6500 Da) molecules that maintain activity against factor Xa with less potential to interact with other molecules, including platelet factor 4. The LMWH enoxaparin has established efficacy in the management of patients with acute coronary syndromes modestly superior to that of heparin, with the advantage of subcutaneous administration and fixed dosing that does not require serial monitoring. LMWH is renally excreted, and its use in patients with severe kidney disease is relatively contraindicated. Like heparin, LMWH is not associated with a high risk for pharmacokinetic drug interactions, but there is potential for pharmacodynamic interactions with antiplatelet and other anticoagulant drugs. In instances where bleeding is severe, the effects of LMWH can be partially reversed by protamine sulfate. LMWH use is associated with a lower risk (but not a 0 risk) for HIT compared with unfractionated heparin. However, because LMWH has been shown to cross-react with HIT antibodies in up to 70% of patients with known HIT, the use of LMWH as a heparin alternative in patients with HIT is not advised.

# ■ DIRECT THROMBIN INHIBITORS

The direct thrombin inhibitor bivalirudin has established efficacy as an alternative to heparin in patients with acute coronary syndromes who require percutaneous revascularization, particularly in the setting of renal insufficiency. Bivalirudin binds directly to thrombin at its catalytic site and reversibly inhibits circulating and clot-bound thrombin. The drug is proteolytically cleaved and excreted in the urine, and its anticoagulation effects resolve within an hour of discontinuation. Bivalirudin is not associated with significant pharmacokinetic interactions. The potential for pharmacodynamic interactions when given with other anticoagulant and antiplatelet agents exists, but bivalirudin use is associated with a lower risk for significant bleeding than the combination of heparin and glycoprotein IIb/IIIa receptor inhibitors.

# ■ ADVERSE DRUG REACTIONS RELATED TO CARDIAC CATHETERIZATION

The majority of patients presenting with acute coronary syndromes will benefit from early invasive management of their disease, and the catheterization laboratory is often the site of first exposure to potentially hazardous pharmacologic agents.

## Radiocontrast Media

Iodinated contrast agents are associated with several potential adverse reactions. Hypersensitivity reactions occur in approximately 1% of patients treated in the catheterization laboratory and can range in severity from a mild rash to airway compromise and hemodynamic collapse. Most severe contrast reactions are anaphylactoid (non–immunoglobulin E mediated) reactions that involve the release of molecules such as histamines from mast cells and tend to occur within minutes of contrast exposure. Pretreatment of patients with a known contrast allergy with oral corticosteroids, at least 6 hours before catheterization, and antihistamines, just before catheterization, may reduce the likelihood of contrast reactions. The efficacy of intravenous corticosteroid administration just before catheterization has not been established, though this is often done in practice. Acute management of hemodynamically unstable patients or those with airway compromise may include intravenous epinephrine or methylene blue. Contrast agents may also produce contrast-induced nephropathy (CIN), which may lead to permanent kidney damage or dialysis in a minority of patients. Underlying kidney disease appears to be the greatest risk factor for CIN, and prophylactic hydration and treatment with *N*-acetylcysteine may have a modest effect on reducing the risk for CIN, although the clinical outcome data are not definitive. Lastly, patients taking metformin for diabetes are at risk for rare but potentially lethal lactic acidosis. Metformin-related lactic acidosis tends to occur most commonly in patients who develop CIN, and it is advisable to withhold metformin for 24 to 48 hours after catheterization because this is the period when CIN typically occurs.

## Drug-Eluting Stents

The introduction of drug-eluting stents (DES) has significantly reduced in-stent restenosis rates, and DES have grown to dominate the market since their debut. However, there is concern over the potential for late stent thrombosis with DES, particularly after antiplatelet agent withdrawal. Although rare, local and systemic hypersensitivity reactions involving DES have been reported and may contribute to late stent thrombosis risk. These factors may result in prolongation of dual antiplatelet therapy after DES deployment and raise concerns about the safe management of patients who require discontinuation of antiplatelet therapy due to bleeding or a compelling indication for surgery.

# RHYTHM DISORDERS

Despite the recent attention given to nonpharmacologic rhythm management options such as device therapy and catheter-based ablation procedures, many patients with rhythm disorders will require some form of antiarrhythmic therapy. The potential for significant adverse drug interactions involving antiarrhythmic drugs is enormous. Antiarrhythmic drugs *in general* function within a narrow therapeutic spectrum; minor alterations in serum levels may result in loss of efficacy or overt toxicity. Many of these agents are dependent on oxidative metabolism via subtypes of cytochrome P450, thus allowing for possible interactions with the ever-growing list of inducers and inhibitors of these enzymes. Additionally, patients with rhythm disorders often have structural heart disease and comorbid conditions that require their own cadre of medications. Avoiding adverse drug interactions in patients with rhythm disorders can be challenging, and this section focuses on the more common or concerning interactions of specific antiarrhythmic drugs, organized by the Vaughn Williams classification scheme.

# ■ CLASS IA ANTIARRHYTHMICS

All class IA antiarrhythmic drugs block membrane sodium channel activity and moderately depress phase 0 of the action potential, slowing conduction and prolonging repolarization. These drugs have utility in treating both atrial and ventricular tachyarrhythmias. A number of cardiac and noncardiac drugs also prolong repolarization, which is manifest electrocardiographically as QT interval prolongation (**Table 58-4**). QT prolongation increases the risk for potentially fatal arrhythmias such as *torsade de pointes* (**Fig. 58-5**); therefore, the use of QT prolonging drugs with class IA agents is contraindicated.

## Quinidine

Quinidine inhibits CYP2D6 and 3A4 and has the potential to interact with a number of cardiac and noncardiac drugs. Coadministration of quinidine with digoxin can result in a rapid, 3-fold increase in digoxin levels, likely due to a reduction in digoxin clearance and displacement of tissue-bound digoxin. Reducing the digoxin dose by half is recommended when starting with quinidine.

## Procainamide

Procainamide is acetylated by the liver to form the active metabolite *N*-acetyl-procainamide (NAPA) and has the distinction of being the only class 1 antiarrhythmic that does not depend on cytochrome P450 for its metabolism. Procainamide use may result in positive antinuclear antibodies and a drug-induced lupus syndrome in 50% and 30% of patients, respectively. Development of lupus-like symptoms should prompt discontinuation of the drug. Procainamide can in rare circumstances produce blood dyscrasias, including severe neutropenia. Procainamide and NAPA levels may be monitored to avoid toxicity.

## Disopyramide

Disopyramide is metabolized by CYP3A4. This drug frequently causes anticholinergic side effects such as dry mouth, urinary retention, and constipation. Disopyramide is also a potent negative inotrope and should be used with extreme caution in patients with left ventricular dysfunction. Coadministration of disopyramide with β-blockers can result in profound bradycardia and may precipitate heart failure. Macrolide antibiotics can also inhibit disopyramide metabolism and precipitate toxicity, QT prolongation, and torsade de pointes. Protease inhibitors, essential for effective HIV management, are all potent inhibitors of CYP3A4 that can promote disopyramide toxicity when these drugs are taken together.

# ■ CLASS IB ANTIARRHYTHMICS

The class IB antiarrhythmics block membrane sodium channels and have little effect on phase 0 of the action potential in normal cardiac tissue. These agents depress phase 0 in abnormal cardiac tissue and can shorten repolarization. Class IB agents are useful for the treatment of arrhythmias but also have analgesic properties. They are frequently used for local injections in pain management or during minor procedures.

**TABLE 58-4.** Drugs That Prolong the QT Interval

### Cardiovascular drugs

| *Class IA Antiarrhythmics* | *Class III Antiarrhythmics* | *Other Cardiac Drugs* |
|---|---|---|
| Disopyramide[a] | Amiodarone | Bepridil[a] |
| Procainamide[a] | Bretylium[a] | Diltiazem |
| Quinidine[a] | Dofetilide[a] | Indapamide |
| | Dronedarone | Isradipine[a] |
| | Ibutilide[a] | Moexipril/HCTZ |
| | Sotalol[a] | Nicardipine[a] |
| | | Ranolazine |
| | | Triamterene |

### Antimicrobial drugs

| *Macrolides* | *Quinolones* | *Other Antimicrobial Drugs* |
|---|---|---|
| Azithromycin | Gatifloxacin | Chloroquine |
| Clarithromycin | Grepafloxacin | Foscarnet |
| Clindamycin | Levofloxacin | Halofantrine |
| Erythromycin | Moxifloxacin | Itraconazole |
| Roxithromycin | Ofloxacin | Ketoconazole |
| Telithromycin | Sparfloxacin | Trimethoprim/sulfamethoxazole |
| | | Voriconazole |

### Psychiatric drugs

| *Antipsychotics* | *Antidepressants* | *Other Psychiatric Drugs* |
|---|---|---|
| Haloperidol[a] | Amitriptyline[a] | Chloral hydrate |
| Lithium | Bupropion | Felbamate |
| Mesoridazine | Citalopram | Fosphenytoin |
| Olanzapine | Clomipramine | Levomethadyl |
| Pimozide[a] | Desipramine[a] | Methadone |
| Quetiapine | Doxepin | |
| Risperidone | Fluoxetine[a] | |
| Thioridazine[a] | Imipramine | |
| Ziprasidone | Maprotiline | |
| | Nortriptyline | |
| | Paroxetine | |
| | Trazodone | |
| | Venlafaxine | |

### Other drugs

| *Gastrointestinal* | *Pulmonary/Allergy* | *Other Agents* |
|---|---|---|
| Cisapride[a] | Albuterol[a] | Amantadine |
| Dolasetron | Astemizole[a] | Arsenic trioxide[a] |
| Domperidone[a] | Fenoterol[a] | Enflurane |
| Droperidol | Fexofenadine | Halothane |
| Famotidine | Salmeterol[a] | Organophosphates (insecticide) |
| Granisetron | Terfenadine[a] | Pentamidine |
| Octreotide | | Propofol |
| Ondansetron[a] | | Quinine |
| | | Tacrolimus |
| | | Tamoxifen |
| | | Vincamine |

[a]Drugs associated with an increased risk for torsade de pointes.

HCTZ, hydrochlorothiazide.

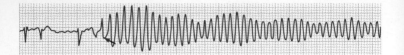

**FIGURE 58-5.** Torsade de pointes. The tachycardia is preceded by a short R-R interval followed by a long R-R interval with a ventricular premature complex (VPC) falling during repolarization; the R on T phenomenon (*arrow*).

## Lidocaine

Lidocaine inhibits CYP1A2 and depends on CYP1A2 and CYP3A4 for its oxidative metabolism. Amiodarone is an inhibitor of CYP3A4 and may increase lidocaine levels and result in toxicity. Because lidocaine is often used to treat ventricular arrhythmias in patients with ischemic heart disease, lidocaine is often used in patients receiving β-blocker therapy. β-blockers as a class may reduce hepatic blood flow and therefore decrease lidocaine clearance. This may occur more frequently with nonselective β-blockers such as propranolol; however, it is reasonable to monitor lidocaine levels in patients receiving any β-blocker.

## Mexiletine

Mexiletine, like lidocaine, inhibits CYP1A2 and depends on this enzyme for oxidative metabolism, along with CYP2D6. Mexiletine levels may fall substantially in the presence of P450 inducers such as rifampicin and phenytoin, and patients may require higher mexiletine doses to achieve efficacy. At the other extreme, CYP2D6 inhibitors such as the widely used selective serotonin reuptake inhibitors (SSRIs) may decrease mexiletine clearance and promote toxicity. Mexiletine can substantially increase serum levels of theophylline, a CYP1A2-dependent drug.

## ■ CLASS IC ANTIARRHYTHMICS

Class IC antiarrhythmic drugs block membrane sodium channels and markedly reduce phase 0 of the action potential, slowing conduction with little effect on repolarization. These drugs can be used to treat ventricular arrhythmias but should not be used in patients with coronary artery disease due to their association with higher rates of arrhythmia-related death in the Cardiac Arrhythmia Suppression Trial (CAST). The class IC drugs also play a role in the management of atrial arrhythmias in patients with non-ischemic, structurally normal hearts. These agents are often given in conjunction with an AV nodal blocking agent to prevent 1:1 AV conduction with development of atrial flutter, though this combination has the potential for pharmacodynamic interactions (see Class II Antiarrhythmic Drugs).

## Flecainide

Flecainide inhibits the enzyme responsible for its oxidation, CYP2D6, and dose reduction should be considered when flecainide is used in conjunction with CYP2D6 inhibitors such as amiodarone and SSRIs.

## Propafenone

Propafenone inhibits CYP2A6 and undergoes oxidative metabolism to variable degrees via CYP3A4, 1A2, and 2A6. This metabolic diversity gives propafenone the potential to interact with a broad array of agents. Propafenone decreases the volume of distribution and nonrenal clearance of digoxin, resulting in increased digoxin levels. It is advised to reduce the digoxin dose by as much as 25% when propafenone is added. Propafenone also interacts with warfarin and may increase the international normalized ratio by 30%.

# ■ CLASS II ANTIARRHYTHMIC DRUGS

The class II agents are β-adrenergic receptor blockers, ubiquitous in cardiovascular medicine due to their broad clinical utility. The pharmacokinetic profiles of these agents are discussed in detail in the hypertension section of this chapter. The pharmacodynamic relationships between β-blockers and other antiarrhythmic drug classes are more clinically relevant, as they tend to have both positive and negative qualities. β-blockers appear to reduce the proarrhythmic potential of the class IC drugs, although the combined negative inotropic and chronotropic properties of these drug classes may become clinically problematic. Similar issues exist when β-blockers are coadministered with class III antiarrhythmics such as sotalol and amiodarone. Clinical trial data suggest that combining β-blockers with class III agents in patients with ischemic heart disease may improve outcomes when compared with either class alone; however, such combinations also carry an increased risk for clinically significant bradycardia, especially among the elderly. The same type of synergy exists between β-blockers and digoxin in the setting of atrial fibrillation.

# ■ CLASS III ANTIARRHYTHMIC DRUGS

The class III antiarrhythmic drugs prolong repolarization and alter membrane potassium channel function. Several class III drugs have sodium channel antagonist properties and some have β-blocker activity. The class III drugs are used to treat both supraventricular and ventricular rhythm disorders. Because they prolong repolarization, all class III drugs have the potential to lengthen the QT interval. Therefore, the use of class III antiarrhythmic agents in combination with drugs known to prolong the QT interval (see Table 58-4) is contraindicated.

## Amiodarone

Amiodarone is among the most widely used antiarrhythmic agents available, but its propensity to interact with other drugs deserves special attention. The new congener of amiodarone, dronedarone, is also discussed in a later section.

## Dofetilide

Dofetilide undergoes oxidative metabolism via CYP3A4 and is excreted in the urine by the renal cation transport system. Potent inhibitors of CYP3A4 such as cimetidine and ketoconazole may increase serum dofetilide levels and precipitate toxicity. Drugs that inhibit the renal cation transport system are also contraindicated with dofetilide and include ketoconazole, cimetidine, trimethoprim, prochlorperazine, and megestrol. Diuretics may alter the renal clearance of dofetilide and reduce serum potassium and magnesium concentrations, both risk factors for dofetilide toxicity. Patients requiring both dofetilide and diuretic therapy should be closely monitored for electrolyte disturbances and ECG changes. Verapamil accelerates dofetilide absorption and increases serum levels substantially; cases of torsade de pointes have been described when these drugs have been used together. Because of these effects, dofetilide can only be initiated in an inpatient setting by physicians who have been specifically trained to monitor the drug.

## *Sotalol*

Sotalol is a class III antiarrhythmic agent with nonselective β-adrenergic antagonist properties. Most of the administered dose is excreted unchanged in the urine. Sotalol has been observed to interact with prazosin, resulting in significant hypotension. The converse has been observed with sotalol and clonidine; significant *hypertension* has been described. Antacids containing magnesium or aluminum salts can decrease the bioavailability of sotalol and should not be given for at least 2 hours after sotalol ingestion.

## ■ CLASS IV ANTIARRHYTHMIC DRUGS

The class IV antiarrhythmic drugs block calcium channels and include verapamil and diltiazem. Verapamil interacts with several drugs, including several antiarrhythmic agents (**Table 58-5**). Like the class II drugs (β-blockers), many of the adverse

**TABLE 58-5.** Significant Drug-Drug Interactions Involving Verapamil

| Drug | Interaction | | Effect | Recommendation |
|------|------|------|--------|----------------|
| Amiodarone | PK<br>PD | ⊗ CYP3A4 | Bradycardia<br>Hypotension<br>Reduced cardiac output | Close clinical<br>monitoring |
| Azole antifungals | PK | ⊗ CYP3A4 | Increased verapamil effects | Avoid concurrent use |
| Barbiturates | PK | ⊕ CYP3A4 | Reduced verapamil effects | Increase verapamil dose |
| β-Blockers | PD | AV node | Bradycardia<br>Hypotension<br>Reduced cardiac output | Close clinical<br>monitoring |
| Calcium | PD | | Reduced verapamil effects | Increase verapamil dose |
| Carbamazepine | PK | ⊕ CYP3A4 | Reduced verapamil effects<br>Carbamazepine toxicity | Avoid concurrent use |
| Cyclosporine | PK | ⊗ CYP3A4 | Increased cyclosporine levels, toxicity, renal failure | Avoid concurrent use |
| Digoxin | PK<br>PD | ⊗ CYP3A4 | Bradycardia<br>Digoxin toxicity | Reduce digoxin dose |
| Grapefruit juice | PK | ⊗ CYP3A4 | Increased verapamil effects | Avoid concurrent use |
| HMG-CoA reductase inhibitors | PK | ⊗ CYP3A4 | Increased HMG-CoA Reductase Inhibitor levels and toxicity | Use pravastatin or fluvastatin |
| Midazolam | PK | ⊗ CYP3A4 | Increased midazolam | Close clinical<br>monitoring |
| Phenytoin | PK | ⊕ CYP3A4 | Reduced verapamil effect | Increase verapamil dose |
| Rifampin | PK | ⊕ CYP3A4 | Reduced verapamil effect | Increase verapamil dose |
| Tacrolimus | PK | | Increased tacrolimus levels | Avoid concurrent use |

CYP, cytochrome P450 enzyme; HMG-CoA, hydroxymethylglutaryl coenzyme A; ⊕, induction; ⊗, inhibition; PD, pharmacodynamic; PK, pharmacokinetic.

interactions involving class IV antiarrhythmic drugs are pharmacodynamic. Please see the section Hypertension in this chapter for more information regarding the calcium-channel antagonists.

## Adenosine

Adenosine enhances permeability of acetylcholine-sensitive muscarinic $K^+$ channels $I_{k(ACh)}$ in cardiac tissue and vascular smooth muscle. Adenosine can be both diagnostic and therapeutic in the management of supraventricular tachyarrhythmias. However, because adenosine is degraded rapidly, it must be administered quickly through a proximal vein in order to reach the heart. Adenosine is also useful as a vasodilator in pharmacologic cardiac imaging. Methylxanthines such as aminophylline and theophylline compete with adenosine for receptor binding and are useful antidotes in patients with adenosine-induced hypotension or flushing. Conversely, dipyridamole slows the breakdown of adenosine and may exaggerate its clinical effects. Adenosine doses should be reduced by 75% or more in patients taking dipyridamole.

# HYPERTENSION

Hypertension, perhaps more than any other medical diagnosis, is associated with an increased risk for adverse drug reactions. The prevalence of hypertension among adults in the United States is approximately 30%, and the incidence of hypertension is increasing. Worldwide, the number of hypertensive individuals is approaching 1 billion. The necessity for multidrug therapy to control hypertension also increases the risk of ADRs. Although the risk for significant pharmacodynamic interactions (principally hypotension) with a multidrug approach to hypertension is obvious, in general, the consequences of untreated hypertension are graver than the risk of adverse drug reactions. Hypertension is associated with substantially increased morbidity and mortality across all age strata, and adequate blood pressure control is achieved in only a minority of treated hypertensive patients. Current management guidelines recommend an aggressive approach to the initiation and titration of antihypertensive therapy. For example, *initial* pharmacotherapy for a patient with stage 2 hypertension (systolic pressure ≥160 mm Hg, diastolic pressure ≥100 mm Hg) should include 2 drugs, and many of these patients will require additional agents for adequate blood pressure control. Thus, for the majority of hypertensive patients, polypharmacy is the standard of care. Finally, by virtue of their collective influence on cardiac output and systemic vascular resistance, antihypertensive drugs can alter hepatic and renal blood flow and set the stage for adverse pharmacokinetic interactions. Awareness of potential adverse drug interactions is therefore mandatory for the safe and appropriate management of hypertension.

## ■ DIURETIC THERAPY

### Thiazide Diuretics

Thiazide-type diuretics are considered first-line agents in hypertension management due to their efficacy and favorable effects on cardiovascular and all-cause mortality. These agents are most effective at lower doses. Higher doses do not result in a substantial increase in antihypertensive effect but have been associated with class-specific adverse events such as hyperlipidemia, insulin resistance, erectile dysfunction, and a very small increase in the relative risk for renal cell carcinoma, particularly in middle-aged women. Thiazide diuretics have the potential to induce clinically relevant hypovolemia and electrolyte disturbances such as hypokalemia and hypomagnesemia. When severe, the latter may result in life-threatening ventricular arrhythmias. Hyponatremia is another potential risk of diuretic therapy. Thiazide diuretics can also promote hyperuricemia and precipitate gout; this is a significant problem among solid-organ transplant recipients. The antihypertensive efficacy of thiazide diuretics is reduced by the concurrent use of nonsteroidal anti-inflammatory drugs (NSAIDs), including cyclooxygenase-2 (COX-2) inhibitors. As a result of their influence on plasma volume and glomerular filtration, thiazide diuretics can interfere with the pharmacokinetics of renally excreted drugs, particularly lithium carbonate. Lithium levels can increase by as much as 40% with the introduction of a thiazide diuretic, potentially resulting in lithium toxicity.

## Loop Diuretics

Concerning their risk for potential adverse drug reactions, the loop diuretics are similar to thiazide diuretics in many respects. One significant difference between these drug classes is that loop diuretics promote renal calcium *excretion*, which can potentially promote nephrolithiasis. Loop diuretics are also used extensively in patients with heart failure and renal insufficiency. These higher-risk patients are susceptible to diuretic-induced hypovolemia and may experience hypotension and worsening renal function with the coadministration of drugs such as ACEIs and ARBs. Loop diuretic–induced renal insufficiency, hypokalemia, and hypomagnesemia can also precipitate digitalis toxicity.

## Potassium-Sparing Diuretics

Triamterene and amiloride are mild potassium-sparing diuretics that are often coadministered with thiazide diuretics for the treatment of hypertension. This combination substantially reduces the risk of thiazide-induced hypokalemia. Although not commonly associated with adverse events, these drugs do promote potassium retention. Thus, their use in patients with renal insufficiency or with agents known to potentiate hyperkalemia should be approached with extreme caution. The aldosterone receptor antagonists, spironolactone and eplerenone, possess the same potential for adverse drug reactions as the other potassium-sparing diuretics. These agents are discussed more extensively in Heart Failure section.

## ■ ADRENERGIC ANTAGONISTS

### β-Adrenergic Receptor Blockers

β-adrenergic receptor antagonists (β-blockers) are commonly used as first-line agents in hypertension and have substantial clinical benefits in patients with heart failure and ischemic heart disease. β-blockers promote peripheral vasodilation, reduce myocardial contractility, and slow electrical conduction through the AV node. Thus, there is potential for significant pharmacodynamic interactions with drugs of similar design. The concurrent use of nondihydropyridine calcium-channel antagonists (diltiazem and verapamil) and β-blockers can precipitate hypotension, heart failure, and profound bradycardia. Synergistic hypotension and bradycardia may also occur when β-blockers are given in conjunction with antiarrhythmic drugs such as amiodarone. β-blocker therapy can result in significant, sometimes life-threatening hypertension via unopposed α-adrenergic stimulation in patients who are beginning therapy with clonidine or methyldopa or who abuse stimulant drugs, particularly cocaine. Previous concerns regarding the risk of β-blocker therapy in patients with lung diseases such as asthma and chronic obstructive pulmonary disease have been greatly diminished, in part because of the introduction of β1-specific agents such as metoprolol. As is the case with many drugs, the antihypertensive effects of β-blockers may be attenuated by the concurrent use of NSAIDs.

Many commonly used β-blockers (carvedilol, metoprolol, propranolol, and labetalol) are metabolized by hepatic CYP2D6 and are therefore susceptible to hepatic pharmacokinetic changes imposed by other drugs. Cimetidine and verapamil inhibit the oxidative metabolism of these β-blockers, leading to increased serum levels and exaggerated clinical effects. In contrast, the hydrophilic, renally excreted β-blockers, atenolol, nadolol, and sotalol, are not influenced by hepatic pharmacokinetic interactions.

## α-Adrenergic Receptor Blockers

The α-adrenergic receptor antagonists (α-blockers) currently play a limited role in hypertension management, largely because of the established efficacy of other agents and concerns regarding the safety of α-blockers in patients with cardiovascular disease. Nonetheless, these drugs still play a role as adjunctive agents in refractory hypertension and in the management of patients with symptomatic benign prostatic hyperplasia. The major pharmacodynamic limitation of α-blocker therapy is postural hypotension, and this may be exacerbated by other antihypertensive agents. Additionally, because benign prostatic hyperplasia, hypertension, and erectile dysfunction become increasingly more common with age, one needs to be particularly cautious when using α-blockers in men taking phosphodiesterase 5 (PDE5) inhibitors. Finally, verapamil alters the pharmacokinetics of terazosin and prazosin, resulting in increased drug bioavailability.

## ■ CALCIUM-CHANNEL BLOCKERS

Calcium-channel blockers are used extensively for the treatment of hypertension. These drugs are uniform with respect to metabolism; all calcium-channel blockers are metabolized via CYP3A4. Therefore, as a drug class, calcium-channel blockers are sensitive to pharmacokinetic alterations in CYP3A4 activity. Grapefruit juice, a known CYP3A4 inhibitor, increases plasma concentrations of calcium-channel blockers and can lead to significant hypotension.

## Verapamil

Verapamil is useful for the treatment of hypertension and angina. Verapamil reduces AV nodal conduction, myocardial contractility, and systemic arterial tone, and it may act synergistically with β-blockers to induce hypotension, heart failure, and bradycardia. Similar pharmacodynamic interactions have been observed between verapamil and antiarrhythmic agents such as amiodarone and flecainide, and the coadministration of verapamil and clonidine can result in significant hypotension and atrioventricular block.

Verapamil is oxidized in the liver by CYP3A4 and inhibits the P-gp–mediated drug transport. This drug also enhances hepatic blood flow and can potentially alter the first-pass metabolism of hepatically modified drugs. Verapamil can increase levels of digoxin by as much as 50% to 90%, likely because of its influence on P-gp. Thus, digoxin dosing should be proportionately reduced if both drugs are required. Other significant drug-drug interactions involving verapamil are listed in Table 58-5.

## Diltiazem

Diltiazem is similar to verapamil in many respects, especially regarding the potential for pharmacodynamic interactions with drugs like β-blockers. Diltiazem does not appear to have the same effect on P-gp as verapamil and does not influence digoxin levels appreciably. Diltiazem, along with verapamil, does reduce the hepatic clearance of cyclosporine, resulting in increased cyclosporine levels. This interaction can be exploited in hypertensive solid-organ transplant patients where diltiazem therapy permits lower cyclosporine doses, reducing cyclosporine-related morbidity and cost of care. Diltiazem also increases serum levels of simvastatin, lovastatin, and atorvastatin. Closer monitoring for signs of statin toxicity and lower statin dosing are advised.

### Dihydropyridines

The dihydropyridine-type calcium-channel blockers such as amlodipine and nifedipine are potent vasodilators with minimal direct effect on myocardial contractility or conduction. These agents are useful in the management of hypertension and angina. Dihydropyridines have the propensity for pharmacodynamic interactions with blood pressure-lowering drugs, leading to significant hypotension. As a consequence of vasodilation-induced inter-compartment fluid shifts, they produce significant leg edema in up to 20% of users. This type of edema may be substantially improved or avoided by coadministration of an ACEI, allowing for balanced venodilation with removal of sequestered fluid. The pharmacokinetic profile for the dihydropyridines is similar to that of diltiazem.

## ■ INHIBITORS OF THE RENIN-ANGIOTENSIN-ALDOSTERONE AXIS

### Angiotensin-Converting Enzyme Inhibitors

ACEIs have widespread applicability in cardiovascular disease and are commonly used in the management of hypertension, heart failure, and coronary artery disease. Thus, the likelihood of encountering an ACEI-related adverse event in clinical practice is high.

All ACEIs have the potential to provoke a chronic, nonproductive cough in 5% to 35% of patients. The associated cough may be due to decreased degradation of bradykinin by ACE resulting in bradykinin-induced sensitization of airway sensory nerves and typically resolves upon discontinuation of the drug. Another rare but potentially fatal adverse reaction to ACEI therapy is angioedema. ACEI-related angioedema is considered a contraindication to future ACEI use, and recent data suggest that patients who experience angioedema with ACEIs are at increased risk for subsequent angioedema if treated with an ARB. The precise mechanism for this interaction is not known, but ARB use in patients with a history of ACEI-related angioedema should be approached with caution.

ACEIs are associated with a number of significant pharmacodynamic and pharmacokinetic drug interactions. ACEIs interfere with the pharmacokinetics of lithium, and concurrent use of both agents results in increased serum lithium levels. If the need for ACEI therapy in a patient taking lithium is compelling, lithium levels should be monitored frequently. ACEIs should be used cautiously with potassium supplements or potassium-sparing diuretic agents to avoid significant hyperkalemia. Similarly, patients with hypovolemia, often a consequence of diuretic therapy, are at increased risk for ACEI-related acute renal failure. The use of NSAIDs may attenuate the antihypertensive effects of ACEIs, and the combination of NSAIDs with a diuretic and ACEI carries a substantial risk for renal failure. The issue of aspirin use in combination with ACEIs is controversial and discussed in Heart Failure section. Finally, the ACEI captopril can increase digoxin levels by as much as 20%. This interaction has not been consistently observed with other ACEIs.

## Angiotensin Receptor Blockers

The ARBs are effective antihypertensive agents that also appear to have benefit in heart failure. ARBs are associated with few adverse reactions relative to other antihypertensive drug classes. Unlike their ACEI cousins, they carry little risk for cough, and angioedema with ARB therapy is extraordinarily rare. Losartan and irbesartan have strong affinity for CYP2C9 and interact to some degree with CYP3A4 and CYP1A2. As a result, the effects of these drugs may be magnified or attenuated in the presence of known inhibitors or inducers of these P450 enzyme subtypes (see Table 58-1). In contrast to losartan and irbesartan, valsartan appears to depend little on oxidative metabolism, but valsartan bioavailability is reduced by approximately half when the drug is taken with food. Patients should be advised to take valsartan 1 to 2 hours before or after meals. Candesartan is converted to its active form within the gastrointestinal tract and is eliminated unchanged in the urine and feces. Eprosartan has a similar pharmacokinetic profile, and neither drug appears to result in clinically significant interactions with commonly prescribed agents such as warfarin, digoxin, or hydrochlorothiazide. Telmisartan is the most lipophilic ARB. Although telmisartan may increase digoxin concentrations by 50%, this change appears to be of little clinical concern.

## Aliskiren

Aliskiren is a potent direct renin inhibitor approved for the treatment of hypertension alone or in combination with other antihypertensive drugs. In the AVOID study, aliskiren reduced albuminuria in patients with hypertension and type 2 diabetes, even in patients already on recommended doses of an angiotensin receptor blocker (losartan). When evaluated in patients with systolic heart failure already on β-blockers and ACEI/ARB, aliskiren had a favorable neurohormonal effect, decreasing plasma N-terminal pro-brain natriuretic peptide, plasma brain natriuretic peptide, and urinary aldosterone levels. Whether adding aliskiren to background medical therapy for heart failure will improve outcomes is still to be determined.

As with other antagonists of the renin-angiotensin-aldosterone axis, potassium levels need to be monitored, particularly with combination therapy, and aliskiren should be used with caution in patients with renal dysfunction. Hypotension can occur when used in combination with other antihypertensives, especially in patients with an activated renin-angiotensin system (volume and salt depletion). Angioedema is a rare complication, and absorption may be decreased by high-fat meals. Aliskiren is a substrate of P-gp; concurrent use of P-gp inhibitors such as cyclosporine is not recommended. In vitro studies indicate metabolism via CYP3A4, and caution is advised when used with strong CYP3A4 inhibitors.

## ■ VASODILATORS

Direct vasodilators such as hydralazine and minoxidil are generally reserved for use in patients with refractory hypertension or in heart failure patients who cannot take ACEIs or ARBs. Hydralazine is a direct arteriolar vasodilator that can produce peripheral edema in a minority of patients. Hydralazine may also induce a lupus-like syndrome with fever, malar rash, malaise, and positive antinuclear antibodies, particularly antihistone antibodies. The syndrome typically resolves several weeks after discontinuation of the drug. Abrupt cessation of hydralazine therapy can trigger a significant reflex tachycardia, and gradual withdrawal of hydralazine is advisable. Hydralazine is acetylated by the liver and is a weak inhibitor of CYP3A4; it can alter hepatic blood flow and increase levels of shorter-acting, hepatically metabolized β-blockers, such as propranolol and metoprolol. Minoxidil is a potent peripheral arteriolar vasodilator that is pharmacodynamically similar to hydralazine.

Thus, the same precautions regarding peripheral edema and reflex tachycardia apply. Minoxidil may cause hypertrichosis, a unique side effect that has been exploited for the benefit of those suffering from alopecia. Rare cases of pericardial effusion and Stevens–Johnson syndrome have been reported with minoxidil.

# PREVENTIVE CARDIOLOGY

Aggressive risk factor modification plays a crucial role in our ongoing attempt to reduce cardiovascular event rates. In parallel with advances in catheter-based technology, advances in biotechnology have allowed us to better understand and modify cardiovascular risk at the molecular level.

## HMG-CoA Reductase Inhibitors

The HMG-CoA reductase inhibitors (statins) have revolutionized preventive cardiology since their introduction in the mid-1980s, and the mortality and morbidity benefits of statins have been firmly established in primary and secondary prevention trials.

## ■ HEPATOTOXICITY

All statins have the potential to cause asymptomatic elevation of serum hepatic aminotransferase levels. Significant (>3× the upper limit of normal) elevations in serum aminotransferase levels occur in 1% to 3% of statin-treated patients, but the clinical relevance of this finding is unknown. Drug-induced liver injury related to statin use is an exceedingly rare, idiosyncratic reaction that occurs in less than 1 in 1 million patient-years of treatment. Although routine monitoring of hepatic aminotransferase levels is presently recommended for patients taking statins, this practice has not been shown to prevent liver injury.

## ■ MYOTOXICITY

Statin use is associated with diffuse myalgias in a minority of patients, but clinically significant muscle injury occurs in only 0.5% of statin-treated patients. The mechanism of statin-induced myotoxicity is unknown but may be related to the depletion of metabolic intermediaries. Low levels of ubiquinone (coenzyme Q) have been reported in patients receiving statin therapy, an observation that has fueled popular interest in coenzyme-Q supplementation. However, based on current evidence, the routine use of coenzyme-Q for the prevention of muscle injury in patients taking statins cannot be recommended.

## Drug-Drug Interactions

Most statins are dependent on CYP3A4 for metabolism and are thus subject to pharmacokinetic interactions with agents that inhibit or induce CYP3A4. One notable exception to this rule is pravastatin, which undergoes hepatic metabolism primarily via non–CYP-dependent mechanisms. Despite the potential for adverse events, relatively few drug-drug interactions involving statins have been described. The use of grapefruit juice in patients taking statins should be avoided. Cases of statin toxicity have also been reported in patients taking cyclosporine. Thus, pravastatin is preferred for the primary and secondary prevention of cardiovascular disease in solid-organ transplant patients.

# ■ OTHER ANTILIPEMIC AGENTS

## Ezetimibe

Ezetimibe is a novel inhibitor of Niemann-Pick C1-like protein, a small bowel transport protein that facilitates the absorption of dietary and biliary cholesterol. Ezetimibe preferentially blocks the absorption of cholesterol while allowing absorption of triglycerides and fat-soluble vitamins. It is metabolized via hepatic glucuronidation and is excreted predominantly in the feces. Ezetimibe does not interact with CYP450 isozymes or P-gp, and thus its use results in relatively few significant pharmacokinetic interactions. Ezetimibe does not interact with statins and does not appear to be affected by food. Any beneficial effect of ezetimibe on clinical outcomes has come into question with the ENHANCE trial, where the combination of ezetimibe and simvastatin failed to show a significant change in intima-media thickness compared with simvastatin alone. Large-scale trials assessing clinical outcomes with ezetimibe are needed and ongoing.

## Niacin

Nicotinic acid (niacin) has a favorable influence on lipid profiles, but drug tolerance is poor secondary to the common reactions of flushing and pruritus. These reactions may be caused by prostaglandin release, and 325 mg of oral aspirin given with niacin greatly attenuates these cutaneous effects. Sustained-release niacin is associated with an increased risk for elevated serum aminotransferases, and fulminant hepatic failure has been described. The potential for hepatotoxicity may be increased when niacin is administered with a statin.

## Fibrates and Bile Acid Sequestrants

Use of fibric acid derivatives is associated with a number of mild complaints, including gastrointestinal upset, headache, and skin reactions such as increased photosensitivity. These drugs may also cause transient elevation of hepatic aminotransferase levels, but overt liver injury is rare. Bile acid sequestrants such as cholestyramine are associated with gastrointestinal bloating and discomfort and may interfere with the absorption of other drugs, particularly warfarin.

## Omega-3-Acid Ethyl Esters

Omega-3-acid ethyl esters, known as prescription fish oil (LOVAZA), is FDA-approved for treatment of hypertriglyceridemia when levels exceed 500 mg/dL. In patients with severe hypertriglyceridemia who are not on a statin, a 45% reduction in triglycerides was observed with omega-3-acid ethyl esters but was associated with 31% increase in LDL levels. Therefore, LDL levels should be monitored periodically with treatment. When used in patients with hepatic impairment, AST and ALT should also be monitored periodically because they may rise with treatment. Bleeding time can be prolonged with omega-3-acid ethyl esters, and caution is advised when used in patients with coagulopathy or on therapeutic anticoagulation. The drug should be used with extreme caution in patients with hypersensitivity to fish or shellfish.

# ■ SMOKING CESSATION

Cigarette smoking directly contributes to 1 of every 5 deaths in the United States and is a potent modifiable risk factor for cardiovascular disease. In addition to direct end-organ toxicity, cigarette smoking induces hepatic CYP1A2 and 2D6, potentially reducing the biologic effect of drugs metabolized by these enzymes.

## Nicotine Replacement

Nicotine replacement therapy (NRT) improves smoking cessation rates and eases the severity of tobacco withdrawal. Despite its established benefit, physicians often do not prescribe NRT for several reasons, including the unwarranted concern that patients receiving NRT who concurrently smoke are at high risk for adverse events. Although certainly not advisable, the use of NRT in the setting of ongoing smoking does not appear to produce clinical toxicity.

## Bupropion

Bupropion hydrochloride is a novel antidepressant that modulates the activity of serotonin, norepinephrine, and dopamine. Bupropion, like NRT, increases the likelihood for sustained smoking cessation by approximately 2-fold compared with placebo, and bupropion and NRT are frequently used in combination. Bupropion is metabolized by CYP2B6 and thus has the potential for pharmacokinetic interactions with CYP2B6 inducers and inhibitors. Because it can lower the seizure threshold, bupropion use should be avoided in patients with a history of seizures.

## Varenicline

Varenicline is a partial agonist at the $\alpha4\beta2$ subunit of the nicotinic acetylcholine receptor. It reduces the symptoms of nicotine withdrawal and reduces the rewarding aspect of cigarette smoking. The efficacy of varenicline for smoking cessation has been shown in multiple trials; it was superior to buproprion with a cessation rate of 33% at 6-month follow-up. The side effects of varenicline include nausea, and slow uptitration of dose and administration with meals minimize gastrointestinal upset. Neuropsychiatric symptoms, including suicidal thoughts and aggressive behavior, have been reported with use as well as after withdrawal of varenicline. In February 2008, the FDA issued an alert stating that varenicline was increasingly likely to be associated with serious neuropsychiatric symptoms. Therefore, patients should be closely monitored for behavioral changes, psychiatric symptoms, and suicidal ideation. Extreme caution should be exercised in treatment of patients with underlying psychiatric conditions. Finally, varenicline is cleared by the kidneys, and dose reduction is needed for severe renal impairment.

# PERIPHERAL VASCULAR DISEASE

Atherosclerotic disease is a systemic illness, and significant coronary artery disease is a strong predictor of the presence of underlying peripheral vascular disease and vice versa. Although pharmacotherapies targeting the primary and secondary prevention of coronary artery disease also benefit peripheral vascular beds, certain agents such as the phosphodiesterase (PDE) inhibitors are used specifically to treat noncoronary arterial disease. PDE breaks down cyclic adenosine monophosphate (cAMP), a ubiquitous molecule responsible for the intracellular signal transduction of numerous cell surface receptors in a variety of tissue types, including myocytes, platelets, and vascular smooth muscle cells. The discovery of tissue-specific PDE subtypes has led to the development of PDE inhibitors that target individual vascular beds with reasonable specificity. PDE inhibitors are presently used to treat leg claudication and erectile dysfunction.

# ■ INTERMITTENT CLAUDICATION

Two PDE3 inhibitors are currently approved for the management of moderate-to-severe leg claudication. The precise mechanism of action of these agents in claudication is not known but is likely due to cAMP-mediated dilation of vascular smooth muscle and inhibition of platelet aggregation.

## Cilostazol

Cilostazol is metabolized by CYP3A4 and CYP2C19 in addition to other isozymes. Moderate inhibitors of CYP3A4 such as erythromycin and diltiazem can increase cilostazol levels by greater than 50%. For this reason, the coadministration of these agents with cilostazol is contraindicated in Europe. In the United States, it is recommended that the cilostazol dose be reduced to 50 mg twice daily. Such is also the case with the CYP2C19 inhibitor omeprazole. The concurrent use of cilostazol with potent CYP3A4 inhibitors such as grapefruit juice, azole antifungal agents, and fluoxetine may also substantially increase cilostazol levels. Cilostazol influences platelet function, and its concurrent use with antiplatelet agents and anticoagulants may theoretically increase the risk for bleeding, although this has not been observed clinically. Similarly, because other PDE inhibitors have been shown to increase mortality in patients with heart failure, the use of cilostazol in patients with heart failure is contraindicated.

# ■ ERECTILE DYSFUNCTION

PDE5 is highly concentrated in vascular smooth muscle cells, particularly the cells of the corpora cavernosa. There are currently 3 PDE5 inhibitors indicated for use in patients with erectile dysfunction: sildenafil, vardenafil, and tadalafil. These agents are generally well tolerated, but, like many vasodilators, these drugs may produce mild flushing and systolic hypotension. The systemic vasodilator effects of PDE5 inhibitors can be dramatically amplified by the coadministration of drugs that inhibit the degradation of cyclic guanosine monophosphate, such as organic nitrates. This interaction may produce dramatic increases in cAMP levels that can precipitate potentially life-threatening hypotension. For this reason, PDE5 inhibitor use in patients taking any nitrate preparation is contraindicated.

# DRUGS WITH HIGH INTERACTION POTENTIAL

## ■ AMIODARONE

Amiodarone has been referred to as a broad-spectrum antiarrhythmic because of its multiple mechanisms of action, established efficacy in treating both ventricular and supraventricular tachyarrhythmias, and applicability across patient populations regardless of left ventricular function. The propensity of amiodarone for end-organ toxicity and significant drug-drug interactions is equally broad.

## Organ Toxicity

Amiodarone has a biologic half-life of approximately 100 days, and clearance after amiodarone discontinuation may take months. The drug is extremely lipophilic and continues to accumulate in tissues after stable plasma levels have been achieved. The likelihood for end-organ toxicity is therefore greater in patients taking higher (≥400 mg daily) doses for longer periods of time. Periodic monitoring for end-organ toxicity in amiodarone-treated patients is recommended.

## Pulmonary Toxicity

The most feared complication of amiodarone therapy is amiodarone-induced pulmonary toxicity (APT). APT is directly related to the total cumulative amiodarone dose and thus tends to present after months or years of drug therapy. The annual incidence of severe APT is approximately 1% for patients taking lower (150-300 mg/d) maintenance doses of amiodarone and may be as high as 5% to 10% among patients taking ≥400 mg/d of amiodarone. The precise pathophysiology of APT is unknown, but direct pulmonary phospholipidosis and immune-mediated hypersensitivity likely play causative roles. The symptoms and signs of APT are nonspecific and include a nonproductive cough, dyspnea, and diffuse inspiratory crackles, findings that are often attributed to underlying heart disease. The only consistent physiologic alteration in patients with APT is a reduction in the carbon monoxide diffusing capacity (DLCO), although moderate (20%) decrease in DLCO may occur in amiodarone-treated patients without symptoms of overt lung toxicity. The treatment of choice for APT is the discontinuation of amiodarone. High-dose corticosteroid therapy may be of benefit in patients with severe APT, although this has not been firmly established in clinical trials.

## Hepatic Toxicity

Mild, transient serum aminotransferase elevation is not uncommon during initiation of amiodarone therapy, but amiodarone should be discontinued in patients who experience more than a 2-fold rise in aminotransferase levels. Overt hepatitis related to amiodarone treatment is uncommon and occurs in fewer than 3% of patients, and rare cases of hepatic failure and cirrhosis have been described.

## Thyroid Toxicity

Amiodarone-induced thyroid disease is common. Abnormal thyroid function is detected in approximately 5% to 20% of amiodarone-treated patients, and the risk for thyroid toxicity is dose-dependent. The clinical presentation of amiodarone-induced thyroid disease depends on the mechanism of thyroid injury and the presence or absence of underlying thyroid dysfunction. Amiodarone may directly injure the thyroid gland, resulting in thyroiditis and clinical hyperthyroidism. Amiodarone metabolism releases approximately 3 mg of iodine for every 100 mg of ingested drug. This resultant iodine excess may inhibit thyroid hormone production and the conversion of thyroxine ($T_4$) to triiodothyronine ($T_3$) in normal or hypoactive thyroid glands, producing clinical hypothyroidism. Conversely, autologously functioning thyroid nodules are not subject to feedback inhibition and will utilize the excess iodine to produce more thyroid hormone, resulting in thyrotoxicosis. Discontinuation of amiodarone often results in normalization of thyroid function; however, this may occur slowly secondary to the long elimination half-life of amiodarone. In patients who cannot safely discontinue amiodarone therapy, hypothyroidism may be successfully treated with thyroid hormone replacement. Amiodarone-induced hyperthyroidism may respond to treatment with methimazole and steroids.

## Ocular and Skin Manifestations

Corneal microdeposits are highly prevalent in amiodarone-treated patients, but only 10% experience visual disturbances, usually described as halos during night vision. The presence of corneal microdeposits without visual changes is not a reason to discontinue amiodarone. Skin reactions are common with long-term amiodarone therapy and may present as photosensitivity or bluish skin discoloration, often involving the face (Blue Man facies, **Fig. 58-6**). Patients with photosensitivity should

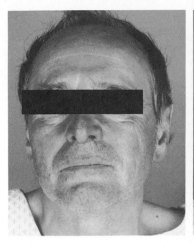
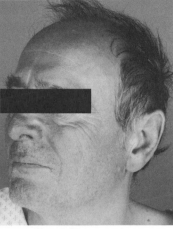

**FIGURE 58-6.** Amiodarone skin discoloration. (Reproduced with permission from Enseleit, et al.)

be advised to avoid the sun and use sun block. Amiodarone skin discoloration may be lessened by dose reduction and can resolve entirely (albeit slowly) after amiodarone discontinuation.

## Pharmacokinetic Interactions

Amiodarone is metabolized by CYP3A4 and inhibits many hepatic oxidative enzymes, including CYP1A2, 2C9, 2D6, and 3A4. Amiodarone also inhibits the activity of the P-glycoprotein transport system. Thus, amiodarone has enormous potential for pharmacokinetic drug interactions. Cyclosporine levels may increase in the presence of amiodarone due to the inhibition of CYP3A4 activity. Similarly, serum digoxin levels can double when the drug is coadministered with amiodarone, possibly secondary to inhibition of P-gp transport in the gastrointestinal tract. Periodic monitoring of cyclosporine and digoxin levels with appropriate dose reduction is recommended. Antimicrobial agents may also interact with amiodarone. Fluoroquinolones can prolong the QT interval and should be avoided in patients taking amiodarone. The HIV protease inhibitors, amprenavir, nelfinavir, and ritonavir, inhibit CYP3A4 and may precipitate amiodarone cardiotoxicity. The anticoagulant effect of warfarin is enhanced by amiodarone secondary to CYP3A4 inhibition, increasing the prothrombin time by more than 40%. This effect may be offset by reducing the warfarin dose by 25% to 50%.

## Pharmacodynamic Interactions

Amiodarone possesses the pharmacodynamic properties of several drug classes, including the β-blockers and calcium-channel blockers. Severe sinus bradycardia and atrioventricular block may result from the concurrent use of amiodarone with β-blockers. Similar pharmacodynamic interactions have been described between amiodarone and diltiazem and verapamil. As is the case with all class III antiarrhythmic drugs, the concurrent use of amiodarone with agents known to cause QT interval prolongation is contraindicated.

# ■ DRONEDARONE

Dronedarone is a noniodinated benzofuran derivative that has similar electrophysiologic effects as amiodarone along with antiadrenergic properties, but a shorter half-life (**Fig. 58-7**). The absence of the iodine moiety was developed to free dronedarone from the pulmonary, hepatic, and thyroid toxicity of amiodarone. Early trials showed that it could be used to prevent recurrent atrial fibrillation/flutter and was safe. In the ATHENA trial of 4628 patients with paroxysmal or persistent atrial fibrillation, dronedarone significantly reduced death and cardiovascular hospitalization by 24%, leading to its approval for the treatment of atrial fibrillation (**Fig. 58-8**). Although an acceptable safety profile was shown in patients with preserved ejection fraction, the ANDROMEDA trial, which included patients with left ventricular systolic dysfunction and NYHA class III to IV symptoms, showed an increased risk of death and heart failure exacerbation with dronedarone (**Fig. 58-9**).

Furthermore, in the recent PALLAS trial of high-risk patients with permanent atrial fibrillation, dronedarone was associated with an increase in the rate of stroke, heart failure, and cardiovascular death. Of note, 54% of the patients in PALLAS had NYHA class II-III heart failure. Given the increased adverse outcomes in ANDROMEDA and PALLAS, dronedarone should not be used in patients with heart failure or in permanent atrial fibrillation. The reason for the drastic differences in outcomes between ATHENA and PALLAS is unclear, but until further information is available, dronedarone should only be considered in selected low-risk patients with paroxysmal/persistent atrial fibrillation.

Dronedarone is also contraindicated with concomitant use of strong CYP3A inhibitors, severe hepatic failure, and concomitant use of drugs that prolong the QT interval. When hepatically cleared statins are used with dronedarone, lower doses of statin should be initiated, with titration as needed. Hepatic function should also be monitored, as there have been several case reports of fulminant hepatic failure with dronedarone. Caution should be exercised when used with other AV nodal blocking agents, including β-blockers and digoxin. Similar to amiodarone, small increases in creatinine have also been observed with dronedarone without significant change in underlying renal function.

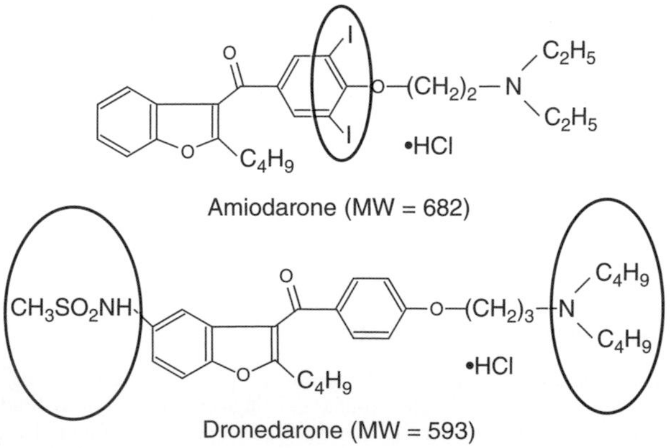

**FIGURE 58-7.** Compared with amiodarone, dronedarone is noniodinated and has butyl group on the terminal nitrogen and an additional methane sulfonyl group on the benzofuran moiety (note colored circles). (Reproduced with permission from Sun et al.)

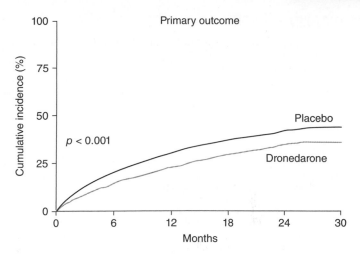

**FIGURE 58-8.** Compared with placebo, dronedarone decreased the primary composite outcome of hospitalization due to cardiovascular events or all-cause mortality by 24%. (Reproduced with permission from Hohnloser et al. Copyright © 2003 Massachusetts Medical Society. All rights reserved.)

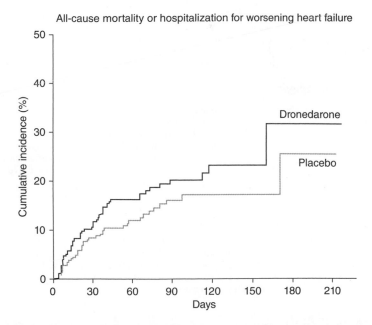

**FIGURE 58-9.** All-cause mortality or hospitalization for worsening heart failure was higher in dronedarone group compared with placebo. (Reproduced with permission from Kober et al. Copyright © 2008 Massachusetts Medical Society. All rights reserved.)

CHAPTER 58

# ■ DIGOXIN

Digoxin is a cardiac glycoside derived from the foxglove plant (*Digitalis purpurea*) that inhibits the sodium/potassium ATPase pump on the myocyte surface. This subsequently results in an increase in intracellular calcium and improves myocardial contractility. Digoxin also reduces conduction through the sinoatrial (SAN) and atrioventricular (AVN) nodes. These properties make digoxin a useful drug for the management of supraventricular tachyarrhythmia and left ventricular failure.

## Digoxin Toxicity

Digoxin toxicity can result in lethal cardiac arrhythmias and should be considered a medical emergency. Ideal serum digoxin levels are in the range of 0.5 to 0.9 ng/mL, and toxicity is more likely to occur when the level is 1.2 ng/mL or greater. Predisposing factors for digoxin toxicity include impaired renal function, hypokalemia, hypercalcemia, hypothyroidism, and advanced age.

The symptoms of digoxin toxicity are fairly nonspecific and include fatigue, nausea, vomiting, diarrhea, dizziness, and confusion. Digoxin at therapeutic levels produces fairly characteristic ECG changes, including PR segment prolongation and lateral ST-segment depression with a "scooped" pattern (**Fig. 58-10A**). Atrial and ventricular ectopy and variable AVN block represent early electrocardiographic manifestations of digoxin toxicity. Another characteristic ECG finding is atrial fibrillation with a slow ventricular response (Fig. 58-10B). The presence of a junctional escape rhythm in a patient taking digoxin is highly suggestive of digoxin toxicity, and the presence of bidirectional ventricular tachycardia is practically pathognomonic (Fig. 58-10C and D). Complete heart block, ventricular tachycardia, and ventricular fibrillation may occur in late-stage digoxin toxicity. The treatment of digoxin toxicity depends on the clinical presentation and degree of ECG derangement. Discontinuation of digoxin along with supportive measures such as telemetry monitoring, electrolyte repletion, and correction of renal insufficiency may suffice in milder cases. More severe cases of digoxin toxicity may require temporary transvenous pacing, intravenous lidocaine, or the infusion of digoxin-specific Fab fragments.

## Pharmacokinetic Interactions

Digoxin is metabolized in the stomach and small intestine by hydrolysis and eliminated by the kidneys. Anaerobic gastrointestinal bacteria contribute to digoxin metabolism in approximately one-third of American patients, although the contribution of gut flora to digoxin metabolism may vary by ethnicity or geography. Verapamil and quinidine increase serum digoxin levels by 60% to 90% by decreasing the renal and extrarenal clearance of the drug, and digoxin doses should be reduced by approximately half. Erythromycin increases serum digoxin levels by eradication of the gut bacteria responsible for digoxin hydrolysis.

## Pharmacodynamic Interactions

Digoxin may produce significant bradycardia when given in conjunction with calcium-channel blockers, β-blockers, and amiodarone. Spironolactone may interact with digoxin indirectly by promoting hyperkalemia, with subsequent attenuation of the effect of digoxin at its binding site on the ATPase pump. Conversely, thiazide and loop diuretics may promote digoxin toxicity by causing hypokalemia.

# ■ WARFARIN

Warfarin is a vitamin K antagonist that inhibits the synthesis of several vitamin K–dependent clotting factors, including factors II, VII, IX, and X. Warfarin has

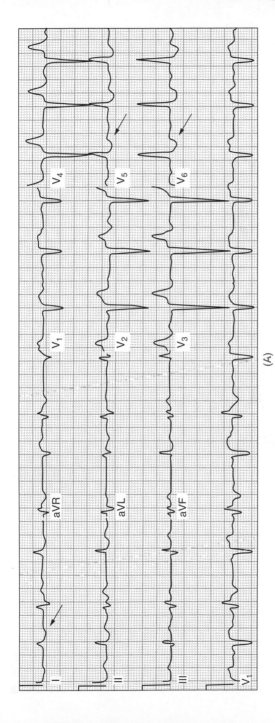

**FIGURE 58-10.** The electrophysiologic effects of digoxin. **A.** Digoxin effect. Please note the scooped ST-segment depressions (*arrows*). **B.** Atrial fibrillation with a slow ventricular response. Note the scooped ST segments (*arrows*) and ventricular premature contractions (VPC) (*star*). **C.** Atrial fibrillation with a junctional bradycardia. **D.** Bidirectional ventricular tachycardia. Note the wide QRS duration and undulating QRS axis (*arrows*). (Reproduced with permission from Kummer JL, Nair R, Krishnan SC. Images in cardiovascular medicine. Bidirectional ventricular tachycardia caused by digitalis toxicity. *Circulation*. 2006;113:e156-e157.)

(A)

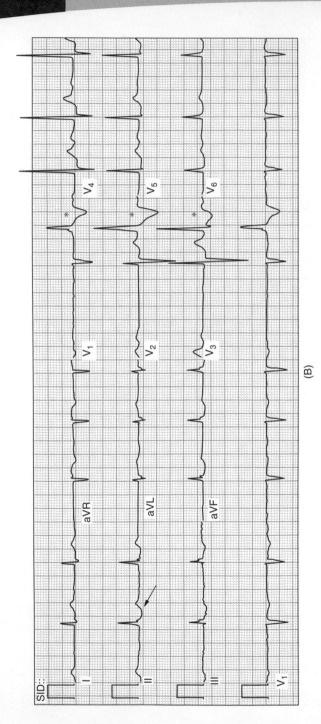

**FIGURE 58-10.** (Continued)

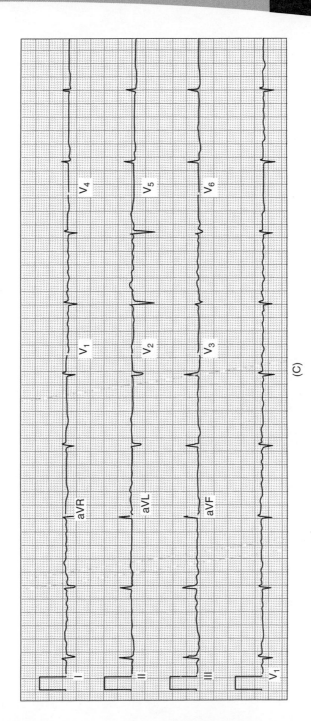

**FIGURE 58-10.** (*Continued*)

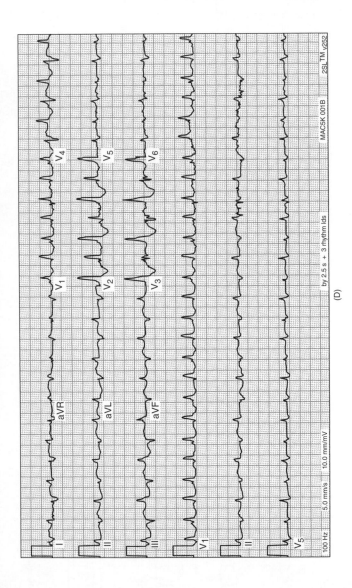

**FIGURE 58-10.** (*Continued*)

established efficacy in the prevention and treatment of thrombosis in atrial fibrillation, venous thromboembolic disease, and in patients with mechanical heart valves. Despite its widespread use, warfarin has a very narrow therapeutic window and carries a substantial risk for bleeding if the drug is not closely monitored. To date, more than 120 separate drug and food interactions involving warfarin have been reported.

## Warfarin Toxicity

The primary manifestation of warfarin overdose is pathologic bleeding. Patients with international normalized ratios (INR) >4 are at increased risk for significant bleeding compared with those with lower INR levels, although the incidence of serious bleeding in warfarin-treated patients presenting with INRs in the range of 5 to 9 was recently shown to be approximately 1%. One rare complication of warfarin therapy is warfarin skin necrosis, which tends to occur more commonly in women treated for deep vein thrombosis.

## Pharmacokinetic Interactions

Warfarin exists as a racemic mixture of 2 isomers, and the potency of the S-enantiomer is 5-fold greater than that of the R-enantiomer. The S-enantiomer undergoes oxidative metabolism via CYP 2C9, whereas the R-enantiomer is dependent on CYP 1A2 and 3A4 for metabolism. Thus, warfarin has the potential to interact with a wide range of CYP 450 inhibitors and inducers. Potent inhibitors of CYP 2C9, such as amiodarone, fluconazole, fluvastatin, sertraline, isoniazid, and lovastatin, reduce warfarin metabolism and contribute to bleeding risk. Closer monitoring of the INR and dose reduction is generally required. Quinolone and macrolide antibiotics also potentiate the effects of warfarin by inhibiting CYP 1A2 and 3A4, respectively. Despite the vast potential for drug-drug interactions, the likelihood and clinical significance of potential warfarin interactions can be difficult to predict. Holbrook and colleagues recently examined the medical literature to document which warfarin-drug and warfarin-food interactions are most probable based on published reports.

## Pharmacodynamic Interactions

The anticoagulant properties of warfarin may be attenuated by increased dietary vitamin K intake with vitamin K–rich foods such as kale, spinach, lettuce, broccoli, liver, avocado, and soy beans. Concurrent use of warfarin with drugs that alter platelet function (aspirin, clopidogrel, NSAIDs) or systemic anticoagulants (heparin, direct thrombin inhibitors) may result in pharmacodynamic bleeding.

## ■ NOVEL ORAL ANTICOAGULANTS

Two oral anticoagulants, dabigatran and rivaroxaban, have recently been approved for the prevention of thromboembolism in nonvalvular atrial fibrillation. A third agent, apixiban, was recently shown to be more effective than warfarin in nonvalvular atrial fibrillation but is not yet approved for clinical use. The advantage of these agents is that they do not require monitoring of the prothrombin time.

## Dabigatran

Dabigatran is an orally active direct thrombin inhibitor. In the RE-LY trial of patients with nonvalvular atrial fibrillation, dabigatran at 2 doses (150 mg twice daily and 110 mg twice daily) was compared to warfarin. The 110-mg dose was associated with similar rates of stroke and embolism as well as lower rates of major hemorrhage as compared to warfarin. The 150-mg dose was associated with lower rates of stroke and embolism but similar rates of major bleeding. In the United States, dabigatran is approved for the treatment of nonvalvular atrial fibrillation at the 150-mg dose. In addition, 75 mg twice daily is approved for patients with renal impairment based on pharmacokinetic modeling. The 150-mg and 110-mg dosages are available in Europe.

Dabigatran was well tolerated in RE-LY, with dyspepsia being the most common adverse reaction (11.8% of patients). Dabigatran does not interact with the cytochrome P450 system, but it is a substrate for the P-gp transporter system. Caution should be used when using drugs that affect the P-gp system such as ketoconazole and verapamil. Dabigatran is primarily eliminated by the kidneys, and patients with a creatinine clearance of <30 mL/min were excluded from RE-LY. In patients with moderate to severe renal dysfunction, dabigatran should be avoided or the dose should be lowered to limit the risk of hemorrhage. In addition, some advocate a lower dose of dabigatran in patients older than 75 years, as there was a trend toward increased bleeding in this population in RE-LY. There is currently no antidote to reverse dabigatran, but hemodialysis and activated factor VII or prothrombin complex concentrates can be considered in the event of life threatening bleeding.

## Rivaroxaban

Rivaroxaban is an oral factor Xa inhibitor that was approved in November 2011 by the FDA for the prevention of thromboembolism in nonvalvular atrial fibrillation. In the ROCKET-AF trial, rivaroxaban at a dose of 20 mg daily (15 mg daily in patients with creatinine clearance 30-49 mL/min) was noninferior to warfarin in preventing stroke and systemic embolism. While there was no difference in the overall rate of bleeding events, rivaroxaban was associated with significantly less intracranial hemorrhage and fatal bleeding. As with dabigatran, coagulation monitoring is not required for rivaroxaban. Of note, at the completion of ROCKET-AF when the blinded study medications were stopped, there were significantly more strokes in the rivaroxaban arm than in the warfarin arm (22 vs 6). Because of the possibility of a rebound phenomenon, the package label contains a black box warning about the possibility of an increased risk of stroke with discontinuation of rivaroxaban and recommends that the administration of another anticoagulant upon discontinuation should be considered.

Rivaroxaban is primarily eliminated by the kidneys, and it should not be used in patients with severe renal dysfunction. The 15-mg dose can be used in patients with moderate renal impairment. Rivaroxaban is metabolized by CYP3A4 and CYP2J2, and its use is contraindicated in patients with moderate to severe hepatic impairment. While drugs that affect both CYP3A4 and P-gp transport should not be used with rivaroxaban, agents that only affect either system appear to be safe for concomitant use. There is no specific antidote to reverse rivaroxaban, but prothrombin complex concentrates may be useful in the event of life-threatening hemorrhage.

# SUGGESTED READINGS

Pina IL, Oghlakian G. Adverse cardiovascular drug reactions and complications. In: Fuster V, Walsh R, Harrington RA, et al. *Hurst's The Heart*. 13th ed. New York, NY: McGraw-Hill; 2011:95:2096-2127.

Anderson JR, Nawarskas JJ. Cardiovascular drug-drug interactions. *Cardiol Clin*. 2001;19:215-234.

Bełtowski J, Wojcicka G, Jamroz-Wiśniewska A. Adverse effects of statins—mechanisms and consequences. *Curr Drug Saf*. 2009;4:209-228.

Enseleit F, Wyss CA, Duru F, Noll G, Ruschitzka F. Images in cardiovascular medicine. The blue man: amiodarone-induced skin discoloration. *Circulation*. 2006;113.

Hohnloser SH, Crijns HJGM, van Eickels M, et al. Effect of dronedarone on cardiovascular events in atrial fibrillation. *N Engl J Med*. 2009;360:668-678.

Holbrook AM, Pereira JA, Labiris R, et al. Systematic overview of warfarin and its drug and food interactions. *Arch Intern Med.* 2005;165:1095-1106.

Kober L, Torp-Pedersen C, McMurray JJV, et al. Increased mortality after dronedarone therapy for severe heart failure. *N Engl J Med.* 2008;358:2678-2687.

Kohler GI, Bode-Boger SM, Busse R, et al. Drug-drug interactions in medical patients: effects of in-hospital treatment and relation to multiple drug use. *Int J Clin Pharmacol Ther.* 2000;38:504-513.

Lazarou J, Pomeranz BH, Corey PN. Incidence of adverse drug reactions in hospitalized patients: a meta-analysis of prospective studies. *JAMA.* 1998;279:1200-1205.

Michalets EL. Update: clinically significant cytochrome P-450 drug interactions. *Pharmacotherapy.* 1998;18:84-112.

Oghlakian G, Klapholz M. Vasopressin and vasopressin receptor antagonists in heart failure. *Cardiol Rev.* 2009;17:10-15.

Page RL, Klem PM, Rogers C. Potential elevation of tacrolimus trough concentrations with concomitant metronidazole therapy. *Ann Pharmacother.* 2005;39:1109-1113.

Pirmohamed M, Breckenridge AM, Kitteringham NR, et al. Adverse drug reactions. *BMJ.* 1998;316:1295-1298.

SI, Cheng A, Frishman WH, et al. Cardiovascular drug therapy in patients with hepatic diseases and patients with congestive heart failure. *J Clin Pharmacol.* 2000;40:11-30.

Sun W, Sarma JS, Singh BN. Electrophysiological effects of dronedarone (SR33589), a noniodinated benzofuran derivative, in the rabbit heart: comparison with amiodarone. *Circulation.* 1999;100:2276-2281.

Trujillo TC, Nolan PE. Antiarrhythmic agents: drug interactions of clinical significance. *Drug Saf.* 2000;23:509-532.

# CHAPTER 59
# AGING AND CARDIOVASCULAR DISEASE IN THE ELDERLY

Wilson Young, Edward G. Lakatta, Samer S. Najjar,
Steven P. Schulman, and Gary Gerstenblith

The world population in both industrialized and developing countries is aging. In the United States, 35 million people are older than the age of 65 years, and the number of older Americans is expected to double by the year 2030. The clinical and economic implications of this demographic shift are staggering because age is the most powerful risk factor for cardiovascular diseases.

The incidence and prevalence of hypertension, coronary artery disease, congestive heart failure, and stroke, the quintessential diseases of Western society, increase steeply with advancing age (**Fig. 59-1**). Although epidemiologic studies have discovered that some aspects of lifestyle and genetics are risk factors for these diseases, age, per se, confers the major risk. There is a continuum of age-related alterations of cardiovascular structure and function in healthy humans. These changes appear to influence the steep increases in hypertension, atherosclerosis, stroke, left ventricular hypertrophy, chronic heart failure, and atrial fibrillation with increasing age. Specific pathophysiologic mechanisms that underlie these diseases become superimposed on cardiac and vascular substrates that have been modified by an "aging process," and the latter modulates disease occurrence and severity. In other words, age-associated changes in cardiovascular structure and function become "partners" with pathophysiologic disease mechanisms, lifestyle, and genetics in determining the threshold, severity, prognosis, and therapeutic response of cardiovascular disease in older persons.

The nature of age-disease interactions is complex and involves mechanisms of aging, multiple defined disease risk factors, and as yet undefined risk factors. The role of specific age-associated changes in cardiovascular structure and function in such age-disease interactions has not been considered in most epidemiologic studies of cardiovascular disease.

Quantitative information on age-associated alterations in cardiovascular structure and function in health is essential to unravel age-disease interactions and to target the specific characteristics of cardiovascular aging that render it such a major risk factor for cardiovascular diseases. Such information is also of practical value to differentiate between the limitations of an older person that relate to disease and those that might be expected, within limits, to accompany advancing age or a sedentary lifestyle. During the past 3 decades, a sustained effort has been applied to characterize the effects of aging in health on multiple aspects of cardiovascular structure and function in a single study population, the Baltimore Longitudinal Study on Aging (BLSA). These community-dwelling volunteers are rigorously screened to detect both clinical and occult cardiovascular disease and are characterized with respect to lifestyle (eg, exercise habits) in an attempt to clarify the interactions of disease, risk factors, and aging itself. Perspectives gleaned from these studies are emphasized throughout this chapter.

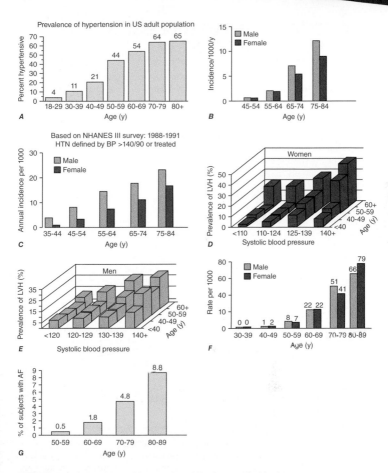

**FIGURE 59-1. A.** Prevalence of hypertension, defined as systolic blood pressure ≥140 mm Hg or diastolic blood pressure ≥90 mm Hg or current use of medication for purposes of treating high blood pressure. Data are based on National Health and Nutrition Examination Survey (NHANES) III (1988-1991). **B.** Incidence of atherothrombotic stroke (per 1000 subjects per year) by age in men and women from the Framingham Heart Study. **C.** Incidence of coronary heart disease by age in men and women from the Framingham Heart Study. **D.** Prevalence of echocardiographic left ventricular hypertrophy (LVH) in women according to baseline age and systolic blood pressure. **E.** Prevalence of echocardiographic LVH in men according to baseline age and systolic blood pressure. **F.** Prevalence of heart failure by age in men and women from the Framingham Heart Study. **G.** Prevalence of atrial fibrillation (AF) by age in subjects from the Framingham Heart Study. (A to C. data compiled from Burt VL, Whelton P, Roccella EJ, et al. Prevalence of hypertension in the US adult population: results from the Third National Health and Nutrition Examination Survey, 1988-1991. *Hypertension*. 1995;25:305-313; Wolf PA. Lewis A. Conner lecture: contributions of epidemiology to the prevention of stroke. *Circulation*. 1993;88:2471-2478; Kannel WB, Wolf PA, Garrison RJ, eds. Framingham Study: An Epidemiological Investigation of Cardiovascular Disease. Section 34. NIH Publication No.87-2703. Bethesda, MD: National Heart, Lung and Blood Institute; 1987. D to G, data compiled from Levy D, Anderson KM, Savage DD, et al. Echocardiographically detected left ventricular hypertrophy: prevalence and risk factors: the Framingham Heart Study. *Ann Intern Med*. 1988;108:7-13; Ho KK, Pinsky JL, Kannel WB, et al. The epidemiology of heart failure: the Framingham Study. *J Am Coll Cardiol*. 1993;22:6A-13A; Wolf PA, Abbott RD, Kannel WB. Atrial fibrillation as an independent risk factor for stroke: the Framingham Study. *Stroke*. 1991;22:983-988.)

# SUCCESSFUL VERSUS UNSUCCESSFUL CARDIOVASCULAR AGING

To define why age (or an aging process × exposure time) is so risky, the specific components of the risk associated with age must be identified. Two complementary approaches have evolved. Epidemiologists search for novel measures of "subclinical disease" (in addition to the more established risk factors that are already well characterized) in large, unselected cohorts composed of persons both with and without cardiovascular disease. In contrast, gerontologists attempt to develop quantitative information on cardiovascular structure and function in apparently healthy individuals to define the specific characteristics of aging that render it such a major risk factor for cardiovascular disease, even in the absence of clinically apparent comorbidity. The latter approach consists of identifying and selecting community-dwelling individuals who do not have (or have not yet experienced) clinical disease and who do not have occult disease that can be detected by noninvasive methods. These individuals are then grouped by age and stratified according to the level of a given variable, which may include some of the novel measures of subclinical disease identified by the epidemiologists. If the variable is perceived as beneficial or deleterious with respect to cardiovascular structure or function, those with extreme measures are considered to be aging "successfully" or "unsuccessfully," respectively. Unsuccessful aging in this context is not synonymous with having clinical disease, because individuals with defined overt or occult clinical disease have been excluded from consideration a priori. Instead, unsuccessful aging, that is, falling within the poorest category with respect to the measure viewed as deleterious, may be viewed as a risk factor for future clinical cardiovascular disease. In this regard, unsuccessful aging is a manifestation of the interaction of the cardiovascular aging process and specific aspects of vascular disease pathophysiology. Thus, gerontologists and epidemiologists have become part of a joint effort in the quest to define why aging confers enormous risk for cardiovascular disease.

# AGE-ASSOCIATED CHANGES IN ARTERIAL STRUCTURE AND FUNCTION

Close examination of the age-associated changes in arterial structure and function may help explain why aging is such a strong predictor of adverse events. Findings from clinical studies show that the age-associated changes in arterial structure and function are risk factors for cardiovascular diseases. These novel risk factors, including intimal-medial thickness, arterial stiffness, and endothelial dysfunction, alter the substrate upon which the cardiovascular diseases are superimposed; therefore, they affect the development, manifestation, severity, and prognosis of these diseases.

Many age-associated changes are seen in the large arteries of humans. Cross-sectional studies show that central elastic arteries dilate with age, leading to an increase in lumen size (**Fig. 59-2A**), which results in increased inertance. In addition, postmortem studies have indicated an age-associated increase in arterial wall thickening, which is caused mainly by an increase in intimal thickening. In cross-sectional studies, carotid intimal-medial thickening increases nearly 3-fold between the ages of 20 and 90 years (Fig. 59-2B). Both the average and range of intimal-medial thickness values are greater at higher ages, suggesting heterogeneity in the magnitude of the age-associated thickening process among older individuals. The increase in arterial wall thickening is accompanied by an increase in arterial stiffening (reduction in compliance) (Fig. 59-2C), which is due to structural changes: increase in collagen content, cross-linking of adjacent collagen molecules to form advanced glycation end products, fraying of elastin, a decrease in the amount of elastin, and deposition of calcium in the medial layer. Functional alterations include an age-associated deterioration in vascular endothelial vasoreactivity.

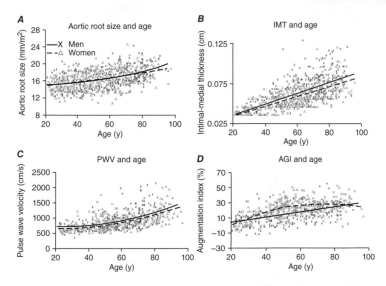

**FIGURE 59-2.** Age-associated changes in arterial structure and function in healthy Baltimore Longitudinal Study of Aging volunteer men (*x*) and women (Δ). Best fit regression lines (quadratic or linear) are shown for men (*solid lines*) and women (*dotted lines*). **A**. Aortic root size, measured via M-mode echocardiography. **B**. Common carotid intimal-medial thickness (IMT) as a function of age and sex. Note that the range of values for IMT is much greater in older individuals than in younger ones. **C**. Carotid-femoral pulse wave velocity (PWV). **D**. Carotid arterial augmentation index (AGI), which is defined as the ratio of the distance from the inflection point to the peak of the arterial waveform, over the pulse pressure. Note that unlike PWV, which increases quadratically with age, the age-associated increase in AGI is linear in men and convex shape in women, suggesting that factors other than stiffness also modulate the origin of reflected waves and the amplitude of AGI. (Reproduced with permission from Najjar SS, Scuteri A, Lakatta EG. Arterial aging: is it an immutable cardiovascular risk factor? *Hypertension.* 2005;46:454-462.)

# ■ BLOOD PRESSURE

Both systolic and pulse pressures increase with age in all adults, whereas diastolic blood pressure increases until the fifth decade of life and then levels off before decreasing after 60 years of age (**Fig. 59-3**). These age-dependent changes in systolic, diastolic, and pulse pressures are consistent with the idea that in younger people, blood pressure is determined largely by peripheral vascular resistance, whereas in older people, blood pressure is determined mainly by the stiffness of central conduit vessels.

In older individuals, isolated systolic hypertension SBP>140 and DBP<90 mm Hg is the most common form of hypertension that may be attributed to arterial stiffening. Even mild isolated systolic hypertension (stage 1) is associated with an appreciable increase in cardiovascular disease risk and is an indication for treatment. Although past guidelines for systolic blood pressure in diabetics <135 mm Hg, JNC guidelines suggest <130 mm Hg.

Systolic blood pressure and pulse pressure in the central aorta may differ from the values that are measured more distally along the arterial tree due to blood pressure amplification across the arterial tree. Even though peripheral systolic and pulse pressure increase with age, the central to peripheral pressure amplification decreases with age. Studies have shown that central blood pressures are independent predictors of

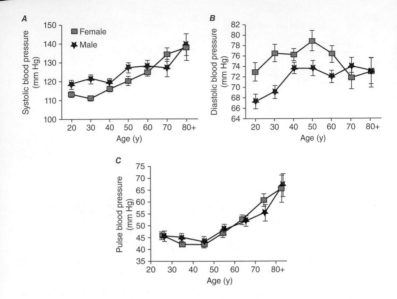

**FIGURE 59-3.** Average systolic (**A**), diastolic (**B**), and pulse (**C**) pressures and age in Baltimore Longitudinal Study of Aging participants stratified by sex. Values are mean ± standard error of mean (SEM). (From Lakatta EG, Levy D. Arterial and cardiac aging: major shareholders in cardiovascular disease enterprises: part I. Aging arteries: a "set up" for vascular disease. *Circulation*. 2003;107:139-146.)

outcomes and may even be better predictors of cardiovascular mortality than peripheral blood pressures. The usefulness and feasibility of integrating measurements of central arterial blood pressures into routine medical practice are areas of intense ongoing research.

## ■ INTIMAL-MEDIAL THICKNESS

Studies of morphologic, cellular, enzymatic, and biochemical changes in animal models have increased our understanding of age-associated arterial remodeling in humans. For example, the age-associated intimal-medial thickening seen in humans is often ascribed to "subclinical" atherosclerosis. This idea has become so well accepted that intimal-medial thickening is used by some investigators as a surrogate measure of atherosclerosis. Intimal-medial thickening, which is usually measured in areas devoid of atherosclerotic plaque, is only weakly associated with the extent and severity of coronary artery disease. Furthermore, findings in rodent and nonhuman primate models of aging clearly indicate that intimal-medial thickening is an age-related process that is separate from atherosclerosis because atherosclerosis is absent in both of these animal models. Thus, excessive intimal-medial thickening is not necessarily synonymous with early or subclinical atherosclerosis.

An association between intimal-medial thickening and atherosclerosis has been documented in humans. In individuals rigorously screened for the absence of clinical cardiovascular disease, excessive intimal-medial thickening at a given age predicts silent coronary artery disease (**Fig. 59-4A**), which, in turn, progresses to symptomatic ischemic heart disease. In the Atherosclerosis Risk in Communities (ARIC) study, which comprised middle-aged adults, intimal-medial thickening was associated with

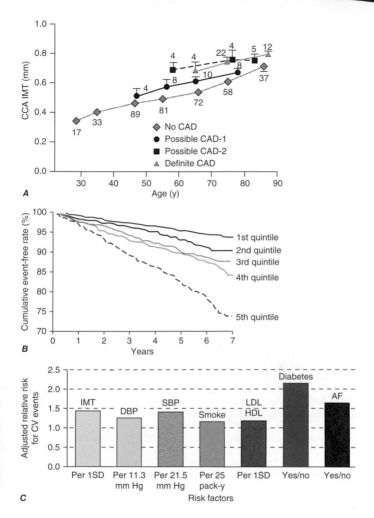

**FIGURE 59-4.** Carotid intimal-medial thickness (IMT) and cardiovascular diseases. **A**. Common carotid artery IMT (CCA-IMT) as a function of age, stratified by coronary artery disease (CAD) classification, in Baltimore Longitudinal Study of Aging subjects. CAD-1 denotes a subset with positive exercise electrocardiogram (ECG) but negative thallium scans; CAD-2 represents a subset with concordant positive exercise ECG and thallium scans. **B**. Common carotid IMT as a predictor of future cardiovascular events in the Cardiovascular Health Study (CHS). Note the nonlinear increase in the risk for cardiovascular event rates with increasing quintiles. **C**. Comparisons of the associations of age- and sex-adjusted cardiovascular risk factors with the combined events of stroke or myocardial infarction in the CHS study, using Cox proportional hazards models. Note that IMT is a potent risk factor for future cardiovascular events. 1SD, one standard deviation; AF, atrial fibrillation; CV, cardiovascular; DBP, diastolic blood pressure; HDL, high-density lipoprotein; LDL, low-density lipoprotein; SBP, systolic blood pressure. (A and C, reproduced with permission from Lakatta EG, Levy D. Arterial and cardiac aging: major shareholders in cardiovascular disease enterprises: part I. Aging arteries: a "set up" for vascular disease. *Circulation*. 2003; Jan 7;107(1):139-146.) (B, reproduced with permission from O'Leary DH, Polak JF, Kronmal RA, et al. Carotid artery intima and media thickness as a risk factor for myocardial infarction and stroke in older adults. Cardiovascular Health Study Collaborative Research Group. *N Engl J Med*. 1999;Jan 8;340(1):14-22.)

a greater prevalence of cardiovascular diseases and was an independent predictor of stroke. In the Cardiovascular Health Study (CHS), which comprised individuals older than age 65 years, intimal-medial thickening was an independent predictor of future myocardial infarction and stroke. In the CHS study, subjects were grouped according to quintiles of intimal-medial thickening, and the results indicated a nonlinear gradation in risk, with higher quintiles conferring a greater risk for cardiovascular diseases (Fig. 59-4B). Compared with the lowest quintile, the fifth quintile had a 3.15 relative risk for cardiovascular events, even after adjusting for traditional risk factors. In fact, the strength of intimal-medial thickening as a risk factor for cardiovascular diseases equals or exceeds that of most other traditional risk factors (Fig. 59-4C).

Thus, intimal-medial thickening is not a manifestation of atherosclerosis but is associated with it. Intimal-medial thickening is an aging-related process that is separate from the pathophysiologic process of atherosclerosis, yet intimal thickening is a risk factor for atherosclerosis.

Studying the relationship between primary age-associated vascular wall remodeling and cardiovascular diseases has led researchers to search for new phenotypic manifestations of arterial remodeling to explore their clinical and prognostic significance. For example, the various carotid geometric patterns that are derived by combining the measurements of vascular mass with wall-to-lumen ratio were recently associated with unique functional and hemodynamic profiles that are largely independent of age and hypertension. These patterns were recently found to have differing prognostic implications.

## ◼ ARTERIAL STIFFNESS

In addition to intimal-medial thickening, increased arterial stiffness has been observed with advancing age in humans and in animal models of aging. Strictly speaking, stiffness and its inverse, distensibility, depend on intrinsic structural properties of the blood vessel wall that relate a change in pressure with a corresponding change in volume. However, in this chapter, the terms *stiffness* and *compliance* are used in a broader sense to denote the overall lumped stiffness and compliance, which include the additional effects of vascular tone, blood pressure, and other modulating factors, all of which impact left ventricular (LV) afterload. Of note, in contrast to central arteries, the stiffness of muscular arteries does not increase with advancing age. Thus, the manifestations of arterial aging may vary among the different vascular beds, reflecting differences in the structural compositions of the arteries and, perhaps, differences in the age-associated signaling cascades that modulate the arterial properties or differences in the response to these signals across the arterial tree.

## ◼ PULSE WAVE VELOCITY

With each systolic contraction of the ventricle, a propagation wave that is generated in the arterial wall travels down the arterial tree. This propagation wave accompanies (and slightly precedes) the luminal flow wave generated during systole. The velocity of propagation of this wave is determined by the intrinsic stress-strain relationship of the vascular wall and by the smooth muscle tone, reflected by the mean arterial pressure.

The availability of noninvasive measures of the velocity of this pulse wave allows for large-scale epidemiologic studies. Pulse wave velocity was assessed in BLSA participants who were rigorously screened for the absence of overt or silent cardiovascular disease and in other populations with varying degrees of prevalence of cardiovascular disease. In all these studies, a significant age-associated increase in pulse wave velocity has been observed in both men and women.

Several clinical studies have recently shown the adverse cardiovascular effects of accelerated vascular stiffening. In the ARIC study, several indices of arterial compliance were predictors of hypertension. In the BLSA, pulse wave velocity was an independent predictor of incident hypertension. In hypertensive patients, pulse wave velocity was a marker of cardiovascular risk and coronary events and was an independent predictor of mortality. In addition, pulse wave velocity was an independent predictor of mortality in population-based studies, in subjects older than 70 years of age and in patients with end-stage renal disease (**Fig. 59-5A**). Other noninvasive indices of vascular compliance, including stroke volume divided by pulse pressure and the incremental modulus of elasticity, are also independent predictors of adverse outcomes. Thus, arterial stiffening, like intimal-medial thickening, should be viewed as another marker of aging, which, when accelerated, also becomes a risk factor for cardiovascular diseases.

The interaction between vascular wall stiffening and cardiovascular diseases may set in motion a vicious cycle. Pulse wave velocity is determined, in part, by smooth muscle cell tone, which, in turn, is partially regulated by endothelial cells. Moreover, endothelial dysfunction occurs early in several cardiovascular disorders including atherosclerosis, diabetes, and hypertension. Thus, in this cycle, alterations in the mechanical properties of the vessel wall contribute to endothelial cell dysfunction and, ultimately, vascular stiffening.

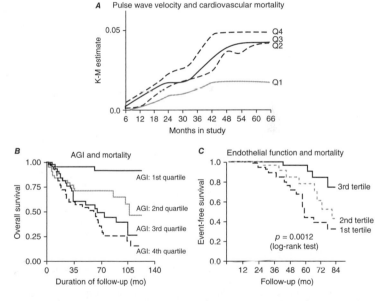

**FIGURE 59-5.** Markers of arterial aging are risk factors for adverse cardiovascular outcomes. **A.** Pulse wave velocity is a predictor of cardiovascular mortality in community-dwelling older subjects. This association remained significant after adjusting for age, sex, race, systolic blood pressure, known cardiovascular disease, and other variables related to events. K-M, Kaplan-Meier; Q, quartile. **B.** Probability of overall survival in patients with end-stage renal failure, stratified by quartiles of augmentation index (AGI). **C.** Probability of event-free survival in never treated hypertensive patients, stratified by tertiles of endothelial dysfunction. (**A,** reproduced with permission from Sutton-Tyrrell K, Najjar SS, Boudreau RM, et al. Health ABC study. Elevated aortic pulse wave velocity, a marker of arterial stiffness, predicts cardiovascular events in well-functioning older adults. *Circulation.* 2005;111:3384-3390.) (**B,** reproduced with permission from London GM, Blacher J, Pannier B, et al. Arterial wave reflections and survival in end-stage renal failure. *Hypertension.* 2001;38:434-438.) (**C,** from Perticone F, Ceravolo R, Pujia A, et al. Prognostic significance of endothelial dysfunction in hypertensive patients. *Circulation.* 2001;104:191-196.)

# ■ REFLECTED WAVES

In addition to the forward pulse wave, each cardiac cycle generates a reflected wave, which travels back up the arterial tree toward the central aorta. This reflected wave, which probably originates in the smaller arteries and arterioles, alters the arterial pressure waveform and is modulated, in part, by nitric oxide. The velocity of the reflected flow wave is proportional to the stiffness of the arterial wall. Thus, in young individuals with compliant vasculature, the reflected wave reaches the large elastic arteries in diastole. With advancing age and vascular stiffening, velocity of the reflected wave increases, and the wave reaches the central circulation earlier systole.

This reflected wave can be noninvasively assessed from the carotid or radial arterial pulse waveforms by arterial applanation tonometry and high-fidelity micromanometer probes. The difference in pressures between those at the inflection point (arrival of reflected wave) and at the peak of the arterial waveform is the pressure pulse augmentation that is due to the early arrival of the reflected wave. Dividing this augmentation by the pulse pressure) yields the augmentation index. The augmentation index (difference in pressure from peak to inflection point divided by pulse pressure), like the pulse wave velocity, increases with age in early and mid-adulthood (Fig. 59-2D). However, unlike pulse wave velocity, the rate of increase in the augmentation index decreases at older age, particularly in women.

Although attention has focused on the transmission velocity of reflected waves as an index of arterial stiffness, evaluation of the pulse wave contour may provide valuable insight into the characteristics and the pathology of more distal vessels, where reflected waves originate.

The pressure pulse augmentation provided by the early return of the reflected wave is an added load against which the ventricle must contract. Furthermore, the loss of the diastolic augmentation present in compliant vessels caused by the late return of the reflected waves decreases diastolic blood pressure and thus has the potential to reduce coronary blood flow. These considerations suggest that excessively early return of the reflected waves may be detrimental to the cardiovascular system. In fact, the augmentation index has been shown to be a predictor of adverse events in end-stage renal disease patients (Fig. 59-5B). Thus, this index is another marker of vascular aging that is a risk factor for cardiovascular diseases.

# ■ PULSE PRESSURE

The combination of arterial wall stiffening and early return of the reflected waves widens the pulse pressure. Age-associated decreased elasticity also increases the systolic pressure for any given volume of ejected blood and lowers diastolic pressure by diminishing elastic recoil. Thus, pulse pressure is a useful hemodynamic marker of the vascular stiffness of conduit arteries. Clinical and epidemiologic studies in several different populations with varying prevalences of cardiovascular diseases have confirmed the prognostic importance of pulse pressure. Furthermore, in several studies, pulse pressure was a stronger predictor of outcome than were systolic or diastolic blood pressures.

# ■ ARTERIAL STIFFNESS AND HYPERTENSION

Recent studies showing that increased vascular stiffness may precede the development of hypertension have underscored the relationship between hypertension and arterial wall stiffening. An increase in mean arterial pressure (or peripheral resistance) can lead to a secondary increase in large-artery stiffness; however, the primary age-associated increase in large-artery stiffness can lead to an increase in arterial pressures. Thus, hypertension can be defined as a disease that is, in part, determined or modulated by properties of the arterial wall.

# ■ ENDOTHELIAL FUNCTION

Endothelial cells are extremely important and powerful regulators of the vasculature (see Chapter 8). Several cardiovascular conditions and risk factors are associated with endothelial dysfunction, including hypercholesterolemia, insulin resistance, cigarette smoking, and heart failure. Endothelial cell dysfunction contributes to the pathogenesis of hypertension and atherosclerosis. In addition, endothelial cells play a pivotal role in regulating vascular tone, vascular permeability, angiogenesis, and the response to inflammation. Endothelial-derived substances (eg, nitric oxide [NO] and endothelin-1) are determinants of large-artery compliance, suggesting that endothelial cells may modulate arterial stiffness. Endothelial function in central arteries, however, has not been directly assessed in humans. In the brachial artery, endothelial function, as assessed by agonist- or flow-mediated vasoreactivity, declines with advancing age. Several studies have demonstrated that impaired endothelial vasoreactivity, in both the coronary and peripheral arterial beds, is an independent predictor of future cardiovascular events (Fig. 59-5C).

# ■ VASOREACTIVITY

With advancing age, NO-dependent mechanical and agonist-mediated endothelial vasodilatation is reduced in humans and animals. This vasoreactivity depends on NO generated by endothelial nitric oxide synthase (eNOS). In aging rats, activity of the eNOS isoform is markedly reduced. In addition, the bioavailability of NO may be reduced due to age-associated increase in the amounts of superoxide and nitrated tyrosine residues of proteins.

# ■ INFLAMMATION

Aging is associated with increased expression of adhesion molecules in rats and increased adherence of monocytes to the endothelial surface in rabbits. Adhesion molecules on the luminal surface of endothelial cells mediate leukocyte binding to endothelial cells and subendothelial migration. This process is probably facilitated by the actions of matrix metalloproteinases (MMPs). Serum levels of adhesion molecules show age-associated alterations in humans. In patients with hypercholesterolemia and ischemic heart disease, serum levels of soluble vascular cell adhesion molecule-1, but not soluble intercellular adhesion molecule-1 (ICAM-1), are positively associated with aging.

# ■ PERMEABILITY

In rat aortas, aging is associated with increased permeability to albumin. Moreover, glycosaminoglycans, which help regulate several arterial properties including vascular permeability, accumulate in greater number in the intima of older rabbits. Within hours of an acute arterial balloon injury to the rabbit carotid artery, the pericellular distribution of glycosaminoglycans is significantly reduced in the arterial wall, associated with a significant expansion of the extracellular space. The glycosaminoglycans are rapidly replaced in the media but not in the developing neointima by smooth muscle cells. Additionally, aging promotes endothelial cell permeability and stiffening of extracellular matrix in in vitro and ex-vivo mouse models.

# ■ ENDOTHELIAL DYSFUNCTION AND CELLULAR SENESCENCE

Telomeres are specialized DNA-protein complexes that form the ends of chromosomes, and they have been proposed as possible indicators of biologic, as opposed to chronologic, aging. Telomeres shorten with each replicative cell division, unless they are rescued by the enzyme telomerase reverse transcriptase. When telomere length reaches a critical size, the cell becomes senescent. Telomere length is inversely associated with atherosclerotic grade and chronologic age in endothelial cells from human abdominal aorta, iliac arteries, and iliac veins. In a study of Danish twins, telomere length of chromosomes in white blood cells was negatively associated with pulse pressure. In a normotensive French cohort, telomere length of chromosomes in white blood cells was longer in women than in men but was associated with variations in pulse pressure and pulse wave velocity only in men. Loss of telomere function induces endothelial dysfunction in vascular endothelial cells, whereas inhibition of telomere shortening suppresses age-associated dysfunction in these cells. The impact of telomere-induced vascular senescence may be accentuated in older individuals, in whom studies indicate that the number and activity of progenitor cells is reduced, suggesting an age-associated diminution in regenerative capacity, which may contribute to the age-associated impairment in angiogenesis.

## ■ ENDOTHELIAL DYSFUNCTION AND ANGIOGENESIS

Endothelial cells play a pivotal role in angiogenesis, in which new vessels grow from the existing microvasculature. Angiogenesis requires the migration and proliferation of endothelial cells in response to cytokines. The age-associated impairment in angiogenesis is partly a result of changes in the levels of extracellular enzymes, matrix proteins, and growth factors that affect endothelial cell migration.

## ARTERIAL AGING IN CARDIOVASCULAR DISEASES

Although the aforementioned changes in arterial structure and function with aging were previously thought to be part of normative aging, this concept was challenged when data emerged showing that these changes are accelerated in the presence of cardiovascular diseases and, as noted earlier, that they are risk factors for cardiovascular morbidity and mortality.

Patients with hypertension exhibit greater carotid wall thickness, central arterial stiffness, and central pressure augmentation than do normotensive subjects, even after adjusting for age. They are thought to have higher central arterial diameters, although this is presently debated. Hypertensive individuals exhibit endothelial dysfunction, and the mechanisms underlying their endothelial dysfunction are similar to the ones that occur with normotensive aging, albeit they appear at an earlier age. Normotensive offspring of hypertensives also exhibit endothelial dysfunction, suggesting that endothelial dysfunction may precede the development of clinical hypertension. Among hypertensive men, shorter telomere length of circulating white blood cells is associated with greater arterial stiffness. Prevalent among older individuals, the metabolic syndrome, is associated with elevated carotid arterial thickness and stiffness. Diabetics also exhibit higher carotid intimal-medial thickness than nondiabetics and accelerated progression of intimal-medial thickness. Although central arterial stiffness is increased, it is not accompanied by an increase in the central pressure augmentation. Diabetics also exhibit endothelial dysfunction, as do their insulin resistant first-degree relatives.

The circulating white blood cells of insulin-dependent diabetics have shorter telomere lengths than those from normoglycemic controls or non–insulin-dependent diabetics. Patients with atherosclerosis have increased thickness and stiffness of their central arterial walls, greater central pressure augmentation, and shorter telomere lengths on their circulating white blood cells. They also exhibit endothelial dysfunction, implicated in the pathogenesis of atherosclerosis and an early pathologic manifestation.

# AGE-ASSOCIATED CHANGES IN CARDIAC STRUCTURE AND FUNCTION IN PERSONS WITHOUT A HEART DISEASE DIAGNOSIS

## ■ LV PRELOAD AND AFTERLOAD

Overall cardiovascular structure and function vary dramatically among older individuals. Rather, interactions among aging, disease, and lifestyle must be considered in interpreting age-associated changes in cardiovascular structure and function as measured in various studies.

A unified interpretation of identified cardiac changes that accompany advancing age, in otherwise healthy persons, suggests that, at least in part, these are adaptive, occurring in response to arterial changes that occur with aging (**Fig. 59-6A**). Central arterial stiffening and an increase in systolic and pulse pressures produce a late increased vascular impedance, moderate increase in LV wall tension, and increase in LV wall thickness (Fig. 59-6A, B), due to an increase in ventricular myocyte size and due to modest increase in collagen levels. Large population studies demonstrate that arterial pressure, varies directly with vascular loading, is a major determinant of LV mass, and the relative impact of age and arterial pressure on LV wall thickness varies with the manner in which study subjects are screened with respect to hypertension. The increase in LV wall thickness with aging reduces the expected increase in cardiac afterload caused by increased LV volume in older persons during stress (**Table 59-1**).

Prolonged contraction of the thickened LV wall maintains a normal ejection time in the presence of the late augmentation of aortic impedance preserving the systolic cardiac pumping function at rest. One disadvantage of prolonged contraction is that, at mitral valve opening, myocardial relaxation is more incomplete in individuals and causes the early LV filling rate reduction (Fig. 59-6C). Structural changes and functional heterogeneity within the LV with aging also contribute to this reduction in peak LV filling rate. Adaptations—left atrial enlargement and an enhanced atrial contribution to ventricular filling (Fig. 59-6D)—compensate for the reduced early filling and prevent reduction in end-diastolic volume. Age-associated changes in tissue levels or responses (to growth factors, catecholamines, angiotensin II, endothelin, transforming growth factor β [TGFβ], or fibroblast growth factor) that influence myocardial or vascular cells or their extracellular matrices (see Lessons Learned About Cardiac Aging From Animal Models) may also have a role in the schema depicted in Fig. 59-6A.

Biologic sex is an important factor in the physiology and pathophysiology of the cardiovascular system, including the aging heart. Postmortem morphometric assessments in nonfailing human hearts showed extensive age-related myocyte loss and hypertrophy of the surviving myocytes in males but preserved ventricular myocardial mass, average cell diameter and volume in aging female hearts. These sex differences stem from differences in the replicative potential of cardiac myocytes. Analysis of gene expression differences by sex and age in LV samples from patients with dilated cardiomyopathy has identified more than 1800 genes displaying sexual dimorphism in the heart. A number of these genes were highly represented in gene ontology pathways involved in ion transport and G-protein–coupled receptor signaling.

Impaired heart rate acceleration and impaired augmentation of blood ejection from the LV, accompanied by an acute increase in LV end-diastolic volume, dramatic changes in cardiac reserve capacity that occur with aging in healthy, community-dwelling persons (see Table 58-1). Mechanisms of the age-associated reduction in cardiovascular reserve are multifactorial and include (1) a reduction in intrinsic myocardial contractility; (2) an increase in vascular afterload (ventricular load is the opposition to myocardial contraction and the ejection of blood; afterload is the component of load that pertains to the time following excitation, as opposed to preload,

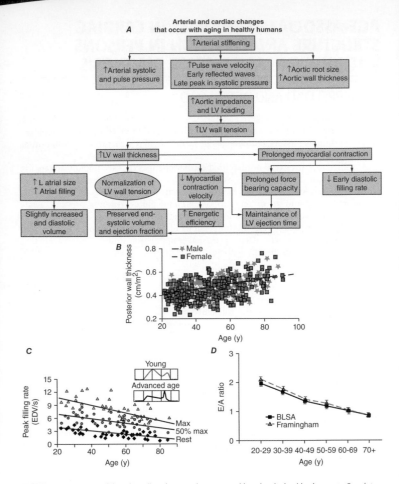

**FIGURE 59-6. A.** Arterial and cardiac changes that occur with aging in healthy humans. One interpretation (flow of arrows) of the constellation is that vascular changes lead to cardiac structural and functional alterations that maintain cardiac function. L, left; LV, left ventricular. **B.** Left ventricular posterior wall thickness, measured by M-mode echocardiography, increases with age in healthy Baltimore Longitudinal Study on Aging (BLSA) men and women. Note that the marked age-associated increase in left ventricular wall thickness in these healthy BLSA participants is within what is considered to be the clinically "normal" range. **C.** Maximum left ventricular filling rate at rest and during vigorous cycle exercise assessed via equilibrium gated blood-pool scans in healthy volunteers from the BLSA. EDV, end-diastolic volume. **D.** The ratio of early left ventricular diastolic filling rate (E) to the atrial filling component (A) declines with aging, and the extent of this E/A decline with aging in healthy BLSA volunteers is identical to that in participants of the Framingham Study. (**A**, from the Merck Manual of Geriatrics, 2nd edition, edited by William B. Abrams, Mark H. Beers, and Robert Berkow. Copyright 1995 by Merck Sharp & Dohme Corp., a subsidiary of Merck & Co, Inc, Whitehouse Station, NJ.) (**B**, reproduced with permission from Gerstenblith G, Frederiksen J, Yin FC, et al. Echocardiographic assessment of a normal adult aging population. *Circulation.* 1977;56:273-278.) (**C**, reproduced with permission from Schulman SP, Lakatta EG, Fleg JL, et al. Age-related decline in left ventricular filling at rest and exercise. *Am J Physiol.* 1992;263:H1932-H1938.) (**D**, reproduced with permission from Lakatta EG, Levy D. Arterial and cardiac aging: major shareholders in cardiovascular disease enterprises: part II: the aging heart in health: links to heart disease. *Circulation.* 2003;107:346-354.)

**TABLE 59-1.** Exhaustive Upright Exercise: Changes in Aerobic Capacity and Cardiac Regulation Between Ages of 20 and 80 years in Healthy Men and Women

| | |
|---|---|
| Oxygen consumption | ⇊ (50%) |
| (A-V)O$_2$ | ⇊ (25%) |
| Cardiac index | ⇊ (25%) |
| Heart rate | ⇊ (25%) |
| Stroke volume | No Δ |
|   Preload | |
|     EDV | ⇈ (30%) |
|   Afterload | ⇈ |
|     Vascular (PVR) | ⇈ (30%) |
|     Cardiac (ESV) | ⇈ (275%) |
|     Cardiac (EDV) | ⇈ (30%) |
|   Contractility | ⇊ (60%) |
| Ejection fraction | ⇊ (15%) |
| Plasma catecholamines | ⇈ |
| Cardiac and vascular | ⇊ |
| Responses to β-adrenergic stimulation | |

EDV, end-diastolic volume; ESV, end-systolic volume; PUr, peripheral vascular resistance.

prior to excitation); (3) arterial-ventricular load mismatching; (4) impaired autonomic regulation; and (5) physical deconditioning. Although these age-associated changes in cardiovascular reserve are insufficient to produce clinical heart failure, they do affect its clinical presentation—the threshold for symptoms and signs or the severity and prognosis of heart failure secondary to any level of disease burden (eg, chronic hypertension that causes either systolic or diastolic heart failure).

Cardiac afterload has two components—one generated by the heart itself and the other by the vasculature. The cardiac component of afterload during exercise can be expected to increase slightly with age because the heart's size increases in older persons throughout the cardiac cycle during exercise. Vascular load on the heart has four components: conduit artery compliance characteristics, reflected pulse waves, resistance, and inertance. Inertance is determined by the mass of blood in the large arteries that requires acceleration prior to LV ejection. As the central arterial diastolic diameter increases with aging (see Fig. 59-2A), the inertance component of afterload also increases likely. Thus, each pulsatile component of vascular load, at rest, increases with age. Hence, the aortic impedance, a composite function of the determinants of vascular afterload, increases with age.

# ARTERIAL/VENTRICULAR LOAD MATCHING

Optimal and efficient ejection of blood from the heart occurs when ventricular and vascular loads are matched. It has been suggested that the precise cardiac and vascular load matching that is characteristic in younger persons is preserved at older ages, at least at rest, because the increased vascular stiffness in older persons at rest is matched by increased resting ventricular stiffness.

During exercise, the LV end-systolic elastance ($E_{LV}$), that is, end-systolic pressure–to–end-systolic volume ratio, must increase to a greater extent than the effective vascular elastance ($E_A$), that is, end-systolic pressure–to–stroke volume ratio.

With increasing age, however, $E_{LV}$ fails to increase in proportion to the increase in $E_A$; hence, the $E_A/E_{LV}$ during exercise in older persons decreases to a lesser extent than it does in younger persons (**Fig. 59-7A**). This is a mechanism for the deficit in the acute LV ejection fraction (LVEF) reserve that accompanies advancing age in many individuals. An acute pharmacologic reduction in both cardiac and vascular components of LV afterload by sodium nitroprusside (SNP) infusions in older, healthy BLSA volunteers augments LVEF (Fig. 59-7B) in these subjects (at rest and exercise). Because of concomitant reductions in preload and afterload during SNP infusion, the LV of older persons delivers the same stroke volume, stroke work, and cardiac output while working at a smaller size (Fig. 59-7C).

Diminished effectiveness of the autonomic modulation of heart rate, LV contractility, and arterial afterload collectively comprise a sizeable component of the age-associated deficit in cardiovascular reserve. Each of the deficient components of cardiovascular regulation with aging (ie, heart rate [and thus filling time], afterload [both cardiac and vascular], myocardial contractility, and redistribution of blood flow) exhibits a deficient sympathetic modulation.

The efficiency of postsynaptic β-adrenergic signaling declines with aging. Observations that cardiovascular responses to beta-adrenergic agonist infusions at rest decrease with age, and acute beta-adrenergic receptor blockade changes the exercise hemodynamic profile of younger persons to make it resemble that of older individuals is evidence of post synaptic beta-adrenergic signaling decline. Significant beta-blockade–induced LV dilatation occurs only in younger subjects (**Fig. 59-8A**). The heart rate reduction during exercise in the presence of acute β-adrenergic blockade is greater in younger versus older subjects (Fig. 59-8B), as are the age-associated deficits in LV early diastolic filling rate, both at rest and during exercise (Fig. 59-8C).

β-adrenergic blockade in younger individuals in Fig. 60-8 causes the stroke volume index to increase to a greater extent than does β-adrenergic blockade in older individuals, suggesting that mechanisms other than deficient β-adrenergic regulation compromise LV ejection. One potential mechanism is an age-associated decrease in maximum intrinsic myocardial contractility. Another likely mechanism is enhanced vascular afterload caused by the structural changes in compliance arteries and possibly also by impaired vasorelaxation during exercise. In this regard, it has been observed that the increase in aortic impedance during exercise in old dogs is abolished by β-adrenergic blockade.

Apparent deficits in sympathetic modulation of cardiac and arterial functions with aging occur in the presence of exaggerated neurotransmitter levels. Plasma levels of norepinephrine (NE) and epinephrine, during any perturbation from the supine basal state, increase to a greater extent in older compared with younger healthy humans). The age-associated increase in plasma levels of NE results from an increased spillover into the circulation and, to a lesser extent, to reduced plasma clearance. The degree of NE spillover into the circulation occurs within the heart. Deficient NE reuptake at nerve endings is a primary mechanism for increased spillover during acute graded exercise. During prolonged exercise, however, diminished neurotransmitter reuptake might also be associated with depletion and reduced release and spillover. Cardiac muscarinic receptor density and function are also diminished with increasing age and might contribute to the decrease in baroreflex activity observed in aged subjects.

Because a marked reduction in physical activity accompanies advancing age in a majority of adults, a reduction in physical conditioning status might be implicated as a factor in the reduced cardiovascular reserve of older, healthy, and sedentary individuals. Aerobic capacity in persons of varying age, estimated by either peak oxygen consumption or work capacity, accompanying the hemodynamic pattern at maximal exercise across the age range (see Table 59-1) declines approximately 50% (**Fig. 59-9A**). In this study population, rigorously prescreened to exclude disease, the age-associated reduction in the cardiac component, exclusively a result of a reduced ability to accelerate the heart rate (Fig. 59-9B), accounts for roughly half of the

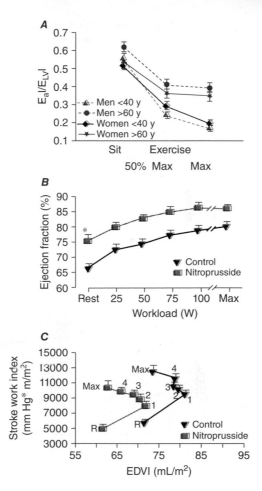

**FIGURE 59-7. A**. Load mismatch during exercise. Effective arterial elastance index ($E_aI$)/left ventricular end-systolic elastance ($E_{LV}I$), an index of arterial-ventricular coupling, in men (dashed lines) and women (solid lines), <40 years of age (solid triangles) and >60 years of age, at rest, submaximal exercise (50% of max), and maximal exercise. In both men and women, $E_aI/E_{LV}I$ decreases with exercise in both age groups, but there is a greater decrease in Fal/Elvl at maximal exercise in younger than in older subjects. **B**. Ejection fraction at seated, at upright rest, at intermediate common submaximal workloads, and at maximum effort in healthy volunteers aged 71 ± 7 years prior to and during sodium nitroprusside (SNP) infusion. At any level of effort, ejection fraction is substantially increased by SNP. **C**. Ventricular function, depicted as stroke work index versus end-diastolic volume index (EDVI) relationship at upright, at seated rest (R), and during exercise in the presence and absence of SNP. The relationship is shifted leftward and downward with SNP, indicating a smaller EDVI and lower stroke work index at any exercise load. (**A**, reproduced with permission from Najjar SS, Schulman SP, Gerstenblith G. Age and gender affect ventricular-vascular coupling during aerobic exercise. *J Am Coll Cardiol*. 2004;44(3):611-617.) (**B** and **C**, reproduced with permission from Nussbacher A, Gerstenblith G, O'Connor F, et al. Hemodynamic effects of unloading the old heart. *Am J Physiol*. 1999;277:H1863-H1871.)

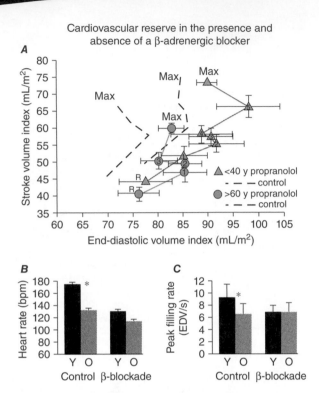

**FIGURE 59-8. A.** Stroke volume index (SVI) as a function of end-diastolic volume index (EDVI) at seated rest (R) and during graded cycle workloads in the upright seated position in healthy Baltimore Longitudinal Study of Aging (BLSA) men in the presence and absence of β-adrenergic blockade. 1-5, graded submaximal workloads on cycle ergometer; max, maximum effort. Stroke volume versus end-diastolic functions with symbols are those measured in the presence of propranolol; dashed line functions without symbols are the stroke volume versus end-diastolic functions measured in the absence of propranolol. Note that in the absence of propranolol, the SVI versus EDVI relation in older persons is shifted rightward from that in younger persons. This indicates that the left ventricle (LV) of older persons in the sitting position compared with that of younger persons operates from a greater preload both at rest and during submaximal and maximal exercise. Propranolol markedly shifts the SVI-EDVI relationship in younger persons (▲) rightward, but does not markedly offset the curve in older persons (●). Thus, with respect to this assessment of ventricular function curve, β-adrenergic blockade with propranolol makes younger men appear like older ones. The abolition of the age-associated differences in the LV function curve after propranolol is accompanied by a reduction in heart rate, which at maximum effort is shown in B. **B.** Peak exercise heart rate in the same subjects as in A in the presence and absence of acute β-adrenergic blockade by propranolol. **C.** The age-associated reduction in peak LV diastolic filling rate at maximum exercise in healthy BLSA subjects is abolished during exercise in the presence of β-adrenergic blockade with propranolol. Y, subjects <40 years old; O, subjects >60 years old. (**A**, reproduced with permission from Fleg JL, Schulman SP, O'Connor F, et al. Effects of acute beta-adrenergic receptor blockade on age-associated changes in cardiovascular performance during dynamic exercise. *Circulation*. 1994;90:2333-2341.) (**B and C**, data from Schulman SP, Lakatta EG, Fleg JL, et al. Age-related decline in left ventricular filling at rest and exercise. *Am J Physiol*. 1992;263:H1932-H1938.)

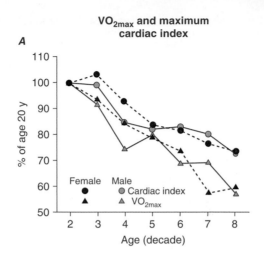

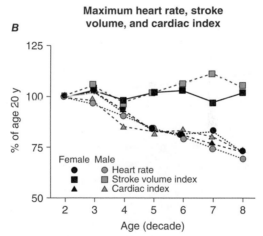

**FIGURE 59-9. A.** Peak oxygen consumption ($VO_2$) and cardiac index at exhaustion during upright cycle exercise. The age-associated reduction in peak $VO_2$ in both males and females is 2-fold greater than the decline in maximum cardiac index. This indicates, via the Fick Principle, that oxygen extraction declines by approximately 25% over this age range. **B.** The age-associated decline in maximum cardiac index is entirely a result of a decline in maximum heart rate. Maximum stroke volume varies little with aging in healthy persons. $VO_{2max}$, maximum oxygen consumption. (Reproduced with permission from Fleg JL, O'Connor FC, Gerstenblith G, et al. Impact of age on the cardiovascular response to dynamic upright exercise in healthy men and women. *J Appl Physiol*. 1995;78:890-900.)

age-associated decline in aerobic capacity, the remainder being attributable to age-associated differences in oxygen use. Such reductions in oxygen use during vigorous exercise result from age-associated reduction in muscle mass and from a reduction in the shunting of blood from viscera to working muscles during exercise, as well as the amount of oxygen use.

Cross-sectional studies, for example, those in Fig. 59-9, have been largely interpreted to indicate that the maximal oxygen uptake ($VO_{2max}$) declines linearly as a function of age. The longitudinal rate of decline in peak $VO_2$ in healthy adults is not constant across the age span in healthy persons but accelerates markedly with each successive age decade, especially in men, regardless of physical activity habits (**Fig. 59-10**). When the components of peak $VO_2$ were examined, the rate

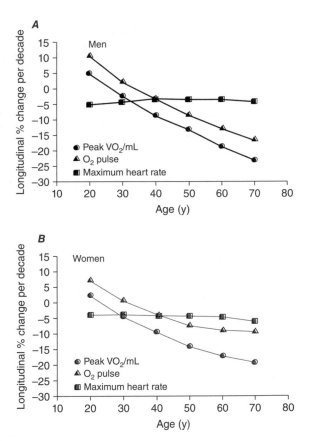

**FIGURE 59-10.** Longitudinal changes in maximal heart rate, oxygen ($O_2$) pulse, and peak oxygen consumption ($VO_2$) by sex, predicted from the mixed-effects model and separated by sex into panels **A** and **B**. Peak $VO_2$/FFM (fat-free mass) declines progressively more steeply with advancing age, with similar declines in men and women. Note that peak $VO_2$ per kilogram FFM is only slightly higher in men than women at younger ages, converging by old age. Declines in heart rate are similar across age in men but steepen modestly with age in women. $O_2$ pulse declines progressively more steeply with age, especially in men, leading to near convergence of $O_2$ pulse in elderly men and women. Note the similarity of these plots to those of peak $VO_2$ in Fig. 102-1A. The longitudinal percent change per decade in maximal heart rate is only 4% to 5% per decade across the age span in both sexes. In contrast, longitudinal decline in $O_2$ pulse accelerates progressively with age, especially in men. Note the similarity in the shape and magnitude of the decline in $O_2$ pulse to that of peak $VO_2$. (Reproduced with permission from Fleg JL, Morrell CH, Bos AG, et al. Accelerated longitudinal decline of aerobic capacity in healthy older adults. *Circulation*. 2005;112:674-682.)

of longitudinal decline of the oxygen pulse (ie, the oxygen use per heart beat) mirrored that of peak $VO_2$, whereas the longitudinal rate of heart rate decline averaged only 4% to 6% per 10 years and accelerated only minimally with age (see Fig. 59-10). The accelerated rate of decline of peak aerobic capacity has substantial implications with regard to functional independence and quality of life, not only in healthy older persons, but also when disease-related deficits are superimposed.

Metabolic debts associated with the performance of dynamic exercise increase with aging. For several minutes after an acute bout of exercise, the body continues to consume oxygen at a rate in excess of the basal rate referred to as an *oxygen debt*. When expressed relative to work performed during the exercise, it can range from 14% to 21% of the total $VO_2$ associated with the performance of and recovery from exercise. This oxygen debt, paid during exercise recovery, is often not factored into estimates of exercise efficiency (calories expended for work performed) and reduces efficiency because it contributes to the total oxygen cost associated with the exercise but contributes no external work.

Although work performed and $VO_2$ during the exercise are lower in most older persons than in younger persons, the $VO_2$ during the exercise, per unit work performed, does not change with age. $VO_2$ during recovery (metabolic debt) from exercise in older subjects, however, exceeds that in younger persons by >30%. This is likely attributable to an inability of the older body to adapt to the energy requirements of exercise. Specific factors include reductions in muscle mass and strength, inadequate blood flow to muscles, and a reduced efficiency of muscle respiration. Excessive elevation of catecholamines and core temperature occurs during exercise in older persons, as do other less well-characterized factors (eg, excessive reactive oxygen species and an exaggerated elevation of inflammatory cytokines). These factors cause muscle fatigue and a shift to anaerobic metabolism. During recovery, excessive catecholamine concentrations and incomplete waning of cell responses to catecholamine drive during exercise might continue to stimulate both muscle respiration in the absence of continued demand for muscle work and the cardiovascular system to dissipate lactate and heat generated during exercise. The physiologic significance of this metabolic debt incurred during exercise is that its underlying factors collectively reduce exercise capacity, with all the attendant health and performance drawbacks of such a reduction.

The issue arises as to whether physical conditioning via aerobic training of sedentary older persons can affect deficits in cardiovascular reserve capacity as a consequence of the aging process. Physical conditioning of older persons can substantially increase their maximum aerobic work capacity and peak oxygen consumption. The extent to which this conditioning effect results from enhanced central cardiac performance or from augmented peripheral circulatory and oxygen use mechanisms, including changes in skeletal muscle mass, varies with the characteristics of the population studied, the type and degree of conditioning, sex, body position during study, and likely genetic factors. A longitudinal study of older men in the upright position indicates that enhanced physical conditioning increases oxygen consumption and work capacity, in part, by increasing the maximum cardiac output by increasing the maximum stroke volume and, in part, by increasing the estimated total-body arteriovenous oxygen use. Conditioning effects to increase LV ejection appear to relate to the reduction in vascular afterload, as reflected in a reduced pulse wave velocity, and to carotid augmentation index in older athletes compared with sedentary controls, as well as possibly to an augmentation of maximum intrinsic myocardial contractility.

Aerobic exercise training in older persons not only improves exercise work capacity but also increases muscle mass; improves capillary density, muscle respiration, mitochondrial enzymes, and muscle oxidative capacity; reduces plasma lactate during exercise; and reduces the oxygen debt. Exercise training benefits on exercise efficiency of oxygen use are more pronounced in older than younger subjects, irrespective of sex. For example, in older subjects, an exercise conditioning program reduced the metabolic debt following exercise by nearly 30%, which translated into an 18% increase in exercise efficiency; but efficiency did not change in younger persons.

# ■ HEART CONDUCTION AND RHYTHM

There is an increase in elastic and collagenous tissue in all parts of the conduction system with advancing age. Fat accumulates around the sinoatrial node, sometimes producing a partial or complete separation of the node from the atrial musculature. A pronounced decrease in the number of pacemaker cells in the sinoatrial node begins at age 60 years, and by age 75 years, the sinoatrial node cell number may become substantially reduced. Calcification of the left side of the cardiac skeleton, including the aortic and mitral annuli, the central fibrous body, and the summit of the interventricular septum, also occurs with aging. Because of their proximity to these structures, the atrioventricular (AV) node, AV bundle, bifurcation, and proximal left and right bundle branches may be affected.

The PR interval increases with aging as a result of a prolongation of the A-H time with no change in the H-V time. Although the supine basal heart rate is not affected by aging, beat-to-beat fluctuation of heart rate, heart rate variability, declines steadily with age. Reduced heart rate variability is an indicator of altered cardiac autonomic regulation commonly found in older people and has been linked to increased morbidity and mortality.

An increase in the prevalence and complexity of both supraventricular and ventricular arrhythmias—occurs in otherwise healthy older, as opposed to younger, persons. Isolated atrial premature beats (APBs) appear on the resting ECG in 5% to 10% of subjects older than 60 years of age and are generally not associated with heart disease. Isolated APBs are detected in 6% of resting healthy BLSA volunteers older than 60 years of age, in 39% during exercise testing, and in 88% during ambulatory 24-hour monitoring. Over a 10-year mean follow-up period, isolated APBs, even if frequent, were not predictive of increased cardiac risk in these individuals.

Short bursts of paroxysmal supraventricular tachycardia (PSVT) were observed in 1% to 2% of apparently healthy individuals older than 65 years of age.

Twenty-four hour ambulatory monitoring studies have demonstrated short runs of this PSVT (usually 3 to 5 beats) in 13% to 50% of clinically healthy older subjects. Although nonsustained PSVT did not predict future coronary events in BLSA subjects, 15% with PSVT later developed de novo atrial fibrillation (AF), compared with <1% of subjects without PSVT. The incidence of asymptomatic PSVT during exercise, typically 3- to 5-beat salvos, increases with age, to approximately 10% in the ninth decade. Ten percent individuals with exercise-induced PSVT developed a spontaneous atrial tachyarrhythmia, compared with only 2% of control. Thus, PSVT at rest or induced by exercise is an early clue that some healthy individuals are at increased risk for future AF. Another risk factor for AF may be the increase in left atrial size that accompanies advancing age in otherwise healthy persons.

In older subjects without heart disease, data support a marked age-associated increase in the prevalence and complexity of ventricular ectopy (VE), both at rest and during exercise, in men. A steep increase in the prevalence of VE with advancing age occurs both in those clinically free of heart disease and in unselected populations. In healthy BLSA volunteers with a normal ST-segment response to treadmill exercise, isolated VE occurred at rest in 8.6% of men older than age 60 years compared with only 0.5% in men 20 to 40 years of age, however there was no age relation in women. Among 98 carefully screened asymptomatic BLSA participants older than 60 years of age, 35% had multiform isolated VE, 11% had ventricular couplets, and 4% had short runs of ventricular tachycardia on 24-hour monitoring; all occurred substantially more commonly in older than in healthy younger persons. Neither the prevalence nor the complexity of resting VE was a determinant of future coronary events over a 10-year mean follow-up period.

Isolated VE during or after maximal treadmill exercise increased in prevalence 5-fold, from 11% to 57%, between the third and ninth decades in apparently healthy BLSA volunteers.

# LESSONS LEARNED ABOUT CARDIAC AGING FROM ANIMAL MODELS

## ■ CARDIAC STRUCTURE

Cellular and molecular mechanisms implicated in age-associated changes in myocardial structure and function in humans have been largely studied in rodents. Many experimental studies have shown that increased activation of the renin-angiotensin-aldosterone system is a prominent feature of age-related cardiac remodeling that may account for many of the phenotypic changes that are observed. The altered cardiac structural phenotype that evolves with aging in rodents includes an increase in LV mass due to an enlargement of myocyte size, and focal proliferation of extracellular matrix may be linked to an altered cardiac fibroblast number or function. The number of cardiac myocytes reduces predominantly because of necrosis and secondarily apoptosis. Stimuli for cardiomyocyte enlargement with aging in rodents include an age-associated increase in vascular load due to arterial stiffening and stretching of cells caused by death of myocytes. Stretch of cardiac myocytes and fibroblasts initiates growth factor signaling (eg, angiotensin II/TGFβ), which modulates cell growth and matrix production, and leads to apoptosis. In mouse heart, activation of the calcineurin-NFAT pathway increases with age. The expression of atrial natriuretic and opioid peptides is increased in the senescent rodent heart. There is evidence that transcriptional events associated with hypertrophic stressors become altered with advancing age (eg, the nuclear-binding activity of the transcription factor nuclear factor-κB is increased and another transcription factor, Sp1, is diminished). A recent proteomic comparison study discovered 117 proteins to be differentially expressed in the aged LV. An increase in oxidative stress is also implicated in age-related cardiac remodeling, and aging is indeed well recognized to be associated with increased production of reactive oxygen species (ROS) in many different tissues.

## ■ CARDIAC MYOCYTE FUNCTION

### Excitation–Ca²⁺ Release–Contraction

Coordinated changes in the function or expression of proteins that regulate several key steps of the cardiac cell excitation-contraction coupling process occur in the rodent heart with aging and result in a prolonged action potential (AP), a prolonged cytosolic calcium ($Ca_i$) transient after excitation, and a prolonged contraction. Both the number and activity of individual cardiac L-type Ca channels increase with age in the rat. L-type current inactivates more slowly in myocytes from older rats versus those in younger rats, and reductions in outwardly directed $K^+$ currents, could account, partly for the prolonged AP of the former. The imposition of a shorter AP to myocytes from the old rat heart reduces the $Ca_i$ transient amplitude, an effect attributable to a reduction in sarcoplasmic reticulum $Ca^{2+}$ load, which is presumably due to a reduced $Ca^{2+}$ influx via L-type $Ca^{2+}$ channel and likely also to an increased net $Ca^{2+}$ extrusion via sarcolemmal $Na^+$-$Ca^{2+}$ exchanger.

The prolonged $Ca_i$ that occurs with aging is partly explained, by a reduction in the rate of $Ca^{2+}$ sequestration by the sarcoplasmic reticulum (SR). This is attributable to a reduced transcription of the gene coding for the SR $Ca^{2+}$ pump, *SERCA2*. The abundance of transcripts of the cardiac $Na^+$-$Ca^{2+}$ exchanger (NCX-1), which serves as the main transsarcolemmal $Ca^{2+}$ extrusion mechanism, is increased approximately 50% in senescent (24-month) compared with the young adult (6-month) rat hearts. The age-associated prolonged $Ca^{2+}$ transience and contraction may impair myocardial relaxation during early diastole and contribute to the reduction in early diastolic filling rate that accompanies advancing age. Studies in rodents that have used gene therapy or exercise conditioning to increase the level of *SERCA2* have demonstrated that impaired relaxation and $Ca^{2+}$ sequestration that occur with aging can be reduced by these interventions.

Marked shifts occur in the cardiac myosin heavy chain (MHC) isoforms in the senescent rat heart, predominance of the beta-isoform myosin $Ca^{2+}$-ATPase activity declines with the decline in alpha-MHC content. *MHC* gene expression is regulated, in part, via binding of thyroid hormone receptors retinoic acid receptors, vitamin D receptors, and retinoid X receptors, to thyroid response elements in gene 5′ flanking regions. A significant reduction (~50%) in the levels of thyroid hormone receptor-β and retinoid X receptor-γ proteins between 6 and 24 months and in mRNA encoding these receptor subtypes has been observed in hearts of senescent rats.

The altered composite cellular profile, which results in a contraction that exhibits reduced velocity and prolonged time due to prolonged elevation of cytosolic Ca after a prolonged AP, can be considered to be adaptive rather than degenerative because myocardial shortening at reduced velocity is energy efficient. This altered pattern of $Ca^{2+}$ regulation and myosin protein expression allows the myocardium of older hearts to generate force and active stiffness for a longer time after. Prolonged isovolumic relaxation in the healthy human heart with aging may be attributable to prolonged contractile protein $Ca^{2+}$ activation, enabling the continued ejection of blood during late systole, a beneficial adaptation with respect to enhanced central arterial stiffness, and early reflected pulse waves.

The age-associated reduction in β-AR signaling may, in part, also be related to upregulation of opioid peptide receptor signaling because of the significant antagonistic effects between stimulation of opioid peptide receptor and β-AR–mediated positive contractile response.

Remarkably, the available examinations of cardiac excitation-contraction coupling in rodents of both sexes or females only show a lack of age-related changes in the $Ca^{2+}_i$ transient in myocytes from female hearts. Findings in aged female myocytes include (1) increase in the SR $Ca^{2+}$ content, (2) lack of effect of the latter on the configuration of the $Ca^{2+}_i$ transients and contraction, and (3) reduction of fractional SR $Ca^{2+}$ release in the presence of unchanged $I_{CaL}$. Nevertheless, these results provide an initial direct demonstration of sexually dimorphic changes in cardiac excitation-contraction coupling associated with normal adult aging.

## Impaired Cellular Reserve During Acute Stress Ca²⁺ Cycling

Aging-associated major changes in heart structure and function place the aged heart constantly "on the edge" and at risk, including the loss of its adaptive response to stress. Reserve cardiac myocyte $Ca^{2+}$ cycling is modulated by β-AR stimulation. Age-associated reduction in the postsynaptic response of myocardial cells to β-AR stimulation is the result of changes in molecular and biochemical steps that couple the receptor to postreceptor effectors. The major limiting modification of acute β-AR signaling with advancing age in rodents is the coupling of the β-AR to adenylyl cyclase via the $G_s$ protein and changes in adenylyl cyclase protein, leading to a reduction in the ability to augment cell cyclic adenosine monophosphate and to activate protein kinase A to drive the phosphorylation of key proteins that are required to augment cardiac contractility. In contrast, desensitization of β-AR signaling with aging is not mediated via increased β-AR kinase (β-ARK) or increased $G_i$ protein activity.

Acute excess myocardial $Ca^{2+}$ loading leads to dysregulation of $Ca^{2+}$ homeostasis, impaired diastolic and systolic function, arrhythmias, and cell death. The cell $Ca^{2+}$ load is determined by membrane structure and permeability characteristics, the intensity of stimuli that modulate $Ca^{2+}$ influx or efflux via their impact on regulatory function of proteins within membranes, and ROS, which affect both membrane structure and function. Excessive cytosolic $Ca^{2+}$ loading occurs during physiologic and pharmacologic stimuli that increase $Ca^{2+}$ influx (eg, neurotransmitters, postischemic reperfusion, or oxidative stress). In older hearts or their myocytes, enhanced $Ca^{2+}$ influx, impaired relaxation, and increased diastolic tone occur during pacing at an increased frequency. The amounts and ratios of each class of proteins involved in cell ion homeostasis, the lipids of plasma membranes (eg, types and amounts of long-chain polyunsaturated fatty acids [PUFAs]), and the threshold to produce ROS and ROS-derived alkenes change with aging and reduce the threshold for acute $Ca^{2+}$ overload that occurs in the older heart.

# ■ MITOCHONDRIAL ROS GENERATION

Mitochondria possess unique $Ca^{2+}$ transport machinery, regulate metabolism under partial control by $Ca^{2+}$, and contribute to cell $Ca^{2+}$ homeostasis. Although multiple enzymes, including nicotinamide adenine dinucleotide phosphate (NADPH) oxidase at the plasma membrane and cyclooxygenases and xanthine oxidase in the cytoplasm, also contribute to the overall oxidative burden, mitochondria contribute the majority of ROS generation as a byproduct of electron transfer and oxidative phosphorylation. Thus, mitochondria appear to play a central role in the reduced $Ca^{2+}$ tolerance observed in aged animals.

Mitochondria undergo aging-related changes that enhance sensitivity to and compromise their response to stress (such as ischemia) and also result in the loss of the ability to trigger cardioprotection mechanisms. Compared with young adult myocardium, the senescent myocardium is more sensitive to ischemia, suggesting that protective pathways in adult myocardium are modified or impaired by aging. Repetitive ischemia is an endogenous cardioprotective mechanism incited by, and this protection is reduced in the older heart. This may relate to diminished heat shock protein 70 expression. NO, which is produced by eNOS or inducible NO synthase (iNOS), plays a role in cardioprotection. However, iNOS and eNOS expression and activity are modified in senescent myocardium. Changes in protein kinase C (PKC) translocation have been described in aged myocardium, leading to certain age-associated changes in the specific sites targeted by each PKC isoform.

Several studies indicate that reperfusion that follows ischemia generates ROS and that exogenous application of ROS to cells causes $Ca^{2+}$ overload, adenosine triphosphate (ATP) depletion, and rigor. Mitochondrial production of ROS in the heart and mitochondrial dysfunction are associated with reperfusion increase with age. ROS and therefore calcium activates the permeability transition pore, a nonselective, high-conductance channel in the mitochondrial inner membrane, causing loss of the proton gradient in the respiratory chain, thus rendering it incapable of generating ATP. Mitochondrial ROS play a role in mitochondrial membrane permeability transition (MPT). The release of mitochondrial contents into the cytosol—resulting from the MPT induction—can lead to high $Ca_i$ and to the generation of additional ROS, initiation of necrosis and/or apoptosis, and eventual death. A phenomenon referred to as *ROS-induced ROS release* ("trigger" ROS generated by mitochondria in response to laser excitation of fluorescent mitochondrial membrane label leads to an amplification of ROS production by the mitochondria) is associated with induction of the MPT and collapse of mitochondrial membrane potential. This renders the mitochondrial membrane permeable to ions, larger molecules, and water between the cytosol and the mitochondrial matrix. Cells from senescent hearts have a substantially lower threshold for the generation of ROS-induced ROS release and more likelihood of the MPT. The hydroxyl radical is highly reactive and short-lived species and causes damage at or near the site of formation. Namely, mitochondrial DNA damage and dysfunction in a feedforward manner, causing functional cellular and organ decline.

# ■ MEMBRANE ω PUFA

Membrane PUFAs undergo lipid peroxidation by ROS, producing aldehydes, alkenals, and hydroxyalkenals, such as malonaldehyde and 4-hydroxy-2-nonenal (HNE). HNE, the most reactive of these compounds, is formed by superoxide reactions with membrane ω-6 PUFAs and reacts with protein sulfhydryl groups to alter protein conformation. An increase in ω-6:ω-3 PUFA that occurs with aging may be a mechanism for increased HNE production following ischemia/reperfusion, but this effect can be markedly attenuated by an ω-3 PUFA–rich diet. Notably, an ω-3 PUFA–rich diet also prevents the age-linked decrement of the mitochondria-specific membrane phospholipid cardiolipin, a crucial cofactor for cytochrome c oxidase and adenine nucleotide translocase activity.

An overview of changes in the aging heart that predispose to a reduced threshold for abnormal $Ca^{2+}$ handling during acute stress are schematically summarized in **Fig. 59-11**. With advancing age, constitutive changes occur in cardiac cells with a substantial impact on cardiovascular function, reducing cellular tolerance and adaptation to stress, ie, ischemia/reperfusion. A relative decrease in the ω-3:ω-6 PUFA content ratio in cellular membranes, increased production of ROS, and alterations in $Ca^{2+}$ mobilization proteins, especially decreased SERCA2 and $Na^+$-$Ca^{2+}$ exchange protein level and function. Disturbances in excitation-contraction coupling (prolonged AP and $Ca^{2+}$ transient) and intracellular $Ca^{2+}$ compartmentalization (abnormal regulation of systolic $Ca^{2+}$, increased diastolic $Ca^{2+}$, and increased mitochondrial $Ca^{2+}$) lead to spontaneous $Ca^{2+}$ oscillations and arrhythmias. Eventual mitochondrial dysfunction impairs energy metabolism (diminished ATP production) along with excessive ROS production. Overproduction of ROS and the inability to scavenge excess ROS lead to damaging lipid peroxidation and more diffusible, potent, reactive

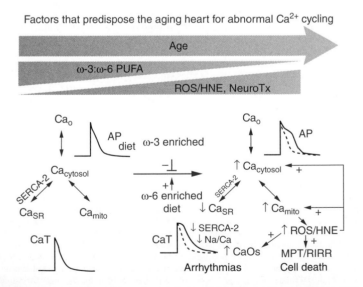

Factors that predispose the aging heart for abnormal $Ca^{2+}$ cycling

**FIGURE 59-11.** An overview of change in the aging heart that predisposes to a reduced threshold for abnormal $Ca^{2+}$ handling during acute stress. See text for details. AP, action potential; Ca, calcium; HNE, 4-hydroxy-2-nonenal; MPT, membrane permeability transition; PUFA, polyunsaturated fatty acid; RIRR, reactive oxygen species (ROS)-induced ROS release; ROS, reactive oxygen species.

intermediates, such as HNE, which affect widespread protein targets and amplify $Ca^{2+}$ dysregulation and mitochondrial abnormalities. Finally, the abnormal $Ca^{2+}$ handling and ROS buildup can induce the MPT with the release of contents that activate a sequence of events leading to cell death. These effects of aging are exacerbated by poor nutritional habits but can be ameliorated by diets rich in ω-3 PUFAs. Other promising avenues to ameliorate these aging changes include gene therapy to restore the expression of $Ca^{2+}$ regulatory proteins and the effective use of antioxidants.

# ■ REDUCED CHRONIC ADAPTIVE CAPACITY OF THE OLDER HEART

Many of the changes in cardiac structure, excitation, myofilament activation, contraction mechanisms, $Ca^{2+}$ dysregulation, deficient β-AR signaling, and altered gene expression of proteins involved in excitation-contraction coupling that occur with aging also occur in the hypertrophied myocardium of younger animals with induced chronic hypertension and in failing animal or human hearts. When chronic mechanical stresses that evoke substantial myocardial hypertrophy (eg, pressure or volume overload) are imposed on the older heart, the response in many instances is reduced. The acute induction of both immediate early genes and later responding genes that are expressed during the hypertrophic response is blunted in hearts of aged rats after aortic constriction. Similarly, the acute induction of heat shock protein 70 genes in response to either ischemia or heat shock is reduced in hearts of senescent rats. A similar loss of adaptive capacity is observed in younger rats that have used a part of their reserve capacity before a growth factor challenge.

Premature development of heart failure or death in males compared with matching females has been documented in rat models of pressure overload and/or myocardial infarction (reviewed in Olivetti et al). Sexually dimorphic cardiac phenotypes have been also discovered in some studies in genetically engineered mice. Transgenic models of heart failure have a more rapid onset and/or a greater severity of cardiac dysfunction in male versus female hearts. Mice with cardiac-specific overexpression of tumor necrosis factor-α (TNF-α) exhibit heart failure and increased mortality in young males than females (~50% and 4%, respectively, by 20 weeks of age). At 12 weeks of age, female mice displayed LV hypertrophy without dilatation and a small reduction in basal LV fractional shortening and response to isoproterenol. Male mice showed a large LV dilatation, reduced fractional shortening relative to both wild-type littermates and transgenic females, and minimal response to isoproterenol. Cardiac myocyte hypertrophy was similar in male and female transgenic mice. Compared with wild-type mice, myocytes from female TNF-α transgenic mice displayed a slower decline of the $Ca^{2+}$ transient but similar amplitudes of $Ca^{2+}$ transients and contractions and the inotropic response to isoproterenol. In contrast, the amplitude and the rate of decline of $Ca^{2+}$ transients and contractions and the response to isoproterenol were significantly reduced in myocytes from male transgenic TNF-α mice.

# ■ MYOCYTE PROGENITORS IN THE AGING HEART

Observations in humans and animals suggest that myocyte maturation and aging are characterized by loss of replicative potential, telomeric shortening, and the expression of the senescence-associated protein/cell cycle inhibitor p16[INK4a]. Telomeric shortening in precursor cells (PCs) leads to generation of progeny that rapidly acquire the senescent phenotype. The activity of telomerase, an enzyme present only during cell replication, was decreased 31% in aging male rat myocytes but increased 72% in female counterparts. The diminished cellular adaptive capacity to increases in pressure and volume loads involves progressive increase in the size of the cell (up to a critical volume beyond which myocyte hypertrophy is no longer possible), deficits in the electrical $Ca^{2+}$ cycling and mechanical properties, and cell death. Cardiac myocytes with senescent and nonsenescent phenotypes already coexist at a young age. However, aging limits the growth and differentiation potential of PCs, thus interfering not only with their ability to sustain physiologic cell turnover, but also with their capacity to adapt to increases in pressure and volume loads.

The loss of PC function with aging is mediated by an imbalance between oxidative stress, telomere attrition, death, and growth, migration, and survival. Recent findings suggest a pre-eminent position of insulin-like growth factor-1 (IGF-1) among factors that interfere with cardiac cellular senescence. Specifically, cardiac-specific overexpression of IGF-1 in transgenic mice delays the aging myopathy and the manifestations of heart failure and restores SERCA2a expression and rescues age-associated impairment of cardiac myocyte contractile function. The latter effect was also partly mimicked by short-term in vitro treatment with recombinant IGF-1. Furthermore, intramyocardial delivery of IGF-1 improved senescent heart phenotype in male Fisher 344 rats, including increased proliferation of functionally competent PCs and diminished angiotensin II–induced apoptosis. Myocardial regeneration mediated by PC activation attenuated ventricular dilation and the decrease in ventricular mass-to-chamber volume ratio, resulting in improvement of in vivo cardiac function in animals at 28 to 29 months of age.

# WHAT TO DO ABOUT "UNSUCCESSFUL" AGING OF THE HEART AND BLOOD VESSELS BEFORE IT'S TOO LATE

Extreme age-associated changes in cardiovascular structure/function that are perceived as deleterious aspects of cardiovascular aging in otherwise healthy persons ought to be interpreted to reflect "unsuccessful" cardiovascular aging. Data from epidemiologic studies indicate that specific aspects of cardiac and vascular aging in otherwise apparently healthy persons confer an increased risk for cardiovascular events.

If cardiac and vascular aging are risk factors for disease, they represent potential targets for treatment and prevention. Lifestyle intervention or pharmacotherapy, to retard the rate of progression of subclinical disease, might be considered before clinical disease becomes manifest. The risk factor of lack of vigorous exercise increases dramatically with age in otherwise healthy persons. Pulse pressure, pulse wave velocity, and carotid augmentation index are lower and baroreceptor reflex function is improved in older persons who are physically conditioned compared to sedentary. Exercise conditioning also improves endothelial function in older persons.

Diets low in sodium are associated with reduced arterial stiffening with aging. Exercise conditioning improves LV reserve function. In the rat model, as well as in elderly patients, physical activity and exercise training restore the cardiac protective effects of ischemic preconditioning and preinfarction angina otherwise lost during aging.

With respect to pharmacotherapy, angiotensin-converting enzyme (ACE) inhibitors retard vascular aging in rodents. Progressive vascular damage can continue to occur even when arterial pressure is controlled. Drugs that retard or reverse age-associated vascular wall remodeling and increased stiffness will be preferable to those that lower pressure without affecting the vascular wall properties. A novel drug that breaks such cross-links has been shown to reduce indices of arterial stiffness measures in rodents, dogs, and nonhuman primates, as well as in humans. Retardation or reduction in intimal-medial thickness in humans has been achieved by drug/diet intervention. It is thus far unproved if such treatment can "prevent" unsuccessful aging of the vasculature in individuals of early middle age who exhibit excessive subclinical evidence of unsuccessful aging.

Accelerated cardiac and vascular aging in apparently healthy younger and middle-aged adults may indicate the need for interventions designed to decrease the occurrence and/or manifestations of cardiovascular disease at later ages. Similarly, exaggerated heart or vascular aging in older persons, such as those with age-associated vascular measurements in the upper tertile, may merit similar consideration. Such a strategy would thus advocate treating "unsuccessful" aging. However, additional studies of the effectiveness of treatment regimens to delay or prevent each change are required for this strategy to be put into practice.

# THERAPEUTIC CONSIDERATIONS IN OLDER PATIENTS WITH CLINICAL CARDIOVASCULAR DISEASES

## ■ ISCHEMIC HEART DISEASE

Increasing age is the most powerful predictor of future coronary artery disease in asymptomatic individuals. Autopsy studies demonstrate that the prevalence of obstructive coronary disease increases from 10% to 20% in the fourth decade to 50% to 70% in the eighth decade. Advancing age is also associated with more severe, diffuse atherosclerosis and more damage to the LV, with prevalence of triple vessel and left main coronary disease doubling between ages 40 and 80 years. Elevated end-diastolic pressure and wall motion abnormalities on left ventriculography are also more common in the elderly patient with coronary artery disease. Almost all clinical manifestations of ischemic heart disease have a higher mortality rate and a worse outcome in the older population. Finally, clinical assessment of the elderly patient with coronary artery disease is often limited comorbidities that make interpretation of ischemic symptoms difficult. Coexisting comorbidities, such as chronic kidney disease, also make certain cardiovascular therapies and diagnostic tests more challenging in the elderly. Thus, in the elderly, a high clinical index of suspicion and careful attention to the appropriate diagnostic tests and therapies are important in assessing, diagnosing, and treating ischemic heart disease.

## ■ ACUTE CORONARY SYNDROMES

People 75 years of age and older account for 6% of the US population but account for >60% of acute coronary syndrome (ACS) mortality. The elderly also have a much greater risk for heart failure, cardiogenic shock, and major bleeding with ACS. Unfortunately, older coronary artery disease patients are severely underrepresented in the randomized controlled trials that resulted in current guidelines for the management of ACS. The incidence of myocardial infarction (MI) has increased in the elderly over the last 15 years, particularly in older women. Older patients with acute myocardial infarction are more likely to be female; have a pre-existing history of angina, heart failure, hypertension, and diabetes; and experience a non–ST-segment elevation MI. Older patients, particularly women and diabetics, are also more likely to present with atypical symptoms of acute myocardial ischemia and infarction such as shortness of breath, confusion, and failure to thrive. Furthermore, older patients with ACS are more likely to have a nondiagnostic ECG compared with younger patients, including a higher incidence of left bundle-branch block. The frequent atypical presentation of ACS and lack of diagnostic ECG findings result in a delay in diagnosis and initiation of treatment in this age group. This delay likely contributes to the high in-hospital mortality in the elderly patient presenting with an acute coronary syndrome.

Age is a powerful independent predictor of short- and long-term mortality in patients with non–ST-segment elevation ACS and ST-segment elevation acute myocardial infarction. In the Global Registry of Acute Coronary Events of 21 000 ACS patients, the adjusted odds ratio for in-hospital death compared with a 40-year-old patient is 5.0 for patients 65 to 74 years of age, 8.0 for patients 75 to 84 years of age, and 15.7 for patients 85 years of age and older. In non–ST-segment elevation ACS, the 6-month death rate in randomized trials increased from 2% in patients who were <50 years old to 11% in patients of age 70 to 79 years and 19% in patients age ≥80 years. In patients admitted with a first ST-segment elevation myocardial infarction and treated with thrombolytic therapy, in-hospital mortality increases exponentially as a function of age from 1.9% among patients 40 years or younger to 31.9% among patients older than 80 years.

Elderly acute infarct patients experience a much greater incidence of heart failure, AF, and cardiogenic shock despite no change in infarct size, cardiac enzymes, and QRS scores, with age. The risks of heart failure and shock increase 3- to 4-fold in patients >85 years old compared with those <65 years old, in both ST-segment and non–ST-segment elevation ACS. Even with a first infarct, the incidence of in-hospital heart failure in the elderly is approximately 37%. Postinfarct heart failure portends a much higher short-term and 5-year mortality in this group. The higher incidence of heart failure and shock may result from age-related changes in diastolic filling, aortic compliance, and decreased sensitivity to catecholamine stimulation, resulting in diminished cardiac reserve and afterload mismatch following ischemic damage. Worse outcomes with AMI result from fewer angiographic collateral vessels to an occluded infarct vessel in older patients with an acute ST-segment elevation myocardial infarction (STEMI) compared with younger infarct patients. This age-related decrease in collateral vessels predicts mortality in elderly infarct patients and may result in less recovery of LV function, especially if reperfusion therapy is delayed. Endothelial repair and angiogenesis arise from bone marrow endothelial progenitor cells. Elderly subjects have a decreased number and function of endothelial progenitor cells. This age-associated decrease in endothelial progenitor cell number and function contributes to the progression of atherosclerosis, impaired ability to heal following AMI, decreased collateral blood vessel development, and poor prognosis in the setting of coronary disease.

Mortality in older patients with myocardial infarction is less likely to result from ventricular fibrillation compared with younger patients, but the former are much more likely to have electromechanical dissociation and cardiac rupture on autopsy. The latter age-associated risk is particularly notable in patients receiving fibrinolytics. The high morbidity and mortality associated with ACS in the elderly dictate an aggressive approach to management. Nevertheless, reperfusion and anti-ischemic therapies and procedures have risks, and these risks are particularly relevant in the elderly due to frequent coexisting morbidity such as renal insufficiency, frailty, and cerebrovascular disease.

# ■ REPERFUSION IN ST-SEGMENT ELEVATION MYOCARDIAL INFARCTION

Most practitioners agree that prompt reperfusion of the infarct-related artery is critical to reducing the high mortality in the elderly patient with acute STEMI. Unfortunately, the delay in hospital presentation and diagnosis of STEMI, along with increased comorbidity, make the elderly patient less likely to be eligible for reperfusion therapy. Large registry data in the United States show that fibrinolytic eligible patients older than 75 years of age are significantly less likely to receive reperfusion therapy than patients younger than 65 years. Fibrinolytic therapy in AMI reduces mortality, and data suggest a benefit in the elderly. In a meta-analysis of large randomized trials of fibrinolytic therapy, subset analyses of 5800 patients older than

74 years of age showed a net saving of 1.0 life per 100 patients treated at 35 days after infarction. The benefit for fibrinolytics is increased in patients >75 years old when these patients presented within 12 hours of symptom onset with ST-segment elevation or left bundle-branch block on their admission ECG (34 lives saved per 1000 patients treated). It is difficult to draw conclusions about the risk:benefit ratio of fibrinolytic therapy in patients 85 years of age and greater, even those without contraindications, because so few of these patients were enrolled into randomized trials and observational studies show no benefit or harm compared to no treatment in this age group.

Fibrinolytic agents are reluctantly used in the elderly because of concerns about intracranial hemorrhage. Age is an important predictor of hemorrhagic stroke with fibrinolytic therapy. Careful dose adjustment of anticoagulation is necessary to limit bleeding risk in the elderly. In considering fibrinolytic therapy, careful risk stratification of the patient with an STEMI above the age of 75 years needs to be considered. These factors include the age and weight of the patient, other comorbidities, the number of leads with ST-segment elevation, the duration of symptoms, and the proximity of a facility with high-volume percutaneous coronary intervention. Lastly, benefit of fibrinolytics decreases if pathologic Q waves are present on the admission ECG versus lone ST-segment elevation.

Primary angioplasty compared with fibrinolytic therapy has beneficial effects on mortality, recurrent myocardial infarction, and recurrent ischemia for percutaneous coronary intervention. A meta-analysis of the 23 randomized trials and 32 observational studies shows a significant reduction in short-term mortality, reinfarction, and stroke in patients receiving percutaneous coronary intervention compared with fibrinolytic therapy. Subgroup analyses show a large survival advantage for percutaneous coronary intervention compared with fibrinolytic therapy in patients $\geq 70$ years old with an STEMI. One randomized trial of 87 patients older than 75 years of age with STEMI showed a significant decrease in death, reinfarction, and stroke 30 days and 20 months following direct angioplasty compared with fibrinolytic therapy. An important caveat to all these comparative trials is that they involve operators with great expertise from high-volume angioplasty centers.

Older patients have a higher risk of cardiogenic shock than younger patients. In a randomized study of early revascularization compared with initial medical stabilization, mean 6-year survival was significantly greater with early revascularization strategy. Survival curves show an absolute 13% long-term survival advantage for an early revascularization strategy. Because there was no age (<75 years vs $\geq 75$ years) × treatment interaction over the long term, these data suggest that elderly acute myocardial infarction patients with cardiogenic shock should receive emergent revascularization therapy if possible.

# ■ MEDICAL THERAPY FOR ACUTE MYOCARDIAL INFARCTION

β-blocker therapy is greatly underprescribed in older post-myocardial infarction patients, despite a significant survival advantage with this therapy. In the Cooperative Cardiovascular Project database of >200 000 Medicare beneficiaries who suffered a myocardial infarction, only 34% of this elderly cohort was discharged home on a β-blocker. Of ideal postinfarct patients >65 years of age with no contraindications to β-blocker therapy, only 50% leave hospital on this therapy. All subgroups in this database had a large survival advantage (~40% relative reduction and 10% absolute reduction in 2-year mortality) with β-blocker therapy. Benefits were seen in Q and non–Q wave infarction, age less than 70 years to greater than 80 years, and any of LV function. The benefits of chronic β-blocker therapy after myocardial infarction in the Cardiovascular Cooperative Project database are similar to subgroup analyses of the placebo-controlled trials of chronic β-blocker therapy after stabilization from myocardial infarction, showing a survival advantage in patients older than 65 years of age.

Aggressive intravenous β-blocker followed by oral therapy on admission to the hospital should be used with caution in elderly patients. The Clopidogrel and Metoprolol Infarction Trial Investigators randomized 45 852 patients with acute myocardial infarction to intravenous followed by oral beta-blockade or matching placebo. Patients with cardiogenic shock, heart rate <50 beats/minute, and systolic blood pressure persistently <100 mm Hg were excluded. Reinfarction or cardiac arrest after 28 days was not significantly different in patients randomized to placebo or β-blocker. Mortality at 28 days was also not different. Although the incidence of reinfarction and ventricular fibrillation was reduced with early β-blockade, this benefit was countered with a higher risk of developing cardiogenic shock. The excess risk of shock with aggressive β-blockade occurred on the first hospital day. Because age is a powerful predictor for the development of cardiogenic shock, this age group should not receive aggressive β-blockade on arrival to the hospital.

Aspirin therapy decreases mortality and reinfarction in elderly infarct subjects. Nevertheless, among 10 000 Medicare beneficiaries with an AMI with no contraindication to aspirin therapy, only 61% of patients received it within the first 2 hospital days. Aspirin therapy in this group of elderly infarct patients was independently associated with a lower 30-day mortality. Furthermore, only 76% of elderly subjects without any contraindications were discharged home on aspirin following an MI. Aspirin use was independently associated with improved 6-month outcome. In a randomized, placebo-controlled trial of 45 852 medically treated patients with acute STEMI, clopidogrel therapy added to aspirin reduced the short-term composite end point of death, reinfarction, or stroke, as well as mortality alone. Therefore, in elderly infarct patients at low bleeding risk, dual antiplatelet therapy should be considered. ACC/AHA guidelines recommend use of aspirin when ACS is suspected.

ACE inhibitor therapy following AMI reduces morbidity and mortality. In the randomized, placebo-controlled clinical trials that involved high-risk patients with LV dysfunction or clinical heart failure, there was a large survival benefit in older patients randomized to ACE inhibitor therapy compared with placebo. A meta-analysis of these trials involving 5966 patients with LV dysfunction (ejection fraction <40%) or heart failure was reported. The mean age of the cohort was 63 years. After a mean follow-up of 31 months, high-risk patients with postinfarction LV dysfunction or heart failure on an ACE inhibitor experienced a 26% reduction in mortality (29.1% placebo vs 23.4% ACE inhibitor; odds ratio = 0.74; 95% confidence interval, 0.66-0.83). Secondary end points were also improved in patients on an ACE inhibitor, including a 27% reduction in heart failure hospitalizations and a 20% reduction in recurrent myocardial infarction. There was no statistical heterogeneity of the ACE inhibitor effect by age (<55 years, 55-75 years, or >75 years).

For lower risk patients without heart failure or left ventricular dysfunction postmyocardial infarction, the benefits of ACE inhibitors are clearly less and individualized treatment, based on factors such as hypotension and renal insufficiency, should be considered. Aggressive ACE inhibitor blockade on arrival to the hospital should be avoided in the elderly. In older postinfarction patients with LV dysfunction, clinical heart failure, or both intolerant of ACE inhibition, high-dose angiotensin receptor blockade is equivalent. The combination of an ACE inhibitor plus an angiotensin receptor blocker does not provide further benefit and results in more adverse effects. Postinfarct patients with LV dysfunction, have enhanced production and impaired hepatic clearance of aldosterone resulting in elevated aldosterone despite ACE blockade. As a result, aldosterone levels are elevated in postinfarction patients with LV dysfunction despite ACE blockade. Elevated aldosterone levels may promote LV fibrosis and progressive remodeling after infarction, and aldosterone blockade in animal models of myocardial infarction prevents this progression. Randomized trial data show that in patients with LV dysfunction plus heart failure in the coronary care unit, the addition of an aldosterone antagonist to standard postinfarction therapy decreases cardiovascular morbidity and mortality. In this study, there was no statistical heterogeneity of benefit between subjects age <65 years and >65 years. These data suggest that in the appropriate older patients with LV dysfunction and heart failure following a large transmural myocardial infarction, one should consider the addition of an aldosterone antagonist to standard postinfarction therapy. An important caveat to adding an aldosterone antagonist to an ACE inhibitor or angiotensin receptor blocker in the older postinfarct patient with LV dysfunction and heart failure is the frequent occurrence of renal insufficiency. Creatinine clearance, renal function, and potassium levels should be followed particularly closely in the elderly when these agents are used.

# ■ NON–ST-SEGMENT ELEVATION ACUTE CORONARY SYNDROME

Large cohort studies show that the majority of patients admitted with non–ST-segment elevation ACS are 65 years of age and older, and >10% of patients are of 85 years of age and older. With advancing age, guideline-recommended medication contraindications are more frequent. Even in patients without recognized contraindications, in-hospital use of aspirin, beta-blockers, and anticoagulation decreases with increasing age. Early invasive management of non–ST-segment elevation ACS is reduced with advancing age as well, with only 40% of patients >75 years of age proceeding to early catheterization. Decreased utilization of medications and procedures in the elderly patient with ACS is mirrored by in-hospital mortality that is 2.5- and 3-fold greater in patients of 75 to 84 years old and >85 years, respectively, compared with patients <65 years. As guideline-recommended therapies are used more commonly, the risk of in-hospital death is lowered in patients >75 years of age. Adherence to guideline recommended therapies in the elderly acute coronary syndrome patient during hospitalization and at discharge can result in a decreased risk of short-term mortality and morbidity in this high-risk group of patients.

In elderly patients with non–ST-segment elevation ACS, antiplatelet therapy decreases events. The thienopyridine derivative clopidogrel was evaluated in 12 562 patients with non–ST-segment elevation acute coronary syndrome, all treated with aspirin. The primary end point of cardiovascular mortality, nonfatal myocardial infarction, or stroke was reduced 20% compared with placebo following a mean of 9 months of therapy. This benefit was evident in the 6208-patient subgroup above the age of 65 years. In elderly patients with low bleeding risk and non–ST-segment ACS, dual antiplatelet therapy with aspirin and clopidogrel reduces future cardiovascular events. Another thienopyridine, prasugrel, when compared with clopidogrel in ACS patients proceeding to coronary intervention, reduced the 15-month primary end point of cardiovascular death, nonfatal MI, or nonfatal stroke. In subgroup analyses, this benefit was seen primarily in subjects <65 years old. Prasugrels benefit in preventing ischemic events was offset by an increase in bleeding risk, especially in the elderly, underweight, and those with prior neurologic disease. Recent data suggest that upstream parenteral glycoprotein IIb/IIIa inhibitor therapy does not reduce ischemic events and increases bleeding compared with selective use of a glycoprotein IIb/IIIa inhibitor at the time of angiography. This study included nearly 2400 acute coronary syndrome patients ≥75 years old. The majority of randomized patients received dual antiplatelet therapy at the time of admission. If a small-molecule glycoprotein IIb/IIIa inhibitor is used in the elderly, creatinine clearance should be calculated prior to dosing due to dose adjustments.

Although antithrombotic and antiplatelet therapies reduce cardiovascular events in elderly patients with ACS, these agents must be used judiciously due to the increased bleeding risk that occurs in this age group. Elderly patients often receive excess anticoagulants and glycoprotein IIb/IIIa inhibitors, resulting in increased major bleeding risk. Assesment of creatinine clearance is crucial in dosing.

Advanced age is a powerful independent predictor of major bleeding. Thirty-day mortality from non–ST-segment elevation ACS increases from 1.2% to 7.3% with the occurrence of a major bleed. Additionally, risk of myocardial infarction, emergency revascularization, and stent thrombosis all increase 3- to 6-fold with a major bleed.

Several randomized trials have compared a conservative medical strategy versus an invasive approach on short-term outcomes of death, MI, and recurrent ischemic events in patients with non–ST-segment elevation ACS. Most studies, including a recent meta-analysis, show a decrease in death or nonfatal MI with initial invasive compared with conservative strategy. The invasive approach benefitted higher risk patients, including those with positive troponin, ST-segment depression on electrocardiography, and patients >65 years old. Subgroup analysis of the randomized elderly patients with non–ST-segment elevation ACS shows a large absolute and relative reduction in death or nonfatal myocardial infarction at 6 months with an invasive compared with conservative approach. These data suggest that because older patients with ACS are often at increased risk for adverse outcomes, an early invasive approach should be considered. Very few elderly subjects were enrolled in these randomized studies, and the vast majority of these subjects had minimal comorbidities and normal renal function. How these data apply to older patients with significant comorbidities or renal insufficiency or to the very elderly is uncertain.

# ■ CHRONIC CORONARY DISEASE

The use of coronary revascularization, both percutaneous coronary intervention (PCI) and coronary artery bypass grafting surgery (CABG), has increased in patients ≥75 years old, with a decline in short-term mortality with both revascularization modalities. The use of PCI has increased significantly along with improved outcomes in elderly patients with chronic CAD, likely due to increased operator experience, new tools such as the introduction of drug-eluting coronary stents, and antiplatelet therapies. Despite increasing age and greater comorbidities, the procedural success rate of PCI in the elderly has significantly improved, with reduction in complications and need for emergent CABG and decreased length of stay.

Use of bypass surgery has also increased in the very elderly. In-hospital mortality is significantly greater in octogenarians undergoing coronary artery bypass surgery than younger patients. In a large cohort of patients undergoing CABG, in-hospital mortality is 8.1% in octogenarians, in addition to increased incidence of postoperative stroke (4%) and renal failure (7%). In a subset of octogenarians without significant comorbidity and undergoing elective CABG, in-hospital mortality was only 4.2%. These data suggest that octogenarians can undergo coronary artery bypass surgery with relatively low short-term mortality, especially if the surgery is elective, a first time CABG, and comorbidities are low. Despite the higher short-term morbidity and mortality in elderly bypass patients compared with younger patients, the 3-year mortality rate of this group was similar to the general octogenarian population.

Studies suggest that older age is a powerful predictor of both short-term and 5-year cognitive decline following CABG. This concern resulted in initial enthusiasm for the treatment of the elderly patient with critical multivessel CAD with off-pump CABG. Because emboli are the main source of strokes following CABG, off-pump bypass may theoretically reduce intraoperative cerebral emboli, resulting in a decrease in perioperative stroke and cognitive decline. A meta-analysis of 9 observational studies comparing conventional CABF with off-pump surgery in patients ≥70 years old suggests that the stroke risk may be lower with off-pump surgery. These data contrast with a recent randomized study in older subjects (mean age, 76 years) undergoing CABG showing similar cognitive function 3 months following surgery in subjects randomized to conventional compared with off-pump CABG. A large, randomized, single-blind trial of 2203 patients (mean age, 63 years) requiring CABG showed that 30-day rates of the composite end point of death or serious complications were similar in off-pump compared with on-pump surgery patients. However, patients randomized to off-pump surgery had less complete revascularization, a higher rate of graft failure at 1 year, and worse 1-year outcomes including death, nonfatal MI, and repeat revascularization. Neuropsychological testing outcomes were similar between the two groups. These data suggest that routine off-pump coronary artery bypass surgery has no advantages over on-pump surgery, with worse graft patency at 1 year.

Previous randomized trials of medical versus revascularization therapy in patients with stable coronary artery disease excluded the elderly. An important recent trial prospectively randomized patients of age 75 years and older (mean, 80 years) with moderate angina on at least 2 antianginal drugs to coronary angiography and revascularization versus optimal medical therapy. The primary end point of this trial was quality of life scores at 6 months. Seventy-four percent of patients randomized to the invasive arm had anatomy appropriate for either percutaneous intervention (54%) or coronary artery bypass surgery (20%). These data dispel the myth that older patients usually have diffuse coronary disease not amenable to revascularization. Quality of life improved in both groups by 6 months, but the invasive therapy had better quality of life. Secondary end points of death, myocardial infarction, or hospitalization for unstable angina, at 6 months, were significantly lower in elderly patients randomized to invasive therapy (19%) versus medical therapy (49%). One-third of patients in the medical arm crossed over to revascularization due to refractory symptomatology. There was no difference in 4 year survival and non-fatal MI. Rehospitalization was significantly higher in the medical therapy group. This suggests that age alone is not a contraindication to proceed with an invasive approach to the treatment of moderate to severe angina that is present despite antianginal therapy.

Although several trials have randomized patients with stable CAD to PCI versus CABG, the elderly were generally excluded. In a recent randomized trial, 454 high-risk veterans with medically refractory angina were randomized to percutaneous coronary intervention with or without stents or coronary artery bypass surgery. High-risk characteristics included age >70 years, prior bypass, LVEF <35%, recent myocardial infarction, and need for intra-aortic balloon pump. Survival at 30 days was excellent in both groups (95% vs 97% for bypass and angioplasty, respectively). Survival up to 3 years remained similar in the 2 groups. Therefore, high-risk elderly patients with medically refractory angina, can undergo revascularization with angioplasty or bypass surgery with excellent survival as well as relief of angina.

# ■ CONGESTIVE HEART FAILURE

In contrast to other cardiovascular disorders, the prevalence of congestive heart failure (CHF) is increasing, with approximately 5.7 million Americans with CHF. The incidence of heart failure doubles with each decade of life, and the prevalence increases to almost 10% >80 years old. Heart failure represents a final common pathway for most other cardiac disorders and, it is more successfully treated with ischemic and valvular disease. These successful treatments increase the numbers of surviving patients, albeit with, or at increased risk for, heart failure.

CHF is a highly lethal condition, with significant mortality, morbidity, and associated costs in the older population. Analyses in >160 000 Medicare recipients with newly diagnosed CHF indicate a median survival of only 2 to 4 years. More than 90% of CHF deaths occur in adults >age 65 years. CHF is also the leading cause of hospitalization in Medicare beneficiaries, with those <65 accounting for 75% of the 1.1 million heart failure discharge diagnoses. Hospitalization in these patients is itself a major risk factor for subsequent rehospitalization, mortality, and functional decline.

Evaluation of the older patient presenting with heart failure symptoms should include a noninvasive study to determine whether the primary problem is impaired systolic function. Although systolic dysfunction is present in half of CHF cases, the presence of a normal or elevated ejection fraction is more common in older heart failure patients with AF and hypertension, particularly women. The number of patients with heart failure and preserved systolic function is increasing and is with the aging of the general population. These patients experience significant limitations in exercise duration and quality of life, increases in neurohormonal activation and CHF markers such as natriuretic peptide, and increased mortality, hospitalization rates, and health care costs when compared with the general population. Rehospitalization rates are similar to patients with primary systolic dysfunction, as is mortality, depending on enrollment in randomized clinical trials; it leads to lower risk because of less comorbidities and better therapy, whether they are drawn from community or referral centers, and the extent to which noncardiac etiologies that might confound the diagnosis of heart failure are excluded. The etiology for heart failure with preserved ejection fraction may be related to abnormalities in diastolic filling including impaired calcium handling, hypertrophy, and/or fibrosis. Hypertension, increased central vascular stiffness and thus impaired ventricular-vascular coupling are present. Evidence of long-standing volume overload and an $S_3$ gallop are less likely in patients with preserved systolic function and exertional symptoms are less common and symptoms related to fatigue and mental status changes are more common. The diagnosis of heart failure with preserved systolic function is primarily one of exclusion in patients with objective evidence of pulmonary vascular congestion without findings of an ischemic, hypertensive, or valvular etiology. Amyloid should also be considered in older patients in the absence of another identifiable cause.

Reversible etiologies in older individuals who present with new-onset or worsening heart failure symptoms, including anemia, infection, thyroid disease, AF, and dietary or medication noncompliance should be ruled out. Common comorbidities should be explored because they are associated with increased hospitalizations and adverse clinical outcomes. Diuretics are useful in older patients with increased vascular stiffness presenting with acute congestive symptoms because significant reductions in pressure occur with relatively small changes in intravascular volume. In patients with systolic dysfunction, sinus rhythm, and CHF, digitalis may improve signs and symptoms of heart failure. However, the maintenance dose should be reduced to 0.125 mg/d because of the age-associated decreased volume of distribution and creatinine clearance. Digitalis does not improve outcomes, in patients with preserved systolic function and sinus rhythm. The Ancillary Digitalis Investigation Group trial reported that in those with mild to moderate failure and preserved systolic function, digitalis had no effect on overall or heart failure mortality and was associated with trends toward lower heart failure hospitalizations but increased unstable angina hospitalizations.

Heart failure with primary systolic and preserved systolic function are both associated with increased sympathetic and rennin-angiotensin-aldosterone activation. In patients with primary systolic dysfunction, β-blockers improve survival and other important cardiovascular outcomes in the older subsets of large randomized trials. Unfortunately, many older individuals with heart failure and systolic dysfunction are receiving no or underdosed β-blocker therapy. There are no reported randomized studies limited to the effects of β-blockers in older individuals with heart failure and preserved systolic function. In a study of patients >70 years old with a recent heart failure hospitalization, nebivolol, a β-blocker with vasodilating properties, was associated with a decrease in the composite end point of all-cause mortality or cardiovascular hospitalization. There was no difference between the relative reduction rates in those with ejection fractions of greater or less than 35%, and no effect in the two individual subsets. Thus, the value, if any, of beta-blockers in the older heart failure group with preserved systolic function is not known.

ACE inhibitors are a cornerstone of therapy in patients with systolic dysfunction, in the elderly. Their benefit in patients with preserved systolic function, however, is less certain. The Perindopril in Elderly People with Chronic Heart Failure (PEP-CHF) study randomized 207 patients >70 years of age with heart failure, normal systolic and valve function, and echocardiographic evidence of diastolic dysfunction to perindopril or placebo. Results were confounded by lower enrollment and outcomes and significant numbers of study patients switching to open-label ACE inhibitor therapy. There was a trend toward reduction in the primary outcome of all-cause mortality and unplanned CHF hospitalization and significant improvement in functional class and the 6-minute walk test in the ACE inhibitor group during the first year. In heart failure patients with systolic dysfunction, angiotensin receptor blockers improve survival. However, there was no survival benefit in patients with preserved systolic function in randomized trials of candesartan and irbesartan that showed no survival benefit although candesartan was associated with decreased heart failure hospitalization. There were no differences between patients randomized to irbesartan or placebo in survival; heart failure or any hospitalization; quality of life scores; and change in N-terminal prohormone brain natriuretic peptide levels. A trial of spironolactone in heart failure patients with preserved systolic function was recently completed, but outcomes data is not yet available.

Devices may significantly improve outcomes in patients with persistent failure despite medical therapy. The use of atrial-synchronized, biventricular pacing in patients with heart failure and evidence of cardiac dyssynchrony improves survival, ejection fraction, functional class, and quality of life, and decreases hospitalization. The use of long-term LV assist devices as "destination therapy" may be particularly useful in older patients without concomitant diseases, an estimated 1-year mortality of >50%, and no other life-threatening illnesses. Complications are frequent, and although age itself does not appear to be a risk factor for early adverse outcomes, renal and pulmonary dysfunction and poor nutritional status, which may be more common in the elderly, are risk factors. The continuous-flow rotary devices are smaller in size and have a simpler design, which may be associated with less malfunction and infection risks. Transcutaneous energy transfer is likely to make these devices safer and applicable to a broader patient population. Recent advances in stem cell treatments raise the possibility that these therapies may improve function and survival and decrease cardiovascular events. Allogeneic, rather than autologous, cells may offer more promise in the older population because of the previously noted age-associated decrease in stem cell function in some animal and human studies. Implantable defibrillators provide primary prevention, reducing total mortality in patients with ischemic and non-ischemic disease and reduced ejection fraction. Current guidelines recommend that implantable defibrillators be placed for primary prevention in patients with an ejection fraction of ≤35% despite beta-blockers and ACE inhibitors (or angiotensin receptor blockers), with mild to moderate heart failure symptoms, and with a reasonable expectation of survival with a good functional status for >1 year. Implantable cardioverter-defibrillators are not recommended for those with refractory heart failure symptoms or with concomitant diseases that would shorten their lives. Discussions in older patients should include complications, including bleeding and infection, and the possibility of inappropriate shocks, particularly with AF, more common in the older population. In older patients with refractory end-stage heart failure, current guidelines also include recommendations for discussion of end-of-life care and of options including inactivating defibrillators and referral for hospice care.

The importance of the individual patient's role as a partner in his/her care and of individualizing treatment and monitoring plans cannot be overemphasized. Although patients may carry the same heart failure diagnosis, they differ markedly in terms of disease severity and complexity, comorbidities, social support, education, ingrained habits, access to medical personnel and knowledge, and understanding of health care information and directions. Noncompliance with medications or diet is often cited as a major factor contributing to hospitalization in heart failure patients. In the older patient, noncompliance is more likely due to social isolation, financial difficulties, limited travel and meal options, decreased tolerability for some medicines, comorbidities, and difficult-to-follow complex medical regimens. A multidisciplinary team approach including simplification of the medical regimen, close monitoring, and intensive patient education can decrease hospital admission and improve quality of life.

# ■ ARRHYTHMIAS

Supraventricular and ventricular arrhythmias increase in frequency with aging and are common in older, apparently healthy individuals. In BLSA participants, 88% of those >60 years of age had isolated supraventricular beats, 13% had paroxysmal atrial tachycardia, 80% had isolated premature ventricular beats, 35% had multiform premature ventricular contractions, and 11% had ventricular couplets during a 24-hour monitoring period. The increase with age is probably due to loss of pacemaker and conducting cells and fibrosis, as well as an increased incidence of mitral annular and aortic calcification. Recent studies describe slowed conduction and decreased voltage in the atria, downregulation of sinus node L-type calcium expression, and loss of connexin-43 expression in the sinus node. Other illnesses may present with arrhythmias in the elderly as well, including pulmonary embolism, pericarditis, myocardial infarction, hyperthyroidism, anemia, hypoxia, electrolyte imbalance, and infection. Age-associated changes in diastolic properties, decreased systolic reserve, may increase the likelihood that the older individual more likely develop hemodynamic compromise and/or ischemia during an arrhythmic episode.

The older patient with arrhythmias should be evalutated for concomitant illnesses and triggers like chest pain, exercise, smoking, caffeine, electrolyte abnormalities, and medicine and alcohol ingestion. Ambulatory ECG monitoring during normal activities is most likely to determine the nature and severity of the arrhythmia. Invasive electrophysiology studies can be used to diagnose the arrhythmia, and determine its mechanism, obtain prognostic information, and determine the suitability of different therapeutic approaches.

Atrial flutter and AF are common in the elderly. Both are associated with structural heart disease, therefore patients with newly diagnosed atrial tachyarrhythmias should undergo echocardiographic evaluation. Patients with atrial flutter who are at increased stroke risk, which includes those >75 years of age, should receive anticoagulation unless there are contraindications. Flutter that is symptomatic should be cardiovered. If flutter recurs, catheter ablation is more successful than pharmacologic therapy in the maintenance of sinus rhythm.

AF is the most common arrhythmia in the elderly, with a prevalence of 8% in those >80 years old and an incidence of 1.5% per year in women and 2.0% per year in men >80 years old. In 5 randomized trials of anticoagulation for the prevention of stroke in AF, the mean age of enrolled patients was 69 years, with 25% over the age of 75 years. AF in the elderly is associated with increasing age, heart failure, valvular heart disease, stroke, diabetes, and hypertension. Older individuals are more likely to experience hemodynamic compromise from any increased ventricular rate and atrial/ventricular dyssynchrony because of age-associated changes in relaxation properties and increased dependence on atrial contribution. Because of increased CAD, the higher rate is also more likely to be associated with MI. AF may cause atrial remodeling, which tends to maintain the arrhythmias, cardiomyopathy and lower output. The risk of embolic stroke in AF also increases with age. The Framingham Study reported that the annual risk of stroke attributed to AF increased from 1.5% in those of age 50 to 59 years to 23.5% in those of age 80 to 89 years.

Therapeutic goals in patients with AF include stroke prevention, rate control, and possibly rhythm control. In randomized trials, anticoagulation prevents embolic strokes in most patients with AF, including those >75 years old. This benefit of anticoagulation is greater than aspirin therapy in the elderly, although there is a higher rate of intracranial hemorrhage. Careful monitoring of the international normalized ratio is important because most embolic strokes in the elderly occur when the ratio is <2.0 and most cerebral hemorrhages occur when the ratio is >3.0.

The risks of major hemorrhage associated with anticoagulation in the older patient were noted in a study of 472 patients >65 years of age, all treated at a major medical center who were followed for 1 year after institution of warfarin for AF. The incidence of major hemorrhage was 4.7% for those age 65 to 80 years and 13.1% for those age ≥80 years. Warfarin was discontinued in 26% of patients ≥80 years old, with safety concerns accounting for 81% of the discontinuations. The authors conclude that risks calculated from noninception studies (eliminating those who experience early adverse bleeding outcomes) and from younger individuals may be underestimated. Bleeding risks are also recognized in the latest guidelines concerning management of AF, wherein it is recommended that patients with a $CHADS_2$ (CHF, hypertension, age ≥75 years, diabetes, and prior stroke or transient ischemic attack) score of 0 be treated with aspirin alone and that those with a score of 1 can be treated with aspirin or warfarin. Although the benefits of aspirin are less significant, aspirin can be used in older patients who have a contraindication to warfarin therapy, including an inability to carefully monitor the international normalized ratio. When the $CHADS_2$ score is 0-1 the $CHA_2DS_2$ VASc score is utilized for stroke risk. Points are assigned for additional risk factors such as age 65-74, or <75, Vascular disease (CAD, MI, PAD, and complex aortic plaque), and female gender (Sc). High risk is a score of 2 or greater requiring anticoagulation, a score of <2 may be treated with aspirin. Direct thrombin inhibitors may achieve results similar or superior to warfarin while avoiding the necessity for frequent clinic visits and dose adjustments. A recent study randomized >18 000 patients with AF to dose-adjusted warfarin, dabigatran 110 mg/d, or dabigatran 150 mg/d. Compared to warfarin over a 2-year follow-up, 110-mg dose of dabigatran had similar stroke and systemic embolization rates and lower rates of major hemorrhage, the 150-mg dose was associated with lower stroke and systemic embolism rates and similar rates of major hemorrhage. An additional approach is obliteration of the left atrial appendage, which is the source of approximately 90% of emboli. This can be achieved during surgery or by the use of presently experimental intravascular catheters. The relative efficacy, safety, and long-term effectiveness of these approaches in the older patient are not yet characterized.

Rate control in patients without systolic dysfunction is achieved with diltiazem, verapamil, and β-blockers; amiodarone or digitalis may be used in patients with systolic dysfunction. A useful goal is a rate of <80/minute at rest and <110/minute on a 6-minute walk test. Patients intolerant of medical therapy or if medical therapy is ineffective, AV node ablation and pacemaker insertion or AV node modification, which results in slowed AV conduction, but not complete heart block of AF ablation should be considered. Cardioversion should be attempted in patients who are hemodynamically compromised, in acute AF, and for those who are at low likelihood of reversion to AF if conversion does occur. This can be attempted with electrical or pharmacologic approaches. A randomized study comparing several weeks of warfarin therapy before cardioversion with more immediate cardioversion if transesophageal echocardiography reveals no atrial thrombi demonstrated similar rates of thromboembolism and maintenance of sinus rhythm but a lower hemorrhage rate in the transesophageal group. Either approach would be reasonable, but it is important to continue warfarin for at least 1 month following cardioversion.

Two studies compared rate control and rhythm control strategies in primarily older (mean ages, 70 and 68 years) patients with AF. In the Atrial Fibrillation Follow-Up Investigation of Rhythm Management (AFFIRM) trial, 5-year estimates indicated that a higher proportion of patients were in sinus rhythm in the rhythm control group (63%) than the rate control group (35%). In the second study, 39% of the rhythm control group and 10% of the rate control group were in sinus rhythm at follow-up. There were no differences in mortality, although subgroup analysis showed a higher mortality in the rhythm control group for those ≥65 years old. Ischemic stroke and thromboembolic events were nonsignificantly higher in the rhythm control group, and were associated with discontinuation of or subtherapeutic anticoagulation. Hospitalizations were higher in the rhythm control strategy group. Thus, rate control is a reasonable strategy in older patients with AF and is not associated with significant symptoms or hemodynamic compromise. Anticoagulation should be maintained regardless of a rate or rhythm control strategy. If rhythm control is attempted, flecainide and propafenone may be used in patients without ischemic or structural heart disease. In patients with ischemic disease, sotalol may be used. In patients with heart failure, dofetilide increases the likelihood of conversion to and maintenance of sinus rhythm without the increase in mortality associated with some other antiarrhythmic agents in patients with heart failure. Amiodarone is useful in nearly all patient populations and, in a randomized trial, was more effective than sotalol or propafenone in preventing recurrences of AF.

The recognition that rapid firing of atrial myocytes located near the pulmonary veins may be responsible for some episodes of AF has led to the use of catheter ablation to terminate AF. Subsequently, it was recognized that foci may propagate from other regions, including the right and left atrium and veins, and techniques were modified. It is possible that this approach may result in improved outcomes compared with pharmacologic therapy and/or a rate control strategy. At present, the long-term success, approaches 70% with repeat procedures, and complications in the older patient are improving. It may be considered for patients with AF associated with significant symptoms who are refractory to or intolerant of medical therapy.

Approximately one-half of pacemakers are placed because of sinus node dysfunction with bradycardia. Pacemakers that appropriately time atrial and ventricular systole may be particularly useful in older patients because diastolic filling and cardiac output are more dependent on atrial contribution. In a randomized trial comparing single- and dual-chamber pacing modalities in patients with sinus node dysfunction, there was no difference in stroke-free mortality, but the risk of new and chronic AF and signs and symptoms of heart failure were significantly reduced and quality of life was higher in patients assigned to dual-chamber pacing.

Ventricular arrhythmias in the elderly are to be approached in the same fashion as in younger individuals; that is, patients who are asymptomatic and have no evidence of cardiac disease can be viewed as less serious than patients with evidence of LV dysfunction and/or ischemia. Both older and younger post-myocardial infarction patients benefit from beta-blocker therapy with a reduction in sudden death. Life-threatening ventricular arrhythmias are common in the elderly patient with severe CAD and LV dysfunction. Aggressive management of elderly survivors of cardiac arrest and of those with hypotensive ventricular tachycardia is justified. In the Multicenter Automatic Defibrillator Implantation Trial II (MADIT-II) trial, patients with an ejection fraction of ≤30% and a prior myocardial infarction randomized to an implantable defibrillator experienced improved survival compared with patients randomized to conventional therapy. For patients ≥70 years old, the hazard ratio of death was decreased by >30%. In the Defibrillators in Non-ischemic Cardiomyopathy Treatment Evaluation (DEFINITE) study of prophylactic implantable defibrillators in patients with nonischemic dilated cardiomyopathy, an ejection fraction of ≤35%, and premature ventricular complexes, the decrease in death from any cause was similar in those older and younger than 65 years of age. In an analysis of >30 000 Medicare beneficiaries who underwent implantable cardioverter-defibrillator placement in fiscal year 2003, 10.8% experienced an in-hospital early complication, which was associated with an adjusted $7251/patient hospital cost and 3.4-day increased length of stay. The most frequent complications were mechanical related to the implantable cardioverter-defibrillator system, hemorrhage, infection, and pneumothorax. It should also be noted that as age increases beyond 75 years, the likelihood of dying from causes other than lethal ventricular arrhythmias increases, and thus the survival benefit is likely less than in younger patients.

# ■ VALVULAR HEART DISEASE

Prevalence of valvular disease increases markedly with age. Based on 12 000 echocardiograms performed in 3 population-based epidemiologic studies in the United States, 9.3% of the population of age 75 years or older has mitral regurgitation and 2.8% has aortic stenosis. The most frequent valvular heart disease in the elderly is calcific aortic stenosis. The development of clinically significant aortic stenosis may be very rapid in this age group because calcification and severe scarring can occur rather abruptly. Evidence suggests calcific aortic stenosis in the elderly is not the result of a degenerative process, but involves an active inflammatory process similar to that present in atherosclerotic vascular lesions. Pathologic findings of lesions containing inflammatory mediators, as well as macrophages that produce osteopontin, a protein that enhances tissue calcification supports this. The presence of calcific disease is also related to traditional atherosclerotic risk factors including cigarette use, diabetes, hypertension, and hyperlipidemia.

Doppler echocardiogram is used to assess aortic valve calcification, mobility, aortic valve area, the transvalvular gradient, the presence of any LV hypertrophy, and LV function. Asymptomatic elderly patients with significant aortic stenosis by echocardiography can be followed carefully without surgical intervention until the first symptoms appear. If the older patient is limited by other disease (eg, arthritis), the patient may not be able to exercise to the point where symptoms occur despite the presence of significant disease requiring surgery. Important factors include the rate of progression, with an increase of >0.1 cm$^2$ per year favoring earlier surgery, and elevated brain natriuretic peptide. Aortic valve replacement is recommended for patients with severe aortic stenosis and an ejection fraction of <50% and in those undergoing bypass surgery or other aortic or valve surgery. A low calculated valve area in the presence of a low cardiac output may be due to incomplete valve opening, rather than severe stenosis. Calculation of the valve area during dobutamine administration in these instances provides a more accurate assessment of valvular stenosis. A recent report classifying the hemodynamic response to dobutamine based on the projected aortic valve area at a common transvalvular flow may be helpful in patients in whom it is difficult to interpret the response to dobutamine, most particularly if the dobutamine-induced increase in flow is small. Significant coronary stenosis increases valvular surgical risk, therefore coronary angiography is usually performed in patients being considered for surgery. Multislice computed tomography may serve as an alternative to the invasive diagnostic procedure in these patients.

Aortic valve replacement often results in marked improvement in symptoms and LV function, expected survival in the older patient. In a recent report, median survival times in patients undergoing isolated aortic valve replacement were 6.8 years for those 80 to 84 years old and 6.2 years for those ≥85 years old, which are similar to life expectancies of the general population. Predictors of surgical mortality with aortic valve replacement include low ejection fraction, CHF, AF, associated surgical procedures, comorbidities including cerebrovascular disease, and an emergency procedure. Moderate mitral regurgitation is also an independent risk factor for poor outcomes following surgery for aortic stenosis, therefore, mitral valve repair or replacement should be considered in those whose regurgitation is due to intrinsic mitral valve disease. Although age is not an independent risk factor in most studies, older individuals are more likely to have the associated conditions that increase operative and postoperative mortality and complications. Percutaneous aortic balloon valvuloplasty in the elderly is associated with poor outcomes including early restenosis, aortic regurgitation, stroke, high mortality, and heart failure. It is useful only for palliation and as a "bridge" to valve replacement in very ill patients. There are several new experimental surgical and percutaneous procedures that may afford a lower complication rate in those with factors that increase the risk of traditional median sternotomy, aortic valve replacement procedures. These include the off-pump ventriculoaortic valved conduit, in which a tract is created from the LV to the descending aorta. It avoids bypass and surgery on a diseased aortic root and thus the associated cerebrovascular and embolic complications. Clinical trials of percutaneous aortic valves are also in progress. In a recent report of 168 patients with severe aortic stenosis and increased surgical risk (median age, 84 years) who underwent transcatheter aortic valve implantation, the overall success rate was 94%, and 30-day mortality was 11.3%. Mortality decreased with increased experience. One-year survival was 74%, structural valve failure did not occur, and the majority of readmissions and deaths were due to comorbidities and not due to the procedure or to valve disease.

Chronic aortic regurgitation may occur in elderly individuals secondary to aortic root dilatation related to long-standing hypertension. Symptoms include angina, without significant coronary disease, and CHF symptoms may not occur until significant LV dysfunction is present; therefore, the onset of dysfunction is sufficient to prompt surgery. Vasodilator therapy is currently recommended only in those with severe aortic regurgitation and with symptoms or LV dysfunction in whom surgery cannot be performed and as short-term therapy to improve the hemodynamic profile in those with symptoms or LV dysfunction prior to surgery. It has a class IIb recommendation for asymptomatic individuals with severe aortic regurgitation, LV dilatation, and normal systolic function, but long-term therapy is not recommended for asymptomatic patients with mild to moderate aortic regurgitation and normal systolic function. Best operative results occur in individuals with no or minimal symptoms, mild to moderate ventricular dysfunction, and a brief duration of LV dysfunction. Current indications include symptomatic severe aortic regurgitation or have an ejection fraction of ≤50%. LV dilatation, defined as an end-diastolic dimension of ≥75 mm or an end-systolic dimension of ≥55 mm, in patients with severe aortic regurgitation has a class IIb indication. Symptoms should be given more importance in older patients with aortic regurgitation because improvements in long-term survival are less realistic in the elderly.

Common causes of mitral stenosis in the elderly are rheumatic disease, which at times may not result in symptoms until the patient reaches old age, obstruction resulting from extensive mitral annular and leaflet calcification, and fibrosis. The diagnosis of mitral stenosis may be more difficult in the elderly because calcification of the valve may decrease the intensity of the first heart sound and the opening sound, and diminished cardiac output may decrease the intensity of the diastolic rumble. Doppler echocardiography is useful in diagnosing the presence of significant disease. If symptoms are more than mild or if pulmonary hypertension develops, surgery or balloon mitral valvuloplasty should be considered. AF often triggers functional deterioration in older individuals because the dependence of filling on atrial contraction is exaggerated in the presence of mitral stenosis. Balloon mitral valvuloplasty compares favorably with open surgical commissurotomy in appropriate candidates (ie, those with minimal calcification, good mobility, little subvalvular disease, and only mild mitral regurgitation) and should be considered for elderly patients with symptomatic mitral stenosis. Periprocedural mortality (3%) and morbidity, including tamponade (5%) and thromboembolism (3%), are higher than in younger patients.

Mitral regurgitation in the elderly is most often related to ischemic heart disease and myxomatous degeneration of the mitral valve. As is true for aortic insufficiency, symptoms may be recognized only after significant LV dysfunction and if cavity dilatation has occurred, then favorable unloading conditions will increase the ejection fraction in the presence of significant mitral regurgitation. Therefore, an ejection fraction of <60% should be considered abnormal and is associated with a poorer postsurgical prognosis. Thus, an ejection fraction of <60% or an end-systolic dimension of ≥40 mm can be considered indications for surgery in asymptomatic patients with severe mitral regurgitation. The prognosis for patients with ischemic mitral regurgitation is significantly poorer than for patients with degenerative etiologies. Nevertheless, operative success has increased in recent years, with some studies reporting survival rates following surgery for degenerative disease similar to those expected in the general population. For elderly patients with non-ischemic mitral regurgitation, mitral valve repair is associated with a lower operative mortality and improved late outcomes, obviates anticoagulation in patients without AF, and produces excellent long-term results. Thus, repair, rather than replacement, should be performed if possible. If repair is not possible, chordal preservation should be attempted. In patients with ischemic mitral regurgitation at least one study showed similar outcomes with repair and replacement procedures. New surgical techniques designed to address the particular anatomic abnormality, often guided by intraoperative transesophageal echocardiography, are likely to result in improved outcomes. Hospital procedural volume has a significant impact on operative mortality for patients undergoing surgery for mitral regurgitation. The risk-adjusted odds ratio for mortality in the highest volume quartile hospitals participating in the Society of Thoracic Surgeons National Cardiac Database was 0.48 that of the lowest quartile. High-volume center surgery was also associated with increased rates of mitral valve repair and use of a bioprosthetic valve for patients >65 years old. Percutaneous approaches may be particularly applicable in patients with ischemic mitral regurgitation who have greater postprocedure adverse outcomes because they also impact annular dilatation and poor leaflet coaptation, the major pathophysiology in patients with this condition.

For elderly patients requiring valve replacement, a mechanical valve with the bleeding risk of lifelong anticoagulation must be weighed against a bioprosthetic valve and risk of structural deterioration. Additional factors in this choice include candidacy for anticoagulation and other requirements for anticoagulation such as AF, age, and valve position. Successful intraoperative AF ablation will enhance the benefit of a bioprosthetic valve. In a series of elderly subjects receiving aortic or mitral mechanical valve replacements, freedom from major anticoagulant-related hemorrhage was 76% at 10 years. A bioprosthetic valve in the mitral position deteriorates more rapidly than in the aortic position. In a large series of elderly patients receiving porcine bioprostheses, freedom from structural deterioration at 10 years was 98% for the aortic valve bioprostheses and 79% for the mitral valve bioprostheses, with excellent long-term survival free of major morbidity.

# SUGGESTED READINGS

Lakatta EG, Najjar SS, Schulman SP, Gerstenblith G. Aging and cardiovascular disease in the elderly. In: Fuster V, Walsh RA, Harrington RG, eds. *Hurst's The Heart*. 13th ed. New York, NY: McGraw-Hill; 2011:102:2196-2225.

Alhusban A, Fagan SC. Secondary prevention of stroke in the elderly: a review of the evidence. *Am J Geriatr Pharmacother*. 2011 Jun; 9(3):143-152.

Alexander KP, Roe MT, Chen AY, et al. Evolution in cardiovascular care for elderly patients with non-ST-segment elevation acute coronary syndromes: results from the CRUSADE national quality improvement initiative. *J Am Coll Cardiol*. 2005;46:1479-1487.

Chrysohoou C, Tsiachris D, Stefanadis C. Aortic stenosis in the elderly: challenges in diagnosis and therapy. *Maturitas*3.2011 Dec;70(4):349-353.

Keller NM, Feit F. Atherosclerotic heart disease in the elderly. *Curr Opinion Cardiol*. 1995;10:427-433.

Lakatta EG. Cardiovascular regulatory mechanisms in advanced age. *Physiol Rev*. 1993;73:413-465.

Lakatta EG, Levy D. Arterial and cardiac aging: major shareholders in cardiovascular disease enterprises: part II: the aging heart in health: links to heart disease. *Circulation*. 2003;107:346-354.

Lakatta EG. Deficient neuroendocrine regulation of the cardiovascular system with advancing age in healthy humans. *Circulation*. 1993;87:631-636.

Najjar SS, Lakatta EG. Vascular aging: from molecular to clinical cardiology. In: *Principles of Molecular Cardiology*. Totowa, NJ: Humana Press; 2002:517-567.

Olivetti G, Giordano G, Corradi D, et al. Gender differences and aging: effects on the human heart. *J Am Coll Cardiol*. 1995;26:1068-1079.

Van Staa TP, Setakis E, Di Tanna GL, Lane DA, Lip GY. A comparison of risk stratification schemes for stroke in 79,884 atrial fibrillation patients in general practice. *J Thromb Haemost*. 2011;9(1):39.

# CHAPTER 60

# COMPLEMENTARY AND ALTERNATIVE MEDICAL THERAPY IN CARDIOVASCULAR CARE

Rajesh Vedanthan, Mitchell W. Krucoff, Rebecca B. Costello, Daniel B. Mark, and John H. K. Vogel

The American College of Cardiology (ACC) recently published a consensus statement on complementary and alternative medicine (CAM) as applied to cardiovascular disease (CVD). Patients are increasingly using CAM therapies, and there is a concomitant growing professional interest in CAM therapies as adjuncts to the high-tech world of cardiovascular care. These developments have generated concerns about exaggerated claims of efficacy and potential toxicity across the largely unregulated pantheon of CAM practices. There is therefore an urgent mandate for cardiologists to become better informed about CAM therapeutics, with the ultimate aim to support more thoughtful and less defensive dialogue between physicians and patients, as well as to encourage novel research directions and more integrated evidence-based clinical strategies.

Although many CAM therapies have been practiced for thousands of years, the evidence-based literature is still not well developed in this arena. Ambiguous nomenclature, lack of practice certification standards, and absence of quantitative profiles of active agents in consumables such as herbal remedies confound evaluation of safety and efficacy in specific heart disease populations. In addition, investigator bias, reporting bias, and publisher bias also confound the interpretation of available data. However, research in CAM therapies in cardiovascular care must balance standards for clinical trial designs or mechanistic studies with sensitivity to the cultural assumptions of how these therapies actually work.

In this chapter, we adopt the framework developed by the National Center for Complementary and Alterative Medicine (NCCAM) at the National Institutes of Health, with a focus specifically on cardiovascular applications across 5 key treatment areas: biologically based practices, manipulative and body-based practices, energy medicine, mind–body medicine, and whole medical systems. We conclude the chapter with a discussion of end-of-life care as relevant for CVD.

## BIOLOGICALLY BASED PRACTICES: SELECTED BOTANICALS AND DIETARY SUPPLEMENTS

### ■ BOTANICALS

The medicinal use of botanicals originated more than 7000 years ago; the written history spans more than 3500 years. Approximately 25% of pharmaceuticals prescribed today are derived from plant sources. In addition, there has been a rekindling of consumer interest in the use of natural whole-plant products. A significant result of this public interest and demand for access to herbal products was the passage of the Dietary Supplement Health and Education Act (DSHEA) of 1994. Herbs, vitamins, minerals, and proteins were classified as dietary supplements. However, neither good manufacturing practices nor labeling certifying concentrations of active ingredients or bioavailability have been required for DSHEA products. As a result, independent examination has revealed inconsistency and variability between product labeling and actual compound concentration. In this setting, safety concerns with potential adulteration of supplements with active prescription compounds, contamination of preparations, and herb–herb and herb–drug interactions are significant. Research into the safety and efficacy of botanical compounds has been hampered by this lack of standardization.

In December 2006, the Dietary Supplement and Nonprescription Drug Consumer Protection Act (the "AER bill," Public Law 109-462) was passed by Congress. This bill requires manufacturers of dietary supplements and over-the-counter (OTC) products to submit serious adverse event reports (SAERs) to the FDA. Under this Act, a *serious adverse event* is defined as any adverse event resulting in death, a life-threatening experience, inpatient hospitalization, a persistent or significant disability or incapacity, or a congenital anomaly or birth defect, as well as any adverse event requiring a medical or surgical intervention to prevent one of the aforementioned conditions, based on reasonable medical judgment. Physicians may also be proactive and report SAERs directly to the FDA MedWatch Reporting system at https://www.accessdata.fda.gov/scripts/medwatch/medwatch-online.htm.

In addition, in July 2007 the Food and Drug Administration (FDA) announced a rule establishing regulations to require current good manufacturing practices (CGMPs) for dietary supplements and finished products. The regulations establish the CGMPs needed to ensure quality throughout the manufacturing, packaging, labeling, and storing of dietary supplements. The aim of the rule is to prevent inclusion of the wrong ingredients, too much or too little of a dietary ingredient, contamination by substances such as natural toxins, bacteria, pesticides, glass, lead, and other heavy metals, as well as improper packaging and labeling.

## Garlic (Allium sativum)

Garlic has long been touted as a natural product useful for the modulation of immune system activity, in the treatment of hyperlipidemia and hypertension, as well as in the primary and secondary prevention of myocardial infarction. Medicinal use of garlic can be traced back to the ancient Babylonians and Chinese, with long-term usage occurring in Western folk medicine as well. Allicin is felt to be the bioactive component responsible for the potential cardiovascular activity of garlic. Allicin content is determined by the nature of the garlic preparation, with raw crushed garlic having the highest concentration. Multiple mechanisms of action have been proposed, including decrease in cholesterol and fatty acid synthesis and cholesterol absorption. Potent antioxidant properties, as well as antiplatelet and fibrinolytic activity with garlic has also been reported.

Clinical studies of garlic have yielded contradictory results, with significant design flaws notable in trials designed to demonstrate garlic's effectiveness. Short-term studies have shown some benefit in the lipid profiles of patients taking garlic, whereas long-term studies of 6 months or more fail to show sustained benefit when garlic is used as a single agent. A recent well-designed randomized controlled trial using highly characterized diet and supplement interventions comparing the effects of raw garlic, powdered garlic supplement, aged garlic supplement, and placebo in 192 moderately hypercholesterolemic adults demonstrated no significant difference in LDL cholesterol between treatment groups. A systematic review of 21 garlic studies to evaluate the reporting quality, safety, and efficacy of randomized controlled trials for lipid lowering demonstrated that 53% of the garlic trials reported positive efficacy, with a mean safety score of 63 of 100.

Studies of garlic's effectiveness in hypertension have also suffered from poor methodology, and results have revealed small, mostly insignificant decreases in blood pressure. A subsequent systematic review of 27 small, randomized controlled trials of at least 4 weeks' duration comparing garlic with placebo, no garlic, or another active agent reported mixed effects of various garlic preparations on blood pressure. Two meta-analyses published in 2008 concluded that compared with placebo, garlic significantly lowered systolic blood pressure in hypertensive individuals but not in normotensive individuals. Evidence for the supplemental intake of garlic for both the primary and secondary prevention of heart disease is not sufficient to recommend its use for this indication.

The anticoagulant properties of garlic can be problematic in the perioperative period and in combination with other anticoagulant compounds. Garlic has also been reported to interact with the P450 enzyme system. Side effects are minor other than occasional nausea with excessive raw intake of garlic and the development of an unpleasant odor.

## Hawthorn (Crataegus species)

Hawthorn species are a group of small trees and shrubs found throughout North America, Asia, and Europe. Preparations made from flowers with leaves are sold as a prescription medication in parts of Europe and Asia. Sales of hawthorn products have increased steadily in the United States for the past 10 years, placing it among the top 40 best-selling botanical products. Purported cardiovascular indications include congestive heart failure (CHF), angina, and arrhythmias. Hawthorn's activity is felt to be related to the presence of a number of key constituents, including flavonoids and oligomeric procyanidins. Animal and in vitro models reveal positive inotropism with a mechanism of action similar to that of digitalis through a cyclic adenosine monophosphate-independent effect. There is also evidence of a direct vasodilating effect.

Literature review reveals evidence for hawthorn's efficacy in the treatment of mild to moderate CHF. Some efficacy has been documented in increasing maximal workload capacity and decreasing symptom severity in patients with CHF. One uncontrolled study also reported an increase in ejection fraction measured by angiography from 30% to 41% in patients with class II to III heart failure. A recent systematic review and meta-analysis of 14 randomized controlled trials in 1110 patients with heart failure treated with standard heart failure medications for up to 26 weeks reported that standardized preparations of hawthorn can increase exercise performance and cardiac oxygen consumption and may improve heart failure symptoms such as dyspnea and fatigue. In the first mortality-driven trial, the SPICE trial, a European multicenter trial randomizing 3601 patients with class II to III heart failure, a standardized preparation of hawthorn had no significant effect on the primary end point of time until first cardiac event compared with standard treatment therapies. Analysis of secondary outcomes, however, suggested benefit in patients with left ventricular ejection fractions between 25% and 35%. The study preparation was well tolerated, and there were no significant adverse events. Post hoc analysis of a smaller but comparably designed clinical trial conducted in the United States suggested that hawthorn did not reduce, but possibly contributed to, early risk of heart failure progression.

The usual dose of hawthorn for CHF is 300 to 600 mg 3 times daily of an extract standardized to contain approximately 2% to 3% flavonoids or 18% to 20% procyanidins. Full effects can take up to 6 months to develop. Combination with cardiac glycosides should be monitored closely, and CNS depressants should be avoided. Side effects are rare but include gastrointestinal upset, sedation, dizziness, vertigo, headaches, migraines, and palpitations.

## Ginkgo biloba

Ginkgo extracts are derived from the leaf of the ginkgo, a botanical tree with a known history dating back 300 million years. Ginkgo is the most commonly purchased herbal remedy in the United States, with sales of more than $150 million. Widely used for its purported benefits in treating nondementia-related memory problems, Alzheimer disease, and vertigo, ginkgo has also been proposed as a treatment for intermittent claudication and peripheral vascular disease. Ginkgo has been documented to inhibit platelet activation factor, decrease blood viscosity, and decrease vascular resistance. The mechanisms responsible for ginkgo's effectiveness in peripheral vascular disease are unknown but can include its ability to scavenge free radicals, promote vasodilatation, and decrease blood viscosity; it also possesses anti-inflammatory and antiplatelet actions.

Individual studies have revealed benefit in increasing mean pain-free walking distance. Two meta-analyses have examined the literature and reported a statistically significant increase in walking distance averaging nearly 25 m (82 ft). A recent randomized controlled trial in 62 adults with peripheral vascular disease confirmed a modest and insignificant increase in maximal treadmill walking time and flow-mediated dilation after 4 months of therapy with 300 mg/d of *Ginkgo biloba*. In addition, the Ginkgo Evaluation of Memory Study (GEMS) enrolled 3069 people of age 75 years and older who were randomized to placebo or ginkgo and followed-up for 6 years to evaluate the effect of the supplement on dementia. Although no effect was found on dementia, and no differences in heart disease or stroke, the investigators did note a possible benefit in the reduction of peripheral vascular events in a small number of subjects, which warrants further study.

The usual dose of ginkgo for the treatment of claudication is 40 to 80 mg 3 times daily of a 50:1 extract standardized to contain 24% ginkgo-flavone glycosides. Caution must be exercised in using ginkgo, as it inhibits platelet aggregation factor and has been reported to increase both spontaneous and trauma-related bleeding, including bleeding during surgery and other procedures. Caution must also be exercised in combining gingko with heparin, warfarin, clopidogrel, and other compounds that can increase the risk of bleeding. Ginkgo has been reported to decrease the metabolism of trazodone in at least 1 case report, perhaps by an inhibition of monoamine oxidase. Side effects are common and include headaches, dizziness, gastrointestinal complaints, and skin reactions.

## Horse Chestnut Tree Extract (Aesculus hippocastanum)

The horse chestnut tree is found worldwide. Its seeds contain active compounds known as saponins, which have mild anti-inflammatory properties. Aescin, a combination of triterpene saponins, appears to be the pharmacologically active component. Its mechanism of action is considered to be sensitization to $Ca^{2+}$ ions and a sealing effect on small vessel permeability to water. Traditionally, this botanical tree has been used for hemorrhoids, rheumatism, swellings, varicose veins, and leg ulcers. Research has focused on horse chestnut tree extract in the treatment of chronic venous insufficiency, and multiple studies have reported the superiority of horse chestnut tree extract over placebo, with equal effectiveness to compression stockings as quantified by significant improvement in objective measurements of leg edema and subjective reporting of pain and sensation of heaviness.

The usual dose of horse chestnut tree extract is 300 mg twice daily, standardized to contain 50 mg of aescin per dose, for a total daily dose of 100 mg of aescin. Aescin binds to plasma protein and can affect the binding of other drugs. Side effects are rare, including headache, itching, and dizziness. Concerns regarding risk of renal impairment do not appear to be warranted.

## Policosanol

Policosanol is a combination of aliphatic alcohols derived most commonly from sugarcane wax, although octacosanol, the predominant active ingredient, is also present in wheat germ oil and other vegetable oils. Policosanol inhibits cholesterol biosynthesis in a step located between acetate and mevalonate and increases low-density lipoprotein (LDL) receptor-dependent processing. There is no evidence for a direct inhibition of hydroxymethylglutaryl coenzyme A (HMG-CoA) reductase. Policosanol has been extensively used clinically and researched in Cuba. These studies suggest a lipid-lowering effect of approximately 15% for total cholesterol and 20% for LDL cholesterol, which can be increased to 30% with higher doses. Maximal effects are seen after only 6 to 8 weeks of use, and benefits have been demonstrated in studies lasting longer than 1 year. In a head-to-head comparison of 10 mg polico-sanol with 20 mg fluvastatin in women with elevated cholesterol, the lipid-lowering effects of policosanol were slightly superior to those of fluvastatin, and policosanol alone significantly inhibited the susceptibility of LDL to lipid peroxidation. The efficacy of policosanol has been noted in a review suggesting a unique role for this natural compound, given the large number of patients desiring a natural alternative to synthetically derived drugs for cholesterol management. However, 3 recent clinical trials found no evidence of beneficial effects on lipid lowering, casting significant doubt on the efficacy of this therapy. There are no data on efficacy determined by clinical end points.

The typical starting dose of policosanol is 5 mg/d, which can be increased to a maximal dose of 20 mg/d. Side effects are infrequent, with weight loss, polyuria, and headache most commonly reported. There is concern that policosanol can potentiate anticoagulant activity; it should therefore be used with caution in combination with any agents known to increase the risk of bleeding. There is also a report of an increased effect of L-dopa when used in combination with policosanol, leading to dyskinesias.

## Gugulipid (Commiphora mukul)

Guggul is a substance derived from the mukul myrrh tree in India. It has played a role in traditional Indian medicine (Ayurveda) for several thousand years. It is used in the treatment of arthritis, and for digestive, skin, and menstrual problems. Today, guggul is used as a lipid-lowering agent that is believed to work by blocking the farnesoid X receptor in liver cells and, as a consequence, altering cholesterol metabolism. Studies of guggul have demonstrated a significant reduction in total cholesterol and LDL-C of 15% to 23% and triglyceride reduction of 20%.

The usual dose is 100 mg of guggulsterone per day. Side effects are usually limited to mild gastrointestinal symptoms. A hypersensitivity rash was reported in a small number of healthy subjects enrolled in a randomized control trial for hypercholesterolemia. There is some evidence that when guggul is used concomitantly with diltiazem or propranolol, there can be a reduction in the bioavailability of those drugs and therefore decreased clinical efficacy. Currently, no clinical studies have been conducted to evaluate the safety of long-term use of guggul or guggulsterone.

## Red Rice Yeast (Monascus purpureus)

Red rice yeast is a product that is derived from a yeast that grows on rice. Red rice yeast has been a food staple and folk remedy for thousands of years in Asia. It was noted in the 1970s that a product of the yeast, monacolin K (lovastatin), was an inhibitor of HMG-CoA reductase. The concentration of lovastatin varies in red rice yeast but averages near 0.4% by weight.

In an early multicenter study of 187 subjects, red rice yeast lowered total cholesterol by 16.4%, LDL-C by 21.0%, triglycerides by 24.5%, and the ratio of total-to-high-density lipoprotein (HDL) cholesterol by 17.7%; it increased high-density-lipoprotein cholesterol (HDL-C) by 14.6%. The China Coronary Secondary Prevention Study randomized 4870 patients with a prior history of myocardial infarction to either a commercial red rice yeast product 600 mg twice daily or placebo for a mean duration of 4.5 years. The primary end points of nonfatal myocardial infarction and fatal coronary events, cardiovascular mortality, and total mortality were significantly reduced in the treatment group. The need for coronary revascularization was similarly reduced. Total cholesterol was reduced by 13% and LDL-C was reduced by 20%, with a noted 4.2% rise in HDL-C. No treatment-related serious adverse events or deaths were reported during the study period.

Although the reported side effects of red rice yeast are few—including mainly gastrointestinal upset, headaches, and dizziness—red rice yeast must theoretically be considered a typical HMG-CoA reductase inhibitor, and caution is advised with regard to potential side effects, including rhabdomyolysis. However, red rice yeast has been successfully used in statin-intolerant patients with dyslipidemia and may provide an alternative treatment for some difficult-to-treat patients. Similarly, drug interactions should be considered to be identical to those with lovastatin, requiring caution when red rice yeast is combined with niacin, macrolides, cyclosporine, ketoconazole, and many other agents. Products range in their recommended dosage from 2.5 to 10 mg of lovastatin equivalent per day. However, red rice yeast is no longer marketed with standardized lovastatin levels in the United States, owing to legal issues, and it is now sold without lovastatin levels declared.

# ■ DIETARY SUPPLEMENTS

A number of dietary components have been postulated to have beneficial effects on cardiovascular disease and have been used therapeutically. These include omega-3 fatty acids, antioxidant vitamins, B vitamins, plant sterols, soluble fiber, soy, and teas.

## Omega-3 Fatty Acids

Omega-3 polyunsaturated fatty acids (FAs) can be derived from either plant or marine sources. The principal plant-based omega-3 FA, alpha linolenic acid (ALA), is found in soy and its derivative tofu, as well as in canola oil, flax seeds, and nuts. Omega-3 FAs derived from the tissues of marine animals (*fish oil*) include docosahexaenoic acid (DHA) and eicosapentaenoic acid (EPA). Typical dietary sources include mackerel, salmon, herring, sardines, anchovies, and albacore tuna.

Several mechanisms of benefit have been proposed for omega-3 FAs. The reductions in sudden cardiac death observed in several studies suggest a direct antiarrhythmic effect. High-dose omega-3 FAs produce a significant reduction in serum triglyceride concentrations and a small drop in blood pressure. They also decrease platelet aggregation. Other suggested mechanisms include an anti-inflammatory effect and enhanced production of nitric oxide. In addition, there are many reports of fish oil ingestion favorably affecting a variety of other intermediate targets believed to be relevant to cardiovascular disease.

Early suggestions that fish oil consumption might provide protective health benefits came from epidemiologic comparisons of Greenland Eskimos, Alaskan Inuits, and Japanese islanders with high fish consumption with other cohorts. Three follow-up epidemiologic studies in the 1980s found that persons who ate fish every week had a lower mortality from coronary artery disease (CAD). More than 40 cohort studies have now examined the effects of fish consumption on CAD outcomes. The best of these suggest a protective effect, with a stronger effect on death (four studies, relative risk [RR] 0.65) than on cardiovascular events (seven studies, RR 0.91).

A systematic review of randomized trials of omega-3 FAs published from 1966 to 2003 involving more than 33 000 patients found a small, nonsignificant reduction in all-cause mortality with a strategy of high omega-3 intake relative to low omega-3 intake (RR 0.87, 95% confidence interval [CI], 0.73-1.03). For cardiovascular events, the RR for high omega-3 was 0.95. Among these trials, the ones with the largest estimated benefit for high omega-3 intake were almost always the smallest trials. The largest of these is the Gruppo Italiano per lo Studio della Sopravvivenza nell'Infarto Miocardico (GISSI)-Prevenzione study, which randomized 11 324 post-myocardial infarction (MI) patients to 1 g/d or usual therapy. The primary analysis showed a 20% reduction in all-cause mortality ($p = 0.01$) and a 45% reduction in sudden death ($p < 0.01$).

The Diet and Angina Randomized Trial (DART) 2 estimated borderline excess mortality from high omega-3 intake (adjusted hazard ratio [HR] = 1.26; $p = 0.047$). This study randomized 3114 men younger than 70 years of age to a factorial design involving advice to eat two portions of oily fish each week (or take 3 g of fish oil capsules daily) versus sensible eating advice. The apparent excess mortality seen in this trial appeared to be driven by results in the subjects given fish oil capsules. The Japan EPA Lipid Intervention Study (JELIS) randomized 18 654 hypercholesterolemic patients to 1800 mg of EPA per day plus statin therapy versus statin therapy alone. After a mean follow-up of 4.6 years, the EPA group had a 19% reduction in composite cardiac events ($p = 0.01$). The two treatment arms had an equivalent reduction in LDL-C of 25%. The magnitude of the treatment effect was similar in the primary prevention and secondary prevention subgroups. One notable aspect of this trial is the fact that it was carried out in a population that typically has a high dietary intake of fish. The GISSI-HF trial randomized 7046 NYHA class II to IV heart failure patients (10% with ejection fraction >40%) to 1 g/d of n-3 polyunsaturated fatty acids (PUFA) or placebo. With median 3.9 years of follow-up, a significant risk reduction in those assigned to the n-3 PUFA group was seen for all-cause mortality (HR = 0.91; $p = 0.041$), cardiovascular deaths (HR = 0.90; $p = 0.045$), hospital admissions for any reason (HR = 0.94; $p = 0.049$), and hospital admissions for cardiovascular reasons (HR = 0.93; $p = 0.026$).

The recently completed Alpha Omega Trial randomized 4837 patients with previous myocardial infarction to 1 of 4 arms: margarine supplemented with a combination of EPA and DHA, margarine supplemented with ALA, margarine supplemented with EPA-DHA and ALA, or placebo margarine. Neither EPA-DHA nor ALA reduced the primary endpoint of major fatal and nonfatal cardiovascular events and cardiac interventions [HR (EPA-DHA) 1.01; $p = 0.93$; HR (ALA) 0.91; $p = 0.20$]. Although the dosages of EPA-DHA and ALA were less than in other trials, the results of this trial cast doubt on the effectiveness of omega-3 fatty acid dietary supplements in the context of state-of-the-art antihypertensive, antithrombotic, and lipid-modifying medical therapy.

Currently, there are strong recommendations for the general public to consume 2 servings of fish (especially fatty fish) per week, as well as vegetables containing ALA, as part of a heart-healthy diet. In Europe, use of fish oil for secondary prevention after myocardial infarction is almost considered routine. Nonetheless, there is still much uncertainty regarding the value of dietary sources of omega-3 FAs compared with supplemental omega-3 FAs, appropriate target populations, and proper dosage. Early concerns about the concomitant use of omega-3 FAs with antiplatelet or antithrombotic medications causing significant bleeding have not been supported by the evidence. Contaminants in dietary sources of fish (particularly farm-raised fish) remain an important concern regarding recommending population-level increases in fish consumption for health reasons. The effect that such recommendations will have on increasing the rate of depletion of the world's fish stores from industrial overfishing is also a significant concern.

## Antioxidants and Antioxidant Vitamins

Despite a large body of epidemiologic evidence suggesting a favorable association between a diet high in antioxidants and reduced risk of coronary heart disease (CHD), the clinical trial evidence related to supplements has failed to confirm the expected benefits.

*Vitamin E* refers to a group of molecules that includes 4 tocopherols and 4 tocotrienols. Several large epidemiologic studies involving more than 170 000 subjects have assessed the association between dietary and supplement-based vitamin E and CHD outcomes. In secondary prevention trials, the Cambridge Heart Antioxidant Study (CHAOS) demonstrated that 400 to 800 IU of vitamin E reduced the combined end point of death or nonfatal MI by 47%. The Heart Outcomes Prevention Evaluation (HOPE) trial, which tested 400 IU of vitamin E in a high-risk secondary prevention population, found no therapeutic benefit on a variety of outcome measures, including disease progression as assessed by carotid ultrasound. The GISSI-Prevenzione trial, which tested 300 mg/d of vitamin E in almost 11 324 patients, also failed to detect a benefit. The HOPE—The Ongoing Outcomes (TOO) trial reported on almost 4000 patients from the original HOPE study with long-term follow-up. As with the original HOPE analysis, there was no evidence of a benefit of vitamin E on cardiovascular outcomes, and there was actually a modest increase in heart failure with active treatment. In primary prevention trials, the collaborative group of the Primary Prevention Project (PPP) found no evidence for a therapeutic benefit for 300 IU of vitamin E in 4495 subjects with one or more major cardiovascular risk factors. The Women's Heath Study of 39 876 apparently healthy women of age 45 years and older found that vitamin E (600 IU on alternate days) reduced cardiovascular death (RR = 0.76; $p = 0.03$) but had no effect on total cardiovascular events, MI, or stroke. In the Physicians' Health Study II randomized trial, no benefit was found for 400 IU/alternate day in 14 641 male physicians with cardiovascular disease over an 8-year follow-up. At present, therefore, the preponderance of the evidence does not support a role for vitamin E supplements in either primary or secondary prevention of CHD.

*Vitamin C* (ascorbic acid) is a strong water-soluble antioxidant. In the Nurses' Health Study, estimated vitamin C intake using questionnaire data was modestly related to incident heart disease events with an adjusted RR of 0.72 ($p < 0.05$). Several randomized trials have tested vitamin C supplements in varying doses for CHD prevention. In the Heart Protection Study, 20 536 patients with CAD or diabetes were randomized to antioxidant vitamins (600 mg of vitamin E, 250 mg of vitamin C, and 20 mg of beta-carotene) versus placebo. Although the vitamin regimen was found to be safe, there was no evidence for a therapeutic effect after 5 years of treatment. In the Antioxidant Supplementation in Atherosclerosis Prevention (ASAP) study, hypercholesterolemic patients were randomized to twice-daily supplements of 136 IU of vitamin E, 250 mg of slow-release vitamin C, both, or placebo only. At 6 years among the 440 subjects completing the study, vitamin supplementation slowed carotid atherosclerosis (judged by common carotid intimal-medial thickness) by 25%. In the Physicians' Health Study II, 500 mg/d of vitamin C provided no significant risk reduction for major cardiovascular events, MI, stroke, or cardiovascular mortality.

*Coenzyme Q10* (CoQ10) is a fat-soluble vitamin-like compound that is involved in mitochondrial adenosine triphosphate generation, serves to protect low-density lipoprotein particles from oxidation, and aids cell membrane stabilization. Some data suggest that this micronutrient is deficient in patients with heart failure. For this reason, several small studies have been conducted to assess its impact in heart failure patients, with improvement seen in a number of markers, including ejection fraction, cardiac output, and pulmonary artery pressures. The ongoing Q Symbio randomized clinical trial is examining 300 mg/d of CoQ10 versus placebo in 550 NYHA class III or IV chronic heart failure patients to assess its impact on cardiovascular morbidity and mortality. A meta-analysis of 3 small trials (total 96 patients) of CoQ10 for lowering blood pressure concluded that there is currently insufficient evidence to determine its effectiveness.

Because statins interfere with the synthesis of CoQ10, there has been speculation that CoQ10 supplementation may prevent or mitigate the effects of statin-induced myopathy. However, a 2007 systematic review found that there is insufficient evidence to support recommending CoQ10 supplementation to statin users and that large, well-designed trials are needed.

*Selenium* (Se) is an essential element with antioxidant properties. Recent studies of selenium supplementation have not shown benefit and some suggest there may be an increased risk of harms at levels higher than 130 ng/mL.

## B Vitamins

Moderate elevations of plasma homocysteine levels have been associated with an enhanced risk for atherosclerotic disease. The metabolism of homocysteine requires several B vitamins as cofactors, specifically vitamins $B_6$, $B_{12}$, and folate. Homocysteine levels can be decreased by the administration of supplemental folate, with or without vitamins $B_6$ and $B_{12}$. Although epidemiologic studies suggested potential cardiovascular benefit with B vitamin supplementation, most trial results have shown no such benefit. A meta-analysis of 4 randomized, controlled trials of B vitamin therapy found no evidence that B vitamin supplements slowed the progression of atherosclerosis. A randomized, placebo-controlled trial with 636 patients found that combined folate, $B_6$, and $B_{12}$ therapy can increase the risk of restenosis and revascularization after coronary stenting. A recent placebo-controlled trial involving 3096 patients undergoing coronary angiography randomized participants to B vitamin and/or folic acid supplementation and found no effect on total mortality or cardiovascular events after a median 38 months of follow-up.

## Vitamin D

Vitamin D refers to a group of fat-soluble vitamins that are critical to body calcium regulation and that must be obtained in the diet in order to prevent a deficiency state. The role of vitamin D in the normal functioning of the cardiovascular system is just beginning to be understood. Recent evidence has suggested that 25-hydroxy-vitamin D [25(OH)D] deficiency may contribute to cardiovascular disease. However, further studies of vitamin D supplementation are needed to clarify its role in the primary or secondary prevention of CVD. The ongoing VITAL trial aims to evaluate the effectiveness of vitamin D supplementation for primary prevention of CVD.

## Soy Protein and Isoflavones

Substitution of soy protein for animal protein can produce significant reductions in LDL-C and triglycerides. Whether this reflects a unique benefit of soy or its isoflavones (weak, plant-derived estrogen compounds) in particular, or merely a reduction in dietary animal protein and fat, is unclear. A review of the benefits of soy protein and isoflavones has been published by the AHA Nutrition Committee. A total of 22 randomized trials tested the effects of soy protein and found a small decrease in LDL-C with no effects on other lipid fractions or blood pressure. Soy isoflavones were tested in 19 studies and had no effects on lipids or blood pressure.

## Flavonols and Flavones

Flavonols and other dietary flavonoids are plant-based metabolites that are believed to provide beneficial effects to the cardiovascular system, although which compounds provide benefit and what the specific benefits are remain controversial. Both tea and chocolate have been postulated to produce cardiovascular health benefits through this group of compounds. Evidence to date in this area is largely observational. In 1 recent study, dietary questionnaires collected from 66 360 women in the Nurses' Health Study showed no association between overall dietary flavonol and flavone consumption and risk of nonfatal MI or fatal coronary heart disease with 12 years of follow-up. However, the highest quintile of kaempferol (a flavonoid found in food sources including broccoli, brussel sprouts, apples, and tea) consumption showed a significant reduction in risk of coronary heart disease death (RR = 0.66; $p$ = 0.04) when compared with those in the lowest quintile. A recent meta-analysis of observational studies reported that highest levels of chocolate consumption were associated with a significant reduction in CVD (RR 0.63 [95% CI, 0.44-0.90]).

### Plant Sterols

Plant sterols and stanols have been persuasively shown to lower cholesterol and are now commercially available in margarine products. Long-term outcome studies with these compounds are needed.

## ■ CHELATION THERAPY

The intravenous infusion of ethylenediamine-tetraacetic acid (EDTA) is used by some CAM practitioners for the treatment of atherosclerotic vascular disease. The original rationale behind this therapy was that EDTA chelation would remove calcium from atheromatous arterial lesions. However, there is little empiric support for this putative mechanism, and other possible benefits such as an antioxidant effect have been proposed.

There have been 4 randomized trials of chelation therapy, all quite small. The most recent is the Program to Assess Alternative Treatment Strategies to Achieve Cardiac Health (PATCH), which randomized 84 stable angina patients and followed them for 6 months. Event rates in this trial were quite low, and there were no differences between the chelation and the placebo arms. The investigators concluded that a much larger trial would be required. The National Institutes of Health has funded a major randomized trial of chelation, the Trial to Assess Chelation Therapy (TACT), which will randomize more than 1600 patients ≥50 years of age with a prior MI to either chelation therapy or placebo; results are expected in 2012.

## ■ ALCOHOL

Mild to moderate alcohol consumption has been associated in a variety of reports with reduction in stroke and rates of MI, functional improvement with claudication, and improved cardiovascular survival. Vasodilating and central nervous system effects, as well as antioxidant compounds in alcohol preparations such as red wine, have all been proposed as potential mechanisms of these benefits. At higher dose in susceptible individuals, alcohol is a well-known myocardial toxin, with equally deleterious potential in other end organs such as the liver, gastrointestinal tract, and central nervous system. A science advisory overview from the AHA was issued on this topic in 2001.

## ■ MANIPULATIVE AND BODY-BASED PRACTICES

Acupuncture, acupressure, and an array of massage techniques represent manipulative and body-based therapies. Of these, the most robust scientific information is available on acupuncture.

## Acupuncture

The ancient Chinese medical therapy acupuncture has garnered growing interest since the early 1970s. In cardiovascular care, there are 3 areas for which acupuncture has been explored: anginal pain, hypertension, and arrhythmias. The rationale for using acupuncture to treat myocardial ischemia, hypertension, and arrhythmias stems from its ability to inhibit autonomic sympathetic outflow. Acupuncture techniques can release opioids in a number of regions in the hypothalamus, midbrain, and medulla concerned with processing information that influences sympathetic neuroactivity. Other neurotransmitters that can also be associated with the cardiovascular effects of acupuncture include gamma-aminobutyric acid, serotonin, and acetylcholine. Because placebo effects can occur in as many as 40% of patients and because acupuncture seems to be efficacious in approximately 70% of patients, actual benefit may represent a narrow window of response.

Studies also suggest that catecholamine reduction with acupuncture can affect myocardial ischemia and stress-induced hypertension. These studies indicate that acupuncture may reduce myocardial oxygen demand rather than increase coronary blood flow. In sham acupuncture placebo-controlled studies of moderate anginal pain and exercise tolerance, Ballegaard was unable to document a decrease in the rate of anginal attacks, consumption of nitroglycerin, or improvement in exercise tolerance, whereas 2 other studies including patients with severe stable angina who had been treated vigorously with medical therapy showed an acupuncture-related improvement in exercise capacity and rate-pressure product, particularly when acupuncture reduced measures of sympathetic tone. There are currently no trials showing reduction in mortality or other clinical outcomes with acupuncture in ischemic heart disease.

Other cardiovascular effects of acupuncture have been studied. Improvement in primary Raynaud cold-induced vasoconstriction by acupuncture compared with sham treatment has been reported. Hypertension can also be improved by acupuncture, although the absolute effects reported are small. Reliable data on arrhythmia control with acupuncture are rare. Acupuncture can inhibit ventricular extrasystoles induced by stimulating the hypothalamus or paraventricular nucleus or after administration of $BaCl_2$. Understanding patient selection and the level of incremental effect in the context of other drug or device therapies will require dedicated research.

Most authorities agree that the risk of an adverse event resulting from acupuncture is small, generally less than 10% when performed by physicians. Pneumothorax, spinal cord lesions, hepatitis, HIV infections, endocarditis, arthritis, and osteomyelitis have been reported but are rare, with an overall rate of less than 2%. The risk of an adverse event for nonphysician acupuncturists is higher (up to 30%), although the risk of serious events is low.

## Energy Medicine

Bioenergetics or energy medicine includes healing disciplines that harness intangible natural forces to influence physiologic, emotional, and spiritual healing. No scientific evidence has demonstrated or characterized actual bioenergy fields associated with many of these techniques, although practitioners claim to see, feel, or otherwise sense the color, alignment, intensity, and flow of such energy in practice. In several ancient Eastern practices, detailed diagrams of energy meridians and chakras are well known. Examples of bioenergy disciplines include therapeutic and healing touch, Qigong, Johrei, Healing touch, Reiki, crystal therapy, and magnet therapy. Energy therapies are generally administered by an active practitioner who conducts both diagnostic and therapeutic functions by *sensing* or *reading* energy patterns and then manipulating or adding to those energy patterns, with the patient in a more passive role.

Practitioners of the ancient Chinese healing tradition of Qigong use deep breathing, meditation, and body movement to capture and focus the vital life energy, Qi. In cardiovascular application, Qigong has been claimed to influence hypertension in patients with heart disease as well as sudden death by accentuating vagal tone, as demonstrated by changes in heart-rate variability. Qigong has also been associated with shorter hospitalization in patients after MI and reduced mortality with stroke. The reproducibility of these findings has not been established.

In hospitalized patients, therapeutic touch has been reported to palliate anxiety, with a potential effect on serum catecholamines before invasive procedures. In a small pilot study of healing touch before urgent percutaneous coronary intervention, this modality was associated with a suggestive trend toward improved short-term outcomes.

In the absence of known mechanisms, the safety assessment of bioenergy practices is problematic. Although bioenergy approaches are widely considered safe by practitioners, careful attention to both safety and efficacy in future research in these areas should be considered mandatory.

## Mind–Body Medicine

A remarkably large and consistent observational literature provides evidence that the presence or absence of acute and chronic stress; emotional states such as obsessive behavior, depression, and hostility; spiritual attitudes such as faith and hope; and interactive support systems such as companionship and community connectedness have significant correlations to cardiovascular outcomes such as hypertension, MI, stroke, and cardiac death. It is possible that these observations may partially reflect genetically driven physiologic responses to stress, with measurable impact on catecholamine levels, cortisol levels, glucose metabolism, autonomic tone, vascular tone, coagulability, pain perception, and immune reactivity. Teleologically the *fight-or-flight* responses are frequently recognized as physiologic survival mechanisms. However, with chronic, repetitive overstimulation, or in the setting of preexistent heart disease, the roles of stress, isolation, anger, and depression can clearly reach pathologic proportions. Also, these states of mind and spirit are frequently paired with behaviors such as smoking, eating disorders, obesity, diabetes, hypercholesterolemia, a sedentary lifestyle, and hypertension. Coping strategies and therapies that address this mind–body axis can be a fertile area to integrate into the current predominantly pharmacologic armamentarium.

Mind–body therapies are generally characterized by learned disciplines that affect both mind and body in a deliberately harmonious or even simultaneous way. Techniques can emphasize the mental component, such as in meditation, mindfulness, relaxation therapy, guided imagery, music, and mirthful laughter, with a *secondary* relaxation, quieting, or energizing of the body, or they can emphasize the somatic component, as in exercise, tai chi, and yoga, with a secondary quieting or energizing of the mind. A strong emphasis on awareness of and control of the breath, generally with attention to moving the locus of the breath from the chest into a relaxed abdominal breathing, is common among many of these techniques.

One area of mind–body therapy that has been reported in application to cardiovascular disorders is relaxation therapy, where triggering of relative bradycardia, vasodilatation, and changes in the electroencephalogram have been described as the "relaxation response." Relaxation therapies generally involve some combination of relaxed abdominal breathing, quieting of the mind with meditation or related techniques, and somatic relaxation of the body. Relaxation therapies are frequently applied for stress reduction, including just before invasive cardiac procedures. Relaxation therapy has been associated with lowering of blood pressure and possibly with better outcomes in men with risk factors for coronary artery disease. Concerns with possibly unanticipated negative effects from changing vascular tone or heart rhythm must also be carefully evaluated for therapies in patients with known heart disease. Although a reduction in premature ventricular contractions (PVCs) has been observed with relaxation therapy, higher mortality rates were associated with relaxation therapy in a female cohort of the MHEART study who had survived MI.

Other mind–body techniques with published experience in cardiology include music and imagery. Anxiety reduction has been observed with music in coronary care unit (CCU) and MI populations, although outcomes benefit has not been established. Imagery techniques usually encourage a patient to envision a beautiful, peaceful place from his or her life or experience, using a relaxed abdominal breath to let the mind dwell in that place. Music is used in the background in some imagery scripts. Imagery has been reported to reduce pain or the need for sedation in patients undergoing catheterization and to shorten hospital stay after bypass surgery.

Meditation and mindfulness constitute a very broad range of disciplines providing tools that, with practice, cultivate personal access to calming of the body and quieting of the mind, with a variety of potential healing effects including reduction of angina and improved quality of life. In addition to the use of these techniques in cardiac rehabilitation programs, they can have a role in lifestyle modification strategies associated with atheroregression in established coronary disease.

The role of spiritual attitudes, mental intentionality, spiritual intervention, and prayer in life process, disease states, and healing have been the subjects of numerous studies, from their effects on microorganisms and cell growth to human clinical trials. The spiritual dimension and the role of spiritual attitudes or interventions across patients, family, community, and medical staff have particular relevance in cardiovascular care, as patients suffering from heart disease are very directly confronted by issues of personal mortality. To date, a total of 6 prospective, randomized clinical trials of distant intercessory prayer in cardiovascular populations have been published in the peer review literature. Data on therapeutic benefit are inconclusive. Attempts to pool or reflect on this literature all indicate that existing data are most useful for hypothesis generation to guide future research.

## Whole Medical Systems

Whole medical systems broadly constitute approaches to diagnostic and therapeutic applications that are based on paradigms conceptually distinct from the Western allopathic paradigm. By and large, whole medical systems are ancient and culturally based and are notable for their holistic character. Typically the allopathic fixation on mechanical processes or selected organ systems is viewed as an "undersampling error" by whole medical systems. In traditional Chinese medicine, for instance, cardiovascular disorders are simply one feature of symptom complexes characterized across 4 relative states of yin deficiency or excess combined with yang deficiency or excess, where both yin and yang energies are associated with a broad range of emotional states and specific body organs. In Ayurvedic medical systems, the body is essentially referenced across 5 inorganic elements constituting the material universe—earth, water, fire, air, and ether. The body itself is envisioned as coarse material, or *maya*, that is structurally configured by vibrational energy conveyed from a collective or cosmic source, or Atma. This coarse material structure rendered by vibrational influences of life energy could be conceptually compared, in a different metaphor, to the modern Western medical understanding of the genome. In both of these paradigms, wellness and illness exist in the individual human being, but they are also structurally shared across populations and beyond. Computationally demanding statistical models being developed for genomic applications might provide some intriguing approaches to novel medical paradigms in whole medical systems.

Although holistic medical systems at first blush can seem radical in their departure from the rigorously articulate Western scientific medical model, current directions in wellness-oriented lifestyle modification strategies for both the primary and secondary prevention of cardiovascular disease represent a movement with a distinctively holistic character in the mainstream of modern practice—a sign of more enlightened approaches from both East and West toward the development of "integrative" medical practices.

## End-of-Life Care

Cardiology training and the use of modern technologies are generally contextualized as a battle against heart disease, frequently as a fight against death. Less time and education is addressed to facing the inevitability of death, or a focus on the end of life. Integration of holistic healing into technology-laden care, including cardiovascular support, has been the central focus of disciplines such as palliative care. Palliative care "seeks to prevent, relieve, reduce or soothe the symptoms of disease or disorder without affecting a cure." Palliative care in this broad sense is not restricted to those who are dying or those enrolled in hospice programs. End of life, palliative care, and hospice are all terms that reflect the time in which the medical team and patient have agreed to move beyond curing, while still focused on healing. Too often, the patient reaches terminal stages of their disease process before this subject is approached.

End-of-life planning begins with patient education and depends on medical staff knowledge. *Five Wishes* provides one of many living will options that may be primarily accessed through the Internet. It helps organize personal expression of treatment preferences and dialogue with health care staff around those issues, specifically:

1. Which person you want to make health care decisions for you when you can't make them.

2. The kind of medical treatment you want or don't want.

3. How comfortable you want to be.

4. How you want people to treat you.

5. What you want your loved ones to know.

Physician input in end-of-life decisions is crucial, as personal scenarios and considerations of what technology or medical support best fits a particular patient's needs cannot be determined using generic tools such as living wills. A physician extender or palliative care coordinator may be a valuable role to allow "high-tech" cardiovascular care to expand into more holistic, humanistic dimensions at the end of life.

## ■ CONCLUSION

CAM therapies in cardiovascular care represent an enormous area of widely practiced therapeutics with insufficient scientific literature, but, in many cases, an ancient and deeply rooted cultural basis. In modern medicine, CAM therapeutics are probably best considered as adjuncts to current standard medical care, whose study provides opportunities to advance more integrative medical practice. Systematic research to uncover mechanisms of action as well as to better profile the actual safety and efficacy of CAM therapies in specific cardiac disorders is both justified and clearly necessary for new paradigms of integrative medical practice to have an impact and be widely adopted by physicians. In addition, the education and familiarity of cardiologists with CAM therapies is likely to promote better dialogue with patients and more awareness of issues of self-empowerment in dealing with heart disease, opening the door to a broadened range of options for optimizing cardiovascular care.

# SUGGESTED READINGS

Krucoff MW, Costello RB, Mark DB, Vogel HK. Complementary and alternative medical therapy in cardiovascular care. In: Fuster V, Walsh R, Harrington RA, et al, eds. *Hurst's The Heart*. 13th ed. New York, NY: McGraw-Hill; 2011;115:2429-2440.

Aging With Dignity. http://www.agingwithdignity.org/five-wishes.php. Accessed December 18, 2011.

Brinker FJ. *Herb Contraindications and Drug Interactions*. 2nd ed. Sandy, OR: Eclectic Medical Publications; 1998.

Buitrago-Lopez A, Sanderson J, Johnson L, Warnakula S, Wood A, Di Angelantonio E, Franco OH. Chocolate consumption and cardiometabolic disorders: systematic review and meta-analysis. *BMJ*. 2011;343:d4488.

Center to Advance Palliative Care. GetPalliateiveCare.org. http://www.getpalliativecare.org. Accessed December 18, 2011.

De Smet PA. Herbal remedies. *N Engl J Med*. 2002;347(25):2046-2056.

Dusek JA, Astin JA, Hibberd PL, Krucoff MW. Healing prayer outcomes studies: consensus recommendations. *Alt Ther Health Med*. 2003;9(3):A44-A53.

Eisenberg, DM, Davis R, Ettner S, et al. Trends in alternative medicine use in the United States 1990-1997: results of a follow up national survey. *JAMA*. 1998;280(18):1569-1575.

Gagnier JJ, Boon H, Rochon P, et al; CONSORT Group. Reporting randomized, control trials of herbal interventions: an elaborated CONSORT statement. *Ann Intern Med*. 2006;144(5); 364-367.

Goldberg IJ, Mosca L, Piano MR, et al. AHA Science Advisory: Wine and your heart: a science advisory for healthcare professionals from the Nutrition Committee, Council on Epidemiology and Prevention, and Council on Cardiovascular Nursing of the American Heart Association. *Circulation*. 2001;103:472-475.

Hover-Krame M, Mentgen D. *Healing Touch: A Resource for Health Care Professionals*. Albany, NY: Delmar; 1996.

Jevning R, Wallace RK, Beidebach M. The physiology of meditation: a review. A wakeful hypometabolic integrated response. *Neurosci Biobehav Rev*. 1992;16:415-424.

Jonas WB, Crawford CC. Science and spiritual healing: a critical review of spiritual healing, "energy" medicine and intentionality. *Alt Ther Health Med*. 2003;9(2):56-61.

Jonas WB, Linde K., Walach H. How to practice evidence-based complementary and alternative medicine. In: Jonas W, Levin J, eds. *Essentials of Complementary and Alternative Medicine*. Philadelphia, PA: Lippincott, Williams & Wilkins; 1999.

Kris-Etherton PM, Harris WS, Appel LJ. Omega-3 fatty acids and cardiovascular disease: new recommendations from the American Heart Association. *Arterioscler Thromb Vasc Biol*. 2003;23:151-152.

Kromhout D, Giltay EJ, Geleijnse JM, et al. n-3 fatty acids and cardiovascular events after myocardial infarction. *New Eng J Med*. 2010;363(21):2015-2026.

Kuller LH. Does *Ginkgo biloba* reduce the risk of cardiovascular events? *Circ Cardiovasc Qual Outcomes*. 2010;3(1):41-47.

Lin MC, Nahin R, Gershwin M, et al. State of complementary and alternative medicine in cardiovascular, lung, and blood research: executive summary of a workshop. *Circulation*. 2001;103(16):2038-2041.

Linde K, Jonas WB. Evaluating complementary and alternative medicine: the balance of rigor and relevance. In: Jonas W, Levin J, eds. *Essentials of Complementary and Alternative Medicine*. Philadelphia, PA: Lippincott, Williams & Wilkins; 1999.

Longhurst JC. Acupuncture's beneficial effects on the cardiovascular system. *Prev Cardiol*. 1998;1:21-33.

MacPherson H, White A, Cummings M, et al. Standards for reporting interventions in controlled trials of acupuncture: the STRICTA recommendations. *Comp Ther Med*. 2001;9:246-249.

Mulrow C, Lawrence V, Ackerman R, et al. *Garlic: Effects on Cardiovascular Risks and Disease, Protective Effects against Cancer, and Clinical Adverse Effects*. Rockville, MD: Agency for Healthcare Research and Quality; 2000. AHRQ publication 01-E023.

National Institutes of Health. National Center for Complementary and Alternative Medicine (NCCAM). http://nccam.nih.gov/health/whatiscam/. Accessed December 27, 2009.

Sacks FM, Lichtenstein A, Van HL, et al. Soy protein, isoflavones, and cardiovascular health: an American Heart Association Science Advisory for professionals from the Nutrition Committee. *Circulation*. 2006;113:1034-1044.

Schulz V, Hansel R, Tyler VE. *Rational Phytotherapy: A Physician's Guide to Herbal Medicine*. 4th ed. Berlin, Germany: Springer-Verlag; 2001.

Singh BB, Vinjamury SP, Der-Martirosian C, et al. Ayurvedic and collateral herbal treatments for hyperlipidemia: a systematic review of randomized controlled trials and quasi-experimental designs. *Altern Ther Health Med*. 2007;13:22-28.

Soukoulis V, Dihu JB, Sole M, et al. Micronutrient deficiencies: an unmet need in heart failure. *J Am Coll Cardiol*. 2009;54:1660-1673.

The Vitamin D and Omega-3 Trial (VITAL). http://www.vitalstudy.org/index.html. Accessed December 18, 2011.

Trial to Assess Chelation Therapy (TACT). http://clinicaltrials.gov/ct2/show/NCT00044213. Accessed December 18, 2011.

Vogel JH, Krucoff MW. *Integrative Cardiology: Complementary and Alternative Medicine for the Heart*. New York, NY: McGraw Hill Medical; 2007.

Vogel JHK, Bolling SF, Costello RB, et al. Integrating complementary medicine into cardiovascular medicine: a report of the American College of Cardiology Foundation Task Force on Clinical Expert Consensus Documents (Writing Committee to Develop an Expert Consensus Document on Complementary and Integrative Medicine). *J Am Coll Cardiol*. 2005;46:184-221.

# INDEX

*Note:* Page numbers followed by *f* or *t* indicate figures or tables, respectively.